FRENCH'S
Index of
Differential
nosis

D0870979

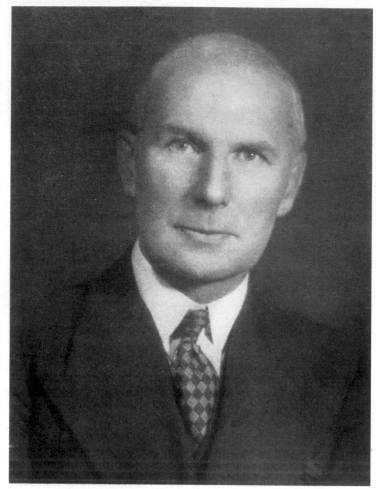

HERBERT FRENCH, C.V.O., C.B.E., M.A., M.D., F.R.C.P.

FRENCH'S
Index of Differential Diagnosis

THIRTEENTH EDITION

EDITED BY

Ian A.D. Bouchier CBE, MD, FRCP, FRCPE,
Hon FCP (SAF), FFPHM, FRSA, FIBiol, FRSE

Professor of Medicine, University of Edinburgh, Department
of Medicine, Royal Infirmary, Edinburgh, UK

Harold Ellis CBE, FRCS, FACS, FRCOG

Emeritus Professor of Surgery, Charing Cross and
Westminster Medical School, London, UK; Clinical
Anatomist, Guy's and St Thomas's Medical School, London,
UK

Peter R. Fleming MD, FRCP, DHMSA

Lately Senior Lecturer in Medicine, Charing Cross and
Westminster Medical School, London, UK; Consultant
Physician, Westminster Hospital, London, UK.

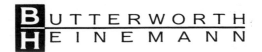

Butterworth-Heinemann
Linacre House, Jordan Hill, Oxford OX2 8DP
A division of Reed Educational and Professional Publishing Ltd

 A member of the Reed Elsevier plc group

OXFORD   BOSTON   JOHANNESBURG
MELBOURNE   NEW DELHI   SINGAPORE

First edition, 1912
Second edition, 1917
Third edition, 1917
Fourth edition, 1928
Fifth edition, 1936
Sixth edition, 1945
Seventh edition, 1954
Eighth edition, 1960
Ninth edition, 1967
Tenth edition, 1973
Eleventh edition, 1979
Twelfth edition, 1985
Thirteenth edition, 1996

British Library Cataloguing in Publication Data

A catalogue record for this book is available from the British
Library

Library of Congress Cataloguing in Publication Data

A catalogue record for this book is available from the Library
of Congress

ISBN 0 7506 1434 X Paper
ISBN 0 7506 2804 9 Cased

Printed in Spain

Preface to the thirteenth edition

The Thirteenth Edition of *French's Index* appears under a new editorial team, and our first duty is to pay homage to Frank Dudley Hart, Physician Emeritus of Westminster Hospital, under whose direction this classic flourished through successive editions. He, in turn, replaced Sir Adolphe Abrahams of Westminster Hospital, who succeeded Dr Arthur Douthwaite of Guy's Hospital who inherited the editorship from the original author, Herbert French.

The aim of the book remains unchanged from the original statement by Dr French in the first paragraph of his preface to the first edition of 1912. It is to help in the differential diagnosis of any condition in medicine, surgery, or any speciality, that may be seen in general or hospital practice. It is essentially, therefore, a book for the clinician. With modern air transport, national disease barriers have broken down. The time taken to get anywhere in the world is considerably less than the incubation period of almost all the infectious diseases. Tropical diseases are no longer confined to the tropics; any country's epidemic may appear anywhere else in the world in record time. This, together with the massive increase in iatrogenic diseases, makes the art of differential diagnosis more interesting today than ever before, and vastly more complex too!

The thirteenth edition has seen the recuitment of numerous new contributors as well as retention of old friends, all chosen for their specialist knowledge and teaching skills. 'French' has now been completely revised, with many sections largely rewritten, illustrations replaced and modern diagnostic methods updated. We hope that this edition will continue to serve the medical profession as it enters the second millennium as well as previous editions have proved of value to most of this, now fading, century.

I.A.D.B., H.E., P.R.F.

Preface to the first edition

This book is a treatise on the application of differential diagnosis to all the main signs and symptoms of disease. It aims at being of practical utility to medical men whenever difficulty arises in deciding the precise cause of any particular symptom of which a patient may complain. It covers the whole ground of medicine, surgery, gynaecology, ophthalmology, dermatology and neurology.

Whatever the disease from which the patient is suffering, the importance of discovering it as early as possible can hardly be over-rated. The present volume deals with diagnosis from a standpoint which is different from that of most textbooks, having been written in response to requests for an *Index of Diagnosis* as a companion to the publishers' *Index of Treatment*, issued in 1907. The book is an index in the sense that its articles on the various symptoms are arranged in alphabetical order; at the same time it is a work upon differential diagnosis in that it discusses the methods of distinguishing between the various diseases in which each individual symptom may be observed. Whilst the body of the book thus deals with *symptoms*, the general index at the end gathers these together under the headings of the various *diseases* in which they occur.

The Editor lays particular stress upon the importance of using these two parts of the book together. Unless reference is made freely to the general index, the reader may miss a number of the places in which is discussed the diagnosis of the disease with which he has to deal; for while each *symptom* is considered but once, each *disease* is likely to come up for discussion under the heading of each of its more important symptoms.

The guiding principle throughout has been to suppose that a particular symptom attracts special notice in a given case, and that the diagnosis has to be established by differentiating between the various diseases to which this symptom may be due. One of many difficulties arising during the construction of the work was that of deciding where to draw the line as regards symptoms themselves. The exclusion of many borderline headings such as 'Dullness at the base of one lung', 'Inability to breathe through the nose', and various signs such as Romberg's, Stellwag's, von Graefe's, and so forth, may perhaps seem arbitrary; but reference to the minor symptoms and physical signs which have not been thought sufficiently important to merit separate articles will be found in the general index at the end of the volume.

Treatment, pathology, and prognosis are not dealt with except in so far as they may bear upon differential diagnosis—the employment of salicylates, for instance, in distinguishing acute rheumatic from other forms of arthritis; the use of the microscope in distinguishing malignant neoplasms from inflammatory or other tumours; the value of the lapse of time in distinguishing between tuberculous and meningococcal meningitis.

Coloured plates and other illustrations have been introduced freely wherever it was thought they might be helpful in diagnosis. Most of them are original, but a few are reproduced from other sources, and thanks are due to the authors and publishers who have kindly lent them.

So far as the Editor is aware, although there exist indexes of symptoms, and medical works in which various maladies are discussed in alphabetical order, the present Index of Differential Diagnosis of Main Symptoms is unique in medical literature. It rests with the medical profession to decide whether it strikes the mark at which it aims. There must be room for improvement in many respects notwithstanding the great amount of time and labour that have been bestowed upon it.

However this may be, the work undoubtedly owes much of what value it possesses to the suggestions and kindly help of the many contributors who have assisted in its making; and to the practitioners and the authorities of various institutions who have generously lent the material for many of the illustrations. Indeed, it is difficult to see how the book could have been produced in its present completeness without their willing collaboration: to all of them the Editor tenders his sincere thanks.

HERBERT FRENCH
62 Wimpole Street, London
March 1912

A note on Herbert French (1875-1951)

It might be of interest to readers to learn a little of the original editor of this volume. Herbert French was a scholar at Christ Church, Oxford and proceeded as a medical student to Guy's Hospital in 1898, with a University Scholarship. He was appointed Assistant Physician at Guy's in 1906 and Full Physician in 1917. He served in the first world war in the Royal Army Medical Corps with the rank of Lieutenant Colonel and was also for many years Physician to the Household of HM George V.

French was a prolific writer, and published *An Index of Differential Diagnosis of Main Symptoms* in 1912. His ambitious aim was to collect all the symptoms and signs that might arise in the course of disease. He was a man of wide erudition and wrote no less than half of the first edition himself, taking the whole of medicine as his province. The book was an immediate success and was reprinted in the same year and again in 1913 with a second edition appearing in 1917.

H.E.

Contributors and their subjects

Paul M. Aichroth MS, FRCS
Consultant Orthopaedic Surgeon, Chelsea
& Westminster Hospital, and The
Wellington Knee Surgery Unit, London
Bone, swelling of
Contractures and deformities of the upper
and lower limbs
Foot and toes, deformities of
Spine, curvature of

David Bates MA, FRCP
Senior Lecturer in Neurology, Royal
Victoria Infirmary, Newcastle on Tyne
Amnesia
Apraxia
Ataxia
Athetosis
Aura
Choreiform movements
Clonus
Consciousness, disorders of
Convulsions and fits
Diplopia

Michael Baum ChM, FRCS
Professor of Surgery, Royal Marsden
Hospital and Past Professor of Surgery,
Kings College School of Medicine and
Dentistry
Breast lumps
Breast, pain in
Nipple, abnormalities of
Nipple, discharge from

Douglas Blackwood MB, ChB, PhD, FRCP,
FRCPsych
Reader in Psychiatry, University of
Edinburgh, Royal Edinburgh Hospital
Confusion
Delusions
Depression
Euphoria
Hallucinations
Memory, disorders of
Obsessions
Overactivity
Paranoid disorders
Sexual dysfunction

Thinking, disorders of
Underactivity

Peter T. Blenkinsopp FRCS, FDS, RCS
Consultant Oral and Maxillofacial
Surgeon, Roehampton, Kingston and St
Helier Hospitals
Gums, bleeding
Gums, hypertrophy of
Gums, retraction of
Jaw, deformity of
Jaw, pain in
Jaw, swelling of
Mouth, pigmentation of
Mouth, ulcers in

Ian A.D. Bouchier CBE, MD, FRCP, FRCPE,
FFPHM, HonFCP(SAF), FRSA, FIBiol, FRSE
Professor of Medicine, University of
Edinburgh, Honorary Consultant
Physician, Royal Infirmary, Edinburgh
Appetite, disorders of
Crepitus
Flatulence
Indigestion
Nausea
Regurgitation
Succussion sounds
Tongue, discoloration of
Vomiting

N.E.F. Cartlidge MBBS, FRCP
Senior Lecturer in Neurology, Consultant
Neurologist, Royal Victoria
Infirmary, Newcastle on Tyne
Hemianopia
Hemiplegia
Monoplegia, upper limb
Muscular atrophy
Muscular tone
Posture, abnormal
Pupils, abnormalities of
Reflexes, abnormalities of
Sensation, abnormalities of
Smell, abnormalities of

Graham Clayden MD, FRCP
Reader in Paediatrics, UMDS of Guys and
St Thomas's Hospitals, London

Contributors and their subjects

Encopresis
Enuresis
Marasmus
Napkin (perineal) eruptions
Pica

Anne Cockcroft MD, FRCP, DIH, FFOM
*Consultant/Senior Lecturer in
Occupational Medicine, The Royal Free
Hospital and School of Medicine, London*
Dyspnoea
Orthopnoea

David P. De Bono MA, MD, FRCP
*British Heart Foundation Professor of
Cardiology, University of Leicester,
Leicester*
Heart, enlargement of
Heart impulse, displaced
Heart, murmurs in
Heart, sounds
Neck, engorged veins in
Thrills

Neil J. Douglas MD, FRCPE
*Professor of Respiratory and Sleep
Medicine, University of Edinburgh, Royal
Infirmary, Edinburgh*
Cyanosis
Fingers, clubbed
Hiccup
Sleep, disorders of

Gordon Duff MA, BM, BCh, PhD, FRCP
*Professor of Molecular Medicine,
Department of Medicine and
Pharmacology, Royal Hallamshire
Hospital and University of Sheffield*
Pyrexia, prolonged
Pyrexia without obvious cause

Lynn Edwards MChir, FRCS (deceased)
*Formerly: Consultant Urological Surgeon,
Westminster Hospital, London*
Dysuria
Micturition, frequency of
Micturition, hesitancy
Pyuria
Urine, incontinence of
Urine, retention of

Harold Ellis CBE, DM, MCH, FRCS, FRCOG
*Emeritus Professor of Surgery, University
of London*

Abdominal pain, acute, localized
Abdominal pain (general)
Abdominal pulsation
Abdominal rigidity
Abdominal swellings
Axillary swelling
Back, pain in
Borborygmi
Constipation
Face, swelling of
Gallbladder, palpable
Gangrene
Kidney, palpable
Leg, ulceration of
Nasal regurgitation
Neck, stiff
Neck, swelling of
Penile sores
Penis, pain in
Perineal pain
Perineal sores
Peristalsis, visible
Pilimiction
Pneumaturia
Popliteal swelling
Priapism
Pruritis ani
Ptyalism
Salivary glands, pain in
Salivary glands, swelling of
Scrotum, ulceration of
Spine, tenderness of
Stomach, dilatation of
Stools, mucus in
Stools, pus in
Strangury
Testicular pain
Testicular swelling
Thyroid enlargement
Thyroid, pain in
Tongue, pain in
Tongue, swelling of
Tongue, ulceration of
Urethra, faeces passed through
Urethral discharge
Veins, varicose abdominal

Peter Emerson MA, MD, FRCP,
FACP(Hon.)
*Honorary Consultant Physician, Chelsea
and Westminster Hospital, London*
Sputum

Peter R. Fleming MD, FRCP
Formerly: Senior Lecturer in Medicine,
Charing Cross and Westminster
Medical School, London and Consultant
Physician, Westminster Hospital,
London
Chest pain
Faints
Haematuria
Leg, oedema of
Oedema, dependent
Oedema, generalized
Oliguria
Polyuria
Pulse, character of
Pulse rate, abnormal
Pulse, rhythm of
Pulses, unequal
Rub, pericardial
Smell as a physical sign
Urine, abnormal colour of
Yawning

William M. Haining MB, ChB, FRCSEd,
FRCOph
Emeritus Head of Department of
Ophthalmology, University of Dundee
Enophthalmos
Eye, pain in
Eyelids, disorders of

T.B. Hargreave MS, FRCS
Western General Hospital, Edinburgh
Impotence

F. Dudley Hart MD, FRCP
Consulting Physician, Chelsea Hospital
for Women, The Hospital of St John
and St Elizabeth, and Westminster
Hospital, London
Face, abnormalities of appearance and
movement
Fatigue
Headache
Leg, pain in

Robert C. Heading BSc, MD, FRCP
Reader in Medicine, Royal Infirmary,
Edinburgh
Dysphagia
Heartburn

M.M. Henry FRCS
Consultant Surgeon, Central Middlesex
Hospital and Honorary Consultant
Surgeon, St Mark's Hospital for Diseases
of the Colon/Rectum, London
Anorectal pain
Faeces, incontinence of
Rectal bleeding
Rectal discharge
Rectal mass
Rectal tenesmus
Rectal ulceration

Edward Housley MB, ChB, FRCPE, FRCP
Royal Infirmary, Edinburgh
Cramps
Fingers, dead (white, cold)

Roland T. Jung MA, MD, FRCP(Edin.),
FRCP
Consultant Physician and
Endocrinologist and Honorary Reader in
Medicine, Ninewells Hospital and Medical
School, Dundee
Weight gain
Weight loss

Andrew Keat MD, FRCP
Reader in Rheumatology, Charing Cross
and Westminster Medical School,
Honorary Consultant Physician, Charing
Cross Hospital, London
Arm, pain in
Joints, affections of
Leg, pain in

Christopher A. Ludlam BSc, PhD, FRCP,
FRCPath
Consultant Haematologist, Director of the
Haemophilia Centre, Royal
Infirmary, Edinburgh
Bleeding
Bruises
Lymphadenopathy
Pallor
Purpura
Splenomegaly

Ian Mackenzie TD, MD, FRCP (deceased)
Formerly: Consulting Physician to the
Department of Nervous Diseases, Guy's
Hospital, London

Contributors and their subjects

Face, pain in
Face, paralysis of
Gait, abnormalities of
Head, retraction of
Taste, abnormal perception of
Trismus (lockjaw)

Charles N. McCollum MD, FRCS
Professor of Surgery, University Hospital of South Manchester
Groin, swellings in

Derek Maclean MB, ChB, PhD, FRCP, FRCP(E)
Ninewells Hospital, Dundee
Hypothermia

A.G.D. Maran MD, FRCS, FRCS(Ed), FRCP(Ed), FACS, FDS(Hon.)
Professor of Otolaryngology, University of Edinburgh, Consultant Otolaryngologist, Royal Infirmary, Edinburgh
Deafness
Earache
Epistaxis
Nasal deformity
Nasal discharge
Nasal obstruction
Otorrhoea
Sneezing
Snoring
Throat, sore
Tinnitus
Tonsils, enlargement of
Vertigo
Voice, disorders of

George Masterton BSc, MD, MRCPsych
Department of Psychological Medicine, Royal Infirmary, Edinburgh
Anxiety
Behaviour, antisocial
Body image, disorders of
Depersonalization
Eating, disorders of
Factitious disorders
Hyperventilation
Hypochondriasis
Hysteria
Irritability
Pain, psychogenic
Panic
Phobias
Self-harm, deliberate

K.R. Palmer MD, FRCP(Ed)
Consultant Gastroenterologist, Western General Hospital, Edinburgh
Jaundice
Liver, enlargement of

Naren Patel MB, ChB, PRCOG
Consultant Obstetrician, University of Dundee, Ninewells Hospital, Dundee
Amenorrhoea
Dysmenorrhoea
Dyspareunia
Frigidity
Infertility
Labour, difficult
Menorrhagia
Metrorrhagia
Oligomenorrhoea
Pelvis, pain in
Pelvis, swelling in
Premenstrual syndrome
Pruritus vulvae
Vagina and uterus, prolapse of
Vagina, discharge from
Vagina, swelling in
Vulva, swelling of
Vulva, ulceration of

Ian D. Ramsay MD(Edin.), FRCP, FRCP(Edin.)
Consultant Endocrinologist, North Middlesex Hospital NHS Trust, London
Gynaecomastia
Hirsutism
Libido, excessive
Libido, loss of
Polydipsia
Puberty, delayed
Puberty, precocious
Pubic hair, loss of
Stature, short
Stature, tall
Testicular atrophy
Tetany

S.T.D. Roxburgh FRCS(Edin) FRCOph
Head of Department of Ophthalmology, University of Dundee
Arcus cornealis
Corneal disease
Cataract
Epiphora
Exophthalmos

Eye, blindness of
Eye, inflammation of
Lacrimation
Nystagmus
Optic fundus, abnormalities in
Photophobia
Ptosis
Squint (strabismus)
Vision, defects of
Vision, subjective disturbances of

Robin I. Russell MD, PhD, FRCP
Head of Department of Gastroenterology,
Royal Infirmary, Glasgow and the
University of Glasgow
Diarrhoea
Faeces, abnormal consistency and shape
Faeces, abnormal contents
Faeces, colour
Haematemesis
Melaena

Peter D. Samman MD, FRCP (deceased)
Formerly: Honorary Consultant
Physician, Dermatology Department,
Westminster Hospital, London and St
John's Hospital for Diseases of the
Skin, London
Nails, affections of

David A. Shaw MB, ChB, FRCP,
FRCP(Edin.)
Emeritus Professor of Clinical Neurology,
University of Newcastle upon Tyne
Drop attacks
Fasciculation
Grip, disturbances of
Muscular hypertrophy
Muscular pain
Paraplegia
Speech, abnormalities of
Tic
Tremor

Richard Staughton MA, FRCP
Consultant Dermatologist, Chelsea and
Westminster Hospital, London
Alopecia
Angioma and telangiectasia
Bullae
Crusts
Erythema
Face, ulceration of

Fingers, skin affections of
Flushing
Foot, ulceration of
Keloid
Lips, affections of
Macules
Napkin (perineal) eruptions
Nodules
Papules
Pruritus, generalized
Pustules
Scalp and beard, fungous affections of
Scaly eruptions
Scrotum, surface affections of
Skin, hardening
Skin, pigmentation of
Skin tumours
Striae atrophicae
Sweating, abnormalities of
Vesicles
Weals

Peter R. Studdy MD, FRCP
Consultant Physician, Harefield Hospital
and Mount Vernon and Watford Hospitals
Chest deformity
Chest, tenderness in
Cheyne–Stokes respiration
Cough
Haemoptysis
Pleural effusion
Pleural rub
Stridor
Tachypnoea
Thoracic wall veins
Tracheal deviation
Wheeze

John D. Swales MA, MD, FRCP
Director of Research and Development,
Department of Health, London
Blood pressure, high
Blood pressure, low

FRENCH'S INDEX OF
DIFFERENTIAL DIAGNOSIS

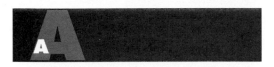

Abdominal pain, acute, localized

A common and extremely important clinical problem is the patient who presents with acute abdominal pain. This may be referred all over the abdominal wall (*see* ABDOMINAL PAIN, general, p. 3) but here we shall consider those patients who present pain localized to a particular part of the abdominal cavity.

The causes are legion and it is a useful exercise to summarize the organs that may be implicated together with the pathological processes pertaining to them so that the clinician can consider the possibilities in a logical manner:

1. Gastroduodenal

Perforated gastric or duodenal ulcer
Perforated gastric carcinoma
Acute gastritis (often alcoholic)
Irritant poisons

2. Intestinal

Small-bowel obstruction (adhesions etc)
Regional ileitis (Crohn's disease)
Intussusception
Sigmoid volvulus
Acute colonic diverticulitis
Large-bowel obstruction due to neoplasm
Strangulated external hernia (inguinal, femoral, umbilical)
Acute mesenteric occlusion due to arterial embolism or thrombosis or to venous thrombosis

3. Appendix

Acute appendicitis
Colic due to faecolith

4. Pancreas

Acute pancreatitis
Recurrent pancreatitis
Pancreatic trauma

5. Gallbladder and bile ducts

Calculus in the gallbladder or common bile ducts
Acute cholecystitis
Acute cholangitis

6. Liver

Trauma
Acute hepatitis

Malignant disease (primary or secondary)
Congestive cardiac failure

7. Spleen

Trauma
Spontaneous rupture (in malaria or infectious mononucleosis)
Infarction

8. Urinary tract

Renal, ureteric or vesical calculus
Renal trauma
Pyelonephritis
Pyonephrosis

9. Female genitalia

Salpingitis
Pyosalpinx
Ectopic pregnancy
Torsion of subserous fibroid
Red degeneration of fibroid
Twisted ovarian cyst
Ruptured ovarian cyst

10. Aorta

Ruptured aneurysm
Dissecting aneurysm

In addition to causes from intra-abdominal, retroperitoneal and pelvic organs, it is important to remember that acute localized pain may be referred to the abdomen from other structures:

11. Central nervous system

Herpes zoster affecting the lower thoracic segments
Posterior nerve root pain (e.g. from prolapsed intervertebral disc or collapsed vertebra from trauma or secondary deposits)

12. The heart and pericardium

Myocardial infarction
Acute pericarditis

13. Pleura

Acute diaphragmatic pleurisy

Occasionally patients are seen, who are often well known in the Casualty Department, presenting with simulated acute abdominal pain due to hysteria or malingering.

Patients with acute abdominal pain present one of the most testing trials to the clinician. In the first place, diagnosis is all important since a decision has to be made whether or not the patient requires urgent laparotomy, e.g. for a perforated peptic ulcer, acute appendicitis or acute intestinal obstruction. The history and examination are often difficult to elicit, particularly in a very ill patient who is in great pain and hardly wishes either to answer a lot of questions or to submit to prolonged examination. Finally, there are very few laboratory or radiological aids to diagnosis. Acute appendicitis, for example, has no specific tests. A raised white blood count suggests intraperitoneal infection but something like a quarter of the cases of acute appendicitis have a white count below 10 000. Plain X-rays of the abdomen may indicate free gas when there is a perforated hollow viscus but this is not invariably so. Intestinal obstruction may be revealed by distended loops of bowel on a plain X-ray of the abdomen but in some 10 per cent of small-bowel obstructions the X-rays are entirely normal, since the distended loops of bowel are filled with fluid only so that the typical gas-distended loops of bowel are not present.

One of the few investigations that the surgeon relies upon heavily is a raised serum amylase. When this is above 1000 units it is almost pathognomic of acute pancreatitis, although every now and then a fulminating case of pancreatitis is seen in whom the amylase is not elevated.

Every effort must therefore be made to establish the diagnosis on a careful history and examination.

One of the important aspects in the assessment of the acute abdomen is the establishment of a trend. Increasing pain, tenderness, guarding or rigidity indicates that there is some progressive intra-abdominal condition. This is also suggested by a rising pulse-rate on hourly or half-hourly observations and it is also suggested by progressive elevation of the temperature. In a doubtful case, repeated clinical examination, together with sequential recordings of the temperature and pulse, will enable the clinician to decide whether the intra-abdominal condition is subsiding or progressing.

GENERAL FEATURES

General inspection of the patient is all important and must never be omitted. The flushed face and coated tongue of acute appendicitis, the agonized expression of the patient with a perforated ulcer, the writhing colic of a patient with ureteric stone, biliary colic or small-bowel obstruction are all most helpful. The skin is inspected for the pallor suggestive of haemorrhage and for the jaundice which may be associated with biliary colic with a stone impacted at the lower end of the common bile duct. In such a case there will also be bile pigment which can be detected in the urine.

ABDOMINAL EXAMINATION

The patient must be placed in a good light and the entire abdomen exposed from the nipples to the knees. The abdomen is inspected. Failure of movement with respiration may suggest an underlying peritoneal irritation. Abdominal distension is present in intestinal obstruction and visible peristalsis may be seen from rhythmic contractions of the small bowel under these circumstances. Retraction of the abdomen may occur in acute peritonitis so that the abdomen assumes a scaphoid appearance, e.g. following perforation of a peptic ulcer.

Guarding, a voluntary contraction of the abdominal wall on palpation, denotes underlying inflammatory disease and this is accompanied by localized tenderness. Rigidity is indicated by an involuntary tightness of the abdominal wall and may be generalized or localized. Localized rigidity over one particular organ suggests local peritoneal involvement, for example in acute appendicitis or acute cholecystitis.

Percussion of the abdomen is useful. Dullness in the flanks suggests the presence of intraperitoneal fluid (e.g. blood in a patient with a ruptured spleen). A resonant distended abdomen is found in obstruction and loss of liver dullness suggests free gas within the peritoneal cavity in a patient with a ruptured hollow viscus.

In intestinal obstruction the bowel sounds are increased and have a particular 'tinkling' quality. In some cases borborygmi may be audible without using the stethoscope. Complete absence of bowel sounds suggests peritonitis.

Examination of the abdomen is not complete until the hernial orifices have been carefully inspected and palpated. It is easy enough to miss a small strangulated inguinal, femoral or umbilical hernia which, surprisingly enough, may have been completely overlooked by the patient.

Rectal examination is then performed. In intestinal obstruction the rectum has a characteristic 'ballooned' empty feel although the exact mechanism of this is unknown. In pelvic peritonitis there will be tenderness anteriorly in the pouch of Douglas. A tender mass suggests an inflamed or twisted pelvic organ and this can be confirmed by bimanual vaginal examination.

THE URINE AND SPECIAL INVESTIGATIONS

The presence of blood, protein, pus or bile pigment in the urine may help to distinguish a renal or biliary colic from other causes of intra-abdominal pain. In obscure cases of abdominal pain, the urine should be examined for porphyrins to exclude porphyria, particularly when the attack appears to have been precipitated by barbiturates.

The clinical assessment of the patient with acute localized abdominal pain, based on a careful history and examination together with examination of the urine, may be supplemented by laboratory and radiological investigations. A full blood count, plain X-ray of the abdomen, estimation of the serum amylase in suspected pancreatitis may all be helpful although, as mentioned above, must be interpreted with caution. Ultrasound of the pelvis may be helpful if a twisted ovarian cyst or some other pelvic pathology is suspected. Ultrasonography is also valuable in demonstrating gall stones in acute cholecystitis. An emergency intravenous urogram is indicated when ureteric stone or some other renal pathology is suspected. An electrocardiogram and appropriate cardiac enzyme estimations are performed if it is suspected that the upper abdominal pain is referred from a myocardial infarction and a chest X-ray may demonstrate a basal pneumonia. It must be stressed, however, that the clinical features take precedence over all other diagnostic aids.

Nothing can be simpler nor more difficult than diagnosing a patient with the so-called 'acute abdomen'. Particular difficulties will be encountered in infants (where the history may be difficult and examining a screaming child most demanding) and in the elderly, where again it is often difficult to obtain an accurate history and where physical signs are often atypical. The grossly obese patient and the pregnant patient are two other categories where particular difficulties may be encountered.

When faced with a patient with severe abdominal pain the main decision that must be taken, of course, is whether or not a laparotomy is indicated as a matter of urgency. If careful assessment still makes the decision difficult, then repeated observations must be carried out over the next hours to observe the trend of the particular case and this will nearly always enable a definite decision as to whether laparotomy or further conservative treatment is indicated.

Harold Ellis

Abdominal pain (general)

(*See also*) ABDOMINAL PAIN, acute localized, p. 1)

Most abdominal pain is localized, for example that due to a renal stone or biliary stone, acute appendicitis, peptic ulceration, and so on. There are, however, a number of causes of generalized abdominal pain, the commonest of which are peritonitis and intestinal obstructions.

ACUTE GENERAL PERITONITIS

Peritonitis must be secondary to some lesion which enables some clue in the history to suggest the initiating disease. Thus the patient with established peritonitis

may give a history of onset which indicates acute appendicitis or salpingitis as the source of origin. Where the onset of peritonitis is sudden, one should suspect an acute perforation of a hollow viscus. The early features depend on the severity and the extent of the peritonitis. Pain is always severe and typically the patient lies still on its account, in contrast with the restlessness of a patient with abdominal colic. An extensive peritonitis which involves the abdominal aspect of the diaphragm may be accompanied by shoulder-tip pain. Vomiting often occurs early in the course of the disease. The patient is obviously ill and the temperature frequently elevated. If initially the peritoneal exudate is not purulent, the temperature may be normal. It is a good aphorism concerning the two common causes of this condition that peritonitis due to appendicitis is usually accompanied by a temperature above 38°C (100°F), whereas the temperature in peritonitis due to a perforation of a peptic ulcer seldom reaches this level. The pulse is often raised and tends to increase from hour to hour. Examination of the abdomen demonstrates tenderness, which may be localized to the affected area or is generalized if the peritoneal cavity is extensively involved. There is marked guarding, which again may be localized or generalized, and rebound tenderness is present. The abdomen is silent on auscultation, although sometimes the transmitted sounds of the heart beat and respiration may be detected. Rectally, there is tenderness of the pelvic peritoneum. As the disease progresses, the abdomen becomes distended, signs of free fluid may be detected, the pulse becomes more rapid and feeble. Vomiting is now effortless and faeculent, and the patient, still conscious and mentally alert, demonstrates the Hippocratic facies with sunken eyes, pale, cold and sweating skin, and cyanosis of the extremities.

X-ray of the abdomen in the erect position may reveal free subdiaphragmatic gas in peritonitis due to hollow viscus perforation (e.g. perforated peptic ulcer), but its absence by no means excludes the diagnosis.

The main differential diagnoses are the colics of intestinal obstruction or of ureteric or biliary stone. Intraperitoneal haemorrhage, acute pancreatitis, dissection or leakage of an aortic aneurysm, or a basal pneumonia are also important differential diagnoses.

TUBERCULOUS PERITONITIS

In Great Britain this is now a rare disease. When it is encountered in this country, the patient is usually an immigrant from the Third World. Usually there is a feeling of heaviness rather than acute pain. The onset of symptoms is gradual, with abdominal distension, the presence of fluid within the peritoneal cavity, and often the presence of a puckered, thickened omentum, which forms a tumour lying transversely across the middle of the abdomen.

INTESTINAL COLIC (*See also* ABDOMINAL PAIN, ACUTE, LOCALIZED)

INTESTINAL OBSTRUCTION

This is a common cause of generalized abdominal pain. In peritonitis there is no periodic rhythm, whereas waves of pain interspersed with periods of complete relief or only a dull ache are typical of obstruction. In contrast to the patients with peritonitis who wish to remain completely still, the victim of intestinal obstruction is restless and rolls about with the spasms of the colic. Usually there are the accompaniments of progressive abdominal distension, absolute constipation, progressive vomiting, which becomes faeculent, and the presence of noisy bowel sounds on auscultation. X-rays of the abdomen usually reveal multiple fluid levels on the erect film together with distended loops of gas-filled bowel which are obvious on the supine radiograph.

LEAD COLIC

Lead colic may cause extremely severe attacks of general abdominal pain. There may be preceding anorexia, constipation and vague abdominal discomfort. The severe pain is usually situated in the lower abdomen radiating to both groins and may sometimes be associated with wrist-drop (due to peripheral neuritis) and occasionally with lead encephalopathy. There may be a blue 'lead line' on the gums if oral sepsis is present, due to the precipitation of lead sulphide. Frequently there is a normocytic hypochromic anaemia with stippling of the red cells (punctate basophilia). Inquiry about the patient's occupation may well be the first clue to the diagnosis. Other signs of lead poisoning are considered on p. 246.

GASTRIC CRISES

Gastric crises may cause general abdominal pain. The patient has other evidence of tabes dorsalis, with Argyll Robertson pupils, optic atrophy and ptosis, loss of deep sensation (absence of pain on testicular compression or squeezing the tendo Achillis), and loss of ankle- and knee-jerks. The pain is severe and lasts for many hours or even days. There may be accompanying vomiting and there may also be rigidity of the abdominal wall. The visceral crisis may be the sole manifestation of tabes. The mere fact that a patient has tabes dorsalis does not, of course, mean that his abdominal pain must necessarily be a gastric crisis. The author has repaired a perforated duodenal ulcer in a patient with

all the classic features of well-documented tabes dorsalis.

ABDOMINAL ANGINA

Abdominal angina occurs in elderly patients as a result of progressive atheromatous narrowing of the superior mesenteric artery. Colicky attacks of central abdominal pain occur after meals and this is followed by diarrhoea. Complete occlusion with infarction of the intestine is often preceded by attacks of this nature. Occlusion of vessels to small or large intestine as is seen in a number of vasculopathies, such as systemic lupus erythematosus or polyarteritis nodosa, may cause generalized abdominal pain and proceed to gangrene, perforation and general peritonitis.

FUNCTIONAL ABDOMINAL PAIN

One of the most difficult problems is the patient, female more often than male, who presents with severe chronic generalized abdominal pains in whom all clinical, laboratory and radiological tests are negative. Inquiry will often reveal features of depression or the presence of some precipitating factor producing an anxiety state. In some cases the abdomen is covered with scars of previous laparotomies at which various organs have been reposited, non-essential viscera removed, and real or imaginary adhesions divided. Some of these patients prove to be drug addicts, others are frank hysterics, others seek the security of the hospital environment, but in still others the aetiology remains mysterious. This forms one type of the so-called 'Munchausen syndrome', described by the late Dr Richard Asher.

ABDOMINAL PAINS IN GENERAL DISEASE

Acute abdominal pain may occur in a number of medical conditions not already considered. These include sudden and severe pain complicating malignant malaria, familial Mediterranean fever, and cholera, or may accompany uncontrolled diabetes with ketosis, that rare condition known as porphyria (*see* p. 757), and any of the blood dyscrasias; the best example is Henoch's purpura in children. Bouts of abdominal pain may occur in the hypercalcaemia of hyperparathyroidism.

Harold Ellis

Abdominal pulsation

A pulsatile swelling in the abdomen may be due to:
(1) a prominent aorta—normal or arteriosclerotic; (2) an abdominal aortic aneurysm; (3) transmission of aortic pulsations through an abdominal mass; or (4) a pulsatile enlarged liver.

1. Prominent aorta

The pulsations of the normal aorta may be felt in perfectly normal but thin subjects along a line extending from the xiphoid to the bifurcation of the aorta at the level of the fourth lumbar vertebra, about 2 cm below and a little to the left of the umbilicus. In the arteriosclerotic and hypertensive subject, it may be difficult to decide whether or not the aorta is merely thickened and tortuous or whether it is aneurysmal. If the two index fingers are placed parallel, one on either side of the aorta, the distance between the fingers can be measured. According to the size of the patient, a gap of 2-3 cm between the fingertips may be considered normal, but any measurement above this is suspicious of aneurysmal dilatation. If in doubt, visualization of the aorta by means of ultrasound or computerized tomography enables accurate measurement of the aorta to be made.

2. Abdominal aortic aneurysm

There is no doubt that arteriosclerotic abdominal aneurysms are becoming more frequently encountered, as is the serious emergency of leakage or rupture of such an aneurysm. The majority of patients are more than 60 years of age and the great majority are men. The aneurysm may be entirely symptomless or the patient may complain of epigastric or central abdominal discomfort which frequently radiates into the lumbar region. The patient himself may actually detect the pulsating mass in the abdomen.

The pulsation may be visible in the upper abdomen, above the umbilicus and, if large enough, may actually appear as a pulsating mass. On palpation, the aneurysm is a midline swelling which bulges over to the left side. If the mass extends below the level of the umbilicus it suggests implication of the iliac arteries. The characteristic physical sign is that the mass has an expansile pulsation. The index fingers are placed one on either side of the mass, which enables the diameter to be assessed. If the diameter is more than 3 cm, this certainly suggests aneurysmal dilatation of the aorta and if above 5 cm, the clinical diagnosis is all but certain. Typically, the fingers are pushed apart with each pulse and not up and down. The latter sign suggests *transmission* of the pulsation (*see section below*).

Usually the aneurysm is resonant to percussion due to overlying loops of intestine. However, an extremely large aneurysm will displace the bowel laterally to reach the anterior abdominal wall and will then give a dull percussion note. Auscultation may reveal bruits over the lower extremity of the aneurysm. This suggests turbulent flow of blood caused by relative stenosis at the aorto-iliac junctions.

Rectal examination may reveal a pulsatile mass when one or both of the internal iliac arteries are involved in the aneurysmal process.

Leakage or rupture of the aneurysm is an acute abdominal emergency. The patient presents with the features of massive blood loss (pale, sweating, clammy skin, a rapid pulse and low blood pressure) together with severe abdominal pain, lumbar pain and marked abdominal tenderness and guarding. Because of the low blood pressure and the associated peri-aneurysmal haematoma, as well as the overlying guarding, the aneurysm may be quite difficult to palpate and, unless sought for carefully, is easy enough to miss.

The diagnosis of aortic aneurysm is readily confirmed by means of a plain abdominal X-ray (*Fig.* A.1) which frequently delineates the aneurysm because of the associated calcification in its wall. Typically the aneurysm is seen to bulge over to the left side of the abdomen. More accurately, an ultrasound or computerized tomogram of the abdomen visualizes the aneurysm and enables its length and diameter to be measured accurately.

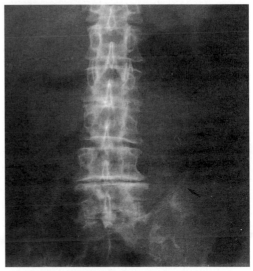

Fig. A.1. Plain X-ray of the abdomen showing a large calcified aortic aneurysm. The outline of the calcified left margin of the sac is indicated by the three arrows.

3. Transmission of aortic pulsations through an abdominal mass

A large intra-abdominal or retroperitoneal solid mass, pressing against the aorta, may exhibit transmitted aortic pulsation. Typical examples are a large carcinoma of the body of the stomach, a carcinoma or cyst of the pancreas and a large ovarian cyst. Indeed, when the whole abdomen is filled by a cystic mass it may be quite difficult to distinguish between such a mass and extensive ascites. Percussion, of course, is helpful since ascites gives dullness in the flanks as compared with the central dullness of a large intra-abdominal mass. The two index fingers, placed on the mass, will perceive that the pulsation is transmitted *directly forwards* from the aorta and is not expansile as would be found in an aneurysm.

4. Pulsatile liver

It is unlikely that an enlarged pulsatile liver will be mistaken for any other kind of pulsatile tumour. It occurs in cases of chronic failure of cardiac compensation, generally from mitral stenosis or tricuspid stenosis. There is associated cyanosis, oedema of the legs and ascites. It is not, however, every liver which seems to pulsate that really presents expansile pulsation. An impression of pulsation may be given by the movements transmitted directly to the liver by the hypertrophied right heart.

Harold Ellis

Abdominal rigidity

Rigidity of the abdomen is a sign of the utmost importance, since in most cases it indicates serious intra-abdominal mischief requiring immediate operation. It is the expression of a state of tonic contraction in the muscles of the abdominal wall. The responsible stimulus may be in the brain or basal ganglia, or in the territory of the six lower dorsal nerves that supply the abdominal wall, but not in the visceral sensory fibres of the sympathetic system. The extent of the rigidity will depend on the number of nerves involved, and its degree on the nature and duration of the stimulus. The analysis in the table on page 7 may be considered.

The patient should be examined lying on the back with the whole abdomen and lower thorax exposed, but the shoulders and legs well covered. The room must be warm. The examiner, seated on a level with the patient, should first watch the abdomen to see whether it moves with respiration or not, and whether one part moves more than another; at the same time he may observe other things which will help in the diagnosis, such as asymmetry of the two sides, local swelling, or the movement of coils of bowel. While watching and later when examining he should engage the patient in conversation, encouraging him to talk in order to allay nervousness and to remove any part of the rigidity which is due to a voluntary contraction. Some nervous patients, especially if the room is cold, hold their abdomens intensely rigid, and can be induced to relax only after gentle persuasion; a request to take a few deep breaths, or to draw their knees up and keep their mouths open, will often help. During this preliminary examination one hand, well

warmed, may be laid gently on the abdomen and passed over its surface with a light touch that cannot possibly hurt; this manoeuvre will help to allay the patient's anxiety still further and give the examiner an idea of the extent, intensity, and constancy of the rigidity which he must later investigate in more detail.

For more exact examination the observer should sit at the patient's side facing his head, and place both hands on the abdomen, examining comparable areas of both sides, simultaneously, and taking in turn the epigastrium, right and left hypochondria, umbilical region, both flanks as far back as the erector spinae (for the rigidity of a retrocaecal appendix may only affect the posterior part of the abdominal wall), the hypogastrium, and both iliac fossae. First, the whole hand should be applied with light pressure; next, the fingers held flat should be pressed more firmly to estimate the extent of the rigidity and to discover deep tenderness; lastly, detailed examination may be made in suspected areas with the firm pressure of one or two fingers. Evidence is not complete without percussion and auscultation. A rectal examination is indispensable.

After a leisurely examination with warm hands in a warm room, during which the physician has also been able to sum up the patient, his temperament, and whether he is really ill or not, the rigidity of anxiety or cold will have been dispelled or recognized. The abdominal rigidity due to a lesion in the chest or chest wall usually involves a wide area limited to one side—a distribution most unusual with intra-abdominal mischief, which, if it has spread widely but not everywhere, tends to be limited to the upper or lower half. The extent and degree of rigidity in chest affections also vary widely during examination. Other things such as a flushed face, rapid respiration, movement of the alae nasi, or a temperature of more than 39°C (102°F), may suggest that the lesion is not abdominal, and a friction rub may be felt or heard in the chest.

Auscultation and rectal examination dispel any remaining doubts, for in chest conditions peristaltic sounds remain normal, and there is no tenderness in Douglas's pouch. Examination of the blood may show a high leucocytosis, up to 30 000 or 40 000, whereas in peritonitis the count is seldom over 12 000. Chest X-rays (including a lateral film) will demonstrate the intrathoracic lesion.

Injuries of the abdominal wall, particularly those caused by run-over accidents, lead to very marked rigidity of the injured segment. Here the rigidity is not necessary to establish a diagnosis, for the injury is already known, but its degree and extent should be carefully noted. There must always be a doubt as to whether abdominal viscera are damaged as well as the

Site of stimulus	Causative agent	Characters of rigidity
Cerebral cortex or basal ganglia	Nervousness, anticipation of pain, cold	Affects the whole abdominal wall; varies in intensity, can be abolished by appropriate means
Dorsal nerve-trunks	Pleurisy; infections of the chest wall	Limited to one side of abdomen; varies in extent and degree
Nerve-endings in abdominal wall	Injury or infection of muscles	Limited to injured or infected segment
Nerve-endings in peritoneum	Irritation by any intraperitoneal foreign substance: infection, chemical irritant, or blood	Degree varies with nature of irritant and suddenness with which stimulus has arrived Extent corresponds to area of peritoneum involved Both degree and extent remain approximately constant during the period of examination

The extent of abdominal rigidity

walls, and this point can only be settled by careful observation. The patient is put to bed and kept warm, the pulse is charted every quarter of an hour, and the abdomen is re-examined from time to time. In the case of a mere contusion collapse will soon disappear, the abdomen will become less rigid, and the pulse-rate will fall. If the contents of a hollow viscus have escaped, rigidity will extend beyond the area of the damaged muscles, and the signs of peritonitis will develop rapidly. An X-ray of the abdomen, in the erect position, will demonstrate free gas beneath the diaphragm. If there is internal bleeding, for example from a ruptured spleen or liver, there is pallor and progressive elevation of the pulse, together with a falling blood pressure. Dullness in the flanks (especially on the left side, in rupture of the spleen) is often detected, as blood collects in the paracolic gutters.

Peritonitis

The commonest and the most important cause of general abdominal rigidity is peritonitis, and it is a safe rule when meeting true rigidity to diagnose peritonitis till it can be excluded. Actually rigidity means no more than that the peritoneum lining the abdominal cavity is in contact with something differing from the smooth surfaces which are its normal environment. The *presence of rigidity* therefore announces a change in the coelomic cavity that is probably infective in origin. When gallstone colic is followed by rigidity of the right rectus, it means, not only that a stone is blocking the cystic duct, but that the wall of the gallbladder is inflamed. Intestinal obstruction of mechanical origin (such as that due to a band or adhesion) gives colic referred to the umbilicus, but no guarding of the muscles; local rigidity accompanying the clinical picture of intestinal obstruction indicates that there is also a local inflammatory focus such as a strangulated loop of bowel, while a more diffuse rigidity suggests changes such as a thrombosis of the superior mesenteric artery, affecting a large segment of bowel. In

appendicitis, rigidity denotes that infection has spread beyond the coats of the appendix.

The *degree of rigidity* varies with the nature of the irritant, the rapidity with which the peritoneum is attacked, and the area involved. At one extreme is the rigidity of a duodenal perforation, where the abdomen is suddenly flooded with gastric contents. Here the whole abdominal wall is fixed in a contraction that can best be described as board-like: there is no respiratory movement, and no yielding to the firmest pressure. At the other extreme is the relatively minor degree of rigidity which accompanies the presence of small amounts of blood or urine in the peritoneal cavity; there is perhaps only a slightly increased resistance when the hands are pressed on the abdomen. Perforation of a gastric or duodenal ulcer produces the most intense rigidity; the escape of pancreatic enzyme in acute pancreatitis leads to less; escape of other sterile fluids, urine for instance, or blood, still less. Bacterial invasion of the peritoneum produces marked rigidity. The degree of muscle contraction also alters during the development of a case. The board-like abdominal wall of a perforation is considerably softer after 3 or 4 hours when the peritoneum has recovered from the shock of the first insult. The slight resistance apparent when sterile urine escapes from a ruptured bladder rapidly increases as infection supervenes.

The *extent of the rigidity* usually corresponds to the area of peritoneum affected. The whole abdomen may be rigid, the upper or lower part only, one side, or a restricted part. Total rigidity should mean a total peritonitis, but because the peritoneum reacts immediately to invasion by forming adhesions which localize the mischief, a general peritonitis is only seen when an irritant or infected fluid is suddenly discharged in large quantities–as in duodenal perforation, pancreatitis, or the bursting of a large abscess or distended viscus–or when the infection is brought by the bloodstream and reaches all parts simultaneously. Occasionally, particularly in children, the reaction to a sudden infection may be excessive and the muscles contract over a wide area in response to a purely local infection, for instance of the appendix, but this exaggerated response rapidly disappears. Conversely the aged, with atrophic abdominal muscles, may exhibit only slight rigidity, even in generalized peritonitis. Local peritonitis starts around some site of infection, and as it spreads is guided by certain peritoneal watersheds, of which the most important is the attachment of the great omentum to the transverse colon, dividing the abdomen into supra- and infra-colic compartments: rigidity accompanies the infection. Thus localized rigidity is found over any inflamed organ, and as the infection and the guarding spread, they tend to involve the upper or the lower half of the abdomen as a whole. When we have mapped out the extent of the rigidity, we should, from a knowledge of the organs at that site and of the watersheds that guide the spread of infection, be able, in conjunction with the history, to make a diagnosis.

The influence of natural subdivisions in guiding intraperitoneal extension must always be taken into account. Infections in the right supracolic compartment tend to pass down between the ascending colon and the right abdominal wall, while one in the pelvis is guided by the pelvic mesocolon to the left side of the abdomen as it ascends. Thus rigidity in the right iliac fossa may indicate a leaking duodenal ulcer, and in the left may be due to a pelvic appendix.

Since the diagnosis of peritonitis in most cases means immediate operation, every endeavour must be made to confirm the diagnosis, particularly by the simple tests of percussion, auscultation and rectal examination. Percussion may reveal the outline of some dilated hollow organ, such as the caecum; it may disclose free gas escaped from a perforation as a shifting circle of resonance or a tympanitic note where liver dullness should be; it may map out an abnormal area of dullness where there is an abscess or a collection of blood; or it may indicate free fluid in the peritoneum. Auscultation is even more important, for with peritonitis peristalsis ceases: in a normal abdomen peristaltic sounds can be heard every 4-10 seconds; in obstruction they are increased in loudness, pitch and frequency; in peritonitis there is complete silence. Rectal examination nearly always reveals tenderness when there is intra-abdominal infection, even if it is distant and localized.

Other signs must be mentioned: the patient lies still, sometimes with the knees drawn up, and resists interference. The abdomen gradually becomes distended, tense and tympanitic. The tongue is brown and dry. Vomiting is to be expected at the onset of any abdominal catastrophe, but except in intestinal obstruction it usually ceases; with advancing peritonitis it reappears, and the vomit becomes first bile-stained, later brownish and faecal smelling, and is allowed to dribble from the corner of the mouth in contrast to the projectile vomiting of obstruction. There may be diarrhoea at first, but absolute constipation soon succeeds it. The temperature tends to fall; the pulse is small and rapid, rising progressively. In late stages the sunken cheeks, wide eyes and anxious expression of the patient form a characteristic feature–the Hippocratic facies.

These signs are indications of a peritonitis discovered too late, and are the heralds of approaching death. Abdominal rigidity, abdominal silence, rectal tenderness and a rising pulse are a tetrad that calls for immediate definitive treatment.

A more detailed diagnosis is usually possible when the history and other signs are taken together, but a consideration of all the alternatives is out of the question in this section. Abdominal paracentesis with a fine needle may clinch the presence of pus, blood or urine in the peritoneal cavity, but a false negative tap may delay rather than aid diagnosis. A list of the more common conditions associated with rigidity may, however, help the inquiry:

STOMACH OR DUODENUM
Perforation of peptic ulcer

GALLBLADDER
Acute cholecystitis
Rupture of gallbladder

PANCREAS
Acute pancreatitis

SMALL INTESTINE
Strangulation of a loop
Traumatic perforation
Mesenteric vascular thrombosis or embolism
Meckel's diverticulitis
Acute ileitis

LARGE INTESTINE
Appendicitis
Volvulus
Diverticulitis with perforation

PERITONEUM
Acute blood-borne peritonitis:
    Streptococcal
    Pneumococcal
    Gonococcal

FEMALE GENERATIVE ORGANS
Twisted ovarian cyst
Ruptured ectopic pregnancy
Acute salpingitis
Torsion or red degeneration of fibroid
Perforation of uterus or posterior fornix of vagina in attempted abortion

SPLEEN AND/OR LIVER
Traumatic rupture

AORTA
Ruptured aneurysm

Perforation of a peptic ulcer is characterized by the most sudden onset, the worst agony and the most extreme abdominal rigidity that the physician is ever likely to see. Radiation of pain to the right shoulder tips (referred pain from diaphragmatic irritation) may be experienced. Immediately afterwards the patient is motionless and speechless, in a state of obvious collapse. A few hours later pain, rigidity and shock have all diminished, and only the dramatic history and persistent abdominal and rectal tenderness may remain to indicate the seriousness of the condition.

Acute pancreatitis is seldom accompanied by the severe pain described in textbooks, or indeed by pain as bad as that of gallstone colic. The abdominal rigidity is more marked in the upper abdomen but is not profound. On the other hand, the patient shows a degree of toxaemia out of all proportion to the physical signs in the abdomen. The diagnosis is confirmed by a considerable rise in the serum amylase.

A *ruptured ectopic pregnancy* may simulate a lower abdominal peritonitis, but the signs of bleeding predominate and rigidity is not well marked. If the patient is a woman of child-bearing age who is known to have missed a period, the onset of abdominal pain and pallor suggest the diagnosis. Extravasated blood will be felt in the pelvis, together with acute tenderness on vaginal and rectal examinations.

Blue discoloration of the skin around the umbilicus, Cullen's sign, may be associated with rigidity. This discoloration is due to extravasated blood coming forwards from the retroperitoneal space. The sign is seen in ruptured kidney, leaking abdominal aneurysm and acute pancreatitis. Occasionally it is seen in ruptured ectopic pregnancy, when the blood gains entry to the subperitoneal space through the broad ligament. Although pancreatitis may produce this sign, it is more common to see a green discoloration in the loins (Grey Turner's sign).

Harold Ellis

Abdominal swellings

(*See also* VARICOSE VEINS, ABDOMINAL.)

This may be acute or chronic, general or local, and caused by abdominal accumulations that are gaseous, liquid or solid. They may arise in the abdominal cavity itself or in the abdominal wall.

A. Swellings in the abdominal wall

Swellings situated in the abdominal wall itself can be recognized by their superficial position, by their adherence to the skin, subcutaneous fascia or muscles, or by their failure to follow the movements of the viscera immediately underlying the abdominal wall (*Fig.* A.2). It may be impossible to differentiate, for obvious reasons, an intra-abdominal mass that has become attached to the abdominal parietes either as an inflammatory or malignant process. A simple test which should be applied to all abdominal masses is to ask the patient to raise either his legs or shoulders from the couch. This procedure tightens the abdominal muscles; if the lump is intraperitoneal it disappears, but if it is situated in the abdominal wall itself it persists.

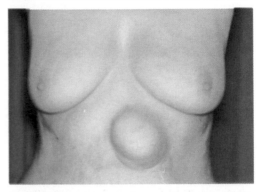

Fig. A.2. Large subcutaneous lipoma in the epigastrium. This moved freely on the abdominal wall even when the underlying muscles were tightly contracted.

Inflammatory swelling of the abdominal wall most commonly complicates a laparotomy incision and the diagnosis is obvious. A superficial cellulitis may complicate infection of a small abrasion or hair-follicle infection. Inflammation of the abdominal wall may be secondary to an extension of an intraperitoneal abscess, particularly an appendix abscess in the right iliac fossa or, on the left side, a paracolic abscess in relation to diverticular disease of the sigmoid colon or to perforation of a carcinoma of the large bowel.

Inflammatory swelling of the umbilicus in newborn infants is rare except in primitive communities where the cord is not divided with the niceties of modern aseptic practice. Suppuration at the umbilicus in adults is not uncommon if the navel is deep and narrow.

A tender haematoma in the lower abdomen may result from rupture of the rectus abdominis muscle or tearing of the inferior epigastric artery which may occur as the result of violent cough.

Tumours of the abdominal wall are usually subcutaneous lipomas. These may be multiple and may be a feature of Dercum's disease (adiposa dolorosa). Lipomas should be carefully differentiated from irreducible umbilical or epigastric hernias containing omentum.

A desmoid tumour may arise in the lower part of the abdominal wall and occasionally malignant fibrosarcomas or melanomas may be encountered. A neoplastic deposit may occasionally be palpated at the umbilicus and represents a transcoelomic seeding, usually from a carcinoma of the stomach or large bowel.

B. General abdominal swellings

Every medical student knows the mnemonic of the five causes of gross generalized swelling of the abdomen: Fat, Fluid, Flatus, Faeces and Fetus.

In *obesity* the abdomen may swell either in consequence of the deposit of fat in the abdominal wall itself or as the result of adipose tissue in the mesentery, the omentum, and in the extraperitoneal layer. In very obese persons it is rarely possible to diagnose the exact nature of an intra-abdominal mass by the usual clinical methods. Indeed, tumours of quite remarkable size, including the full-term fetus, may remain occult to even the most careful examiner.

Distension of the intestines with gas occurs in *intestinal obstruction* and is particularly marked in cases of volvulus of the sigmoid colon, chronic large bowel obstruction and megacolon. It also occurs in a dynamic ileus. The whole of the abdomen, or, in special cases, some part of it, is distended and gives on percussion a highly resonant or tympanitic note. The outlines of the gas-distended viscera are often visible; loops of dilated small bowel, one above the other, may produce a characteristic 'ladder pattern'. The increased size of the inflated intestine may produce displacement of the other viscera; the dome of the diaphragm is pushed up into the chest, shifting the apex beat of the heart upwards. The liver is similarly displaced. The distended *stomach* may occasionally be gross enough all but to fill the abdomen in very advanced cases of pyloric stenosis and in acute gastric dilatation.

The causes producing an accumulation of liquid in the peritoneal cavity can be listed as: congestive cardiac failure, cirrhosis, the nephrotic syndrome, carcinomatosis peritonei and tuberculous peritonitis.

In severe cases of *chronic constipation*, abdominal distension may result from accumulation of faeces in the large intestine, particularly where megacolon exists. The scybala may be felt, usually soft and plastic in the region of the ascending colon, and hard and nodular in the descending and sigmoid colon. Rectal examination often reveals an enormous accumulation of faeces. In some cases of tuberculous peritonitis semisolid inflammatory masses may bring about a general swelling of the abdomen. General swelling of the abdomen may occur in *malignant disease involving the peritoneum* due to the growth of numerous secondary nodules in addition to a concomitant ascites. *Pseudomyxoma peritonei* may follow rupture of a pseudomucinous cystadenoma of the ovary or of a mucocele of the appendix. The whole abdominal cavity becomes distended with gelatinous material.

C. Local intra-abdominal swellings

These may be due to some general cause or to a mass arising in a specific viscus.

1. Due to general causes

Causes which ordinarily produce general swelling of the abdomen may sometimes give rise to only a local swelling. Thus with *encysted ascites* left after an acute diffuse peritonitis or accompanying tuberculous peritonitis, an accumulation of fluid bounded by adhesions between the adjacent viscera may be found in any part of the peritoneal cavity, most often in the flanks or pelvis. A reliable history may be a clue to the nature of such a mass although its cause may not be revealed until a laparotomy has been performed.

Abdominal swellings may occur in *tuberculous peritonitis* resulting from the rolled-up, matted and infiltrated omentum, doughy masses of adherent intestine, or enlarged tuberculous mesenteric lymph nodes. The amount of ascites in such cases varies considerably from a gross degree to almost complete absence (the obliterative form). Discovery of a tuberculous focus elsewhere in the body is support for the diagnosis.

Hydatid cysts may occur in any part of the abdominal cavity. They are usually single. The liver, particularly the right lobe, is the most common situation; more rarely the spleen, omentum, mesentery or peritoneum. The cyst grows slowly and is spherical except in so far as it is moulded by the pressure of adjacent structures. It contains a clear fluid in which may be found hooklets, scolices and secondary or daughter cysts detached from the walls of the parent cyst. Unless large enough to cause mechanical pressure, the single hydatid cyst gives rise to little pain or indeed to any complaint of any kind. It may produce a smooth, rounded, tense bulging of the overlying abdominal wall. It is dull on percussion, and it may yield a 'hydatid thrill' as may any other cyst; this thrill is the vibratory sensation experienced by the rest of the hand when, with the whole hand laid flat over the tumour, a central finger is percussed. Occasionally there may be pain and fever due to inflammation within these cysts, and rupture into the peritoneal cavity may cause a severe anaphylactic reaction. Rupture of a hydatid cyst of the liver into a bile duct may cause jaundice due to biliary obstruction by daughter cysts. Hydatid disease is rare except in countries where the inhabitants live in close association with dogs that are the hosts of *Taenia echinococcus* (Australasia, South America, Greece, Cyprus, and, in the British Isles, North Wales). About one-quarter of patients demonstrate ecosinophilia. A complement fixation test gives a high degree of accuracy. X-rays of the abdomen may reveal calcification of the cyst wall in long-standing cases.

Any part of the abdomen may swell from the formation of an *abscess*. A subphrenic abscess following a general peritonitis is occasionally large enough to produce an upper abdominal swelling. The patient is usually seriously ill with a swinging fever, rapid pulse, leucocytosis and all the general manifestations of toxaemia. However, in this antibiotic era, more and more examples are being seen of a more insidious and chronic progress of the disease, with onset delayed weeks or even many months after the initial peritoneal infection. X-ray examination together with screening of the diaphragms is extremely useful and at least 90 per cent of patients with subphrenic infection have some abnormality on this investigation. On the affected side the diaphragm is raised and its sharp definition is lost. Its mobility on screening is diminished or absent. There is frequently a pleural effusion, collapse of the lung base or evidence of pneumonitis. About 25 per cent of patients have gas below the diaphragm, frequently associated with a fluid level. This gas is usually derived from a perforated abdominal viscus but occasionally is formed by gas-producing organisms. On the left side, gas under the diaphragm may be confused with the gastric bubble. An important differential feature is that the gas shadow of the stomach rarely reaches the lateral abdominal wall, but if there is doubt, a mouthful of barium is given in order to demarcate the stomach. Ultrasonography and computerised tomography usually clinch the diagnosis.

Pus may localize in either the right or left paracolic gutter or iliac fossa. On the right side this commonly follows a ruptured appendix or occasionally a perforated duodenal ulcer. On the left, a perforation of an inflamed diverticulum or carcinoma of the sigmoid colon is the usual cause. A large pelvic abscess frequently extends above the pubis or into one or other iliac fossa from the pelvis and can be palpated abdominally as well as on pelvic or rectal examination. About 75 per cent result from gangrenous appendicitis and the rest follow gynaecological infections, pelvic surgery, or any general peritonitis.

2. The regional diagnosis of local abdominal swellings

For clinical purposes the abdomen may be subdivided into nine regions by two vertical lines drawn upwards from the mid-inguinal point midway between the anterior superior iliac spine and the symphysis pubis, and by two horizontal lines, the upper one passing through the lowest points of the 10th ribs (the sub-

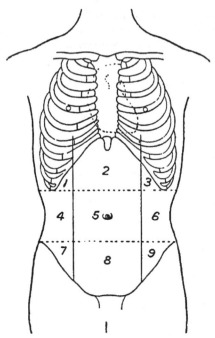

Fig A.3. The regions of the abdomen, for the significance of the numerals, *see* on page 12.

costal line), the other drawn at the highest points of the iliac crests (*Fig.* A.3).

The three median areas thus mapped out are named, from above downwards, the epigastric, umbilical and hypogastric (or suprapubic) regions; the six lateral areas are, from above downwards, the right and left hypochondriac, lumbar and iliac regions.

The viscera, or portions of viscera, commonly situated in the areas thus demarcated are given in the accompanying table.

The abdominal swellings that may be felt in and about these nine regions, excluding the tumours situated in the abdominal wall itself that have already been described, are as follows:

A. RIGHT HYPOCHONDRIAC REGION

Most tumours in this area are connected with the liver or gallbladder and their differential diagnosis is discussed under LIVER, ENLARGEMENT OF (p. 396) and GALLBLADDER, PALPABLE (p. 233)

A mistake easily made is to regard the firm and rounded swelling produced by the upper segment of the right rectus abdominis muscle, especially in a well-developed subject, as a tumour of the liver or gallbladder.

Tumours in connection with the hepatic flexure of the colon, scybalous collections in the hepatic flexure region, or the head of an intussusception may present as masses in this area.

The normal contents of the abdominal regions

1. Right hypochondriac	2. Epigastric
Liver	Liver
Gallbladder	Stomach and pylorus
Hepatic flexure of colon	Transverse colon
Right kidney	Omentum
Right suprarenal gland	Pancreas
	Duodenum
	Kidneys
	Suprarenal glands
	Aorta
	Lymph nodes

3. Left hypochondriac	4. Right lumbar
Liver	Riedel's lobe of the liver
Stomach	Ascending colon
Splenic flexure of colon	Small intestine
Spleen	Right kidney
Tail of pancreas	
Left kidney	
Left suprarenal gland	

5. Umbilical	6. Left lumbar
Stomach	Descending colon
Duodenum	Small intestine
Transverse colon	Left kidney
Omentum	
Urachus	
Small intestine	
Aorta	
Lymph nodes	

7. Right iliac fossa	8. Hypogastric
Caecum	Small intestine
Vermiform appendix	Sigmoid flexure
Lymph nodes	Distended bladder
	Urachus
	Enlarged uterus and
	adnexa

9. Left iliac fossa	
Sigmoid flexure	
Lymph nodes	

B.   EPIGASTRIC REGION

Enlargement of the *liver* may be felt in this area, and indeed it is common to feel the normal liver in this region, especially in infants and in adults with an acute costal angle. The dilated *stomach* produced by pyloric stenosis in either children or adults may present as a visible swelling demonstrating waves of peristalsis travelling from left to right. A succussion splash is usually elicited. Tumours of the stomach, apart from malignant growth, are rare. At the turn of this century a hair ball or trichobezoar was frequently encountered as an epigastric mass in hysterical girls who chewed and swallowed their hair, which then formed an exact mould of the stomach. Hairballs are only rarely encountered these days and modern textbooks hardly mention them; however, as fashions and hair styles change they

may reappear on the clinical scene (*Fig.* A.4). Other foreign bodies are sometimes ingested by mental defectives and form a palpable mass. In congenital pyloric stenosis a tumour the size of a small marble is palpable at the right border of the right rectus.

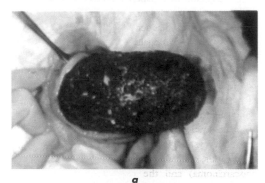

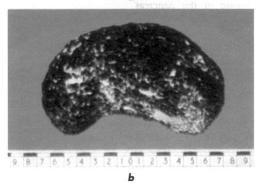

Fig. A.4. Gastric hairball. This formed a large, mobile epigastric mass in a young married woman with long hair, *a*, shows the mass being removed at gastrotomy. *b*, Demonstrates the specimen.

The *transverse colon* usually passes across the upper part of the umbilical area and may be palpated when it is the site of a carcinoma, when it is impacted with faeces, or when it is distended by a large-bowel obstruction placed distal to it.

Swellings in connection with the *omentum* may be due to tuberculous peritonitis or, more commonly, due to infiltration with secondary malignant deposits.

Swellings arising from the *pancreas* push forward from the depths of the abdominal cavity towards the epigastric and the upper part of the umbilical areas, and present themselves as vaguely palpable deeply seated masses. They have the stomach, or the stomach and colon, in front of them and are fixed to the posterior abdominal wall, thus moving but little on respiration. They may transmit a non-expansile pulsation from the subjacent aorta. Unless extremely large, such swellings are resonant on percussion, due to the overlying air-filled gut. A pancreatic swelling may be carcinomatous, in which case wasting, anaemia, and jaundice are likely to be observed. There may be clay-coloured stools and dark urine and it is important to note that frequently the onset of jaundice is preceded by deeply placed abdominal pain, or pain in the back. Glycosuria of recent origin in an elderly patient also raises suspicion of a pancreatic carcinoma. In about half the patients with jaundice due to carcinomatous obstruction the gallbladder is palpably distended (Courvoisier's law). Occasionally the mass may result from chronic pancreatitis; the swollen pancreas of acute pancreatitis has only exceptionally been palpated before laparotomy.

Pancreatic cysts are the pancreatic swellings which are most commonly palpable. Only 20 per cent are true cysts; these are either single or multiple retention cysts which usually result from chronic pancreatitis, neoplastic cysts (cystadenoma and cystadenocarcinoma) and the rare congenital polycystic disease of the pancreas and hydatid cyst of the pancreas. Far more often the cysts are not in the pancreas itself but comprise a collection of fluid sealed off in the lesser sac due to closure of the foramen of Winslow (pseudocyst of the pancreas). This may occur after trauma to the pancreas, following acute pancreatitis, or, less commonly, resulting from perforation of a posterior gastric ulcer. They may reach an enormous size and fill the whole upper part of the abdomen.

Retroperitoneal cysts are rare. The majority arise from remnants of the mesonephric (Wolffian) duct and occur in adult women. Others are teratomatous, lymphangiomatous or dermoid.

Retroperitoneal tumours (apart from those arising in the pancreas, suprarenal or kidney) originate in the mesenchymal tissues, the sympathetic chain and the para-aortic lymph nodes.

Swellings in connection with the *duodenum* are excessively rare. They may result from an inflammatory mass developing around a penetrating duodenal ulcer or be due to a duodenal malignant tumour, but the latter is a pathological curiosity. Those in connection with the *kidneys* and *suprarenal glands* are found in the epigastrium only if very large. Their diagnosis is considered below.

Enlargement of the *spleen* may bring its notched anterior edge into the epigastric area; a splenic swelling always lies in contact with the anterior wall of the abdomen (*see* SPLENOMEGALY p. 615).

Lymph nodes, which are numerous in the para-aortic retroperitoneal tissues and in the mesentery, may become palpable in reticuloses, tuberculous peritonitis, or malignant disease as nodulated chains or masses.

C. LEFT HYPOCHONDRIAC REGION

An abnormal lobe or a tumour in the left lobe of the *liver* may appear as a superficial tumour in this area.

Much of the *stomach* normally lies in the left hypochondrium; the diagnosis of gastric swelling has been considered above and a gastric tumour is commonly felt in this region. On physical signs alone it must be differentiated from a swelling of the adjoining *spleen*. A barium-meal X-ray examination, ultrasound or CT scan help considerably in differentiating between a gastric and a splenic swelling.

The diagnosis of a tumour of the splenic flexure of the *colon*, whether scybalous or malignant, is arrived at in the same way as a case of a tumour of the hepatic flexure or transverse colon (*see* (A) and (B)).

The diagnosis of the various causes of enlargement of the *spleen* is discussed under SPLENOMEGALY (p. 615). The distinguishing features are that it comes down from under the left costal margin in direct contact with the anterior abdominal wall (and is therefore dull on percussion), descends on inspiration, has a smooth surface, and a notch may be palpable on its inner margin. A splenic swelling may be identified on a plain X-ray of the abdomen and differentiated from a renal mass by means of pyelography. A barium-meal examination may show displacement and indentation of the adjacent stomach. Ultrasound or CT scan will clinch the diagnosis.

Tumours of the *pancreas* may project into the left hypochondrium as may retroperitoneal tumours and cysts (*see* (B)).

Tumours of the left *kidney* and *suprarenal gland* have the stomach and colon in front of them and therefore, unless extremely large, are resonant on percussion. Since they arise in the loin, these masses can usually be balloted by bimanual palpation.

D. RIGHT LUMBAR REGION

Occasionally a congenital projection of the *liver*, known as Riedel's lobe, may appear as a superficial tumour continuous with the liver above it in this zone. It may be mistaken for a dilated gallbladder.

The *ascending colon* may be palpable due to contained faecal masses, owing to thickening as a result of long-standing colitis, Crohn's disease or hyperplastic tuberculosis, or due to malignant disease.

The ascending colon can be felt in acute or chronic *ileocaecal and ileocolic intussusception* as a sausage-shaped tumour, at first situated in the right flank, then moving across the abdomen above the umbilicus and finally down the left flank into the pelvis. The vast majority of these cases occur in infants or young children commonly aged between 3 and 12 months. Boys are affected twice as often as girls. The history is of paroxysms of abdominal colic typified by screaming and pallor. There is vomiting and usually the passage of blood and mucus per rectum, giving the characteristic 'red-currant-jelly stool'. Rectal examination nearly always reveals this typical feature and rarely the tip of the intussusception can be felt. In infants there is usually no obvious cause, but the mesenteric lymph nodes in these cases are invariably enlarged. In adults a polyp, carcinoma or an inverted Meckel's diverticulum may form the apex of the intussusception.

Tumours in connection with the *right kidney* and *suprarenal gland* usually appear deep down in this region, having the ascending colon and small intestine in front of them. They can be lifted forwards *en masse* from behind by a hand placed at the back of the loin and thus palpated bimanually. For their diagnosis *see* KIDNEY, PALPABLE (p. 360). The lower pole of the right kidney can be felt in many normal persons on deep abdominal palpation, especially in thin females. When abnormally low and mobile, the whole of the otherwise normal kidney may be palpable. Its shape and consistency are characteristic. Renal swellings move on respiration and, unless very large, are resonant on percussion due to the anteriorly related gut. However, Riedel's lobe of the liver, an enlarged gallbladder, masses in the ascending colon and secondary deposits in the omentum have all been mistaken for it, although they are more superficially placed and lie in contact with the anterior abdominal wall. Other wandering masses, e.g. those arising from the ovary, Fallopian tube and mesentery, as well as hydatid cysts, are all liable to the same error of identification.

Imaging, by means of ultrasound or CT scanning, is invaluable in assistance with the differential diagnosis.

E. UMBILICAL REGION

The grossly dilated *stomach* resulting from long-standing pyloric obstruction may occupy the umbilical region; indeed it may descend below it down into the pelvis.

Tumours in connection with the *transverse colon* have been considered in (B) and (D) above.

Tumours in connection with the *omentum* are common in this region; those arising from the *small intestine* are much rarer, although the thickened small bowel in Crohn's disease may form a palpable mass.

Swellings arising from the *kidneys*, *suprarenals*, *pancreas*, *retroperitoneal tissues*, *para-aortic nodes* and *mesentery* may all present themselves in the deeper parts of the umbilical region, usually as more or less fixed masses arising from or connected with the posterior wall of the abdomen.

The *aorta* bifurcates half an inch below and to the left of the umbilicus (at the level of the 4th lumbar vertebra). In thin patients, pulsation of the normal aorta can often be felt and indeed seen in this region and may lead to the incorrect diagnosis of an abdominal aneurysm. Careful examination, however, will show that this pulsation is no more than a throbbing, an up-and-down movement, and is not laterally expansile. Aneurysm of the abdominal aorta forms an expansile mass situated above the umbilicus itself and may be accompanied by pain in the back from erosion of the bodies of the lumbar vertebrae. Often X-rays of the abdomen in such cases will reveal calcification in the aneurysmal wall. Ultrasound and computerized tomography enable accurate delineation of the size and extent of the aneurysm. They are also valuable in the visualization of the other retroperitoneal masses enumerated above.

F. LEFT LUMBAR REGION

An enlarged *spleen* (*see* (C)) may protrude into this area. It forms a firm mass in contact with the abdominal wall and its dullness to percussion continues with its thoracic dullness which extends back up into the axilla along the line of the 9th or 10th ribs. Tumours in connection with the *right kidney*, the *right suprarenal gland* and the *descending colon* give similar features to those considered in (C) above.

G. RIGHT ILIAC FOSSA

An inflammatory mass in this region is most commonly associated with an *appendix abscess*. Less commonly there may be a *paracaecal abscess* in relation to a perforated carcinoma of the caecum or a solitary caecal benign ulcer. A *pyosalpinx* may result from salpingitis and rarely, inflammatory swellings may arise in connection with suppurating *iliac lymph nodes* or a *psoas abscess*.

An important differential diagnosis is between an appendix mass and a carcinoma of the caecum. Usually in the former there is a preceding episode of an acute abdominal pain, typical of appendicitis, with fever and leucocytosis. The inflammatory mass subsides progressively over 2 or 3 weeks and the occult blood test in the stools is negative. A carcinoma of the caecum may be suspected if there is a preceding history of bowel disturbance in a middle-aged or elderly patient, if the mass fails to resolve rapidly, and if the occult blood test in the stools is repeatedly positive. If there is any clinical doubt, a barium-enema X-ray examination should be carried out and, if necessary, resort made to laparotomy.

It is not at all rare for a soft 'squelchy' caecum to be palpable in a perfectly normal thin, usually female, subject.

Occasionally a grossly distended *gallbladder* may project down as far as the right iliac fossa and a low-lying *kidney* may form a palpable mass in this region. An *ovarian tumour* or *cyst* or a pedunculated *fibroid* of the *uterus* may project into this area.

H.   HYPOGASTRIC REGION

The commonest mass to be felt in this region is the distended *bladder*. This may reach as high as, or slightly above, the umbilicus. Not uncommonly this midline structure tilts over to one or other side. A distended bladder has been tapped as ascites, operated upon as an ovarian cyst or fibroid, or mistaken for the pregnant uterus. No diagnostic opinion should be advanced, and no operative procedure undertaken respecting a tumour in this situation, until the bladder has been emptied, either by voluntary micturition or by the passing of a catheter.

Abdominal swellings arising from the *uterus, ovaries, Fallopian tubes* and *uterine ligaments* may all rise up out of the pelvis and present themselves as swellings in this region; as they grow larger they may be spread into any part of the abdomen. While they remain comparatively small and are manifestedly connected with some intrapelvic organ, their origin, is not difficult to determine (*see* PELVIS SWELLING IN, p. 489). However, when they have extended into the abdomen or have acquired a long pedicle, or have become fixed by adhesions to some distant part of the abdominal wall or to some other viscus, these pelvic tumours may give rise to signs and symptoms which bear no relation to pelvic disease. In such cases they may only be correctly diagnosed at laparotomy. The discerning clinician will always remember the possibility of pregnancy in every female patient between the menarche and menopause.

Tumours of ileal Crohn's disease arising in the *small intestine* may be felt in the hypogastric area.

The *urachus* is a fibrous cord running in the middle line in front of the peritoneum from the fundus of the bladder to the umbilicus. Occasionally it becomes the seat of cyst formation, more often in women than in men. The urachal cyst is a rounded tumour lying between the umbilicus and the pubic symphysis, which occasionally becomes infected.

I.   LEFT ILIAC FOSSA

The *pelvic colon* can often be felt in normal subjects as a tube-like cord either when empty and in spasm or else when disintended with faecal masses. This region is a common site for carcinoma of the colon and there are usually symptoms of chronic intestinal obstruction, or bowel disturbance with the passage of blood and mucus in the stools. It is clinically impossible to differentiate between such a mass and that associated with diverticular disease of the sigmoid colon.

Similarly a paracolic abscess in this region may equally well be associated with suppuration of an inflamed colonic diverticulum or a perforating carcinoma. Rarely such an abscess may be due to perforation of the tip of a long *appendix* passing over the left iliac fossa, or as an extreme rarity due to local perforation of a left-sided appendix in transposition of the viscera. The diagnosis would be suggested by finding the cardiac apex beat to lie on the *right* side.

Harold Ellis

| Alopecia

Although hair may not have an essential biological role for humans, the psychological significance of hairfall is often ignored by doctors. When an increase in hairfall occurs, men may become anxious, fearing loss of potency, and women may be appalled at the cosmetic disaster that they foresee. Convenient clinical division of the possible causes of alopecia can be made by considering: (i) whether obvious scalp skin abnormality is present or not (*Table A1*); (ii) the distribution of hair thinning or baldness (patchy, diffuse or male pattern).

1. Patchy hair thinning/balding accompanied by obvious scalp skin disease

Eczematous inflammation of scalp skin can cause hairfall and there is usually accompanying scaling or weeping. In the majority of such patients there will be signs of dermatitis elsewhere, usually *seborrhoeic dermatitis* (*Fig.* A.5). Here pink greasy-scaled patches are seen in the seborrhoeic distribution, in and behind the ears, in the nasolabial folds, at the anterior hairline, in the eyebrows and on mid-chest and back. *Contact dermatitis* of the scalp is a much less common cause of hair loss. Swelling of eyelids or ears usually accompanies this, e.g. hair dye dermatitis.

The important differential diagnosis, especially in children, is that of tinea capitis (*see* SCALP AND BEARD, FUNGOUS AFFECTIONS OF, p. 582), where the patchy balding is due to hairs breaking off just above the surface, giving a stubbled appearance. The degree of surrounding inflammation and scaling depends on the fungus responsible. *Microsporum canis* and *Trichophyton mentagrophytes* tend to be more inflammatory than *Microsporum audouinii* and *Trichophyton violaceum*. Microsporum infections fluoresce green under ultraviolet (Wood's) light, and microscopical examination and subsequent cultural identification confirms the diagnosis. *Bacterial folliculitis*, if extensive enough, sometimes perpetuated by infestation with head lice, can cause patchy hairfall. Pustules should be easily found, and there will be draining lymphadenopathy (*Fig.* A.6). A sterile inflammatory folliculitis (*folliculitis*

Table A.1. Alopecia

	Scalp skin abnormal	Scalp skin normal

Patches of hair thinning/balding	Dermatitis
	  seborrhoeic
	  contact allergic
		Alopecia areata
		Secondary syphilis

	Tinea capitis	Trichotillomania

	Folliculitis
	  bacterial
	  decalvans
		Traction alopecia

	Lupus erythematosus Lichen planus Morphoea Hot-combing Radiotherapy Lupus vulgaris Pseudo-pelade	
Diffuse hair thinning/balding		Alopecia totalis Telogen effluvium: 3/12 post-trigger event Anagen effluvium: drugs and poisons Endocrinopathy
Male-patterned hair thinning/balding		Androgenic alopecia

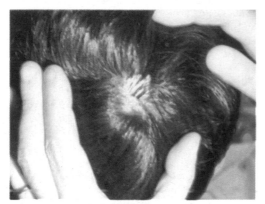

Fig. A.5. Seborrhoeic dermatitis of scalp. (*Dr Richard Staughton.*)

decalvans) is a rare cause of patchy balding in middle-aged scalps.

SCARRING ALOPECIA

Should the scalp skin be obviously tethered and scarred around the balding area, a search should be made for signs of *lupus erythematosus* (*Fig.* A.7) (fixed, sharply demarcated patches of erythema, scaling with follicular plugging and telangiectasia, often with marginal activity and central depigmentation), or *lichen planus* (flat-topped papules on the wrists, lace-like white areas on the buccal mucosae). More esoteric causes of scarring alopecia include radiotherapy, lupus vulgaris, hot-combing in Negroes and pseudo-pelade of Brocq. If scarring is linear, especially if it extends to the forehead and has a violaceous edge, then localized *scleroderma* (*morphoea*) may be the cause. The whole lesion has

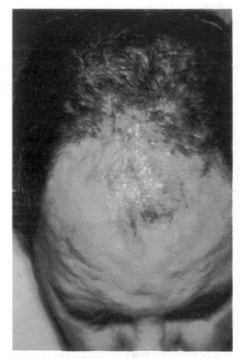

Fig. A.6. Bacterial folliculitis. (*Westminster Hospital.*)

the appearance of an exaggerated scar—*en coup de sabre* (*Fig.* A.8).

2. Patches of hair thinning/balding with normal underlying scalp skin

Alopecia areata is the commonest cause of patchy baldness (*Fig.* A.9). Patches are asymptomatic and are often discovered by relatives or hairdressers. Patients

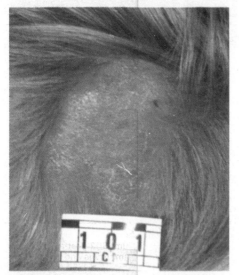

Fig. A.7. Scarring alopecia due to discoid lupus erythematosus. (*Westminster Hospital.*)

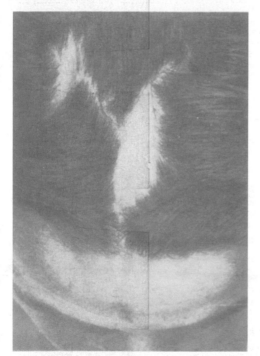

Fig. A.8. Scleroderma—coup de sabre. (*Dr Peter Hansell.*)

are lost. The course and prognosis are highly variable but generally good. On average two or three patches appear, remain stable for anything up to 6 months and then regrow without trace within 12 months. Initially regrowth is often white. The cause is unknown. There is a family history in 30 per cent of cases and it is occasionally associated with autoimmune diseases such as vitiligo, thyrotoxicosis, myxoedema, pernicious anaemia or Addison's disease. Down's children are liable to alopecia areata. A convincing preceding history of emotional shock is given by a proportion of patients and may be a permissive trigger factor.

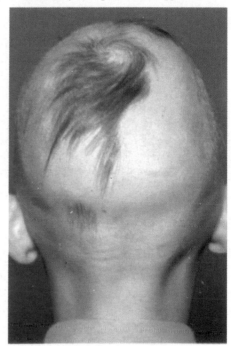

Fig. A.9. Alopecia areata. (*Westminster Hospital.*)

Syphilis is again becoming more common and during the secondary phase alopecia can occur. The appearance is of an asymptomatic patchy 'moth-eaten' baldness. On examination there is no scaling or obvious scalp disease and, in contrast to alopecia areata, baldness is partial rather than complete. Exclamation-mark hairs are not seen, and the patches are more numerous and accompanied by fever, sore throat and lymphadenopathy. The serology is positive and the hair regrows after antibiotic treatment.

Trichotillomania is the rather cumbersome title given to what often amounts to only a 'habit tic'. If hair is twirled between the fingers it eventually breaks, leaving patches of shortened hairs. Microscopic examination reveals obvious fractured ends to affected hairs. Some psychiatrically disturbed individuals pursue hair pulling and produce bald patches. The fractures may be seen at the scalp surface, or even at the roots.

of any age are affected, especially those in late childhood or early teens. The hallmark of this disease is a neat sharply localized patch of billiard-ball baldness with no obvious inflammation or scaling at the edge of lesions, where the diagnostic exclamation-mark hairs should be searched for. There are usually two or three patches and sometimes these coalesce at an alarming rate and may even cause *alopecia totalis* of the scalp, or *alopecia universalis* where beard and all body hairs

Traction alopecia is seen at the hair margins and is due to regular hair-dressing techniques pulling on hairs, e.g. rollers, braiding, ethnic plaiting, tight pony tails (*Fig.* A.10).

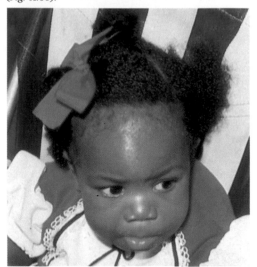

Fig. A.10. Traction alopecia. (*Dr Richard Staughton.*)

3. Diffuse alopecia without scalp disease

Telogen effluvium. A growing (anagen) hair has a large bulb easily seen with a hand lens on plucking. When growth ceases the bulb shrinks and the hair enters a resting (telogen) phase for 3 months before falling (catogen). In healthy adults some 50–100 hairs enter telogen daily and thus fall some 3 months later. Not surprisingly certain events upset the hair cycle, whereupon a larger number of hairs cease growing and enter telogen. Three months later they will fall as a so-called 'telogen effluvium'.

Triggering events include childbirth, stopping the contraceptive pill, a febrile illness, blood loss, an operation, myocardial infarction, stroke, rapid weight loss, bereavement or other psychological stress. The patient often complains of a worrying increase in hairfall but on examining the scalp no obvious abnormality is seen although if the hair is gently grasped between thumb and finger many telogen hairs may be detached. Further evidence can be obtained by asking patients to collect their daily hairfall from hair brushes and pillow. Normally some 50–100 hairs can be collected, 300–400 can fall daily in telogen effluvium. The prognosis is excellent.

Anagen effluvium. Fall of growing hairs also causes diffuse hair shedding, and may occur after exposure to certain drugs or poisons, e.g. cytotoxics, 13-*cis* retinoic acid (Roaccutane-Roche), thiouracil, anticoagulants, excess vitamin A and thallium poisoning.

Diffuse hairfall occurs in endocrinopathy, e.g. myxoedema, hypopituitarism and hypoparathyroidism. Myxoedema is regularly accompanied by hair thinning. The mechanism is unknown and may not be directly related to serum thyroxine level as adequate replacement therapy may fail to reverse the process.

4. Male pattern baldness without obvious scalp disease

Male pattern baldness is not a disease, but an accelerated physiological process. Males and females progressively lose androgen-dependent scalp hairs with increasing age—in males with successive thinning of bitemporal, occipital and pate areas, and in females with a more diffuse patterned thinning over most of the vertex. Some individuals have increased sensitivity of their hair follicles to normal levels of circulating androgens and lose their androgen-dependent hair earlier. Such hairfall does not occur in castrates and oestrogens and anti-androgenic drugs appear to have a protective effect. The prognosis for regrowth is poor.

Richard Staughton

ACID-BASE HOMEOSTASIS
See APPENDIX.

ACROPARAESTHESIAL
See SENSATION, ABNORMALITIES OF.

ADRENAL STEROIDS AND RELATED AMYLATES
See APPENDIX.

Amenorrhoea

The age at which menstruation first appears is variable, being influenced by climatic and racial peculiarities; in UK about 13 years may be taken as the average. About one girl in a hundred does not menstruate until the age of 16 years and it is usual to wait until then before becoming concerned. When the menstrual flow has not become established it is usual to speak of 'primary amenorrhoea', while premature cessation of the flow after it has once been regularly established is known as 'secondary amenorrhoea'. From the table of the causes of amenorrhoea below it will be seen that some of them must of necessity give rise to the primary variety, while others more commonly produce the secondary. In investigating a case one should ascertain first whether the condition is primary or secondary, and next whether it is real or only apparent. The latter condition, known as *cryptomenorrhoea*, implies that the menstrual flow takes place but is unable to escape externally because there is some closure of a part of the genital canal. The congenital form of cryptomenorrhoea is the only variety met with commonly, acquired closure of a part of the genital canal being very rare. Stenosis of the vagina may result from injury or infection, but a small sinus is usually left which suffices for the escape of the menstrual fluid. We are led to suspect cryptomenorrhoea when the patient volunteers the statement that she has pelvic pain, headache, and possibly vomiting, of monthly occurrence-in fact the usual menstrual symptoms, unaccompanied by any visible flow. Secondary sexual development is normal. A not uncommon deciding symptom is the occurrence of acute retention of urine, the result of elongation and stretching of the urethra by a haematocolpos. A physical examination should be made, including abdominal palpation, inspection of the vulva and a recto-abdominal bimanual examination. The common form is that in which the lower end of the vagina is imperforate, the hymen usually being visible on the outer side of the occluding membrane through which a dark blue cystic swelling protrudes. The complete examination will reveal a fluctuating swelling reaching from the vulva to the pelvic brim, above which the uterus can often be palpated and moved about. Distension of the vagina or *haematocolpos* is complete in this case, but may be partial where the lower part of the vagina is absent, and then is likely to be accompanied by distension of the uterus (haematometra) and haematosalpinx. It is important to make out whether the uterus and Fallopian tubes are distended with menstrual products along with the distended vagina, for in the presence of haematosalpinges the uterus and tubes may take longer to recover following surgical drainage. Congenital absence of the vagina can only be inferred from local physical examination. Since the vulva is normally formed and a slight depression is present, only a careful examination, if necessary under anaesthesia, will reveal absence of the vagina. Very often the patient only presents at the time of marriage, complaining of dyspareunia. Complete absence of the vagina is nearly always associated with the absence also of the uterus which means that amenorrhoea will be permanent and there is no hope of child-bearing.

Acquired cryptomenorrhoea produces the same symptoms and requires the same kind of investigation as the congenital cases. Acquired closure of the vagina following the vaginitis of specific fevers may occur in infancy, and then produces primary amenorrhoea.

Causes of apparent amenorrhoea

CONGENITAL
Imperforate vagina
Imperforate hymen
Absence of the vagina
Imperforate cervix
Double uterus with retention
Haematocolpos
Haematometra
Haematosalpinx

ACQUIRED
Closure of the vagina
Due to specific fevers
Due to injury
Closure of the cervix
Due to injury
Following operations

Causes of real amenorrhoea

PHYSIOLOGICAL
Before puberty
After the menopause
During pregnancy
During lactation

PATHOLOGICAL
Generative system
Congenital absence of uterus
Congenital absence of ovaries (rare)
Uterine hypoplasia of infantile type
Uterine hypoplasia of adult type
Ovarian agenesis
Gonadal dysgenesis (Turner's syndrome)
Destruction of both ovaries by double ovarian growths, pelvic inflammation, operation irradiation
Hysterectomy
Circulatory system
Anaemia
Leukaemia
Hodgkin's disease
Wasting conditions
Malignant growths
Tuberculosis
Prolonged suppuration
Diabetes
Late stages of nephritis
Late stage of some forms of heart disease
Late stage of cirrhosis of the liver
Nervous system
Cretinism
Various forms of insanity
Suggestion-fear of pregnancy (pseudocyesis)
Anorexia nervosa or loss of weight
Altered internal secretions
Primary hypothalamic-pituitary failure
Following oral contraceptives (post-pill)
Anterior pituitary failure (Simmond's disease)
Absence of ovarian hormones
Certain rate functioning tumours of the ovary: arrhenoblastoma; granulosa-cell tumour
Stein–Leventhal syndrome (polycystic ovary)
Myxoedema
Addison's disease
Thyrotoxicosis
Adrenal hyperplasia
Adrenal cortical tumours
Acromegaly
Obesity
Dystrophia adipose-genitalis (Fröhlich's syndrome)
Change of habits and environment causing emotional strain
Climatic changes
Dietetic deficiencies, the result of attempts to slim

Toxic

During and after specific fevers

Chronic poisoning by lead, mercury, morphine, alcohol

Real amenorrhoea may be: (1) Primary with delayed onset; (2) Primary and permanent; (3) Secondary. If menstruation has once been established regularly, it is clear that there cannot be any serious congenital anomaly of the generative system; the uterus and ovaries must at least have been present and functioning. We must then make a systematic examination of the generative, circulatory, nervous and endocrine systems, in order to learn by a process of exclusion which group of causes we have to deal with. If, however, the amenorrhoea is primary and real, that is, the patient has no symptoms, our examination must first be directed towards finding out whether the essential organs, namely uterus and ovaries, are present, and are normal in size and shape as far as a bimanual examination can ascertain. If necessary, an anaesthetic may be given for this purpose. In doubtful cases laparoscopy with ovarian biopsy may by helpful.

Certain rare inter-sex cases may present with primary amenorrhoea. They include Turner's syndrome (gonadal dysgenesis) in which there is also dwarfism, web-neck, cubitus valgus, and an XO sex-chromosome pattern; testicular feminization (which is in reality androgen insensitivity) in which the form is female with well-developed breasts but absent or sparse pubic and axillary hair and the gonad, which may be found in the groin or in the abdomen, is a testicle that should be removed because of the risk of malignancy; and ovarian dysgenesis in which there are streak ovaries, an infantile uterus and absent secondary sexual characteristics (*Figs.* A.11–A.14). In these cases a buccal smear for sex chromatin and a chromosome analysis on a sample of peripheral blood are indicated. In ovarian dysgenesis there is a chromatin negative smear but only 45 chromosomes, a single X chromosome (XO); in testicular feminization the smear is also chromatin negative but there are 46 chromosomes, XY. Gonadal biopsy is also helpful in diagnosis. When the secondary sexual development is absent or very poor and there is no chromosome abnormality, further investigation becomes necessary. This includes assay of gonadotrophin and adrenal excretion and of thyroid function.

Apart from congenital anomalies remarkably few lesions of the generative organs produce amenorrhoea; only those diseases which destroy both ovaries completely or render the uterus functionless can cause amenorrhoea, and under this heading we find only bilateral malignant ovarian growths and complete removal of the endometrium by too vigorous curetting (Asherman's syndrome). A tumour destroying one ovary has no effect on menstruation, provided the other is present and functioning. The presence of two tumours in the abdomen symmetrically arranged with regard to the uterus will sometimes permit of the diagnosis of double ovarian destruction if there is amenorrhoea in addition, especially in the case of malignant growths, but commonly one tumour is much larger than the other and the double nature of the lesion cannot be established until the abdomen is opened. The common benign tumours, cystic adenomas, even if bilateral, do not destroy the ovarian tissue and consequently do not produce amenorrhoea. On rare occasions bilateral fibromas of the ovaries may destroy all ovarian tissue and therefore be the cause of amenorrhoea.

In the absence of the above-mentioned gross lesions, which are rare causes of amenorrhoea, most cases, other than those due to pregnancy, will be found to be the result of deficient secretion of gonadotrophins by the anterior pituitary lobe or failure of the ovaries to secrete oestrogen and progesterone (ovarian failure). Pituitary failure may be due to a tumour but is more commonly due to inhibition of hypothalamic releasing factor from extreme loss of weight as the result of severe dieting or anorexia nervosa, from emotional disturbances, or from taking the combined oestrogen–progestagen contraceptive pill. The thyroid, or more rarely the adrenal glands, may be at fault. In some cases the evidence of the failure of certain glands is clear, in others it is difficult to be sure. Such investigations as endometrial biopsy, blood and urine hormone estimations, basal temperature charts, vaginal smear tests, the basal metabolic rate estimation, sugar tolerance tests and X-ray examination of the pituitary fossa may all be useful in determining the main gland at fault. The details of the estimations are dealt with elsewhere.

Gonadotrophin estimations in the urine indicate premature ovarian failure when the gonadotrophins (particularly FSH) reach menopausal levels. If gonadotrophin excretion is low or normal, the ovaries are probably still responsive and induction of ovulation is likely to be successful. Although severe loss of weight is associated with amenorrhoea, young women who are subjected to emotional strain may suffer temporarily from amenorrhoea and suddenly gain in weight. Women who have long intervals between periods (oligomenorrhoea) from puberty are particularly liable to have prolonged amenorrhoea, and therefore inability to conceive, when they stop taking the contraceptive pill, which, for them, is contra-indicated (post-pill amenorrhoea).

Amenorrhoea may be associated with galactorrhoea. Typically the syndrome occurs postpartum but it may follow the contraceptive pill or arise without

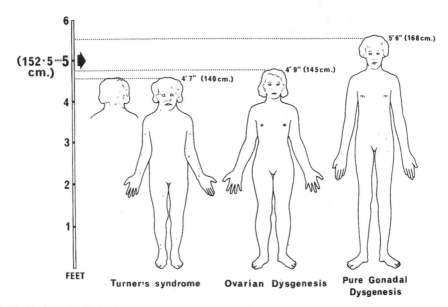

Fig. A.11. (*Professor Paul Polani.*)

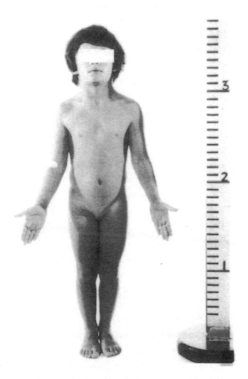

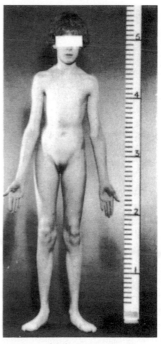

Fig. A.13. Pure gonadal dysgenesis. (*Professor Paul Polani.*)

Fig. A.12. Turner's syndrome. (*Professor Paul Polani.*)

an apparent cause. Raised serum prolactin levels are found probably because of a lowered secretion by the hypothalamus of prolactin-inhibiting factor.

Simmonds' disease (or Sheehan's syndrome) is a rare cause of pituitary failure. It commonly follows very severe postpartum haemorrhage causing necrosis

of most of the anterior pituitary gland through venous thrombosis. It is accompanied by failure of lactation, loss of body hair, wasting and lowered basal metabolism, and the periods fail to be re-established.

An arrhenoblastoma is a very rare ovarian tumour causing virilism in the female, often a young adult women. In addition to amenorrhoea and atrophy of the breasts, there is growth of hair on the face, chest

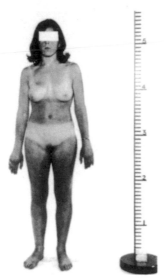

Fig. A.14. Testicular feminization. (*Professor Paul Polani.*)

and abdomen, deepening of the voice and enlargement of the clitoris. 17–Ketosteroid excretion is normal. Granulosa cell tumours of the ovary secrete oestrogen which gives rise to bouts of amenorrhoea interpersed with prolonged irregular vaginal bleeding.

The various disorders of the circulatory, nervous and other systems that may be associated with amenorrhoea are discussed under the headings of other symptoms. With regard to pregnancy, which is the commonest of all causes of secondary amenorrhoea, it may be formulated as an axiom that an otherwise healthy woman who has had perfectly regular menstruation is probably pregnant if she suddenly gets amenorrhoea. Nevertheless, the presence of pregnancy must never be assumed without careful consideration of the history, combined with a complete physical examination. The diagnosis of pregnancy is made upon a complex of symptoms rather than upon any one; but the combination of amenorrhoea, secretion to be squeezed from the breasts, morning sickness, vaginal discoloration and uterine enlargement can only mean pregnancy in the majority of cases; the addition of fetal movements and the fetal heart sounds makes the diagnosis absolute. Immunological pregnancy tests and ultrasound examination are essential when the diagnosis is in doubt.

Summary of the investigation in a case of amenorrhoea

Amenorrhoea may arise in any one of four levels in the body. They are: (1) the hypothalamus; (2) the anterior pituitary; (3) the ovary and (4) the uterus and vagina. To discover at which level lies the cause a careful history and thorough clinical examination

should first be done. Next the endogenous blood oestrogen and the serum prolactin levels should be measured. A progestational agent which has no oestrogenic activity, such as 200 mg progesterone in oil, should be given intramuscularly or 10 mg medroxyprogesterone acetate (Provera) by mouth for 5 days. If bleeding occurs within 2–7 days after cessation of the treatment it shows that there is a functional uterus with reactive endometrium and a patent cervix and vagina. Providing there is no galactorrhoea and the serum prolactin is normal (100–620 mU/1) no further investigation is necessary. Galactorrhoea or a raised serum prolactin means that a CAT scan should be taken or that the sella turcica should be X-rayed for evidence of prolactinoma. If bleeding does not follow the giving of progestagen, there may be an abnormality of the uterus or vagina, such as congenital absence, vaginal atresia, testicular feminization or Asherman's syndrome. Confirmation of these conditions is obtained by priming the endometrium with oestrogen (20 μg ethinyl oestradiol daily for 21 days) before adding progestagen and no bleeding will occur. If bleeding takes place with oestrogen and progestagen, but not with progestagen alone, the fault may lie in the ovary, pituitary or hypothalamus. Now the serum gonadotrophins should be measured by radio-immunoassay. The normal range of FSH is 0.5–5 U/1 and for LH 3–12 U/1. A raised FSH and LH level indicates ovarian failure with absent follicles from a premature menopause, Turner's syndrome, other forms of ovarian dysgenesis, ovarian agenesis (very rare) or the resistant ovary syndrome, a rare condition in which the gonadotrophins are raised, there is amenorrhoea and the ovary contains follicles which do not react to gonadotrophins. The most common situation is that in which the pelvic organs, prolactin level, skull X-ray and gonadotrophins are normal, the condition then being hypothalamic in origin. This commonly follows weight loss or the contraceptive pill. No treatment is needed. Ovulation can be induced in order to produce pregnancy, but not otherwise.

N. Patel

Amnesia (loss of memory)

The function of memory is essential for mental development and the capacity to learn, calculate and speak. For something to be remembered it first has to be appreciated by the cortex of the brain, then be retained or stored, and finally be susceptible to recollection or retrieval. The conscious registration of information occurs in the cerebral cortex with a topographical representation; thus visual information is appreciated in the occipital lobes, tactile memories in the parietal lobes and auditory memories in the temporal lobes.

The retention of memory is divisible into three sections. *Immediate* or working memory is concerned with moment to moment handling of information for transfer to other systems. *Short-term memory* is the processing of this same information into a form suitable for storage, but it remains vulnerable to disruption and therefore may be forgotten. *Long-term memory* is a consolidated form of information in store and this storage is also topographically organized such that auditory memories in relation to language are selectively retained in the dominant temporal lobe and those related to music in the non-dominant temporal lobe. The process by which memory is changed from short-term to long-term memory, suitable for storage, is called encoding.

The neural basis for short-term memory probably involves the medial aspects of both cerebral hemispheres and a neural circuit, called the Papez circuit, which includes the mamillary bodies, the fornices, the hippocampus, the anterior thalamic nuclei and the cingulum. The bilateral representation of these structures means that bilateral damage is necessary to produce a severe amnesic syndrome.

Memory disturbances present commonly in clinical practice and, since the process of memory depends upon attention, retention and recall, it follows that amnesia may be a symptom when attention is diverted in anxiety states, psychotic conditions or lack of interest, when there is structural damage to the memory circuits in the brain, or when general malaise, fatigue or toxaemia cause problems with recall.

Defects in memory may usefully be divided into those which are pure amnesic syndromes and those which are associated with more diffuse cerebral disease resulting in dementia.

1. Pure amnesic syndromes

A. KORSAKOFF'S SYNDROME

Korsakoff's syndrome is a chronic amnesic syndrome, usually related to thiamine deficiency and commonly associated with long-term alcohol abuse. It is sometimes seen with other causes of thiamine deficiency such as persistent vomiting, intestinal obstruction, malabsorption, puerperal sepsis and metastatic carcinoma. The definition of Korsakoff psychosis includes the requirement that the patient is awake and attentive, responsive, and capable of understanding the written and spoken word and of making appropriate deductions and solving problems. Immediate memory should be intact and remote memory may be relatively unaffected, but there is a total loss of memory for recent events and disorientation for time and place. Confabulation, that is falsification of memory, may also be seen

as part of the syndrome. The syndrome may be heralded by an acute confusional state with ophthalmoparesis and ataxia, termed Wernicke's encephalopathy, and the combination of the two phenomena is sometimes referred to as the Wernicke-Korsakoff syndrome.

If recovery occurs, the loss of memory will be as long as the period of illness, and there may be some loss of memory for events prior to the illness, referred to as retrograde amnesia. Neuropathological studies have shown degeneration of neurones and loss of myelin in the mamillary bodies, the anteroventral and pulvinar nuclei of the thalamus and the fornix.

B. TRANSIENT GLOBAL AMNESIA (TGA)

This rare syndrome occurs in middle-aged and elderly patients who develop sudden amnesia and are obviously bewildered. They typically ask questions about their circumstances over and over again: 'Where am I?', 'What should I be doing?', 'What time is it?'. Normal memory function will return within minutes to hours of the onset, and the patient has no subsequent recall for the period of amnesia. Most patients suffer only a single attack but one in five may have recurrent episodes. The cause of this syndrome is uncertain. Most cases are assumed to have a vascular aetiology in which there is posterior ischaemia affecting both medial temporal lobes. Despite this presumed pathology, patients with transient global amnesia do not seem to have an increased risk of stroke. Some TGA attacks occur in patients who suffer temporal lobe epileptic seizures. An epileptic aetiology is more common in those who have more than one episode of transient global amnesia.

C. HEAD INJURY

A severe head injury, sufficient to impair consciousness, will invariably result in amnesia for that period of unconsciousness. It will also be liable to cause the phenomena of *retrograde amnesia*, extending for seconds, minutes or sometimes hours prior to the injury, and *post-traumatic amnesia* (PTA), which always lasts longer than the retrograde amnesia, follows the period of unconsciousness, and lasts for days, weeks or rarely, months.

The duration of the retrograde amnesia will tend to shrink with the passage of time whereas that of post-traumatic amnesia is more constant. Retrograde amnesia is not a reliable guide to the severity of the head injury, but post-traumatic amnesia is of considerable value in this respect; the longer the post-traumatic amnesia the more severe the head injury. Patients who have recovered consciousness following a closed head injury, may appear capable of conversing and carrying out normal activities yet be unable to recall these activities later when recovery is complete because they are still in a state of post-traumatic amnesia. Following recovery from post-traumatic amnesia, patients may be forgetful and may complain of problems with memory for 2 or 3 years after the head injury. A residual defect remaining this long is likely to be permanent. Assessment of memory loss after head injury is difficult and is sometimes influenced by litigation. Formal psychometric assessment of memory function should therefore be undertaken.

Head injuries which do not cause loss of consciousness are unlikely to result in amnesia. Penetrating wounds of the head, unless they specifically injure the medial temporal lobes, are likewise unlikely to cause problems with memory.

Permanent memory defects may follow single severe acute head injuries or repeated minor traumas, as in the case of boxers (dementia pugilis). The pathology of memory loss after closed head injury varies. Trauma can result in cerebral oedema followed by infarction of the hippocampus and cingulate gyri. Again memory loss may be due to diffuse microscopic injuries causing axonal tearing and neuronal degeneration in the medial temporal lobes.

D. EPILEPSY

Memory disturbances are common in the epilepsies. They may occur as part of the seizures or remain as a fixed interictal abnormality.

i. *Ictal amnesia*

Amnesia for the duration of the seizure is inevitable in tonic clonic seizures and in complex partial and absence seizures (petit mal). There may be brief retrograde amnesia prior to attacks and also a period of postictal amnesia. Memory loss may occasionally be the only symptom of an epileptic seizure, though observers can usually describe speech or motor arrest, or automatic behaviour as having occurred. The brief episodes of memory disturbance seen in classic 'petit mal' in childhood may cause problems with learning and behaviour. Rarely, complex partial seizures in adults may result in prolonged subclinical states which have the appearance of 'fugues' and which may last for days or weeks for which the patient is subsequently amnesic.

Amnesia during a seizure is assumed to be due to interference with normal electrophysiological processes by the seizure activity itself. This may be generalized, as in tonic clonic seizures and petit mal, or focal and confined to the temporal lobes in complex partial seizures.

ii. *Interictal memory loss*

Memory problems which persist between seizures are relatively uncommon, though they may be seen both with primary generalized epilepsy and with focal epilepsy. They are most common when seizure discharges arise in one or both temporal lobes. The reason for such memory problems may relate to frequent subclinical seizure discharges, to underlying cerebral pathology, repeated minor head trauma, the use of anticonvulsant drugs, or the depression and social isolation that commonly afflict those that suffer from epilepsy.

iii. *Focal pathology*

Patients who have seizures as a manifestation of focal cerebral pathology in the temporal lobes or who undergo surgery for treatment of epilepsy may present with specific memory defects.

iv. *Anticonvulsant medication*

Several anticonvulsant drugs, particularly phenytoin and the barbiturates, have deleterious effects on memory in normal volunteers and in patients with epilepsy.

E. VASCULAR DISEASE

Apart from the classical syndrome of transient global amnesia, other forms of stroke disease may result in specific memory disorder.

i. *Medial temporal lobe infarction*

Bilateral medial temporal lobe infarction due to posterior cerebral ischaemia is a cause of persistent amnesia, and unilateral infarction in the dominant hemisphere may occasionally cause problems with memory. Most patients with amnesia due to stroke have neurological signs to indicate a posterior circulation infarct, including visual disturbances, cortical blindness, aphasia or alexia.

ii. *Thalamic infarction*

Rarely patients may suffer bilateral thalamic infarction which results in a severe amnesic syndrome. It is assumed that this occurs only when both paramedial and thalamic arteries arise from a common trunk.

iii. *Anterior communicating artery aneurysm*

Patients who suffer rupture of an anterior communicating artery aneurysm, or undergo surgical treatment for such a lesion, may suffer cerebral artery vasospasm and consequent infarction in the distribution of the small penetrating branches of the anterior communicating artery. This results in damage to posterior inferior medial frontal areas and to the anterior portion of the fornix and corpus callosum. These patients may present with an acute amnesia, which may recover in those in whom the ischaemia is due only to vasospasm.

F. HERPES SIMPLEX ENCEPHALITIS

Patients with this severe illness normally present with seizures, dysphasia and hemiparesis; they may develop diffuse signs of dementia, but occasionally, because of the predilection of the temporal lobes for haemorrhagic infarction in this condition, there may be a specific amnesic syndrome.

G. CEREBRAL TUMOUR

Amnesic syndromes are rare as the presentation of cerebral tumours. They may occur with bilateral temporal lobe damage related to tumours arising deep in the midline, within the third ventricle, or involving the third ventricle as in craniopharyngiomas.

H. ELECTROCONVULSIVE THERAPY

Temporary impairment of memory is almost invariable following electroconvulsive therapy. It may be retrograde as well as anterograde. Unilateral ECT has much less effect on memory than has bilateral ECT.

2. Other causes of memory loss

A. MEMORY LOSS ASSOCIATED WITH DEMENTIA

Memory loss is the most common presenting symptom in the diffuse dementing illnesses such as Alzheimer's disease and it becomes increasingly prevalent and severe as the condition progresses. There may be focal elements in the initial symptomatology, but the progression of memory loss is associated with intellectual, perceptual, linguistic, praxic, attentional, personality and mood disturbances indicating the diffuse nature of the condition.

B. PSYCHOGENIC AMNESIA

Complaints of memory impairment are common in depression and anxiety but formal assessment with psychometry will usually reveal that reduced attention or motivation is the cause for the symptom. More florid psychogenic amnesic states do occur but differ from organic amnesia in the pattern of the memory defect and in the time-course of onset and recovery. Loss of personal identity is common in psychogenic amnesia, but extremely rare in organic amnesia. The common setting of the 'psychogenic fugue', in which the patient is discovered wandering, often long distances from home, is associated with loss of personal identity and amnesia for the event. Recovery of normal learning and alertness is often sudden, but loss of personal identity and profound retrograde amnesia may persist. These syndromes occur in a setting of psychopathology and a precipitating cause will usually be identified.

Retrograde amnesia, without anterograde amnesia, after head injury is usually psychogenic. The retrospective forgetting of circumscribed periods from the past is often found to encompass particularly distressing events, as in wartime, but may include periods of alleged criminal activity in malingerers. Feigned amnesia may be detected by the 'two choice' recognition test of memory. Genuine amnesics, operating on chance, will obtain 50 per cent of right answers. Malingerers, being unaware of probability, will score significantly worse than they would by chance.

C. DRUGS

Many drugs impair memory as part of their sedative effect, but others have a more specific effect. The latter include cannabis, organic solvents, heavy metals, such as lead and mercury, anticonvulsant drugs, anticholinergic drugs, benzodiazepines, digoxin and clioquinol. It is inevitable that general anaesthesia will impair memory and this may persist even after apparent recovery. Problems may arise thereby in patients undergoing surgery as day cases.

D. HYPOXIA

An acute hypoxic cerebral insult, such as that resulting from cardiac or respiratory arrest, or after carbon monoxide poisoning, may produce an irreversible amnesic syndrome because of selective involvement of the medial temporal lobes.

E. MULTIPLE SCLEROSIS

Cognitive decline frequently occurs in multiple sclerosis and in rare cases may specifically affect memory.

F. PARANEOPLASIA

In patients with carcinoma of the bronchus there is a specific form of 'limbic encephalitis' in which memory defects occur as a non-metatastic manifestation of cancer.

G. SARCOIDOSIS

A rare form of sarcoidosis affecting the nervous system may present with a specific amnesic syndrome.

D. Bates

ANGINA
See CHEST PAIN.

Angioma and telangiectasia

An angioma is a proliferation of blood vessels and occurs as a developmental or an acquired vascular abnormality (*see Table A.2*).

Table A.2. Angioma and telangiectasia

Developmental
Vascular birthmarks
  Naevus flammeus
  Cavernous haemangioma (strawberry naevus)
  Capillary haemangioma (port wine stain)
Blue rubber-bleb naevus syndrome
Hereditary haemorrhagic telangiectasia (*Fig. A.15*)
Generalized essential telangiectasia
Ataxia-telangiectasia

Acquired
Cherry angiomas (Campbell de Morgan spots)
Venous lakes
Angiokeratoma
  of Fordyce (scrotum and vulva)
  Anderson–Fabry disease
Pyogenic granuloma
Glomus tumour
Kaposi's sarcoma
Acquired telangiectases (spider naevi)
  Pregnancy
  Thyrotoxicosis
  Liver disease
  Carcinoid
  Systemic mastocytosis
  X-radiation skin damage
  Topical corticosteroid abuse
  Rosacea
  Poikiloderma
  Scleroderma (matt telangiectases)
  Dermatomyositis
  Lupus erythematosus

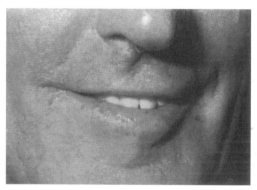

Fig. A.15. Hereditary haemorrhagic telangiectasia. (Osler-Rendu-Weber syndrome). (*King Edward VII Hospital, Windsor.*)

Developmental vascular abnormalities

Vascular birthmarks. Transient small salmon-pink macular birthmarks—naevus flammeus—are remarkably common and are thought to occur in over 50 per cent of live births, affecting the sexes equally. They are most commonly on the nape of the neck, forehead or eyelids. Those on the face usually resolve within months, but the flame naevus on the nape of the neck more often persists into adult life. More significant and disfiguring vascular malformations are also common (approximately 1 in 10 live births). They are often not apparent at birth but develop during the first month of life. Further classification is made

depending on the size of blood vessels affected (capillary or cavernous haemangiomas) but in practice the lesions are often of mixed type.

Cavernous haemangioma (Fig. A.16) or 'strawberry naevus' comprises large vessels proliferating in the dermis and protruding, sometimes alarmingly, from the skin surface. The overlying epidermis may ulcerate with minor trauma, causing brisk bleeding. A strawberry naevus may become very large and disfiguring. It usually appears within or just after the first month of life and undergoes a growth phase for 6-12 months and thereafter gradually shrinks. By the age of 8 a white redundant skin fold is usually all that remains. If sited near the eye a large strawberry naevus may interrupt the development of binocular vision. Rarely a massive cavernous haemangioma may sequestrate platelets and lead to a bleeding tendency (Kasabach-Merritt syndrome).

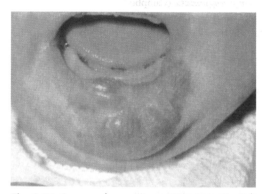

Fig. A.16. Cavernous haemangioma. (*Westminster Hospital.*)

The *capillary haemangioma* (port wine stain) (*Fig.* A.17) is less frequent, but more significant, as the lesions show little tendency to fade with time. They vary in colour from pale pink to deep purple and in size from a few millimetres to lesions which cover very large areas. They seldom cross the midline, and localized tissue hypertrophy may accompany large lesions. A port wine stain in a trigeminal distribution may signal underlying intracranial angiomatosis, especially where ipsilateral ocular abnormalities are also present—the *Sturge-Weber* syndrome.

In the *blue rubber-bleb naevus syndrome* large rubbery cutaneous angiomas of the extremities are associated with bleeding, vascular ectasia in the respiratory and gastrointestinal tracts, beginning with recurrent epistaxis in early adult life. In *generalized essential telangiectasia* the mucosae are spared but the body is more widely affected with telangiectases, which are arborizing rather than spider. *Ataxia-telangiectasia* (Louis–Bar syndrome) is a recessively inherited immunodeficiency syndrome. Affected children are small of stature, and develop progressive cerebellar

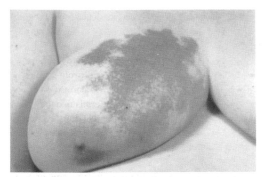

Fig. A.17. Port wine stain. (*Dr Richard Staughton.*)

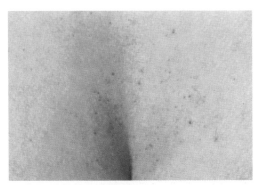

Fig. A.18. Anderson-Fabry disease. (*Westminster Hospital.*)

ataxia from the age of 2; telangiectases appear on bulbar conjunctivae, ears and cheeks from the age of 3.

Acquired vascular abnormalities

Cherry angiomata (Campbell de Morgan spots) develop on the trunks of almost all persons past middle age. They are usually small, from 1 to 3 mm in diameter, bright red, globular and soft. They are of no systemic significance but are said to involute spontaneously should the 8th decade be reached. Larger cavernous lesions, especially on the lower lips, are common in old age (*venous lakes*). Small angiomas surmounted by a variable amount of hyperkeratosis (angiokeratoma) are common on the scrotum (angiokeratomas of Fordyce) but also occur scattered in the bathing trunk area in the extremely rare *Anderson–Fabry disease* (*Fig.* A.18). This is an important diagnosis to make, often delayed due to the inconspicuous nature of the angiokeratomas, because internal organ involvement can lead to early death. *Pyogenic granuloma* has a characteristic morphology, growing on a stalk surrounded by a collarette of normal skin. These rapidly growing angiomas are seen on the chest and extremities of young people and because of their tendency to bleed they are often the cause of alarm. A *glomus tumour* (glomangioma) also occurs on the extremities, often beneath a nail, and is composed of a bluish-red, rounded firm papule a few millimetres in diameter. Lesions can be excruciatingly painful on pressure. *Kaposi's sarcoma* (*Fig.* A.19) is a form of angiosarcoma, which in its classical form grows indolently on the extremities of elderly Jewish or Southern Italian persons. An *endemic* form, more aggressive and metastasizing, was described in younger people in subequatorial East and Central Africa in the 1950s. The *epidemic* of similarly aggressive Kaposi's sarcoma in homosexuals, chiefly though not exclusively with HIV infection, has spread alarmingly from New York since the late 1970s. It has been seen in occasional transplant recipients. The sarcoma waxes in people with decreased immunity, and wanes should this improve.

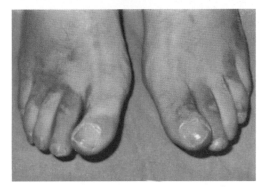

Fig. A.19. Kaposi's sarcoma. (*Westminster Hospital.*)

Acquired telangiectases are common. Isolated spider naevi appear on children's faces, and during late pregnancy over half of the mothers develop several scattered over the face, upper chest, arms and hands. These usually disappear within 6 weeks of delivery. Similar lesions appear in *thyrotoxicosis and liver disease*, and also in two conditions where vasodilatory chemicals are released into the circulation intermittently—the *carcinoid syndrome* and *systemic mastocytosis*. Telangiectasia on exposed skin is related to the gradual disappearance of support tissue that occurs with age and more particularly with cumulative sun exposure. This is extremely rare in older Negroes. Similar mechanisms cause telangiectasia after X-radiation, and abuse of *topical corticosteroids*. They are also seen in localized skin disorders such as *rosacea*, and *poikiloderma*, as well as in collagen-vascular disorders, e.g. *scleroderma* (matt-telangiectases), *dermatomyositis* and *lupus erythematosus*.

Richard Staughton

ANKLE
See JOINTS, AFFECTIONS OF.

Anorectal pain

Where there is an evident cause, the history of anorectal pain is usually of relatively short duration and treatment is frequently successful in relieving symptoms. A small subgroup exists, however, in whom symptoms are longstanding and no orgc cause is found; these patients present a major therapeutic challenge to the clinician.

Anorectal pain: classification of major causes

ACUTE CAUSES
Anal fissure
Anal haematoma/thrombosis
Infection
   Perianal abscess
   Intersphincteric abscess
CHRONIC CAUSES
Proctalgia fugax
Coccygodynia
Idiopathic
   Sometimes associated with descending perineum
   syndrome
Gynaecological disorders
   Ovarian cyst or tumour
   Endometriosis
Anorectal malignancy
Presacral tumours or cysts
Cauda equina lesions
   Tumours
   Trauma
Chronic perianal sepsis
   Anal fistula
   Crohn's disease
   Anorectal tuberculosis

Short history of pain

Acute disorders in the perianal region usually give rise to severe pain because of the profusion of sensory nerve endings prevalent in the squamous epithelium at and below the level of the dentate line. A sudden onset of pain in association with a dark blue oedematous perianal swelling are the characteristic features of either a *perianal haematoma* or *perianal thrombosis*. The two conditions are now generally considered to have the same cause, which is thrombosis of a large venous dilatation in the external venous plexus. A history of anal pain initiated by defaecation and lasting for a variable period up to an hour afterwards is usually diagnostic of an *acute anal fissure*. The lesion is observed on inspection of the anus usually in either the anterior or posterior midline positions and may be associated with an oedematous 'sentinel' skin tag at its more caudal margin. Digital examination or instrumentation of the anal canal causes severe pain and tenderness associated with marked spasm of the internal anal sphincter. Chronicity or multiplicity of a fissure observed in unusual sites around the circumference of the anal canal should arouse suspicions of underlying *Crohn's disease*.

The association of a short history of pain with fever and purulent anal discharge usually signifies *peri-anal sepsis*. The primary source is usually an infected anal gland and if the sepsis remains localized an intersphincteric abscess is the result. The diagnosis can be notoriously difficult because there may be no overt signs of infection; exquisite tenderness on digital examination of the anal canal may be the only physical finding. Usually pus in the infected anal gland extends to the surface (i.e. to the perineum or buttock) in which case a fistula opening will be clearly visible and an area of induration corresponding to the fistula track will be palpable.

Pain of chronic duration

Patients with chronic perineal pain may be found to have organic disease but in many, after exhaustive investigation, no cause is apparent. *Proctalgia fugax* is a common source of perineal pain in which no structural abnormality is apparent. The pain is spasmodic with episodes lasting up to 30 minutes and is probably the consequence of paroxysmal contraction of the levator ani musculature. *Coccygodynia* is a rather loose term applied to a history of vague tenderness and ache in the region of the sacrum and coccyx. Sometimes the pain radiates to the back of the thighs or buttocks and is usually provoked by sitting. Symptoms, without any convincing evidence, have been considered to arise from the coccyx. Idiopathic perineal pain is sometimes associated with the *descending perineum syndrome*, a disorder of the pelvic floor in which the pelvic floor becomes denervated and on examination the perineum is seen to 'balloon' well below the bony pelvis as represented by the level of the ischial tuberosities. The pain, in these patients, may arise from stretching of the pudendal nerves or alternatively from the mucosal prolapse which occurs secondarily to loss of muscle tone. Characteristically the pain is provoked by prolonged standing or walking and is relieved by lying flat.

Of the treatable underlying disorders, malignancy in the rectum or anus must be excluded early on by digital examination and sigmoidoscopy. Gynaecological and presacral pathology should be excluded by ultrasound and CT scanning of the pelvis. If the history of pain accompanies motor disorder of the anorectum and bladder, a cauda equina lesion should be suspected and excluded by lumbar myelography or MRI examination. Finally, chronic perianal sepsis should always suggest a possible inflammatory disorder such as Crohn's disease or anorectal tuberculosis.

M. M. Henry

ANOREXIA
See APPETITE, DISORDERS OF.

ANOSMIA
See SMELL, ABNORMAL PERCEPTION OF.

ANURIA
See OLIGURIA.

Anxiety

Anxiety is a universally experienced emotion whose presentations require understanding of both its adaptive role and the relationship between personality and coping.

Anxiety is the emotional component of the *fight or flight reaction*, the physiological response to threat. Fight *or* flight: the individual has both a choice to make and to prepare for taking either option. Once fight or flight are enacted anxiety subsides, its job done; thus anxiety is the emotion of indecision or conflict and of preparation for action. Anxiety contrasts with fear which is the emotion of a non-conflictual, known, threat and it precedes depression, the emotion of loss, which develops when the consequences of the threat become evident. In daily living anxiety enhances both physical performance, e.g. in sport, and mental performance, e.g. in examinations. Being anxious occasionally makes the difference between surviving or not, but often facilitates action to ward off potential threats like illness, pain, helplessness, punishment, separation, or to one's status or social functioning.

How the anxiety that is generated to deal with a potential menace, internal or external, real or imaginary, great or small, is disposed of depends upon the individual's personality attributes, and especially the array and efficiency of *mental defence mechanisms* that have been developed. To simplify, the 'normal', mature, balanced personality deals with anxiety effectively, either through initiating appropriate actions or through the utilization of various defence mechanisms that produce an adaptive response, for instance a student who feels anxious about a romance may settle their uncertainty or sublimate this emotion by intensifying studying. The immature or disordered personality cannot handle anxiety either because the correct, relieving actions are not undertaken, or because a dearth, imbalance or inadequacy of defence mechanisms lead to a maladaptive response. In such a case the student who feels anxious about a romance may take an overdose or dissociate from this emotion by becoming severely depersonalized and so unable to work. Defence mechanisms therefore are unconsciously operated mental tricks for disposing of anxiety that might otherwise overwhelm the individual. There are at least 30 mechanisms described, and both heredity and upbringing are involved in determining their presence and application: common examples are regression, repression, denial, rationalization, projection and introjection. It follows that many types of psychological

problem can develop from the failure to manage anxiety—from the interaction of personality and stress, and from the combination of coping strategies and defence mechanisms that are employed (*Fig. A.20*).

It should be evident that excessive amounts of anxiety may be generated in spite of a sound personality if the stress is great enough. This is the origin of neurotic reactions named by their association with major life-threatening events like accidents and war—shell shock, battle neurosis, post-traumatic stress disorder—how the ordinary individual copes with the extraordinary event.

Excessive stress is also the basis of the *adjustment reaction*, a common phenomenon in medical practice when patients face the threats and uncertainty of illness cancer or not, transplant or not, survival or not. These reactions tend to follow the pattern of the illness, being florid and severe in acute, life-threatening illness and persistent and less severe in chronic disabling disorders. In adjustment reactions anxiety figures predominantly in the early stages, and depression latterly as the uncertainty becomes certainty and the loss apparent. Sometimes there is an unwelcome tendency for any overt emotional response to be interpreted as pathological and so to be treated with drugs: in adjustment reaction the best approach is inquiry and explanation, exploring the patient's concerns, reassuring when appropriate, expediting investigations and treatment when appropriate, being a good listener. Minor tranquillizers or hypnotics help to relieve the symptoms of anxiety should they become too distressing or burdensome for the patient to cope with during this period of vulnerability—but it is the talking and action that are the key to resolution. Indeed this is an excellent opportunity to forge a therapeutic alliance with the patient that facilitates not only in the recognition and prevention of further emotional distress but also in coping with developments, setbacks and even mistakes as the illness unfolds.

It is when anxiety is *inappropriate in degree or duration* that the basis for diagnosing *generalized/ chronic anxiety disorder* is established. Maladaptive responses to anxiety are topics of other sections.

The *diagnosis* of generalized anxiety disorder rests upon: (1) excessive anxiety and worry; (2) other clinical features (*Table A.3*); and (3) the exclusion of underlying physical or mental disorders.

In addition to the emotion being excessive for the circumstances, anxiety states are characterized by *generalization of worries*—the patient may or may not be concerned about everything, but their anxieties will certainly extend beyond the single issue worry which is more typical of phobias, obsessive compulsive disorder, anorexia nervosa, panic disorder and hypochondriasis.

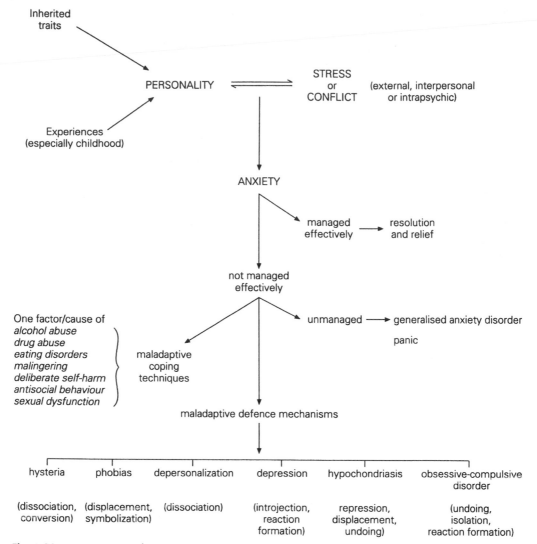

Fig. A.20. Anxiety: origins and outcome.

The features of anxiety are direct consequences of increased activity of the autonomic nervous system. The symptom pattern varies considerably from patient to patient, but physical symptoms are frequently presented as the primary complaint with anxiety and other psychological concomitants interpreted as a secondary response.

Somatization, the presentation of psychological distress with physical symptoms which are attributed to organic disease, takes this process further with the emotional origins of the presentation denied or further still when all emotional aspects are denied—even overt depression and anxiety. Somatization arises partly from the misinterpretation of altered or amplified physiological functions, but there are other important elements—the stigma of mental illness, the belief that doctors are more interested in and sympathetic towards

physical disorders, the inability to express emotions either because of lack of awareness of emotional responses or inarticulateness (alexithymia) and sociocultural factors such as older age, lower social class, Third World culture, and previous physical illnesses. Doctors too play their part in promoting somatization through neglecting to consider and pursue the emotional dimension and by overzealous physical investigations.

Any feature in *Table A.3* may be the presenting complaint, but particularly common are headaches, dizziness, chest pain, palpitations, gastrointestinal symptoms, tremor, fatigue and emotional upset. Of course likely physical illnesses have to be excluded, even in the overtly anxious patient, and the very act of treating the symptom seriously can be therapeutic, for anxious people usually respond to reassurance (*Table A.4*).

Table A.3. Clinical features of anxiety

Somatic
Breathlessness
Palpitations
Accelerated heart rate
Sweating but cold and clammy
Dry mouth
Lump in the throat
Nausea
Butterflies in the stomach
Diarrhoea
Urinary frequency, hesitancy, urgency
Dizziness
Faintness
Lightheadedness

Motor tension
Tension headache
Musculoskeletal aches
Restlessness
Coarse tremor
Trembling, shakiness
Easily fatigued

Hyperalertness
Feeling keyed-up, on edge
Feelings of dread or threat
Irritability
Increased sensitivity to stimuli
Poorly sustained concentration
Inability to relax
Insomnia

Table A.4. Causes of anxiety

Commonest
Normal/stress related
Adjustment reaction
Generalized or chronic anxiety state

Less common
Drugs
  Stimulants—cocaine, amphetamines, caffeine
  Sympathomimetics
  Hallucinogens
Drug withdrawal
Physical disorders
  Thyroid dysfunction
  Hypoglycaemia
  Hyperventilation
  Migraine
  Temporal lobe epilepsy
  Brain tumour
  Head injury
Psychiatric disorders
  Depression
  Mania
  Schizophrenia
  Phobias
  Hysteria
  Malingering
  Obsessive-compulsive disorder
  Post-traumatic stress disorder
  Panic
  Depersonalization
  Hypochondriasis

Rare
Drugs
  Antihypertensives
  Penicillin
  Sulphonamides
  Cannabis
  Nicotine
  Inhalers
  Anticholinergics
Endocrine disorders
  Pituitary dysfunction
  Parathyroid dysfunction
  Adrenal dysfunction
Neurological disorders
  Cerebrovascular disease
  Subarachnoid haemorrhage
  Encephalitis
  Neurosyphilis
  Multiple sclerosis
  Wilson's disease
  Huntington's chorea
Gastrointestinal disorders
  Hiatus hernia
  Peptic ulcer
  Ulcerative colitis
  Crohn's disease
Cardiorespiratory disorders
  Congestive cardiac failure
  Chronic respiratory failure
  Cardiac arhythmias
  Myocardial infarction
  Hypertension
  Anaemia
  Emphysema
  Asthma
Auto-immune disorders
  SLE
  Rheumatoid arthritis
  Polyarteritis nodosa
  Temporal arteritis
Toxicological disorders
  Benzene and derivatives
  Carbon disulphide
  Mercury
  Arsenic
  Lead
  Organophosphates
Other causes
  Vit B_{12} deficiency
  Pellagra
  Aspirin intolerance
  Brucellosis
  Infectious mononucleosis
  Carcinoid syndrome
  Systemic malignancy
  Porphyria
  Uraemia
  Electrolyte disturbances
  Anaphylaxis
  Premenstrual tension syndrome

The differential diagnosis of anxiety is lengthy and complicated by the fact that anxiety frequently overlaps other disorders. This is particularly true when considering the psychiatric differential diagnoses, with *panic* and *hyperventilation* both being cause and effect, and *phobias* and *hysteria* sometimes termed phobic anxiety states and anxiety-hysteria because anxiety figures so prominently—indeed excessive anxiety is more or less invariable in all neuroses. The most important practical distinction is from *depression*, although once again anxiety and depression frequently co-exist particularly in the less severe forms of emotional disorder typically met in general practice. The crux is to identify major depressive states in which agitation is marked. Usually patients with agitated depression have developed typical biological and cognitive depressive changes; but if there is doubt then it is preferable to err on the side of misdiagnosing an anxiety state as an agitated depression than vice versa.

Medical disorders that may cause or present with physical or psychological manifestations of anxiety are numerous (*see Table A.4*). Within this list there are several conditions which merit further discussion. *Hyperthyroidism* is justifiably the best-known differential diagnosis, firstly because the state of metabolic overactivity induced by thyroxine is similar in many respects to primary anxiety, and secondly because anxiety is a common emotional presentation of the disorder. Symptoms that point towards hyperthyroidism are increased cold tolerance, increased appetite and significant weight loss, while distinguishing signs (in addition to the classical findings in the eye and neck) are warm extremities and fine (vs coarse) finger tremor. The time-honoured sign of sleeping pulse rate being maintained at a high level in hyperthyroidism is of little clinical value even when the circumstances are conducive for its accurate measurement; the whole issue should usually be settled biochemically although borderline results require re-evaluation of the clinical presentation. Excluding thyroid disorder is also desirable when no obvious stressor can be established and there is no evident predisposition to anxiety.

Drugs, both stimulants (especially caffeine) and abstinence from alcohol or minor tranquillizers, are another common factor: a detailed inquiry into drug taking habits and recent changes is essential—and this should include coffee and tobacco consumption.

In general an anxiety state arising without adequate explanation in a middle-aged or elderly person is highly suspicious of either an underlying physical disorder or depressive illness.

Finally, and central to the whole issue of diagnosing anxiety disorders, it is usually not the illness that is masked but the doctor that is blind. By confining inquiries to physical systems the right questions are not asked and consequently the correct diagnosis is missed. Perhaps the doctor may justifiably feel sometimes that a psychological line of inquiry could upset the patient and might damage their relationship but there are usually ways round this either by exercising tact and judgement as to how far and fast to make the approach, or by speaking to and involving relatives. Undue delay or inappropriate referrals, investigations and treatments aggravate rather than ameliorate anxiety states, and hence makes the task of helping the patient more difficult.

George Masterton

APHASIA
See SPEECH, ABNORMALITIES OF.

APHONIA
See VOICE, DISORDERS OF.
APPETITE, DECREASED
See APPETITE, DISORDERS OF.

Appetite, disorders of

Loss of appetite

Loss of appetite is so common and non-specific that its presence is rarely of assistance in making a diagnosis. It can be a feature of many physical or psychological disorders, as well as a transient phenomenon in stress or even ordinary living. When a patient complains of diminished appetite, a useful pointer to the importance and clinical significance is the presence and amount of accompanying weight loss. Without confirmed weight loss or other evidence of illness it is inappropriate to pursue investigations of loss of appetite.

Gastrointestinal disorders which are characteristically associated with loss of appetite include the *prodromal stage of viral hepatitis, gastric carcinoma, gastric ulcer* and *coeliac disease*. In coeliac disease, however, the patient may occasionally compensate for the malabsorption with an increase in appetite and under these circumstances, loss of weight is not a problem. Patients with *roundworm* infestation may also have a loss of appetite but, uncommonly, the patient may have an increase in appetite.

Anorexia maybe a prominent feature of chronic diseases such as *advanced malignant disease, chronic alcoholism, uraemia, severe congestive heart failure, chronic pulmonary disease*, and *cirrhosis of the liver*. *Adrenal insufficiency* is constantly associated with anorexia and loss of weight. On the other hand, both *thyrotoxicosis* and *diabetes mellitus* may have marked loss of weight in the absence of any impairment of appetite.

Anorexia may feature prominently in patients with psychiatric illness including *anxiety, stress*, and *depression*. However, there are two psychiatric illnesses in which a disorder of eating features prominently, *anorexia nervosa* and *bulimia*, which may affect as many as 5–10 per cent of adolescent girls and young women with a significant morbidity and mortality. It is rare for these syndromes to occur in males. *Anorexia nervosa* usually begins in teenage in a girl who is either overweight or believes herself to be so. There is a refusal to maintain normal body weight, a loss of more than 25 per cent of original body weight, a disturbance of body image, an intense fear of becoming fat, and there is no associated medical illness leading to weight loss. There are many accompanying physical abnormalities in the patient with established anorexia nervosa. These include amenorrhoea, osteoporosis, abnormal temperature regulation, bradycardia and hypotension, decreased glomerular filtration rate, renal calculi, oedema, constipation, and abnormality of liver biochemistry. The patient will become anaemic with leucopenia and thrombocytopenia.

Increased appetite

An increase in appetite will occur normally in individuals exercising strenuously and transiently in those recovering from an illness. An increased appetite can occur in *mania* and *hyperthyroidism*. *Hypoglycaemia*, such as occurs with an insulinoma, may be associated with an increased appetite but this is an uncommon manifestation of the disease. Occasionally the *depressed* or *hysterical* patient may eat to excess.

Bulimia is characterized by recurrent episodes of binge eating. There is consumption of high calorie easily ingested foods taken in a binge and terminated by abdominal pain, sleep or vomiting. In between binges, there are repeated attempts to lose weight and weight can fluctuate rapidly over short periods of time by more than 5 kg. The patient usually is aware that there is an abnormal eating pattern but she fears that she will not be able to stop voluntarily. After the eating binge the patient becomes depressed. Physical features in bulimia include menstrual abnormalities, hypokalaemia, acute gastric dilatation, parotid gland enlargement, dental-enamel erosion, the risk of Mallory–Weiss tears, and aspiration pneumonia.

Perverted appetite (pica)

A perverted appetite may be a striking manifestation of *iron deficiency anaemia*. Affected individuals may crave earth or clay (geophagia), starch (amylophagia) or ice (pagophagia). Perversion of the appetite is also seen in other psychiatric disorders. Pica may also occur in the course of *pregnancy* and is of no special significance.

Ian A.D. Bouchier

Apraxia

The term was first used by Liepmann in 1900. It applies to a patient with intact sensation, without weakness, ataxia or other extrapyramidal abnormality, who loses the ability to execute previously learned skilled movements and gestures. It is suggested that three types of apraxia may be identified. The initial planning of a voluntary action is developed in the parietal lobe of the dominant hemisphere where visual, auditory and kinaesthetic information is integrated. The engrams of skilled movements are formulated here and, if damaged, planned action cannot be conceptualized with resulting *ideational apraxia*. From the parietal lobe

connections flow, possibly via the arcuate fasciculus, to the premotor cortices of both cerebral hemispheres where the execution of patterns of movement is initiated. Patients with damage in this situation know and remember the planned action but are unable to execute it and have *ideomotor apraxia*. The lowest level of apraxia, *kinetic apraxia*, refers to a clumsiness of the limb in the performance of a skilled act that cannot be accounted for by paresis, ataxia or other abnormality of movement. Several different forms of apraxia are identified clinically:

1. LIMB APRAXIA

Limb apraxia may be recognized by asking the patient to demonstrate how to undertake gestures or to use a particular tool or instrument. There may be an improvement in the performance when the patient attempts to imitate the examiner or when the actual object is used, but the performance will be most defective when the patient attempts to demonstrate the manoeuvre. Such problems are most commonly seen in patients who have lesions in the dominant parietofrontal region and they may often be associated with a speech disturbance, a right hemiparesis and a visual or inattention defect.

2. GAIT APRAXIA

This is probably the most common of all apraxias and refers to patients who walk with a 'marche-à-petit-pas'. Their walking may be improved by cueing each step so that the patient follows a pattern on the floor rather than relying on the natural sequence of walking. This disorder is a feature of normal pressure hydrocephalus, where it is usually associated with dementia and incontinence. It is most frequently seen in elderly patients with bilateral frontal lobe damage.

3. FACIAL APRAXIA

Facial apraxia may be seen with lesions that affect the dominant motor association cortex. Patients will be unable to lick the lips or pretend to blow out a match, though they will be able to perform these tasks if there is jam on the lips or if a lighted match is held in front of them.

4. APRAXIA OF SPEECH

Some patients who have disturbances of motor speech are considered to show an apraxia of buccolingual movements, though the distinction between this and a true Broca's aphasia may be difficult to establish. Both are due to lesions in the dominant frontal lobe.

5. DRESSING AND CONSTRUCTIONAL APRAXIA

In patients who suffer lesions of the non-dominant parietal lobe there may be problems in dressing, such as inability to put on clothes in the correct order, or to identify items which have been turned inside-out. They may therefore put socks on over shoes or fail to find their way into a shirt or coat. Such patients will also show constructional apraxia; that is they will have difficulty in copying a diagram, drawing a clock or constructing a figure from matchsticks.

Such problems of praxis may also occur with dominant parietal lobe lesions but usually they are overshadowed by the attendant dysphasic syndrome; the phenomenon is therefore more apparent in patients with non-dominant hemisphere lesions with intact speech and comprehension.

D. Bates

Arcus cornealis (arcus senilis)

Arcus cornealis is an extremely common bilateral peripheral corneal condition. It is a type of degeneration which is found in 60 per cent of people between the age of 40 and 60 years. It is more common in blacks than other races and increases in frequency with age. If present under the age of 40 years hypercholesterolaemia must be considered and plasma lipid levels should be tested.

The opacity (*Fig.* A.21) is due to deposition of lipid droplets in the superficial and deep layers of the cornea forming a yellowish-white ring about 2 mm in width with a clear space between it and the junction of the cornea and the sclera (the limbus). It first appears in the inferior cornea, then in the superior cornea and then enlarges to encircle the entire cornea. There are no symptoms and no treatment is necessary.

S. T. D. Roxburgh

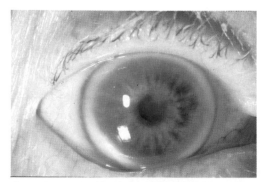

Fig. A.21. Opacity seen in arcus cornealis.

ARM, OEDEMA OF
See Oedema generalized.

Arm, pain in

This section deals primarily with pain referred into the arm from the neck and thorax. In addition, pain arising in the brachial plexus and peripheral nerves is included as also are lesions at the shoulder, elbow, wrist and hand which specifically or characteristically affect the upper limb. The causes of such pain are summarized in *Table A.5*.

Table A.5. Causes of pain specific to the arm

Lesions in the neck
Disc prolapse
Spondylosis
Syringomyelia
Fracture dislocations
Post-herpetic neuralgia
Radiculitis—paralytic/viral
  (Neuralgic amyotrophy)
Spinal abscess—Tuberculous
             —brucella
             —pyogenic
Epidural abscess
Pachymeningitis cervicalis
Tumours—spinal cord
      meninges
      nerve roots
      vertebrae—primary
             —secondary

Lesions of the brachial plexus
Cervical rib
Malignant infiltration
Costoclavicular compression
Subclavian aneurysm
Scalenus anterior syndrome

Lesions of the thorax and thoracic spine
Cardiac ischaemia
Syphilitic aortitis
Thoracic disc
Oesophagitis

Lesions at the shoulder
Periarthritis/capsulitis
Subacromial bursitis
Calcific tendonitis
Bicipital tendonitis
Shoulder-hand syndrome

Lesions at the elbow
Epicondylitis
Olecranon bursitis

Lesions of the forearm, wrist and hand
Carpal tunnel syndrome
Tenosynovitis
Ulnar neuritis
Trigger finger
Algodystrophy
Hypertrophic osteoarthropathy
Pachydermoperiostitis
Repetitive strain injury (RSI)
  e.g. Writer's cramp

Lesions which may arise at any site such as arthritis, bone tumours, injuries and skin disease are excluded.

Pain referred into the arm falls into two major categories. Sharp, well localized neuralgia often associated with paraesthesiae is usually attributed to nerve root or trunk compression. Dull diffuse discomfort in the limb, which is often difficult for the patient to describe and which may be accompanied by changes in skin temperature, vascularity and sweating is often ascribed to involvement of autonomic pathways. In the case of this 'cylindrical' limb pain an origin within the thorax or the thoracic spine should be considered.

Lesions in the neck

X-ray changes of cervical spondylosis are a normal finding after the age of 40. Over the age of 60, neurological symptoms and signs referred from the cervical roots are common. Great care must be taken, therefore, before ascribing patients' symptoms to spondylosis.

Cervical spondylosis can produce three clinical syndromes which may occur alone or in combination. First, pain and stiffness of the neck, which is often recurrent and may be aggravated by tension, anxiety and posture. Secondly, radicular pain radiating down one or both arms and which may or may not be associated with muscle wasting, weakness and reflex changes referred to as brachial neuralgia. Thirdly, compression of the cervical cord may produce three sets of symptoms and signs:

1. Weakness, wasting and fibrillation in the upper limbs with reduction or loss of the tendon reflexes at the level of the compression.
2. Paraesthesiae in the arms and legs with or without impaired sensation in the hands and feet.
3. Pyramidal involvement with weakness, spasticity, hyperreflexia and extensor plantar responses in the legs.

The combination of weakness and wasting in the arms and spastic weakness in the legs resembles amyotrophic lateral sclerosis; spondylosis may usually be distinguished from this by the history of paraesthesiae, evidence of sensory impairment and radiographic or MRI evidence of cord compression. L'Hermitte's sign may be demonstrable.

Disc herniation at the C5/6 and C6/7 intervertebral spaces is a common cause of pain in the upper limb. Onset may be acute with well localized pain radiating from the back of the neck across the back of the shoulder down the arm and forearm to the wrist or fingers; more commonly onset is less dramatic, often after a period of recurrent aching and stiffness in the neck. Pain may be aggravated by movements of the neck, by downward pressure on the head and by changing position of the arm. Pain may radiate downwards into the scapular region and to the upper chest. Sensory disturbances are uncommon though may be detected in a dermatomal distribution (*Fig.* A.22) and muscle weakness may be detected in the appropriate muscles. The clinical signs associated with the most common root lesions are indicated in *Table* A.6. Depression of the biceps jerk may indicate a lesion of the

C5 root, paraesthesiae in the thumb and index finger with depression of the supinator jerk indicate a lesion at the C6 root and paraesthesiae in the index and middle fingers with loss of the triceps jerk are associated with a lesion of the C7 root. Paraesthesiae in the feet with spasticity in the legs and extensor plantar responses indicate pyramidal damage associated with cord compression. X-rays of the cervical spine may show disc space narrowing especially at the C5/6 or C6/7 levels with lipping of the adjacent margins of the vertebral bodies. In the acute stage X-rays may not reveal a relevant abnormality, disc space narrowing in the lower cervical spine being an extremely common appearance in normal individuals over the age of 40. Protrusion of a disc may be demonstrated by contrast myelography, CT or MRI being especially helpful in the demonstration, herniation into the lateral recess. Spinal fluid examination is usually normal though with large herniations the protein content may be raised, especially in the presence of cord compression.

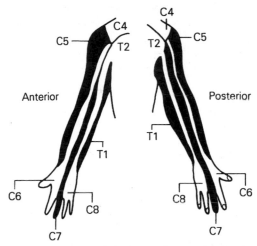

Fig. A.22. Dermatomal distribution of pain referred to the arms. (Redrawn with permission from Doherty, MacFarlane and Maddison (1985), *Rheumatological Medicine,* Churchill Livingstone, Edinburgh.)

Other causes of brachial neuralgia are uncommon. Viral, bacterial and fungal infections should be considered. Herpes zoster may give rise to persistent pain in the arm, especially in the elderly. The history of a vesicular rash and residual pigmented scars in dermatomal distribution is usually diagnostic; weakness of one or more muscles in the limb with cutaneous hyperalgesia or hypoaesthesia may also be present in a minority of cases. Acute viral radiculitis (paralytic brachial radiculitis, neuralgic amyotrophy) produces severe pain in the shoulder and upper arm, often with rapid onset of muscle wasting and weakness. Symptoms usually subside after a few days though there may be some persisting weakness and ache.

Table A.6. Signs and symptoms associated with common nerve root lesions affecting the arms

Root	Paraesthesiae/numbness	Muscle weakness	Reflex change
C5	Radial aspect of forearm	Shoulder abduction Elbow flexion	Biceps jerk diminished
C6	Thumb and index finger	Wrist extension and pronation	Supinator jerk diminished
C7	Middle finger, back of hand	Elbow extension and finger extension	Triceps jerk diminished
C8	Little finger, ulnar border of hand	Finger and wrist flexion	
T1	Ulnar border of forearm (see *Fig.* A.22)	Intrinsic muscles of hand	

Vertebral and paravertebral abscesses may result from tuberculosis or brucellosis or be caused by more common pyogenic organisms such as *Staphylococcus aureus*. In drug addicts and immunocompromised individuals, including those with AIDS, fungal or parasitic lesions may occasionally develop. Such lesions may or may not be accompanied by fever and initial symptoms may closely resemble cervical disc prolapse. Occasionally there are no other pointers to a septic lesion so that severe root symptoms in the arms in the absence of clear radiographic abnormalities should prompt CT or MRI examination of the neck. Pachymeningitis cervicalis hypertrophicia is a rare condition, sometimes syphilitic in origin, which causes diffuse pain in both arms together with paraesthesiae, widespread atrophy, loss of reflexes and variable sensory loss; more than one root is implicated. Positive syphilitic serology should not be taken to indicate this rare condition in the absence of other diagnostic features. Primary or secondary neoplasms of the vertebral bodies may give rise to root pain with or without motor, sensory and reflex changes. X-ray examination is usually diagnostic though isotope bone scanning may also be helpful. Spurious hot spots may be seen in the presence of marked degenerative disease of the spine and it is important to bear in mind that plasmacytomas and myeloma deposits may not be detected by this technique. CT scanning may be helpful in early lesions. Tumours of the meninges and roots usually cause symptoms in the legs, from compression of the pyramidal and sensory tracts, as well as pain in the arm. Root lesions in the presence of multiple cutaneous neurofibromata (von Recklinghausen's disease) should raise the possibility of the development of a neurofibrosarcoma. Specialized spinal imaging is necessary for diagnosis. Where a neural tumour is suspected MRI scanning may provide the most sensitive diagnostic information. *Syringomyelia* occasionally causes pain in the arm but only as a late feature. By this stage the classical features of dissociated sensory loss, muscle wasting and hyporeflexia in the arms with pyramidal signs below the level of the lesion are likely to be apparent. Fracture dislocations of the cervical spine

are especially likely in the presence of rheumatoid arthritis or ankylosing spondylitis. In the former atlantoaxial and/or subaxial subluxation of the spine may lead to upper and lower limb symptoms and fused segments of spondylitic spine are particularly at risk of fracture with or without displacement. Fractures of cervical vertebrae due to osteoporosis are unusual.

Lesions of the brachial plexus

Compression of the neurovascular bundle including the brachial plexus may occur at several sites giving rise to characteristic features classified as thoracic outlet syndromes. Symptoms include paraesthesiae of the fingertips, especially in the night or early morning; the ulnar border of the hand is typically affected (in contrast to carpal tunnel syndrome which affects the radial border) but numbness on waking may extend to the distal forearm. Symptoms may be aggravated by carrying heavy weights though this is not diagnostic. The diagnosis is usually based on induction of paraesthesiae and numbness by abduction of the arm to 90° with external rotation, detection of an arterial bruit in the supraclavicular fossa during this manoeuvre and disappearance of symptoms and bruit with return of the arm to the neutral position. Finding a position of the arm in which the radial pulse is obliterated has been considered a key diagnostic finding. However, this may be demonstrated in normal subjects and symptoms may be due to compression of the brachial plexus without involvement of the subclavian artery. The diagnosis is not, therefore, dependent on demonstration of arterial compression. When chronic or recurrent subclavian artery compression is present this may lead rarely to the development of aneurysmal dilatation of the subclavian artery; such aneurysms may lead to emboli producing digital infarcts.

Compression of the neurovascular bundle may be due to the position of the scalenus anterior muscle, presence of a cervical rib and stretching of the plexus over a normal first rib by drooping of the shoulder, which may occur in middle life. Typically pain is felt behind the clavicle and down the inner aspect of the arm and there may be atrophy of the hypothenar eminence and interossei. Paraesthesiae and hypo-aesthesia in the C8 and T1 dermatomes with associated vasospastic features are common findings. In a few patients the accessory rib may be palpable and visible on X-ray (*Fig.* A.23); not infrequently the rib is vestigial, occuring as a fibrous band which cannot be detected. In the majority of instances in which the diagnosis of thoracic outlet syndrome is considered an alternative cause such as cervical spondylosis, cervical disc lesion or peripheral nerve lesion will be detected.

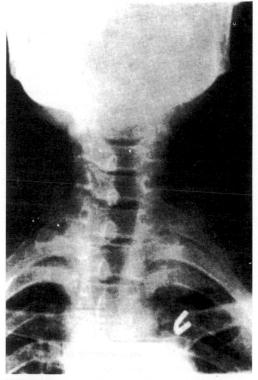

Fig. A.23. Radiograph of cervical ribs in an adult. These are bi-lateral but more fully developed on the left.

Pain in the arm is occasionally due to pressure on, or infiltration of, the brachial plexus by malignant tumours. Lymphadenopathy associated with lymphomas or carcinoma will usually be detectable by palpation of the axilla and of the posterior triangle of the neck though infiltration of the plexus by metastatic carcinoma especially from the breast may take a long time to become detectable. Involvement of the plexus by upward spread of an apical bronchial carcinoma (Pancoast tumour) or more rarely by apical inflammatory lung disease may produce unilateral Horner's syndrome in addition to arm pain. Such lesions can usually be detected on a chest X-ray. In each of these conditions pain may be very severe without any accompanying signs in the early stages. Further infiltration usually leads to paralysis with relative sparing of sensation.

Lesions of the thorax and thoracic spine

In contrast to the characteristically searing localized pain of nerve root involvement, pain in the arm originating in the chest has a dull poorly localized quality, sometimes described as cylindrical. Such pain may also be associated with alterations in autonomic functions including temperature of the limb and sweating.

Pain associated with myocardial infarction and the exercise or stress-related pain of angina pectoris is usually readily recognized and confirmed by ECG or exercise testing. Syphilitic aortitis may induce similar referred pain. Oesophagitis may also produce cylindrical arm pain with or without more classical 'heartburn'. Such pain may also be accompanied by ECG abnormalities so that accurate distinction from myocardial ischaemia may rest upon exercise testing, trial of glyceryl trinitrate and visualization of the upper GI tract. Referral from the thoracic spine is a major but little recognized cause of aching in the arm or 'fibrositis'. Thoracic disc prolapse usually leads to benign thoracic pain though it may also cause referral to the upper limb. Onset is usually insidious and back pain may not be present. However, physical examination of the spine usually reveals local thoracic spine tenderness, often with rib and sternal tenderness and pain on thoracic rotation. Other causes of stiffness of the thoracic spine including spondylosis may lead to similar symptoms.

In a minority of instances myocardial infarction leads to the development of pain and stiffness at one shoulder with varying degrees of pain, swelling, osteoporosis and vasomotor disturbance more distally in the limb. This 'shoulder-hand syndrome' is discussed further below.

Lesions around the shoulder, elbow and wrist

In the absence of swelling, many painful lesions in the arm are referred from the spine even in the presence of local tenderness. Thus even apparently discrete lesions of the shoulder and elbow may originate from spinal lesions.

Degenerative arthritis at the shoulder joint is unusual. Pain around the shoulder radiating to the outer aspect of the upper arm with pain and reduction of glenohumeral movement in all planes is referred to as capsulitis or peri-arthritis. A painful arc on abduction of the shoulder, especially with tenderness at the shoulder tip is typical of supraspinatus tendonitis or subacromial bursitis. Transient calcification around the supraspinatus tendon may be seen on X-ray (*Fig.* A.24). Similarly, tenderness of the long head of biceps (bicipital tendonitis) may be noted usually in association with capsulitis of the shoulder. The pain of tendonitis at the shoulder is usually exacerbated by resisted movement of the appropriate muscles: (a) Supraspinatus—abduction; (b) Infraspinatus—external rotation; (c) Subscapularis—internal rotation; (d) Biceps—supination and flexion of elbow.

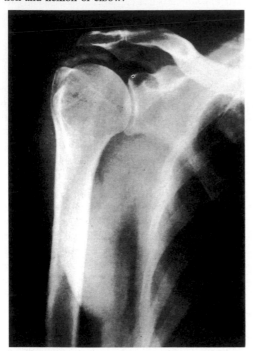

Fig. A.24. Calcific supraspinatus tendonitis. The calcification is seen on a plain AP radiograph of the shoulder.

Epicondylitis is a misnomer for a group of non-inflammatory conditions at the elbow. The cause of such lesions is not usually established, though in a minority, trauma may play a part. Tenderness over the lateral epicondyle sometimes extending to involve the superior radioulnar joint is referred to as 'tennis elbow' and over the medial epicondyle as 'golfer's elbow'. Swelling of the olecranon bursa, due to trauma, gout or infection, may produce pain over the extensor aspect of the elbow with limitation of movement.

Inflammatory or traumatic lesions at the medial aspect of the elbow may lead to ulnar neuritis with characteristic pain, tingling and numbness radiating down the ulnar border of the forearm and hand with impaired intrinsic muscle function. This is especially common after prolonged bed rest where prolonged pressure is applied to the elbows. Radial nerve injury, producing wrist drop with pain, numbness or tingling over the back of the hand is more likely to result from pressure or trauma above the elbow where the nerve runs around the posterior aspect of the humerus in the radial groove. Median nerve dysfunction produces characteristic pain, numbness and tingling in the thumb, index and middle fingers. Symptoms are often worse at night and first thing in the morning. This is most commonly caused by carpal tunnel syndrome, especially in the presence of hypothyroidism, pregnancy or inflammatory arthritis at the wrist. Pressure may also be exerted on the median nerve where it passes between the two heads of pronator teres in the forearm. A positive Tinel's sign with wasting and weakness of abductor pollicis brevis and slowed median nerve conduction on electromyography confirm the diagnosis.

A variety of repetitive strain syndromes are now described. These soft tissue syndromes relate to repeated or sustained actions of the upper limb and produce local pain, fatigue and decline in performance. Symptoms are commonest in young adults especially keyboard workers and a variety of factors including poor posture, stress, inadequate rest periods, poor training and worker's compensation may contribute to their development. Both work and recreational activities may be implicated. Writer's cramp, with pain in the wrist and shoulder associated with an excessively tight grip of the pen and a tense posture whilst writing, may be a related condition.

Tenosynovitis of flexor tendons in the hand may occur as part of generalized arthropathies but also in isolation and in association with diabetes mellitus. The combination of nodular degeneration of a flexor tendon and stenosing tenosynovitis usually at the level of the metacarpophalangeal joint gives rise to 'trigger finger' with pain on flexing the finger followed by inability to extend the finger actively.

MISCELLANEOUS CONDITIONS

Reflex sympathetic dystrophies may affect the upper limb being usually referred to as shoulder-hand syndrome, causalgia or algodystrophy. This condition is characterized by pain, swelling, vasomotor disturbances and trophic skin changes usually affecting the distal part of the limb. This may follow peripheral nerve injury or myocardial infarction, though in at least 50% of cases no cause is demonstrable. In the later stages contractures may also develop.

Hypertrophic (pulmonary) osteoarthropathy (HPOA) may affect many sites but in particular the elbows, wrists, and fingers. Onset of joint pain is often acute with stiffness and weakness and there may be marked tenderness of distal long bones associated with radiographic appearances of periostitis (*Fig.* A.25). Clubbing of the fingers is also present. HPOA is usually associated with malignancy of the lung, pleura or diaphragm though may occasionally be benign or hereditary; it is usually bilateral and symmetrical. Only the upper limbs are affected in association with Pancoast's syndrome and aortic aneurysms. Similar changes of

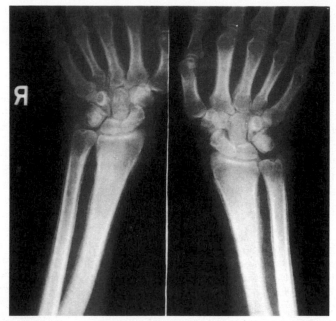

Fig. A.25. Pseudohypertrophic pulmonary osteoarthropathy of the raduis and ulna showing new periosteal bone deposition. (*Dr T.H. Hills.*)

periostitis and clubbing associated with thickening of the skin, especially in the scalp, may develop soon after puberty in the syndrome of pachydermoperiostitis. The condition is benign and gradually becomes inactive after a few years.

Andrew Keat

Ataxia

The coordination of voluntary movement implies the execution of that movement against normal tonus and it demands integration of afferent impulses from the rest of the body so that the movement may occur in a stable organism. Coordination may be affected by muscular weakness, alteration in tone, involuntary movements. disturbance of afferent impulses and by damage to the cerebellum which is the organ of integration of information allowing the coordination of movement. In clinical practice the term ataxia is usually restricted to in-coordination resulting from damage to the afferent sensory inputs or to the cerebellum and its connections. The former is termed sensory ataxia and the latter cerebellar ataxia.

Cerebellar ataxias

The cerebellum is involved in the regulation of muscle tone, the coordination of movement and the control of posture and gait. The cerebellum may be divided into three parts: *the flocculonodular lobe*, which is the oldest part of the cerebellum, *the anterior lobe*, which consists of the anterior vermis and adjacent

cortex, and the *posterior lobe*, or neocerebellum, which is the major portion of the cerebellar hemispheres and the middle of the vermis. These anatomical subdivisions correspond to the functional subdivisions of the organ, the flocculonodular lobe relating, predominantly, to the vestibular nerves and nuclei and concerned with the equilibrium of the body, the anterior lobe receiving fibres from the proprioceptors in muscles of the limbs and therefore involved in the maintenance of posture and tone, and the neocerebellum which derives its fibres from the cerebral cortex and is concerned predominantly with the coordination of skilled movements.

Lesions of the cerebellum and its connections may give rise to loss of muscle tone, incoordination of volitional movement (true ataxia) and disorders of equilibrium and gait, sometimes referred to as truncal ataxia or gait ataxia. The cerebellar hemispheres relate ipsilaterally to the limbs and therefore unilateral lesions of the cerebellar hemisphere will result in ataxia which is most marked on the same side of the body.

Hypotonia is characterized by a decrease in the normal resistance of muscles to passive movement. It may be difficult to appreciate in some patients and is most apparent with acute lesions affecting the cerebellum and its connections. It may most usefully be tested by asking the patient to hold the arms outstretched and then displacing the wrists and noting the range through which the limb is displaced before the patient corrects the posture. This is increased in patients with cerebellar lesions. In addition the knee jerk may be pendular.

The most important manifestation of cerebellar disease is *ataxia*, which may be appreciated by the patient and described as clumsiness or tremulousness. It may be manifested by slurring of speech (ataxic dysarthria), incoordination of the tongue, an intention tremor in the upper limbs and evidence of dysdiadochokinesis on rapid alternating movements of the upper and lower limbs. In the lower limbs, use of the heel–knee–shin test will normally demonstrate a degree of incoordination. The patient may be unsteady whilst sitting (truncal ataxia) and may demonstrate unsteadiness when walking (gait ataxia). The latter, in severe cases, will readily be apparent but, when mild in degrees may only be evident on heel–toe walking (tandem walking) or on rapid turns. True *nystagmus* is not a feature of cerebellar ataxia, but eye movements may be disturbed by *dysmetria* of the eyes wherein voluntary gaze is accomplished by a series of jerky movements which sometimes over-shoot the mark.

Cerebellar ataxia may be seen in patients with lesions in many sites, including the prefrontal area of the cerebral hemispheres, the brain-stem, the cerebellum itself, the vestibular system and the spinocerebellar tracts. It follows that there are many different pathologies which may result in ataxia. In establishing the aetiology of ataxia in the individual patient, it is important to consider the pattern of evolution of the ataxia, its distribution and the associated clinical features.

1.   ATAXIA OF ABRUPT ONSET

The sudden onset of cerebellar ataxia implies an aetiology which is inflammatory, demyelinating or vascular. Multiple sclerosis is one of the most common causes of ataxic syndromes. Involvement may be limited to a single limb or it may be devastatingly extensive with inability to stand or walk and with problems in speech and swallowing.

Infarction or haemorrhage within the posterior cerebral circulation may similarly produce ataxic symptoms of abrupt onset. These may be temporary, as in transient ischaemic attacks (TIA), or more persistent in the case of completed strokes.

2.   SUBACUTE EVOLUTION OF ATAXIA

The subacute evolution of an ataxic syndrome should raise the possibility of a mass lesion within the posterior fossa; gliomas, haemangioblastomas and secondary tumours are among the most frequent. Cerebellar abscesses are relatively rare except in patients with evident infection in the middle ear; encephalitides are extremely uncommon.

In some patients with lung cancer there is a form of paraneoplastic cerebellar ataxia which develops subacutely and which affects particularly the limbs.

3.   CHRONIC CEREBELLAR ATAXIA

The slow development of a cerebellar ataxia is seen not uncommonly in the context of the hereditary ataxias. These may begin in childhood, as in the congenital cerebellar ataxias, and may be associated with discrete metabolic disorders, such as a betalipoproteinaemia, selective vitamin E deficiency, hexosaminidase deficiency and some storage disorders. They may occur intermittently with hyperammonaemia, aminoaciduria and some pyruvate and lactate disorders and they may be associated with other genetic defects such as defective DNA repair in the syndrome of ataxia telangiectasia.

Progressive cerebellar ataxia may develop during adolescence in Friedreich's ataxia, in which it is frequently associated with scoliosis and an axonal sensory neuropathy, in hypogonadism, in the progressive ataxia described by Holmes, or in the Ramsay–Hunt syndrome, in which it is associated with myoclonus.

Late onset cerebellar ataxia occurs in adults and is seen in families with an autosomal dominant pattern, associated with pigmentary retinopathy or with myoclonus.

Other causes of chronic progressive cerebellar ataxia include chronic alcoholism. Acute alcoholic intoxication can produce a cerebellar syndrome which is reversible, but chronic alcoholism may be associated with a permanent ataxia. Severe hypothyroidism may be associated with the development of cerebellar ataxia and overdosage of phenytoin in the treatment of epilepsy can cause profound cerebellar ataxia. Carbon monoxide poisoning has also been reported as a cause of ataxia. Other causes are barbiturate poisoning and prolonged anoxia. The aftereffects of a severe head injury may include ataxia, particularly in those patients who have suffered trauma to the posterior fossa or who have had a head injury complicated by severe anoxia. The chronic progressive traumatic encephalopathy of boxers (dementia pugilis) may also be associated with marked ataxia, hence the name 'the punch drunk syndrome'.

Sensory ataxia

The term 'sensory ataxia' is used to describe the incoordination that is seen in patients who have lost proprioception in a limb or limbs. Afferent proprioceptive impulses travel from the muscles and joints providing information to the cerebellum and cerebrum about the movements of muscles. In the absence of this sensory information, or if it is distorted, the corticospinal system is unable to coordinate normal movements. Such proprioceptive sensory loss may be seen in patients with disease of the peripheral nerves, the posterior nerve roots, the posterior columns of the spinal cord and in lesions of the medial lemniscus, the thalamus and sensory cortex. The resulting ataxia is characterized by symptoms of clumsiness, unsteadiness and incoordination which are most apparent when visual guidance is removed, in the dark or with eyes closed, or when attempting to feel for something in a pocket or handbag.

The gait is typically wide-based and the feet may strike the ground with extreme force causing a *stamping gait*. When asked to stand with the feet together and the eyes closed, the patient will sway (Rombergism). In the upper limbs the phenomenon may be demonstrated by asking the patient to hold the arms out-stretched and to close the eyes. Fine wandering movements of the fingers will develop which are referred to as *pseudoathetosis*. The patient is likely to have great difficulty in undertaking fine movements which are outside the normal range of vision such as fastening the top button of a shirt or tying a tie. The confirmation of the diagnosis is dependent upon the demonstration of loss of proprioceptive sensation in fingers and toes, often associated with loss of vibration sensation.

The differential diagnosis of sensory ataxia will include such conditions as peripheral neuropathy, particularly when the large fibres carrying proprioception are involved, post-infective polyradiculopathy, as in the Guillain–Barré syndrome, and the rare hereditary sensorimotor peripheral neuropathy. But sensory ataxia is most commonly seen in disorders of the spinal cord, classically in subacute combined degeneration associated with vitamin B_{12} deficiency, and frequently in multiple sclerosis where is it particularly common to see patients with deafferentation of both upper limbs, the so-called 'useless hands of Oppenheim'. Other causes in the spinal cord are tumours, transverse myelitis and cervical myelopathy due to disc degeneration or ischaemia. The distinction between those patients with peripheral neuropathic problems and those with dorsal column damage is usually made on the basis of the reflexes.

Hysteria

Ataxia is one of the common somatic symptoms demonstrated in hysteria. The diagnosis may be difficult and depends upon the demonstration of inconsistencies in the degree of ataxia from time to time and from task to task. Most difficulty arises when there is a degree of genuine ataxia on top of which there is hysterical exaggeration. It is important to recognize that prob-

lems due to ataxia are greatly magnified by other motor difficulties; thus the patient with a relatively mild degree of ataxia in multiple sclerosis may be greatly disabled because of an associated spasticity. Similarly, the problems in Friedrich's ataxia due to the ataxia itself are greatly worsened by the peripheral weakness caused by the neuropathy.

D. Bates

Athetosis

The word 'athetosis' derives from the Greek for 'unfixed' or 'changeable'. It is characterized by an inability to sustain the position of the fingers, toes, tongue or any other part of the body in one position. The normal posture is interrupted by slow, sinuous, purposeless movements which are continuous and writhing. They are often confined to the upper limb and are most pronounced in the digits and hands. The face and tongue may be involved; indeed no group of muscles is spared. Within the patterns of movement it is possible to identify extension, pronation and flexion-supination of the forearm, and flexion-extension of the fingers with the thumb often being trapped by the flexed fingers as the hand closes.

In the lower limbs there may be, most typically, eversion-inversion of the foot; in the face, retraction and pursing of the lips and alternate constriction and relaxation of the forehead with opening and closing of the eyes. The neck and torso are prone to rotatory twisting movements.

In general the movements of athetosis are slower and less jerky than those described in chorea but gradations between the two forms of involuntary movement are seen; in some cases the distinction is impossible and the term 'choreoathetosis' is used. Discrete movements of the affected limb are possible, but are performed slowly, and attempted voluntary movements usually worsen the spasms.

In children, particularly after hemiplegia, athetosis may be unilateral, though rarely congenital double athetosis may occur. Both arms and face are involved; speech and swallowing are also affected. Such children are usually slow in gaining their motor milestones and have a degree of mental handicap. Athetosis appearing early in life is usually the result of congenital or postnatal injury, such as hypoxia or kernicterus, and postmortem examinations in some affected children have disclosed a presumed posthypoxic cerebral appearance termed status marmoratus, in which the corpus striatum is broken up into cellular masses separated by a fine network of nerve fibres. In others, probably after kernicterus, there is demonstrable damage to myelin, status dysmyelinatus.

In adults, athetosis may occur as an episodic or

permanent abnormality in hepatic encephalopathy, as a manifestation of chronic intoxication with phenothiazines or haloperidol, and, most commonly, as an effect of excess dosage with L-dopa in patients undergoing treatment for Parkinson's disease. Athetosis is part of the involuntary movement seen in patients with Huntington's chorea and may also be seen in patients with Wilson's disease, Hallervorden–Spatz disease and Leigh's disease.

Athetosis, like most forms of involuntary movement, ceases during sleep.

D. Bates

Aura

An aura may be defined as a premonitory symptom which is commonly related to an epileptic attack. The term may also be used to describe the prodrome occurring before the development of headache in some migraine sufferers.

One of the main differentiating features between the aura of an epileptic seizure and the aura of migraine is its length. The aura in migraine may last from a few minutes to an hour or more, that in epilepsy is usually more transient.

THE EPILEPSIES

An aura in a seizure has been defined as that part of the seizure which occurs before consciousness is lost or an automatism begins and which can be remembered subsequently. It is most commonly seen in patients who have complex partial seizures arising in one portion of the brain, and the aura, which may incorporate any of the symptoms described in simple seizures, tends to indicate the site of the brain in which the seizure begins. Thus *a motor aura* may include an involuntary movement of a limb or part of a limb, or occasionally a more coordinated movement such as walking or running. *A sensory aura* is more common and may be described as discomfort, numbness, tingling or occasionally a more complex sensation such as that of a small animal walking along the limb. A *visual aura* may be disorganized and simply have the appearance of shimmering lights or colours within the field of vision, implying an origin in the occipital lobes; or it may be organized as a formed visual hallucination such as flowers on a brightly coloured background which suggests an origin in the temporal lobes.

Seizures arising in the temporal lobes are those most likely to be associated with a *psychical* aura, involving feelings of apprehension, a sense of unreality or a vision or feeling of something having happened, or a *visceral* aura in which there may be an abnormal sensation beginning in the stomach and welling up into the throat and head, or an olfactory, auditory or gustatory sensation in which patients may describe quite clearly disturbances of smell, hearing or taste.

The most important aspect of the aura in epilepsy is in relation to the diagnosis of the seizure type. It implies that the epilepsy is arising at a focus within the brain and is therefore a form of partial seizure. Thus a patient who describes an aura consisting of a sensory disturbance in the left hand will be likely to have a lesion in the contralateral parietal lobe; one who describes an aura beginning in the right visual field will be likely to have a lesion in the left occipital lobe. An aura of movement beginning in the right thumb and spreading in Jacksonian fashion up the arm implies a lesion in the precentral gyrus of the left frontal lobe.

The second importance of an aura in epilepsy is that it provides evidence of continuing activity of the focus. Patients with seizures may be able to describe minor episodes in which their usual aura does not proceed to a full attack, thus indicating to the physician that, although control is partially achieved in reducing the severity of the attacks, the epileptogenic focus continues and the patient requires an increase in therapy. The main characteristics of an aura are that it shall be spontaneous, normally in the context of good health, and it begins abruptly and lasts for seconds only.

THE AURA IN MIGRAINE

Migraine is a common illness which affects approximately 10% of the population. Most of those afflicted suffer from *common migraine*, that is *migraine without aura*, in which they have episodes of headache, usually unilateral, associated with nausea, photophobia, phonophobia and occasionally vomiting. One in ten patients with migraine will have *classical migraine*, or *migraine with aura*, in which a proportion of the attacks will be preceded by a visual sensation, usually zig-zag lines in black and white in half the field of vision, or, less commonly, by more complex disturbances of function such as loss of vision, loss of speech, numbness or paralysis of part of the body. These syndromes may evolve and continue over a few minutes but occasionally are more prolonged. They are usually, but not always, followed by a typical migraine headache. Whether they are due to vasoconstriction or electrical cortical depression remains uncertain.

D. Bates

Axillary swelling

Swelling in the axilla is due in the great majority of cases to enlargement of the lymph nodes. If the enlargement is inflammatory, a subsequent abscess, either acute or chronic, is frequent. Any form of tumour other than involvement of the nodes by secondary deposits is distinctly rare, but unfortunately it is common to find the axillary nodes to be the seat of metastases from carcinoma of the breast.

Acute abscess

Acute abscess may be recognized at once by the well-marked signs of local inflammation and the general febrile disturbance. There is one form of acute abscess that may not be obvious, namely one situated in the upper part of the axilla and covered by the pectoral muscles. On account of its distance from the surface the local signs of inflammation may not be great, though the general signs are marked. There will be great disinclination to move the arm on account of pain, and there is usually some cause, such as a whitlow on the finger, to account for the trouble. It must be remembered, however, that the abscess may be 'residual'; that is to say, the original source of infection, such as the whitlow, may have healed completely 2, 3 weeks or even longer before the axillary abscess declares itself. Rarely an empyema points in the axilla; there are generally, but not always, abnormal lung signs to suggest the diagnosis.

Chronic or tuberculous abscess

Chronic or tuberculous abscess (*Fig.* A.26) forms a single fluctuating swelling which, if large, may extend upwards under the pectoralis major. Owing to the fact that few, if any, of the local signs of inflammation may be present, difficulty may arise in distinguishing this form of abscess from a soft lipoma. The duration and the rapidity of growth of the swelling are good guides, for though the duration of a chronic abscess may run into months, it does not exist for years, as does a lipoma. Aspiration will settle the difficulty.

Enlargement of the lymph nodes

Next, supposing that examination proves that the swelling is not an abscess, attention should be directed to ascertain whether it arises from lymph nodes, which may present as a single enlarged node, a number of discrete individual nodes or as a mass of matted glands. For the differential diagnosis of nodular swelling, *see* LYMPHADENOPATHY (p. 402). It is sufficient here to enumerate the principal causes. These are: acute infection, chronic infection with tuberculosis; rheumatoid arthritis, lymphatic leukaemia, Hodgkin's disease and non-Hodgkin's lymphoma; malignant glandular metastases. The first and the last are far the most common in the axilla (*Fig.* A.27).

Occasionally a node or group of nodes in the axilla appears malignant and on being removed for histological section is found to be infiltrated with

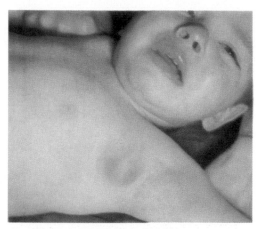

Fig. A.26. Tuberculous abscess in a child.

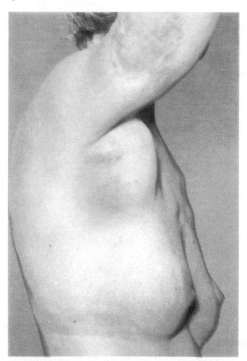

Fig. A.27. Huge mass of melanotic deposits in the axillary nodes following previous resection of malignant melanoma of the upper arm (note the skin graft at this point).

metastatic carcinoma, and yet no source for the primary can be found. The most likely site for such a hidden primary is undoubtedly the breast and, next to this, the lung, so that an energetic search should be instituted by clinical examination, chest X-ray and mammography (in the female), as well as by bronchoscopy to incriminate or exculpate these two organs. Other less common possibilities are the stomach and the ovary, and if all investigations have so far been negative, expert pelvic examination and a complete investigation of the gastro-intestinal tract are called for. If, after careful search in this way, no primary can be detected it may be assumed that this is within the breast. The introduction of mammography has helped to reveal very small breast carcinomas presenting as enlarged axillary nodes.

Primary tumours of the axilla

Primary tumours of the axilla are distinctly rare, but it is a possible site for an accessory breast, the nipple of which will provide the diagnosis.

LIPOMA is the most common tumour (*Fig. A.28*). It may attain a large size and extend up under the pectoral muscles. It should be diagnosed by its long history, slow growth, definite outline and free mobility. When very soft, the tumour may give the feeling of fluctuation, and so be mistaken for a chronic tuberculous abscess, and as it consists of large lobules of fat, some degree of translucency may be present. The skin wrinkles when one attempts to raise it away from the tumour.

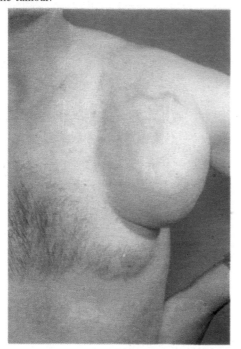

Fig. A.28. A massive but entirely benign lipoma of the axilla.

CYSTIC HYGROMA of the axilla is rare. It is usually congenital, but apparently similar cystic swellings may appear in adult life. It forms a soft, fluctuating, quite translucent and painless swelling, which sometimes grows rapidly. It may be mistaken for a lipoma, and the diagnosis may not be certain until excision and microscopical examination are completed.

PRIMARY MALIGNANT TUMOURS may arise, but are of extreme rarity.

ANEURYSM OF THE AXILLARY ARTERY does occur, but is very uncommon. It is recognized easily because

it is comparatively superficial and it gives an expansile pulsation synchronous with the heart's beat; the veins of the forearm may be distended on account of pressure on the axillary vein, and the radial pulse on the affected side is diminished in size and delayed. There may be a definite history of local injury, or in cases of apparently spontaneous aneurysm there may be signs or symptoms of bacterial endocarditis.

Harold Ellis

Back, pain in

Pain in the back is one of the commonest complaints in general and specialist practice, and no specialty is immune from it. The differential diagnosis therefore covers most of medicine. The first important subdivision is into acute and chronic back pain.

ACUTE SELF-LIMITING PAIN IN THE BACK

This may occur in any febrile condition. A striking though rare, example is dengue or 'break-bone fever'. It may also result from soft-tissue injury: any gardener, spring-cleaning house-cleaner or horse rider knows how common such minor insults are. Such pains usually rapidly settle either when the cause is removed or as the injured tissues heal. Only when the back aches and pains persist after several days does one look further into the possible causes.

CHRONIC BACKACHE

In any backache lasting more than 2–3 weeks the conditions listed in the table below should be considered. By far the commonest are the first four mentioned (1(*a*)–(*d*)), sometimes associated with depression or anxiety.

THE CAUSES OF CHRONIC BACKACHE
1. *Traumatic, mechanical or degenerative:*
(*a*) Low back strain; fatigue; obesity; pregnancy. (*b*) Injuries of bone, joint or ligament. (*c*) Degenerative disease of the spine (osteo-arthritis) including ankylosing hyperostosis. (*d*) Intervertebral disc lesions. (*e*) Lumbar instability syndromes, e.g. spondylolisthesis. (*f*) Scoliosis: primary and secondary. (*g*) Spinal stenosis

2. *Metabolic:*
Osteoporosis. Osteomalacia. Hyper- and hypoparathyroidism. Ochronosis (*Figs.* B.1, B.2) Fluorosis. Hypophosphataemic rickets

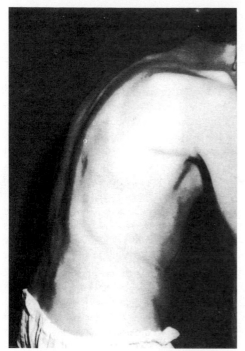

Fig. B.1. Rigid spine due to ochronosis. (*Courtesy of General Raji Al Tikriti of Baghdad.*)

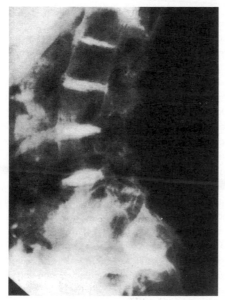

Fig. B.2. Radiograph showing calcification of intervertebral discs in ochronosis. (*Courtesy of the Arthritis and Rheumatism Council.*)

3. *Unknown causes:*

Inflammatory arthropathies of the spine, such as ankylosing spondylitis and the spondylitis of Reiter's syndrome, psoriasis, ulcerative colitis, Whipple's and Crohn's diseases. Rarely polymyositis and polymyalgia rheumatica. Paget's disease of bone. Osteochondritis—(Scheuermann's disease)

4. *Infective conditions of bone, joint and theca of spine:*

Osteomyelitis. Tuberculosis. Undulant fever (abortus and melitensis). Typhoid and paratyphoid fever and other *Salmonella* infections. Syphilis. Yaws. Very rarely Weil's disease (leptospirosis icterohaemorrhagica). Spinal pachymeningitis. Chronic meningitis. Subarachnoid or spinal abscess

5. *Psychogenic:*

Anxiety. Depression. Hysteria. Compensation neurosis. Malingering

6. *Neoplastic—benign or malignant, primary or secondary:*

Osteoid osteoma. Eosinophilic granuloma. Metastatic deposits from primary carcinoma of bronchus, breast, prostate, kidney, thyroid and rarely, from other primaries. Direct invasion from carcinoma of the oesophagus. Myeloma. Primary and secondary tumours of spinal canal and nerve roots: ependymoma; neurofibroma; glioma; angioma; meningioma; lipoma; rarely chordoma. Reticuloses, e.g. Hodgkin's disease

7. *Cardiac and vascular:*

Subarachnoid or spinal haemorrhage. Luetic, degenerative or dissecting aneurysm. Grossly enlarged left atrium in mitral valve disease. Rarely myocardial infarction

8. *Gynaecological conditions:*

Tuberculous disease. Rarely prolapse or retroversion of uterus. Dysmenorrhoea. Chronic salpingitis. Pelvic abscess or chronic cervictis. Tumours

9. *Gastrointestinal conditions:*

Perforating posterior gastric or duodenal ulcer. Pancreatitis, acute or chronic. Referred pain from biliary calculi. Retroperitonial neoplasms (particularly pancreatic carcinoma).

10. *Renal and genito-urinary causes:*

Carcinoma of kidney. Calculus. Hydronephrosis. Polycystic kidney. Necrotizing papillitis. Pyelitis and pyelonephritis. Perinephric abscess

11. *Blood disorders:*

Sickle-cell crisis. Acute haemolytic states

12. *Drugs:*

Corticosteroids. Methysergide. Compound analgesic tablets

13. *Normality:*

(Non-disease)

The list is probably incomplete but covers most of the likely causes. In eliciting the cause a full history is essential, with particular reference to factors operating at the time of onset and factors known to ease or aggravate the condition. On examination the way a patient moves, walks, sits or lies, and how he rises from sitting and lying positions may be highly informative. Spinal range of movement may be measured by various instruments such as Dunham's spondylometer (*Fig.* B.3) or Loebl's inclinometer. Another method is that of Schober, which depends on stretching of the skin over the lumbar spine in spinal flexion. More sensitive and accurate is Macrae's modification of the same method which measures stretching of the skin in spinal flexion between a point 10 cm above the

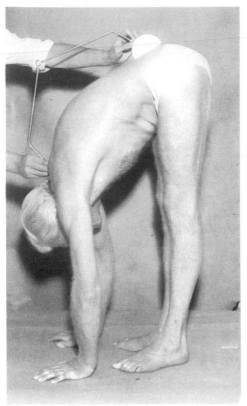

Fig. B.3. Ankylosing spondylitis. The patient can touch the floor easily with his hands as he has very supple hips, but measurement with a spondylometer shows spinal movement to be restricted to 60 per cent of normal.

lumbosacral junction and a spot 15 cm below over the sacrum. Ability to touch the toes is a poor measure of spinal movement as it depends greatly on hip flexion; these methods eliminate the hip component. They also enable the examiner to give a positive figure for the spinal range of movement, which can be measured repeatedly to assess progression or regression of the spinal disorder. Radiography often helps in diagnosis, but even more often does not. The fact that there are radiological changes does not mean that these are the cause of the symptoms. Radiologically speaking, there is no such thing as a normal spine after middle age is passed. Nevertheless, many diagnoses of chronic backache are dependent on radiography, and computed tomography (CT scanning) also helps in the diagnosis of certain back pains due to trauma, malignancy or spinal stenosis, where the degree of stenosis can be assessed. A virtue of computed tomography is that the vertebrae, spinal cord, subarachnoid space and nerve root sleeves can be shown without the use of a contrast medium given intrathecally. Magnetic resonance imaging, where available, gives extremely accurate visualization of this region.

1. Non-infective traumatic and degenerative disorders

Non-infective traumatic and degenerative disorders arising in the bones, joints and soft tissues of the spine are extremely common. In a structure of such complexity as the human spine, with so many joints, ligaments and cartilages at risk, it is no wonder that aches and pains are commonplace. Too-easy chairs at home, badly placed and badly shaped car seats, and unsatisfactory chairs at work are often the cause of postural strain. Fixed unnatural positions held for hours on end are highly productive of symptoms. Bad posture and fatigue act together to produce one of the most common of backaches. The postural back pain of pregnancy usually goes soon after childbirth but is sometimes replaced by one of lumbosacral origin due to the childbirth itself. Obesity is an aggravating factor rather than a sole cause, but chronic backaches may not infrequently be improved or cured by the loss of 30–90 kg (1–3 stones) or more in weight.

Degenerative changes of the spine are almost always present after the age of 45 years, but only sometimes are they accompanied by symptoms, and these in turn are often due to some of the factors mentioned above. *Ankylosing hyperostosis*, a condition often associated with diabetes mellitus, is characterized by coarse bridging along the anterior borders of the lower dorsal vertebrae, seen well in lateral radiographs. Degenerative changes in the *intervertebral cartilages* may be associated with chronic backache, and such changes may be localized, usually to lower cervical and lumbar areas, or may extend widely throughout the entire spine. More severe symptoms of compression may occur when a disc herniation protrudes through a tear of the posterior longitudinal ligament and presses on root and/or cord causing symptoms and signs of sciatica, femoral neuropathy or brachialgia, depending on the site of the lesion. Such lesions can cause severe and prostrating pains which may be aggravated by coughing and straining. A sudden strain, such as lifting a heavy weight with the spine flexed, is often the precipitating cause. Paraesthesia in the distribution of the affected nerve is common and the appropriate reflex may be diminished or absent (*see Table* B.1).

In lumbar lesions the normal lumbar lordosis may be lost; stooping causes great pain but lateral spinal movement may be painless. The so called 'sciatica scoliosis' is a lumbar scoliosis with a limping gait in an attempt by the patient to avoid pain. The back is held stiffly and painfully, the patient feeling the need to press it on to a hard, flat surface for support and pain relief. Stiffness and pain are often worst in the morning when rising from bed and may be agonizing.

Table B.1.   Neurological signs of lumbar disc lesions

Root	Pain reference	Motor weakness	Sensory changes	Reflex changes	Muscle wasting
L2	Anterior upper thigh	Flexion and adduction of hip	None or upper thigh lateral and anterior	None or reduced knee reflex	None
L3	Anterior thigh and knee	Knee extension. Hip flexion and adduction	None or lower thigh medial and anterior	Reduced knee reflex	Thigh
L4	Lateral thigh. Median calf	Foot inversion and dorsiflexion. Knee extension	Antero-medial calf and shin	Reduced or absent knee reflex	Thigh
L5	Buttock, back and side thigh. Lateral lower leg	Extension and abduction of hip. Flexion knee. Dorsiflexion foot and toes. Foot eversion	Lateral calf, dorsal and medial foot, especially hallux	None or (rarely) reduced ankle reflex	Calf
S1	Buttock. Back of thigh and calf to heel	Flexion knee, foot eversion and plantar flexion	Lateral foot, ankle and lower calf, back of heel and sole of foot	Reduced or absent ankle reflex	Calf

Straight-leg raising may cause pain. But not always; pulling the bent knee backwards while pushing the buttocks forwards with the other hand, the patient lying half prone with his back to the examiner, may give a more positive result as it stretches the femoral nerve and puts tension on the upper lumbar roots. A large disc protrusion may not only press directly on nervous tissue but also interfere with its blood supply. Cerebrospinal fluid may show an increase of protein, often with an increase of lymphocytes and perhaps some red blood cells, and the fluid pressure may be altered. Radiographs of the spine after introduction of a contrast medium may occasionally be necessary to localize the obstruction, as is shown in *Fig.* B.4, although CT scans and MRI are more appropriate as non-invasive investigations (*Fig.* B.5).

Many disc protrusions are posterior rather than posterolateral. In the former case they cause back pain only, rarely cord compression. There may be tenderness over the affected area, in some cases referred to paravertebral muscles or buttocks.

Spondylolisthesis, usually in the lower lumbar spine, occurs as a result of the bilateral lesion in the pars interarticularis, i.e. that bony bridge which unites the superior articular facet and pedicle to the lamina and inferior articular process. A forward or backward (retrospondylolisthesis) displacement may also occur as a result of the degeneration of an intervertebral disc ('pseudospondylolisthesis') resulting in instability of the upper vertebra and narrowing of the intervertebral foramina. Well-centred radiographs taken in full flexion and extension will show the lesion. There may be no symptoms in some cases, others have low backache and aches extending round into the groins; unilateral or bilateral sciatica is rare, as is a cauda equina lesion. This (cauda equina) lesion, partly due to compression, partly due to traction, the severest of the syndromes

associated with spondylolisthesis, is more often seen in adolescent children. Physical signs are often non-existent, but the visible and palpable prominence of the spine of the affected vertebra may become more obvious as the patient flexes his spine. Cervical spondylolisthesis is much less common than lumbar.

Scoliosis is a lateral deviation of the spine from a straight line. When the subject flexes his spine a functional scoliosis will disappear but a structural one will persist or even increase. A scoliosis may be compensatory to a short leg, painful hip or knee or any other cause of a pelvic tilt, but if the iliac crests are level the cause of the 'scoliosis' is in the spine itself. Pain may arise from an idiopathic adolescent scoliosis but in most adults arises from factors outside the spine.

Spinal stenosis. The spinal canal can be narrowed by degenerative changes and/or developmentally either centrally or laterally, damaging nervous tissue directly or by leaving less space for a prolapsed disc or osteophyte. Narrowing of the spinal canal may also interfere with the blood supply to the cauda equina causing weakness, burning or numbness on exertion eased by resting, a kind of intermittent claudication without muscle cramps and with normal peripheral pulses (*see* MUSCULAR PAIN). This claudication is present, however, only in a minority of cases and degenerative (acquired) cases are more common than developmental, though both factors may be present. Lumbar stenosis often presents as a nerve root compression distinguished from root compression by a disc by the absence of abnormal straight-leg raising and spinal stiffness. Spinal stenosis may be: (1) congenital—idiopathic or associated with achondroplasia; (2) acquired—degenerative (osteo-arthritic, discogenic, spondylolytic or spondylolisthetic); (3) postoperative or post-traumatic; (4) due to Paget's disease; or (5) fluorosis, but may be due to combinations of the above.

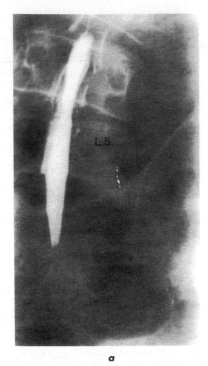
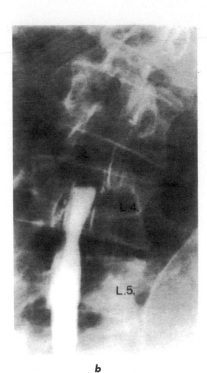

a

b

Fig. B.4. *a.* Radiograph (patient supine) after intraspinal injection of lipiodol showing narrowing of the oil column at the level of the interspace between the 4th and 5th lumbar vertebrae and scoliosis due to muscular spasm. A protruded portion of disc was removed with complete relief of pain in the back and sciatica. (*Dr H.M. Worth.*) *b.* Radiograph in same case with the patient prone.

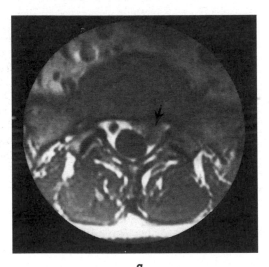
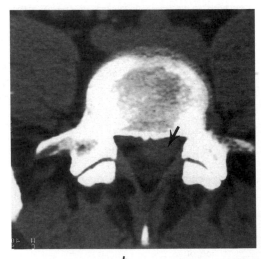

a

b

Fig. B.5. *a.* CT scan. *b.* MRI scan. Both scans demonstrate prolapsed L5/SI disc (arrowed). (Films supplied by Prof. Adrian Dickson, Addenbrookes Hospital, Cambridge.)

2. Crushed or wedged vertebrae

Crushed or wedged vertebrae due to osteoporosis are seen in radiographs to be part of a diffuse thinning of the texture of the bone without lytic lesions or condensation. There is often wedging of several vertebrae from previous crushes and the back is usually rounded. The patient is in most cases an elderly woman. Blood chemistry (serum alkaline phosphatase, calcium and plasma phosphate) is typically normal, though hypocalcaemia often occurs. In a spine painful from malignant deposits there is actual destruction of bone tissue in the radiographs and porosis is patchy and not generalized; if due to carcinoma of the prostate the bone shadow may be denser and dead-white in the radiographs in the affected areas. The serum alkaline phosphatase is elevated in metastatic malignant disease but normal in myelomatosis. In both cases the sedimentation rate is raised, usually in carcinomatosis, invariably and to a high figure around 80-100 mm in 1 hour (Westergren) in myelomatosis; marrow biopsy and electrophoretic studies clinch the diagnosis. The commonest source of spinal malignant deposits today is carcinoma of the breast in the female and the bronchus and prostate in the male, but multiple myeloma should always be kept in mind in any unexplained backache. *Osteomalacia* differs from osteoporosis in that there is often a history of dietetic and/or intestinal insufficiency or of chronic disease and sometimes of a previous gastrectomy. The serum alkaline phosphatase is often elevated, serum calcium and plasma phosphate normal or decreased. Urinary 24-hour calcium output is low. The aches are more diffuse and are not centred on the crushed vertebra, as in osteoporosis; they are nagging and unremitting, are eased by rest, and aggravated by activity. Pain in osteoporosis appears to be due to local fracture of a brittle non-tender vertebral body, in osteomalacia to strain of the tender soft bones of the spine. Radiographs may show stress fractures (pseudo-fractures) and Milkman's lines or Looser zones in pelvis or ribs, rarefied areas consisting of uncalcified osteoid. In *hyperparathyroidism* there may be generalized osteoporosis in the radiographs. Bone cysts may occur; subperiosteal resorption of phalanges and of the distal ends of the clavicles is characteristic. There may be generalized backache and tenderness. Serum calcium is raised, but repeated estimates over a period of time may have to be done to demonstrate this. Plasma phosphorus may be low, though it rises with renal failure, and the alkaline phosphatase is usually but not invariably raised. There may be other features of hypercalcaemia, such as nausea and vomiting, muscle weakness or a true myopathy, corneal calcification (band keratitis) and nephrocalcinosis. Peptic ulceration and pancreatitis may occur. The syndrome is usually due to primary hyperparathyroidism, from hyperplasia or adenoma of the parathyroid gland, but it can occur as secondary to renal and other diseases in which case the serum calcium may be normal. The finding of plasma chloride levels consistently less than 100 mmol/l in the presence of hypercalcaemia virtually excludes the diagnosis of primary hyperparathyroidism. Back pains may also rarely occur in *idiopathic hypoparathyroidism* associated with the hypocalcaemia, cataracts, fits, tetany and rashes.

Paget's disease of bone is often an incidental radiological finding in a patient with no symptons. It can occasionally, however, cause quite severe back-

ache. Diagnosis is made on X-rays and an elevated serum alkaline phosphatase. The disease may extend throughout the pelvis and spine or involve one or two vertebral bodies only. A small number of the lesions become sarcomatous, and severe pain should arouse suspicions of malignant change.

Scheuermann's osteochondritis is a condition of unknown aetiology predominantly affecting adolescent males. There is irregular ossification of the vertebral epiphysial end-plates of the lower dorsal but also the upper lumbar spine, the disc spaces becoming narrowed and the vertebral bodies wedged anteriorly, the patient developing rounded shoulders, a smoother dorsal kyphosis and flat chest.

3. Inflammatory arthropathies of the spine

The best example is idiopathic ankylosing spondylitis (*Fig.* B.6). Here the patient is usually a male aged

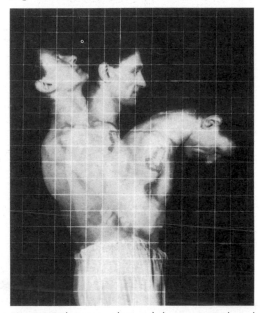

Fig. B.6. Triple-exposure photograph showing restricted spinal extension and flexion in a young man with ankylosing spondylitis.

between 16 and 36, and in the large majority of cases he is of tissue type HLA-B27 (*see Figs.* B.3, B.6, B.7). His spine is stiffened and restricted in movement *in all planes*. Neck movements are often restricted and intercostal expansion at nipple level reduced from the normal 5-7·5 to 2·5 cm or less. This intercostal restriction occurs early in the course of the disease and is not a late complication but an essential and early part of the clinical picture. Diaphragmatic movement is normal. Evidence of active or old iridocyclitis is present in over 20 per cent of the patients, in most cases seen as iritic adhesions or dark spots in the anterior chamber on the posterior surface of the cornea. Tender heels or tender areas over the pelvic brim, ischial tuberosities, or greater trochanters are not uncommon. Peripheral arthritis occurs in some 25 per cent of cases initially and hydrarthrosis of knees in about 7 per cent of cases. The sedimentation rate is elevated in almost all cases, but sheep-cell agglutination and latex tests are negative. Nodules do not occur, nor does lymphadenopathy or splenomegaly. The commonest initial symptom is aching in the buttocks, the patient drawing his hand down the back of the buttocks and thighs at the site of discomfort, but lumbar backache and stiffness soon occur and may be the initial symptoms. Two radiographs help in early diagnosis, a posteroanterior view of the sacro-iliacs and an anteroposterior of the dorsolumbar spine D 8–L 3, but X-ray changes may not be present until symptoms have been present 2–3 years or more. The earliest radiological sacro-iliac changes are blurring of the joint outlines with paraarticular ilial sclerosis, erosions and apparent widening, gradually giving way over the years to narrowing and obliteration of the joint. Small syndesmophytes, resembling bony 'stalagmites and stalactites', are usually seen first along the edges of the intervertebral cartilages between the vertebral bodies of D 10 and L 2; this is where the 'bamboo spine' usually first becomes evident. Lytic lesions with periosteal elevation and 'whiskering' may be seen in the pelvis or in the spine, most commonly in the ischial tuberosities. Ankylosing spondylitis affects the spine primarily (*Fig.* B.7), girdle joints (hips and shoulders) secondly, and peripheral joints least often, in contrast to the distribution of joint involvement seen in rheumatoid arthritis, where initial involvement is usually feet, hands and wrists. The spondylitic pattern of disease may also be seen occasionally in Reiter's syndrome, or in association with psoriasis, ulcerative colitis, Crohn's disease, and occasionally Whipple's disease and Behçet's disease and, very rarely, polymyalgia rheumatica. Some male cases of juvenile chronic polyarthritis progress to the spondylitic picture. In the diagnosis of ankylosing spondylitis these variants should always be considered.

4. Infective conditions

Infective conditions of bones and joints are uncommon and the history will often give a lead to the diagnosis. The *Staphylococcus aureus* is the most common causative organism. The lesions tend to be lytic and abscesses may form and discharge. The final picture may resemble osteoarthritis or even ankylosing spondylitis. *Tuberculosis* of sacro-iliac joint or spine is more painful than these conditions, however, and more incapacitating. The dorsal spine is the most commonly affected portion of the spine, the vertebral bodies being most

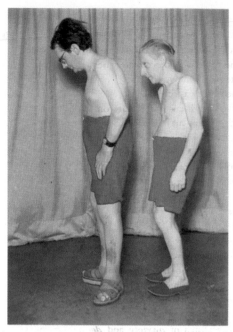

Fig. B.7. Two patients with severe ankylosing spondylitis both of whom have had wedge lumbar osteotomies to straighten the previously grossly flexed spine.

commonly involved though the disease may start in the intervertebral disc. Collapse of vertebral bodies leads to angulation of the spine. Cold-abscess formation and paresis are much less common today than 30 or more years ago. There is pain and weakness in the back and tenderness and muscle spasm in the affected area, the spine being held rigidly. Sacro-iliac disease is usually unilateral in tuberculous disease, bilateral in ankylosing spondylitis.

In brucellosis contracted from *Br. abortus* in cattle, *melitensis* in goats and *suis* in pigs, generalized aches, fever, sweats, anorexia and other features of a febrile infective process may coexist with backache and joint and bone pains; signs of actual joint inflammation are rare. The lesion is essentially an osteomyelitis of the spine or pelvis; both bone and disc may be involved, only occasionally with pus formation. Localization in the spinal column may occur many weeks or months after the original infection, which may have been overlooked and undiagnosed at the time. The same delay of months, or even years, before the advent of spinal symptoms is also seen with typhoid and paratyphoid fevers. *Weil's disease* (leptospirosis icterohaemorrhagica), characterized by fever and high leucocytosis, haemorrhagic manifestations and jaundice, may give rise at the time to acute backache and later to destructive and degenerative changes in the spine with chronic symptoms.

5. Psychogenic

The essence of hysteria is the theatrical nature of the symptoms it causes. This is true of the hysterical spine. The spine is held elaborately bent (camptocormia), all attempts at movement being resisted with great drama and much expression of suffering. The back, nevertheless, straightens out readily on bed, couch or floor. The patient may be able to flex his spine painlessly, but will not straighten it. Palpation or attempts at movement by the examiner may produce much louder groans, grimaces and excessive reactions than in a patient with a true acute inflammatory spondylitis. It is this 'over-reaction' which is typical of the hysteric. Watched closely, movements previously impossible are later made without discomfort and areas previously acutely tender touched without complaint. *Malingering* may give a similar picture though usually less dramatic. In both cases spinal movements are often more grossly restricted than in severe spinal disease. *Compensation neurosis* tends to improve when the case is settled, whatever the legal decision. The history and features of *anxiety* and *depression* are usually apparent in a well-taken history. Backache may be entirely due to either or both, or features of these disorders may become superimposed on an organic cause. Such a picture is common in the overworked, harassed, anxious housewife.

6. Spinal tumours

Spinal tumours may be divided into extradural and intradural, the latter being further subdivided into those outside and those within the cord, i.e. extra- or intramedullary. Meningiomas and neurofibromas are the commonest extramedullary growths, the latter usually arising from spinal roots, the posterior more often than the anterior. They may be single or multiple and may or may not be part of a generalized neurofibromatosis.

Benign tumours of the spine are uncommon. Bone cysts, giant-cell tumours, osteochondroma and chondroma may occur but more common are haemangiomas, aneurysmal bone cysts and osteoid osteomas. Not all haemangiomas are benign; some lead to extensive destruction of bone. X-rays show vertical striations in the vertebral body which may be partially crushed. Aneurysmal bone cysts form large paraspinal masses, usually posteriorly, with scattered calcific deposits. The osteoid osteoma is a painful lesion in which new bone is formed leading to considerable surrounding bony sclerosis. Tomograms may be necessary to demonstrate the lesion well, a zone of dense bone encircling a small radiolucent centre. The pain is often severe and worse at night.

7. Backache caused by cardiovascular and intrathoracic disorders

Backache may be caused by cardiovascular and intrathoracic disorders, of which a good example is the intense, demoralizing, boring pains of an aneurysm invading the spine. Features of luetic aneurysm of the arch and early descending aorta will probably be present with signs of an aortic reflux, collapsing arterial pulses, and possibly signs of neurosyphilis also. Dissecting aneurysms of the descending aorta below the arch are less apparent; unequal or delayed pulses in arms and legs should be noted. An arteriosclerotic aneurysm of the abdominal aorta may cause pain in the lower part of the back as well as in the upper abdomen, the groin, and occasionally in the testicles; a pulsating mass may be felt in the abdomen. A carcinoma of the bronchus or oesophagus may cause backache, myocardial infarction only rarely. *Fig.* B.8 shows a rare cause, enormous enlargement of the left atrium in mitral disease. The pain in such cases is usually relieved by leaning forwards and to the left.

8. Gynaecological conditions

Gynaecological conditions are, on the whole, a rare cause of low lumbar and sacral backache. Disease of the ovaries and tubes may be responsible in a few cases, prolapse or retroversion of the uterus occasionally, but the cause commonly lies elsewhere and correcting the gynaecological condition leaves the backache in most cases unrelieved. If backache worsens during the menses this may suggest a gynaecological cause, but may also suggest a change in pain threshold at this time. Tuberculous endometritis may cause backache which is relieved by appropriate therapy.

9. Gastrointestinal conditions

There are gastrointestinal conditions from which backache may be referred. Chronic pancreatitis and carcinoma of the pancreas may cause a dull, persistent, upper lumbar ache, usually but not always associated with upper abdominal pain and discomfort. Relief of pain may be obtained by leaning forwards. A penetrating ulcer on the posterior wall of the stomach or first part of duodenum quite characteristically gives a boring pain in the upper lumbar region which is related to meals and which may be relieved by antacid therapy. Enlargement of the liver from any cause may give a dull ache felt to the right of the lower dorsal spine, but aches are usually felt also elsewhere in the abdomen and lower chest. The pain of cholecystitis or cholelithiasis may be experienced posteriorly over the liver, or a little higher, in addition to the upper abdomen.

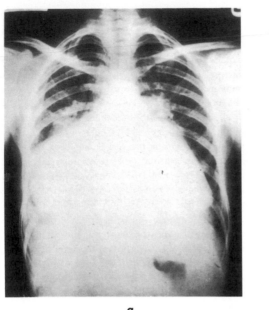
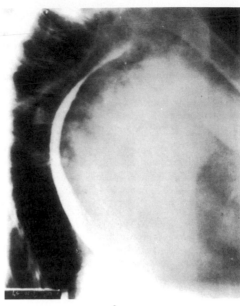

| a | b |

Fig. B.8. *a.* A case of backache due to enormous enlargement of the left atrium in mitral stenosis. The heart shadow to the right of the spine is due to superimposed right and left atrium. *b.* The same case showing scythe-shaped oesophagus from left atrial pressure. (*Dr A. Schott.*)

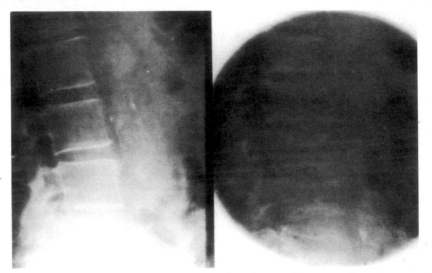

Fig. B.9. Rapid advance of spinal osteoporosis over a 1-year period in a rheumatoid patient on prolonged corticosteroid therapy.

10. Renal and genitourinary causes

Renal and genitourinary causes are not uncommon. Pyelitis and pyelonephritis may cause lower dorsal and lumbar backaches; the diagnosis is usually evident. It is less obvious with renal tumours such as carcinoma, which may remain largely silent since haematuria and the finding of a palpable mass in the flank may only occur late in the course of the disease. Prostatic inflammatory or neoplastic disease may be associated with backache, usually low lumbosacral, but occasionally higher.

Renal papillary nacrosis occurs as a complication of pyelonephritis, particularly in diabetics and particularly if there is urinary obstruction: it is also a feature of analgesic nephropathy.

11. Blood disorders

Severe attacks of backache, often with fever, may occur in sickle-cell disease and haemolytic crises in other disorders. Backache may also be a manifestation of acute or chronic leukaemia.

12. Drugs

Corticosteroids may increase osteoporosis due to other causes and help to precipitate crush factures (*Fig.* B.9). Methysergide taken over long periods to prevent migraine may cause backache from retroperitoneal fibrosis.

13. Normality (*non-disease*)

A chronic backache may be an expression of frustration, unhappiness, or strain and fatigue. The back is a sounding-board for many persons' dissatisfaction with their lives, and no organic or psychiatric disease need be present.

Harold Ellis

Behaviour, antisocial

Antisocial behaviour is behaviour which society regards as disagreeable or unacceptable, and may deem criminal through legislation. The role of the doctor is to determine when such behaviour arises from mental, or less often, physical disorder and to advise upon management or to initiate treatment of the cause.

Society and behaviour

What constitutes antisocial behaviour varies from one society to another, from one section of society to another—and in any society changes over time: attitudes to drinking alcohol and drunkenness exemplify all three aspects. As society's views change so the role of the doctor is altered, either becoming more involved as in the management of therapeutic abortion, or disengaged as in the 'correction' of homosexuality.

The doctor as an agent of societal control occasionally becomes unquestionably corrupted, for instance political objectors being 'treated' in mental hospitals, and doctors getting involved in torture or the disposal of unwanted people such as the 'useless eaters' of Nazi Germany. However the distinction between the proper and improper use of medicine in the interests of society as well as the individual is usually much less apparent. In the 'mad versus bad' debate about criminal behaviour the argument is over treatment/rehabilitation or custody/punishment of offenders and this has its ebbs and flows altering the boundary of medical involvement. Factors like treatment and sentencing fashions and the availability of suitable facilities exert an influence, but the key element is society's attitude to the criminal—mad or bad, gullible or wicked, forgiveness or revenge, and this in turn is determined by issues like the perceived threat of the breakdown of law and order or outrage at a particularly horrible crime.

JUVENILE ANTISOCIAL BEHAVIOUR (DELINQUENCY)

Antisocial behaviour in adolescence is commonplace, and often indicates normal, healthy development. The teenager who never challenges authority nor tests limits may be destined to experience psychological problems in adult life with particular difficulties in relating to others or self-assertion.

In evaluating any adolescent's presentation three special factors must be borne in mind:

i *Maturational tasks of adolescence.* Adolescence is a time of rapid physical, psychological and social change with growing up entailing the resolution of such issues as independence through separation from parents and the formation of identity. This may become expressed in teenage subculture manifestations like clothes, music, causes and behaviour.

ii *Peer group habits and pressure.* A sapling ego requires support hence being acceptable as one of the group or attractive to the opposite sex act as crucial pressures on teenagers. This may provoke youngsters to conform with non-conformity, to indulge in under-age drinking, drug abuse, truanting, promiscuity and offending.

iii *Family circumstances and dynamics.* Within any family teenage years can be times of great stress and unhappiness as parental values and limits are tested; most families survive bruised but unbroken! However where there are other pressures or difficulties operating within the family system the adolescent is often unable to accomplish normal maturational tasks, and resultant problems may be broadly classified as either overcontrolled/unable to separate, or underparented/unable to be checked. The adolescent may be sucked into a pathological role within the family fulfilling a dynamic requirement such as the family's scapegoat, sacrifice, peacekeeper or mascot. Given the limited self-awareness and expression that accompany immaturity, behaviour frequently represents the only available form of self-expression, and such behaviour may therefore be the presenting symptom of a 'sick family'.

Bearing these factors in mind the differential diagnosis of juvenile delinquency can be summarized (*Table* B.2).

Table B.2. Causes of delinquency

Commonest
Normal
Socially determined

Less common
Neurotic
Stress reaction
Conduct disorder (antisocial personality)

Rare
Organic, especially epilepsy
Psychotic, especially schizophrenia
Mental impairment

There are some acts that almost always denote a significant underlying disturbance and the need for professional help. These include fire setting, repeated major or unprovoked acts of violence directed towards other people (may indicate organic or psychotic delinquency), sexual assaults, self-destructive behavior and repeated absconding.

However for most behaviours it is a matter of judgement whether and when to intervene. Two common problems illustrate the principles of assessment to apply.

Glue sniffing usually occurs as a fleeting craze among groups of typically 13–15-year-old males, and no intervention is needed beyond disapproval and education. However the background should be explored more thoroughly if the presentation is unusual, for example if the glue sniffer is a girl or older boy who sniffs repeatedly, secretly or alone, and if the purpose is for psychic escape rather than thrills or showing off.

Not attending school may represent culturally normal behaviour sanctioned by parents, for example in final year pupils without academic aspirations who may have found work already. Truanting can also occur as one facet of a delinquent peer group engaged in activities such as vandalism, joy-riding and drug abuse. This group may disregard all forms of authority and share contempt for an affluent society from which they consider themselves excluded. The pervasive roots of such socially determined delinquency are anchored in factors like poverty, unemployment, poor housing and amenities, endemic criminality, unstable family life and a lack of consistent, effective parenting. Alternatively not attending school can be the behaviour of the inhibited, clinging adolescent who constantly seeks attention from parents and may present repeatedly to the family doctor with a series of inexplicable physical complaints. Although the terms school phobia and school refusal are used, this condition's basis is primarily a fear of separation from parents and home rather than a fear of school. Unlike the truant who is usually found wandering the streets, the school refuser is invariably confined to their home with their parent(s) in attendance. Finally the adolescent who is not going to school may be neither willing truant nor school phobic, but might be obliged to behave in this manner to meet the family's needs. This could involve activities such as looking after a younger sibling while mother is working, caring for an ill or disabled parent, or compensating for an agoraphobic mother by doing the shopping.

Generally, the more acute and unexpected the behaviour or the more closely associated with an important event within the family, then the more likely the problem has remediable elements that would indicate professional intervention.

ADULT ANTISOCIAL BEHAVIOUR

As a rule behaviour conforms increasingly as age advances, and deviation from the norm becomes more likely to be symptomatic of an underlying medical disorder, especially if it arises *de novo*. Apart from alcohol-related convictions in men, rates of all offences fall rapidly in middle age, while criminal behaviour in the elderly is quite unusual. It is a moot point whether the mentally ill and handicapped are more likely to offend than other sections of society; their undoubted overrepresentation in prison populations is probably because they are more likely to be apprehended, less likely to have their case presented well and more likely to be given a custodial sentence when convicted. A mental health policy which curtails bed availability also results in less opportunity to be admitted to hospital for treatment and consequently more likelihood of imprisonment. Certainly the notion that being mentally ill or handicapped is tantamount to being dangerous or disturbed is daft.

Assessment of antisocial behaviour

When assessing an adult who has behaved antisocially the doctor must first establish what has occurred from the patient as well as from eyewitnesses, relatives or involved professionals. Evidence of planning, reasons for behaving in this way and behaviour afterwards require to be considered while how the individual views their behaviour (and themselves) can be important. The standard psychiatric history should be taken, slanted towards issues that might be relevant given the perpetrator's action, age, sex and background. In evaluating the mental state it is helpful to search for specific abnormalities that may have triggered the event—these include disturbances of mood, overactivity, disinhibition, reduced impulse control, impaired judgement and, less often, delusions, hallucinations and clouding of consciousness.

Causes of antisocial behaviour (Table B.3)

There is no action invariably associated with a particular diagnosis, although links between murder-suicide and psychotic depression, matricide and schizophrenia, and infanticide and postnatal depression are well recognized. Other crimes where major mental disorder is likely include arson and attacks upon famous people but of much greater numerical significance is the association between shoplifting and depression (5–10 per cent of cases). The direct and indirect consequences of problem drinking and drug abuse including motoring offences, theft, fraud, child abuse, assault and murder, form the largest area of overlap, and perhaps raise the issues of greatest contention about responsibility for actions, mitigating factors and the purpose of the sentence.

In making an assessment of criminal behaviour in particular, the doctor needs to remain aware that the individual may present an account or express a

Table B.3. Differential diagnosis of antisocial behaviour in adults

Commonest
No medical or psychiatric component

Less common
Stress reaction
Adjustment reaction
Neurological disorders
  Cerebrovascular accident
  Encephalitis
  Neurosyphilis
  AIDS
  Multiple sclerosis
  Subdural haematoma
  Head injury
  Epilepsy
  Dementia
  Delirium
Alcohol
Illicit drugs
  Stimulants
  Opiates
  Hallucinogens
Prescribed drugs
  Benzodiazepines
  Barbiturates
Drug withdrawal
Mental impairment
Major psychiatric disorder
  Schizophrenia
  Paranoid psychosis
  Schizoaffective disorder
  Mania
  Major psychotic depression
Antisocial personality disorder
  (Psychopathy/sociopathy)

Rare
Prescribed drugs
  Tricyclic antidepressants
  Monoamine oxidase inhibitors
  Anticholinergics
  L-tryptophan
  Dopaminergics
  H₂-receptor blockers
  Corticosteroids
  Narcotic analgesics
Psychiatric disorders
  Hysteria
  Malingering
  Post-traumatic stress disorder
Other conditions
  Premenstrual tension syndrome
  Diogenes syndrome
  Hypoglycaemia

ponsibility, remorse and guilt, or feelings of love and pity. They use people (including doctors) for their own ends and wreak havoc in the lives they touch as well as their own. Three consistent features are: (1) an onset before adulthood; (2) *persistent* antisocial behaviour; and (3) a range of problems-features which distinguish antisocial personality disorder from overlapping conditions such as primary alcoholism or drug dependence, stress-related behaviours, and the occasional manic, schizophrenic or epileptic patient who may display superficially similar traits.

As with juvenile delinquency a medical or psychological basis should be suspected when antisocial behaviour represents an acute or unexpected development, and when there has been a recent stress, loss or change in life. Behaviours that sporadically recur in bursts or seem unmotivated, blatant, reckless or otherwise senseless are suspect, while perpetrators who are female, middle-aged or elderly and without a criminal record or family proclivity for crime merit particular consideration. A psychiatric or medical history may be relevant, but current drug treatment and psychiatric or neurological symptoms or abnormal signs are especially important. If there is doubt the individual should be thoroughly assessed and investigated, under Mental Health legislation or by remand from the court if necessary.

When confronted with an antisocial person the doctor's task remains the elucidation and treatment of psychiatric or physical disturbance in his patient—it is up to the legal system to determine charge, guilt and sentence and up to society at large to influence such policy through parliament. It is when the doctor confounds his professional duty with his beliefs (and prejudices) as a member of society that the doctor–patient relationship in these presentations is liable to be subverted by inappropriate moral judgment.

George Masterton

motivation to alter habits which has more to do with avoiding a conviction or stiff sentence than reflecting a genuine wish. This seems particularly likely when problem drinking or drug abuse is involved and contrasts with the depressed shoplifter who frequently accepts or occasionally even welcomes punishment.

Attempts to deceive also characterize psychopathic or sociopathic personality disorder which is now termed dissociated personality. This has proved to be an elusive concept to define and is perhaps best recognized by its core personality traits of guiltlessness and lovelessness. These individuals lack empathy, res-

Bleeding

(*See also* BRUISES, PURPURA)

Excessive haemorrhage may be observed in many different circumstances. In the presence of a normal haemostatic system it may arise secondary to a structural lesion, e.g. peptic ulcer, and if recurrent bleeding is observed predominantly from a single locus a local pathological lesion may be present. More generalized bleeding may arise either due to an isolated coagulation defect, e.g. haemophilia, or platelet disorder, e.g. thrombocytopenia. Many medical disorders, e.g. liver disease, are often associated with a haemorrhagic state which is usually multifactorial in origin. The severity of the haemorrhagic diathesis is usually proportional to the severity of the underlying disorder.

The maintenance of blood within the vascular system depends upon the integrity of the coagulation mechanism, the presence of a reasonable number of functional platelets as well as endothelial-lined vessels capable of constriction when severed.

Platelets are responsible for controlling the initial onset of haemorrhage by adhering to subendothelial components, e.g. collagen and microfibrils, and forming a plug in the severed vessel. After release from bone marrow megakaryocytes platelets circulate for 7–10 days. They have a complex structure which is adapted to responding rapidly to breaches in vascular integrity. In addition to cell surface receptors for various activated components of the coagulation cascade, e.g. thrombin, they possess delta granules which contain vasoactive amines e.g. ATP and 5-HT, as well as alpha granules containing proteins which are components of the haemostatic system, e.g. vWF and factor V. Failure of either platelet function or the presence of thrombocytopenia may result in characteristic bleeding e.g. purpura, easy bruising, epistaxis, gastrointestinal haemorrhage or menorrhagia.

The von Willebrand factor is an important plasma protein, secreted by endothelial cells, which promotes adhesion of platelets to damaged vessel walls. It also acts as a carrier protein for factor VIII; hence in von Willebrand's disease the plasma level of factor VIII is often reduced because without its carrier it is unstable and has a reduced plasma half-life. In von Willebrand's disease bleeding is similar to that in individuals with platelet functional disorders, e.g. mucosal haemorrhage, because the von Willebrand factor is essential for the adhesion of platelet to traumatized vessels.

The coagulation cascade consists of a series of proenzymes; each acts initially as an enzyme substrate and after activation itself has enzymic activity and activates a subsequent proenzyme in the cascade (*Fig. B.10*). Although the reactions can take place in plasma the rates of many of the individual steps can be greatly enhanced if they occur on the platelet surface. This procoagulant property of platelets is due to their possession of specific receptors for components of the coagulation cascade.

Conventionally the coagulation system is considered to be composed of two parts, the intrinsic and extrinsic components although recent research has revealed that the system is considerably more complicated than is illustrated in *Fig*. B.10.

Deficiencies in the coagulation system may be either single, e.g. haemophilia, or multiple, e.g. warfarin therapy. Bleeding can occur due to the presence

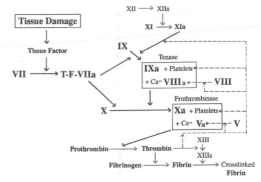

Fig. B.10. The coagulation cascade.

of an inhibitor (usually an IgG antibody) against one or more of the coagulation factors or platelets, e.g. idiopathic thrombocytopenic purpura (ITP).

Bleeding manifestations of isolated deficiencies tend to cause haemarthrosis or muscle haematoma but multiple abnormalities may cause almost any bleeding manifestation. As the primary haemostatic mechanism involving platelets is normal in haemophilia the bleeding often stops immediately after trauma; however haemorrhage may start several hours later because the platelet plug is not consolidated by the deposition of fibrin.

When clinically assessing a patient presenting with possible excessive bleeding it is important to know the following:

1 The duration of symptomatology may indicate whether the possible haemorrhagic predisposition is congenital or acquired.

2 The sites of bleeding may allow assessment of the component of the haemostatic system which is deficient; thrombocytopenia and platelet disorders give rise to purpura and bleeding into mucosal surfaces. A coagulation defect usually results in muscle and joint haemorrhage.

3 Bleeding that starts at the time of trauma, e.g. dental extraction, indicates failure of platelet plug formation due to a platelet disorder or von Willebrand's disease.

4 Haemorrhage which occurs spontaneously is indicative of a more severe bleeding disorder than that which is only provoked by trauma.

5 Dental extractions, tonsillectomy and circumcision are all potent stresses of the haemostatic mechanism. A patient that has had any two of these procedures without loss of excessive blood is unlikely to have a clinically significant bleeding problem.

6 A family history is important as many congenital conditions have a familial predisposition.

7 A drug history is essential because almost all medicines can, by one mechanism or another, predispose to bleeding. Ingestion of warfarin or aspirin are often overlooked. Exposure to toxins or solvents at work or with hobbies may result in hypoplastic anaemia.

8 A general medical history is also essential because many disorders can result in thrombocytopenia or coagulation disturbances, e.g. liver disease or renal failure.

On examination it is important to assess fully the sites of haemorrhage. Examination of the buccal cavity and optic fundi should be carried out in all individuals as superficial bleeding at these sites is indicative of severe platelet dysfunction. It may be necessary to use imaging procedures, e.g. CT scanning or ultrasound to fully document the extent of internal haematoma formation.

Initial screening tests include a complete blood count, examination of a blood film, bleeding time, activated partial thromboplastin time (APTT) (intrinsic system), prothrombin time (extrinsic system), fibrinogen and D-dimers (measure of fibrinolysis).

Observer error

This may be due to instrument design and maintenance, inadequate cuff size, technique of measurement and criteria used for determining systolic and diastolic pressure.

Faulty or inappropriate apparatus

Incorrect readings may be obtained if, in the case of a mercury sphygmomanometer the mercury column does not read zero before inflation. Aneroid sphygmomanometers lose accuracy with time and require regular calibration. Dirt in the escape valve may cause irregular

	Platelet count	Bleeding time	APTT	Prothrombin ratio	Fibrinogen	D-dimer
Thrombocytopenia	↓	↑	N	N	N	N
von Willebrand's disease	N	↑	N or ↑	N	N	N
Haemophilia A or B	N	N	↑	N	N	N
Warfarin/liver disease	N	N	N	↑	N	N
Disseminated intravascular coagulation	↓	↑	↑	↑	↓	↑

If a coagulation deficiency is suspected because of a prolongation of either the APTT or PT it is essential to repeat the test after addition of normal plasma when the test time will become normal. Failure to normalize the clotting time should raise the suspicion of the presence of an inhibitor.

Any patient with thrombocytopenia for which the cause is not immediately and unequivocally apparent should have a bone marrow aspirate and/or trephine performed. This will allow assessment of megakaryocytic numbers; reduced in conditions of under production of platelets, e.g. hypoplastic anaemia, or increased when there is increased destruction and/or pooling of platelets in the circulation, e.g. splenomegaly. A trephine biopsy is particularly useful, for assessing whether the bone marrow is infiltrated with carcinoma cells.

C. A. Ludlam

Blood pressure, high

An isolated (casual) elevated blood pressure reading can have three possible explanations. These are: (1) An error due to either faulty or inappropriate apparatus or faulty technique (observer error); (2) Temporary elevation of blood pressure at the time of measurement (elevation due to biological variability); (3) Sustained blood pressure elevation in the subject not attributable to environmental stimuli (elevated basal pressure).

deflation and add to inaccuracy of reading. If the mercury column is not vertical, readings will overestimate bloodpressure.

If the rubber bladder contained within the sphygmomanometer cuff is too short, blood pressure will be overestimated as pressure is not fully transmitted to the artery. The bladder should therefore cover at least 80 per cent of the circumference of the arm. A 35-cm bladder is recommended for normal or lean arms and longer bladders (up to 42 cm) are necessary for heavily muscled or obese arms. Too narrow a bladder also leads to overestimation of blood pressure although this causes fewer problems than too short a bladder. The width of the bladder should be at least 40 per cent of the circumference of the arm.

Faulty Technique

The cuff should be inflated to at least 30 mmHg above the point at which the radial pulse disappears. The cuff should then be deflated at a rate of 2–3 mmHg per second over the critical points. The eye should be level with the meniscus otherwise parallax will give rise to erroneous readings. Rapid re-inflation of the cuff or failure to deflate properly before repeating blood pressure measurement may increase the level at which the Korotkoff sounds appear and so overestimate systolic blood pressure level. Rounding up or down to the nearest figure ending in a zero or five (digit preference) may make a small contribution to erroneous readings. Normally readings can be rounded to the nearest even number. Pre-determined threshold for the diagnosis of hypertension or for treatment may also unconsciously influence the observer's record (observer bias). In clinical trial work, observer bias is eliminated by the use of special sphygmomanometers (e.g. the Hawkesley random zero sphygmomanometer or the London School of Hygiene and Tropical Medicine sphygmomanometer). In both cases blood pressure is measured without the observer being aware of the true final value. The arm should be supported at the mid-sternal level. If the arm is held in a dependent position diastolic and systolic blood pressures can be overestimated by up 10 mmHg.

Where the phase of muffling (phase IV Korotkoff sounds) is used for estimating diastolic blood pressure levels, values 5–10 mm higher are obtained than when the point of disappearance of the Korotkoff sounds is used (Phase V Korotkoff). Generally phase V values correlate better with intra-arterial pressures and reproducibility between observers is superior.

Subject (biological) variability

Anxiety, recent physical activity, recent cigarette smoking, cold temperature and physical pain all cause elevation of blood pressure through activation of the autonomic nervous system. The first reading obtained by a doctor is usually higher than subsequent readings either on the same occasion or on later occasions. Thus, significant blood pressure falls have been recorded with the passage of time in placebo-treated patients in clinical trials. These important pressor effects can be minimized by careful explanation of the procedure to the patient beforehand, a comfortable environment, and allowing a 2–3-minute period of rest before blood pressure is measured. Final decision about the presence or absence of hypertension should not normally be made before blood pressure has been measured on three or more occasions unless other evidence such as the presence of significant target organ damage is found or unless very high blood pressure levels are observed. Some patients show a consistent pressor response to the presence of a doctor or to blood pressure recording ('White coat' hypertension). This should be suspected where high blood pressure levels are repeatedly recorded in the absence of any fundal, electrocardiographic or echocardiographic evidence of hypertensive organ damage. It should also be suspected in patients who appear consistently tense or anxious during the measurement procedure. Under these circumstances ambulatory monitoring of blood pressure or self-monitoring at home using an electronic digital device should be used.

Blood pressures should, on the first occasion, always be measured in both arms since minor degrees of inequality are quite common. If there is a reproducible difference of 20 mmHg for systolic blood pressure and 10 mmHg for diastolic blood pressure, simultaneous measurements should be carried out: the higher values should be taken as more representative for clinical management for the patient. The time at which antihypertensive drugs are taken may also influence blood pressure. For patients receiving once daily treatment it is probably best to measure blood pressure just before the patient takes his daily dose.

Raised blood pressure—assessment

In unselected populations blood pressure is distributed as a smooth unimodal curve. There is therefore no natural line of demarcation between normal and abnormal blood pressures in unselected subjects. The incidence of cardiovascular disease (i.e. stroke, ischaemic heart disease and peripheral vascular disease) is related to blood pressure level in a curvilinear fashion with no evidence for a threshold. It is impossible therefore to define hypertension by reference to a value above which a patient is at risk. The level of blood pressure at which drug treatment is indicated also provides uncertain guidance since practice in this respect varies considerably not only from one country to another but between different clinicians in the same country.

There are nevertheless great clinical advantages in selecting an arbitrary criterion. The most commonly used criteria are those of the World Health Organisation (5th Korotkoff phase). These are: (1) *Normal range*: equal to or below 140/90 mmHg; (2) *Hypertensive range*: 160/95 and above; (3) *Borderline or intermittent*: 140–159/90–94 mmHg.

Since both systolic and diastolic blood pressures rise with age (*Fig. B.11*), the apparent prevalence of hypertension will also rise with age. Further, where a single reading is used rather than average reading over several measurements, the apparent prevalence of hypertension will be much higher since blood pressure tends to fall with repeated measurements (*see above*). Thus approximately 40 per cent of untreated middle-aged and elderly men will have a diastolic blood pressure of 90 mmHg or over on single readings, but this figure will fall to 15–20 per cent on repeated measurement.

There is little justification in taking age into account in defining hypertension in the adult population since the risks of high blood pressure at least up to extreme old age (i.e. 80 years and above) are related to absolute blood pressure level. In children, however, the same criteria used to define hypertension in adults clearly cannot be applied. Blood pressure rises rapidly in the first few days of life, slightly more slowly over the next few weeks and then shows little change

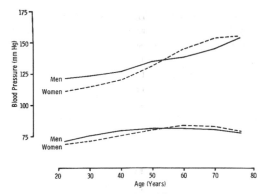

Fig. B.11. Blood pressure levels at different ages in American men and women.

between 6 weeks and 6 years of age when blood pressure begins to rise again slowly. Thus in infancy blood pressures of 80-90/50-60 are observed and in children aged 10, blood pressures of 90-100/60-70. Blood pressure levels which would be acceptable in adults are poorly tolerated by children and the arbitrary values used in adults therefore have to be adjusted and related to age. The American Task Force on Blood Pressure Control in Children has recommended that sustained blood pressure levels (obtained on at least three separate occasions) above the 95th centile for age should be considered abnormal in this context.

The malignant or accelerated phase may occur in hypertension from any cause. Whilst the term malignant hypertension was previously reserved for patients with papilloedema, it is now recognized that, when untreated, the prognosis is just as bad in patients who show hypertensive haemorrhages or exudates (Grade III retinopathy) and it is now customary to term hypertension associated with Grade III or IV retinopathy as malignant. Malignant hypertension is more common in males. It is usually associated with a diastolic blood pressure of 130 mmHg or more and, compared with other hypertensive patients, these patients are relatively young (most usually 40-50 years of age). The clinical picture of malignant hypertension reflects the pathological process, i.e. acute severe vascular damage. Symptoms are much more frequent than with 'benign' essential hypertension. They include blurring of vision, mental impairment, haematuria or haematospermia and clinical features of target organ damage.

Hypertensive haemorrhages in malignant hypertension are of two sorts. Flame-shaped haemorrhages are more superficial and owe their character to constraints imposed by nerve fibres. Dot and blot haemorrhages are deep to the nerve fibres and so are not limited in the same way. Haemorrhages are a sign of recent severe vascular damage and usually disappear after a few weeks of effective blood pressure control. Exudates are of two types. Hard or waxy exudates

represent the end result of fluid leakage into the fibre layers of the retina from damaged vessels often with associated nerve fibre damage. Fluid is reabsorbed leaving a protein lipid residue which is slowly removed by macrophages finally leaving a hyaline deposit which may sometimes persist. Like retinal haemorrhages, hard exudates are forced into a radial spoke-like distribution by the nerve fibres around the macula ('macular star'). Soft exudates or cotton wool patches are quite different aetiologically and ophthalmoscopically. They are usually larger than hard exudates and have a woolly ill-defined edge. They are not true exudates but nerve fibre infarcts caused by hypertensive vascular occlusion. Unlike hard exudates these lesions disappear within a few weeks of establishing adequate hypertensive therapy. Papilloedema is associated with increased pressure within the optic disc secondary to severe vascular damage. Venous distension is followed by increased vascularity of the optic disc which has a pink appearance with blurring of the disc margins and loss of the optic cup. Raising of the optic disc with anterior displacement of the vessels occurs later. Often the surrounding retina shows oedema, small radial haemorrhages and cotton-wool exudates.

Raised blood pressure—causes

ESSENTIAL HYPERTENSION

No identifiable cause can be found in the vast majority of patients who present with sustained blood pressure elevation (essential hypertension). High blood pressure in such individuals is believed to be multifactorial with a substantial contribution from both genetic and environmental factors. Studies of hypertension prevalence in families and in monozygotic and dizygotic twins have confirmed the importance of the genetic factor. Epidemiological studies have also emphasized the importance of other factors which are associated with blood pressure elevation. These include obesity and heavy alcohol intake. In addition, higher blood pressure levels are noted in American (although probably not British) blacks. Extensive investigation of patients with essential hypertension may show a variety of minor changes, e.g. slight elevation in haematocrit, increase in renal vascular resistance, decreased renal plasma flow and increased filtration fraction. All these changes are, however, probably secondary to structural changes induced in the blood vessels by hypertension. One possible clue to the aetiology is provided by evidence for sympathetic nervous systemic activation in young hypertensives, who often have a cardiac output in the upper part of the normal range, increased heart rate and slightly elevated circulating noradrenaline levels. Later in the course of hypertension this evidence for increased nervous system activity disappears and blood pressure is maintained by elevated peripheral resistance alone. There is no evidence that other powerful pressor systems, e.g. the renin–angiotensin system or sodium retention are responsible for blood pressure elevation in essential hypertension.

The vast majority of patients with essential hypertension are diagnosed either at routine examination or incidentally when attending a doctor for other medical problems. The early stages of hypertension are in most cases asymptomatic. Occipital headaches which are throbbing in nature and worse in the morning are described as classical but are only seen in a small minority of patients. In most cases headaches are probably unrelated to hypertension although the frequency of headaches in a hypertension clinic decreases with effective blood pressure control. Epistaxes are more frequent in hypertensive patients but are an unusual manifestation. The other manifestations of hypertension are due to target organ damage. Dyspnoea due to left ventricular failure is a very late manifestation. Besides reflecting increased load against which the left ventricle works, it may also be due to associated ischaemic heart disease which is of course more common in hypertension. Visual disturbances are only seen with advanced (Grade III or Grade IV) retinopathy, although, occasionally, arteriovenous nipping, seen in less severe retinopathy, can cause a branch retinal vein occlusion. Renal impairment is extremely rare in patients who only have Grades I or II retinopathy (so-called benign essential hypertension). Nocturia is, however, frequently seen in hypertension of all grades reflecting a disturbance in the normal circadian rhythm of urine formation. Focal neurological signs may reflect either a cerebrovascular accident (cerebral haemorrhage or thrombosis) or be due to focal oedema (hypertensive encephalopathy). This disorder is characterized by transient focal neurological signs associated with very high blood pressure levels. It is due to systemic blood pressure exceeding the upper autoregulatory range of cerebral blood flow control so that focal hyperaemia and oedema occur. Peripheral vascular disease is due to hypertension-induced atheroma in the large arteries and aorta.

Secondary hypertension

In a minority of patients, high blood pressure can be attributed to a specific disorder or drug. The quoted incidence of secondary hypertension has been as high as 20–30 per cent. However, such figures come from specialist clinics where patients are referred because of the high suspicion of secondary hypertension. The true incidence of secondary hypertension in unselected populations is much lower. Where such populations have been screened intensively for renal or adrenal hypertension, the observed prevalence in patients with elevated blood pressure has been less than 1 per cent. The incidence of iatrogenic hypertension is more difficult to assess since drugs may contribute to hypertension in individuals already predisposed to essential hypertension. It seems likely however that oral contraceptive pill hypertension is more frequent than either renal or adrenal hypertension. Other causes of hypertension are rarer still. A list of the causes of secondary hypertension is given in the *Table* B.4.

RENAL HYPERTENSION

There are three different groups of disorders which cause renal hypertension. These are diseases of the renal artery or its smaller branches (renovascular hypertension), diseases of the renal parenchyma, and renin-secreting tumours which are derived from the cells of the juxtaglomerular apparatus. The last named is an extremely rare cause of hypertension occurring in children or young adults. There are also case reports of hypersecretion of renin by Wilms' tumour, renal carcinoma, bronchial carcinoma and pancreatic adenocarcinoma. Hypertension is caused by the high renin levels, with associated secondary aldosteronism, although structural changes in the resistance vessels help to maintain blood pressure when hypertension has been maintained for prolonged periods. Renovascular and renoparenchymal hypertension are not entirely discrete categories. Thus, renal parenchymal disease such as pyelonephritis or glomerulonephritis gives rise to renal ischaemia and frequently hypersecretion of renin can be demonstrated. The other known factor which plays a role in some patients with bilateral renovascular or renoparenchymal disease (or disease in a single kidney) is sodium retention. This is particularly notable in acute glomerulonephritis and in advanced renal failure where oedema is often associated with hypertension. Unfortunately, from the diagnostic point of view, in many patients with renovascular or renoparenchymal disease there are neither high renin levels nor evidence of sodium retention. In some cases it seems likely that chronic hypertension has given rise to structural changes in the resistance vessels which then maintain blood pressure even after the precipitating factor is no longer in evidence. It also seems likely, however, that the kidney regulates blood pressure in other less well understood ways. For instance, the renal medulla secretes vasodepressor material and this mechanism may be impaired in some forms of renal hypertension.

Because of the multiplicity of renal mechanisms and because secondary changes may maintain blood

Table B.4. Causes of secondary hypertension

Renal
Ischaemia
Atheroma
Fibromuscular dysplasia
Extrinsic pressure by tumour or muscular or fibrous
  bands
Renal emboli
Renal artery thrombosis
Congenital stenosis and other anomalies of renal artery
Intrinsic pressure from tumours or cysts
Parenchymal disease
Glomerulonephritis
  Acute
  Chronic
Chronic pyelonephritis (including hypoplastic kidney)
Polycystic kidneys
Collagen disease
  Polyarteritis nodosa
  Scleroderma
  Systemic lupus erythematosus
Analgesic nephropathy
Hereditary nephritis
Gouty (tophaceous) nephropathy
Diabetes
Irradiation
Amyloidosis
Urinary tract obstruction (unusual)
Renal tuberculosis
Heavy metal poisoning (lead and cadmium)
Renin-secreting tumours (very rarely extra-renal—
  ovary, pancreas, bronchus)

Endocrine
Mineralocorticoid
Primary aldosteronism
Isolated secretion of deoxycorticosterone
                   corticosterone
                   18-hydroxy-deoxycorticosterone
Ovarian dysgenesis and mineralocorticoid excess
Inborn errors of adrenal steroid metabolism
  17α-Hydroxylase deficiency
  11β-Hydroxylase deficiency
  Liddle's syndrome
Glucocorticoid
  Cushing's syndrome
Phaeochromocytoma
Acromegaly
Myxoedema

Other causes
Coarctation
Pregnancy
Pre-eclamptic toxaemia
  Eclampsia
Neurological
Bulbar
  Raised intracranial pressure
Spinal
Iatrogenic

pressure even after the initial mechanism has ceased to act, the diagnosis of renal hypertension is frequently extremely difficult. Clinical and biochemical features are often conspicuous by their absence. Certain clues may however be suggestive. Thus, severe hypertension presenting in a young patient (e.g. below the age of 30) in the absence of a family history of hypertension

makes a renal cause more likely. A renal cause is more likely to be found in patients with malignant hypertension and in patients whose blood pressure rises rapidly. A renal bruit, particularly when it occurs both in diastolic and systolic phases, is more suggestive of a renovascular cause although such bruits are frequently heard in the absence of any lesions of the renal arteries. Generalized oedema suggests acute glomerulonephritis. This may be poststreptococcal or may be a manifestation of systemic disease such as Henoch–Schönlein purpura, Goodpasture's syndrome, polyarteritis nodosa or Wegener's granulomatosis.Clinical evidence of uraemia, perhaps associated with dependent oedema, suggests advanced renal disease, most probably due to end-stage chronic glomerulonephritis or chronic pyelonephritis. It has to be borne in mind, however, that severe hypertension can give rise to hypertensive nephropathy and renal failure so that uraemia can be an effect rather than a cause of hypertension. This is more likely in patients with Grade III or IV retinopathy. Whilst a history of urinary tract infections, perhaps in childhood or many years previously, may suggest chronic pyelonephritis, in the majority of cases of chronic pyelonephritis and hypertension there is no previous history of urinary tract infection. In some patients there may be a history of previous reflux uropathy in childhood. A history of renal disease in the family suggests polycystic kidneys or, less commonly, hereditary nephritis. Relevant features in the history may less commonly indicate such causes as gouty nephropathy, diabetes, irradiation nephritis, amyloidosis, renal tuberculosis or heavy metal poisoning.

In only a minority of cases with renal hypertension will the history and examination yield the diagnosis. Measurement of serum electrolytes, urea and creatinine may indicate the presence of renal disease in a few patients but otherwise is fairly unhelpful. Plasma renin and aldosterone are often normal and may indeed be subnormal where renin secretion has been suppressed by sodium retention. In addition, severe and malignant hypertension often is associated with elevated plasma renin levels even where there is no primary renal disease. If it is felt that it is in the patient's interests for a renal cause to be found (e.g. where hypertension cannot be controlled medically), renal imaging is essential. The first investigation of choice is renal ultrasonography. Intravenous urography will provide the diagnosis in the majority of patients with renal artery stenosis and with renoparenchymal disease although the false negative rate with renal artery stenosis is 20–30 per cent. In renal artery stenosis the affected kidney is usually smaller than that on the opposite side and excretion is delayed, but the dye is more concentrated on the affected side. Because delay in appearance of the dye may be missed with conventional techniques, the first film should be taken 1–2 minutes after injection of the dye (rapid sequence pyelography). Isotope renography has now replaced intravenous urography in most specialist centres. Isotope uptake is measured after administration of an angiotensin converting enzyme inhibitor. This lowers glomerular filtration on the affected side. Definitive diagnosis of the lesion in renovascular hypertension demands renal angiography (*Fig.* B.12). Intravenous digital subtraction angiography is extensively used as an alternative to selective renal angiography. Arteriography may show localized plaques of atheroma or fibromuscular dysplasia. The measurement of renin output in the two renal veins has been advocated as a definitive technique for demonstrating renovascular hypertension which can be corrected by surgery. Whilst some groups have reported nearly 100 per cent accuracy of prediction using this test, in the hands of most groups there is a substantial false positive and false negative outcome from renal vein renin measurements and this technique is now not widely used.

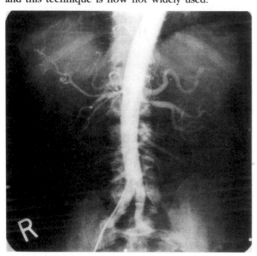

Fig. B.12. Renal angiogram in a patient with a tight left renal artery stenosis. Blood pressure was later restored to normal by venous bypass grafting.

PREGNANCY-INDUCED HYPERTENSION

Pre-eclamptic toxaemia is unique in being a self-limiting form of hypertension. Classical pre-eclamptic toxaemia occurs for the first time during the third trimester of pregnancy and blood pressure falls immediately after delivery. Blood pressure elevation is associated with significant proteinuria and oedema. Classically pre-eclamptic toxaemia is observed during the first pregnancy only and is more common in older women, diabetic patients, multiple pregnancies, and hydatidiform mole. It has to be differentiated from essential hypertension which has been exacerbated by pregnancy. In this case hypertension occurs during the first trimester and becomes progressively worse with successive pregnancies. The difference between the two conditions is often not clear-cut and diagnosis may have to be delayed until the course of blood pressure after gestation can be observed.

ENDOCRINE HYPERTENSION

Primary aldosteronism is associated with either a single adenoma or bilateral hyperplasia of the adrenal cortical zona glomerulosa. The latter may take the form of diffuse hypertrophy or there may be multiple small adenomata (micronodular hyperplasia). It is important to distinguish between a single adenoma and hyperplasia as the treatment of the first is surgical and the second medical. Very rarely the lesion may be carcinomatous and occasional cases have been described with no histological lesion. Primary aldosteronism probably accounts for less than 0·1 per cent of cases of hypertension. The clinical picture may be indistinguishable from essential hypertension. The most characteristic symptom is generalized muscle weakness although cramps, tetany and polyuria occasionally occur. Malignant hypertension is comparatively rare in primary aldosteronism perhaps because the rise in blood pressure is gradual rather than rapid. The biochemical features which suggest primary aldosteronism are a low serum potassium associated with serum sodium which is in the upper part of, or just above, the normal range. Further investigations will demonstrate suppression of plasma renin and elevation of blood and urinary aldosterone. It is important to differentiate primary and secondary aldosteronism (which is frequently seen in severe hypertension or in diuretic treated patients). In secondary aldosteronism the serum sodium is low and plasma renin elevated. Tumours may be visualized by CT scanning although external isotope scanning of the adrenal glands after administration of technetium or iodine-labelled cholesterol is probably the imaging method of choice. If uncertainty still exists, differential adrenal venous sampling should be carried out.

Very rarely, cases have been described with isolated secretion of other mineralocorticoids such as deoxycorticosterone. 11β-Hydroxylase deficiency occurs in children and is associated with virilization (adrenogenital syndrome). 17α-Hydroxylase deficiency is associated with sexual immaturity as the production of sex hormones is impaired. In all these conditions, mineralocorticoid-induced sodium retention and hypokalaemia occur with suppression of plasma renin. Liddle's syndrome is characterized by increased sodium-retaining and potassium-secreting activity by the distal tubular exchange site. Thus, although the biochemical features of primary aldosteronism are present with a low potassium and renin level, aldosterone is also very low. Dexamethasone—suppressible hyperaldosteronism has the biochemical features of primary aldosteronism but the biochemistry is corrected by suppressing ACTH with dexamethasone. It is due to a mutation producing a chimeric gene linking ACTH responsive and aldosterone synthetic activity.

The hypertension of Cushing's syndrome is usually associated with hypersecretion of glucocorticoids although mineralocorticoids such as deoxycorticosterone may also occasionally be elevated. Renin activity is normal or high indicating that sodium retention is not a feature.

Phaeochromocytomata are tumours of sympathetic tissue which produce hypertension by the secretion of catecholamines (adrenaline, noradrenaline and, occasionally, dopamine). They are probably responsible for hypertension in less than 0·1 per cent of hypertensive patients. Although the tumours usually originate in the adrenal medulla (when adrenaline secretion tends to predominate) they may also arise from sympathetic ganglia associated with the abdominal, and rarely thoracic, aorta and the bladder wall. Tumours are frequently multiple and occasionally malignant. Classically, suspicion of phaeochromocytoma is raised on clinical grounds. The patient has short periods of high blood pressure associated with other features of sympathetic activity. These include sweating, flushing and throbbing headache, abdominal or chest pain and weight loss. The anxiety usually associated with such attacks is presumably a manifestation of visceral feedback. Examination during attacks usually shows either tachycardia or bradycardia and severe hypertension. Attacks may be provoked by specific movement, exercise, micturition or by abdominal palpation or at surgery (*Fig.* B.13): indeed occasional fatalities have been described during clinical examination. In addition, some patients have a low standing blood pressure and this may cause symptoms of postural hypotension. Occasionally very high circulating catecholamine levels have been associated with a condition which resembles cardiogenic shock and postmortem focal myocardial lesions have been observed. Glucose tolerance is frequently impaired, basal metabolic rate elevated and free fatty acids raised. In some cases the tumour is associated with neurofibromatosis (von Recklinghausen's disease). A rare combination of endocrine disorders is inherited as an autosomal dominant: this comprises multiple phaeochromocytomas, medullary carcinoma of the thyroid and hyperparathyroidism (Sipple's syndrome or multiple endocrine adenomatosis Type II). Other associations

are tuberose sclerosis and the Sturge–Weber syndrome. Diagnosis is made by finding either unchanged catecholamines or catecholamine metabolites (such as vanillyl mandelic acid or normetadrenaline and metadrenaline) in the urine. Significant numbers of false negatives occur particularly if the urine collection does not coincide with a pressor attack. For this reason, if the diagnosis is seriously being considered, multiple urine collections are necessary. Additionally, plasma catecholamines can be measured while the patient is under observation. Elevated levels associated with tachycardia and raised blood pressure are suggestive. The main differential diagnosis here is anxiety. Administration of clonidine results in a lowering of plasma catecholamine levels in patients with anxiety but has no effect upon the high catecholamine levels observed in phaeochromocytoma. Tumours can be imaged either by CT scanning or by isotope studies using metaiodobenzguanidine (MIBG). If no adrenal tumour is seen, venous sampling for catecholamines at different levels in the inferior and superior vena cava may help to locate an ectopic tumour.

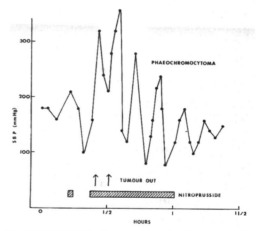

Fig. B.13. Systolic blood pressure fluctuation during manipulation of the tumour at operation in a patient with phaeochromocytoma.

Blood pressure is elevated in about 30 per cent of patients with acromegaly. Growth hormone induces sodium retention which may play a role; consistent with this view is the observation that plasma renin is often suppressed in acromegalic patients. There is also an association between adrenal adenomata and acromegaly which may be relevant in some patients.

High blood pressure is approximately twice as common in hypothyroid patients as in the general population. In most cases blood pressure falls when thyroid deficiency is corrected. Hypertension cannot be clearly related either to increased renin secretion or to sodium and water retention. It has been suggested that there may be an abnormality in vascular smooth muscle produced by thyroid hormone deficiency.

OTHER CAUSES OF HYPERTENSION

In coarctation of the aorta there is narrowing usually situated distal to the origin of the left subclavian artery at or near the insertion of the ligamentum arteriosum. The so-called infantile type of coarctation in which the ductus is patent is irrelevant to hypertension. Uncomplicated coarctation may present as mild blood pressure elevation in childhood and occasionally hypertension becomes suddenly more severe. Infants with other cardiac lesions present with congestive failure. The young adult usually presents with asymptomatic hypertension or with the complications of hypertension. Unless there is an associated cardiac lesion, the clinical symptoms are usually indistinguishable from those of essential hypertension beginning at an unusual age, although diminished circulation through the legs may cause cramps. Physical signs which suggest the diagnosis are: raised blood pressure in the arms associated with normal or low blood pressure in the legs (a wide-leg cuff has to be used to determine this), delayed, weak or absent femoral pulses, an ejection systolic murmur heard best posteriorly between the left scapula and the spine, and pulsatile collateral vessels situated around the scapulae and in the posterior intercostal spaces: these are more noticeable on sitting the patient forward. There are usually associated bruits. There may also be an aortic systolic ejection murmur due to a biscuspid aortic valve which is present in 50 per cent of cases. A firm diagnosis can often be made from the chest X-ray. The characteristic double aortic knuckle is made up of the dilated left subclavian artery and poststenotic dilatation of the descending aorta. Another almost pathognomonic sign is notching of the lower borders of the ribs. These are not to be confused with defects of an erosive nature in the superior margins of the ribs seen rarely in poliomyelitis, hyperparathyroidism, rheumatoid arthritis and scleroderma. The diagnosis can finally be confirmed and the extent of the coarctation delineated by aortography.

Neurological disease causes hypertension only very rarely. Raised intracranial pressure probably causes hypertension through brain stem compression and ischaemia activating sympathetic efferent outflow from the vasomotor centre. Transient blood pressure elevation may be seen after head injury, presumably for the same reason. Vascular disease, brain stem encephalitis and poliomyelitis also occasionally produce hypertension through involvement of the brain stem centre.

Lesions of the upper part of the spinal cord may cause severe hypertension through interference with cardiovascular reflexes. Such hypertension may be paroxysmal, as a result of an acute pressor response to stimulation of viscera such as the bladder or rectum.

Surgical destruction of the nerves supplying both carotid sinuses gives rise to temporary hypertension, although it has been claimed that chronic hypertension can be produced. Variability of blood pressure is certainly increased by this manoeuvre, however, and so, unless resting pressures are measured, an erroneous impression of the blood pressure may be obtained. Peripheral neuropathy has been reported as causing hypertension and this has been attributed to interruption of pathways through the vagus and glossopharyngeal nerves.

In addition to the contraceptive pill and adrenal steroids, certain drugs can either cause hypertension or exacerbate pre-existing hypertension. Non-steroidal anti-inflammatory drugs raise blood pressure probably through inhibition of renal prostaglandin synthesis, which plays a role in the regulation of sodium and water output. Usually the degree of blood pressure elevation is mild but administration of non-steroidal anti-inflammatory drugs may cause loss of blood pressure control in patients on antihypertensive therapy. Severe paroxysmal hypertension is produced by the combination of monoamine-oxidase inhibitors (e.g. phenelzine and tranylcypromine) and tyramine-containing foods of which mature cheese is the most important. The combination of amphetamine and monoamine oxidase inhibitors has the same effect. Clinically the resulting syndrome resembles that observed in phaeochromocytoma. Sympathomimetic amines (e.g. amphetamine, ephedrine, metaraminol and other synthetic agents) are often used as nasal decongestants and may cause significant hypertension. Liquorice and carbenoxolone raise blood pressure through inducing a syndrome which resembles primary aldosteronism with a hypokalaemic alkalosis; in addition the patients may be oedematous. Although this was once believed to be due to a direct mineralocorticoid action, it is now known that these compounds inhibit the steroid dehydrogenase which converts cortisol to cortisone in the kidney and therefore high concentrations of cortisol accumulate and cause sodium retention. Cyclosporin and erythroprotein cause high blood pressure by mechanisms which have not been elucidated. Withdrawal of the centrally acting antihypertensive agent clonidine causes paroxysmal hypertension due to increased efferent sympathetic nerve activity. Clinically the syndrome resembles phaeochromocytoma with sweating and tachycardia. Certain medical preparations contain large amounts of sodium. These include resonium A, paraminosalicylate, sodium carbenicillin and some antacid mixtures. Whilst these have no effect on blood pressure in healthy individuals, hypertension may be caused in patients with renal failure.

Systolic Hypertension

Elevated systolic blood pressure can occur without any elevation of diastolic pressure. The risks of systolic hypertension are just as great as those of diastolic hypertension and indeed in elderly subjects the risks are rather greater. Isolated systolic hypertension is frequent in the elderly and, in healthy populations, the rise in systolic blood pressure with ageing exceeds the rise in diastolic so that pulse pressure naturally widens. The cause of isolated systolic hypertension in the elderly is believed to be loss of elasticity in the aorta and large arteries (the Windkessel vessels). In other situations, a high systolic blood pressure may be associated with a low diastolic blood pressure and increased left ventricular stroke volume. Wide pulse pressure under these circumstances may be due to a large persistent ductus arteriosus, arteriovenous fistulas and high output states, e.g. in hyperthyroidism, pyrexia or Paget's disease. It is also seen in bradycardia from any cause when cardiac output is maintained by increased stroke volume. A wide pulse pressure is also, of course, a feature of aortic regurgitation.

J. D. Swales

Blood pressure, low

The lower half of the blood pressure distribution curve in healthy unselected populations is just as smooth as the upper half with no evidence for a discrete group of hypotensive subjects (*see* BLOOD PRESSURE, HIGH, p. 57). The diagnosis of low blood pressure is therefore just as arbitrary as the diagnosis of high blood pressure. The clinical significance of the diagnosis is, however, quite different. Both high and low blood pressure are most commonly multifactorial i.e. the result of the interaction of genetic and environmental factors (biological variability). High blood pressure carries an increased cardiovascular risk although it is only infrequently due to a specific disease. Low blood pressure, however, when it is attributable only to biological variability carries a lower risk of cardiovascular disease than the population average. Its only clinical significance therefore is when it causes symptoms (*see* FAINTS) or when it is a manifestation of disease. In epidemiological studies it has been associated with increased prevalence of psychoneurotic symptoms. Additionally, in some studies, low diastolic blood pressure in treated hypertensive patients has been associated with an increased risk of cardiac death. Whether this is a result of treatment or not is controversial. The causes of low blood pressure are listed in the *Table B.5*.

Table B.5. Causes of low blood pressure

Cardiac
Disturbances of rate and rhythm
Heart block
Dysrhythmias
Obstruction to flow
Aortic or pulmonary valvular stenosis
Hypertrophic obstructive cardiomyopathy
Atrial myxoma
Primary pulmonary hypertension
Pulmonary embolism
Cardiac tamponade
Mitral and tricuspid stenosis
Cor triatriatum
Tetralogy of Fallot
Eisenmenger's syndrome
Impaired ventricular function
Myocardial infarction
Cardiomegaly

Impaired vasomotor control
Vasovagal syncope
Glossopharyngeal neuralgia
Micturition, deglutition or post-tussive syncope
Baroceptor dysfunction in the elderly
Autonomic degeneration (Diabetes and Shy–Drager
    syndrome)
Carotid sinus hypersensitivity

Impaired venous return
Haemorrhage and dehydration
Muscle wasting and prolonged bed-rest

Metabolic and endocrine
Phaeochromocytoma
Serotonin-secreting tumours
Hyporeninaemic hypoaldosteronism

Drugs
Antihypertensives (particularly centrally acting
    agents, ganglion-blockers, post adrenergic
    ganglion blockers, alpha-blockers and diuretics)
CNS depressants
Quinidine and other cardiac depressant drugs

Low blood pressure can result from underactivity of any of the systems which maintain blood pressure. Since these systems assume particular importance when the subject stands, postural hypotension may be the only manifestation of low blood pressure. It is seen commonly, therefore, when fluid is lost from the gastrointestinal tract as a result of vomiting or diarrhoea, when renal fluid losses occur as in the excessive use of diuretics, Addison's disease or in some patients with chronic pyelonephritis and a sodium-losing tendency. It is observed when fluid is lost as a result of bleeding or burns. In wasting conditions or after prolonged bedrest, venous return to the heart and cardiac output may be reduced as a result of loss of skeletal muscle bulk; a low blood pressure is therefore frequently seen in this situation. Hypotension may result less commonly when cardiac output is reduced as a result of primary cardiac disease or cardiac tamponade, or as a result of obstruction to outflow of blood from the right or left side of the heart from, for example, valvular lesions.

Impairment of autonomic circulatory reflexes is often observed in diabetics and elderly patients with postural hypotension. In the latter case this is probably due to rigidity of the carotid artery and aorta in the region of the baroreceptors. Lesions of central pathways less commonly cause hypotension. Efferent pathways are interfered with particularly by ganglion-blocking drugs and alpha-blocking agents such as prazosin or terozsin. Degeneration of sympathetic pathways occurs in the rare Shy–Drager syndrome. The renin–angiotensin system does not assume great importance in blood pressure control unless patients are fluid depleted, so inhibition of this system does not normally cause a low blood pressure. However, a syndrome of hyporeninaemic, hypoaldosteronism has been described in elderly subjects with postural hypotension.

J. D. Swales

Body image, disorders of

Broadly, disorders of body image can be divided into two categories differentiated by whether or not the problem is the presenting complaint for which the patient seeks correction (*Table* B.6.)

Table B.6. Causes of disorders of body image

A. Not the presenting complaint
Commonest
Anorexia nervosa
Bulimia nervosa
Parietal lobe lesions
Temporal lobe epilepsy
Rare
Migraine
Depersonalisation
Schizophrenia
Drugs
  LSD
  Mescaline

B. The presenting complaint
Common
Dysmorphophobia
  Personality disorder (body dysmorphic disorder)
  Stress reaction
Rare
Transsexualism
Schizophrenia
Monosymptomatic hypochondriacal psychosis
Major depression

Not the presenting complaint

The classical organic presentation is *hemiasomatognosia*, the unilateral misperception of one's own body which is associated with parietal lobe lesions. There is a conscious form of hemiasomatognosia occasionally found in epilepsy or migraine when the disturbance is transient and may be related to lesions in either cerebral lobe. Much more common and spectacular is unconscious hemiasomatognosia when the patient believes and behaves as if half the body no longer exists. This can be subdivided into three forms: (1) anosognosia for left hemiplegia, the denial of the existence of paralysis which is usually confined to the first 2 weeks after onset (right parietal lobe); (2) neglect syndromes, hemi-inattention and spatial neglect which is permanent (either parietal lobe); (3) Gerstmann's syndrome which consists of finger agnosia, acalculia, agraphia and right/left disorientation and is associated with autopagnosia, the failure to localize, recognize or name parts of the body (left parietal lobe).

Macro or microsomatognosia, the experience that parts (or the whole) of the body have enlarged or shrunk is associated most notably with temporal lobe epilepsy, but may also occur in depersonalization, migraine, schizophrenia and LSD or mescaline abuse. Similarly changes in body shape, weight, colour or familiarity may occur in any of these conditions.

Overestimation of body width is a recognized feature of both anorexia nervosa and bulimia nervosa. The patient's overestimation of size does not involve their height or other people's body width. It is an inconsistent finding among patients although characteristic of the group, while its clinical significance lies in the observations that it is a useful indicator of treatment response and the likelihood of relapse. This phenomenon has been reported to a lesser extent in young women without eating disorders and it is postulated that overestimation of body width reflects the degree of personal value attached to body shape and size.

The presenting complaint

In *transsexualism* the individual's dissatisfaction with their body stems from a deeply held belief that they belong to the opposite gender from their physical sexual characteristics. Sex reassignment surgery is sought so that the external sexual characteristics of the desired sex may be acquired. These patients usually live, dress and act as if they belong to their chosen gender, and may 'shop around' for hormonal and surgical correction. Prolonged specialist assessment is always required before proceeding to definitive surgery.

A commoner presenting complaint of body image disorder is *dysmorphophobia*, when the patient asserts to being physically misshapen or defective in some way which cannot be substantiated or is grossly exaggerated upon objective examination—and seeks cosmetic surgery. The most frequent sites for complaint are the nose or breasts, but ears, chin, other facial features and genitals are not uncommon. While recognizing a dysmorphophobic presentation is usually straightforward it can be difficult—and sometimes impossible—

to determine whether the belief is held with delusional conviction or is an overvalued idea. Generally, the more unusual the site and the more bizarre the belief the more likely the presentation is a delusion, occasionally in the setting of major depression but more often as a feature of schizophrenia or monosymptomatic hypochondriacal psychosis. When doubt exists about whether the presentation is delusional, a treatment trial with a neuroleptic has been advocated and reported to be effective, although many patients will baulk at the prospect of this management approach.

The second problem is to determine whether cosmetic surgery will help the patient whose dysmorphophobia is neurotically or personality based. It used to be considered that surgical correction in dysmorphophobic patients was inappropriate as it would neither affect their beliefs nor prevent the psychological problems that many of them subsequently suffered. However it has become apparent that following corrective surgery for minor deficits the level of psychological disturbance falls and the change in appearance is frequently regarded as satisfactory by the patient. This has led to an important distinction developing between patients who have trivial deformities and those who have none, notwithstanding such a delineation can prove difficult to define.

In patients who have minor defects the key is to understand the significance of the problem from the patient's perspective. A middle-aged male doctor is likely to view a small bump on the nose quite differently from a teenage girl, and it is important to acknowledge it is her viewpoint that should be the more relevant. Sometimes minor physical defects can have major cultural, social or financial implications for the patient. Even certain types of personality disorder may be favourable indicators for a surgical course of action, for example the narcissistic individual will attach much greater importance to a minor imperfection.

Patients who should not be operated upon are firstly, of course, those in whom corrective surgery is technically inappropriate either because there is no defect, or the likelihood is that surgery will make matters worse or unchanged, or these is no corrective procedure for the patient's complaint. Secondly, patients who have vague complaints and no specific treatment in mind yet expect surgery both to be performed and to create perfection should not be operated upon; most of these individuals suffer fundamentally from personality disorders—oversensitive, insecure, schizoid, narcissistic and obsessional traits are all described. Thirdly, seeking corrective surgery following a major life event is likely to be a method of coping maladaptively with adjustment and loss; a characteristic presentation is the middle-aged woman wanting mammoplasty

after her successful husband has left her for a younger women. For this group of patients psychiatric intervention can prove particularly helpful, but although psychiatric treatment has been advocated generally for dysmorphophobic patients in whom surgery is considered inappropriate, in practice this is rarely acceptable to the patient, and even when it is, successful interventions are the exception rather than the rule.

George Masterton

Bone, swelling of

A simple emuneration of the more important conditions to be considered will indicate the complexity of this subject:

Subperiosteal haematoma (calcified or ossified)
Callus following fracture
Acute osteomyelitis
Chronic osteomyelitis (including Brodie's abscess)
Tuberculous disease of bone
Syphilitic disease of bone
Typhoid (periostitis)
Rickets (*Fig.* B.14)
Scurvy
Leontiasis ossea
Acromegaly
Generalized fibrocystic disease (von Recklinghausen)
Paget's disease of bone
Osteoma
Chondroma
Localized fibrocystic disease (or solitary bone cyst)
Giant-cell tumour (osteoclastoma)
Aneurysmal bone cyst
Non-osteogenic fibroma
Benign chondroblastoma
Osteosarcoma
Fibrosarcoma
Chondrosarcoma
Angiomas and angiosarcoma
Ewing's tumour
Myeloma
Metastic tumours

Joint conditions such as Charcot's disease and osteoarthritis give rise to swelling of the ends of the bones involved, but these lesions are more properly considered in the discussion on joints.

This list includes diseases which are prevalent at certain ages and it can be simplified for diagnostic purposes by sifting the conditions into approximate age-groups:

From birth until 5 years

Intra-uterine fracture with callus, including those due to osteogenesis imperfecta
Battered baby syndrome
Rickets (*Fig.* B.14)
Scurvy
Congenital syphilitic epiphysitis
Acute osteomyelitis

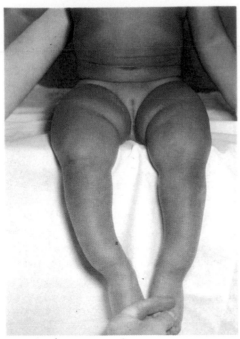 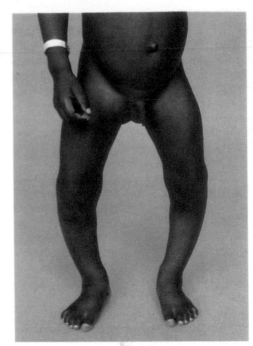

Fig. B.14. Rickets: Note bow legs and swelling in the region of the epiphyses at the knee. (*Courtsey of the Gordon Museum, Guy's Hospital.*)

From 5 until 15 years

Fracture
Calcified subperiosteal haematoma
Acute osteomyelitis
Tuberculous disease
Congenital syphilitic periostitis
Localized fibrocystic disease
Multiple exostoses usually come under observation at this age
Ewing's tumour
Aneurysmal bone cyst
Non-osteogenic fibroma
Benign chondroblastoma
Osteosarcoma

From 15 until 25 years

Fracture
Calcified subperiosteal haematoma
Chronic osteomyelitis
Tuberculous rib and cold abscess
Osteoma, osteochondroma, chondroma
Chondrosarcoma
Angioma
Osteosarcoma
Ewing's tumour

From 25 until 40 years

Fracture
Onset of acromegaly
Tuberculous rib and cold abscess
Acquired syphilitic disease of bone
Osteoclastoma
Fibrosarcoma
Chondrosarcoma
Generalized fibrocystic disease (von Recklinghausen)

From 40 onwards

Fracture
Acquired syphilitic disease of bone
Paget's disease (in the upper years of age-group)
Acromegaly
Myeloma
Metastitic tumours

Although these groups are obviously very elastic there are only a certain number of possibilities at any given age and the field is therefore restricted a little. The difficulties of diagnosis lie not only in distinguishing the varieties of bone swelling, but also in deciding whether the condition is arising from the bone or not, which may be particularly difficult in the case of inflammatory lesions where there is surrounding oedema of soft parts and very little enlargement of the bone itself. If careful palpation fails to reveal alteration in the normal bony contour in a patient where a bone lesion is suspected, the character of any overlying soft-tissue swelling that may be present will sometimes act as a guide. If present it involves all layers, arising from the deep tissues and radiating more or less symmetrically outwards. A central bone lesion will result in swelling of the whole contour of the limb in the area at fault. Pain originating in bone is deep and boring in character and often very intense.

Special investigations

In all cases a radiograph is essential and the differential diagnosis of many of these conditions often resolves itself into a question of interpreting the radiograph. The definite diagnosis of a bone abnormality is now frequently made on isotope bone scanning. In acute osteomyelitis the radiographic evidence of infection is not revealed until the 10th–12th day. An isotope scan, however, will show at the earliest stage an increased bone blood flow and this is indicated by an increased uptake of the isotopic material. Isotopic technetium and gallium are used and both these indicators will show tumours (*Fig*. B.15) and infections in bone.

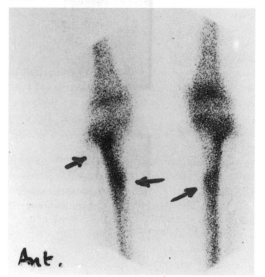

Fig. B.15. Radio-isotope bone scan showing increased uptake in both tibial shafts in a patient with metastic bone disease.

Computerized tomography (CT) is able to show clearly the gross anatomy and the detailed architecture of bone in transverse section. The surrounding soft tissues are also demonstrated (*Fig*. B.16). With the appropriate computer software, these CT sections may be brought up into a three-dimensional reconstruction and this is of great help to the surgeon in planning operative procedures.

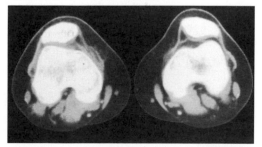

Fig. B.16. CT scan of the knees in an 18-year-old girl with a history of recurrent bilateral subluxation of the patellae.

Magnetic resonance imaging (MRI) will show sections in any plane of altered anatomy of the bone and surrounding soft tissues. Enhanced signals are also seen where there is alteration of blood flow and also of chemistry (*Fig*. B.17). The combination of several of these investigations may be necessary in order to elucidate fully the nature of an obscure bone swelling.

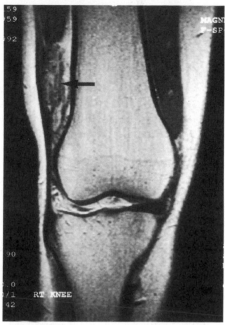

Fig. B.17. Coronal view of magnetic resonance image in a 32-year-old patient, showing cavernous haemangioma in the inferior part of the vastus lateralis muscle (arrowed).

It must be stressed that biopsy of the swelling is the only technique that will give the definitive histological diagnosis.

Bone swellings prevalent in infancy

Fractures rarely occur at the time of birth. In breech deliveries, fractures of the lower limbs may be sustained with the usual signs of fracture—swelling, pain, tenderness and loss of function. In oestogenesis imperfecta, rickets, scurvy and syphilis the bone lesions are multiple and in scurvy and rickets they are symmetrical.

INTRA-UTERINE FRACTURE

This occurs in osteogenesis imperfecta. The disease may be familial and is characterized by blue sclera, multiple fractures which result in limb deformity, broadness of the skull base and poor and retarded dentition. In severe cases the child may be stillborn. If the child lives then deformity may be very severe in the overt case but in the 'tarda' variety fractures will be less problematic and later surgical treatment by means of internal fixation rods will control the bone fragility.

THE BATTERED BABY

The battered baby may have multiple fractures and there is usually evidence of repeated external injury in association. Whole body X-rays are required, for multiple fractures in various healing phases may be seen.

RICKETS (*Fig.* B.14)

Rickets is rarely recognized before the age of 6 months and more usually at a year to 18 months. General backwardness often calls attention to the disease, the child being late in sitting up and in dentition, and making little attempt to walk. Restlessness, fretfulness, sweating of the head and abdominal distension are other features. The bone swellings occur in the region of the epiphyses and are often most marked in the lower end of the radius. The ribs are another situation where the deformity occurs, with resulting 'rickety rosary'. Bossing of the frontal and parietal bones leads to the 'hot-cross bun' head. Bowlegs, sinking in of the ribs at the costochondral junctions, and other bending deformities are due to softening of the bones. The history may reveal that the diet has been inadequate in vitamin D and that there has been a lack of fresh air and sunlight. Radiographic examination shows general osteoporosis with considerable broadening and cupping of the metaphyses, which have a hazy irregular margin as if the bone had melted away. The lower end of the radius is usually the best area to choose to obtain a good radiograph. The diagnosis is not difficult except in the mildest cases.

SCURVY

Scurvy is commonly manifest about the age of 12 months or later. The child is restless and irritable and develops extreme tenderness of the affected bones. These are usually the lower end of the femur and upper end of the tibia, and to touch them or even to approach the infant results in paroxysms of screaming. The bone lesion is one of subperiosteal haemorrhage, to which the swelling is due. The overlying skin may become glossy although signs of inflammation are absent. The gums may become swollen and dusky, and haematuria is an occasional feature. In the radiograph the bones show loss of cancellous structure and extreme thinning of the cortex. The haematoma calcifies, beginning at the deep surface of the periosteum; as soon as this has occurred the haemorrhages can be delineated on the radiograph. Here as in rickets a history of inadequate nutrition (vitamin C deficiency) may be obtained.

CONGENITAL SYPHILITIC EPIPHYSITIS

This appears earlier than rickets or scurvy and can sometimes be demonstrated radiographically as early as the second month. The bones of the knee- and wrist-joints are the commonest to show the characteristic changes, and the pain of the lesion is such that the affected limb is often held quite still (syphilitic pseudo-paralysis). The pseudo-paresis which accompanies syphilitic epiphysitis can be distinguished from that occurring in rickets or scurvy by the younger age of onset in the syphilitic form and by other stigmata of congenital syphilis (*see below*). The radiograph shows broadening and irregularity of the metaphysis which is quite different from rickets in that the outline, although irregular, is dense and sclerosis is predominant, whereas in rickets the outline is hazy and ill defined and osteoporosis is marked. Typically the layer of dense irregular bone capping the metaphysis is bounded on the shaft side by a thin layer appearing translucent in the radiograph, while the cortical region of this part of the bone shows punched-out areas of subperiosteal erosion. Other bone manifestations present in syphilis of infancy include areas of periosteal new-bone formation, syphilitic dactylitis, and also Parrot's nodes. These last are bosses on the bones of the vertex of the skull which results in a 'hot-cross bun' head often of more exaggerated shape than in rickets. Syphilitic dactylitis is discussed with tuberculous dactylitis in the next section. Other signs of syphilis will of course aid the diagnosis. Pemphigus and other skin eruptions, snuffles, condylomas, mucous patches and fissures at the corners of the mouth are all stigmata to be looked for, while in any suspicious case the VDRL reaction will be tested both in the infant and the parents.

NEONATAL SEPTIC ARTHRITIS OF HIP (TOM SMITH'S DISEASE)

The hip of an infant may become infected at the 7th–10th day of life. The infection is blood-borne with the portal of entry usually being an infected umbilical remnant. The diagnosis is frequently made late, as there are no external signs. However, the child becomes ill, feverish and fretful and is in obvious pain. The affected hip becomes immobile and then, after a day or two, there is a marked swelling around the hip and upper femoral region. There are no early radiological signs but later the joint becomes distended and the femoral head may actually dislocate. Early surgical treatment is imperative.

Bone swellings prevalent in childhood and early adolescence: 5–15 years

Fractures and subperiosteal haematoma are considered in the next age group.

ACUTE OSTEOMYELITIS

This occurs in this period in the great majority of cases. The diagnosis does not present itself as a bony swelling of doubtful nature, but as an acute inflammatory condition whose anatomical origin is the matter for decision. A history of sepsis such as boils or tonsillitis is frequently obtained. The lesion is usually found at one end of a long bone and the severe pain with which it is accompanied causes the child to cry when the limb is touched or moved. There is hot tender brawny oedema of the part, with subsequent reddening and glossiness of the skin; the temperature and the leucocyte count and the ESR are high and the patient is very toxic. The differential diagnosis is from cellulitis of soft parts and from an acute joint lesion. Cellulitis does not usually result in such severe toxaemia as does osteomyelitis and there may be a skin lesion such as a septic abrasion over the area of cellulitis to indicate its origin, in which case the diagnosis will be rendered much easier. The swelling of a cellulitis tends to be localized at least in the early stages to one aspect of the limb and its limits can be approximately gauged, whereas the swelling over an osteomyelitis is more generalized and less defined. Furthermore, cellulitis is usually accompanied by lymphangitis and lymphadenitis, whereas osteomyelitis, unless it has extended through the periosteum and invaded the soft tissues around, is not commonly associated with these complications. The diagnosis from a joint lesion such as an acute infective arthritis is made more difficult by the frequent presence of a sympathetic effusion into the joint in cases of oestomyelitis. The maximum swelling in the bone lesion, however, is not over the joint but over the end of the bone, and gentle passive movements of the joint are just possible; in the primary arthritic condition movement is exquisitely painful and the maximum swelling is confined to the joint. Rheumatic fever is differentiated by the unusually rapid pulse-rate as compared with the rise in temperature, by the 'flitting' nature of the pains, and by the response to salicylate therapy.

Osteomyelitis is diagnosed by these clinical features in the early stage together with a positive blood culture. The early X-ray is negative but the gamma scan is intensely positive. A combination antibiotic therapeutic course of high dose is started as soon as the blood culture has been taken. This antibiotic is changed to the appropriate drugs as soon as the culture and sensitivity is available. If the antibiotic regime is not successful in reducing the fever and the acute symptoms within 48 hours, then surgical decompression must be undertaken without further delay.

CHRONIC OSTEOMYELITIS

This may follow acute osteomyelitis, the infection persisting and chronic discharging sinuses developing as a result of sequestra still present. A subacute or chronic abscess may also form as a metastasis in another bone or may arise as a chronic infection from the beginning. A Brodie's abscess, as it is called, is usually found near the end of a long bone and is evidenced by palpable thickening of the bone. Radiographs show a central area of rarefaction with more or less surrounding sclerosis, with a deposition of subperiosteal new bone and sometimes with a sequestrum in the cavity. The diagnosis is chiefly from a tuberculous lesion. This may be impossible without exploration, although sclerosis and subperiosteal new bone are in favour of pyogenic infection. On opening a Brodie's abscess, pus and granulation tissue, usually not exuberant, are found. A tuberculous abscess contains caseous material and the granulations are thick and juicy. If microscopy does not reveal tubercle bacilli in a suspicious case, bacteriological culture is essential. It may not be possible to distinguish radiologically a Brodie's abscess in an older patient from a central gumma. Other signs of syphilis and the serological reactions will give help in this direction.

There are two likely situations for *tuberculosis* to present itself as a bony swelling of doubtful origin. One is the digits, when one or more of the phalanges, metacarpals or metatarsals may be the subject of tuberculous dactylitis; and the other is the ends of the long bones where a focus may remain localized for some time before spreading, as eventually it frequently does, into the joint. Tuberculous dactylitis begins early in life, usually before the age of 5, and results in a spindle-shaped swelling of the affected segment of the digit. Radiography shows central erosion with deposition of subperiosteal new bone with consequent expansion (*Fig.* B.18). The erosion may spread outwards, destroying the new bone laid down, and finally breaking through the skin already red and shiny. At the stage when the original cortex has been destroyed and there is just a shell of the new bone left the appearance in the radiograph is of the shaft distended as if by gas bubbles, to which the term 'spina ventosa' has been applied. Pain is not a marked feature of the disease. The diagnosis is from syphilitic dactylitis. This latter condition occurs at an even earlier age than tuberculosis, usually before 12 months. Other signs of syphilis (skin rashes, snuffles, thick mop of coarse hair, oral fissures, etc.) and positive serological tests of infant and parents will in most cases aid the diagnosis. Locally the distinction is difficult; there is not the same tendency in syphilis to erosion of the bone or the formation of sinuses, and the new bone is usually thicker and denser, but these slight differences are unreliable. Sarcoidosis of the phalanges may produce a similar radiographic appearance and only biopsy will confirm. Enchondromas should not enter into the differential diagnosis as they occur in adult life, rarely in childhood, never in infancy; and the radiograph shows clear-cut central rarefaction without erosion, and expansion without new bone formation. The only other site of bone tuberculosis where periosteal new bone formation is common is in the ribs. This is a disease of adult life and is not usually presented as a bony swelling but as a cystic swelling, the result of abscess formation. Tuberculosis of the ends of long bones results in an ill-defined swelling with slight pain and some evidence of loss of function, for example a persistent slight limp if the lower limb is involved. Clinically some thickening can be detected, but the diagnosis really rests on the radiograph, which shows an area of rarefaction sometimes containing an ill-defined sequestrum and with little or no new bone formation. The differential diagnosis is from a lesion due to non-specific pyogenic organisms and is discussed under *chronic osteomyelitis* above. Tuberculosis of bone is a condition insidious in onset and chronic in progress: there may be slight pyrexia, there is no increase in polymorph leucocytes, but usually a slight lymphocytosis. Abscess formation is common in the late stages; the abscess is of the cold variety and tends to break down through an indolent undermined opening on to the skin. Wasting, reflex guarding and starting pains are marked only when the adjacent joint is invaded.

SPYHILITIC PERIOSITIS

At about the age of 9 or 10 congenital syphilitics are liable to develop local or diffuse deposition of dense periosteal bone. This typically occurs in the tibias, which also undergo some elongation resulting in the well-known sabre shape. Other signs of congenital syphilis appear at this age, including Clutton's joints, interstitial keratitis and Hutchinson's teeth (affecting the permanent incisors), and these, together with signs present since infancy (rhagades, saddle-shaped nose, etc.), and the positive serology will give the diagnosis.

LOCALIZED FIBROCYSTIC DISEASE OR SOLITARY BONE CYST

Commonly occurs between the ages of 10 and 15 and usually arises in the upper ends of the humerus, femur or tibia, the patient most often coming under observation for a pathological fracture. The fracture is notably caused by comparatively slight violence, and the radiograph shows the well-defined outline of a cyst with cortical thinning but no erosion. There are usually trabeculae running across the cyst cavity which may

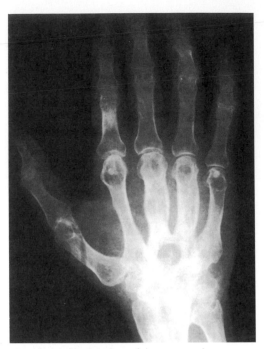

Fig. B.18. Old tuberculosis of the carpus and metacarpus. (*Dr T.H. Hills.*)

lead to confusion with a giant-cell tumour, but the simple cyst occurs at a younger age, does not invade the epiphysis, and does not expand to the same extent as an osteoclastoma and therefore does not perforate the cortex. The clear-cut margins and the absence of erosion or melting away of the bone differentiate the condition from a sarcoma. Following a fracture, healing may occur.

FIBROUS DYSPLASIA (*Figs.* B.19, B.20)

Fibrocystic disease may extend through much of the diaphysis and metaphysis of a long bone in a child of this age. The extension of the fibrous infiltration continues up to maturity and again the commonest presenting feature is a pathological fracture. The mechanical weakness produced by this fibrous lesion may require exploration of this area of bone, curettage of the fibrous area, cancellous bone grafting and sometimes strengthening by internal fixation. This will also allow adequate biopsy material to be taken.

MULTIPLE CARTILAGE-CAPPED EXOSTOSES (DIAPHYSIAL ACLASIA)

A hereditary disease where multiple bony outgrowths may be accompanied by dwarfing, curved and deformed limbs. The radiographs are typical (*Fig.* B.21).

EWING'S TUMOUR (*Fig.* B.22)

This is a sarcoma of small, round progenitor cells in the bone. The characteristic site of this tumour is the diaphysis of a long bone but no area of the skeleton is exempt. The tumour classically metastasizes to bone and it is highly malignant. The clinical presentation is frequently one of an inflamed area of the bone with localized tenderness, swelling, heat and redness. The child may become systemically ill. Radiographs show increased density and width of the cortex with some mottling of the medulla and later some erosion and destruction of bone. The characteristic feature of the radiological diagnosis is, however, the multiple periosteal layers of new bone which are built up around this mid-diaphysial region and the classic radiological appearances are often described as resembling 'onion skins'. As the tumour metastasizes to other bones a full skeletal survey must be undertaken together with an isotope scan. Biopsy is necessary and this is best undertaken through a small puncture with a trocar and cannula and appropriate biopsy forceps. In the past there has been some confusion between this tumour and secondary deposits from a medulloblastoma, but it is now accepted that this is a sarcoma, primarily from bone and it is not a metastasis.

ANEURYSMAL BONE CYSTS

These may occur in any bone but mainly in the axial skeleton. The affected bone is expanded, the cyst thinning and distending the cortex. Pathological fractures may occur through this lesion which frequently requires biopsy for its final diagnosis. The gross appearance of the aneurysmal bone cyst resembles that of the giant-cell tumour in later life and the histological features are very similar including many giant cells. The aneurysmal bone cyst, however, only occurs in the immature skeleton and remains benign.

NON-OSTEOGENIC FIBROMA

This lesion is usually an incidental X-ray finding in the long bones, particularly of the lower limb. However, it may affect any area of the immature skeleton and is seen incidentally on radiographs as a 'bubble' in the cortex. At the time of skeletal maturity these fibromas disappear but their site may be marked by a little sclerosis, sometimes called a 'bone island'. Non-osteogenic fibromas may become large and again may be the site of a pathological fracture.

BENIGN CHONDROBLASTOMA AND OSTEOBLASTOMA

There are rare, benign tumours affecting the epiphysis. The osteoblastoma resembles the osteoid osteoma when it affects the spine and particularly its lamina

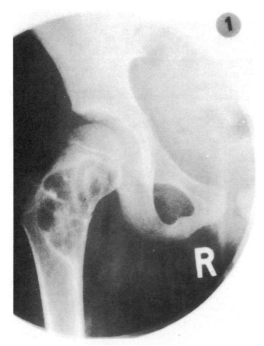

Fig. B.19. Fibrous dysplasia of the femoral neck.

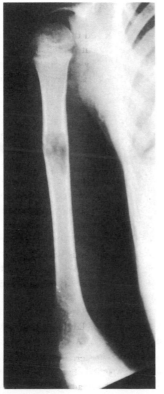

Fig. B.20. Bone cyst in fibrous dysplasia.

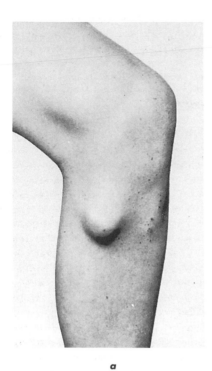

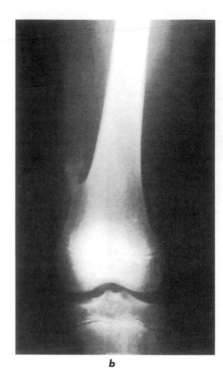

a

b

Fig. B.21. *a.* Cartilage-capped exostosis of the tibia. *b.* Exostosis of the lower end of the femur. (*Dr T.H. Hills.*)

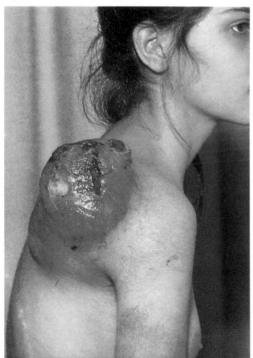

Fig. B.22. Fungating Ewing's tumour of the scapula.

and pedicle. Diagnosis is made on radiological features with a rarefied zone in the epiphysis; final biopsy is essential.

OSTEOSARCOMA

Although the osteosarcoma is the most common of the primary malignant bone tumours, it is still seen as a rare event and it is calculated that in Britain each general practitioner will see one new case in his professional lifetime. The tumour affects the young person between the age of 5 and 25, but it may be seen *de novo* in the elderly person in an area of Paget's disease (Paget's osteosarcoma). It is a highly malignant tumour with early metastases to the lungs. It develops in the metaphysis of the long bone, but again no area of the skeleton is exempt. The most common sites are around the knee where the lower femur and upper tibial metaphyses are involved (*Fig.* B.23). The lower forearm and upper arm are again the most specific sites in the upper limb. The clinical presentation is frequently insidious and the symptoms and signs may be those of an inflammatory condition. The area around the knee joint may become a little swollen, inflamed, red and hot and pain is frequently delayed. Differential diagnosis at this early stage may be that of a cellulitis, an inflammatory arthropathy or even an internal derangement of the knee, and for this reason the diagnosis may be sadly delayed. The radiological appearance, however, is characteristic and is characterized by new bone formation with sclerosis of the metaphysical region and osteogenic bone spreading out in a radial fashion (sun-ray spicules) (*Fig.* B.24). Periosteal new bone at the end of the tumour area may form a small triangle known as 'Codman's triangle'. Radiologically there is a soft tissue mass in continuity and the tumour may produce bone rarefaction in its destructive area.

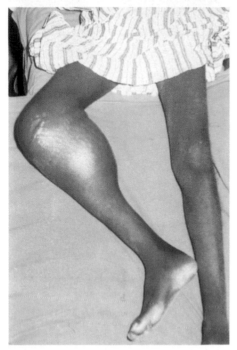

Fig. B.23. Osteosarcoma of the upper tibia.

wound a trocar and cannula is inserted under image intensification X-ray control and appropriate biopsy forceps are inserted to take representative portions of this tumour for histological assessment.

Bone swellings seen from 15 until 25 years

FRACTURE

That *fracture* is a possible diagnosis can usually be suspected from the history. It is uncommon for patients to present themselves with a bony swelling without having had pain dating from definite trauma. Occasionally, however, a fracture has occurred without very much being noticed at the time and as the lack of immobilization may cause excessive formation of callus, the consequent swelling, possibly associated with some continued slight weakness or discomfort, is the symptom for which the patient seeks advice. Likely situations for this to occur are in a metatarsal ('march fracture') and at the upper end the tibia ('recruits' fracture'). Both these fractures are stress fractures and the radiological diagnosis may be delayed. At a later stage (after 3 weeks) a little sclerosis of the cortex may be seen and the only way to make a diagnosis before this time is to undertake an isotope bone scan which clearly shows increased bone blood flow. There is also some possibility of confusing the mass of callus with a bone sarcoma but it is only rarely necessary

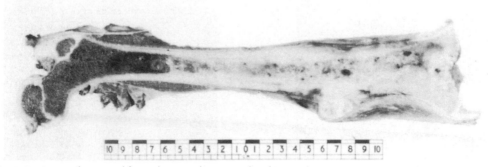

Fig. B.24. Section of amputated femur showing a lower metaphysial osteosarcoma.

A full radiological review of the patient's skeleton should be made together with detailed radiographs of the lungs, to include either tomography or CT scanning. An isotope bone scan of the body is also required to determine 'skip' lesions in the same bone or rarely distant metastases to other bones.

The final diagnosis is by biopsy. Although the material submitted to the pathologist must be adequate, it should be remembered that a puncture over the tumour is ideal and a longer incision may be regretted for this highly malignant sarcoma may rapidly fungate through such a wound. Through a small puncture

to biopsy this area if doubt persists. A spontaneous pathological fracture is more properly considered with the appropriate cause. Radiologically there is usually some abnormal rarefaction around the fracture site and on isotope scanning other multiple deposits may be detected.

A SUBPERIOSTEAL HAEMATOMA

This is formed as the result of a blow. Calcification and subsequent ossification may follow, leaving a small permanent thickening. Such nodes are found not infrequently on the shins of football players. The diagnosis should present no difficulty, the swelling is quite local-ized and the radiograph shows normal dense bone causing a slight increase in the thickness of the cortex.

OSTEOCHONDROMAS (CANCELLOUS EXOSTOSES)

These are found most commonly in the bones forming the knee joint, the upper end of the tibia and the lower end of the femur. The upper ends of the femur and humerus and the small bones of the foot are the other common sites. Typically the outgrowth is pedunculated and projects from the metaphysis over-hanging the shaft away from the epiphysis (*see Fig. B.21*). The base is osseous and is capped by cartilage—the extent of each and the degree of pedunculation being variable. The patient usually seeks advice because he has noticed the swelling, there may be some discom-fort, or some injury may have drawn attention to the outgrowth. The only likely cause for confusion is myositis ossificans, particularly if the lesion is found around the elbow or hip, but differentiation should not be difficult as it can be demonstrated on the radiograph that the bony swelling of traumatic myositis is not continuous with the bone.

OSTEOMAS (IVORY EXOSTOSES)

These are hard sessile growths, densely opaque to X-rays, which occur in the membrane bones, notably the vertex of the skull and the maxillae. On the inner surface of the skull bones they may give rise to signs resembling a cerebral tumour.

PURE CHONDROMAS

These occur in the great majority of cases in the fingers, the only other common sites being the toes and the chondrosternal junctions (*Fig. B.25*). They cause a painless expansion of the bone and the patient again comes for advice for the tumour. Radiographs (*Fig. B.26*) show a clear cut translucent central space with thinned cortex predisposing to pathological frac-ture. Trabeculae traverse the cavity and the general picture somewhat resembles a giant-cell tumour or a bone cyst, but neither of these conditions occurs in the small bones of the hand or foot or in the sternum.

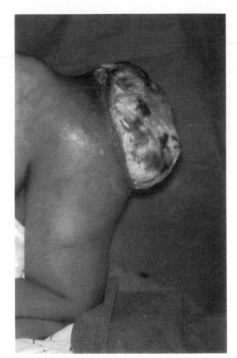

Fig. B.25. Fungating chondrosarcoma of the scapula.

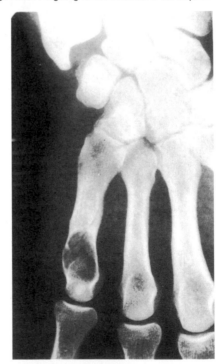

Fig. B.26. Enchondroma of 5th metacarpal. (*Dr John D. Dow.*)

CHONDROSARCOMA

This is the commonest primary malignant tumour of bone. Any age between 20 and 60 may be affected. The pelvis, ribs, sternum, scapula and femur are common sites. A useful aphorism is that "the nearer a cartilaginous tumour is to the axial skeleton and the larger it is, the more likely it is to be malignant". Macroscopically it is a bulky tumour which extends away from the bone to invade adjacent soft tissues (*Fig.* B.25). Blood spread occurs to the lungs, X-rays of the tumour reveal an expanding lesion with irregular mottling and calcification, often with frank destruction of cortical and trabecular bone.

Microscopically, the tumour shows cellular atypical cartilage with irregular cells, many of which have double nuclei. There may be areas of cystic change and calcification or ossification is frequently seen in the stroma.

ANGIOMA

Angioma is a very rare condition, as a rule only diagnosed by microscopy. The skull and vertebrae are occasionally subject to this tumour. Radiography shows a spongy honeycombed appearance at the site of the lesion.

OSTEOID OSTEOMA

This is a rare tumour of the adolescent and young adult. It is considered to be a primary bone tumour arising from osteoblasts, usually in the cortex of a bone. Osteoid is laid down within this cortex and soon comes under substantial pressure, producing severe pain. Although it is considered to be a neoplasm there has been considerable debate over the past few years as to the exact nature of this lesion. The symptoms are those of severe pain both day and night. The night pain is frequently so disturbing as to make the patient haggard and ill and the most effective analgesic is aspirin. The specific relief of painful symptoms with pure aspirin may be considered a diagnostic feature. There is usually an area of tenderness of the bone at the site of this osteoid osteoma but if the lesion is hidden in an inaccesible part of the skeleton, pain may be present over a much wider area.

Radiologically the features are those of a peaked-up area of sclerotic cortical bone with a central translucent nidus. At the early stages in the life of this lesion the minor radiological changes may be missed but an isotope bone scan is again characteristic, showing the localized hot spot. Tomography may assist the localization of the nidus when X-ray changes are present. Simple local excision of the lesion is curative.

Bone swellings from 25 until 40 years

ACROMEGALY is discussed on p. 631. It is a general disease affecting the skeleton symmetrically, particularly the bones of the head, face and hands, which undergo together with the adjacent soft tissues a tremendous hypertrophy. The condition is unlikely to be presented as a doubtful bony swelling.

Leontiasis ossea is of unknown aetiology. Here again there is a generalized overgrowth of the bones of the head and face, but without changes in the soft tissues or in other areas.

ACQUIRED SYPHILITIC DISEASE OF BONE

Most commonly presents in the form of circumscribed gummas, which may appear in the cancellous tissue or subperiosteally. The skull is a common site, the bone being eroded by gummatous infiltration, leaving a worm-eaten defect of serpiginous outline with areas of dense sclerosis and irregular sequestra. The ulceration involves the scalp, and the typical 'wash-leather' base to the ulcer is observed. The sternum, clavicle and ribs are the subject of subperiosteal lesions of bone which tend to be accompanied by dense sclerosis, limiting the outline of the punched-out area of gummatous formation and piling up under the periosteum at the edges of the lesion. Central gummas may appear at the end of a long bone in the form of localized areas of rarefaction. The diagnosis is aided by the presence of other signs of tertiary syphilis, including skin lesions, scarring and perforations of the palate, testicular swelling and loss of sensation, and sometimes the presence of cerebrospinal syphilis or rarely tabes and general paralysis of the insane, and in all cases of bone lesions the serological reaction should be tested. This rule has saved needless amputations, although of course syphilis and malignant disease can be present together, but in the case of a purely syphilitic lesion the administration of anti-syphilitic treatment will cause regression of signs (*Fig.* B.27).

GIANT-CELL TUMOUR OR OSTEOCLASTOMA

This occurs, as do so many bone lesions, most commonly around the knee joint, but a second common site, not so frequently shared with other conditions, is the lower end of the radius (*Fig.* B.28). Pain and tumour formation are the symptoms for which the patient seeks advice, and these are often preceded by a history of injury. The swelling is usually easily palpable and in advanced cases the shell of bone becomes so thin that 'egg-shell cracking' can be elicited. Early perforation of the expanded cortex is common. This is seen on radiographic examination (*Fig.* B.29), the radiograph showing the trabeculated translucent growth so typical of the condition, expanding the cortex asymmetrically at first and later generally. The epiphysis is involved in the process but the articular cartilage is seldom perforated. There is complete absence of new bone formation, which helps to distinguish

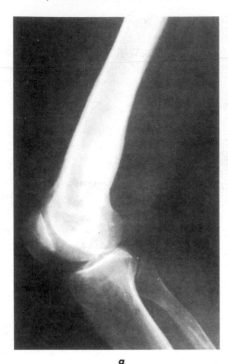

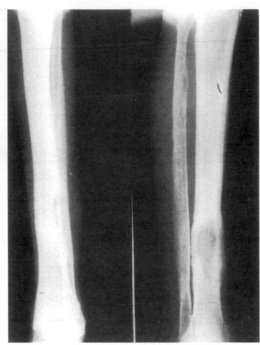

a   *b*

Fig. B.27. *a.* Syphilitic osteitis of the femur, showing sclerosis and periosteal new bone formation. *b.* Gumma of the tibia, showing dense sclerosis around area of rarefaction. (*Dr T.H. Hills.*)

the condition from sarcoma. The characteristic radiograph does not usually suggest confusion with a malignant lesion but rather with simple bone cysts. In the latter case the age of onset is earlier and the bone expansion and destruction much less marked. Microscopy of a giant-cell tumour shows the typical picture of a round celled stroma densely packed with giant cells each with a large number of crowded nuclei. However, careful histology is needed for differentiation from the three other giant-cell tumours.

PERIOSTEAL FIBROSARCOMA

This is characterized by a very large usually asymmetrical clinical swelling often out of all proportion to the radiographic evidence of disease. The lower end of the femur is the site of predilection and the patients are older, often by more than a decade, than those suffering from osteogenic sarcoma. Once more pain and tumour formation are the symptoms and microscopy as well as radiography may be necessary for diagnosis. The earliest sign on a radiograph is a little thin line of bone just where the periosteum begins to be raised; later erosion of the bone gradually takes place from without inwards.

GENERALIZED FIBROCYSTIC DISEASE (VON RECKLINGHAUSEN)

A rare condition sometimes associated with hyperparathyroidism due to adenoma or hypertrophy of these

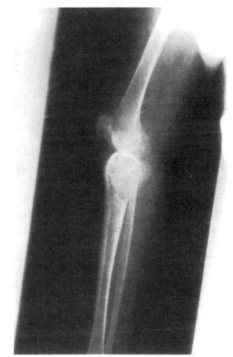

Fig. B.28. Giant-cell tumour of the upper tibia.

glands. There is widespread resorption of the skeleton resulting in softening and bending of the bones. X-ray shows diminished density, areas of fibrocystic forma-

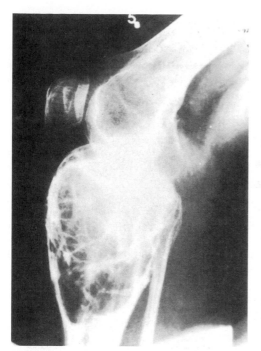

Fig B.29. Osteoclastoma (giant-cell tumour) of the tibia. (*Dr John D. Dow.*)

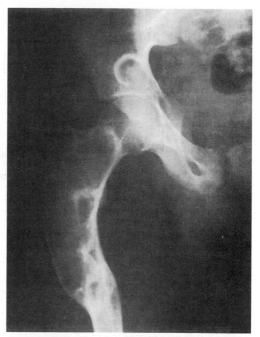

Fig. B.30. Fibrocystic disease of the upper end of the femur and ilium. (*Dr T.H. Hills.*)

tion (*Fig.* B.30), and the presence of bone cysts in varying numbers and sizes. The diagnosis is clinched by the increased serum-calcium and urinary-calcium output, the diminished plasma-phosphorus and the increased plasma-phosphatase (normals—serum calcium 9-11 mg per cent (2·25-2·75 mmol/l), often raised to 12-15 mg (3-3·75 mmol/l); phosphate 3·5 mg per cent (1·15 mmol/l), often lowered to below 2 mg (0·65 mmol/l).

Bone swelling prevalent in advancing years

PAGET'S DISEASE

Paget's disease (osteitis deformans) is a generalized condition occurring in old age and resulting in progressive enlargement of the long bones and the skull. The normal architecture is lost and there is deposition of soft porous bone both inside and outside the cortex, the whole bone becoming very much broadened.The skull may show the most marked increase in size, rendering necessary the wearing of a progressively larger size in hats. The long bones tend to bend and the femurs to become bowed, which, together with the kyphosis which develops, causes the hands to hang at a very low level; the large head is thrust forward and the whole attitude is 'simian'. Radiography show a genarlized thickening of the cortical bone without increased density. The tibia, femur, pelvis,

skull and spine are the bones most commonly affected, occasionally asymmetrically, while in rare cases one bone is affected for a long period before any others. Sarcoma may develop in a bone affected by Paget's disease (*Fig.* B.31).

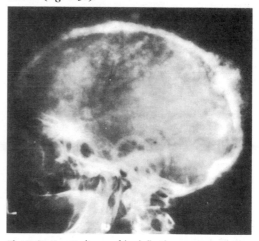

Fig. B.31. Paget's disease of the skull with sarcomatous change.

MULTIPLE MYELOMA

Multiple myeloma is a disease of older life, being commonest in males between the ages of 40 and 60. The outstanding symptom is pain, beginning intermittently and wandering and becoming so severe as to cause the patient to shrink back as the clinician approaches to carry out his examination. A severe

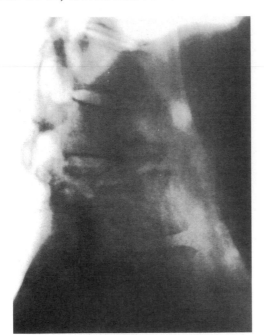

Fig. B.32. Destroyed vertebral bodies with secondary deposits.

rounded, punched-out holes occurring in the marrow, varying in size greatly, but usually between 0·5 and 2·5 cm. In their characteristic form they are unmistakable. Microscopy shows the majority of the cells to be oval with eccentric nuclei, so-called plasma cells. Another diagnostic point is the presence in about 60 per cent of cases of Bence-Jones protein in the urine. A light cloud of protein is precipitated as the urine is heated between the temperatures of 50 (122°F) and 60°C (140°F); as the temperature is raised the cloud goes into solution again, to reappear on cooling. Bence Jones protein is also present in a number of other conditions involving bone marrow, as for example malignant metastases, which is the only condition likely to be confused with multiple myeloma. Electrophoretic study of the serum shows a 'spike' close to the gamma position and this is highly distinctive of multiple myeloma.

METASTATIC TUMOURS

These are liable to occur in the bones when the primary lesion is in the breast, lung, prostate, kidney, thyroid and uterus. The appearance of the secondary tumours

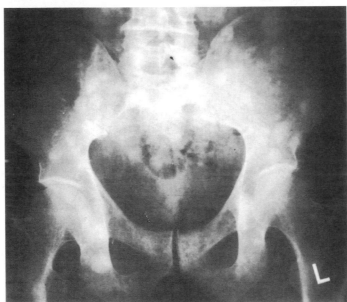

Fig. B.33. Secondary deposits of carcinoma of the prostate, showing discrete osteoblastic areas. (*Dr T.HY. Hills.*)

bout of pain may leave the patient exhausted and collapsed. The ribs and vertebrae and skull are the most frequent sites, followed by the upper end of the femur, the upper end of the humerus and the pelvic bones. The lesions are almost without exception multiple, and therefore in any suspicious case the ribs, spine and skull should all be radiographed. There is frequently a palpable mass, fairly often a pathological fracture. Radiography shows the typical lesions as

varies according to the primary conditions (*Fig.* B.32). The three liable to produce multiple lesions are the breast, lung and prostate; in the former particularly the appearances can simulate those of multiple myeloma, but fortunately the breast being so easily accessible the primary (or an operation scar) is usually readily detectable to suggest the diagnosis. Metastates from a prostatic carcinoma tend to be osteoblastic and the radiograph shows diffuse mottling, usually of the pelvic bones, with general increase in density (*Fig. B.33*).

Paul Aichroth

Borborygmi

'Borborygmi' is the term applied to rumbling noises of varying quality and intensity produced by peristaltic movements of the bowel propelling mixed gaseous and liquid contents.

These sounds, although normally inaudible to the patient or to other persons, and detected only by auscultation by means of a stethoscope, may occasionally be annoyingly obtrusive. They may occur in perfectly normal people, especially when the alimentary canal is relatively empty, for instance when a meal is overdue, and they may occur as a result of nervous air-swallowing. They may be due to excessive ingestion of aperients or may complicate the excessive fermentation within the bowel that may occur in steatorrhoea. In other cases they may be due to the powerful peristaltic waves of a bowel that is hypertrophied and dilated above a slowly developing obstruction of the large bowel; here there will usually be accompanying progressive constipation, colicky abdominal pains and distension. Some people are able to produce a loud sound by forcibly contracting the muscles of the anterior abdominal wall and splashing the fluid content of the stomach. Avery Jones reports one patient who could be heard the whole distance across a large outpatient clinic.

The *carcinoid syndrome* may feature loud borborygmi as well as flushing of the face, trunk and limbs, pulmonary stenosis, cramping abdominal pains and diarrhoea. In the *Peutz-Jeghers* syndrome (adenomatosis of the small intestine) borborygmi are common, the intenstinal polyps causing increased peristalsis and sometimes intussusecption.

The absence of borborygmi, resulting in complete silence in the abdomen on auscultation for several minutes, is seen in adynamic ileus and peritonitis.

Harold Ellis

BOWEL SOUNDS
See BORBORYGMI.

Breast lumps

(*See also* NIPPLE, ABNORMALITIES OF)

Method of examination

The patient should sit stripped to the waist, so that a clear view of both breasts, the thorax, axillae and supraclavicular fossae may be obtained. The surgeon should sit with his eyes level with the nipples. Both breasts should first be looked at as a whole, to see whether they are symmetrical in size, contour and level, and whether the two nipples are in the same site and of the same circumference, prominence and inclination. One breast may always have been smaller or one nipple inverted, but any recent change is highly significant. The patient should then lie on a couch and the breasts be studied in detail for the evidence of local enlargement or shrinking, and for abnormalities such as redness of the skin, dilatation of veins, tumour or ulcer. If no difference is at first noticed, the patient should be asked to raise both arms slowly above the head and bring them down again to the side, since differences previously invisible, particularly dimpling of the skin from attachment of a lump, may come into view as the breast glides over the chest wall. Next the breasts are felt, using first the flat of the hand, passingly systematically over all parts, examining comparable sectors on the two sides simultaneously; afterwards the fingers are used for more detailed examination of any irregularity that may have been discovered or suspected. The axillae should also be palpated carefully for enlarged nodes, particular attention being paid to the inner wall, along the pectoralis minor and to the apex. In cases of suspected cancer the supra and infraclavicular fossae should also be examined for fullness or enlarged nodes, and the chest and liver should be investigated for signs of secondary growth. Examination from behind with the patient sitting may be used to check any abnormalities seen, felt or suspected in the lying position.

ALTERNATIVE POSTURE FOR 'DIFFICULT' OR PENDULOUS BREASTS

When dealing with a woman with large, obese or pendulous breasts, the conventional posture for examination is often unsatisfactory. An alternative posture is to arrange the woman in a semi-recumbent position, rotated obliquely with a pillow behind the scapula of the side under examination and the shoulder fully abducted, with the hand tucked behind the head. This fixes the pectoralis major and allows the breast disc to 'float' over a rigid base (*Fig.* B.34).

Classification

SWELLINGS OF THE WHOLE BREAST
Bilateral
Pregnancy
Lactation
ANDI (abnormalities of normal development and involution)
Hypertrophy
In males from stilboestrol administration.
Acute mastitis
Unilateral
Fibro-adenosis of the newborn
Puberty
Unilateral hypertrophy

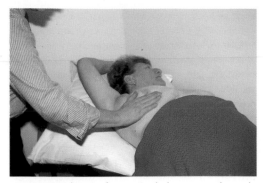

Fig. B.34. Technique of examining the breast in an obese subject.

DISCRETE LUMPS IN BREAST

Benign
Fibro-adenoma
Simple cyst
Galactocele
Lipoma
Plasma cell mastitis
(Rare fat necrosis
   Tuberculous abscess)
   Phylloides tumour

Malignant
Carcinoma
(Rare sarcoma
   Lymphoma)

MULTIPLE SWELLINGS, USUALLY
INVOLVING BOTH BREASTS
ANDI
Multiple cysts

SWELLINGS THAT ARE NOT OF THE BREAST
Retromammary abscess:
   From disease of rib
   Chronic empyema
Chondroma of chest wall
Deformities of the ribs
Mondor's disease

Swelling in pregnancy and lactation

Swelling in these cases is normal, and only liable to cause confusion when the patient is unaware of her condition. Both breasts are enlarged equally and feel tense and nodular. The superficial veins are usually prominent, and on gentle squeezing a few drops of milk are discharged from the nipple. Montgomery's tubercles will be evident.

True hypertrophy

True hypertrophy is rare. The enlargement is of two types; the commoner where multiple fibro-adenomas cause a bilateral enlargement of varying consistency, and the less common consisting in a diffuse lipomatosis of both breasts sometimes attaining prodigious proportions (*Fig.* B.35). The condition is usually bilateral, but may be one-sided, in which case it is very disfiguring.

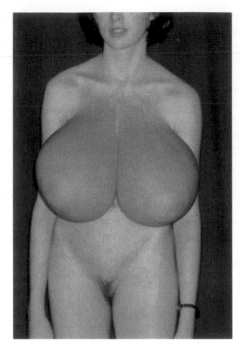

Fig. B.35. Enormous bilateral breast hypertrophy in a teenaged girl.

Unilateral enlargements

These are usually found in the undeveloped breast. In the *newborn* one breast is often enlarged to the limits of its infantile size, and may discharge a little serous fluid from the nipple. The enlargement used to be attributed to the manipulation of midwives, but it is more probably due to an endocrine imbalance consequent on the withdrawal of the maternal hormones in the fetal circulation, and subsides rapidly. In girls at *puberty* one breast may enlarge several months before the other, and may distress a solicitous mother; unless there are obvious signs of an inflammatory change, no notice need be taken of unilateral enlargement of the breast in girls from 10 to 13. Uniform enlargement of one breast also occurs in *men* usually after the age of 40, and nodular plaques may appear in both sexes at puberty as a result of endocrine disturbance.

On no account should the breast disc of an adolescent girl be biopsied, as this may cause failure of either a quadrant or the whole breast to develop and would be a legitimate reason for litigation.

Acute mastitis

Actue mastitis usually occurs during lactation, occasionally during pregnancy, and is most often due to infection with pyogenic organisms which have gained entrance through cracks in the nipple. At the beginning of the illness there is shivering, followed by fever and a feeling of weight and pain in the breast; the pain soon becomes very acute. In the early stages the swelling is limited to one part of the breast, which feels more resistant than normal; the skin is not reddened at first, nor are the lymphatic nodes enlarged. Pressure over the swelling may cause extrusion of a drop of pus from the nipple, and this is distinguished from milk by its viscidity and yellow colour. Later, fluctuation may become evident and, as the inflammation approaches the skin, this becomes red and oedematous, and ultimately an abscess may point and burst through it; at the same time other foci of suppuration form, until the breast may be a bag of pus. The presence of fever and the intense tenderness of one portion of the breast are sufficient to distinguish acute mastitis from physiological engorgement.

It is not uncommon to find a small *areolar abscess*, which represents an infected gland of Montgomery.

Duct Ectasia/Plasma Cell Mastitis (Periductal Mastitis)

There is a common group of diseases which are generally poorly recognized, that cluster together under this heading. Their aetiology is unknown. For example, it is even uncertain whether the inflammatory process comes first, followed by ectasia of the duct, or whether ectatic ducts are the primary phenomena with sloughing duct epithelium responsible for initiating the process of periductal mastitis. Assuming the latter sequence of events, then the cycle of clinical features may develop in the following way. The terminal lactiferous ducts dilate and often become hugely ectatic. As a consequence of this, the epithelial lining loosens and liquifies, causing plugs of cellular debris to fill up the ectatic ducts. The first clinical symptom of this condition is the extrusion of viscous multicoloured discharge from multiple duct orifices on the nipple surface. The milk ducts then become permeable to cellular and lipid contents normally contained within the lumina and these then excite a chemical periductal inflammatory process, which is characterized - by infiltration with plasma cells and foreign body giant cells. At this stage, a hard indurated mass with overlying inflammation may appear at the areolar margin. Commonly this condition resolves spontaneously within a week or two. Less often, the inflammatory mass becomes secondarily infected with anaerobic organisms liquifying to produce a periareolar abscess. This may point at the areolar margin and spontaneously discharge. If the condition is not recognized and treated appropriately, then a pathological communication between the ducts of the nipple and the skin develops, forming a so-called mamillary duct fistula. Over the

years, a series of clinical or subclinical episodes of periductal mastitis produces fibrosis along the ducts, causing them to shrink and pull in the nipple, producing a typical slit-like indrawing at the centre (*Fig.* B.36). Ultimately the condition burns itself out with age. This complex of conditions is most common postmenopausally but, if it occurs in premenopausal women, tends to be more florid, often bilateral, leading to multiple abscesses and fistulae. The mammillary duct fistula should be treated by laying open the fistula track and excising the chronic inflammatory tissue. Recurrent episodes of periductal mastitis and troublesome nipple discharge should be treated by removing surgically the whole of the subareolar system, according to Hadfield's procedure.

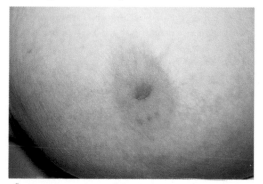

Fig. B.36. Duct ectasia of the nipple.

Tuberculous abscess

Tuberculous abscess is rare, but a certain number of cases of chronic mastitis and chronic abscess are really tuberculous, particularly in developing countries. The disease is insidious, starting as a painless irregular swelling, the periphery of which is hard and the centre soft. Later, the skin becomes reddened, and an abscess forms which may burst and leave a sinus. It differs from an acute abscess in that the duration is much longer, there is little or no pain or fever, and the pus, if examined, reveals no organisms on culture unless there has been secondary infection; direct examination of stained films of the pus may show tubercle bacilli. The facts that the history is a long one, that the swelling or the edges of it are hard, and that the axillary nodes may be enlarged, render this condition liable to be confounded with carcinoma of the ordinary form, or one in which suppuration has occurred.

Local fat necrosis

If this follows a blow on the breast it may give rise to a tumour almost indistinguishable from cancer. It is hard, irregular in outline, and fixed to the skin. Points of distinction are the previous history of severe injury at the exact spot where the swelling lies, the impression given on palpation that the lump is *on* rather than *of* the breast, and the absence of hard nodes in the axilla. Sometimes a period of 2 to 3 weeks observation is justifiable, in which time a traumatic swelling should decrease in size, but if there is any real doubt about its nature it should be excised and submitted to section.

Contrary to popular myth this is a rare condition of the breast. It is usually wise to ignore a history of trauma to the breast and fully investigate the lump with mammography and biopsy.

Galactocele

A cyst containing milk, this is formed by dilatation of one of the larger ducts owing to obstruction. Galactoceles occur only during lactation and very rarely in the later months of pregnancy; they form oval fluctuating swellings lying in the central zone of the breast just outside the areola, and on pressure milk can sometimes be squeezed out of the nipple. Aspiration both confirms the diagnosis and cures the condition.

Single cysts

These usually lie on the deep surface of the breast, so that their outline is obscured and they bear a considerable resemblance to carcinoma. The absence of skin dimpling and of any alteration in the size or shape of the breast as a whole or in the appearance of the nipple, and a sensation of elasticity when the swelling is pressed firmly, suggest the diagnosis.

Innocent tumours

A fibro-adenoma is the only common innocent tumour of the breast. It is an encapsulated tumour, generally single, but sometimes multiple, and varying in size. It is more common (and often multiple) in Afro-Carribean women. It is firm, with the consistency of hard rubber, rounded, or with irregular rounded projections, and clearly outlined. Most characteristic is the ease with which it can be moved under the skin and in the substance of the breast, to neither of which does it appear to have any attachment, hence the term 'breast mouse' which is applied to this lesion. These tumours generally occur between the ages of 18 and 30 and, though they are quite painless, they are so firm that they are usually discovered by the patient. Although a carcinoma of the breast is rare in this age group, it is wise practice to remove all such lumps for urgent microscopic examination. A *lipoma* may occur in the breast as elsewhere, and has the same characters.

However, always beware the 'pseudolipoma' which may be the earliest sign of a small invasive duct cancer, which by infiltrating Cooper's ligaments may extrude fatty lobules forming a mushroom-like umbrella over the primary focus.

Malignant tumours

Malignant tumours of the breast are nearly always primary. Sarcoma is very rare, but *carcinoma* is common and the most important tumour that affects the breast. It is essentially a disease of the female breast, only about 1 per cent of the cases occurring in males. It is common in both married and unmarried women, and may occur at any age after puberty, though the majority are in women between 35 and 60. In advanced cases the disease is obvious (*Fig.* B.37); the tumour is large and hard, attached to and ultimately, if not removed, fungating through the skin and becoming fixed to the chest wall; the axillary nodes are enlarged and hard. Such cases are beyond any but palliative treatment, and the importance of diagnosis lies in the recognition of the early case, where the only sign is a small lump which the patient has probably discovered accidentally. Usually there is no pain and the patient looks and feels perfectly well. The lump may lie in any part of the breast, but typically is intermediate between the nipple and the periphery, and is more commonly in the upper and outer quadrant than in the other three. It can usually be felt with the flat of the hand. These lumps may be stony hard, but any consistency may be met with. Its outline is usually not sharply defined. In the early stage it is freely movable over the pectoral muscles and under the skin, but it is not so movable in the breast substance as is a fibro-adenoma. Very soon bands of fibrous tissue that connect the breast with the skin become involved, and by their contraction prevent free movement of the skin over the swelling, and cause first dimpling when the tumour is displaced, later puckering visible all the time. If the tumour is anywhere near the centre of the breast, the nipple becomes retracted (*Fig.* B.38); a nipple may have been always depressed, but if one previously well formed becomes retracted the sign is of serious import. Fixation to the deep fascia, which usually comes later, can be demonstrated by making the patient press her hands on the iliac crests to fix the pectoralis major, when the involved breast will be found to move less on the muscle than the normal one. Many cancerous tumours, even when extensive infiltration has occurred, cause shrinkage, so that the affected breast may appear smaller than the healthy one, and in the atrophic form it may almost disappear (*Fig.* B.39). In the ordinary form it will be rare to find any discharge from the nipple. After a while the axillary nodes become enlarged and hard. Too much attention should not be given to the absence of palpable nodes; in a fat patient they may be enlarged but impalpable,

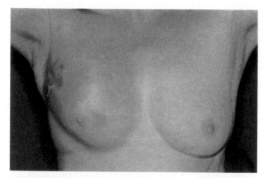

Fig. B.37. Massive carcinoma of the right breast. Note incipient skin ulceration and the elevation and retraction of the nipple.

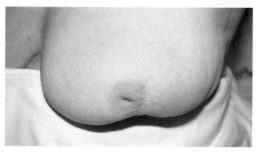

Fig. B.38. Recent nipple inversion in carcinoma of the breast.

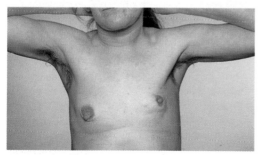

Fig. B.39. Shrinkage of the breast in an advanced scirrhous cancer.

and in any case it is hoped to recgonize cancer before the nodes are involved.

DUCT CARCINOMA IN SITU

The earliest premalignant condition affecting the breast ducts is referred to as duct carcinoma-in-situ (DCIS). Rarely the condition starts within the lobules, where it is referred to as lobular carcinoma-in-situ. In most cases the condition is impalpable and may only be discovered at a chance biopsy of a coincidental benign lump. More commonly these days DCIS may be discovered as a result of a breast screening programme, where the condition shows itself as a cluster of micro-calcifications on mammography. Rarely a large mass of duct carcinoma *in situ* of the comedo variety may present as a clinical mass or, if the *in situ* disease is close to the nipple, may present as a bloody nipple

discharge or Paget's disease (*see* NIPPLE, ABNORMALI-TIES OF).

Sarcoma of the breast is rare. It generally occurs in women under the age of 40. In the early stages it is not easily distinguishable from a fibro-adenoma, particularly one which is enlarging rapidly on account of a cyst or intracycstic growth. It is soft, vascular, grows quickly, at first seems to push the breast aside, but later infiltrates its tissues and eventually fungates through the skin.

PHYLLOIDES TUMOUR

A phylloides tumour is a rare clinical and pathological entity which presents with all the features of a giant fibroadenoma. In the past this condition was referred to as a cystosarcoma phylloides. However, the majority of these lesions are completely benign. The term phylloides means 'leaf-like'. This refers to the slit-like clefts arranged in a 'botanical' manner when viewed on cut section. Rarely the stromal elements of these tumours become hyperplastic and atypical, adopting some of the features of a sarcoma. This tumour is then referred to as a malignant phylloides tumour. They have a tendency to recur locally if not widely excised at the first attempt and, with each recurrence, their malignant potential is more pronounced.

Abnormalities of normal development and involution (ANDI)

When a woman presents at the clinic complaining of a lump in the breast, the first step on clinical examination is to distinguish between a discrete lump and an area of lumpiness or nodularity. Although these lumpy areas in the breast of a young woman are extremely common (perhaps affecting 30 per cent of the female population), there is enormous confusion amongst the medical profession as to the correct terminology. In the past these lumpy areas have been referred to by a series of terms, such as fibrocystic disease, fibroaden-osis, mammary dysplasia, cystic hyperplasia, Schimmel-busch's disease, chronic cystic mastitis, cystic mastopathy, Koenig's disease and masoplasia. What-ever name is given to these lumpy breasts, there are no consistent pathological features which explain the varying textures palpable in different quadrants of the breast. For that reason, a group of clinicians in the University Hospital of Wales headed by Professor Hughes has come up with a rational description of these conditions, which can be grouped together under the catchy acronym ANDI, standing for abnormalities of normal development and involution. These abnorm-alities vary in extreme from normal physiological pro-cesses, which may be considered as benign disorders of little significance, to the other extreme where the pathology can produce particular problems of discomfort or anxiety to the young woman. For example, during the developmental phase of the breast architecture, duct lobular overgrowth can lead to a fibroadenoma, which may cease growing at 2 cm or continue to grow to the extreme of a giant fibroadenoma, reaching sizes of 4 or 5 cm. Normal cyclical changes can produce premenstrual swelling and epithelial hyperplasia. Physiological abnormalities in sensitivity of the duct epithelium to the cyclical hormone changes can lead to cyclical mastalgia, nodularity and intraduct papilloma. Taken to its extreme, the intraduct epithelial hyperplasia can progress to atypia which is known as a risk factor predicting the development of breast cancer. Finally, normal lobular involution may progress to the formation of cysts, sclerosing adenosis and duct ectasia. If a lumpy area of breast tissue is biopsied, almost all these features can be seen under the microscope to one extent or another. Accepting that these conditions are aberrations of normal physiological developments or involution, it can be accepted that in most cases the woman with a lumpy breast or a painful lumpy breast can be reassured. However, if the condition extends beyond the menopause into the cancer age group, clinical diagnosis can be extremely difficult and it is in this area that X-ray mammography is of great value. In younger women, where there is great uncertainty as to the presence of a discrete lump within a diffuse area of nodularity, ultrasound scanning is proving to be a useful complementary investigation.

Multiple cystic disease

Multiple cystic disease of the breast is usually regarded as a variety of ANDI. One breast, sometimes both, becomes filled with cysts, some microscopic, others as large as walnuts, with all intermediate sizes, so that the organ has a bossy appearance. The diagnosis is usually simple but can be confirmed by aspiration of the cysts—a simple outpatient procedure, which is also curative, although several aspirations may sometimes be necessary.

The diagnosis of a single lump in the breast, where cancer must be taken into consideration, may cause considerably difficulty. A lump definite enough to be felt with the flat of the hand and hard enough to resemble cancer is a fibro-adenoma or a tense cyst or a carcinoma. A fibro-adenoma is usually found in women under 30, is less hard than a carcinoma, and is of rounded outline, but its contour may be obscured by surrounding fibro-adenosis. A cyst is usually round and elastic, but if it is deep its outline is obscured, and if it is tense it may feel hard. A carcinoma is undoubtedly solid, and has an ill-defined outline; where these characters are present or where there is the

slightest suggestion of skin dimpling, local flattening of the breast or alteration in the nipple, cancer must be diagnosed.

The diagnosis of cancer at this early stage is intensely important, for only then is the prospect of cure high. If there is the possibility that the lump is a cyst this can easily be confirmed by ultrasound scanning, then aspiration is attempted under local anaesthetic. If clear fluid is obtained and the lump disappears, then we can be certain that the diagnosis is one of simple cyst. If no fluid is obtained, or only a few drops of blood, smears should be made for cytological examination, a core-cut biopsy taken or arrangements must be made for urgent excision and microscopic examination of the specimen. Local resection of a doubtful lump is imperative. It is important that this procedure should be carried out in an institution where, should the lump turn out to be a cancer, there will not be delay of more than a day or two before definitive treatment is carried out.

Swellings pushing the breast forwards

There are often mistaken by the patient for breast tumours. *A retromammary abscess* is most commonly tuberculous, arising in an underlying rib or in a mediastinal abscess that has tracked along a branch of the internal thoracic artery. Sometimes an empyema points beneath the breast, usually in the 5th or 6th intercostal space in the midclavicular line. A *chondroma* is a hard nodular swelling springing form one of the ribs and tilting the breast or pushing it aside. More common is a swelling of one or more of the costal cartilages, especially the 2nd and 3rd, which may be bilateral. This condition, *Tietze's syndrome*, is entirely benign and requires no treatment.

Deformities of the ribs may also cause confusion; the commonest is a prominence of the costochondral junction of the 3rd rib, which may be forked and join two cartilages. The condition is often bilateral, and may be associated with other abnormalities of the ribs or vertebrae.

Role of X-ray mammography and ultrasound scanning

It is now well established that routine X-ray mammography for women over the age of 50 who are otherwise asymptomatic may be of value in preventing premature death from breast cancer by the detection of subclinical cancers (*Fig.* B.40). In addition, no patient with breast cancer should be managed without mammography, as this will describe the extent of the disease within the ipsilateral breast and exclude the presence of synchronous contralateral cancers. Ultrasound scanning may help distinguish a solid from a cystic lump

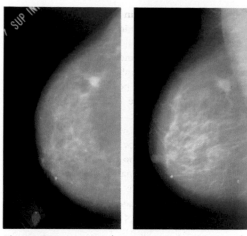

Fig. B.40. Mammogram demonstrating a dense shadow of a carcinoma in the upper outer quadrant of the breast.

and may help define a discrete lump within an area of diffuse nodularity (*see section on* ANDI above).

MONDOR'S DISEASE

Although strictly speaking not a lump in the breast, it is difficult to know how to classify this condition. If a woman presents with characteristic guttering over the surface of the breast, this a pathognomonic sign of Mondor's disease, which is due to spontaneous thrombophlebitis of a superficial vein coursing over the thorax and breast. It has an indurated feel and can be mistaken for the dimpling of an underlying cancer except for its linearity. The author has reported a case where Mondor's disease was the only presenting sign of a cancer, which was detected on mammography. Other such cases have been reported but it is unsure whether this may be coincidental or casual.

Michael Baum

Breast, pain in

Pain in the breast (*mastalgia*) is a common symptom encountered in general surgical practice.

When pain in one breast is the chief symptom the first step is to palpate both breasts with a view to detecting any abnormality which might suggest an early carcinoma. The methods of such examination are described on p. 81. Unfortunately, pain does not occur as an early symptom in carcinoma of the breast, and by the time it is pronounced there may be an obvious stony-hard tumour.

Other causes of pain in the breast are:

Pregnancy
Menstruation (cylical mastalgia)
The onset of puberty
Lactation
Cracked nipple
Inflammation of the nipple
Cyst of the breast
Galactocele
Breast abscess
Submammary abscess
Mastitis, acture mastitis, periductal
Epithelioma of the nipple
Tuberculous disease of the breast
The after-effects of a blow or injury
Anxiety state
Angina
Cervical spondylosis
Herpes zoster

The differential diagnosis of most of these conditions is discussed under the heading of BREAST LUMPS.

Pain in the breast due to intrauterine or to ectopic *pregnancy* will generally be bilateral and will be associated with the other signs of pregnancy. Suggestive indications are the dark brown colour of the nipples, and the broad secondary areola and swollen Montgomery's glands.

The pains in the breast which precede *menstruation* are also bilateral, and their relationship may be indicated by their development synchronously with the first menstruation or their periodic recurrence before each menstrual period. This common condition is best described as pronounced cyclical mastalgia.

Pronounced cylicial mastalgia

Most young women notice some soreness and discomfort in the outer quadrants of their breasts in the week preceding a period and this is a normal consequence of cyclical changes in their hormonal environment. In about one in ten women, this condition is sufficiently pronounced to cause anxiety, distress and insomnia. Characteristically the pain is felt in the upper outer quadrants of both breasts, reaching a crescendo 2 or 3 days before the menses. Immediately after this, 2 weeks of comfort are experienced and then the pain starts building up during the luteal phase of the cycle. The cyclical mastalgia may or may not be associated with lumpiness and the two conditions should be considered separately. In the majority of such cases simple reassurance with advice on mild analgesia is all that is needed. However, in severe cases, it is worth asking the woman to keep a diary and if the pattern is clearly cyclical, then a 6-month course of prolactin inhibitors can be prescribed (bromocriptine, danazol). In addition there is some circumstantial evidence that oil of evening primrose and the withdrawal of caffeine may benefit the condition, although it is notorious for this self-limiting disease to respond remarkably well to suggestion or placebo. By common consent, cyclical mastalgia has nothing to do with water retention and therefore diuretics are not indicated. The underlying pathology is thought to relate to a hypersensitivity of the duct epithelium to biologically active prolactin.

Mammography is only indicated in women over the age of 35 or if pain is non-cyclical and localized to one area of the breast.

Michael Baum

Bruises

Subcutaneous bleeding may present as bruises (ecchymoses) which will vary in colour from dusky red to green, yellow, purple or black depending on the duration of the bruise and the various haemoglobin breakdown products. Superficial crops of small capillary haemorrhages are called petechiae and are best seen in the skin, mucous membranes and retina, although they also occur on the internal organs. Ecchymoses result from the confluence of petechiae or from haemorrhages from vessels larger than capillaries. Multiple bruises characterize bleeding disorders (q.v.) whereas petechaie suggest an abnormality of either the platelets or the vessel wall. However bruising frequently occurs after trauma which may be minimal (or unobserved) in the elderly, and isolated ecchymoses are normal in women and young children. Multiple skin petechiae and ecchymoses are collectively referred to as purpura (q.v.).

C. A. Ludlam

Bullae (blisters)

Bullae or blisters can be diagnostic of important and serious diseases (*see Table* B.7).

Table B.7. Bullae (blisters)

Trauma
   Friction, thermal, caustic
Insect bites
Jelly-fish
Dermatitis artefacta
Bullous impetigo
Lyell's syndrome
Eczema
   Contact dermatitis, pompholyx
Fixed drug eruption
Erythema multiforme
Porphyria cutanea tarda
Epidermolysis bullosa
Pemphigus
Pemphigoid
Dermatitis herpetiformis

Normal skin is a cohesive multilayered tissue remarkably resistant to friction and only neonatal skin blisters easily. In adults localized blistering of the skin occurs following thermal (*Fig.* B.41) or chemical burns and sometimes frost bite. Friction due to ill-fitting footwear may cause blistering of the feet, likewise palmar blisters follow unaccustomed manual toil. Sometimes the bites and stings of insects (*Fig.* B.42) cause bullous reactions and present as discrete large blisters on the lower legs, especially in children. The sting of jelly-fish produces a bullous reaction. In *dermatitis artefacta* bullae may be artificially induced by patients themselves, e.g. with acids, alkalis and phenolics.

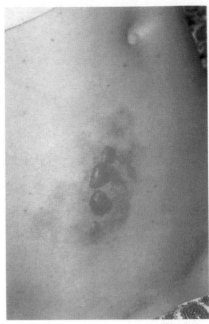

Fig. B.41. Thermal burn (hot-water bottle).

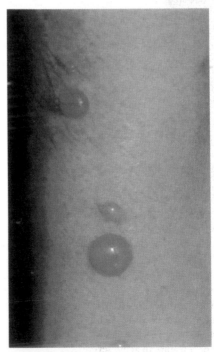

Fig. B.42. Insect bites. (*Westminster Hospital.*)

In *bullous impetigo*, mostly due to staphylococcal infection, the initial lesion is usually a blister appearing on the normal skin and surprisingly containing clear fluid. Blisters occur usually on the face around the mouth, on the hands, elbows and knees and are fragile. Within 24–48 hours they break, leaving crusted weeping erosions. Pus may at this stage accumulate beneath the crusts and typically new lesions appear nearby or spread more distantly.

Toxic epidermal necrolysis (scalded skin syndrome) (*Fig*. B.43) is a serious variant of bullous impetigo, where a certain phage type of *staphylococcus aureus* produces a powerful exotoxin into the circulation. This causes breakdown of cohesiveness within the upper layers of the epidermis, such that with minimal friction large sheets separate off, resembling scalds. Similar but deeper widespread toxic epidermal necrolysis (Lyell's syndrome) can be seen as a drug allergy (e.g. following non-steroidal anti-inflammatory drugs, carbamazepine, sulphonamides and others) or rarely as a graft-versus-host reaction after bone marrow transplantation.

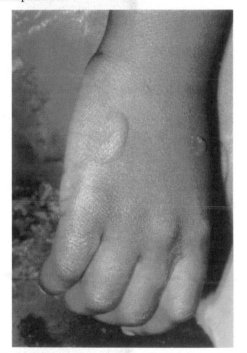

Fig. B.43. Toxic epidermal necrolysis (Lyell's syndrome). (*Westminster Hospital.*)

There is fairly artificial separation between vesicular (*see*. p. 700) and bullous skin diseases—lesions smaller than a pea are usually called vesicles—however, it is not uncommon for such lesions to coalesce. This is particularly the case in severe *eczema*. Thus bullae can be a feature of acute severe eczema of any cause. This is seen on the palms, sides of fingers and soles in *pompholyx* (*Fig*. B.44) and in acute contact dermatitis. For example, in a *plant dermatitis*, streaky blis-

tering on exposed surfaces is highly characteristic. In the USA, poison ivy and poison oak are the chief culprits; in the UK, primulae and umbelliferae such as giant hogweed or cow parsley. Sometimes the vesicles of *herpes zoster* or *herpes simplex* form bullae.

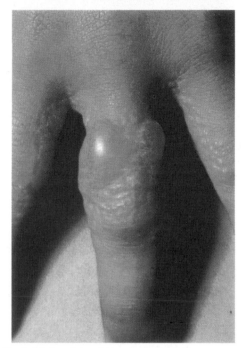

Fig. B.44. Pompholyx. (*Westminster Hospital.*)

The *fixed drug eruption* (*Fig*. B.45) is a dramatic and intriguing condition where blisters on an erythematous base recur in exactly the same location (commonly including the orogenital mucosae) each time affected individuals are exposed to certain medicaments, e.g. phenolphthalein laxatives, codeine, tetracyclines and sulphonamides. It is remarkable how rarely patients associate the recurrent painful blistering with taking the offending medication.

Erythema multiforme (*see Fig*. E.11) is a fairly similar reaction pattern, and likewise can be due to drugs. The characteristic 'target' lesions on the dorsa of hands and feet, over knees and elbows, and sometimes more widely, owe their pattern to two erythematous rings of different shade, surrounding a central blister. In severe cases blistering may be extensive and associated with fever, prostration and occasionally pneumonitis (Stevens–Johnson syndrome). Patients with *porphyria cutanea tarda* form blisters on exposed surfaces, in response both to sun exposure and minor trauma. Blisters heal with pigmentation, scarring and milia formation. Localized hypertrichosis is common. Similar blisters occasionally occur in patients with renal failure on haemodialysis.

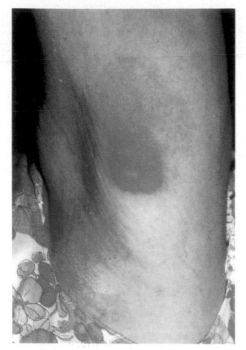

Fig. B.45. Fixed drug eruption. (*Dr Paul August.*)

In *epidermolysis bullosa* there is an inherited lack of cohesion between certain layers of the skin, which blisters in response to minor trauma. In the mildest varieties blistering only occurs during the summer months in response to the friction of walking, but in severe varieties blistering begins *in utero* and infants may be stillborn or rapidly succumb in the neonatal period. Electron microscopic and immunofluorescent examination of skin biopsies (some taken *in utero*) is currently achieving better classification of the many varieties described. The recessively inherited dystrophic varieties cause scarring and early loss of finger- and toenails, and sometimes syndactyly. Blistering and scarring may extend to mucosae of mouth and oesophagus and thus prejudice nutrition. The diagnosis is simple when family history, reaction to trauma and involvement of the extremities are taken into consideration.

The principal blistering skin disorders are pemphigus, pemphigoid and dermatitis herpetiformis. The first two illnesses gained their sinister reputation in the pre-antibiotic era when the extensive blistering was often complicated by fatal cellulitis. More recently the high dose corticosteroids and cytotoxics necessary to suppress blistering can themselves be a cause of morbidity and mortality. *Pemphigus* comprises a group of disorders, most common in semitic peoples, characterized by the formation of blisters *within* the epidermis. Both skin and mucous membranes are affected. *Pemphigus vulgaris* begins in the 3rd and 4th decades

with equal sex incidence. The mucosa of the mouth is affected (*Fig.* B.46) before the eyes, anus and genital tract. Fragile intraepidermal cutaneous blisters occur at any site and quickly become erosions. These are often extensive, slow to heal and become secondarily infected. The uncomfortable oral lesions are the most constant, persisting even when blistering elsewhere is controlled, and making eating difficult. The blistering is thought to be due to a circulating auto-antibody directed against the intercellular substance. This is detectable in the blood by an indirect immunofluorescence technique on a suitable substrate tissue, e.g. primate oesophagus, and the titre of this antibody is related to the severity and progress of blistering. Affected patients also have a higher incidence of organ specific autoimmune diseases, and thymoma. A milder form of pemphigus with positive immunofluorescence may arise in patients under treatment with penicillamine.

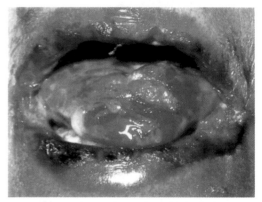

Fig. B.46. Pemphigus vulgaris. (*Dr Richard Staughton.*)

Chronic familial benign pemphigus (Hailey–Hailey disease) is unrelated but has histological similarities. Affected family members show a vulnerability of flexural skin to friction, producing characteristic fissured erosions on the sides of neck, axillae, perineum and oral and vulval lips (*Fig.* B.47). Circulating auto antibodies have not been detected.

Bullous pemphigoid is usually a disease of the over sixties. Bullae 2–5 cm in diameter arise on an erythematous urticated background on the limbs which later becomes generalized: 200–300 blisters can appear within a few days. They are thick roofed and can last many days; initially their constituent fluid is clear but soon becomes cloudy or haemorrhagic. Scratching may lead to extensive erosions which unlike pemphigus heal fairly rapidly. Once the multiple large blisters occur the diagnosis can be easily made. However, widespread pruritus, erythema and urticaria may precede the blistering by several weeks or months, and at this stage diagnosis is difficult. There is also a

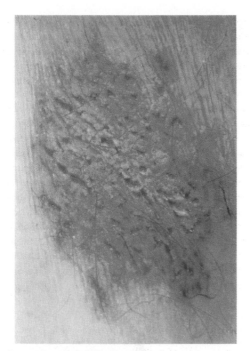

Fig. B.47. Hailey–Hailey disease: familial benign pemphigus. (*St Stephen's Hospital.*)

circulating autoantibody, but in this case directed at the dermo-epidermal junction. The mucosae can be affected with similar tense bullae, but this is a much less constant feature than in pemphigus.

Cicatricial pemphigoid (benign mucous membrane pemphigoid) is a variant where the blister forms just below the dermo-epidermal junction, so that healing takes place with scarring. Blisters appear on mucosae rather than skin, particularly the eyes, frequently causing blindness.

In *dermatitis herpetiformis* blisters are subepidermal and tend to be short-lived, as, being intensely pruritic, they are quickly excoriated. The condition chiefly affects the extensor surfaces of shoulders, buttocks, knees, forehead and scalp, sparing the mucosae. There appears to be a related gastrointestinal gluten hypersensitivity and direct immunofluorescence of frozen skin reveals diagnostic deposits of IgA in the dermis. The condition responds dramatically to the antileprosy drug dapsone, its action being anti-inflammatory rather than antimicrobial.

Richard Staughton

Cataract

A cataract is an opacity within the lens of the eye. Most are associated with ageing but cataract may be due to a wide variety of causes. Cataract may be congenital or acquired and sometimes complicates other eye disease such as iritis, glaucoma and trauma and may be a feature of some systemic disorders, e.g. diabetes mellitus, hypoparathyroidism and Down's syndrome.

Table C.1. Causes of cataract

1. *Senile cataract*
2. *Cataract associated with ocular disease*
   a. Congenital disorders
   b. Acquired disorders
      Uveitis
      Glaucoma
      Neoplasia
      Topical drug therapy—steroids and miotics
      Trauma—mechanical, chemical or radiation
2. *Cataract associated with systemic disease*
   a. Maternal infection
      Rubella
      Cytomegalovirus
      Toxoplasmosis
   b. Chromosomal abnormalities, e.g. Down's syndrome and Turner's syndrome
   c. Hereditary disorders, e.g. Marfan's syndrome
   d. Systemic drugs, e.g. steroids, antimitotics, chlorpromazine
   e. Metabolic disorders, e.g. diabetes mellitus, galactosaemia, mannosidosis, Fabry's disease, Lowes syndrome, Wilson's disease, hypocalcaemia (hypoparathyroidism)
   f. Muscular disorders, e.g. myotonia dystrophica
   g. Skin disorders, e.g. atopic dermatitis, ichthyosis

Most cataracts are not visible to the casual observer until they are advanced and causing profound visual loss (*Fig.* C.1). In its early stages it is best diagnosed by examining the red reflex of the fundus with an ophthalmoscope through a well dilated pupil or by slit-lamp examination. The most common symptom caused by cataract is decreased visual acuity. Other symptoms may also be increasing myopia (this allows the elderly patient to read without glasses—so-called 'second sight'), monocular diplopia, and glare where vision is much worse in conditions of bright illumination.

The rate of progression of cataract is very variable and when the visual loss is interfering significantly with the patient's requirements, surgery is indicated. Lens extraction followed by the insertion of an intra-ocular lens restores vision very successfully. On rare occasions it is not possible to implant a lens and in these cases either contact lenses or cataract spectacles

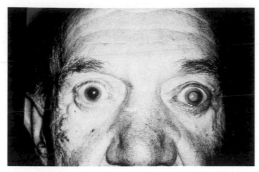

Fig. C.1.

will be prescribed. Cataract surgery has dramatically changed over the last 20 years. Nowadays almost all patients will have an intra-ocular lens implanted after the cataract is removed (*Fig*. C.2). Such lenses are now extremely refined and there is a very low complication rate. Implants have considerable optical advantages over cataract glasses, which are associated with disturbing problems of image magnification, lens aberrations and limited visual field. Contact lenses overcome these optical problems but many elderly patients are unable to tolerate them.

S. T. D. Roxburgh

CEREBROSPINAL FLUID
See APPENDIX.

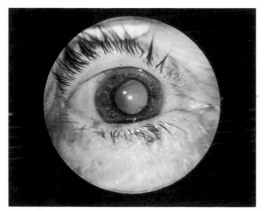

Fig. C.2.

Chest Deformity

The chest wall is an integral part of the 'pump' that ventilates the lungs. Minor chest wall deformities with no significant effect on respiration may cause concern and are relatively common. These are described together with the infrequent but more serious conditions which adversely affect cardiorespiratory function.

The normal configuration of the chest is influenced by age, sex and physical build of the individual. It is determined by the condition of the spine,

ribs and sternum, the overlying muscles and soft tissues, and the underlying lung and pleura. In infants the chest wall is almost circular in cross-section, the ribs lie horizontally and the anteroposterior and transverse thoracic diameters are similar. With growth the chest becomes flattened anteroposteriorly, wider transversely and the ribs adopt an oblique downward sloping position.

The shape of the adult chest is dependent upon body build. In stocky mesomorphic individuals the chest wall tends to be circular with relatively deep posteroanterior and wide transverse diameters. The heart may lie horizontally. The vertical height from sternal notch to the diaphragm is proportionally reduced (*Fig*. C.3). In contrast, the chest in ectomorphic individuals is long in proportion to the overall width, shallow anteroposteriorly and the heart adopts a more vertical position (*Fig*. C.4). Variation in normal body build is not associated with predisposition to respiratory disease, although morbid obesity may cause respiratory failure either directly by influencing chest wall function or indirectly by provoking obstructive sleep apnoea.

Congenital defects

1. RIB ABNORMALITY

a. Bifid ribs are common, particularly in the upper six ribs and may cause confusion if the abnormality is not appreciated on the chest radiograph.

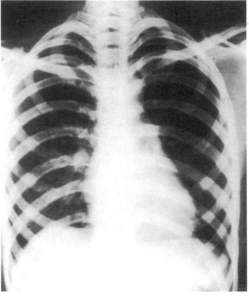

Fig. C.3. Radiograph of normal chest. Patient of stocky build with transversely disposed heart.

b. Cervical ribs, usually arising from the seventh cervical vertebra occur in 0.5 per cent of the popula-

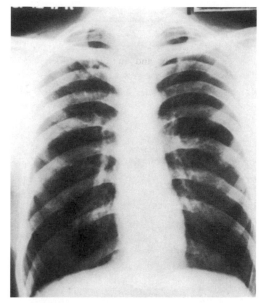

Fig. C.4. Radiograph of normal chest. Patient of tall thin build with vertically disposed heart.

tion, in 80 per cent are bilateral and vary greatly in size and shape. They are seldom a cause of symptoms and often are a chance discovery on either routine chest radiograph or at physical examination when a deep bony mass is discovered in the supraclavicular fossa. Symptoms due to compression are more prevalent in females and commoner on the left side. Neurological symptoms include pain and weakness in the arm with paraesthesiae of the fingers and wasting of the intrinsic muscles of the hand. Vascular symptoms may mimic Raynaud's phenomenon and subclavian artery obstruction or thrombosis may cause distal gangrene.

2. PECTUS CARINATUM OR PIGEON-CHEST DEFORMITY

The sternum is prominent forming an anterior ridge and the ribs inclined forwards causing a greatly increased anteroposterior diameter. The condition can be acquired (asthma), but if congenital is due to premature obliteration of the sternal sutures during growth or to malattachment of the anterior portion of the diaphragm to the posterior portion of the rectus sheath rather than, as normally, to the xiphoid process, with consequent distorting mechanical effects.

3. PECTUS EXCAVATUM OR FUNNEL CHEST DEFORMITY

The costal cartilages are prominent, curve inwards and the body of the sternum is depressed backwards towards the spine from the manubrio-sternal joint downwards with maximum recession at the xiphoid.

In severe cases the lower sternum forms a deep concavity and may almost touch the spine. The heart is displaced to the left side of the chest. Radiographic displacement of the heart to the left and rotational changes of the electrocardiogram may be wrongly interpreted as evidence of heart disease. The electrocardiogram may show persistence of the juvenile pattern with T wave inversion in the right precordial leads, incomplete right bundle branch block and right axis deviation. Because of cardiac rotation there may be P wave inversion and a QR pattern in lead V1. Minor lung function abnormalities occur with reduced total lung, maximum breathing and vital capacities. The condition does not predispose to cardiac or respiratory disease in later life. Surgery is rarely required because of symptoms but is occasionally sought for cosmetic reasons.

4. INCOMPLETE FUSION OF THE STERNUM

An unusual abnormality, apparent at birth, producing the appearance of a split sternum with indrawing of the soft tissue over the central fissure during inspiration and bulging on expiration. This paradoxical respiratory movement is much increased when coughing or in the presence of respiratory obstruction.

5. PARTIAL OR COMPLETE ABSENCE OF THE PECTORAL MUSCLE

A rare congenital abnormality, usually unilateral and mostly involving the lower portion of the pectoralis major. The condition produces no symptoms, but if it is of a severe degree the rib cage is deformed and the anterior chest wall on the affected side is underdeveloped and shrunken because it is not subject to the lateral pull of the pectoral muscle. The chest radiograph may show abnormal transradiancy of the affected side which may give rise to an erroneous impression of pulmonary disease (*Fig.* C.5).

6. THE STRAIGHT BACK SYNDROME

This is an absence of the normal physiological dorsal kyphosis of the spine associated with a reduced anterioposterior diameter of the chest. A mild insignificant restrictive defect of lung function may be present, but cardiac complications are more likely to occur. Examination may reveal a palpable left parasternal systolic impulse and exaggerated splitting of the second heart sound on auscultation, presumably caused by compression of the pulmonary outflow tract and great vessels between the spine and sternum. The ECG may show an RSR pattern in V1.

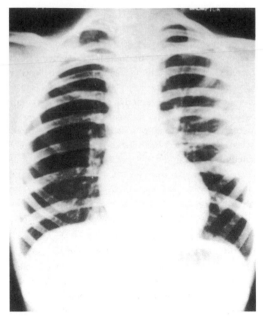

Fig. C.5. Radiograph of chest of a patient with congenital absence of the right pectoral muscles. Note the greater transradiancy of the right side.

Acquired skeletal deformities of the chest

1. SCOLIOSIS

Acquired abnormalities of the vertebral column may directly impair respiration should they interfere with the mechanical action of the ribs and diaphragm or prevent full expansion of the lungs.

Scoliosis is a lateral curvature of the vertebral column, sometimes accompanied by abnormal flexion (kyphoscoliosis) or by rotation of the spine and adjacent viscera. In about 80 per cent of cases the cause is obscure—*idiopathic scoliosis*. In the remainder it is secondary to a variety of conditions (*see Table* C.2).

Scoliosis may be functional (non-structural or postural) or structural. Functional scoliosis is reversible, the curvature being abolished by forward flexion of the spine whereas in structural scoliosis the deformity persists on forward flexion. Idiopathic scoliosis may be seen at any age during growth and at all spinal levels. It occurs most frequently in girls from 10–15 years of age who most commonly present with midthoracic scoliosis to the right. The sideways curvature is usually accompanied by some spinal rotation. The vertebral bodies of the most prominent part of the curve rotate to a greater extent than is indicated by external inspection of the line of spinous processes and this rotation is the cause of the significant rib displacement that so often accompanies apparently moderate spinal scoliosis. The ribs are prominent posteriorly on the convex side of the curvature and bulge anteriorly on the concave side. The shoulder tends to droop on the concave side. If there is a double thoracic spine curve the chest wall deformities are more complex.

The higher the structural curve in the spine the worse the outcome, for the prognosis depends upon the angle of the curvature. This is measured as shown in (*Fig* C.6): lines are drawn parallel to the upper and lower vertebral bodies lying beyond the structural curvature and the angle of curvature measured where the perpendicular lines intersect.

In scoliosis the total lung volume is reduced and, if the deformity has been present since infancy, the alveolar growth may also be deficient. The spectrum of symptoms varies from none in young mild scoliotics to severe disability and chronic respiratory failure in those with high curves greater than 100 degrees leading to chronic hypercapnia, pulmonary hypertension, right heart failure and death.

Neuropathic (poliomyelitis) and myopathic conditions are usually associated with a worse prognosis for a given degree of curvature due to associated muscle weakness causing ventilatory problems.

Table C.2.   Causes of scoliosis

Idiopathic—80 per cent

Secondary scoliosis—20 per cent
Non-structural (postural)
  Compensatory (short leg)
  Sciatica
  Hysterical
  Postural
Structural
  Idiopathic
  Bone disorders
    Congenital hemivertebra
    Osteogenesis imperfecta
    Osteoporosis
    Bone lysis
    Tuberculosis
    Malignancy
    Spondylolisthesis
Neurological disorders
  Syringomyelia
  Friedreich's ataxia
  Neurofibromatosis
  Poliomyelitis
Muscular disorders
  Duchenne's muscular dystrophy
  Faciohumeroscapular dystrophy
Connective tissue disease
  Marfan's syndrome   ⎤ Dominant
  Ehlers–Danlos syndrome   ⎦ inheritance
  Homocystinuria   ⎤ Recessive
  Morquio's syndrome   ⎦ inheritance
Thoracic disorders
  Thoracoplasty
  Fibrothorax (secondary to empyema)
  Lung fibrosis
  Pneumonectomy
  Thoracic burns
  Chest irradiation

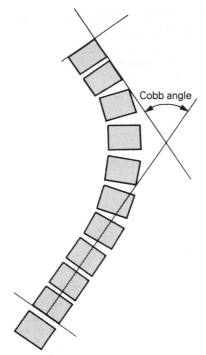

Fig. C.6. The measurement of a thoracic scoliosis by Cobb's angle.

2. ANKYLOSING SPONDYLITIS

This is an inflammatory arthritis, affecting the axial skeleton of young men the great majority of whom are HLA-B27 positive. The condition results in the fusion of costotransverse and vertebral joints with relative fixation of the rib cage in an inspiratory position. Sternomanubrial and sternoclavicular joints may also be affected. Clinical examination of the chest may reveal a dorsal kyphosis and diminished chest expansion with corresponding increase in abdominal expansion. Changes in the relative proportion of diaphragmatic and chest wall movement alter the normal relationship of ventilation to perfusion in the upper lobes. Most of the ventilatory movement is performed by the diaphragm and abdomen. With advanced disease signs of apical fibrosis, consolidation or cavitation may be present. The PA chest radiograph may demonstrate the characteristic bilateral apical cavitating lesions and the lateral radiograph the classical 'bamboo' calcification of the anterior spinal ligaments. The clinical picture is completed if there is an aortic diastolic murmur and cardiac failure due to aortic valve disease.

3. RICKETS (OSTEOMALACIA)

Rickets, either nutritional, due to renal disease or inherited enzyme defects (1-alpha-hydroxlase), may cause important skeletal deformity with disorganiza-tion of the bone growth plate and faulty replacement of calcified cartilage. In active childhood rickets the costochondral junctions enlarge producing the so-called 'rickety rosary'. The soft plastic ribs are readily moulded. The upper ribs tend to be indrawn by inspiratory forces while the lower chest is supported at the costal margins by the underlying abdominal viscera. A depression is produced above the costal margins with a flaring outwards of the costal margin itself. This deformity may remain and is known as Harrison's sulcus.

4. PIGEON-CHEST

This condition may be congenital (rare), due to rickets or most commonly accompanies chronic bronchopulmonary disease in childhood. This is most frequently seen as a skeletal manifestation of severe uncontrolled asthma. It is, to a considerable extent, reversible if the asthma is treated adequately and sufficiently early. It should be a rarity. Pigeon-chest deformity may also occur in bronchiectasis.

5. BARREL CHEST

Barrel chest is the name given to the deep chest, in which the anteroposterior diameter is increased often to equal the transverse diameter, the subcostal angle is abnormally wide and the horizontal position of the ribs is accentuated. This appearance is most constantly related to over-inflation of the lungs and may be observed in acute attacks of asthma and in chronic obstructive pulmonary disease usually associated with irreversible structural emphysema, especially when associated with alpha-1 protease deficiency. Radiologically the lungs are hyperinflated and hypertransradiant, the heart is narrow and lies vertically and the diaphragm adopts a low position.

6. GENERAL EXPANSION OF ONE SIDE OF THE CHEST

General expansion of one side of the chest is unusual. It may occur in children and young adults but is unlikely in older subjects with more rigid chest walls. Clinically detectable expansion of one hemithorax may accompany large rapidly accumulating pleural effusions, large tension pneumothoraces, especially in patients undergoing assisted ventilation, or unilateral obstructive emphysema associated with partial bronchial obstruction causing a check valve effect allowing air to enter the lung segment and preventing its escape, and to over-expansion of giant air-containing cysts in the lung.

7. GENERAL CONTRACTION OF ONE SIDE OF THE CHEST

General contraction of one side of the chest is due to loss of volume of the underlying lung. This may follow lung collapse, lung fibrosis, surgical resection of the lung tissue or pleural thickening preventing inflation of the underlying lung. Pleural thickening may result from chronic empyema (bacterial and tuberculous) and malignant infiltration from adenocarcinoma or mesothelioma. Unilateral pulmonary fibrosis may result from lung inflammation due to pulmonary tuberculosis, chronic lung abscess or organizing pneumonia (*Fig.* C.7). The whole hemithorax may appear shrunken with abnormalities most apparent in the upper anterior chest showing obvious flattening and reduced respiratory excursion (remember the adage 'flattening equals fibrosis'). The contracted fibrotic lung due to chronic pulmonary suppuration is frequently the site of bronchiectasis (*Figs* C.8, C.9).

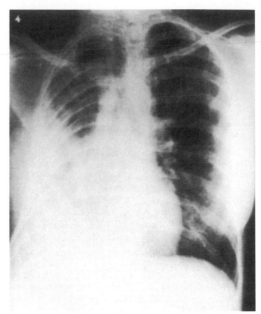

Fig. C.8. Radiograph of chest showing contraction of the right side due to fibrosis of the lung, pleural thickening and bronchiectasis.

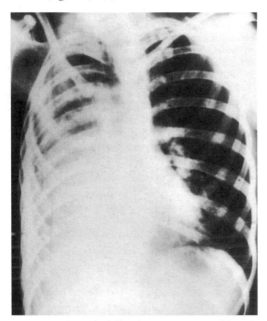

Fig. C.7. Radiograph of chest showing contraction of the right side with gross pleural thickening due to a chronic empyema. Note the scoliosis and the periosteal thickening of the ribs on the affected side.

When unilateral contraction of the chest with gross pleural thickening arises from any cause during childhood or adolescence, the resulting scoliosis may become extreme as growth proceeds.

Localized chest wall disease

Table C.3 lists disorders of the chest wall which may present as localized swellings.

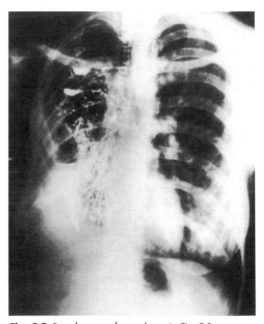

Fig. C.9. Bronchogram of case shown in *Fig.* C.8.

TUBERCULOSIS OF THE CHEST WALL

Tuberculosis of the chest wall usually arises from breakdown of intercostal lymph nodes and presents as a painless fluctuating cold abscess that may be mistaken for a lipoma. Diagnosis is made by aspiration of caseous pus or during histological examination. There are two main groups of intercostal lymph nodes. The first lie at the angle of the ribs from which pus may

Table C.3. Causes of localized swelling of the chest wall

Infectious inflammations

Tuberculosis of the chest wall	—see text
Osteomyelitis	—in children—staphyloccal infection involving the ribs
	—in adults—usually staphyloccal in drug addicts following a blow
Osteochondritis of costochondral junction	—Tietze's syndrome (uncommon)—see text
	—typhoid fever (very rare)—see text
Syphilitic gumma	—starts in anterior mediastinum and presents at the front of an intercostal space. Now very rare
Actinomycosis	—see text
Fungal infections	—blastomycosis, coccidiodomycosis and cryptococcosis can cause osteolytic rib lesions

Benign soft tissue tumours

Lipoma	—commonest benign tumour of the chest wall. CT scan confirms the presence of fat
Haemangioma	—mass may pulsate. Bruit heard. Phleboliths in the tumour on chest radiograph diagnostic
Cystic hygroma	—a rare hamartomatous lymphatic malformation producing a thin-walled cystic tumour lined with endothelium
Neurofibromatosis	—multiple fibromas present in one or more intercostal spaces. *Café au lait* patches, etc

Malignant soft tissue tumours

Fibrosarcoma	—commonest malignant soft tissue primary tumour of the chest wall; can arise in soft tissues in older women many years after radiotherapy to the breast

Benign bony tissue tumours

Osteochondroma (exostosis)	—small hard tumour fixed to a rib or the sternum in children and young adults. May cause severe pain
Chondroma	—tends to become sarcomatous—see Chondrosarcoma
Diaphysial aclasis	—generalized disorder of skeleton. The rib excrescences resemble chondromas but are not potentially malignant
Osteoclastoma	—rarely affects ribs. About 10 per cent can become malignant

Malignant bony tissue tumours

Metastases	—primary is usually in lung, breast, prostate, thyroid or kidney in adults and is usually a neuroblastoma in children
Multiple and solitary myeloma	—monoclonal hypergammaglobulinaemia
Chondrosarcoma	—initial silent painless growth—may stop growing for a time only to become painful and invasive
Ewing's sarcoma	—aggressive, commonest in those under 30 years of age. Involves the ribs and rarely scapula or sternum
Osteogenic sarcoma	—may occur in rib of a patient with Paget's disease or in a woman many years after radiation therapy to the breast

track backwards with the posterior primary division of the intercostal nerves to present near the erector spinae muscles or forwards with the anterior division of the intercostal nerve to present in the lateral chest wall. Abscesses may arise from nodes in the region of the internal mammary artery from which pus may present near the costochondral junction.

Tuberculosis of the sternum can cause a cold abscess over the anterior chest wall. Rib tuberculosis is rare but may give rise to local pain, swelling and sinus formation. Radiologically there is an initial small area of bone destruction which progresses to periosteal elevation and soft tissue swelling. Multiple cold abscesses of the ribs may accompany spinal tuberculosis (Potts disease) with paravertebral abscess formation pointing over the back and lower ribs.

TIETZE'S SYNDROME (COSTOCHONDRITIS)

This condition of obscure aetiology results in pain, swelling and tenderness of one or more of the upper six costal cartilages. The second costal cartilage is most often affected. It may present at any age but is most common in young adults. The onset may be insidious or abrupt, the pain variously described as aching, gripping, sharp or dull, and the condition, which is self-limiting, can persist for weeks, months or rarely years. It has been suggested that asymmetrical rib growth, prolonged coughing or hyperventilation may be the cause but it is often idiopathic.

OSTEOMYELITIS OF THE RIBS, SPINE OR STERNUM

Osteomyelitis is a well known, albeit rare, consequence of bacteraemia. Classically difficult to diagnose, patients present with chronic symptoms of pain, fever, thoracic cage swelling and radiographic evidence of erosion and bony sclerosis. *Staphylococcus aureus* is the most common agent. *Staphylococcus epidermidis* has emerged in recent years as a frequent cause from infected intravenous lines and prosthetic implant material. Gram-negative organisms are often responsible for haematogenous vertebral osteomyelitis, especially in patients with sickle cell anaemia. Intravenous drug abusers are especially susceptible to a wide range of bacterial and fungal causes of osteomyelitis.

ACTINOMYCOSIS

Thoracic actinomycosis may spread from the lungs to cause a diffuse indurated swelling of the chest wall; if the condition is undiagnosed and untreated it progresses to destructive rib lesions associated with periostitis and multiple sinuses discharging 'sulphur-granule pus'.

EMPYEMA NECESSITATIS

A localized swelling of the chest wall may be caused by a neglected empyema pointing externally to produce a soft diffuse fluctuant swelling which sometimes gives an impulse on respiration or coughing.

TUMOURS

Tumours may originate or metastasize to the chest wall (*Table* C.3).

AORTIC ANEURYSMS

Aortic aneurysms involving the ascending part of the aorta may cause pulsating swellings over the upper anterior chest; they should be easily recognizable by the characteristic expansile pulsation and by other signs and symptoms of aneurysm. The commonest situation for such a swelling is to the right of the sternum at the first, second and third intercostal spaces. In the presence of a grossly enlarged heart the precordium may become prominent, a condition most often seen in children suffering from severe rheumatic or congenital heart disease.

P. R. Studdy

Chest pain

Pain in the chest is one of the commonest of all complaints. However slight it may be, it only too often conjures up in the mind of the sufferer a vision of serious organic disease of the lungs or, more often, of the heart. Accurate diagnosis depends, to a considerable extent, on physical examination and special investigations but, most of all, on a detailed and precise history of the site and radiation of the pain, of its character and duration, and of factors by which it is aggravated or relieved. A useful clinical classification of pain in the chest is into pain felt mainly in the centre of the chest or in its lateral aspects; each of these categories can be further subdivided into pain of sudden onset, often presenting as an emergency, and pain which, on presentation to the physician, has

been present for several days or weeks. The common, and some of the less common, causes of chest pain are listed in this way in *Table* C.4. Pain in the precordium will be included in the discussion of central chest pain. The adjectives 'central' and 'precordial' are not, of course, synonymous—the precordium being that area of the anterior chest wall circumscribed by the surface markings of the heart—but the two sites are naturally associated in the diagnosis of pain which arises, or is thought to arise, from the heart. Before proceeding to the main discussion, a brief account will be given, for the sake of completeness, of several causes of chest pain which are immediately obvious on superficial examination.

Table C.4. Causes of chest pain

Acute	*Chronic*
Central or precordial	
Common	*Common*
Myocardial infarction	Angina of effort
Unstable angina	Oesophageal spasm or
Pericarditis	reflux
Dissecting aortic aneurysm	Cervical spondylosis
Massive pulmonary	Prolapsed mitral cusp
embolism	Da Costa's syndrome
Less common	*Less common*
Upper abdominal	Pulmonary hypertension
catastrophe	Peptic ulcer
Precordial catch	Gallbladder disease
Acute anxiety	Chronic pancreatitis
Tracheitis	Ankylosing spondylitis
Mycoplasma pneumonia	Tietze's disease
Pericardial fat necrosis	Lesions of sternum
	Mediastinal tumour
Lateral	
Common	*Common*
Pleurisy: infection, infarction,	Spinal disease: infection,
connective tissue disease	tumours, spondylosis
Trauma, e.g. fractured rib	Chronic trauma
	Bronchial carcinoma
Less common	*Less common*
Superficial lesions, e.g.	Rib metastases
herpes zoster	Aortic aneurysm
Bornholm disease	Aortic aneurysm
Trichinosis	

1. Pain due to superficial lesions

Pain due to *inflammation of the superficial tissues* of the chest wall poses no great diagnostic problem. It is important to remember, however, that the inflammation may have spread from a deeper lesion such as an empyema. *Herpes zoster*, which involves thoracic nerve roots in at least 50 per cent of cases, is also obvious once the eruption has appeared but pain and paraesthesiae may be present for a few days before this and cause temporary diagnostic confusion. The vesicles are implanted on an erythematous base and may be discrete or confluent; they are strictly unilateral and occupy the area of one or more dermatomes (*Fig.* C.10). Fever and malaise occur in a few patients and the axillary lymph nodes may be enlarged. Scabs form and the lesions heal in a week or two, without scarring unless they have become secondarily infected. Post-herpetic neuralgia may, occasionally, cause severe pain for a long period after the eruption has disappeared, especially in the elderly. Very rarely *Mondor's disease*, which is phlebitis of the subcutaneous anterior thoracic veins, produces pain, either pleuritic in type or provoked by raising the arms. The inflamed vein may be palpable as a tender cord. Resolution occurs in a few weeks or a month or two.

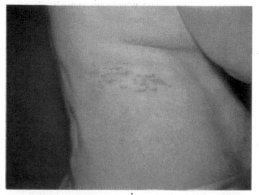

Fig. C.10. Intercostal herpes zoster.

2. Central chest pain

Much the most important cause of central chest pain is myocardial ischaemia. Three separate clinical syndromes are recognized—angina of effort, unstable angina and myocardial infarction—although there is some overlap, at least between the first two.

The diagnosis of *angina* turns, in the great majority of cases, on an accurate history. The pain is typically symmetrical in the chest, or nearly so, being felt in the region of the sternum, or slightly to the left, and radiating laterally towards the axillae and down the inner sides of the arms; the left is involved a little more often than the right but this is of no diagnostic importance as bilateral radiation is the rule. Radiation to the epigastrium, the side of the neck, jaw and tongue also occurs. Very occasionally the pain is felt in the midline of the back or in one or other scapular region. The pain is described as 'tight', 'gripping' or 'like indigestion', or the patient may deny actual pain and describe only a feeling of pressure or of tightness. A particularly revealing gesture is the clenched fist placed on the sternum to indicate both the site and, presumably, the character of the sensation. A pain described as 'stabbing' is probably not angina, but patients do not always choose their words with care and each statement must be carefully analysed to ascertain the patient's meaning exactly. Certainly a

pain which comes in sharp jabs, lasting a second only, is not angina and adjectives such as 'shooting' and 'stabbing' are suspect on this account. The typical duration of an attack is a few minutes only and a pain lasting for a much longer or shorter time than this is unlikely to be angina; there are exceptions, however, which will be discussed. Perhaps the most important aspect is the relationship to exertion. A pain in the anterior part of the chest which is consistently provoked by effort and relieved by rest must be presumed to be angina unless there is overwhelming evidence to the contrary. The pain may be provoked more easily after meals or in cold weather, but it is the relationship to effort which is of paramount importance provided that the pain develops *during* the exercise; a pain starting *after* exercise is not angina. The effect of sublingual trinitrin may be of diagnostic importance but, again, the time relationship is important. If the pain is relieved within a minute by trinitrin, angina is probable; patients are, however, unfamiliar with such a rapid effect from oral medication and may claim that trinitrin relieves their pain, omitting the essential fact that the pain does not cease until, perhaps, half an hour after the tablet was taken. Occasionally variants of angina are seen such as pain felt only in one of the distal sites of radiation; even 'tennis elbow' and 'toothache' may prove to be angina if the constant relationship to exertion can be elicited.

Apart from exercise, angina may be precipitated by sympathetic overactivity. This is the mechanism of angina provoked by emotion as in the case of John Hunter who said, some time before he died after an acrimonious Board Meeting, 'My life is in the hands of any rascal who chooses to annoy and tease me.' Nocturnal angina is also related to sympathetic overactivity as it has been shown to occur after a period of REM (rapid eye movements) sleep which is associated with dreaming. Angina decubitus, provoked by lying down, is probably due to the increase in cardiac output in this posture; it is rather characteristic of syphilitic aortic valve disease. In general, angina which is easily provoked or occurs, apparently spontaneously, at rest is associated with severe disease involving all three coronary arteries (right, left circumflex and anterior descending).

In the majority of cases of angina no abnormal physical signs are found but two important signs should be specifically sought. A left atrial impulse may be palpable at the apex and an atrial gallop rhythm heard particularly during an actual attack of pain. Paradoxical splitting of the second heart sound is less common and is difficult to elicit but, if present, implies prolongation of left ventricular systole and a serious disturbance of left ventricular function. The electrocardiogram is usually normal at rest but the typical depression of the RS-T segment may be present to confirm the diagnosis of ischaemia (*Fig.* C.11); evidence of previous infarction may also be present or non-specific changes such as bundle-branch block. Recording the electrocardiogram during exercise to demonstrate RS-T depression (*Fig.* C.12) and, sometimes, other changes is a reliable method of confirming the diagnosis of myocardial ischaemia; after many years of uncertainty this technique is now established as a routine procedure. Radio-isotope scanning of the myocardium using, for example, thallium-201 is also helpful in delineating areas of ischaemia which develop during exercise. In the majority of patients with angina and a positive exercise test, coronary angiography will show occlusive lesions of one or, usually, several coronary arteries. In a few, however, the arteries are normal or nearly so and, in such cases the most likely cause of the ischaemia is coronary artery spasm. This concept is an old one but was convincingly revived by Maseri et al. It can occur in otherwise normal arteries or in association with occlusive disease of any degree of severity.

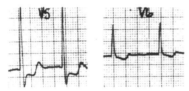

Fig. C.11. RS-T segment depression. The record on the left (V5) is from a patient with severe ischaemic heart disease causing angina on the slightest exercise. Depression of the whole of the RS-T segment, which remains horizontal, should be compared with the downward sloping RS-T segment due to digitalis seen in the record, from another patient, on the right (V6).

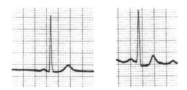

Fig. C.12. Positive exercise test. The complex on the left was recorded at rest from a patient with chest pain suspicious of angina. The complex on the right from the same lead, recorded after exercise, shows depression of the whole RS-T segment which remains horizontal. The diagnosis of myocardial ischaemia is confirmed.

In a large majority of cases of angina the underlying lesion is coronary atherosclerosis. In addition, other forms of arterial disease can, occasionally, cause ischaemia. Angina is a well-recognized, though rare, symptom of polyarteritis nodosa and giant-cell arteritis; smaller vessels may be involved in rheumatoid arteritis and in association with livedo reticularis. Another inflammatory cause of angina is involvement of the coronary ostia in syphilitic aortitis; the attacks of pain

tend to last longer and occur rather characteristically at night although the relationship to effort is as in other varieties of angina. Ischaemic pain is aggravated by left ventricular hypertrophy due to hypertension and, particularly, aortic valve disease. In these conditions, and in hypertrophic obstructive cardiomyopathy, the disease of the coronary arteries themselves may be trivial and the pain due to relative ischaemia of the hypertrophied muscle. Severe anaemia, for example pernicious anaemia or following gastrointestinal haemorrhage, thyrotoxicosis and rapid ectopic tachycardia can also cause angina in patients with minor coronary disease only. All these factors must be borne in mind particularly when dealing with a case of angina in a premenopausal woman. Coronary atherosclerosis is rare in such patients and angina is likely to be due to one of the precipitating factors mentioned or to premature atherosclerosis resulting from hyperlipidaemia, as in diabetes, myxoedema or hereditary hypercholesterolaemic xanthomatosis (Type II hyperlipidaemia in Fredrickson's classification) (*Fig.* C.13).

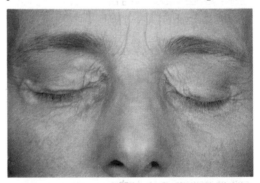

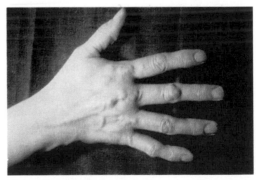

Fig. C.13. Xanthelasma palpebrarum and xanthomas on the hand of a female aged 52 with angina of effort. The serum cholesterol was 15·5 mmol/l.

Unstable angina is the least common clinical variety of ischaemic heart disease. This is one of a number of terms used to describe cases in which prolonged cardiac pain occurs at rest without evidence of myocardial necrosis. Other terms used include 'acute coronary insufficiency', 'preinfarction angina' and 'crescendo angina' which carry the, often correct, implication that myocardial infarction is imminent. A variant of this condition is the so-called 'angina inversa', described by Prinzmetal, in which RS-T *elevation* occurs briefly in association with ischaemic pain at rest or on exercise; this is believed to be due to severe ischaemia of a rather localized area of myocardium due to severe arterial disease or, sometimes, spasm (*Fig.* C.14). RS-T depression can also occur in similar circumstances and it is probable that the elevation of 'angina inversa' is produced merely by the relationship of the site of the ischaemia to the position of the electrode.

complication, especially if it develops in a case of anterior infarction. Congestive heart failure or frank pulmonary oedema occur from time to time but lesser degrees of left ventricular failure are common. As a result of the consequent pulmonary venous congestion, with the probable addition of multiple alveolar collapse, mild arterial hypoxaemia is seen very frequently, the arterial PO_2 being around 9 kPa; this often causes sufficient hyperventilation to reduce the arterial PCO_2 to about 5 kPa. The term 'cardiogenic shock' should be reserved for cases with severe hypotension, cold, clammy skin, oliguria and clouding of consciousness. Less common complications include rupture of

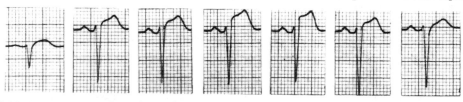

Fig. C.14. 'Angina inversa'. Male aged 50, with angina at rest. RS-T elevation appeared and disappeared over a period of about 2 minutes. Recorded via a monitoring chest electrode.

Myocardial infarction is nearly always due to occlusion of a coronary artery by atherosclerosis, with or without superadded thrombosis; a much rarer cause is coronary embolus in association with, for example, atrial fibrillation or infective endocarditis. The pain of myocardial infarction has exactly the same character and areas of radiation as angina. It is not, however, related to exercise and typically lasts for several hours, if untreated, rather than the few minutes of an anginal attack. Myocardial infarction can, rarely, be painless, especially in the elderly in whom it may manifest itself as syncope or a dysrhythmia or as otherwise unexplained left ventricular failure. In contrast to the paucity of physical signs in angina, it is unusual to find no abnormal physical signs in a case of myocardial infarction provided that frequent examination is carried out as many of the signs may be very transient. Some fall in blood pressure is common but may not be detected if the previous level is unknown. Slight elevation of the jugular venous pressure is seen in many cases and an audible or palpable atrial gallop is found even more frequently. Paradoxical splitting of the second sound may occasionally be detected and, after a day or two, a pericardial rub may be heard.

The three most common complications are dysrhythmias, cardiac failure and shock, in that order. Continuous monitoring has demonstrated that over 90 per cent of cases of myocardial infarction have some form of dysrhythmia, of which ventricular extrasystoles are the most common and may presage ventricular tachycardia and fibrillation. Supraventricular dysrhythmias also occur, often in association with cardiac failure. Atrioventricular block is an ominous

the infarct which will usually cause rapidly fatal haemopericardium or, if a papillary muscle is involved, acute mitral regurgitation with pulmonary oedema; rupture of the interventricular septum causes acute right ventricular failure. Systemic embolism from a mural thrombus is not uncommon; pulmonary embolism arises most often from phlebothrombosis of the calf veins secondary to enforced recumbency. Later sequelae are ventricular aneurysm, which may rarely calcify (*Fig.* C.15), Dressler's syndrome of recurrent pericarditis and pleurisy and the shoulder-hand syndrome, which consists of 'frozen shoulder' and Raynaud's phenomenon, usually on the left.

Electrocardiography remains the most commonly used method of confirming a diagnosis of myocardial infarction but estimation of various serum enzymes is also valuable particularly in the, not infrequent, cases in which the electrocardiographic signs are equivocal. There are three cardinal electrocardiographic signs of myocardial infarction; a pathological Q wave, at least a third the amplitude of the R wave in the same lead and at least 0·04 second in duration; RS-T segment elevation with an upward convexity; and T wave inversion which may not be seen until the RS-T segment is returning to the iso-electric line as it does during the first few weeks after the episode. The T wave may also return to, or towards, normal after some months, but the Q wave, the sign of irreversible muscle necrosis, virtually always remains indefinitely. These changes are seen in leads whose positive terminals face the infarcted area of myocardium; in leads 'facing' the diametrically opposite part of the heart reciprocal changes are seen which may, occasionally, be of diagn-

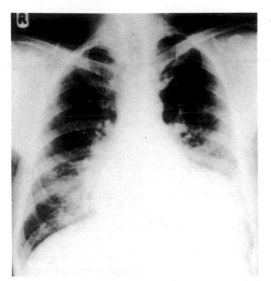

Fig. C.15. Left ventricular aneurysm. Male, aged 48, who had an anterior myocardial infarction 6 months previously.

circulation from the infarcted myocardium and the rise and fall of their serum levels can be of great diagnostic value. Those most commonly estimated clinically are aspartate amino-transferase (previously known as 'glutamic-oxalacetic transaminase'), creatine phosphokinase and lactate dehydrogenase. The first two remain elevated for 3 or 4 days only but elevation of the serum lactate dehydrogenase persists for up to 2 weeks. Greater specificity for myocardial damage can be achieved by estimating the iso-enzymes of lactate dehydrogenase separately; the iso-enzyme released in largest amounts from the myocardium also acts upon hydroxybutyrate and can be conveniently estimated as hydroxybutyrate dehydrogenase. Apart from the changes in the serum enzymes, non-specific evidence of tissue necrosis is also present following myocardial infarction; such evidence includes pyrexia, leucocytosis and raised sedimentation rate. Such changes, although characteristic, are of little or no diagnostic value.

ostic significance. For descriptive purposes, infarcts are subdivided into anterior, inferior (or diaphragmatic) and 'true' posterior. Originally the term 'posterior' was applied to the diaphragmatic surface of the heart but, now that it is possible to diagnose infarction of the small part of the left ventricle which lies posteriorly, the anatomically more correct term 'inferior' is preferred. To avoid confusion with the older nomenclature, infarcts at the back of the left ventricle are designated *true* posterior (*Figs.* C.16–C.19).

Many intracellular enzymes are released into the

The pain of *pericarditis* is, in some respects, similar to that of myocardial infarction and, as localized pericarditis is common in the latter, the differentiation may present some difficulty. Pericardial pain is felt in the sternal region and towards the left and may radiate to the epigastrium, neck, back, shoulders and, occasionally, to the arms. The severity varies markedly, from a mild discomfort to extreme agony and the pain is described either as 'stabbing' or 'like a knife' or in terms very reminiscent of those used to describe the pain of myocardial ischaemia. It is aggravated by deep

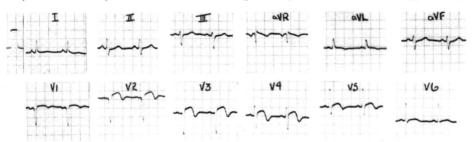

Fig. C.16. Anteroseptal myocardial infarction. Pathological Q waves are present in V1 and 2 and RV3 is diminutive RS-T elevation is seen in V1–6 and aVL. The T wave is inverted in V1–5 and in aVL.

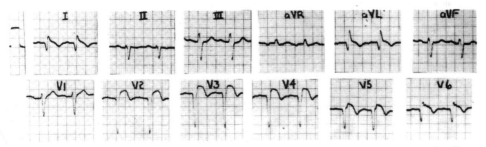

Fig. C.17. Anterolateral myocardial infarction. Pathological Q waves are present in 1, aVL and V2–6 with RS-T segment elevation and T inversion.

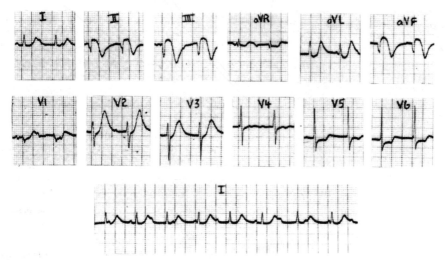

Fig. C.18. Inferior myocardial infarction. Pathological Q waves. RS-T elevation and T wave inversion are present in II and III and aVF. The tall T waves in V2 and V3 and the RS-T depression in V5 and V6 are probably reciprocal to the primary inferior changes. Atrioventricular dissociation is also present.

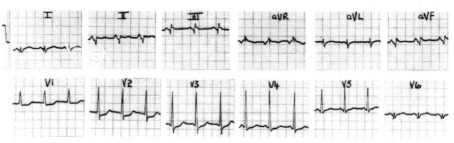

Fig. C.19. Posteroinferior myocardial infarction. The pathological Q waves in II, III and aVF are evidence of infarction of the inferior (diaphragmatic) surface of the left ventricle. The dominant R wave and RS-T depression in V1–3 were known to have been absent before the episode of pain. This pattern is reciprocal to a, presumed pathological Q wave and RS-T elevation which would have been recorded from an electrode diametrically opposite to V1–3. These changes, in this context, are those of true posterior infarction but the pattern of V1–3, taken alone, is also compatible with right ventricular hypertrophy.

breathing, coughing and by twisting movements involving the muscles of the chest wall. There is therefore some relationship with exertion, on account of the associated hyperventilation, but the aggravation by specific movements such as turning over in bed serves to distinguish it from angina. The pain is also worse in the recumbent position and is relieved by sitting up; it may also be aggravated by swallowing. The characteristic physical sign is the friction rub, heard over all or part of the precordium (see RUB, PERICARDIAL). The third cardinal feature of pericarditis is the electrocardiogram. RS-T elevation is seen in all epicardial levels, that is in all the leads of a conventional 12-lead record except a VR (*Fig.* C.20). The RS-T elevation is concave upwards unlike that of myocardial infarction; pathological Q waves are, of course, absent. Later in the course of the disease, T-wave inversion appears and, at this stage, the differentiation from myocardial ischaemia may be difficult. The diagnosis of pericarditis is incomplete unless the aetiology is determined. Common causes include virus infection

(often Coxsackie B), connective-tissue disorders such as systemic lupus erythematosus, rheumatic fever, rheumatoid arthritis, bacterial infections and Dressler's and other similar syndromes. Chronic renal failure is a well-known cause but the commonest cause of all is myocardial infarction; in that condition the pericarditis probably contributes little to the pain.

Pericardial fat necrosis is a rare cause of pain simulating that of pericarditis. No friction rub can be heard and the electrocardiogram is normal. A paracardiac mass may be visible in the chest radiograph.

Dissecting aneurysm causes very severe anterior chest pain radiating to the neck, back and, later, to the abdomen; it rarely spreads to the arms. With dissection of the descending thoracic aorta the pain may begin in the back. The resemblance to myocardial infarction is close and, indeed, if the dissection involves a coronary artery, infarction may, in fact, occur and confuse the diagnostic issue further. Important differentiating features include the absence of one or more peripheral pulses, particularly if a pulse disappears

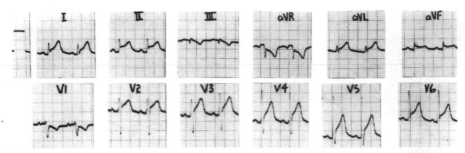

Fig. C.20. Acute pericarditis. RS-T elevation, concave upwards, is present in I, II, aVL, aVF and V2–6. There are no pathological Q waves and the T waves are upright in most leads. These features, together with the *widespread* RS-T elevation, confirm the diagnosis of pericarditis.

while the patient is under observation, or other evidence of arterial occlusion such as hemiparesis, blindness in one eye, or haematuria. The development of aortic regurgitation, due to involvement of the aortic valve ring by the dissection, is a valuable diagnostic feature. Also the blood pressure is little changed compared with the fall commonly seen in myocardial infarction. The severity of the pain is of some diagnostic significance; chest pain which is hardly influenced by morphine or diamorphine may well be due to a dissecting aneurysm. The electrocardiogram is normal unless a coronary artery is involved or pre-existing hypertensive changes are present. Much reliance is placed on radiography in diagnosis: gross dilatation of the thoracic aorta may be seen but this is not always easy to distinguish from unfolding unless a previous film is available. Also the dilatation may not be very marked in the early stages. In practice, a firm diagnosis is rarely possible from the plain radiograph. If available, MRI is the investigation of choice; otherwise the definitive diagnosis can only be made by aortography and even this can be misleading at times (*Fig.* C.21).

Another important cause of sudden anterior chest pain is massive *pulmonary embolism*. Smaller pulmonary emboli cause pulmonary infarction which is discussed below among the causes of lateral, pleuritic chest pain. Pulmonary embolism occurs commonly in the postoperative period or during a period of enforced recumbency associated with a low cardiac output, as after myocardial infarction or in cardiac failure; in young women, oral contraceptive agents have been incriminated as the cause of the initiating venous thrombosis. The same complication may, of course, occur in pregnancy. The source of the embolism is commonly thrombosis in veins of the leg or pelvis but this may not have been clinically manifest except, perhaps, as a small 'spike' of temperature. The patient rapidly becomes severely ill with central chest pain, nearly identical to that of myocardial infarction, breathlessness and, often, faintness or even loss of consciousness. Peripheral cyanosis is present, the pulse is rapid, and the blood pressure very low. Elevation of the

jugular venous pressure is nearly always present; it is usually a good deal higher than in myocardial infarction causing a comparable degree of hypotension. Gallop rhythm may be heard over the right ventricle. The chest radiograph may show dilatation of one or both main branches of the pulmonary artery, and one lung, or part thereof, may appear unusually translucent. Pulmonary angiography, which is less hazardous than might have been expected in this situation, may show the occlusion of the pulmonary artery clearly. In the electrocardiogram the appearances may simulate those of antero-inferior infarction with a Q wave and inverted T in lead III and T inversion in leads V1–4; right axis deviation, with a prominent S wave in lead II, and clockwise rotation, causing an RS pattern from V1 to V5, are other common features.

Chronic *pulmonary hypertension*, as in mitral stenosis or the Eisenmenger syndrome, can produce a pain indistinguishable from angina. The cause, indeed, is almost certainly myocardial ischaemia as a result of the severely limited cardiac output. Severe *pulmonary stenosis* can cause a similar pain.

The anterior chest pain associated with *prolapse of a mitral valve cusp* is not usually ischaemic in origin. This lesion, which is not very rare, is often associated with a mid-systolic click and late systolic murmur. The diagnosis can be confirmed by echocardiography or angiocardiography. The pain is very variable in site, duration and severity and has no clear-cut diagnostic features.

Pain arising from the oesophagus is felt in the midline of the chest with radiation to the jaw, back, shoulders and, to a small extent, down the inner sides of the arms. The resemblance to angina is close and oesophageal pain may even have some relationship to exertion although this is never constant. The pain may be due to *oesophageal spasm* without any other lesion, it may occur early in the evolution of *achalasia of the cardia* or it may be due to *hiatus hernia* with oesophageal reflux and oesophagitis. Heartburn, with radiation of sternal pain upwards from the xiphoid, is very characteristic of the last. Helpful diagnostic feat-

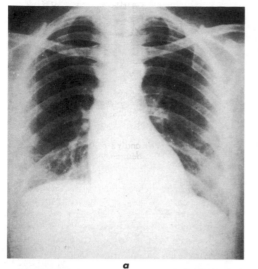

a

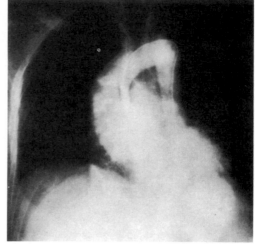

b

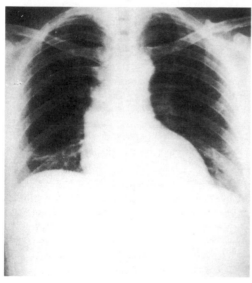

c

Fig. C.21. Dissecting aneurysm of the aorta. Male, aged 39, admitted with severe central chest pain. *a* As late as 6 weeks after admission a chest radiograph showed very little cardiac enlargement or widening of the mediastinum. *b*. Aortography, however, showed dissection of the ascending aorta and gross aortic regurgitation. *c*. A month later the mediastinal shadow was a good deal wider and the heart was considerably enlarged. The patient was in left ventricular failure and died following surgical repair.

ures include the association of the pain with taking food and relief from belching; the pain of oesophageal reflux is commonly worse in the recumbent position or in other postures favouring regurgitation, such as bending forward or the cramped position of the driver of a small car, especially if wearing a tight safety belt. If the pain can be reproduced by the instillation of 0·1 *N* hydrochloric acid into the lower oesophagus, this is good evidence that it is due to reflux. The demonstration of a hiatus hernia by a barium swallow is only too easy. Most hiatus hernias produce no symptoms at all and chest pain in a patient in whom such a lesion has been demonstrated is as likely to be due to myocardial ischaemia or other conditions as to the hernia. There is no substitute for a detailed analysis of the symptoms.

Other upper abdominal lesions can cause pain felt in the midline of the front of the chest. The frequency with which angina is regarded as 'indigestion' even by experienced physicians suffering from this condition bears witness to this. Catastrophes such as perforated peptic ulcer and acute pancreatitis must be remembered in the differential diagnosis of myocardial infarction. Gastric distension due to aerophagy or other causes can cause substernal discomfort, but peptic ulcer and chronic relapsing pancreatitis are less common causes of confusion; in the former, the relationship of the pain to meals is obviously important.

Finally, there is the, almost mystical, association of gallbladder disease with ischaemic heart disease. Both conditions are common and can certainly coexist. Much debate has centred around whether this coexistence occurs more commonly than would have been expected by chance; many experienced clinicians have a strong impression that this is so but none of the theories to account for it are very convincing. Suffice it to say that gallbladder pain can certainly radiate into the front of the chest and simulate angina; also, central chest pain with a constant relationship to exertion must be regarded as angina even if gallbladder disease is present in addition.

There are numerous musculoskeletal causes of anterior chest pain. Local *trauma* is usually obvious but recurrent mild trauma, for example in some particular occupation, may not be mentioned by the patient as a possible cause for his pain. The pain may be a dull ache on one or other side of the chest, rarely exactly in the midline, or it may be possible to relate it to particular movements if anterior thoracic muscles are the site of origin. Pain from *spondylosis* or spondylitis of the thoracic, or even the cervical, spine can be referred to the front of the chest. The distribution can occasionally simulate that of angina and radiological proof of the spondylosis is of little diagnostic significance. Relief of the pain from wearing a cervical collar is, however, good evidence of a skeletal origin. Less obvious spinal disease may also be a cause of pain felt diffusely over the precordium or in the corresponding area on the right. Experimentally, the injection of hypertonic saline into an interspinous ligament produces pain referred to the anterior part of the corresponding dermatome with some radiation upwards and downwards. It is difficult to prove this aetiology in any particular patient but it has been suggested that chronic mild trauma to interspinous ligaments, for example due to scoliosis, may be a cause of otherwise unexplained precordial pain.

Less common musculoskeletal lesions include *Tietze's disease*. This causes pain of sudden or gradual onset in one or more upper costal cartilages. The pain is worse on coughing or deep breathing and the affected cartilage is swollen and tender. *Xiphoidalgia* is a similar condition involving the xiphisternum which is possibly a variant of Tietze's disease or, more likely, due to recurrent mild trauma. Ankylosing spondylitis can cause a diffuse pain in the anterior chest wall often associated with local tenderness over the sternum and costal cartilages. Pain arising in the sternum itself may be due to *myelomatosis, metastases, ankylosing spondylitis, osteomyelitis* or *fracture*. The sudden, sharp pain at, or near, the cardiac apex, known as *precordial catch*, is probably quite common although

rare as a spontaneous complaint. There is rarely any diagnostic confusion with other causes of chest pain as the history is quite characteristic. The pain occurs most often when the subject is seated and lasts for a few minutes only. It can be relieved by a single, painful, deep inspiration.

Respiratory disease most often causes pain, if at all, in one or other side of the chest, but *trachetis* should be mentioned as a cause of upper sternal pain. It is aggravated by the hyperventilation of exercise and may thus, very occasionally, have to be distinguished from angina. *Mycoplasma pneumonia*, unlike other varieties of pneumonia, is never associated with pleurisy but may cause a substernal pain aggravated by coughing. *Dyspnoea* itself, especially if it is associated with obstruction of airways, may be described as 'tightness in the chest' and an injudicious series of leading questions may persuade the patient that he has a 'tight pain' across his chest and lead to an erroneous diagnosis of angina.

Two psychological conditions are important in the differential diagnosis of anterior chest pain. The terrifying panic of an attack of *acute anxiety* can be confused with a myocardial infarction or other intrathoracic vascular catastrophe. The patient, very often a woman, complains of dizziness, palpitations, dyspnoea and precordial oppression or pain. Angor animi—the fear of impending death—is a prominent feature, much more so than in genuine myocardial ischaemia, and further exacerbates the anxiety. The circumstances in which the attack occurs and the complete absence of objective evidence of organic disease are important distinguishing features, and doubt about the nature of the condition should rarely persist for long. Chronic anxiety is the commonest underlying disorder in *Da Costa's syndrome*; the non-committal eponymous title is preferred to the numerous other terms, such as 'effort syndrome', 'cardiac neurosis' and 'disordered action of the heart', which have been used—with no great semantic accuracy—to describe this condition. Apart from the pain, the features of the syndrome are dyspnoea, palpitation, fatigue and dizziness. The pain is most commonly felt in the left submammary region although it may be nearer the midline or, indeed, anywhere on the left side of the chest, even radiating into the left arm. In character it is sharp and stabbing, with occasional momentary twinges superimposed on a dull ache which persists for many hours at a time. It often occurs *after*, rarely during, exertion; this important point may be elicited only after careful questioning. In summary, it differs from angina in almost all respects except in the rare, difficult case in which it has a more constricting quality and is felt near the left border of the sternum. The mechanism of the pain is unknown but it seems likely that, in some cases at least, the original cause was a minor musculoskeletal abnormality. The pain convinces the patient that his heart is diseased and is perpetuated by the anxiety engendered by this conviction.

3. Lateral chest pain

Almost all the tissues of the lateral chest wall, the pleura, muscles, ribs and intercostal nerves, can be the site of painful lesions. Frequently the pain is closely related to respiration as exemplified most clearly in *pleurisy*. The visceral pleura is insensitive but the parietal pleura is plentifully supplied with pain fibres from the intercostal nerves. The pain is felt, therefore, in the cutaneous areas supplied by these nerves which, it is important to remember, include a large area of the anterior abdominal wall. Apart from inflammation of the pleura itself, there is some evidence that spasm of the intercostal muscles may be a factor in producing the pain. The pain is characteristically sharp, superficial, of any degree of severity and is aggravated by deep breathing and by coughing. Inspiration is abruptly halted by the pain so that respiration is often very shallow. Holding the breath in expiration will usually relieve the pain completely and a change in the patient's posture in bed can produce considerable relief or exacerbation. The only physical sign of pleurisy, in the absence of effusion, is the pleural friction rub, a characteristic creaking sound present during inspiration and expiration. The sound is difficult to describe but easy to recognize with a little experience although a coarse rhonchus may sometimes be mistaken for a rub. The pain is not at all closely related to the rub as one may be present without the other; neither alone is essential for the diagnosis of pleurisy. The pain of diaphagmatic pleurisy is typically referred to the shoulder; this is a common feature of pleurisy due to subdiaphragmatic lesions such as liver abscess or subphrenic abscess.

Pleurisy may be due to pulmonary infections such as lobar pneumonia or tuberculosis, to vascular lesions such as pulmonary infarction, or to connective-tissue disorders such as systemic lupus erythematosus. In many of these conditions, the clinical picture is modified by the development of an effusion which usually results in the disappearance of the pain and the rub.

A pain identical to that of pleurisy is felt in epidemic pleurodynia or *Bornholm disease*, due to Group B Coxsackie viruses. The pain is the presenting symptom and may be extremely severe; fever quickly develops and headache and malaise are common. Recovery is usually rapid but relapses are frequent and may continue for several weeks. *Trichinosis*, involving the intercostal muscles, can also produce pleuritic pain; the diagnosis would be supported by finding periorbital or generalized oedema and by eosinophilia in the peripheral blood. Pain arising from the capsule of the spleen is also related to respiration; it is commonly due to *splenic infarction* and may be accompanied by a friction rub so that the resemblance to pleurisy is very close. Splenic pain is not uncommon in Hodgkin's disease and in other similar conditions.

The pain of *spontaneous pneumothorax* is usually abrupt in onset and pleuritic in type. Some patients, however, complain only of a dull ache or a sense of tightness and a few have no pain at all. The typical physical signs are a diminution in movement and in breath-sounds on the affected side, often with a hyperresonant percussion note and, especially if the pneumothorax is under tension, deviation of the trachea towards the normal side. Dissection of the air into the mediastinum may cause central chest pain and the patient may notice a 'crunching' sound over the heart which is also audible on auscultation. The diagnosis of spontaneous pneumothorax can be confirmed by radiography but careful study may be needed if the pneumothorax is shallow; a film taken in expiration will show the lesion more clearly.

Involvement of the intercostal nerves in many pathological processes can cause pain in the corresponding areas of the chest wall. *Spinal disease* has already been mentioned as a cause of referred pain in the anterolateral regions of the chest. Direct pressure on nerves may occur in fracture of the thoracic spine, from malignant metastases in that region or in tuberculosis of the spine. Spondylosis with disc protrusion is not common as a cause of nerve-root compression in the thoracic spine. Neurofibromatosis may affect the thoracic nerve roots but does not often cause pain.

Aortic aneurysm is not a common lesion although, in former years, it was an important cause of chest pain. Aneurysm of the ascending aorta may cause chest pain by eroding the sternum but much more often causes no symptoms at all. Aneurysm of the arch and descending thoracic aorta can cause very severe radiating pain by vertebral erosion and pressure on nerve roots (*Fig. C.22*) Other symptoms and signs result from pressure on mediastinal structures. Thus, pressure on the left recurrent laryngeal nerve will cause paralysis of the left vocal cord, cough and stridor may follow pressure on the trachea, and dysphagia results from pressure on the oesophagus. Pressure on the left main bronchus may cause collapse of the left lung with subsequent infection; a tracheal tug is a well-known physical sign of aneurysm depressing the left main bronchus.

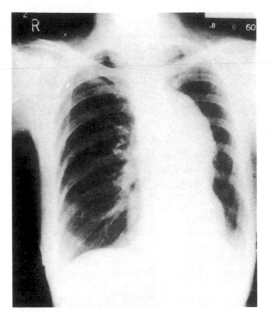

Fig. C.22. Aortic aneurysm. Female, aged 67, complaining of pain in the left side of the chest. Autopsy confirmed a huge aneurysm involving the arch and most of the descending aorta. (*Dr Basil Strickland.*)

Primary or secondary intrathoracic *malignant disease* may cause pain in various ways. Direct invasion of the pleura by a bronchial carcinoma can cause pleurisy, often with effusion; more often pleural pain occurs as a result of infection in the lung distal to a blocked bronchus. Primary tumours of the pleura, such as mesothelioma, cause pleuritic pain directly. Apart from the pleura, the ribs and intercostal nerves may be involved by tumour with the production of severe pain. Metastases in the thoracic spine have been mentioned as a cause of intercostal pain; secondary deposits in the ribs can also be extremely painful. Rarely, tumours in the mediastinum can apparently cause a poorly localized central chest pain without other pressure symptoms; the mechanism is not known.

Peter R. Fleming

Chest tenderness in

Chest pain is one of the most common symptoms given for seeking medical advice. Because there is no clear relationship between the intensity of discomfort and aetiology, all complaints of chest pain must be considered carefully. (*See also* CHEST PAIN). This section deals exclusively with tenderness which is, in fact, rarely complained of in the absence of pain.

Tenderness in the chest, an ache or discomfort perhaps with increased sensitivity and often accompanied with pain, can be difficult for the patient to describe. It is best classified according to the situation or character of the responsible lesion. Pains referred

from visceral lesions may sometimes be associated with local tenderness in the chest wall. The parietal pleura is exquisitely sensitive to painful stimuli and unpleasant sensations may also arise from lesions in the tracheobronchial tree.

1.   LESIONS OF THE CHEST WALL:
Inflammation of the skin and underlying tissues including the breasts
Intercostal myositis
Myalgia
Inflammation of the ribs and sternum
Blood diseases
Intercostal neuritis and neuralgia
Injury of the intercostal nerves
Ankylosing spondylitis
Herpes zoster
Tietze's syndrome

2.   LESIONS OF THORACIC AND
      ABDOMINAL VISCERA:
Lungs
Heart and aorta
Diaphragm
Stomach and oesophagus
Liver/gallbladder

1.   Lesions of the chest wall

Discomfort in the chest wall can result from respiratory diseases as well as from primary musculoskeletal lesions. Patients with chronic cough, dyspnoea or asthmatics subject to chest tightness often complain of anterolateral chest wall tenderness.

Tenderness is always present in *superficial inflammatory lesions* of the chest wall, such as bruises, burns, cuts, mastitis and superficial infections the diagnosis of which will usually be evident on examination.

Pain will be the chief complaint in the so-called *intercostal myositis* that occurs after injury or strain of an intercostal muscle, the affected muscle being tender to deep pressure. The condition is also known as *intercostal myalgia* or *pleurodynia*. It is distinguished from pleurisy by the absence of a pleural friction rub. Similar but more transient pain with a variable degree of tenderness may accompany the *stitch* to which some athletes are prone.

The acute pain of Bornholm disease, epidemic myalgia due to Coxsackie virus B infection, may be accompanied by hyperaesthesia of skin but less often by muscle tenderness. The myalgia of Phlebotomus (Sandfly) fever and dengue may also be accompanied by tenderness, often mild.

Tenderness of the *breasts* in the absence of mastitis is a common occurrence at or just before the menstrual periods and with high-dosage oestrogen therapy. Gynaecomastia in males, whatever the cause, is accompanied by tenderness of the breasts. It is not uncommon in chronic male alcoholics with cirrhosis of the liver.

Tenderness in the chest may result from *disease or injury of a rib or the sternum* when it will be localized to the injured spot; fracture, inflammation, tuberculosis or new growth may be the immediate cause. If *fracture* is present, X-rays may show the lesion or crepitus between the fragments on movement may be obtainable. *Sternal* or *costal osteitis* or *periostitis* may follow injury and may also occur in such diseases as typhoid or paratyphoid fever, tuberculosis or pyaemia. The local signs of inflammation (pain, redness, heat, swelling) will usually but not invariably be present. The chest wall may be invaded by local extension of a peripheral primary bronchial carcimoma or secondary tumour. Tenderness in the chest due to *new growth* in a rib or in the sternum—such as multiple myeloma, sarcoma, secondary deposit from carcinoma—is generally a late occurrence, the existence of malignant disease elsewhere having usually been established. Tenderness of the ribs and sternum occurs in certain *blood diseases* such as leukaemia. Diagnosis depends on examination of the blood and marrow biopsy. Tenderness over the sternum and ribs also occurs as part of the clinical picture of ankylosing spondylitis. In this disease the sternomanubrial and sternoclavicular joints may become acutely swollen and tender, causing considerable discomfort.

The particularly tender spots in the course of an *intercostal nerve* are three in number, corresponding to the points at which the posterior, the lateral cutaneous and the anterior cutaneous branches are given off, near the spinal column, in the midaxillary line and at the sternal margin respectively. Such tenderness may be marked in so-called *intercostal neuritis*, when some intrathoracic disorder such as pneumonia or pleurisy is present and in cases of pressure on an intercostal nerve, as for example by *abscess* about the spinal column, *aneurysm* of the descending aorta or *new growth* invading the spinal canal. Local tenderness may more commonly result from external pressure by, for instance, the buckle of the braces or some tool carried in a breast pocket, a simple detail but one not infrequently overlooked.

Pain and tenderness along an intercostal nerve are common in *herpes zoster* and may be present before, during and after the appearance of the characteristic rash. Tenderness can often be elicited at the three spots mentioned above; it is particularly when it occurs past middle age that herpes may be followed by a long period of pain and tenderness along the course of the affected nerve. The rash, once seen, can hardly be mistaken; to anticipate it on the type and site of the pain is a diagnostic *tour de force*. Similar pain and tenderness may follow thoracotomy and occasional patients experience intractable postoperative discomfort.

Tietze's syndrome is an unexplained disorder in which pain and swelling are found in the upper costochondral junctions of the anterior chest wall. Biopsies of costal cartridges show nothing characteristically abnormal. One or more costal cartilages, usually on one side only, the 2nd and 3rd most often, may be affected. Spontaneous remission occurs in weeks, months or, occasionally years.

2. Lesions of the underlying viscera

Tenderness in the chest may sometimes be a symptom of disease in the thoracic or abdominal viscera. The tenderness is as a rule superficial, confined to the skin and subjacent areolar and fatty tissues. Tactile hyperaesthesia or the production of unpleasant sensations or pain by the lightest touch may occur in neuralgia, neuroses, following thoracotomy or in cases of referred pain. A similar hyperaesthesia for cold or less often for heat sometimes occurs in the chest of tabetic patients. Hyperalgesia, where a normally painless stimulus becomes transformed into an acutely painful sensation, may be regarded as a form of 'tenderness' in the chest. This occurs in patients suffering from anxiety states, often with added depression. Further, perversions of sensation sometimes occur in organic nervous diseases, such as syringomyelia or tabes.

Tenderness of the chest may occur in *pleurisy*. The tenderness is as a rule deeply seated and not in the skin and subcutaneous tissues. However, chest wall pain can mimic pleurisy and conditions in the chest wall can cause confusion. Tenderness due to strain or tearing of thoracic muscles can be severe and painful, may be exacerbated by coughing and confused with pleurisy.

The sternum may be tender as the result of *mediastinal inflammation, tumour* or *aneurysm*. The diagnosis in these cases is made by physical and X-ray examination. Tenderness with pain over the precordium may occur in *pericarditis*, accompanied usually by a pericardial rub. It may be so severe as to preclude percussion or even the application of a stethoscope. Similar pain and tenderness may also be found in the epigastrium and upper costal angles.

Chest tenderness is sometimes found in cases of *acute* or *chronic disease of the lungs*, particularly *tuberculosis*. The tenderness may be either superficial or deep. It is generally felt most about the region of the apices of the lungs, the curve of the shoulder or the scapula. Similar tenderness is met with occasionally in *acute bronchitis* or in *chronic bronchitis* and *emphysema*. Tenderness along the lower chest wall anteriorly may be found after vigorous coughing, probably from trauma in the soft tissues, the muscles particularly. A rib may be fractured by vigorous coughing.

Direct tenderness about the precordium is almost never due to *heart disease*. It is more generally associated with cardiac neurosis than with organic heart disease. Tenderness at the area of the apex beat is common in the Da Costa syndrome ('soldiers' heart' or 'neurocirculatory asthenia'), a nervous condition in which there is no cardiac abnormality. The tenderness, which may be extreme, felt by some patients with heart disease, such as mitral stenosis, at the cardiac apex is due to anxiety rather than to an organic lesion.

Tenderness in the right side of the chest near the costal margin is not rare in *diseases of the liver* and *gallbladder* corresponding to the cutaneous distribution of the D7, D8 and D9 nerves; for the most part, however, the pain and tenderness are in the epigastrium and the right hypochondrium. The right phrenic nerve (C3–5) sends branches to the liver and gallbladder so that tenderness and pain may also be felt in the right shoulder as in the case of disorders of the diaphragm. It is particularly in cases of gallstone or biliary colic that these areas of tenderness are likely to be found. In patients with hepatic abscess the spread of inflammation to the chest wall may give rise directly to pain and tenderness.

P. R. Studdy

Cheyne–Stokes Respiration

This well-known abnormality of respiration, described independently by John Cheyne in 1818 and William Stokes in 1846, is probably referred to in the Hippocratic writings in an account of a patient whose breathing was 'like that of a man recollecting himself, and rare and large'.

Cheyne–Stokes respiration, the commonest form of periodic breathing, consists of alternating periods of apnoea and hyperventilation, beginning with hardly perceptible movements, gradually increasing until the tidal volume is much above normal, and then dying away to end in apnoea (*Fig.* C.23). The apnoeic period lasts for 10–30 seconds or more and the hyperpnoeic phase comprises thirty or more breaths and usually lasts between 1 and 3 minutes. The condition is obvious to the experienced observer but an untrained person will often describe the hyperpnoeic phase as 'breathlessness'. The patient may be unaware of the breathing abnormality. As Cheyne–Stokes breathing is accentuated during sleep the hyperpnoea may disturb the patient's sleep and the symptoms may be confused with those of paroxysmal nocturnal dyspnoea due to cardiac failure.

The mechanism responsible for Cheyne–Stokes breathing is complex. In health there is an oscillating balance between changes in arterial blood gas tensions and respiratory drive. The system is controlled by peripheral and central chemoreceptors whose rate of response is dependent upon the time it takes the circulation to carry arterial blood from the lungs to the carotid bodies and to the brain. The effect of these functional changes is most apparent when the predominant regulator for breathing is by the chemical control system that occurs in non-REM sleep. Thus in stages 1 and 2 of non-REM sleep periodic breathing is normal and is initiated by a change in the homoeostatic set point for ventilation induced by the onset of sleep. Physiological periodic breathing is accentuated at altitude.

Pathologically Cheyne–Stokes respiration, which is an extreme form of periodic breathing, occurs almost exclusively during non-REM sleep and typically ceases during REM sleep. Periodic breathing commonly signifies cerebral or cardiac disease and is most common following a stroke or in cases of left ventricular failure. At least three mechanisms have been postulated. Firstly, in patients with an increased respiratory drive due to chronic hypoxaemia, a further fall in arterial oxygen gas tension (PaO_2) at the onset of sleep may result in periodic breathing by a mechanism analogous to that occuring in healthy subjects at altitude. Secondly there is an inevitable circulatory delay in $PaCO_2$ changes produced by altered ventilation and the detection of blood gas changes by the central chemoreceptors. The lung to brain circulation time may be prolonged in certain cardiac or cerebrovascular diseases. Thirdly the chemoceptors may be over-responsive to changes in PaO_2 due to loss of normal inhibitory influences on the metabolic control system, such as may occur in bilateral pyramidal tract destruction.

Thus in normal subjects, voluntary hyperventilation with air will lead to a short period of apnoea followed by a few cycles of Cheyne–Stokes breathing. It is therefore possible to reduce the $PaCO_2$ to such a level that even a healthy respiratory centre fails to discharge normally; this does not occur after hyperventilation with 5 per cent CO_2. The slow decline in arterial oxygen saturation and rise in carbon dioxide during the apnoea begins to stimulate the respiratory centre and respiration is resumed either normally or leading to a second fall in $PaCO_2$ with repetition of the cycle. The changes in the blood gases during the cycle are shown in *Fig.* C.24.

Cheyne–Stokes respiration occurs in normal subjects not only after hyperventilation but also at high

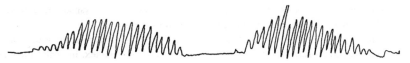

Fig. C.23. Spirogram from a patient with severe cerebral vascular disease. Two cycles of Cheyne–Stokes breathing are shown, over a period of 143 seconds.

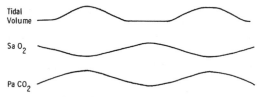

Fig. C.24. Diagram of changes in tidal volume, arterial oxygen saturation (SaO_2) and partial pressure of carbon dioxide in arterial blood ($PaCO_2$) over two cycles of Cheyne–Stokes breathing.

altitude where the hypoxic stimulus to respiration reduces the $PaCO_2$. It may also be seen in apparently healthy elderly subjects during sleep; it is difficult however to exclude minor degrees of cardiac or cerebrovascular disease causing depression of the respiratory centre in such cases. In clinical practice the commonest cause is left ventricular failure; hyperventilation is the mechanism. Periodic breathing occurs especially in patients with degenerative arterial disease in whom the blood supply to the brainstem may be reduced as a result of the low cardiac output and local arterial disease. Cheyne-Stokes respiration is commonly regarded as indicating a poor prognosis in left ventricular failure, but it may disappear with treatment for the failure and, rarely, may persist for many months in patients in whom the other symptoms and signs of failure are unimpressive.

Bronchopneumonia or other respiratory infections may also precipitate Cheyne-Stokes breathing in the elderly. However, it must be realized that in chronic respiratory failure in which a raised rather than a lowered $PaCO_2$ is the rule, Cheyne-Stokes respiration does not occur. Occasionally there may be a few cycles in the recovery period following a Stokes–Adams attack. Respiration continues during the period of circulatory arrest and the first blood to enter the cerebral circulation after cardiac action is resumed contains very little carbon dioxide. The sensitivity of the respiratory centre is reduced by hypoxia during the circulatory arrest and this combines with the hypocapnia to cause Cheyne-Stokes breathing. Rarely Cheyne-Stokes breathing is complicated by cardiac dysrhythmias, including junctional rhythm and atrioventricular block, which occur intermittently in phase with the respiratory dysrhythmia; the mechanism is unknown.

Primary depression of the respiratory centre in the absence of much change in the $PaCO_2$ can also cause Cheyne-Stokes respiration. Thus it occurs in many diseases of the central nervous system. These include cerebral vascular disease with or without hae-

morrhage or thrombosis, cerebral tumours especially those involving the brainstem, and severe head injuries. Cheyne-Stokes respiration is always more prominent during sleep and can be precipitated by the administration of narcotic hypnotic drugs such as morphine or occasionally benzodiazepines. It is also seen quite often in uraemia but is probably not due to the renal failure *per se*. Hyperventilation in renal failure is caused by acidosis, the effect of which persists despite the fall in $PaCO_2$. Left ventricular failure resulting from renal hypertension may be responsible for Cheyne-Stokes breathing in this situation although it may occur in patients whose blood pressure is normal.

Cheyne-Stokes respiration may be confused with other periodic breathing patterns which typically show a shorter, less symmetrical, and regular contour. In pontine brainstem lesions or if the intracranial pressure is raised abrupt short clusters of hypernoiec breathing may be interrupted by abrupt spasms of apnoea (Biot's breathing). Ataxic respiration may be seen with medullary lesions which can provoke a grossly irregular breathing pattern. Respiratory apraxis is recognised by a monotonously regular pattern of breathing which cannot be modified and is seen in the 'locked in' syndrome when subjects suffer bilateral pyramidal lesions. Central neurogenic hyperventilation is seen occasionally in midbrain lesions.

P. R. Studdy

Choreiform movements

Chorea is derived from the Greek word for 'dance' and refers to involuntary arrhythmic movements of a forceful, rapid and jerky type, in contrast to the slow writhing and repetitive spasms of athetosis. The movements may be simple or elaborate and may vary in site. They are purposeless, but the patient may be able to incorporate them into a deliberate movement, as if to make them less noticeable, when they are called 'semipurposive'. The movements may affect the face, causing grimacing; there may be movements of the tongue and also peculiar grunting sounds on respiration. Normal volitional movements are possible but frequently are interrupted by the involuntary movement. Muscle tone is often reduced and reflex testing may be interrupted by involuntary movements.

It is frequently difficult to dissociate chorea from the slower, writhing movements of athetosis, and the term 'choreoathetosis' is sometimes used to describe involuntary movements which have characteristics of both. It is also important to differentiate chorea from myoclonus, the distinguishing features being that myoclonus is much more rapid than chorea and that it involves single muscles or part of a muscle as opposed to groups of muscles as in chorea.

Chorea is classically seen in *Sydenham's chorea*, a disease associated with rheumatic fever and with the finding of Aschoff nodules within the deep grey matter of the brain. The involuntary movements, which may affect any of the muscles of the body, are made worse by attempted voluntary movement, excitement and by the maintenance of posture. Testing of the upper and lower limbs may appear to demonstrate marked incoordination, but the differentiation from true cerebellar ataxia is evident from the absence of intention tremor. *Chorea gravidarum* is a form of chorea which occurs during pregnancy and which has been reported in patients taking oral contraceptives. It may have some relationship to Sydenham's chorea and may be a manifestation of an earlier episode of rheumatic fever.

Huntington's Chorea is an inherited autosomal dominant disorder in which patients show dementia and involuntary movements. The latter tend to be a mixture of chorea and choreoathetotic posturing. Intoxication with *phenothiazine* drugs or haloperidol is another, although relatively rare, cause of chorea. *Hyperthyroidism* and *cerebral arteritis* are other rare causes.

The involuntary movements seen in patients with Parkinson's disease on treatment with L-dopa may also resemble chorea, though again the movements are more typical of choreoathetosis than of true chorea.

Chorea of a peculiarly violent type in its initial stages, and limited to the proximal muscles of one side of the body, is called *hemiballismus*. It is seen in elderly patients, frequently with diabetes mellitus, who suffer small vascular lesions within the contralateral subthalamic nucleus of Luys. The syndrome begins abruptly but the movements tend to decrease in magnitude and the patient may be left only with minor irregular flexion or extension movements of the wrists and fingers.

Senile chorea is sometimes used to describe the development of involuntary movements in the sixth and seventh decades. Patients do not show any evidence of dementing illness and although it is possible that this represents a forme fruste of Huntington's chorea, it carries a more benign prognosis.

Congenital chorea is sometimes seen in association with congenital hemiplegia and diplegia, but is less common than congenital athetosis. Choreoathetosis in the young may be seen in the rare familial Lesch-Nyhan syndrome in which involuntary movements are associated with spasticity, mental handicap, aggressive behaviour, self-injury and hyperuricaemia.

Choreiform movements are rare in hysteria except in young adults who have previously suffered from Sydenham's chorea. Psychogenic tics may occasionally be mistaken for chorea, but the former are repetitive and stereotyped unlike the constantly changing pattern of the latter.

The anatomical basis of chorea is not certain. In Huntington's disease there are obvious lesions in the caudate nucleus and putamen, but other patients may be seen with pathological damage to the same nuclei and yet without chorea. It is assumed that chorea and hemiballismus are related to disorders of the same neuronal system.

D. Bates

CLAUDICATION, INTERMITTENT
See LEG, PAIN IN.

Clonus

Clonus refers to a series of rhythmic, monophasic contractions and relaxations of a group of muscles. Myoclonus is the term used to describe abrupt contractions of a group of muscles which are irregular in rhythm and amplitude and usually asynchronous and asymmetrical. If such contractions occur singly, or only a few times, in a restricted group of muscles, they are referred to as segmental myoclonus; but if they are widespread and repetitive they are called polymyoclonus or myoclonus multiplex.

1. Clonus in Upper Motor Neurone Lesions

The hyperreflexic state that characterises spasticity after damage to the upper motor neurones of the corticospinal tract is due to sustained hyperexcitability of alpha and gamma motor neurones below the site of the lesion. Clonus, a series of rhythmic involuntary muscle contractions occurring at a frequency of 5–7 Hz in response to an abruptly applied and sustained stretch stimulus, is frequently seen at the ankle and may also be elicited at the patella. It depends for its elicitation upon voluntary relaxation of the muscles, the integrity of the spinal stretch reflex mechanisms, sustained hyperexcitability of the alpha and gamma motor neurones, and synchronization of the contraction-relaxation cycle of the muscle spindles.

Several beats of clonus (less than 5 or 6) may be elicited normally at the ankle by abrupt dorsiflexion of the foot. More numerous beats, or sustained clonus, imply an upper motor neurone lesion above the level of the first sacral segment and it will usually occur in association with an extensor plantar reflex. When the upper motor neurone lesion is above the third and fourth lumbar motor neurone pool, patellar clonus may also be elicited.

2. Palatal Myoclonus

This rhythmic clonus causes rapid elevation of the uvula and palate between 60 and 100 times per minute. Sometimes muscles of the pharynx, face and eyes may also be involved, and rarely the diaphragm and vocal cords. The condition is seen when lesions interrupt the central tegmental tracts in the brainstem, presumably disinhibiting the inferior olivary nucleus. It has recently been suggested that palatal myoclonus occurs when denervation affects the nucleus ambiguus and the dorsal lateral reticular formation adjacent to it. The cause may be vascular or demyelinating.

3. Epilepsia Partialis continua (EPC)

Epilepsia partialis continua is another form of rhythmic clonus in which one group of muscles is involved in a series of monophasic contractions which may continue for weeks, months or years. The disorder is believed to be cerebral in origin and is commonly vascular in aetiology. It may be associated with EEG abnormality and is usually resistant to therapy.

4. Opsoclonus and Body Tremulousness

There is a condition in which clonus or marked dysmetria of the eyes is associated with unsteadiness and often extreme tremulousness. This syndrome is believed to be postviral in origin, though it may occur in the young as a paraneoplastic complication of neuroblastoma, and it has also been reported in adults as a paraneoplastic complication of breast malignancy.

5. Myoclonus Simplex

This is either a single contraction or several rapid contractions of muscles in a part of the body and may occur physiologically just before sleep or may be seen in patients with seizures. In one form of childhood epilepsy, benign Rolandic epilepsy, myoclonic jerks occur unilaterally. Myoclonus may also be seen with petit mal and akinetic seizures in the Lennox-Gastaut syndrome in children.

Monophasic myoclonus involving the legs may occur frequently during the night and disturb sleep; this situation is distinct from the physiological nocturnal startle and from the restless legs syndrome of Ekbom.

6. Myoclonus Multiplex

A. PARAMYOCLONUS MULTIPLEX

This condition, first described by Friedreich, is a sporadic form of widespread muscle jerking in adult life. The twitches may be symmetrical, may vary in site and commonly occur when the patient is at rest in bed. They are usually prevented by voluntary movement and may vary from being almost unnoticed to being severe enough to throw the patient to the floor. The condition may rarely occur as a familial illness with an autosomal dominant mode of inheritance and it is occasionally progressive.

B. MYOCLONIC EPILEPSY

Myoclonus associated with epilepsy may be seen in several different conditions. Some patients have a progressive illness associated with dementia as in the familial myoclonic epilepsy of *Unverricht* and *Lundborg*. Similarly, myoclonus and epilepsy occur together in childhood and adolescence in *Lafora body* disease. In so-called *Baltic myoclonus*, patients have progressive ataxia accompanied by light sensitive myoclonus and epilepsy.

Some of the storage diseases may cause syndromes which include myoclonus and epilepsy. In children the development of myoclonus, epilepsy and dementia should raise the possibility of *subacute sclerosing panencephalitis* which is a subacute or chronic form of postmeasles encephalitis. In the adult, myoclonus may be seen together with epilepsy and dementia in the spongiform encephalopathies such as *Cruetzfeldt-Jakob* disease. Myoclonus may also be seen with or without epilepsy and altered consciousness in a variety of presumed viral encephalitides.

D. Bates

COMA
See CONSCIOUSNESS, DISORDERS OF.

Confusion

Confusion is the term used to indicate that a subject is temporarily unable to think in a clear and logical fashion. The value of the term in diagnosis is however much diminished by imprecise definition. In a confusional state some or all of the following features are found: an impairment of concentration and attention span with an inability to shift attention to new external stimuli; memory impairments; disorientation in time, space or person; speech which is rambling, irrelevant or incoherent; an impaired ability to properly grasp the meaning or significance of surrounding events. These features are extremely common and are found in a wide range of disorders which fall into the following main categories: *acute confusional states* or *delirium*; *chronic confusional states* (chronic organic reactions or the dementias); *the functional psychoses*; *dissociative states* and other neurotic conditions where features of confusion are brought on by strong emotions in the absence of brain pathology. The term should therefore be considered not as a syndrome but as a convenient clinical description of a certain qualitative change in consciousness. Organic confusional states are usually subdivided according to their mode of onset and duration into acute and chronic conditions.

Acute confusional states

The term acute confusional state and acute brain syndrome should be considered synonymous with delirium even though that term has sometimes been reserved for the more severe forms of confusional states such as those presenting with vivid visual hallucinations. The speech of the delirious person is incoherent and rambling indicating disordered thinking. Questions have to be repeated because the subject's attention is poor. There is a reduced level of consciousness short of actual coma. The onset is usually rapid, the course often fluctuating and the total duration of delirium is brief rarely lasting for as long as a week. There is a disturbance of the sleep–wake cycle. Fearfulness and rapid swings of mood are common. Random picking and plucking bed clothes is often in response to vivid illusionary experiences.

The range of possible causes of delirium is too large to be summarized in detail. These causes frequently lie outside the nervous system and include infectious, metabolic and toxic states. A careful history, complete physical examination and laboratory investigations suggested by the features of the case will generally be sufficient to identify the cause (*Table* C.5).

Chronic confusional states (chronic organic reactions) (*see also* MEMORY, DISORDERS OF)

These are sometimes broadly defined as 'the dementias' and, like acute confusional states, may result from many different pathological processes. The majority of cases are due to diffuse widespread brain pathologies which are often progressive although they may be static following head injury, stroke or subarachnoid haemorrhage, or sometimes reversible if due to a metabolic cause, a benign intracranial tumour or subdural haematoma evacuated surgically (*Table* C.6).

Table C.5. Causes of acute states of confusion (delirium)

Common
Hypoxia (due to cardiac and respiratory disorders)
Metabolic disorders
  Electrolyte imbalances
  Hypoglycaemia
  Uraemia
  Hepatic failure
Systemic infections
  Septicaemia
  Bronchopneumonia
  Urinary tract infections
  Malaria
Cerebral infections
  Meningitis
  Encephalitis
  Brain abscess
Non-infective cerebral causes
  Head injury
  Raised intracranial pressure
  Hypertensive encephalopathy
  Tumours
  Cerebral haemorrhage
  Cerebral embolism
Endocrine disorders
  Diabetic keto-acidosis
  Myxoedema
Thiamine deficiency (Wernicke's encephalopathy)
Vitamin B_{12} deficiency
Substance intoxication and withdrawal
  Alcohol (delirium tremens)
  Barbiturates
  Heroin
  Opiates
  Stimulants (amphetamine, cocaine)
  Digoxin
  Lithium
  Steroids
  L-dopa
Postictal state

Less common
Focal lesions of right parietal lobe
Porphyria
Hyperparathyroidism
Hypoparathyroidism
Hypopituitarism
Cushing's disease

The commonest presenting feature is impairment in short and long-term memory often accompanied by other features of higher cortical dysfunction such as impairment of abstract thinking and judgement. Relatives may notice a gradual personality change and a depressive, irritable, disinhibited or euphoric mood disturbance. The memory loss initially may be mild and most marked for recent events. The person forgets names, loses objects round the house or experiences distressing confusion in unfamiliar surroundings due to loss of spatial memory. As the condition progresses new information is not retained, the person may become forgetful enough to become a danger to themselves leaving tasks undone, taps and switches left on. Impairment in abstract thinking is suggested when the patient cannot cope with new tasks, thinking becomes

Table C.6. Causes of chronic states of confusion

Common
Vascular brain disease
  Subarachnoid haemorrhage
  Subdural haematoma
  Infarct (multi-infarct dementia)
Head injury
Intracranial space occupying lesion
Brain degenerative diseases
  Alzheimer's type dementia
  Huntington's disease
Infections
  Viral encephalitis (including HIV encephalopathy)
Systemic
  Myxoedema
  Anoxia (anaemia, cardiac and respiratory failure)
  Vitamin deficiency (B$_{12}$, folate, thiamine)

Less common
Parkinson's disease
Multiple sclerosis
Pick's disease
Normotensive hydrocephalus
Depressive pseudodementia

Uncommon
Binswanger's leucoencephalopathy
Tertiary syphilis

more literal and concrete and the repertoire of conversation is narrowed. There may be impaired judgement, the person becoming disinhibited with inappropriate behaviour in social situations. Marked disinhibition can be a feature of frontal lobe impairment. Other neurological deficits including aphasias and apraxias are common as are changes in mood usually to depression and irritability.

It is important to consider the onset and course of the illness carefully since the features of acute confusional states (delirium) may overlap with and coexist with chronic states (dementias). Of the chronic progressive conditions usually starting after the age of 40 the most common are Alzheimer's-type dementia and multi-infarct dementia. Alzheimer's-type dementia is diagnosed by the clinical findings and the exclusion of other causes of a progressive dementia. In multi-infarct dementia there may be hypertension and a stepwise progression of impairment with a history of transient ischaemic episodes. CT scan may show old infarcts whereas in Alzheimer's dementia the CT scan may be either normal or show cerebral atrophy and ventricular enlargement.

Metabolic disorders giving rise to chronic confusional states include B$_{12}$, folate and thiamine deficiency. The latter (Wernicke–Korsakoff syndrome) is commonly associated with chronic alcoholism but may be due to gastric carcinoma or malabsorption. Cerebral anoxia due to anaemia, respiratory or cardiovascular disease also causes symptoms of confusion.

Brain degenerative conditions giving rise to dementia include Huntington's chorea, which is an autosomal dominant condition usually presenting, in the age range 35–45 years, with involuntary movements and cognitive changes. A proportion of patients with *multiple sclerosis* develop a steadily progressive illness with severe impairment of higher cortical function. There are usually other signs and symptoms disseminated in time and place. In *normotensive hydrocephalus* a dementia is typically accompanied by apraxic gait and urinary incontinence. *Pick's disease* is a rare condition developing usually in older patients typically with a marked personality change consistent with frontal lobe impairment and a speech disorder which progresses to mutism. Signs of cognitive impairment are found in *Parkinson's disease* especially in older patients who have had the condition for a long time. *Binswanger's leucoencephalopathy* is a very rare progressive degenerative disease with focal signs and hypertension.

Central nervous system infections which give rise to features of dementia include viral encephalitis. The human immunodeficiency virus is neurotropic as well as lymphotropic and people with AIDS may develop a confusional state with fever leading to a state of lethargy, apathy and ataxia due to a subacute encephalopathy. *Tertiary syphilis* is now quite uncommon. *Creutzfeldt–Jakob spongiform encephalopathy* caused by a transmissable agent is also quite rare and has features including limb weakness with spasticity, myoclonus and other movement disturbances. EEG changes are common.

Psychiatric illness can present as confusion. Schizophrenia which may remain undiagnosed until relatively late in life can present with a degree of intellectual deterioration, impaired volition, disordered thinking and confused speech. A detailed history may reveal a family history or earlier episodes of psychotic illness and memory loss is not a feature. The condition of patients with major depressive illness presenting with poor memory, impoverished thinking and reduced intellectual abilities may mimic an organic dementia. This condition of *pseudodementia*, diagnosed by careful history taking care from the patient and relatives, should be born in mind in every case of 'dementia' as it is often completely treatable by conventional anti-depressant therapy. Very rarely a *factitious disorder* may mimic acute or chronic confusional states, but careful assessment will usually reveal inconsistencies in the patient's account of symptoms and their performance in tests of higher cerebral function. Epileptic *twilight states* and automatisms are characterized by an abrupt onset and ending, a duration of hours or rarely days and the occurrence of apparently purposeless acts. The subject has impaired consciousness. A history of seizures and EEG evidence of epileptic activity should be sought and would be essential evidence for a patient facing prosecution for offences claimed to have been perpetrated during a state of epileptic automatism.

D. Blackwood

Consciousness, disorders of

Consciousness is the state of awareness of the self and the environment when provided with adequate stimuli. Patients who are in normal wakefulness will be fully responsive to stimuli and will display correct behaviour and speech in response to these stimuli. Physiological changes in consciousness occur during sleep when the patient may be easily aroused by external stimuli. Pathological impairment of consciousness occurs in states of injury, disease or intoxication.

A useful measure to assess level of consciousness is the Glasgow Coma Scale (*Fig.* C.25). It is based on observation of levels of response to graded stimuli in three modes—eye opening, motor function and verbal utterance. In the first, spontaneous eye opening and blinking score the highest grade, eye opening in response to voice the next highest, eye opening in response to painful stimuli the next, and finally no response of eye opening to stimuli the lowest. The highest motor response is voluntary movement to command, followed by localizing response to painful stimuli, withdrawal from painful stimuli, a pathological flexor response, sometimes called decorticate, a pathological extensor response sometimes called decerebrate, and finally no response at all to pain. In terms of verbal response, the highest level is orientated conversation, the next disorientated conversation, followed by the use of occasional recognizable words, no recognizable words but groaning in response to pain, and finally no response of a verbal nature. By allocating a score in each of these categories the level of consciousness of the individual patient may be recorded and monitored in order to measure progress.

Several terms are used to define altered states of consciousness:

1. Confusion

Confusion, or clouding of consciousness, is characterized by an impaired capacity to think clearly and to perceive, respond to and remember current stimuli. There is usually disorientation. There may be a gradation between an initial clouding of consciousness and a more profound confusional state in which the main elements are reduced attention, an inability to express thoughts clearly together with a defect in memory and drowsiness. The differential diagnosis is from patients with dysphasia, an amnesic syndrome, an acute psych-

Eyes open
- Spontaneously
- To speech
- To pain
- Never

Best verbal response
- Orientated
- Confused
- Inappropriate words
- Incomprehensible sounds
- None

Best motor response
- Obeys commands
- Localizes pain
- Flexion to pain
- Extension to pain
- None

Fig. C.25. Glasgow Coma Scale

osis or severe retarded depression. Patients with confusion frequently have a generalized disturbance of cerebral function which may be associated with widespread EEG changes. A reduction in cerebral oxygen consumption, has been demonstrated in such patients. Confusion is most commonly the result of toxic or metabolic abnormalities and it occurs particularly in the elderly.

2. Delirium

A state of severely disturbed consciousness with motor restlessness, disorientation and delusions. Patients are out of touch with reality, frightened, irritable, and frequently have visual hallucinations. Delirium is associated with a diffusely abnormal EEG and is commonly seen with toxic and metabolic disorders. It may be mimicked by degenerative brain disease, acute psychosis or hypomania, but patients with these conditions do not usually show the depressed alertness which is a cardinal feature of delirium. Both confusion and delirium are more common in the elderly. They are more likely to occur when there is underlying degenerative disease and may be the precursor of coma.

3. Stupor

The patient, though not unconscious and still rousable, exhibits little or no spontaneous activity. The patient may seem to be asleep but will not respond to vigorous stimulation and will show relatively limited motor abilities, tending to lapse back into sleep when the stimulus ceases. The differential diagnosis is from catatonic schizophrenia and severe depression; the finding of catatonia, posturing of the limbs or flexibilitas cerea is more common with psychiatric disturbances. In organic stupor the EEG is invariably diffusely abnormal whereas in psychiatric disease it will usually be normal. The exception to this is Gjessing's syndrome in which periodic stupor may occur with minor EEG abnormalities.

4. Coma

This is a condition of absolute unconsciousnesses judged by the absence of any psychologically understandable response to external stimulus or internal need. It may more simply be defined as a state of 'unrousable unconsciousness'. The patient will appear to be asleep but is incapable of sensing or responding normally to external stimuli. The condition may vary in depth from the deepest levels in which there will be no eye opening, motor or verbal response, to a level in which there may be eye opening to pain, a weak flexor response of the limbs to pain and groaning, without recognizable words, in response to pain.

States of altered consciousness will be seen in patients who have suffered from *head injury*, *intoxication* with drugs or alcohol, *metabolic* disturbances, *infections* or *vascular* disturbances, and as the result of *hypoxic* or *ischaemic injuries*.

Rarely patients without evident organic illness may appear to have disturbances of consciousness, or pseudocoma. The distinction between pseudocoma and organic disease may be established by testing the oculo-vestibular reflex in response to the instillation of ice water into the external auditory meatus. In patients in organic coma, the normal reaction of nystagmus will not been seen, but in patients with pseudocoma, nystagmus will occur and the patients will usually reveal their responsiveness.

D. Bates

Constipation

A. Acute

Acute constipation may be: (1) due to acute intestinal obstruction; (2) a symptom of some general disease or of some other acute abdominal disease; or (3) due to a sudden alteration in daily habits, e.g. admission to hospital.

1. Acute intestinal obstruction

The following points help in the distinction between acute intestinal obstruction and severe cases of acute constipation of other origin:

a   In other conditions the constipation is incomplete, in that flatus, and even a small quantity of faeces, may be passed spontaneously. A rectal examination should always be made. In organic intestinal obstruction the rectum is usually empty. If it contains faeces these may be present below an obstruction or, if impacted, may themselves be responsible for the occlusion, but it is exceedingly rare for faecal impaction to produce symptoms quite comparable in severity with those due

to acute obstruction. In doubtful cases, it used to be the custom to carry out the two-enema test; the first enema generally brought away a certain amount of faeces even if obstruction was complete; the second, given at an interval of half to one hour, resulted in the passage of faeces or flatus if obstruction was incomplete, whereas, in complete obstruction, the second enema was either retained or expelled unaltered. This test should never be employed; it is exhausting to the patient, time wasting, and the information obtained is often equivocal. Diagnosis can usually be made on clinical grounds supplemented by abdominal radiographs.

b   Vomiting is rarely a feature of constipation, whereas it is frequently present in small-bowel obstruction, and in late cases becomes faeculent.

c   Visible peristalsis, accompanied by noisy borborygmi, is never present except in obstruction.

d   Obstruction is accompanied by progressive distension of the abdomen.

e   Pain is usually the first symptom of intestinal obstruction and is colicky in nature; its severity is out of all proportion to the mild abdominal discomfort that may accompany simple constipation.

Plain radiographs of the abdomen are essential in the diagnosis of intestinal obstruction and in attempting to localize its site. A loop or loops of distended bowel are usually seen, together with multiple fluid levels. Small bowel is suggested by a ladder pattern of distended loops, by their central position, and by striations which pass completely across the width of the distended loop and which are produced by its circular mucosal folds (*Fig.* C.26). Distended large bowel tends to lie peripherally and to show the corrugations produced by the taenia coli (*Fig.* C.27). A small percentage, perhaps 5 per cent of intestinal obstructions, shows no abnormality on plain radiographs. This is due to the bowel being completely distended with fluid in a closed loop and thus without the fluid levels which are produced by coexistent gas.

AETIOLOGY OF ACUTE INTESTINAL OBSTRUCTION

The causes of intestinal obstruction may be classified as:

a. In the lumen—faecal impaction, gallstone ileus, pedunculated tumour and meconium ileus.

b. In the wall—congenital atresia, Crohn's disease, tumours, diverticular disease of the colon and tuberculous stricture.

c. Outside the wall—strangulated hernia (external or internal), volvulus, intussusception, adhesions and bands.

Before considering any other possibility, all the hernial apertures should be examined, even in the absence of local pain, as a small strangulated femoral hernia in an obese woman, for example, may easily be overlooked.

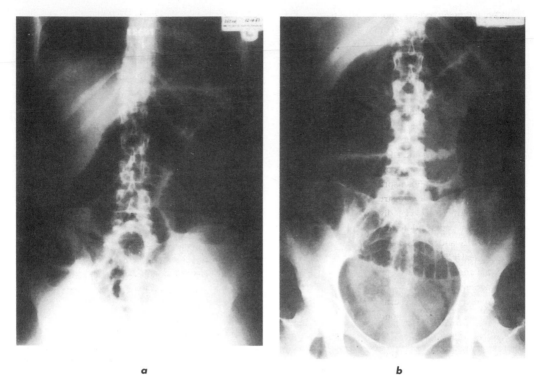

a   *b*

Fig. C.26. Small bowel obstruction due a band. *a* Erect showing fluid levels. *b* Supine showing ladder pattern of distended small bowel loops, the valvulae conniventes make complete bands across the width of the gut.

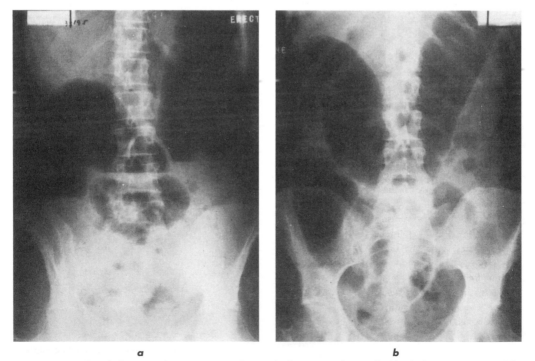

a   *b*

Fig. C.27. Large bowel obstruction due to carcinoma of sigmoid colon. *a* Erect showing fluid levels. *b* Supine gas distend the colon and caecum, the haustrae make incomplete bands across the width of the gut.

The following points should be considered in determining the cause of the acute intestinal obstruction.

i. Age

Intestinal obstruction in the newborn should always be suspected in the presence of bile-vomiting; the rectum should be examined first for the presence of an imperforate anus; other possibilities are congenital atresia or stenosis of the intestine, volvulus neonatorum, meconium ileus and Hirschsprung's disease. In infants the commonest cause of intestinal obstruction is intussusception, but Hirschsprung's disease, strangulated inguinal hernia, and obstruction due to a band from the tip of a Meckel's diverticulum should be considered. In young adults and patients of middle age, adhesions and bands from previous surgery or intraperitoneal inflammation are common, but strangulated hernia and Crohn's disease are also encountered. In older patients strangulated hernias, carcinoma of the bowel and diverticular disease, as well as postoperative adhesions, are all common conditions.

ii. History

The history of a previous abdominal operation, or of inflammatory pelvic disease in females, suggest the possibility of bands or adhesions. A history of biliary colic or of the symptoms which may result from cholecystitis may suggest that obstruction might be due to impaction of a gallstone in the ileum. Obstruction following a period of increasing constipation, perhaps with blood or slime in the stools or spurious diarrhoea, in a middle-aged or elderly patient, suggests cancer or diverticular disease of the colon. The history in an infant or child that blood and mucus have been passed per rectum is suggestive of an intussusception.

iii. Abdominal examination

We have already mentioned the importance of searching specifically for a strangulated hernia. The presence of a recent or old laparotomy scar always raises the possibility of postoperative adhesions. Gross distension generally means that the obstruction is in the colon; if occurring very soon after the onset of symptoms it suggests volvulus of the sigmoid or, less commonly, the caecum. If distension has been present to a less extent for some time before the onset of acute symptoms, a growth is likely. In infants and small children great distension suggests Hirschsprung's disease. Slight distension occurs when the obstruction is in the duodenum or high in the jejunum.

The diagnosis of intussusception can be made with certainty only when the characteristic sausage-shaped tumour situated somewhere in the course of the colon is felt. In acute obstruction due to cancer the tumour is often not palpable as it may be disguised by the dilated intestine; however, large masses are sometimes felt, especially when present in the right or left iliac fossa. On the right side, they are generally due to cancer of the caecum, on the left to cancer of the sigmoid colon or diverticular disease.

iv. Rectal examination

A growth of the rectum should be recognized easily, although this is rather unusual as a cause of obstruction. Sometimes a growth of the pelvic colon can be felt through the front wall of the rectum. In infants, the tip of an intussusception may be felt in the lumen of the rectum and the typical red-current jelly stool (a mixture of blood and mucus) will be seen on the examining finger. Occasionally the mother will report that a sausage-like structure actually prolapses from the child's anal verge during the attacks of colic accompanying the intussusception. I have only seen this on one occasion. A much-ballooned rectum suggests obstruction in the colon; this is an undoubted fact but its cause is obscure.

v. Vomiting

The more frequent the vomiting and the earlier the onset of faeculent vomiting the higher in the intestine is the obstruction likely to be. Its onset is later and its occurrence less frequent in cases of colonic obstruction.

2. Symptomatic

A. In acute general diseases

Constipation beginning acutely is a frequent symptom of a large variety of acute infective and other diseases. It is never so severe as to become a presenting symptom and the other features in the majority of cases are so much more striking that the presence of constipation has little influence on making a diagnosis.

B. In acute abdominal conditions

Constipation is a conspicuous symptom in most acute abdominal conditions. However, once again, other symptoms are often so well marked that the question of intestinal obstruction hardly arises. Thus it frequently accompanies acute appendicitis, salpingitis, perforation of a peptic ulcer, and biliary and renal colic. In lead colic the constipation is not absolute and the occupation of the patient, the blue line on the gums, and the presence of punctate basophilia point to the diagnosis.

3. Changes of daily routine

These may precipitate constipation as in patients admitted to hospital, children going to boarding school, or patients suddenly being confined to bed from illness.

B. Chronic

Constipation can be defined as delay in the passage of faeces through the large bowel and is frequently associated with difficulty in defecation. Most people empty the bowel once in every 24 hours, but there is a considerable range of variation in perfectly normal individuals; in one study of a large working population this varied from three bowel actions daily to one act every three days.

The abnormal action of the bowel in constipation may manifest itself in three different ways:

1   Defecation may occur with insufficient frequency.
2   The stools may be insufficient in quantity and a certain amount of faeces is retained although the bowels may be opened once daily or more often (cumulative constipation).
3   The bowels may be open daily yet the faeces are hard and dry owing to prolonged retention in the bowel, dehydration, or insufficient residue in the food consumed.

The commoner causes of constipation are as follows:

1   Organic obstructions, for example carcinoma of the colon or diverticular disease.
2   Painful anal conditions, e.g. fissure in ano or prolapsed piles.
3   Adynamic bowel as may occur in Hirschsprung's disease, senility, spinal cord injuries and diseases, and myxoedema.
4   Drugs which decrease peristaltic activity of the bowel—including codeine, probanthine and other ganglion-blocking agents, and morphine.
5   Habit and diet, for example dehydration, starvation, lack of suitable bulk in the diet, and dyschezia.

It is comparatively rare for a patient to consult a doctor on account of constipation without having already attempted to cure himself with aperients. The symptoms generally ascribed to 'auto-intoxication' caused by intestinal stasis are usually really caused by the purgatives themselves, which may produce depletion of sodium and potassium in the resultant watery stools, or from the abdominal colic and flatulence produced by powerful aperients.

In spite of his probable protests, the patient is instructed to see what happens if no drugs are taken for a few days, an attempt being made to open the bowels each morning on a normal diet containing plenty of fruit and vegetables. In most cases he loses his abdominal pains and so-called 'toxic' symptoms. During this test the bowels are often opened daily, in which case a diagnosis of functional pseudoconstipation can be made, the patient having suggested to himself, as a result of faulty education combined with advice of his friends and with the reading pernicious advertisements, that he was constipated and required aperients to keep himself well; whereas a little psychotherapy in the form of explanation of the physiology of his bowels and the origin of his symptoms, and persuasion to try to open his bowels each morning without artificial help results in a cure.

The investigation of constipation entails a careful and accurate history, full examination including, of course, examination of the rectum and sigmoidoscopy, followed, in some cases, by special laboratory tests and a barium-enema X-ray examination.

Organic obstructions

The two common causes of narrowing of the lumen of the large bowel are diverticular disease and carcinoma of the colon. Other non-malignant strictures are rare but include Crohn's disease of the large bowel, stricture complicating ulcerative colitis and tuberculous stricture.

Organic stricture of the colon is most commonly due to carcinoma. The possibility of cancer should always be considered when an individual above the age of 40, whose bowels have been regular previously, without change of diet or habit develops constipation of increasing severity, or when a patient who is habitually constipated becomes more so without obvious reason. The constipation is at first intermittent and may alternate with diarrhoea, or rather with a frequent desire to go to stool without effective evacuation. Aperients become steadily less helpful. There may be colicky pain and episodes of distension and the patient may notice blood, pus, and mucus in the faeces. Examination of the abdomen may reveal a palpable mass due to the presence of the tumour itself or to inspissated faeces which have become impacted above a cancerous stricture which is itself impalpable. Progressive loss of weight and strength, anorexia and anemia are rather late features of the disease. A rectal examination reveals a usually empty rectum but not infrequently a carcinoma in the sigmoid colon can be felt through the rectal wall as the mass in this loop of bowel prolapses into the pelvis. An occult blood test on any faecal material is often positive. Sigmoidoscopy or colonoscopy may visualize the tumour and its nature can be confirmed by biopsy and histological examination. A barium-enema examination is invaluable (*Fig. C.28*).

DIVERTICULAR DISEASE of the sigmoid colon can mimic carcinoma exactly and indeed the surgeon, even at laparotomy, may not be able to differentiate between the two conditions. The barium-enema examination (*Fig. C.29*) is often helpful, but the radiologist may have difficulty himself in distinguishing a stricture due to one or other cause; indeed not infrequently these two common diseases may co-exist. Again, colonoscopy will often be useful in making the differential diagnosis.

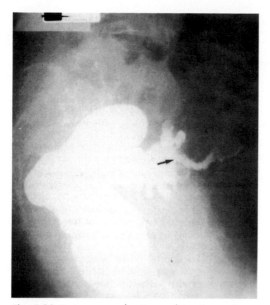

Fig. C.28. Barium enema showing an obstructing carcinoma of the sigmoid colon (arrowed). Note that the patient also has diverticulosis—not an uncommon combination.

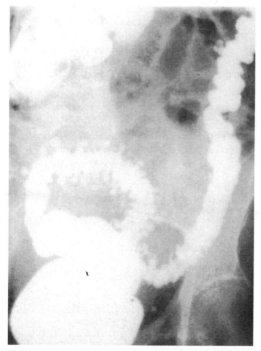

Fig. C.29. Extensive diverticulosis of the sigmoid colon.

Occasionally extracolonic masses may press upon the rectum or sigmoid colon with resultant constipation; for example, the pregnant uterus, a mass of fibroids, a large ovarian cyst or other pelvic tumours.

Painful anal conditions

When defecation is painful, reflex spasm of the anal sphincter may be produced with resultant acute constipation. A local cause of the pain such as a fissure in ano, strangulated haemorrhoids or a perianal abscess is obvious on careful local examination of the anal verge and surrounds.

Adynamic bowel

In Hirschsprung's disease there is always a history of constipation dating from the first few months of life. The abdomen becomes greatly enlarged soon after birth and the outline of distended colon can be seen, often with visible peristalsis. The abdomen finally becomes enormous and it is then tense and tympanitic. There may be eversion of the umbilicus and marked widening of the subcostal angle. The condition is due to the absence of ganglion cells in the wall of the rectosigmoid region of the large bowel, although in some cases a more extensive part of the colon may be involved. Males are affected more often than females.

A barium-enema examination reveals gross dilatation of the colon leading down to a narrow funnel in the aganglionic rectum (*Fig.* C.30).

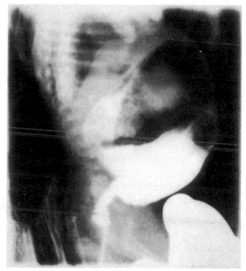

Fig. C.30. Barium enema in a case of Hirschsprung's disease showing enormous dilatation of the pelvic colon proximal to the narrow aganglionic segment of rectum (*Dr T.H. Hills.*)

Deficient motor activity of the bowel may be due to senile changes in the elderly and may be a prominent feature of myxoedemic patients. Constipation may occur in the course of organic nervous diseases, including tabes dorsalis, spinal compression from tumour, transverse myelitis, and disseminated sclerosis, as well as cord transection in trauma. This is due to disturbance of the motor and sensory pathways responsible for defecation.

Drugs

Many commonly employed drugs have a constipating effect on the bowel; these include codeine, morphine and the ganglion-blocking agents. Constipation accompanied by abdominal pain may be a feature of lead poisoning.

Habit and diet

By far the greatest number of patients complaining of constipation fall into this group. When the faeces are abnormally hard as a result of dehydration, inadequate liquid intake or inadequate cellulose material in the diet, rectal examination will reveal impacted faeces of rocklike consistency. This may occur as an acute phenomenon following barium-meal examination when masses of inspissated barium may lodge in the rectum.

Dyschezia

Dyschezia is the term applied to difficulty in defecation due to faulty bowel habit. The patient ignores the normal call to stool, the rectum distends with faeces with eventual loss of the defecation reflex. The very same patient who gets into this habit is probably one who lives on the modern synthetic diet grossly deficient in roughage. As we have mentioned above, the so-called symptoms of constipation usually result from the purgatives that the patient ingests when he becomes anxious about the scarcity of his bowel actions. Rectal examination in such individuals often reveals large amounts of faeces in the rectum and more scybala may be palpated in the sigmoid colon. Dyschezia is, of course, present in those patients who have to remove faeces from the rectum digitally.

Harold Ellis

Contractures and deformities of the upper and lower limbs

(*See also* FOOT AND TOES, DEFORMITIES OF)

Lower limb

Lower limb contractures occur in:

1   Post-trauma states,
2   Spastic conditions—upper motor neurone lesions
3   Flaccid paralysis—lower motor neurone lesions and peripheral nerve injuries
4   Joint disease and injury
5   Growth disorders
6   Muscle dystrophies and primary muscle disease and damage.

1. Trauma

Malunion of fractures may leave a deformity. The femur may be left in varus, the tibia may be bowed into any deformity and fractures malunited around the knee and ankle are potent causes of joint deformity.

2. The spastic lower limb

Cerebral palsy due to birth trauma will produce spasticity in the limbs—quadriplegia, diplegia or a monoparesis. Contractures frequently follow (*see Fig.* F.259). Treatment is by stretching and physical therapy, splintage with orthoses and sometimes surgical releases. Upper motor neurone lesions producing similar spastic states may occur in postmeningitis syndromes, post-intracerebral haemorrhage, intracerebral tumours and other space-occupying lesions.

3. Flaccid paralysis

Poliomyelitis is the most common condition producing muscle weakness and subsequent contracture when the world scene is observed. Muscle imbalance will produce contractures of any type and in any area of the body. The most frequent are flexion contractures of the hips and knees, together with equinus deformities of the feet and ankles. Treatment depends upon appropriate surgical correction of deformities with muscle transplants and transfers. Calliper or orthosis splintage is frequently required.

PERONEAL MUSCULAR ATROPHY (CHARCOT MARIE TOOTH DISEASE)

This produces wasting, particularly below the knee. The lower limbs appear like inverted champagne bottles (*Fig.* C.31). Contractures of the feet and ankles occur—equinovarus deformities together with a pes cavus and claw toes (see *Fig.* F.45). The upper limbs show wasting of the hand intrinsic muscles.

SPINA BIFIDA

The neurological abnormality is complex, for although most contractures are due to lower motor neurone paralysis, there is a frequent spastic element due to cord lesion or hydrocephalus. Contractures are often gross and extremely disabling and are resistant to treatment (*Fig.* C.32).

4. Joint disease

Any destructive joint disease will produce contractures if severe. Septic arthritis may leave a contracted articulation with a fibrous ankylosis and may eventually fuse the joint (*Fig.* C.33). Rheumatoid arthritis and other inflammatory arthropathies produce joint contracture of any part of the body (*Fig.* C.34). Degenerative joint disease such as osteoarthrosis may produce contractures or deformity due to bone collapse.

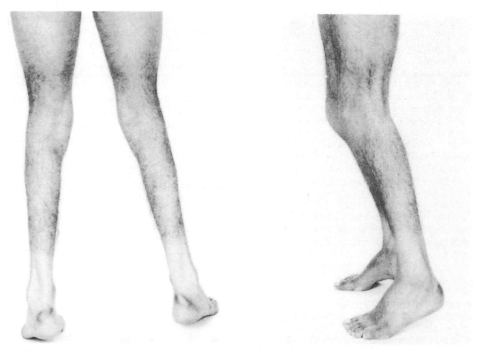

Fig. C.31. Contractures due to peroneal muscular atrophy sent to the author as an old poliomyelitis.

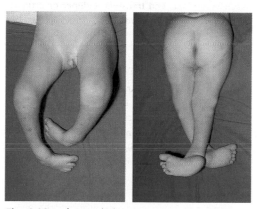

Fig. C.32. *a, b* Lower limb contractures in spina bifida.

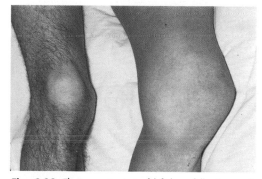

Fig. C.33. Flexion contracture of left knee following septic arthritis.

5. Growth disorders

These are due to:

1 Primary epiphyseal dysplasia,
2 Metabolic abnormalities such as rickets (*see Fig.* B.14) and
3 Injury to the epiphyseal plate.

6. Muscle dystrophy

Duchenne-type muscle dystrophy produces initially an enlargement of the muscle bulk in the child ('infantile Hercules') but there is progessive weakening of all muscle groups and contractures may eventually develop. Diagnosis is made from the clinical state and increased level of creatinine phosphokinase (CPK).

Muscle injury may occur in severe trauma and acute pyogenic infections may produce a septic myositis.

Muscle Ischaemia

This occurs in the lower limb when traumatized. A closed compartment syndrome with muscle ischaemia may occur in trauma with or without a fracture. The most common deformities are those of an equinus ankle and foot with clawing of the toes and weakness, or frank paralysis of the ischaemic musculature (*see* VOLKMANN'S ISCHAEMIC CONTRACTURE, p. 126).

Primary muscle contracture

Arthrogryphosis multiplex congenita is a congenital abnormality due to non-differentiation of mesenchymal

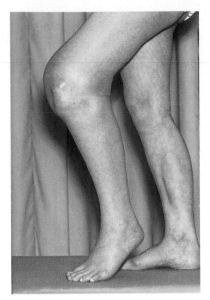

Fig. C.34. Flexion contracture of left knee in rheumatoid arthritis.

tissue. There is frequently a neurogenic element (lower motor neurone) with severe weakness. The combination produces gross contracture.

Upper limb

The general causes of upper limb contractures are similar to those described in the lower limb (*see* p. 122).

1 Post-trauma states
2 Spastic conditions—upper motor neurone lesions
3 Flaccid paralysis—lower motor neurone lesions and peripheral nerve injuries
4 Joint disease and injury
5 Growth disorders
6 Muscle dystrophies and primary muscle disease and damage.

Peripheral nerve injuries

THE ULNAR NERVE

The ulnar nerve may be divided or compressed at the elbow, or in the forearm and wrist. The hand intrinsic muscles are paralysed with gross wasting of the interossei and a claw hand results. The thenar eminence musculature is variably innervated by the median nerve and abductor pollicis brevis is always preserved. There is anaesthesia over the little finger and ulnar border of the hand together variably with the ring finger—part or whole.

THE RADIAL NERVE

The radial nerve may be divided or compressed in the arm producing paralysis of the wrist and forearm

extensors. A wrist drop develops and anaesthesia is present over the dorsal surface of the hand in an area usually confined to the first web space.

THE MEDIAN NERVE

The median nerve may be divided or compressed at the elbow or above producing a 'pointing hand'. The thenar eminence is wasted due to paralysis of abductor pollicis brevis and, variably, the other short thenar muscles. The index and middle fingers are weak in flexion and are therefore kept extended in repose by the unopposed action of the finger extensors. The ring and little fingers are held in some flexion for the deep flexor muscles to these digits are innervated by the ulnar nerve. Anaesthesia is over the palmar surface of the radial three-and-a-half digits.

Carpal tunnel syndrome

The median nerve at the wrist is compressed within the carpal tunnel which results in wasting of the thenar eminence. There is always abductor pollicis brevis wasting, for this muscle is autonomously supplied by the median nerve and the other short thenar muscles are variably supplied by the ulnar nerve. Anaesthesia may eventually involve the whole radial three-and-a-half digits but initially there is hypoaesthesia together with tingling, numbness and some pain over the tips of the thumb, middle and index fingers. The symptoms are very specific to the night hours or at the time of awakening with exacerbation by hand exercise. The majority of cases are in women at or just beyond the menopause. Compression in the carpal tunnel may occur also in pregnancy, following a Colles' fracture, in myxoedema and in situations where ganglia or other space-occupying lesions are present around the median nerve at the wrist.

The rheumatoid hand

Rheumatoid synovium may produce swelling of the synovial sheath in the hand and this leads to destruction of extensor tendons with the fingers 'dropping'. The metacarpophalangeal joints are involved at an early stage and the fingers drift into ulnar deviation (*Fig. C.35*). As the disease progresses, mutilation and destruction of all finger joints may occur. Swan neck deformities occur due to intrinsic muscle spasm and then contracture. Psoriatic arthropathy produces inflammation of the distal finger joints together with characteristic pitting of the finger nails.

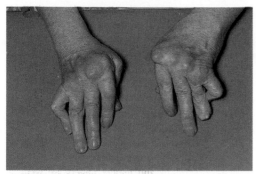

Fig. C.35. Contractures of the hands in severe rheumatoid arthritis.

The osteoarthritic hand

The terminal phalangeal joints are primarily affected. The distal joint osteophytes are nodular and are called 'Heberden's nodes'. There are sometimes small retention cysts in association with these.

De Quervain's stenosing tenosynovitis

The thumb tendons at the wrist may become inflamed and stenosed. Abductor pollicis longus and extensor pollicis brevis run over the radial styloid in their sheaths and here there is localized tenderness, severe pain on thumb movement and eventual stenosis, which results in an extension and adduction contracture of the thumb.

Mallet finger

This is otherwise known as a cricket or baseball finger. The distal phalanx of one finger remains flexed following a stubbing injury. The distal insertion of the extensor tendon to the phalanx is ripped and the finger tip drops.

Dupuytren's contracture

A fibrotic nodule in the palm fascia is frequently felt or seen in the older man. This nodule may then extend

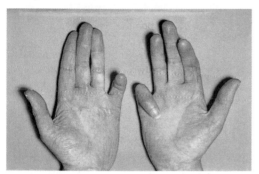
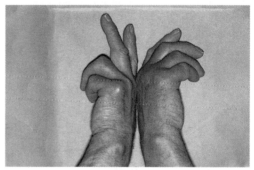

Fig. C.36. Dupuytren's contractures: a, affecting the little fingers; b severe deformities.

Trigger finger

When the flexed fingers are extended one digit may remain flexed. It may be manually extended with a snap and this phenomenon is termed 'trigger finger'. It is due to localized stenosis of the fibrous flexor sheath opposite the metacarpophalangeal joint. The poststenotic swelling of the tendon is pulled into the sheath in flexion and remains stuck until forcibly extended. It is due to an idiopathic stenosis in most cases. Diabetics may develop one or more trigger fingers. The stenosis may also occur in rheumatoid arthritis.

Snapping thumb

The same triggering phenomenon may occur in the thumb. The child may be affected by a congenital stenosis of the sheath of the flexor pollicís longus. The continued flexion contracture of the thumb interphalangeal joint is rarely noted until the child is a year old. Similar surgical release is required.

and produce skin puckering with subsequent contracture of the palmar aponeurosis. The thickening and contracture then extends to the digits and the little, ring and middle fingers contract in that order. No digit is exempt. The contracture may become severe and disabling and surgical treatment should be undertaken before the deformity becomes gross (*Fig.* C.36). The ideal time for release is when the finger metacarpophalangeal joints present a flexion contracture of some 30 degrees. Garrod's pads occur in Dupuytren's disease and the lump on the dorsal aspects of the knuckles contains Dupuytren's tissue. In 5 per cent of patients Dupuytren's contracture occurs on the foot with the planar aponeurosis involved.

The aetiology of Dupuytren's contracture is unknown but there is a very definite genetic association. Although far commoner in men, it does occur in women. Patients with liver disease have a higher incidence and epileptics on Epanutin medication have a predisposition.

Volkmann's ischaemic contracture

Contracture of the hand may occur in unrecognized avascularity of the upper limb after fracture. The supracondylar fracture in the child is the most commonly associated injury. The displacement of the lower humeral fragment compresses, or in some cases lacerates the brachial artery. The large associated haematoma may similarly compress the vessel which easily goes into spasm.

The damage to forearm muscles and nerves occurs in the first few hours. It is usually identified by the absence of the radial pulse, but this is not always the case. The most important early sign is the inability to extend the patient's fingers without severe pain and the possibility of this diagnosis must be based on this sign. The features of an avascular extremity will then progressively follow and at this stage it is too late to reverse the damage (*Fig.* C.37). In the full Volkmann's contracture the claw fingers become more flexed with the wrist extended and the fingers extend as the wrist flexes. The median, ulnar and sometimes the radial nerves are frequently damaged by this ischaemia.

Paul Aichroth

Convulsions and fits

(*See also* TETANY, TICS, VERTIGO)
The words 'convulsion', 'fit' or 'seizure' are used to describe attacks of involuntary tonic or clonic movements of the limbs, trunk and face with or without incontinence. They include genuine epileptic seizures, pseudo-seizures, tetanus, tetany, rigors and strychnine poisoning. This section is concerned solely with epileptic convulsions of cerebral origin; the others are described in their respective sections.

The phenomena which control the seizure threshold at a neuronal level in the cerebral cortex are now reasonably well understood. Normal neurones have both inhibitory and excitatory influences which cause inhibitory and excitatory postsynaptic potentials (IPSP and EPSP). Once a critical level of membrane depolarization is achieved, an action potential develops and is propagated leading to the firing of individual neurones in a repetitive fashion with intervals between the action potentials. Neurones in epileptic foci behave abnormally. They have a shift in the depolarization level which results in 'burst' firing of action potentials; they fire for a time and then become refractory. Such neurones are found in the centre of an epileptic focus and they fire spontaneously, acting as the epileptic pacemaker. Adjacent to this are more normal neurones which are triggered by the burst firing of the primary neurones and which act to ensure propagation of the epileptic stimulus.

Two patterns of physiological organization of epileptic discharge are recognized: those arising from a focal cortical disturbance and those characterized by immediate synchronous spike-wave discharge in both hemispheres. These patterns correspond to focal and generalized seizures and the focal and generalized forms of epilepsy. The latter pattern is occasionally termed 'centrencephalic' epilepsy and is thought to originate from a primary discharge in the brainstem reticular formation.

Classification of seizures

The major division in classifying seizures is between those which are partial and those which are generalized. *Partial seizures* begin locally in the cortex and include an aura which reflects the functional role of that part of the cortex in which the discharge begins. These seizures may also be associated with a postictal focal disturbance (Todd's phenomenon). *Generalized seizures* begin bilaterally, consciousness is lost suddenly and the patient does not therefore experience an aura. Any partial seizure may spread to become generalized as a secondary tonic-clonic (grand mal) seizure.

1. Partial seizures

A. SIMPLE PARTIAL SEIZURES

i. Frontal lobe seizures
Frontal lobe seizures are commonly seen as 'adversive' attacks in which there is tonic or clonic deviation of the head and eyes to one side—the side opposite the focus of origin—sometimes associated with jerking of the arm or the adoption of a raised flexed posture of the arm on the side to which the head turns. This form of frontal lobe seizure is more common than the classical Jacksonian motor seizure with a march of movement beginning in a digit and spreading up a limb. Both of these forms of motor seizure may be followed by a Todd's paresis and involvement of the frontal speech areas may cause speech arrest.

ii. Temporal lobe seizures
Seizures beginning in the temporal lobe may create sensations of taste or smell, usually unpleasant, epigastric disturbances and pallor, flushing or changes in the heart rate. In addition there may be psychic phenomena such as '*déjà-vu*' and '*jamais-vu*' and patients may also identify auditory or visual hallucinations which are like 'memory playback'.

iii. Parietal and occipital lobe seizures
These are less common. They may be associated with positive sensory disturbance such as pins and needles, or with distortions of light and colour, usually confined

to the contralateral half of the visual field and not comprising any form of structured image.

B.   COMPLEX PARTIAL SEIZURES

Complex partial seizures, previously termed psychomotor or temporal lobe seizures, are differentiated from simple seizures by varying degrees of impairment of consciousness. Such disturbance of consciousness may be preceded by symptoms of simple partial type, but there may not be an aura. Occasionally seizures are associated with automatism, frequently stereotyped such as smacking of the lips, fidgeting or picking at the clothes, but occasionally with more complex behaviour which can lead to problems such as shoplifting or indecent exposure.

2.   Generalized seizures

A.   THE TONIC-CLONIC SEIZURE (GRAND MAL)

The most common form of generalized seizure is the tonic-clonic grand mal seizure. When this is of primary origin there is no preliminary aura. The patient initially cries out during a tonic phase of extension and opisthotonus, with subsequent respiratory arrest and cyanosis. There is reflex emptying of the bladder and occasionally of the bowel. The patient then enters a clonic phase of generalized jerking, lasting for a variable length of time and followed by deep coma and then a gradual return of consciousness with postictal confusion and sometimes automatic behaviour.

B.   SIMPLE ABSENCE (PETIT MAL)

The most classic form of childhood generalized seizure is the petit mal seizure. This is an absence which is usually momentary in which a child loses contact with his or her surroundings. There may be minor myoclonic activity around the eyelids. The attacks may be very frequent and the child may not be aware of their occurrence. They may present as problems with learning at school.

C.   MYOCLONIC JERKS

Brief myoclonic jerks occur in numerous epileptic syndromes. They may be associated with an absence but more commonly occur without impairment of consciousness. The arms are more frequently involved than the legs.

3.   Status epilepticus

Most epileptic seizures are self-limiting but rarely they follow one another in close succession resulting in *status epilepticus*. This is described as a state of recurrent tonic-clonic seizures without recovery of cons-

ciousness. It is a medical emergency with a high morbidity and mortality. It is seen in about 3 per cent of epileptic patients, most commonly in those with severe epilepsy and those who have problems with compliance in drug taking. It may be seen with acute alcohol withdrawal, meningitis or encephalitis, and with other metabolic disturbances. *Absence status* is occasionally seen in children. They present with confused behaviour, often with blinking or small myoclonic jerks. *Complex partial status* may cause confusion and disorientation, sometimes with automatic behaviour. Epilepsia partialis continuans is a repetitive rhythmic jerking of a group of muscles. It is most commonly seen in association with vascular disease and rarely with cerebral tumours.

The investigation of the epilepsies

The diagnosis of epilepsy is ultimately clinical and based on the history obtained from the patient and witnesses. An electroencephalogram may add weight to a clinical diagnosis but can never prove or disprove the clinical diagnosis of epilepsy. The value of interictal recordings in the diagnosis of epilepsy is limited, mild non-specific abnormalities being found in up to 10 per cent of the normal population and many patients with seizures having a normal interictal EEG. The use of ambulatory monitoring or video telemetry EEG recording does improve the yield of positive diagnosis, and the principal role of the EEG, particularly in the young, is to help to differentiate between the different types of epilepsy.

The need for investigations other than an EEG in patients with epilepsy depends upon various factors: the age of the patient, the type of epilepsy and the presence of neurological signs. It may be argued that all patients presenting with epilepsy require biochemical and haematological screening together with exhaustive neuroradiological investigation to determine a cause for their epilepsy, but this would be difficult to defend in view of the low rate of detection of conditions requiring treatment other than anticonvulsant drugs. It is important to remember that a careful history and physical examination may be sufficient to reveal the cause of the seizure disturbance.

The differential diagnosis of patients presenting with epilepsy is considerable and includes *generalized epilepsies* which may be idiopathic or symptomatic, *partial epilepsies* which may also be idiopathic or symptomatic, specific *epileptic syndromes* and *unclassified seizures*. The *idiopathic epilepsies* include childhood absence seizures, benign myoclonic epilepsy of adolescence and the tonic-clonic epilepsy seen in the young adult. Partial epilepsies which are idiopathic include benign focal motor epilepsy of childhood, sometimes called Rolandic epilepsy, and benign occipital epilepsy of childhood. Symptomatic seizures may be indicative of a systemic disturbance such as fever, hypoxia, hypoglycaemia, electrolyte imbalance, renal failure, hepatic failure or respiratory failure. They may be due to toxins, such as drugs, particularly tricyclic agents, alcohol, heavy metals, or those derived from poisonous insects and snakes. Pyridoxine deficiency, porphyria, some inborn errors of metabolism and drug withdrawal are other possible causes of symptomatic seizures.

Central nervous system diseases that may also cause symptomatic epilepsy include the following: congenital disorders such as birth trauma, tuberose sclerosis, arteriovenous malformation, lipid storage diseases, leucodystrophies, Down's syndrome, microcephaly and hydrocephalus; infective conditions such as meningitis, encephalitis, cerebral abscess, neurosyphilis and, more rarely, fungal, HIV and herpes simplex infection; trauma, either due to diffuse brain injury, penetrating brain injury or depressed skull fracture, or resulting in anoxia or the formation of a haematoma; cerebral tumours, particularly gliomas, meningiomas and secondary carcinomas; vascular disturbance such as atheroma, arteritis and aneurysm; and degenerative conditions such as Alzheimer's disease and Pick's disease. Rarely multiple sclerosis may present with seizures when a plaque is close to the grey matter of the cortex.

The investigations of the various causes of symptomatic seizures will depend upon the presentation and the likelihood that the individual patient may be suffering from one of these primary diseases. It is apparent that the plan of investigation will vary. It may be restricted to biochemical and haematological investigation or may include, imaging with CT or MRI, and possibly CSF examination—whatever is appropriate in order to reach a diagnosis.

Pseudo-seizures are increasingly recognized as an important consideration in the differential diagnosis of convulsions. They may occur classically in the hysterical subject and will rarely involve self-injury or incontinence of urine or faeces. If witnessed, it is usually possible to demonstrate that there is no alteration in neurological signs; the plantar responses remain flexor and ice water calorics remain intact. These tests will be abnormal in the presence of genuine seizures. The management of the patient with pseudo-seizures is extremely difficult, and even with modern technology including EEG telemetry, it is often not possible to exclude completely the possibility that some genuine seizures are also occurring in a patient with obvious pseudo-seizures.

D. Bates

Corneal disease

The main symptoms of corneal disease are pain, reduced vision, haloes, photophobia and lacrimation. The cornea has a rich sensory nerve supply from the ophthalmic division of the trigeminal nerve, stimulation of which can result in severe pain with secondary excess lacrimation. Reduced vision is due to loss of corneal transparency which may be secondary to corneal oedema, cellular infiltration, or scarring. Haloes are due to epithelial oedema producing diffraction of light.

The cornea is examined by ophthalmologists using the slit-lamp (biomicroscope) but may be examined by the naked eye by the non-ophthalmologist, using focal illumination and magnification (pen torch and magnifier). Corneal epithelial defects (such as ulcers or abrasions) can be most easily detected by instilling sodium fluorescein which will stain any epithelial defects, e.g. corneal abrasions secondary to trauma.

Corneal disease can be classified into ulcers which may be infective or immune, nutritional and metabolic disorders and corneal degenerations.

Corneal degeneration

The commonest *degenerative condition* of the cornea is *arcus senilis*, a concentric yellowish-white crescent of lipid deposition in the peripheral cornea, which, through time, completely encircles the cornea. It has no clinical importance except, perhaps, in younger patients in whom it may be associated with serum lipid abnormalities. *Band keratopathy* (Fig. C.38), extending over the area of cornea normally exposed between the eyelids, is rarely found in otherwise healthy eyes, but occurs frequently in blind, shrunken eyes and following prolonged uveitis. *Keratoconus* or conical cornea is due to an abnormal thinning of the central cornea resulting in a cone-shaped cornea. It starts around puberty and progresses slowly, although sometimes develops an acute progressive phase causing sudden visual deterioration and eye discomfort.

Corneal ulcer

The cornea can be infected by viruses, bacteria or fungi. The herpes simplex virus is a common pathogen, producing the typical dendritic ulcer. Early lesions comprise opaque epithelial cells which later desquamate to form the branching pattern of the *dendritic ulcer* which can be demonstrated by fluorescein staining.

The ulcer is frequently recurrent with repeated relapses. In many cases a stromal scar results which will produce visual impairment if it is centrally located. The virus remains dormant and is easily reactivated in

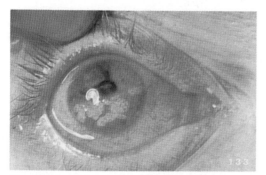

Fig. C.38. Band-shaped degeneration of cornea.

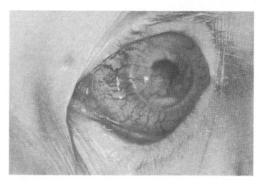

Fig. C.39. Hypopyon ulcer (see p. 188). (Institute of Ophthalmology.)

future by a variety of trigger factors such as poor general health or exposure to excessive sunlight or topical steroids.

The herpes zoster virus when involving the ophthalmic nerve also produces corneal lesions in the form of microdendritic ulcers and corneal opacities. Both herpes simplex and herpes zoster infection reduce corneal sensation, which can be tested by touching the cornea with a wisp of cotton-wool and comparing the blink reflex of the two eyes. Damage to the corneal sensory nerves can result in ulceration of neurotrophic keratitis. The corneal epithelium requires an intact sensory nerve supply to permit normal healing and neurotrophic ulcers show little tendency to heal often requiring a tarsorrhaphy.

Bacterial ulcers or abscesses often follow minor trauma to the cornea. The most common pathogens are *Streptococcus pneumoniae* and *Straphylococcus aureus* but β haemolytic streptococcus, *Pseudomonas, Proteus, Klebsiella, Escherichia coli* and *Neisseria* can also be causative. Clinically the ulcer appears as a yellowish irregular opacity associated with corneal stromal necrosis. It is usually associated with reactive iritis with outpouring of white blood cells into the anterior chamber which settle inferiorly to form a pus level or hypopyon (*Fig.* C.39). The causative organism is identified and the appropriate antibiotics given. The ulcer may heal without perforating, but if the resulting scar is both large and centrally placed ultimately the vision is often much impaired. If perforation does occur the underlying iris may adhere to the site of perforation with subsequent dense corneal scar formation, which may then distend to form a bulging anterior staphyloma.

Marginal ulcers situated around the periphery of the cornea with a clear zone between the ulcer and the limbus, tend to remain superficial. They most commonly follow *Staphylococcus aureus* conjunctivitis or blepharitis and are produced as an immunological reaction against staphylococcal exotoxins.

Interstitial keratitis is a late manifestation of congenital syphilis producing stromal corneal opacities with associated stigmata as discussed on (p. 188).

Keratomalacia due to vitamin A deficiency is characterized by desiccation and subsequent necrosis of the cornea and conjunctiva. It affects undernourished infants and is extremely rare in the UK. Urgent administration of vitamin A is required together with attention to the corneal hydration.

S. T. D. Roxburgh

Cough

Healthy persons seldom cough; their scant bronchial secretions result in a thin sheet of mucus constantly carried up the tracheobronchial tree towards the larynx by the action of cilia. On reaching the pharynx the secretions raised in this way are disposed of into the alimentary tract by unconscious acts of swallowing.

Coughing is an essential defence mechanism that protects the airways from the adverse effects of inhaled noxious substances and also serves to clear them of retained secretions. Patients recognize that coughing indicates an abnormality and this symptom is one of the most frequent reasons given for seeking medical advice.

Coughing may be produced voluntarily, but more often it results from reflex stimulation. To a lesser extent it can be suppressed voluntarily. The involuntary initiation of a cough takes place in a reflex arc. Extrathoracic cough receptors are present in the nose, oropharynx, larynx and upper trachea. Intrathoracic irritant receptors are located in the epithelium of the lower trachea and large central bronchi, which are the air passages from which coughing effectively expels retained secretions or foreign material. Efferent pathways include the recurrent laryngeal nerves to cause closure of the glottis, and the cortico-spinal tract and peripheral nerves to cause contraction of the thoracic and abdominal musculature. The cough receptors may accommodate to repeated stimuli, as they often do in cigarette smokers who may only cough after the first cigarette of the day. The cough reflex becomes less sensitive in the elderly and is lost in anaesthesia and unconsciousness leading to an increased danger of aspiration pneumonia.

The act of coughing occurs in three phases. The first is a preliminary deep inspiration, the second is closure of the glottis, relaxation of the diaphragm and contraction of the thoracic and abdominal expiratory muscles generating a positive pressure of 100–300 mmHg within the thorax. Because the positive pressure in the pleural space is higher than the luminal pressure in the trachea and central bronchi, a pressure difference is created that causes the posterior membranous portion of the airway walls to fold inwards and partially obliterate the lumen. When the third event occurs, namely sudden relaxation of the glottis the linear velocity of airflow through the narrow channels is markedly increased creating forces that dislodge secretions and particles from the mucosal surface. During cough the volume rate of flow out of the lungs (l/sec) is very similar to that obtained during a forced expiratory manoeuvre, a fact that is not always appreciated. In patients with severe airflow obstruction, high rates of flow cannot be generated because the airways are already narrowed; such patients may have prolonged wheezy coughs which sometimes cause the involuntary effects of a valsalva manoeuvre and resultant cough syncope which occasionally is accompanied by convulsions mimicking epilepsy.

In general the diagnosis of the cause of cough depends not only on an analysis of the cough itself but on the other symptoms and physical signs and, above all, the chest radiograph. When the chest radiograph shows a significant abnormality such as bronchiectasis (*Fig*. C.40), lobar collapse (*Figs*. C.41–C.43), carcinoma (*Fig*. C.44), bronchopneumonia (*Fig*. C.45), or pulmonary tuberculosis (*Figs*. C.46, C.47), the reason for the cough is established and the next step is to initiate appropriate treatment. Diagnostic problems arise in those patients in whom the chest radiograph appears normal. *Table* C.7 lists the disorders that need to be considered. Some helpful diagnostic clinical clues and signs and further investigations are listed in the same table. Enquiry about the presence or absence of sputum, whether the cough is occasional or persistent, provoked by any activity or situation and especially where there is disturbed sleep will provide helpful pointers to diagnosis. When the causes of the chronic cough are analysed, asthma frequently heads the list and indeed chronic non-productive cough, especially at night, may be the sole presenting complaint of patients subsequently proven to have bronchial asthma.

Dry cough is also a feature of lung fibrosis from any cause. Typically the chest radiograph will be

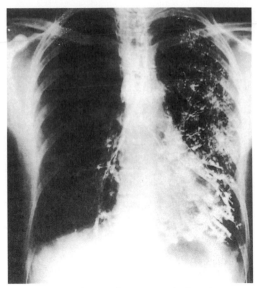

Fig. C.40. Bronchogram showing saccular bronchiectasis in the left lower lobe.

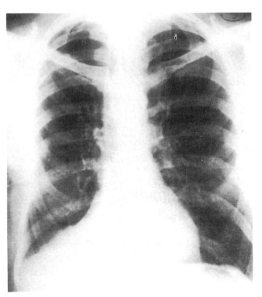

Fig. C.41. Radiograph of chest showing collapse of the right lower lobe, due to carcinoma of the bronchus. Note the roughly triangular shadow filling the right cardiophrenic angle, with slight displacement of the heart to the right.

abnormal but, if equivocal, thoracic high resolution CT scanning is helpful in confirming or refuting the presence of structural lung disease. An intractable dry cough is now recognized as an important side-effect of angiotension-converting enzyme inhibitors.

In *pertussis* the characteristic cough is paroxysmal and occurs in bouts which may last for a minute or two and culminate in vomiting, in addition to a characteristic terminal inspiratory whoop. In severe paroxysms the child may become cyanosed. On exam-

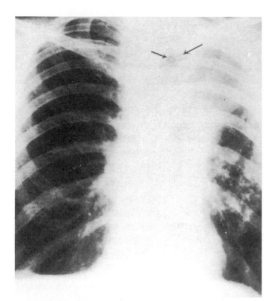

Fig. C.42. Radiograph of chest showing collapse of the left upper lobe due to carcinoma. Note the uniform shadow of the upper part of the left lung with gross displacement to the left of the trachea (indicated by an arrow). The shadows in the lower part of the left lung are due to residual-iodized oil.

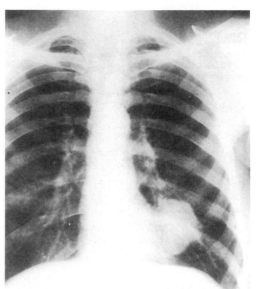

Fig. C.44. Radiograph of chest showing an isolated well-defined shadow in the lower part of the left lung. This was due to carcinoma of the bronchus giving rise to a well-defined tumour without obstruction of a major bronchus.

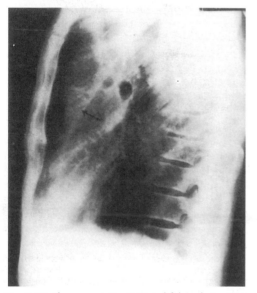

Fig. C.43. The same as *Fig.* C.42, in left lateral view. Note the displacement forwards and upwards of the interlobar fissure delimiting the contracted upper lobe.

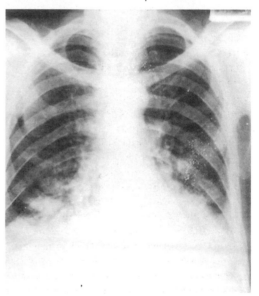

Fig. C.45. Radiograph of chest showing bilateral basal bronch-opneumonia (postoperative).

ination the most striking finding in the chest is a negative one, the rhonchi characteristic of ordinary acute bronchitis being generally absent. A sublingual ulcer on the fraenum linguae due to the friction of the protruding tongue on the lower front teeth during long paroxysms of coughing is a helpful finding, as is a history of exposure to infection.

A cough which an adult patient has had intermit-tently since childhood is more likely to be associated with bronchiectasis than one the onset of which can be dated more recently.

In children and even young adults with a persis-tent or recurrent cough, the possibility of cystic fibrosis must be borne in mind; the presence of associated bowel symptoms should lead to an estimate of sweat sodium level.

A cough appearing and persisting for the first time in a young adult, especially if an Asian, must give

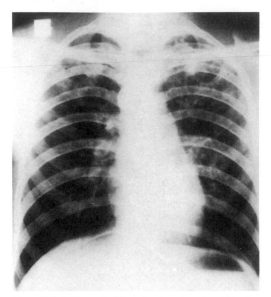

Fig. C.46. Radiograph of chest showing tuberculous infiltration of the upper parts of both lungs, with a moderate-size cavity on the left.

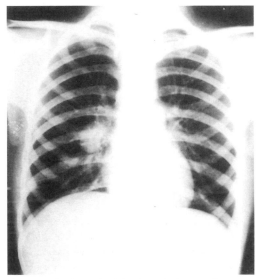

Fig. C.47. Radiograph of the chest of a boy aged 11 years showing a primary tuberculous complex in the right lung with gross enlargement of the hilar lymph nodes.

rise to suspicion of pulmonary tuberculosis, and calls for complete investigation including a chest radiograph and sputum examination. Similarly a cough appearing for the first time in middle age, especially in a man, must raise suspicion of bronchial carcinoma which should only be dismissed after a complete investigation.

The characteristic morning cough of the cigarette smoker is due to a chronic pharyngotracheobronchitis; many cigarette smokers regard it as a normal part of their lives and refer to it as 'clearing the throat'. It is in fact the first symptom of chronic bronchitis. The frequency with which chronic bronchitis and bronchogenic carcinoma coexist, both directly associated with tobacco consumption, has lead to the important axiom that any change in the character or pattern of a chronic cough warrants investigation for carcinoma of the lung. Chronic nasal sinusitis may produce or contribute to this symptom, secretions which have trickled down into the trachea during sleep being expelled when the patient wakes. A cough which appears on first lying down at night or on some other changes of posture is suggestive of localized bronchiectasis or chronic pulmonary suppuration. In older people, recurrent aspiration is a not uncommon cause that is often overlooked. It may be related to oesophageal regurgitation, stricture or neurological disease affecting swallowing. Asthma and cardiac failure also commonly cause cough in the elderly but this may be especially prominent at night. Asthmatic patients sometimes complain of cough as a predominant feature of their attacks and wheezing and dyspnoea may be relatively trivial. In typical asthma, cough may also occur on exercise or nocturnally, waking patients from sleep. A cough with dyspnoea or orthopnoea waking the patient from sleep may also be due to pulmonary congestion or oedema due to left ventricular failure in hypertension, aortic valvular disease, or disorders of the myocardium. Because such nocturnal attacks of paroxysmal dyspnoea in these conditions may be accompanied by wheeziness they are sometimes referred to as 'cardiac asthma'. _Table_ C.8 lists the important findings that might help to differentiate bronchial and cardiac asthma.

The presence or absence of expectoration and the quality of expectoration are important diagnostic features of any cough. It should be remembered that many patients find it difficult to expectorate and habitually expel small amounts of secretion through the larynx by cough and then swallow it. This is the rule in children. A dry cough or one producing only scanty mucoid sputum may be due to inflammation or tumour of the larynx when there will be associated hoarseness. Laryngeal involvement in syphilis is a very unusual cause of a dry cough with hoarse voice. Another cause of cough associated with a weak voice often described as 'hoarseness' is carcinoma of the bronchus with recurrent laryngeal nerve involvement. A dry cough may be a manifestation of nervousness but should not be accepted as such without proper investigations. A dry cough may also be due to external pressure on a bronchus by a mediastinal mass such as benign or malignant tumour or by enlarged mediastinal lymph nodes due to reticulosis or tuberculosis; the latter should be particularly considered in Asians. Cough due to external pressure on the trachea is usually described as 'brassy' or 'bovine'.

Table C.7. Causes of cough to be considered when the chest radiograph does not show any gross abnormality

Acute conditions	Helpful diagnostic clinical clues
Acute specific fever, e.g. measles, typhoid or paratyphoid	Other features, e.g. Koplik's spots and rash of measles
Whooping cough (pertussis)	Characteristic cough and whoop (see text)
Acute laryngitis	Associated with hoarseness
Acute tracheobronchitis	Painful cough with retrosternal soreness
Exposure to noxious gases	Obvious history
Inhaled foreign body	Usually a young child, usually no history

Chronic or recurrent conditions	Diagnostic investigations
Chronic sinusitis	Sinus radiographs
Chronic laryngitis	
Laryngeal papilloma, carcinoma, tuberculosis, syphilis	Laryngoscopy
Cystic fibrosis	Chest radiograph may be characteristic
	Sweat test
Chronic bronchitis	PEFR or FEV$_1$ measurement
Bronchial asthma	
Bronchiectasis	Bronchoscopy, CT scan of lungs
Carcinoma or adenoma or foreign body only partly obstructing the trachea or main bronchus	Flow volume loop may be characteristic Bronchoscopy
Mediastinal lymphadenopathy or tumour pressing on a bronchus	Tomography and/or mediastinoscopy
Diaphragmatic irritation due to subphrenic abscess or hepatic abscess	Ultrasound and fluoroscopy

Table C.8. Differentiation of bronchial and cardiac asthma

Bronchial asthma	Cardiac asthma
History of previous bronchial asthma	History of hypertension, valvular or ischaemic heart disease
Often young—sometimes old	Rarely young—usually old
Expiratory wheezing	Sometimes also expiratory wheezing
No crackles	Many basal crackles
Cardiac examination normal	Gallop rhythm/cardiac failure
	Evidence of pre-existing cardiac disorder
ECG normal	ECG often abnormal
Chest radiograph shows hyperinflation of lungs	Chest radiograph shows enlargement of left ventricle, Kerley's septal lines and other evidence of pulmonary venous congestion and/or pulmonary oedema
Bronchial hyperactivity (PEFR measurements)	No evidence of bronchial hyperactivity
Methacholine or histamine challenge	

If a cough is productive the quality and mode of production of the sputum should be noted. Frankly purulent sputum suggests bronchiectasis, lung abscess, primary or secondary to bronchial obstruction by new growth, foreign body, or cavitating pulmonary tuberculosis. The odour of the sputum is important, a malodorous sputum almost invariably indicates infection with anaerobic organisms and suggests bronchiectasis, inhalation pneumonia, lung abscess or bronchopleural fistula with expectoration of a putrid empyema. See also SPUTUM. Cough due to a bronchopleural fistula is characteristically dependent on position; the cough is worse when the patient lies on his good side and it is relieved by lying on the side of the lesion.

Coughing seems to provoke more coughing. Paroxysms of coughing as in pertussis may terminate in vomiting which seems to break the cycle. Paroxysmal attacks may also terminate in syncope. At times, severe coughing attacks have continued to the point of utter exhaustion. The muscular force developed during coughing may be sufficient to cause occasional fractures of ribs (cough fractures) and even compression fractures of vertebral bodies. In some cases no physical cause for the cough may be detected and in some of these patients psychogenic factors are important.

P. R. Studdy

Cramps

Cramps are irrational, involuntary, often painful, contractions of voluntary muscles which become hard and 'knotted'. They may be initiated by a sudden voluntary contraction but usually occur at rest. They may persist for seconds or minutes and can generally be relieved by a slow passive extension of the affected muscle. Electromyography of a muscle in cramp shows fluctuating high frequency bursts of motor unit activity.

Cramps are very common in patients in general practice and in such patients there is usually no definable cause for the condition. In hospital patients some cause such as a metabolic or neurological disorder is often found.

Although the idiopathic variety may occur at any age they are more common in the elderly suggesting a degenerative neurological basis for the condition. They often occur in the night, waking the patient from sleep. The foot and calf muscles are most commonly affected and the thighs less often. In my experience patients with unilateral disease of the leg arteries commonly complain of cramps occurring more often in the diseased leg than in the healthy leg.

Certain physiological, rather than disease, states are associated with cramps. They often occur during *pregnancy*. Excessive *unaccustomed exercise* can cause cramps, thus athletes and swimmers commencing training are often affected, the cramps disappearing with increasing fitness. Cramp of intercostal muscles (stitch) may occur during and after exercise in untrained individuals. Excessive use of combinations of small muscle groups can cause cramps, e.g. writers' and musicians' cramp. In these subjects *psychological factors* appear to play a part though possibly a *neurological disorder*, dystonia, may be present in some cases.

Metabolic disorders may cause cramp. A low plasma ionized calcium causes cramp. This is most strikingly seen in the forearm and hand muscles as carpopedal spasm. *Hypoparathyroidism, malabsorption* and *inadequate dietary calcium intake* can cause hypocalcaemia. *Acute alkalosis* from hysterical hyperventilation may lower the ionized calcium in the plasma and cause carpopedal spasm. *Chronic renal failure* may also result in hypocalcaemia and, with hypomagnesaemia, be a cause of cramp. In these patients cramps may be particularly troublesome during dialysis. *Severe salt and water depletion* as a result of hard physical work in a hot environment causes cramps, i.e. 'Stoker's cramp' or 'heat cramp'. Cramps may occur in the recovery phase from severe gastrointestinal disease with diarrhoea causing salt and water imbalance.

Neurological diseases cause cramps. Extensive cramp of the flexor muscles of the legs ('flexor spasms') may be seen in patients with *cord transection* and cord involvement in muscle sclerosis. *Diseases of the peripheral nerves* such as alcoholic or diabetic neuropathy tend to cause cramps of the legs and feet.

Drugs such as *diuretics* are often associated with cramps presumably by causing alteration in electrolyte and water balance. *Beta adrenoreceptor stimulating drugs* such as terbutaline, *calcium channel-blocking drugs* such as nifedipine and *phenothiazine-type* drugs may also cause cramps, the latter causing a particular form of cramp and spasm of the facial and neck muscles 'orofacial dyskinesia'.

Very rarely cramps may be due to *enzyme disorders of muscles* e.g. phosphoglycerate mutase, phosphoglycerate kinase and adenylate deaminase deficiency.

Tetanus is a form of cramp due to infection by the *Clostridium tetani*. The spasm appears first in the facial muscles and then spreads over the body.

Cramps due to *lead poisoning or strychnine* are rarely seen and only of historical interest.

E. Housley

Crepitus

Crepitus is a term generally used to denote the grating or crackling sensation and noise produced when two rough substances rub together, as for instance the grating that can be felt and heard between the fractured ends of a bone. Crepitus from within a joint should be distinguished from sharp cracking sounds occurring in normal or abnormal joints after temporary immobility and from the slipping of tendons and ligaments over bone surfaces on movement.

Articular crepitus arises most commonly from osteoarthrotic degenerative changes in joints, most commonly the knee, where subpatellar fine friction can be felt with the hands in many cases, often early in the degenerative process. The patient should be reassured that it is not a serious finding and is felt by most middle-aged or elderly persons at some time in their lives.

A common and unimportant observation after middle-age is the awareness of a grating sensation in the neck, apparent to both patient and clinician. In acromegaly gross crepitus throughout the full range of articular movement is often found in large peripheral joints as it may in other syndromes be associated with hypermobile joints, such as Marfan's and Ehlers–Danlos syndromes. A coarser crepitation may be felt after trauma and in chondromalacia patellae. Coarse crepitation or 'crackling' may be felt with the hands or heard with the ear wherever degenerative changes occur, for instance in the neck or shoulder, but is more common in the more mobile weight-bearing joints, where cartilage has become worn and degenerated, as in, most commonly, the knee.

In rheumatoid arthritis a fine 'rubbing' crepitus occurs which can be felt over the joints in relatively early cases; this may become coarser as the disease advances. At the shoulder inflammatory or degenerative processes may produce crepitus at scapulohumeral or acromioclavicular joints, and a peculiar sensation may be experienced with the hand over the scapular border as though the bone were moving over soft marbles; this, again, is not a sign of serious disease and the patient can in most cases be fully reassured.

On palpation of a joint with hydrarthrosis, the so–called 'silken crepitus' can occasionally be felt, as if two silken surfaces were being rubbed together by the examiner's hands. *Tenosynovitis*, especially around the flexor tendons at the wrist, can also produce a feeling of crepitus, to patient and examiner.

When there is an enlargement of a bone without fracture, and when on palpation a feeling of crepitus or eggshell crackling is obtained, it indicates that some tumour is eroding the overlying cortex. A radiography will be necessary to establish the diagnosis.

Rarefraction of the bones of the skull, either as the result of syphilitic lesions in adults, or of *hydrocephalus* or *craniotabes*, especially in the occipital region of congenitally syphilitic and rickety infants, may make the skull bones so thin that they bend readily on pressure, and sometimes the result is a sensation of crepitus. The diagnosis is generally obvious. The condition is very rare.

Apart from bony, arthritic, or synovial changes, a characteristic feeling of crepitus may be felt beneath the skin when gas or air has accumulated in the subcutaneous tissues as the result of surgical emphysema.

Ian A. D. Bouchier

Crusts

Crusts or scabs are secondary skin lesions formed when serum, blood, sebum, purulent exudate or a mixture of these dries on the surface of the skin. In addition, they may contain dirt and the remains of local applications (e.g. calamine lotion). Scabs often constitute the last stage of vesicles (*see* p. 700) and blisters (see p. 88).

They can result from scratching, or the application of irritant or caustic chemicals. They vary considerably in thickness, from the light crust of dermatitis to the thick barnacle-like scabs seen in keratoderma blennorrhagica. It may sometimes be necessary to remove crusts by prolonged soaking to make a diagnosis of the underlying lesion. This is particularly important when a crust overlies a neoplasm, e.g. rodent ulcer on the scalp. (*See also Table* C.9.) *Impetigo* is the classic cause of golden-coloured crusts on the skin (*Fig.* C.48). These are commonest around the mouth and face of children, but can be very widespread or affect any age group. Acute vesicular 'wet' *eczema* results in crust formation (*Fig.* C.49), usually with a brownish colour, and should this become golden-coloured, secondary impetiginization should be suspected. Crusting rapidly follows secondary degree

burns, or chemical burns, which may on occasion be factitial. *Herpes simplex* (*see Fig.* P. 48) sores become crusted on the fourth or fifth day, and crusting is prolonged if there is a secondary impetigo. The same may occur in *herpes zoster*, but here crusts are often haemorrhagic. In *eczema herpeticum* (*Fig.* C.50) (Kaposi's varicelliform eruption) crusting can be very extensive and pose a difficult nursing problem.

Table C.9. Crusts

Impetigo
Eczema
Trauma—thermal, chemical, factitial
Herpes simplex, eczema herpeticum
Herpes zoster
Pemphigus
Stasis ulcers
Pyoderma gangrenosum
Keratoderma blennorrhagica
Syphilis—rupial
Yaws

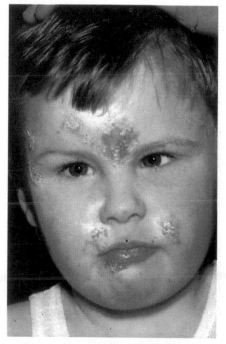

Fig. C.48. Impetigo. (*Westminster Hospital.*)

Pemphigus is the bullous disorder that is characterized by crusting and erosions because the blisters are superficial and therefore very fragile (*see Fig.* B.46). Search should be made for the characteristic mucosal erosions. These crusts are notoriously slow to heal and are probably the only situation where the application of a potent topical corticosteroid can speed re-epithelialization.

Scabbing can be profuse around stasis ulcers, particularly if a *dermatitis medicamentosa* (e.g. to

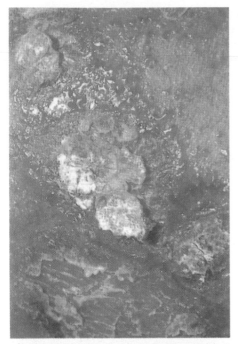

Fig. C.49. Acute crusted eczema. (*St Stephen's Hospital.*)

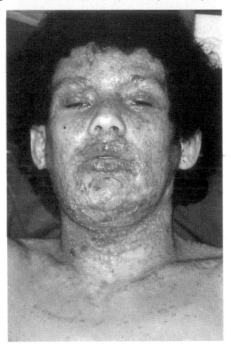

Fig. C.50. Eczema herpeticum. (*Westminster Hospital.*)

lanolin or topical antibiotic) has developed. The crusting over *pyoderma gangrenosum* overlies the characteristic cribriform fibrous scarring.

In *keratoderma blennorrhagica*, the skin eruption of Reiter's syndrome, crusty rupioid nodules may be seen on the limbs accompanying the pustular

crusted lesions of palms and soles. In the rupial form of secondary *syphilis* the crusts are greenish or blackish and consist of several layers, each smaller than the one immediately below it, so that a pyramidal structure is formed resembling a barnacle. Removal of these crusts exposes a foul-smelling ulcer. One of the features of yaws (framboesia, *see* p. 716) is heavily encrusted flexural granulations.

It should not be forgotten that scabbing ulcers and erosions which fail to heal with appropriate anti-infective treatment may be self-inflicted—*dermatitis artefacta* (*see Fig. F.23*).

Richard Staughton

Cyanosis

Cyanosis is an abnormal blue discoloration of the skin and mucous membranes seen whenever the cutaneous and subcutaneous vessels contain an excess of reduced haemoglobin. There is wide interobserver variation in the detection of mild cyanosis. The long held belief that cyanosis was detectable when 5 g/dl or more of reduced haemoglobin was present is not consistently true.

Cyanosis can either be *central* or *peripheral*. Central cyanosis is due either to arterial hypoxaemia or to the presence of the abnormal pigments methaemoglobin or sulphaemoglobin. Central cyanosis is seen in the mucous membranes, particularly the lips, and tongue, as well as on the skin and in good lighting can be identified by most observers when the arterial oxygen saturation falls below about 87 per cent. In anaemia greater desaturation will occur before cyanosis is apparent as less reduced haemoglobin will be present at a given saturation.

Peripheral cyanosis is due to reduced blood flow in the skin, allowing more oxygen to be extracted than normal. Peripheral cyanosis may result from local vasoconstriction, from a low cardiac output or from a combination of both. It is apparent in exposed areas such as fingers, ears, nose and cheeks but not in mucous membranes or the warmer parts of the skin.

Central cyanosis

1. Respiratory disease

The commonest mechanism for arterial hypoxaemia due to respiratory disease is the impairment of matching of ventilation to perfusion. Poorly ventilated but well perfused alveoli will have a low oxygen tension and will contribute poorly oxygenated blood to the systemic arterial circulation. Alveolar hypoventilation will also result in arterial hypoxaemia, usually in association with hypercapnia.

Virtually any diffuse lung disease, if sufficiently severe, will result in central cyanosis. The commonest respiratory cause of central cyanosis is chronic bronchitis and emphysema (chronic obstructive lung disease). Central cyanosis is the hallmark of the 'blue and bloated' form of chronic bronchitis and emphysema (*Fig.* C.51), and is then due to a combination of ventilation/perfusion mismatching and hypoventilation. Patients with the 'pink and puffing' form of chronic bronchitis and emphysema have impaired ventilation/perfusion matching but avoid marked arterial hypoxaemia by maintaining adequate ventilation at the cost of developing dyspnoea. Central cyanosis is a feature of advanced pulmonary fibrosis from whatever cause, when it results from ventilation/perfusion mismatching. Ventilation/perfusion mismatching is also the cause of cyanosis in pulmonary embolism, pulmonary oedema and pneumonia.

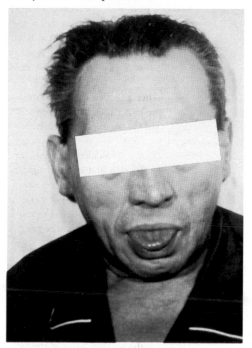

Fig. C.51. Central cyanosis in a 'blue bloater'.

Alveolar hypoventilation is the cause of central hypoxaemia following excess sedation and in patients with ventilatory failure due to impaired chest wall movement. Impaired chest movement may result from kyphoscoliosis or from paresis of respiratory muscles. Alveolar hypoventilation may also cause cyanosis in patients with the sleep apnoea/hypopnoea syndrome, a condition characterized by daytime sleepiness and loud snoring (*see* SLEEP, DISORDERS OF). Patients with severe long-standing sleep apnoea/hypopnoea may develop the 'Pickwickian syndrome' and become cyanosed due to alveolar hypoventilation; this is caused by blunting of respiratory drive by long-term recurrent nocturnal hypoxaemia as a result of repeated obstructive apnoeas. Alveolar hypoventilation also occasionally occurs following obstruction to a major airway. For example, the larynx may be obstructed by aspiration of a foreign body, by laryngeal oedema (usually due to angioneurotic oedema), or bilateral abductor paralysis following thyroidectomy. Tracheal obstruction from thyroid carcinoma, haemorrhage into a thyroid cyst, malignant lymph nodes, primary tracheal tumours or benign tracheal stenosis following tracheostomy or intubation are all rare causes of cyanosis due to alveolar hypoventilation.

2. Cardiovascular disease

Although the commonest cardiac cause of mild hypoxaemia is left heart failure, usually on the basis of ischaemic heart disease, this is rarely severe enough to cause cyanosis except during acute attacks of pulmonary oedema. Although cyanotic congenital heart disease is a less common cause of hypoxaemia, it is a much more common and more dramatic cause of cyanosis (*Fig.* C.52). An important point differentiating cyanosis due to a central veno-arterial shunt from that due to lung disease is the response to breathing oxygen. In lung disease, cyanosis will disappear and arterial hypoxaemia greatly improve as a result of breathing 100 per cent oxygen, unless many perfused alveoli are completely unventilated. In cyanotic congenital heart disease, oxygen produces little change in arterial oxygen saturation as the blood in the shunt does not participate in gas exchange. Other features common to all types of cyanotic congenital heart disease are clubbing of the fingers and toes and polycythaemia. In severe cases the haemoglobin concentration may be well over 20 g/dl.

Fallot's tetralogy is by far the most common congenital cardiac lesion to cause cyanosis. The four classic features are pulmonary stenosis, ventricular septal defect, overriding aorta, and right ventricular hypertrophy; of these, the last is the direct haemodynamic consequence of the pulmonary stenosis; the overriding aorta, although characteristic, is not a major factor in determining the presence or severity of cyanosis. An associated anomaly in several cases is a right-sided aortic arch; this must not be confused with dextro-position of the aorta—a synonym for overriding. Cyanosis is not often present at birth but develops, with clubbing, during the first year or two of life. The symptoms include dyspnoea, relieved by squatting, and syncope associated with deepening of the cyanosis (*see* DYSPNOEA and FAINTS). The arterial and venous pulses are unremarkable except for, occasionally, a dominant 'a' wave in the jugular venous pulse. The

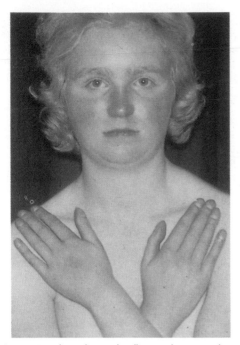

Fig. C.52. Girl, aged 18, with Fallot's tetralogy. Central cyanosis and finger clubbing.

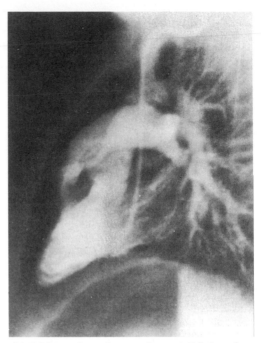

Fig. C.53. Lateral view of angiocardiogram in Fallot's tetralogy. The contrast medium has been injected into the right ventricle and has passed both into the pulmonary artery via an infundibular stenosis and into the overriding aorta via a large ventricular septal defect. The normal pulmonary valve can be seen just distal to the infundibular stenosis. (*Film by courtesy of Dr Basil Strickland.*)

apex beat is little displaced and there may be a slight or moderate right ventricular impulse at the left sternal border. The systolic murmur is rather short and often loud enough to be accompanied by a thrill; the second sound is single. The definitive diagnosis can be made by angiocardiography (*Fig.* C.53).

Pulmonary atresia is embryologically related to Fallot's tetralogy and usually produces very severe cyanosis. The differentiation is easily made by the absence of the systolic murmur of pulmonary stenosis in atresia and its replacement by a subclavicular continuous murmur, usually bilateral, due to large anastomoses between the bronchial and pulmonary arteries. Other conditions which may be more difficult to distinguish clinically from Fallot's tetralogy are pulmonary stenosis with reversed interatrial shunt and Eisenmenger's complex, properly so-called, that is pulmonary hypertension with reversed interventricular shunt. Tricuspid atresia is another cause of cyanosis, characterized by an unusual electrocardiographic pattern suggesting right atrial and left ventricular hypertrophy.

Transposition of the great arteries is a relatively common form of cyanotic congenital heart disease in infancy although few untreated patients survive. The aorta arises from the right ventricle and the pulmonary artery from the left, and clearly, communications between the two circulations, at atrial or ventricular level, must also be present if life is to be maintained. Pulmonary stenosis or pulmonary hypertension may also be present to complicate the haemodynamic situation. The physical signs vary with the associated abnormalities but the X-ray may be of diagnostic value. The vascular pedicle of the heart is rather narrow in the postero-anterior view and pulmonary plethora is nearly always present. As oligaemia of the lung fields is the rule in most types of cyanotic congenital heart disease, the association of cyanosis with plethora is very suggestive of transposition. Angiocardiography is diagnostic, showing, in the lateral view, the aorta arising anteriorly from the right ventricle and the pulmonary artery posteriorly from the left (*Fig.* C.54). Very rare types of cyanotic congenital heart disease include drainage of the superior or inferior vena cava into the left atrium and some cases of Ebstein's anomaly of the tricuspid valve with reversed interatrial shunt.

Pulmonary arteriovenous malformations may cause central cyanosis if the shunt is large enough. They are frequently associated with cutaneous telangiectases, especially on the lips, and may occur in the familial condition, hereditary haemorrhagic telangiectasia. Continuous murmurs may be heard over the aneurysms, which may be multiple. In the radiograph one or more round opacities are visible and tomography will often reveal the feeding artery and draining vein (*Fig.* C.55).

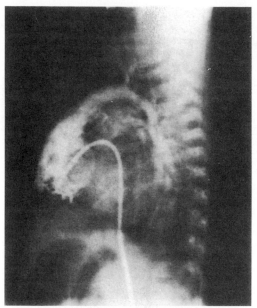

Fig. C.54. Lateral view of angiocardiogram in transposition of the great arteries. The contrast medium has been injected into the right ventricle and has passed into the anteriorly placed aorta. The pulmonary artery, lying posteriorly, has been opacified via a ductus which is visible. (Film by courtesy of Dr Basil *Strickland*.)

3. Pigmentary cyanosis

Cyanosis is a major feature of a group of conditions in which ferric (Fe^{+++}) rather than ferrous (Fe^{++}) iron is present in haemoglobin, producing methaemoglobin. Sulphaemoglobin is a poorly characterized substance which can be produced by the action of hydrogen sulphide on haemoglobin. Small amounts of these pigments, for example, 1·5 g methaemoglobin or 0·5 g of sulphaemoglobin, are said to produce as marked cyanosis as 5 g of deoxygenated haemoglobin.

Methaemoglobinaemia may be congenital or acquired. *Congenital methaemoglobinaemias* due to deficiency of NADH-methaemoglobin reductase have a recessive inheritance. Methaemoglobinaemia may also result from congenital abnormalities of the alpha or beta globin chain of haemoglobin rendering the molecule unresponsive to methaemoglobin reductase, and these varieties may be inherited as autosomal dominant characteristics. Acquired methaemoglobinaemia can result from the ingestion of a large group of chemicals including oxidizing agents such as nitrites and chlorates. Nitrates can be converted to nitrites in the bowel and cyanosis has been reported in infants in association with a high nitrate content of drinking water. Poisoning with potassium chlorate can also produce methaemoglobinaemia apart from its more serious effects. Aniline dyes have also been incriminated: these compounds can be absorbed through the intact skin. Phenacetin

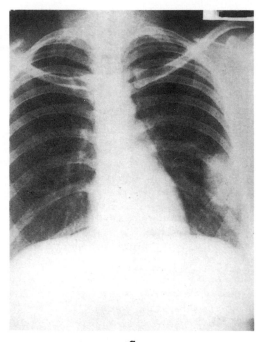

a

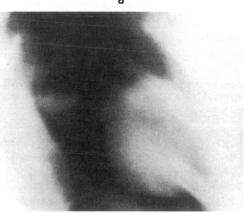

b

Fig. C.55. Pulmonary haemangioma in a case of hereditary haemorrhagic telangiectasia. *a*, In the plain film large vessels can be seen passing to and from the tumour. *b*, These are shown more clearly in the tomogram. (*Films by courtesy of Dr Basil Strickland.*)

can also cause methaemoglobinaemia and cyanosis, although due to declining use of this preparation, this is now rare. The symptoms of methaemoglobinaemia are those of severe anaemia to which the condition is closely analogous, namely dyspnoea on exertion and dizziness. The diagnosis can be confirmed by spectroscopic analysis which will detect a band at 630 μm which disappears with the addition of a reducing agent.

Sulphaemoglobinaemia is a poorly defined condition which may occur in conjunction with methaemoglobinaemia following ingestion of nitrates, nitrites, aniline dyes and phenacetin. It has also been reported in conjunction with chronic constipation and with malabsorption. There is no congenital form of this condition. Sulphaemoglobinaemia is usually asymptomatic.

Peripheral Cyanosis

When red cell transit through cutaneous vessels is delayed, continued oxygen extraction will decrease the oxygen saturation of the haemoglobin and cyanosis will appear. This may result either from increased resistance to blood flow, from decreased cardiac output or from increased blood viscosity.

1. Increased resistance in blood flow

The commonest cause of peripheral cyanosis is the transient and appropriate vasoconstriction in response to cold. The best-known medical conditions associated with peripheral cyanosis are *Raynaud's disease* and *Raynaud's phenomenon* which are described in detail in the section on FINGERS, DEAD.

Acrocyanosis is a relatively benign condition due to spasm of smaller cutaneous arteries and arterioles. The hands and fingers are cold and mottled red and blue but pain is not a feature. Arteriolar spasm is also the mechanism of *erythrocyanosis*, a disease almost confined to young women in which cyanotic blotches are seen in the lower parts of the legs. Cyanosis of the affected leg or legs occurs occasionally following deep venous thrombosis, particularly if collateral drainage is poor. This condition has been termed 'phlegmasia caerulea dolens'. Similarly, cyanosis of the face may occur, together with gross venous engorgement and oedema, as a feature of *superior vena caval obstruction* from whatever cause. This mechanism may contribute to the so-called *traumatic* cyanosis following crush injury to the chest although hypoxaemia due to lung trauma may contribute.

2. Decreased cardiac output

The ashen grey appearance of patients with severe shock is a typical example of peripheral cyanosis due to a marked fall in cardiac output and occurs irrespective of the cause of the shock. The low cardiac output and vasoconstriction which occur with left ventricular failure can also cause peripheral cyanosis, although central cyanosis will usually coexist. Similarly, cyanosis in massive *pulmonary embolism* is usually both central and peripheral. The classical malar flush in mitral stenosis is an example of local peripheral cyanosis but why this should be so sited is unknown.

3. Increased blood viscosity

Cyanosis may occur in *polycythaemia rubra vera* despite a normal arterial oxygen saturation. This is presumed to result from decreased cutaneous blood flow due to increased viscosity.

Neil J. Douglas

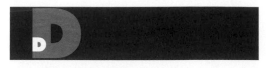

Deafness

Deafness is one of the major handicaps suffered by mankind and is inevitable with the ageing process. There are many causes of deafness in the younger years and, of these causes, 99 per cent are peripheral. If information reaches the acoustic nerve, it is very rare for there ever to be any lesions beyond the acoustic nerve which can cause deafness. Peripheral causes of deafness can be classified as:

Conductive
These are obstructive lesions in the external and/or middle ear which prevent sound from reaching the cochlea.
Sensorineural
These are lesions in the cochlea or acoustic nerve which prevent sound from reaching the brain-stem.
Mixed
Combined conductive and sensorineural lesions.

Hearing Tests

These are carried out to diagnose the cause of the deafness and also to ascertain its severity. We will list them in ascending order of complexity.

Voice tests

In the clinical situation, a good idea of the severity of the deafness can be gained from these simple clinical tests. The patient sits facing a wall at one end of the room and occludes one ear pressing a finger against the tragus. He is instructed to repeat after the examiner whatever the latter says.

The examiner stands behind the patient and whispers test words. He increases the distance between him and the patient until the patient is no longer able to repeat the words accurately. The same process is repeated with the use of the conversation voice. Someone with normal hearing should be able to hear both a whispered and a conversation voice at 20 ft with each ear. Someone who is able to hear a conversation voice at 20 ft but a whispered voice only at say 6 ft is suffering from a sensorineural deafness. Patients with conductive loss will have a diminished but equal response to both conversation and whispered voice tests. In assessing medicolegal cases, malingerers quite often show a discrepancy between the assessment by voice test and by more complex tests.

It is important that lip-reading is avoided and so the patient should never be allowed to see the examiner's lips.

Tuning-fork tests

These have been used for over a century for the purpose not only of measuring the degree of deafness but also to subdivide it into sensorineural or conductive. The tuning-fork should either by a 256 cps or a 512 cps fork and should be big enough so that its note lasts at least 60 seconds after being sounded.

THE RINNE'S TEST

Someone with normal hearing will hear the tuning-fork better by air-conduction than by bone-conduction. This, unfortunately, is the same in someone with sensorineural deafness and so the test does not have a diagnostic specificity. It can, however, distinguish between sensorineural and conductive deafness because, in conductive deafness, the patient hears bone-conduction better than air-conduction, the so-called Rinne negative test. There is no logical reason why one response is called Rinne positive and the other Rinne negative. It is only by convention that the conductive deafness response is known as a negative Rinne.

The base of the tuning-fork is held on the patient's mastoid process until he says he can no longer hear the sound. The fork is then rapidly transferred so that the vibrating forks are close to the external auditory meatus. If the patient continues to hear the sound then it is considered that he hears better by air-conduction than by bone-conduction.

If there is a big difference between the ears then an extraneous sound should be introduced into the non-tested ear to prevent a false response.

WEBER'S TEST

In the Weber test, the sound is heard either in the better ear if there is a sensorineural deafness present or in the worse ear if it is a conductive deafness. The normal response is to hear the sound equally in both ears. Again, the test does not have a diagnostic specificity unless it is lateralized. The tuning-fork is placed in the middle of the forehead and the patient is asked to signify in which ear he hears the sound clearly.

ABSOLUTE BONE-CONDUCTION TEST

In this test an assessment is made of the patient's ability to hear by bone-conduction. This is a measure of sensorineural deafness and the patient's response is compared to the examiner's response. If the examiner has roughly normal hearing then the patient ought to hear a tuning-fork placed on his mastoid as long as

the examiner does. If he hears it for less time then it is considered that his bone-conduction is diminished and, thus, he has a sensorineural deafness.

Audiometry

PURE-TONE AUDIOMETRY

A pure-tone audiometer produces tones of varying intensity (0–100 db) and frequency (250 cps to 8000 cps). The test is carried out by the patient wearing earphones. Test sounds at different intensities and frequencies are introduced via the earphones and the patient is asked to indicate when he hears the sound. The sounds are produced at the threshold of hearing and this is marked on a graph producing an audiogram (*Fig. D.1*). A normal person should hear between 0–10 dB over the full frequency range.

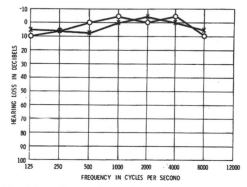

Fig. D.1. Audiogram showing hearing that is within 'normal limits'. It is conventional to represent hearing by air-conduction in the right ear by O—O, and in the left ear by X—X.

Bone conduction is tested by putting an applicator in contact with the patient's mastoid process. The test is then carried out in the same manner and the threshold of hearing indicated on the audiogram. In this way it can be seen if bone-conduction is better than air-conduction (conductive deafness) or if bone-conduction and air-conduction are roughly equal (normal or sensorineural deafness).

SPEECH AUDIOMETRY

It is possible for a patient to have a normal pure-tone audiogram because for this he only requires to have about half of the acoustic nerve functioning. A more discriminatory test of hearing is a speech audiogram where the patient has to respond to a list of test words played at threshold through earphones. Either a graph can be made of the patient's speech responses or a simple raw speech discrimination score can be recorded.

A difference between the speech audiogram and the pure-tone audiogram is indicative of malingering.

TYMPANOMETRY

This is carried out by an Impedance Meter and two tests are possible with this. In the first, the pressure in the middle ear is measured as is the compliance of the drum. A graph is produced and it is possible to diagnose Eustachian tube obstruction, fluid in the middle ear, otosclerotic fixation and ossicular discontinuity. The stapedius muscle reflexes can also be measured and this is of diagnostic importance in otosclerosis, ossicular discontinuity and in facial palsy.

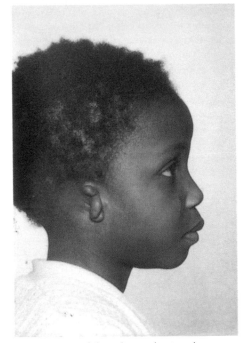

Fig. D.2. Atresia of the right ear showing absent external auditory meatus and deformed auricle.

TESTS FOR RECRUITMENT

In the space available it is not possible to give an explanation of the phenomenon of recruitment. Suffice it to say that this is a very important test of hearing because it can distinguish between lesions of the acoustic nerve and lesions of the cochlea. It is a simple test to do and is carried out with a pure-tone audiometer.

EVOKED RESPONSE AUDIOMETRY

This can be done as cortical evoked response audiometry, electrocochleography or brainstem-evoked audiometry. It is now the main test of hearing after pure-tone audiometry. It is invaluable in assessing medico-legal problems and the brainstem-evoked response audiogram can clearly indicate whether or not there is a lesion in the acoustic nerve.

Evoked response audiometry is of enormous importance in the testing of infants, young children and people with multiple handicaps.

Hearing tests in children

Deafness should be diagnosed in infants as early as possible. The earlier deafness is diagnosed, the more chance there is of the child developing normal lingual language as opposed to sign language.

Every child now born in the UK has a hearing test by specially trained nurses at 6 weeks and at the end of the first year of life. Where the nurse does not receive an unambiguous response indicating normal hearing from her simple clinical tests, the child is referred to special children's speech and hearing clinics. There, further clinical tests will be carried out and probably evoked response audiometry.

If the child is found to be deaf then special education is set in hand at a very early age and amplification devices are fitted to the child, depending on the severity of the deafness.

CONDUCTIVE DEAFNESS

The causes of conductive deafness may be summarized in *Table* D.1.

Conductive deafness is often less severe than sensorineural deafness and it has a maximum of 60 dB. Very frequently medical or surgical procedures can be carried out either to arrest the process or to cure it. In some cases, such as serious otitis media or otosclerosis, there can be a dramatic restoration of hearing with relatively simple surgery.

It is relatively easy to establish whether a deafness is conductive or sensorineural with the tests listed above. In certain cases of conductive deafness, radiography has to be used, especially in the assessment of congenital syndromes or ossicular discontinuity. In this, CT scanning is extremely helpful.

There are a very considerable number of congenital syndromes associated with deafness; mostly sensorineural in character. Where conductive lesions occur there is often an inner ear lesion so that a mixed deafness is the result. It is quite impossible to list all the possible recorded combinations of congenital abnormalities, but the golden rule is that if one abnormality is observed a careful search for others must be made and, during this search, deafness must never be forgotten.

Some of the more common are listed. The Treacher Collins syndrome (*Fig.* D.3) comprises micrognathia, depressed malar bones, eyes sloping downwards and outwards with notched lower lids, ptosis of the auricles and middle-ear abnormalities with deformed ossicles. The Crouzon deformity is craniofacial dysost-

Table D.1. The causes of conductive deafness

Congenital lesions
1. Atresia of the external meatus and middle ear usually with microtia (*see Fig.* D.2.)
2. Atresia associated with other facial defects
3. Middle-ear deformities
   Some syndromes (frequently associated with sensorineural loss in addition to the conductive loss)
       Mandibulofacial dysostosis (Treacher Collins)
       Crouzon deformity
       Marfan's syndrome
       Klippel–Feil syndrome
       Trisomy D and E
       Cretinism
       Cleft palate
       Submucous cleft palate
       Osteogenesis imperfecta (van der Hoeve–de Kleyn triad)
       Thalidomide
       Rubella

External auditory meatus
    Wax
    Foreign bodies
    Otitis externa
    Exostoses (Diver's ear) (Wet ear)

Middle-ear lesions
    Trauma
        Blood
        Ossicular disruption
        Perforated tympanic membrane
    Acute otitis media
    Eustachian malfunction
        Atelectasis of middle ear
        Serous otitis ('Glue ear')
    Otitic barotrauma
    Chronic otitis media
    Haemotympanum
    Malignant disease
    Glomus tumour
    Otosclerosis

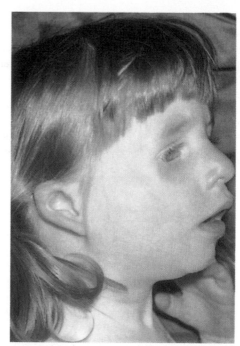

Fig. D.3. Treacher Collins syndrome showing typical appearance of eye, micrognathia, depressed malar bone and ptosis of the ear.

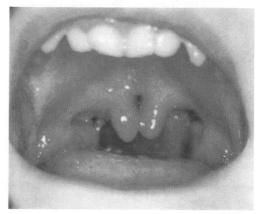

Fig. D.4. Submucous cleft palate with deeply bifid uvula typical of this rare condition.

osis. Marfan's syndrome comprises an inherited collagen disorder—abnormally long extremities, subluxation of the lens, cardiovascular abnormalities and deafness. In the Klippel–Feil syndrome there are malformed cervical vertebrae and a webbed neck.

Chromosomal disorders in the trisomy D and E cause very marked ossicular abnormalities. Thyroid deficiency leads more often to cochlear end-organ damage as do rubella and the thalidomide abnormality, but in all these middle-ear deformities are found.

The van der Hoeve–de Kleyn triad of deafness, due to stapedial fixation (otosclerosis), blue sclerotics and fragile bones is uncommon with a frequency of 2–3/100,000. It is a strongly familial disorder.

Cleft-palate (*Fig.* D.4), with a frequency of about 1/1000, is much more common and is an important cause of deafness. Since it is the palatal muscles (tensor palati and levator palati) that control the Eustachian tube it is not surprising that nearly every cleft-palate child before closure of the cleft is deaf to some degree due to failure of tubal opening and atelectasis or fluid in the middle ear. After operation a considerable but

reducing number of children are still deaf, often to some 30 dB.

A submucous cleft-palate, where the muscle layer is separated under intact mucosa, has the same effects on the ear but is not easy to recognize. The uvula is deeply bifid and a notch instead of a tubercle may be palpated in the centre of the free border of the hard palate.

Diseases of the external auditory meatus rarely cause deafness as hearing is retained while there is the smallest airway past the obstruction to the drum.

Sudden deafness results from closure—often as wax swells on contact with water.

Middle-ear lesions causing deafness are often easily identified by thorough and careful otoscopy with a good light. Two of those listed deserve special mention: serous otitis and otosclerosis.

Serous otitis, otherwise known as 'secretory otitis media' or 'glue ear', is extremely common and is present in 4 per cent of all children between the ages 5 and 15. This means that almost every classroom in the country will contain one child deaf to a level of 20 dB or more. Detection and treatment of deafness in these children is very important because it has been shown that it can hold up progress at school.

The changes in the drum are fairly typical. There can be a dark appearance or a yellowish glaze. Occasionally, fluid levels and bubbles can be seen through the drum membrane but in other instances there may be no observable clinical signs. The diagnosis is primarily by tympanometry where a negative middle-ear pressure is found together with an increased drum compliance.

In adults, serous otitis media may be the first sign of Eustachian tube obstruction by a nasopharyngeal carcinoma. Although not so important in the European, it is of very definite clinical significance in the Chinese where nasopharyngeal carcinoma is the commonest head and neck tumour.

Otosclerosis occurs in young adults with females being more commonly afflicted than males. In females the deafness is often made worse by pregnancy. Patients very often hear better in noisy environments (paracusis). Audiometry shows a conductive loss with bone-conduction being better than air-conduction. Depending on the so-called 'air–bone gap', decisions regarding surgery can be made. When the air–bone gap is more than 30 dB then the patient stands to gain from surgery but, until then, should probably use a hearing aid.

SENSORINEURAL DEAFNESS

Though there may be some overlap it is probably better to separate those conditions chiefly arising in childhood (*Table* D.2) from the adult deaf.

The importance of early testing and the identification of the profoundly deaf child has already been mentioned. Normal development of an infant is greatly dependent upon hearing, the understanding of speech being the one function of human behaviour which sets man apart from animals. Failure to hear speech not only prevents the development of language but inhibits formation of personal and social relationships. Since nearly all deaf children have some residual hearing it is of vital importance to pick out the deaf

Table D.2. Causes of deafness in children

1. *Prenatal*
    a. Genetic
        Scheibe type
        Bing–Siebenmann type
        Waardenburg's syndrome
        Pendred's syndrome
        Mondini-Alexander type
        Michel type
        Usher's syndrome
        Endemic cretinism
        Klippel–Feil syndrome
    b. Non-genetic
        Diseases occurring in pregnancy
        Rubella and other viral
            illnesses
        Toxaemia
        Diabetes
        Syphilis
        Nephritis
        Drugs taken in pregnancy
        Streptomycin
        Quinine
        Salicylates
        Thalidomide
2. *Perinatal*
    Prematurity
    Jaundice—haemolytic disease and kernicterus
    Anoxia due to birth trauma
3. *Postnatal*
    a. Genetic
        Familial degenerative deafness
        Otosclerosis
        Alport's syndrome
    b. Non-genetic infectious diseases
        Measles
        Mumps
        Meningitis
            Meningococcal
            Pneumococcal
            Viral
            Tuberculous
        Trauma
        Otitis media
        Ototoxic antibiotics
            Streptomycin
            Neomycin
            Gentamicin

and maximize the use of the hearing they have as early as possible, at least by 6 months of age, and before they have developed into 'fixed visualizers'.

Infants who have a family history of deafness, maternal infections during the pregnancy or perinatal problems, who are late to talk or who have other congenital defects, must be considered as being 'at risk' and should be carefully tested. The frequency of sporadic cases of deafness makes testing of all babies important. In this respect the mother's views should never be ignored; if she thinks her child is deaf the diagnosis should be presumed correct until firmly proved otherwise. It must be remembered, also, that mild or moderate conductive deafness may be an additional handicap and even a small amount of additional deafness is significant when the base line is already low.

There are many more genetically determined syndromes involving sensorineural deafness than conductive; a number of examples from the main groups have been listed. The Scheibe abnormality shows a normal vestibular mechanism with failure of sacculo-cochlear development; in the Mondini type of deficiency both vestibular and cochlear structures are deformed. The Bing type has a normal bony labyrinth but the membranous labyrinth is malformed or degenerate in both cochlea and vestibule; in addition there may be central nervous system abnormalities. The fourth member of this group where abnormalities are mainly in the otic capsule, the Michel type, shows almost complete lack of development of the inner ear and often associated mental retardation.

Waardenburg's syndrome is an example of the group of integumentary system disease and deafness. A white forelock and heterochromia of the iris are combined with familial genetic deafness.

Pendred's syndrome comprises a congenital goitre, hypothyroidism with severe abnormalities of the labyrinth, both vestibular and cochlear parts.

A large group of abnormalities is described where hearing loss is associated with eye disease, retinal abnormalities, myopia, optic atrophy and corneal degeneration. Usher's syndrome is deafness combined with retinitis pigmentosa.

Cretinism is associated with deafness which may respond to early and intensive treatment.

The Klippel–Feil syndrome has been mentioned above.

Non-genetic prenatal influences are well known from the rubella story. A careful history may implicate one or other factor. It should be noted that, with regard to rubella, the virus may persist after birth and deafness may develop as a late-onset problem in childhood.

Perinatal causes of deafness are important and preventable. The resulting deafness is in general less severe than that arising from rubella which is characteristically very profound.

Late-onset genetic deafness is now considered to be a much more important cause of deafness in childhood and later life than previously thought. Alport's syndrome is an example of this and is also representative of a group of syndromes where genetic hearing loss is associated with nephritis. Otosclerosis as a cause of mixed deafness is included here as well as elsewhere.

Of the non-genetic group the diagnosis will be arrived at from the history or from consideration of the disease. Mumps deafness is usually very profound but, curiously, is nearly always unilateral and this serves to identify it on occasion.

The proportion of the various groups of conditions causing congenital deafness has been estimated as one-quarter each of genetic, maternal rubella, perinatal causes and unknown. Genetic causes, either alone or as a contributory factor by increasing the liability to other influences, are being increasingly implicated. In areas of the world where consanguineous marriages are common—and in expatriate communities of those peoples—genetic sensorineural deafness is reported to comprise 70–80 per cent. A careful family history is most important in making a probable diagnosis.

A different scheme of classification is appropriate for adults (see Table D.3).

Many conditions in this list of the causes of sensorineural deafness in adults have been considered above. Some, however, require more attention.

Refsum's disease is yet another syndrome combining eye disease (retinitis pigmentosa), polyneuritis, cerebellar ataxia and a genetic late onset deafness. The inheritance is autosomal recessive.

Acoustic trauma from noise is wholly preventable and entirely untreatable. It may be diagnosed from the history and the audiogram which shows a typical curve, sharply falling in the higher frequencies with a dip at 4 kHz. As the lesion is at the end-organ, recruitment of loudness is present and patients are intolerant of amplification and often have little benefit from hearing aids. Noise-induced hearing loss may be demonstrated audiometrically as temporary (Noise-Induced Temporary Threshold Shift—NITTS) or permanent (Noise-Induced Permanent Threshold Shift—NIPTS) and may be caused by sudden loud sounds such as gunfire or by continuous trauma such as traffic noise, industrial noise, agricultural noise or 'pop' music.

Compensation is now being offered on a very large scale to workers exposed to noise in industry. This affects mainly shipyard and railway workers, motor car industry workers and miners. In the early stages these men show a dip at 6 kHz. With long exposure to noise, the dip widens and affects 3, 4 and 6 kHz. It is usually hearing maintained at 8 kHz until the late stages of deafness. Tinnitus is very frequently present in noise-induced hearing loss.

Vascular lesions of the inner ear are the cause, or part cause, of many cases of deafness. Sudden, small vascular accidents in the end-arterioles may cause deafness by damaging part or the whole of the organ of Corti. Immediate treatment with vasodilators may restore the whole circulation, so early diagnosis is important.

The cause of Menière's disease (Fig. D.7) is not fully known and is probably multi-factorial, but failure of vasomotor control and vasoconstriction of the vessels of the stria vascularis play an important part.

Table D.3. Causes of deafness in older children and in adults

1. Cochlear lesions
    Late-onset genetic deafness
        Familial degenerative
        Alport's syndrome
        Refsum's syndrome
        Otosclerosis (later cochlear effects)
    Inflammatory (labyrinthitis)
        Bacterial
        Late-onset rubella
        Syphilis
        Mumps
        Herpes
        Measles
    Trauma
        Fracture of temporal bone
        Acoustic trauma—temporary
                        permanent
    Vascular lesions
        Atherosclerosis
        Hypertension
        Vascular accident of end-artery
        Menière's disease (labyrinthine hydrops)
        Lermoyez's syndrome
        Leukaemia
        Malaria
    Degenerative (partly vascular)
        Presbyacusis (*Figs* D.5, D.6)
    Vitamin deficiency
        Vitamin B deficiency
    Dietary
        Tropical ataxic neuropathy
    Hormonal
        Myxoedema
        Pregnancy
    Drug-induced deafness
        Antibiotics
            Aminoglycosides
                Streptomycin
                Neomycin
                Gentamicin
            Others in large doses
        Aspirin (reversible deafness)
        Quinine
        Chloroquine
        Chemotherapeutic agents for malignant
            disease
    Unknown

2. Retrocochlear lesions
    a. Neural   Acoustic neuroma
                     (8th nerve neurilemmoma)
                  Meningitis
                    Leptomeningitis
                    Syphilitic
                    Tuberculous
                  Cerebello-pontine angle tumour
                  Trauma
                  Carcinomatous neuropathy
                  Vogt–Koyanagi syndrome
                  Harada's disease
                  Unknown

    b. Central   Multiple sclerosis
                  Encephalitis
                  Meningomyelitis
                  Pontine glioma
                  Concussion
                  Vascular accidents
                  Brainstem damage from head
                    injury
                  Psychogenic—hysterical
                  Unknown

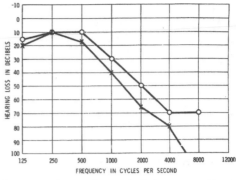

Fig. D.5. Audiogram showing the fairly symmetrical hearing loss for high tones in presbyacusis.

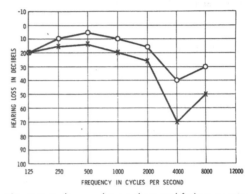

Fig. D.6. Audiogram showing the typical findings in noise-inducing hearing loss. In this case the patient had been shooting for some years with a 12-bore gun and the left ear, being nearer the muzzle, has sustained greater damage than the right.

Diagnosis is made from the typical history of fluctuant sensorineural deafness with a gradual increase in severity, combined with tinnitus and prolonged and severe attacks of vertigo with vomiting. The disease shows periods of remission between groups of attacks. There is a psychological component as well. Depressed vestibular function and an end-organ deafness together with the history serve to identify this disease. Lermoyez's syndrome is a variant where the hearing improves very suddenly after an attack of vertigo and tinnitus. It is thought that the membranous labyrinth ruptures releasing the endolymphatic pressure and restoring cochlear function.

    Leukaemia causes haemorrhage in the inner ear and in malaria the destruction of the blood cells leaves pigment in the cells. Deafness in this disease may also be caused by antimalarial drugs.

    Presbyacusis (senile deafness) is common to mankind and loss of hearing in the higher frequencies is almost invariable with age though the rate is dependent upon genetic background, exposure to noise (city dwellers lose their hearing more rapidly than country dwellers) and vascular changes of atherosclerosis. The audiogram shows an increasing depression in the high

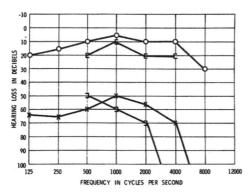

Fig. D.7. Audiogram in a case of Meniére's disease affecting the left labyrinth. Careful investigations are required to exclude acoustic neuroma if unilateral sensorineural deafness such as this is found.

frequencies. Failure to hear speech ('I can hear you talking but I cannot hear what you say'), in background noise especially, results from the high tone loss and inability to hear the consonants which carry the meaning in speech.

Diet is important. Vitamin B deficiency leads to dermal, mucosal and aural damage. It has been shown that hearing loss stemming from other causes is always worse in those with a B-deficient diet. Cassava, which contains cyanides and is an important part of the diet of Africans and some Caribbeans, allied to genetic factors it is thought, causes tropical ataxic neuropathy, an oto-ophthalmo-neuropathy described in tropical regions.

The deafness of myxoedema, the occasional deafness of pregnancy and aspirin deafness are unusual among the causes of sensorineural loss in that they are reversible.

With regard to drug-induced deafness it must be noted that ototoxicity results not only from systemic treatment but also from the use of antibiotics locally in the ear to treat otitis media—chloramphenicol, neomycin and gentamicin may all act in this manner.

Among the neural and central lesions acoustic neuromas are important because they are silent, slow growing, difficult to diagnose and potentially lethal if not found in a small and easily operable state. They may be solitary or occur as a manifestation of familial neurofibromasosis (von Recklinghausen's disease), when other fibromas will be seen. The presentation is usually with increasing, unilateral, non-recruiting sensorineural deafness often accompanied by tinnitus. Vertigo is not intermittent and severe as in Meniére's disease but it is often present in the form of a vague unsteadiness. Vestibular function is affected and there is a canal paresis on the side of the tumour. Fifth nerve symptoms are often early with loss of homolateral pain and temperature sensation on the face due to pressure

on the descending tract of the 5th nerve. The best clinical method is to test the corneal reflex as an indicator of pain sensation. Nowadays it is hoped to find these tumours before they have extended beyond the internal auditory meatus to impinge on the brainstem.

Diagnosis of acoustic neuroma, after clinical, audiometric and vestibular tests, requires an MRI to show any enlargement or erosion of the internal auditory meatus, as little as 1-2 mm of difference being significant.

The Vogt-Koyanagi syndrome, from which it is thought that the artist Goya suffered, is a sudden and rare illness with severe headache and malaise which goes on to uveitis, alopecia, vitiligo and deafness. Harada's disease is very similar but with retinal detachment instead of uveitis. The deafness is usually permanent but the uveitis recovers. The depressing effects of sudden complete deafness on a sensitive artist such as Goya explains his change of style from brightly coloured, happy pictures of handsome men and pretty girls to those of his later 'Black Period' and the 'Disasters of War'. This is an indication of the severe psychological effects that deafness may bring.

A.G.D. Maran

Delusions

A delusion has been defined as a false unshakeable conviction which is out of keeping with the patient's educational, cultural and social background. It is a belief which is held with great certainty and patients themselves may not complain of this symptom but will come to medical attention because they have acted on a delusional belief or relatives have become aware of their unusual or bizarre content. A delusion should be distinguished from an *overvalued idea* which is a comprehendable conviction held beyond the bounds of reason. For example, morbid jealously is an overvalued idea when a spouse who is unduly preoccupied by thoughts of their partner's suspected infidelity can be reassured after lengthy persuasion that their belief is irrational. In delusional jealousy on the other hand such reassurance would not be possible because the spouse would be convinced of infidelity in the face of all evidence to the contrary. Delusions are also to be distinguished from obsessional ideas which may be bizarre but trouble the patient and are seen by them as intrusive, unwanted and requiring some response (*see* OBSESSION). Similarly, religious and political nonconformity, however extreme, does not represent delusional belief when it is in keeping with the culture to which the patient belongs.

Delusions may be caused by organic disease, by drug or substance abuse or may be signs of a functional psychotic illness (*Table* D.4).

Table D.4. Delusions

Common causes
Schizophrenia
Depression
Mania
Paranoid illnesses
Substance abuse
  Alcohol
  Amphetamines
  Methylphenidate
  Cocaine
  Cannabis
  Hallucinogens (e.g. LSD)
  Phencyclidine
Delirium (*see* p. 114)
Drugs
  Bromocriptine
  L-dopa
  Corticosteroids
Alzheimer's-type dementia
Multi-infarct dementia
Huntington's chorea
Temporal lobe epilepsy
Hyperthyroidism
Hypothyroidism
Encephalopathies
Head injury

Rarer causes
Neurosyphilis
AIDS
Cerebral abscess
Multiple sclerosis

Organic delusional state

Delusions may be a prominent feature of a number of quite diverse conditions and organic causes should be considered in any patient particularly if delusions arise for the first time in someone over the age of 35. Substances such as amphetamines, cocaine and phencyclidine, if taken intravenously, cause an initial feeling of well-being and confidence. Intoxication with high doses may however lead to an episode of paranoid delusions with visual, auditory and tactile hallucinations, incoherent speech and anxious mood. Associated with these mental phenomena are tachycardia, pupillary dilatation, elevated blood pressure, sweating and sometimes nausea. Full recovery is usual within 48 hours but cessation of regular heavy use may lead to a withdrawal state which again may be associated with paranoid delusions and suicidal ideation, fatigue, depression and agitation persisting for several days. Cocaine, shortly after intake, leads in some users to the rapid onset of a delusional disorder which can persist for over a week and occasionally for several months. Delusions are usually persecutory, and other features are body image distortion, the feeling of insects on the skin (cocaine bug) and sometimes aggression

directed against imagined persecutors. Cannabis and hallucinogens such as LSD may also cause paranoid delusions in some users.

An organic delusional state may develop in some subjects with temporal lobe epilepsy who show interictal features similar to schizophrenia. Huntington's chorea and space-occupying cerebral lesions may also cause a similar picture.

Delusions in functional psychoses

In the absence of organic causes delusional thinking is commonly a symptom of *schizophrenia*, the *paranoid states*, *mania* or *depression*. To distinguish these possibilities considerable stress is placed on whether or not the content of the delusions are congruent or incongruent with the prevailing mood of the patient. For example, when a depressed patient expresses the delusion that there is a plot to kill him this is in keeping with the depressed mood as is the case with a manic patient who believes he has been invested with special powers and has a mission to save the world. These delusions are said to be secondary because an understandable connection can be made between the patient's mood and the content of the delusion. Moreover these beliefs will disappear when the mania and depression have responded to treatment. In schizophrenia, by contrast, the content of delusional thinking is often bizarre and out of keeping with the patient's mood state, and the beliefs often persist. *Primary delusions* describe those beliefs which take the form of sudden convictions which come into the patient's mind in response to what the ordinary observer would consider a totally unrelated experience. For example, a patient when reading the number plate of a passing car suddenly became convinced that the driver was accusing him of being a homosexual. Primary delusions of this sort are observed more often in schizophrenia than affective illness. Schizophrenic patients may also experience *delusional mood* when they are perplexed, unsettled and convinced that something self-referential is occurring but are unable to understand what it is. There is no hard and fast distinction between the types of delusions found in schizophrenia, mania and depression but clinical observation suggests that certain types of delusion are more commonly associated with schizophrenia. These include the delusion that the body is being influenced by outside forces and the subject is being 'made' to perform certain acts, think certain thoughts or, rarely, to feel certain emotions. The patient may complain that alien thoughts have been inserted into his head or that his own thoughts have been removed. Some commonly encountered delusions which may occur just as frequently in schizophrenia as affective illness include paranoia, persecutory beliefs, grandiose delusions and delusions of guilt, poverty, worthlessness and hypochondriacal beliefs. Both *grandiose* and *depressive delusions* are often set in a religious context although beliefs in influence by radio, radar and other real or imagined physical forces are also common.

Monosymptomatic delusions sometimes occur in a patient whose thinking, mood and behaviour show none of the disturbances normally associated with schizophrenia or affective psychosis. Morbid jealously, the total conviction of the spouse's infidelity although sometimes associated with the psychoses, alcohol abuse or psychopathic personality, may also occur as the only symptom when it must nevertheless be taken seriously by the clinician as a significant cause of domestic violence and even homicide. Other delusions which occur in isolation as well as in the context of major psychotic illness include delusions of love (*de Clerambault's syndrome*) in which the patient believes that some person, usually an authority figure, is in love with them, and delusions of misidentification (*Capgras syndrome*) in which the patient believes that someone close to them, for example a wife, has been replaced by an imposter pretending to be that person. *Somatic* (*hypochondrical*) delusions take several forms. The person may be convinced that certain parts of the body (brain, intestine, stomach) are not functioning or in extreme cases are not there at all. There may be conviction of an internal parasite or infestation on or in the skin. The body may be held to be misshapen or ugly or there may be a belief that a foul smell is emanating from it. Hypochondriacal delusions are frequently found in depression and may include the belief that the patient is dying from an incurable disease such as cancer. However, such beliefs may also occur in the absence of other overt psychiatric abnormality. Delusions concerning the face, mouth, teeth and gums may be accompanied by frequent and persistent demands for medical and dental investigations and be the basis for litigation. Some patients with monosymptomatic delusions are considered depressed or schizophrenic but in others the conditions is ill-understood and difficult to treat.

Delusions on their own have little diagnostic significance and their assessment must take account of all aspects of the patient's physical and mental state as well as their cultural background. Brief delusional ideas may develop in normal people following severe sleep deprivation and delusions often of a persecutory nature will develop in a person in strange or unusual surroundings especially when under stress. Examples of this may be found in immigrants during the first few months living in a strange culture. In delirium, delusions develop when consciousness is clouded and

the cause of the condition may be apparent. Similarly in chronic organic states, delusions will rarely be the only presenting feature and the diagnosis will be suggested by the memory disturbance and other cognitive and deficits. The differential diagnosis of substance abuse, schizophrenia and mania gives most difficulty particularly because drug abuse is common in patients with functional psychosis and may be the precipitant as much as the cause of the delusional state (*see also* HALLUCINATIONS). A careful history and urine drug screen should elucidate the role of stimulants and hallucinogens in a psychotic episode.

D. Blackwood

Depersonalization

Depersonalization is the experience of losing the accustomed sense of one's own reality, and should be distinguished from the very much rarer delusion of not being real occasionally elicited in schizophrenia. There are a variety of unusual phenomena which can accompany depersonalization—*derealization* (a sensation that the outer world is not real), *emotional numbing*, *bodily change* (particularly enlargement of head or limbs, lifelessness, unfamiliarity), *autoscopy* and *doubling* (perceptions linked to an independently existing double), *automaton experience* with self or others appearing to act or think in a contrived, forced fashion, and *disturbance of time sense*. Dizziness is a particularly common associated symptom. Typically depersonalization is alarming and distressing, which contrasts sharply with the subjective inability to feel emotions: insight is invariably retained. (*Table* D.5).

Depersonalization can be a *normal experience*, occurring in 30–70 per cent of the population. It is commonest in late adolescence and early adulthood, when it is usually mild, transient, associated with fatigue and of no clinical significance. Depersonalization also occurs physiologically in the rare states of sleep deprivation, sensory deprivation and the near-death experience.

Depersonalization can be generated by the mental mechanism of dissociation as an anxiety reducing response in stress hence *dissociative depersonalization* tends to be less unpleasant or alarming, and not a focus for complaint. This process permits a temporary emotional respite and better coping in circumstances like battle, accident, admission to hospital or appearance in court, and during the early stages of grief. It can also precede anticipated trauma, and indeed in deliberate self-injury (especially multiple cutting) may even facilitate the act through diminution of pain. If the stress is prolonged then dissociative depersonalization can persist equally long, for months or even years as

Table D.5. Causes of depersonalization

Commonest
Normal
Stress reaction (dissociative depersonalization)
Anxiety

Less common
Drugs
  Alcohol
  Hallucinogens
  Stimulants
  Cannabis
  Anticholinergics
  Benzodiazepines
Drug withdrawal
Fever
Neurological disorders
  Head injury
  Brain tumour
  Encephalitis
  Multiple sclerosis
  Epilepsy
Psychiatric disorders
  Phobia
  Panic
  Depression
  Obsessive compulsive disorder
  Schizophrenia
  Post-traumatic stress disorder
Insomnia
Primary depersonalization syndrome

Rare
Psychiatric disorders
  Hysteria
  Malingering
Sleep deprivation
Sensory deprivation
Near-death experience
Brain washing

recounted in the experiences of concentration camp survivors.

Depersonalization in the setting of *psychological disorders* is also common but it is unusual for this feature to persist or to be the main complaint. The commonest primary conditions are *anxiety*, *agoraphobia*, and *depression*. In anxiety, agoraphobia, panic disorder and chronic hyperventilation syndrome depersonalization is rarely intense or accompanied by associated experiences apart from derealization, while the amount of anguish and self-concern is substantial with the fear of going mad frequently expressed. In depression and post-traumatic stress disorder emotional numbing characteristically accompanies depersonalization and can even be the predominant feature—bodily change especially physical lifelessness may be reported in severe depression. In schizophrenia, depersonalization is usually an early, transient phenomenon with more typical disturbances of identity either present or emergent soon afterwards—autoscopy, often with emotional detachment, tends to occur when the illness is acute and established.

Drug intoxication or withdrawal can precipitate depersonalization, the commonest associations being

reported with *LSD*, *mescaline*, *cannabis* and *anticholinergics*. *Brain disease or damage* may precipitate or even present with depersonalization. Postconcussional syndrome is usually apparent from the history and accompanying features. However in temporal lobe disease and/or epilepsy depersonalization may not only be the prime symptom but can also precede positive findings upon neurological examination and investigation. This possibility ought to remain under consideration when the state of depersonalization is severe and persistent, autoscopy or perceptual distortions are present, and there are no apparent stressors or evidence of a primary emotional illness.

Primary depersonalization syndrome is an uncommon condition which presents abruptly in early adulthood with recurrent bouts of severe depersonalization, usually with many of the concomitant features. There are characteristic personality traits associated with this condition, the typical sufferer being described as intelligent, obsessional, introspective, sensitive, hypochondriacal. These patients often have particular difficulty in establishing personal relationships and coping with the general upheaval of adolescence. Their disorder tends to be chronic, readily precipitated by stress and anxiety but with minimal impairment in social functioning—they are prone to hypochondriasis in later life.

George Masterton

Depression

Depressed mood is one of the commonest conditions for which patients seek help. Most frequently unhappiness is an understandable response to loss of any sort. Depression refers to a more severe mood change when the patient may describe feelings of hopelessness, misery, tiredness and fatigue and the mood state is communicated by facial expression, gesture, posture, tone of voice and general demeanour. However, not infrequently one has to rely on a history from the patient, their friends and employers to recognize severe depressive illness often associated with a high risk of suicide in some people who do not themselves acknowledge mood change (smiling or masked depression). For cultural and other reasons some patients have no words for moods and may communicate their distress by hypochondriacal complaints or by seeking advice for marital, employment or a variety of other difficulties.

In uncomplicated bereavement a patient responds to loss by an initial experience of shock, numbness and feelings of emptiness. There is an initial tendency to deny that the loss has occurred but this gives way to a depressed mood often with symptoms of anxiety and panic. There may be poor appetite with weight loss, insomnia, impaired concentration and feelings of guilt surrounding the death. Auditory and visual hallucinations of the deceased are commonly reported. The state of grief is resolved as the person accepts the loss and begins to redirect their life and activities. Many cases of depression follow a real or imagined loss or threatening situation and symptoms are not dissimilar to those of bereavement. However, *major depressive illness* may develop without any clear-cut relation to loss or helplessness and classification may be based on symptoms, severity and outcome without making any aetiological assumptions. In *endogenous depression* (melancholia) there is a distinct quality of depressive mood which is perceived by the patient as being distinctly different from the feelings of loss experienced in bereavement. These patients describe a loss of pleasure in all their activities (*anhedonia*) and they cannot be even temporarily cheered out of their depression by something good happening in their life. This type of depressive illness is often associated with diurnal variation of mood, the depression being worse in the morning; early morning wakening; psych-omotor retardation or agitation; significant appetite impairment; and excessive guilt. In the most severe forms the patient may express delusions of poverty, ill health and persecution congruent with depressed mood and hallucinations which are often voices critical of the patient. There is a high risk of suicide and suicidal ideation must always be specifically asked about. There is frequently a family history of depression and although the illness may develop suddenly without a recognizable precipitant adverse stressful life events will often have occurred during the weeks preceding the onset of the illness. Major depressive illness can be usefully subdivided into *bipolar depression* (patients have at some stage in their lives experienced an episode of mania) and *unipolar depression* (patients have bouts of depression without mania). *Cyclothymia* describes a type of bipolar illness where patients have frequent mood swings from depression to elation with only brief periods of normality between episodes. Recurrent mild unipolar depression sometimes described as *depressive neurosis* or dysthymia is a chronic depressed mood persisting for most of the time for 2 years or more. Such patients may present with inability to cope with everyday life, low self-esteem, tiredness, sleep disturbance, somatic complaints and frequently symptoms of anxiety.

Difficulties may arise in the diagnosis of depression especially when a patient presents with physical symptoms such as headache, low back pain, weight loss, constipation, loss of libido, loss of energy or anorexia. Some patients are worried that they may have cancer, venereal disease, angina or memory loss and the physician's attention is directed towards an investigation of these physical conditions. Some patients with 'no words for moods' present with physical symptoms or difficulties in their marriage, occupation or with their children but the underlying depression may be diagnosed by sympathetic listening and a careful history. In the elderly, depression may present as a *pseudodementia* which may be initially hard to distinguish from dementia but which should respond well to standard anti-depressant measures.

Depression in other psychiatric illnesses

Depression is a common accompaniment of almost all other psychiatric disorders. An episode of depression may herald the onset of a schizophrenic illness and schizophrenic patients are more prone to suffer from depression perhaps because of the unpleasantness of the symptoms, the social and other handicaps of the illness or perhaps because mood change is an integral part of the disease itself. Depression is particularly common and difficult to treat immediately following the resolution of an acute exacerbation of schizophrenia. Anxiety may be a principal feature of depressive illness and such cases may be termed *agitated depression*. The patient may be restless and unable to relax during the interview wringing hands, pulling hair, shifting legs or pacing around the room. *Obsessional symptoms* can develop during a depressive illness and these symptoms will generally improve when the depression is treated. However patients with obsessive personality or obsessive compulsive disorder are also very prone to develop depressive episodes. Depressed mood is a frequent complaint in patients with most *personality disorders* including those of the histrionic type and in anorexia nervosa and bulimia.

Physical disease and depression (Table D.6)

A number of possible mechanisms account for the very high instance of depression in almost all types of physical disease. Pain, incapacity and loss of health, independence and social status are entirely understandable causes of depression during and following illness. Some illnesses, however, are more specifically linked with depression. A marked mood change during a *viral* infection is frequent and out of keeping with the incapacity caused by the infection. *Brucellosis* may cause a prolonged depressive illness. Several endocrine disorders may present as depression including *hypothyroidism, hypo-* and *hyperadrenocorticolism, hypoparathyroidism* and *hypopituitaryism*. Certain forms of *carcinoma*, particularly those of the pancreas, the thyroid and the lung may cause depression months before other symptoms of the tumour are manifest,

Table D.6. Physical causes of depression

1. Physical diseases which may cause depression

Infections
Influenza
Hepatitis
Infectious mononucleosis
Brucellosis
Toxoplasmosis

Endocrine disorders
Hypothyroidism
Hyperadrenocorticalism
Hypoadrenocorticalism
Hypoparathyroidism
Hypopituitarism

Pancreatic, pulmonary, thyroid carcinomas.

Acute intermittent porphyria
Disseminated lupus erythematosus
Folate, B_{12} deficiency

Neurological diseases
Multi-infarct dementia
Alzheimer's dementia
Pick's disease
Huntington's chorea
Multiple sclerosis
Parkinson's disease
Temporal lobe epilepsy
Head injury
Cerebrovascular disease and stroke
Subdural haematoma
Subarachnoid haemorrhage
Cerebral tumour
Encephalitis
Neurosyphilis
AIDS

2. Drugs which can cause depression
Reserpine
Alphamethyl dopa
Beta blockers
Corticosteroids
Oral contraceptives
L-dopa
Indomethicin
Isoniazid
Cycloserine
Withdrawal from alcohol
Withdrawal from amphetamine and related drugs
   (fenfluramine, diethylproprion)
Withdrawal from cocaine and phencyclidine
Use of hallucinogens
Opioid intoxication

possibly due to brain active peptides synthesized and released from the tumour. With most central nervous system diseases depression is a common accompaniment. In multi-infarct and Alzheimer's-type dementia, depressive symptoms may arise because the patient is aware of their failing powers but direct cerebral damage may also be implicated. An interaction between a normal response to incapacitating illness and the direct effects of brain damage probably account for mood disturbances found in Huntington's chorea, multiple sclerosis, Parkinson's disease, temporal lobe epilepsy, certain types of head injury and cerebral vascular disease.

Drugs which can cause depression (Table D.6)

These include both therapeutic agents and drugs of abuse. The former include antihypertensive agents (e.g. reserpine, steroids), anti-inflammatory drugs (e.g. indomethacin), and antibiotics (e.g. isoniazid and cycloserine). Withdrawal from alcohol is a very common cause of depression; withdrawal from amphetamines, the appetite suppressants fenfluramine and diethylpropion, cocaine and phencyclidine may precipitate mood change particularly in chronic users. Intoxication with opioids and the use of hallucinogens may trigger severe mood disturbance.

Depression may present at any age including infancy and the diagnosis in children is more difficult. In prepubertal children there may be somatic complaints, agitation, anxiety disorders, avoidance behaviour and phobias. In adolescents a mood disturbance may be accompanied by negativistic or antisocial behaviour, abuse of alcohol and illicit drugs and feelings of restlessness, aggression, withdrawal from social activities, poor school performance and complaints of not being understood.

D. Blackwood

Diarrhoea

Diarrhoea is defined as increased frequency, fluidity or volume of bowel motions. It is commonly, but not exclusively, associated with an increase in faecal excretion of water and electrolytes, with consequent increase in faecal weight. In some instances there is frequent passage of bowel motions of normal consistency and weight, or of blood and pus (exudative diarrhoea).

In an assessment of the many differential diagnoses of diarrhoea, it is important to consider the possible mechanisms which may be involved. Diarrhoea may be classified as being due to reduced fluid reabsorption (osmotic effects, mucosal defects, motility abnormalities), increased fluid secretion (bacterial toxins, hormones and neurotransmitters, prostaglandins, bile acids and fatty acids, detergent laxatives, immature enterocytes and secretion), and exudative diarrhoea.

As diarrhoea is a symptom, and not a disease in itself, it is important that in every patient the underlying cause is identified. After routine history and physical examination (including rectal examination), investigations of importance include examination of the stools by naked eye, by the microscope and by microbiological investigation, sigmoidoscopy and possibly colonoscopy, radiological examination (barium enema and small-bowel enema) and analyses of stools for lipids, bile acids and osmolarity. Tests of absorption, digestion, nutritional deficiency possibly associated with abnormal absorption, and tests such as jejunal biopsy, bacteriological studies of the small and large bowel, and intestinal permeability may all be helpful.

Although there is overlap, it is convenient to consider the causes of diarrhoea into those affecting infants and young children and those occurring in adults.

Diarrhoea in infancy and early childhood

Diarrhoea, with or without vomiting, is a presenting feature of a wide variety of conditions which may occur in infancy. The most important of these are: infantile gastroenteritis, systemic infections, unsuitable foods, carbohydrate intolerance, malabsorption, with or without steatorrhoea—coeliac disease, pancreatic disease, giardiasis, protein-losing enteropathy, drugs, ulcerative colitis or Crohn's disease (both rare in childhood), or Hirschsprung's disease.

Diarrhoea may be mimicked by the blood and mucus associated with intussusception (redcurrent-jelly stools) or by pseudo-diarrhoea associated with constipation.

Infantile gastroenteritis, although less common than previously, still remains a serious problem in many parts of the world and is a prominent cause of mortality and morbidity in infants. In developed countries, infantile gastroenteritis still remains a common cause of diarrhoea in infants and young children and is epidemic in some areas. A wide variety of pathogenic organisms may be responsible, including *Salmonella*, *Shigella*, and enteropathogenic *E. coli*. More rarely, other organisms such as *staphylococci*, are involved. In mild cases there may be diarrhoea without systemic disturbance but in more severe cases the infant passes watery green stools, which may be accompanied by vomiting and may rapidly develop a state of shock due to water and electrolyte depletion.

All other causes of diarrhoea in infancy and childhood must be considered in every case of acute or chronic diarrhoea in young children, possibly associated with failure to thrive. Diarrhoea may be the first sign of a disease such as coeliac disease or cystic fibrosis. *Coeliac disease* (gluten-induced enteropathy) may present in early childhood with acute or chronic diarrhoea. Failure to thrive, abdominal pain and distension may occur. The diagnosis is made by jejunal biopsy showing subtotal villous atrophy. The patient generally responds rapidly and effectively to the exclusion of gluten from the diet.

Cystic fibrosis may be manifested by meconium ileus in the neonatal period and thereafter children develop steatorrhoea with pale, bulky and offensive stools, failure to thrive and marked abdominal distension. The condition is associated with frequent respiratory infections. The prognosis of cystic fibrosis has much improved with nutritional support, pancreatic supplementation and control of repeated chest infections.

TODDLER DIARRHOEA

Toddler diarrhoea is defined as recurrent passage of frequent loose stools by a child who is thriving (maintaining a normal growth pattern compared to children of the same age). By thriving, the children can be distinguished, without full investigations, from those suffering from other causes of chronic diarrhoea such as coeliac disease, cystic fibrosis, secondary lactose intolerance, and severe cows' milk protein intolerance. By being healthy and active children, they can be reasonably distinguished from children with giardiasis or inflammatory bowel disease such as Crohn's disease or ulcerative colitis. There is a gradual improvement in the frequency and consistency of the stool with age although the age at which faecal continence is achieved may be significantly delayed (*see* ENCOPRESIS).

Diarrhoea in adults

The following causes should be considered:

Specific bacterial or viral infections, e.g. *Salmonella* gastroenteritis, dysentery (amoebic or bacillary), cholera, viral infections, AIDS

Inflammatory bowel disease, e.g. ulcerative colitis, Crohn's disease

Malabsorption/maldigestion, e.g. coeliac disease, loss of damage to the absorptive surface of the small intestine (due to resection and short-bowel syndrome), extensive Crohn's disease of the small intestine, progressive systemic sclerosis, vascular insufficiency, lymphoma, lymphangiectasia, bacterial overgrowth, radiation damage, Whipple's disease

Following gastric resection, gastroenterostomy and vagotomy

Pancreatic dysfunction, e.g. chronic pancreatitis, cystic fibrosis, carcinoma of pancreas, pancreatic resection

Tumours of the intestine, e.g. lymphoma of the small intestine, carcinoma of colon or rectum, Zollinger–Ellison syndrome, carcinoid and other hormone-producing tumours

Diverticular disease of the colon

Irritable bowel syndrome

Anxiety states, associated with generalized diseases

Other systemic disease such as hyperthyroidism, diabetes mellitus

Drugs, antibiotics (including pseudomembranous colitis), cytotoxic agents, abuse of laxatives, alcohol, neomycin, mefanamic acid, magnesium-containing antacids, arsenic, colchicine and others

It is helpful to subdivide the causes of diarrhoea into acute and chronic diarrhoea, although many causes of chronic diarrhoea may have acute episodes.

ACUTE DIARRHOEA

Acute diarrhoea in adults is most likely to be due to infection—bacterial or viral, but a detailed history may elicit dietary indiscretion, or the ingestion of a drug which may be the responsible factor.

In dysentery there are generally symptoms of tenesmus, with blood and mucus in the bowel motions. In *amoebic dysentery*, *Entamoeba histolytica* may be found in the stools, and multiple, small, pitted ulcers may be seen at sigmoidoscopy. An amoebic cyst may be found in the mucosa on rectal biopsy. In *bacillary dysentery* agglutination may be positive and the organism recovered from the stools; the incubation period is 1–5 days. *Salmonella infection* has a shorter incubation period (8–24 hours or at the most 2 days) and presents with acute vomiting and diarrhoea, frequently associated with pyrexia.

'*Traveller's diarrhoea*', sometimes also associated with vomiting, may be due to specific *E. Coli* or digestive infections, but is probably caused in many cases by alteration of the normal bacteria of bowel. The diagnosis is generally suggested by a recent history of travel abroad and can be confirmed by the finding of *E. Coli*, or other pathogens including *Giardia lamblia*, campylobacter, salmonella or shigella in the stools.

Infection may trigger an acute exacerbation of ulcerative colitis or Crohn's disease in individuals afflicted by these conditions.

CHRONIC DIARRHOEA

There are many interrelated causes of chronic diarrhoea, associated with a large number of diseases of all parts of the gastrointestinal tract, and sometimes found in non-gastrointestinal conditions.

In *ulcerative colitis* stools are frequent, and often watery, blood is generally present and mucus and pus are often a feature. The disease is confluent and distal, the diagnosis being made in most patients at sigmoidoscopy, which reveals a red, oedematous, friable mucosa. Histological confirmation can be obtained by rectal biopsy.

Crohn's disease affecting small or large intestine, is frequently associated with bouts of diarrhoea. Frequent bowel motions are common, mucus and pus may occasionally be present, but blood occurs in only 10 per cent of cases. It is to be noted that although ulcerative colitis is still commoner than Crohn's disease, Crohn's disease has markedly increased in incidence in Western countries in recent years. Both ulcerative colitis and Crohn's disease may present with acute diarrhoea due to an exacerbation of the disease. Such an episode may be triggered by an acute infection; thus stool cultures should be performed in all patients suspected of having ulcerative colitis or Crohn's disease, or if an exacerbation of these inflammatory bowel diseases is present. Colonoscopy may be of value in confirming the diagnosis, and in determining the extent, and the degree of activity throughout the bowel.

Chronic dysentery may occur in tropical countries and the diagnosis can be made by bacteriological examination of the stools. These conditions may give rise to watery diarrhoea or the passage of pale, white or yellow, bulky, strong-smelling stools, which are often difficult to flush away. There may be abdominal distension and discomfort, and deficiency states leading to anaemias, angular stomatitis, muscle weakness, skin rashes, etc., depending upon the single or multiple deficiencies which may be present. The presence of diarrhoea and/or steatorrhoea may be characteristic of these syndromes, but not diagnostic. It is not possible on clinical grounds to establish the basic cause of these lesions.

Malabsorption may be due to gastric or pancreatic causes; gastric causes include gastric resection, gastroenterostomy and total vagotomy; pancreatic causes include chronic pancreatitis, carcinoma, cystic fibrosis of the pancreas, resection, hypoplasia (Schwachman's syndrome), or congenital enzyme defects. Diarrhoea secondary to pancreatic maldigestion is often associated with marked steatorrhoea, and other aspects of pancreatic disease may be present, such as jaundice.

Diarrhoea associated with malabsorption may be due to a wide range of small intestinal diseases. Damage to the small intestinal mucosa with associated abnormalities of mucosal transport may occur in coeliac disease, dermatitis herpetiformis, tropical malabsorption, Crohn's disease, Whipple's disease, radiation damage to the small intestine, lymphoma, tuberculosis, or damage due to drugs such as neomycin. Other causes include vascular abnormalities of the small intestine, gangrene, abnormalities of the intestinal lymphatics, intestinal resections (tumours, vascular abnormalities, Crohn's disease), endocrine abnormalities, immunodeficiency syndromes, or drug-induced damage. Bacterial overgrowth may also result in malabsorption and diarrhoea, and be due to progressive systemic sclerosis, the short-bowel syndrome following surgical intervention, strictures or the presence of jejunal diverticulosis. Crohn's disease can also cause small intestinal damage with malabsorption and diarrhoea, or lead to small intestinal resection or bacterial overgrowth following the development of strictures. Disaccharidase deficiency may also be a cause of diarrhoea; this may be primary, or secondary to a range of disorders affecting the small intestine.

If maldigestion or malabsorption is suspected as a cause of diarrhoea, the following investigations are appropriate; jejunal biopsy with disaccharidase assay; small intestinal radiology (small-bowel enema), studies of bacterial status of the small bowel with collection and culture of aspirated fluid, or H_2 breath tests, pancreatic function tests, ultrasound and CT scanning.

Tumours of the alimentary tract can also lead to diarrhoea. Carcinoma of the colon is classically associated with alternating constipation and diarrhoea, or the passage of small frequent narrow stools. Tumours of the small intestine may follow coeliac disease and are most commonly lymphomas. Radiological investigations (barium enema or small-bowel enema) are of most value in diagnosing these lesions, although a suspected lesion in the colon may be diagnosed by colonoscopy and biopsy.

Diarrhoea associated with increased excretion of bile acids (cholerrheic diarrhoea) is generally associated with damage to bile acid absorbing mechanisms in the terminal ileum in Crohn's disease or in tumours. Liver disease may also be associated with diarrhoea due to bile acid abnormalities. The diagnosis is confirmed by measuring faecal bile acid excretion or by assessing bile acid absorption using the Se HCAT test; radiology of the terminal ileum may also be helpful.

Other colonic diseases may be associated with diarrhoea; these include diverticular disease of the colon characterized by watery diarrhoea, sometimes containing blood, and the irritable bowel syndrome in which motility disturbance may occur in both large and small bowel; in this condition, alteration of bowel habit may occur with diarrhoea or constipation, associated with lower abdominal pain.

Some generalized diseases may be accompanied by diarrhoea; these include hyperthyroidism, hypothyroidism and diabetes mellitus. Tumours associated with abnormal production of hormones such as the carcinoid syndrome, vipomas (Verner–Morrison syndrome) or gastrin-producing tumour (Zollinger–Ellison syndrome) may present with diarrhoea. A number of drugs have now been recognized as causing diarrhoea. Abuse of laxatives is perhaps the most common cause of diarrhoea due to drugs; antibiotics such as ampicillin and tetracycline may alter gut flora resulting in diarrhoea; neomycin and PAS cause mucosal damage and diarrhoea and pseudomembranous colitis is commonly associated with the use of antibiotics with the production of clostridium difficile toxin. Ethanol in excess is also a common cause of diarrhoea. An accurate drug history should be sufficient to confirm the drug-related nature of diarrhoea in patients although measurements of chemicals associated with laxatives in faeces or urine may be required.

R. I. Russell

Diplopia

Diplopia, or double vision, is the earliest symptom apparent to the patient with dysconjugate gaze of the two eyes. It is seen with ocular paresis or following loss of normal binocular control. It is usually binocular in nature and is rarely described in monocular form. Usually an object is seen singly with each eye separately but appears double when both eyes are open.

1. Binocular diplopia

A. PHYSIOLOGICAL DIPLOPIA

This is a normal phenomenon in all binocular vision. Since the two eyes observe an object from different directions, the retinal images differ, but the double vision is not apparent since the dissimilar images are combined by the visual centres in the brain to form a single solid conception of the object viewed. This physiological appearance of the two retinal images is called 'disparateness'. Such physiological diplopia is sometimes noticed by an individual who realizes that when fixing on a particular object, other objects which are closer or further away than the object of fixation may be seen double. Patients who are anxious or unduly introspective may need reassurance about this normal phenomenon. If the centre in the brain which controls the fusion of the two images is disturbed, as after the excessive consumption of alcohol, the normal balance of the muscular mechanisms of the eyes may be lost and diplopia experienced.

B. PATHOLOGICAL DIPLOPIA

In normal binocular vision both eyes are aligned so that the image of the object fixated falls upon the central and most sensitive part of the retina. Other objects form images upon more peripheral areas of the retina and are less well observed. When an individual is looking at a particular point ahead, the image of any object lying to the right of the eyes will fall upon the nasal side of the right retina and the temporal side of the left retina, and these different areas of the retinae will always correspond and, in normal circumstances, will always be stimulated simultaneously. If the relative position of the two eyes is upset, the image of an object no longer falls upon the two corresponding areas of retina, erroneous forms of projection occur and there is consequent diplopia. An examination of this diplopia leads to the ascertainment of the type of displacement of the eye.

In a paralytic strabismus where one of the eyes is not able to move normally in one direction, the image seen by the affected eye, lying away from the macula of the retina, is usually less distinct. A more reliable way of distinguishing which image is the false one is by finding the direction of gaze in which the images are most displaced, and then doing a 'cover test' in which each eye is alternatively covered; the eye which subtends the more distal image is the one which has the paralysed muscle. Alternatively the use of a red glass test or a Maddox rod test, the former to create red and white images with white light, the latter to create a white pin-point image and a red line image, may be used to identify the images arising from the different eyes. For example, if the greatest horizontal separation of images is on looking to the right, either the right lateral rectus or the left medial rectus is weak. The image which is projected farther from the centre is that arising in the paretic eye and by covering one eye after the other this may be determined.

Binocular diplopia may be caused by paralysis of any extraocular muscle and it will also be seen when there is displacement of one of the globes as with an *intraorbital tumour, abscess, haemorrhage* or *cavernous sinus thrombosis*. It may also be seen following an operation on the *extraocular muscles* if the excursion of one eye is limited by scarring. Binocular diplopia arising from disease within the orbit will frequently be associated with *pain or discomfort* and often with *proptosis*. The investigation of such syndromes is optimally undertaken with a CT or MRI scan of the orbits.

Double vision may be seen in the elderly after *local cerebral ischaemic events*; it is usually thought to be of intrinsic-brain stem origin, and it is often temporary.

Patients with true paralytic strabismus will be identified as having lesions affecting the third, fourth or sixth cranial nerves, singly or in combination, and investigations of the relevant areas may then be undertaken with CT or MRI imaging, CSF examination and possibly angiography.

Rarely *orbital myositis* will cause problems in eye movement and result in diplopia. Occasionally neuromuscular junction disorders will affect the eye as in ocular myasthenia. The diagnosis may be confirmed by the use of intravenous edrophonium and by single fibre EMG studies.

Diplopia may occasionally be seen in patients with *pituitary exophthalmos* or with *thyroid disturbances* resulting in dysthyroid eye disease.

Ocular palsies may be central, that is due to a lesion of the nucleus or of the parenchymal portion of the cranial nerve; or they may be peripheral, arising along the tract of the cranial nerve within the posterior or middle fossa or in the orbit itself. Lesions which can damage individual cranial nerves subserving eye movement include *posterior communicating artery aneurysm*, classically causing third nerve palsy, aneur-

ysms within the *cavernous sinus, raised intracranial pressure*, resulting in sixth nerve palsy, and *vascular lesions* of the trunk of the nerve; these are the commonest cause of fourth nerve palsy. The sixth nerve may also be affected near the *apex of the petrous bone* when involvement with a local infective process or a nasopharyngeal tumour have to be included in the differential diagnosis.

The rare occurrence in children of episodes of ocular palsy in conjunction with unilateral headache may be recognized as *ophthalmoplegic migraine*. There is a rare condition in which an inflammatory or granulomatous process in the anterior portion of the cavernous sinus or superior orbital fissure may involve any one of the nerves responsible for eye movement (*Tolosa–Hunt syndrome*).

The acute development of a bilateral ophthalmoplegia is most commonly seen in brainstem lesions or in *postinfective cranial neuropathies* (Guillain-Barré syndrome), whereas the chronic development of a bilateral ophthalmoplegia is most often seen with ocular myopathy, as in one of the *mitochondrial cytopathies*.

There are rare examples of pseudoparalysis of ocular muscles. In dysthyroid eye disease a tight inferior or superior rectus muscle may limit upward and downward gaze respectively and occasionally muscle enlargement may be demonstrated by CT scan. The Duane syndrome, due to congenital fibrosis of the lateral rectus, causes retraction of the globe on adduction, giving rise to diplopia though, since it is life-long, it is rarely a symptom to the patient and is more likely to be discovered by the unsuspecting examiner.

2. MONOCULAR DIPLOPIA

This is infrequently found, and may be due to early cataract, or irregularity of the corneal surface, e.g. following inflammation.

D. Bates

DIZZINESS
See VERTIGO.

Drop attacks

The term 'drop attack' is applied to a fall occurring without warning and without loss of consciousness or postictal confusion. The patients are usually elderly and female. They suddenly drop to the floor whilst walking or standing; the knees buckle, there is no dizziness and they usually fall forwards, striking the knees and sometimes the nose upon the ground. Some patients will describe loss of power in the legs, and they are unable to raise their hands to stop the face hitting the ground, implying that normal tonus may be lost in both the lower and the upper limbs. After the episode the patient is able to rise and move immediately though the attacks often cause considerable embarrassment. Not infrequently they result in lacerations to the knees and abrasions to the face. Attacks without apparent cause may occur for a few weeks and then stop. They have a benign prognosis and there is no effective therapy.

Elderly people are liable to fall for many reasons other than 'drop attacks', causes such as *postural hypotension, lack of concentration*, the *effects of sedating medicines, disturbances of vision, tripping* and *postural instability* must be excluded from the diagnosis.

It is probable that most 'drop attacks' occur as a result of *brainstem ischaemia*, though a relationship to cardiovascular or cerebrovascular disease is not striking. The fact that some patients describe episodes of double vision and that some identify weakness and inability to move the arm in association with attacks suggests involvement of the brainstem, and a form of vertebro-basilar insufficiency is an attractive though unproven theory of causation.

It is important that such attacks be differentiated from those in patients who have marked *weakness of the quadriceps* and who fall simply due to the knees flexing; such patients can usually identify the weakness in the lower limb muscles and they are able to protect the face by using the arms. 'Drop attacks' may of course occur in patients who have acute *cardiac dysrhythmias* and the elderly may suffer painless *myocardial infarction*. *Orthostatic hypotension* should be differentiated.

'Drop attacks' can occur rarely in the presence of *hydrocephalus* or a *third ventricular tumour*. These, though important in the differential diagnosis, are uncommon in the elderly group who are the most liable to 'drop attacks'.

D. Shaw

DYSARTHRIA
See SPEECH, ABNORMALITIES OF.

Dysmenorrhoea

The causes may be tabulated as follows:

1 SPASMODIC OR PRIMARY
Uterine hypoplasia (small, acutely anteflexed uterus, long conical cervix, stenosed os)
Congenital malformations
Ovarian dysfunction
Psychogenic
2 CONGESTIVE OR SECONDARY
Arising from infection:
Pelvic peritonitis, salpingo-oophoritis, parametritis, cervicitis
Arising from endometriosis:
Chocolate cysts of ovary, adenomyoma
Retroversion of the uterus
Uterine fibroids
If complicated by pelvic infection or endometriosis
Psychogenic
3 MEMBRANOUS

The distribution of the cases into these three classes is often easy; in the first place, spasmodic cases are practically always *primary*, that is they begin when ovulation first takes place, i.e. within 2 or 3 years of the onset of the periods; while congestive cases are *secondary*, that is, acquired later as a result of some definite lesion. Further, the nature of the pain is often characteristic of the type of case, for in spasmodic cases the pain begins with the flow or only just before. It is aching in character, often with griping or colicky exacerbations felt in the midline above the symphysis pubis and passing down the anterior aspect of the thighs. It is associated with prostration, pallor, headache and vomiting. It usually continues for 6–12 hours until the menstrual flow is well established. In the congestive cases, on the other hand, the pain is continuous and aching, begins some hours or days before the flow, and in typical cases is relieved by the flow. In the membranous cases, which may complicate either primary or secondary dysmenorrhoea, the nature of the pain partakes of the characters of both the former types, being aching and continuous first, then becoming colicky and spasmodic when the uterus is attempting to expel the characteristic membrane or cast, and being finally relieved when this comes away.

Many cases are met with in which the pain partakes of the nature of both the congestive and spasmodic types. This usually means that a woman who originally had spasmodic dysmenorrhoea acquires some lesion which in its turn gives rise also to the congestive type of pain.

Having settled that a case belongs to one of the three main types, it is possible to work out the actual causation. This is more difficult in the spasmodic cases than in the congestive, because the latter depend upon well-defined lesions, and the former do not.

1. Spasmodic cases

The causation of the pain in this type of case is obscure because the physical signs are essentially normal. Not infrequently the uterus may be small with a long conical cervix and an exaggerated anterior bend (the 'cochleate' uterus of Pozzi). A sound may pass with difficulty into such a uterus giving rise to the suggestion that there is a stenosis of the internal os. These findings are common in young adult women, however, and are more likely to be a manifestation of their immaturity than a cause of the spasmodic dysmenorrhoea, because they are found just as often in girls of the same age who do not suffer from dysmenorrhoea.

Many cases with spasmodic dysmenorrhoea, moreover, appear to have a normal uterus. In such cases evidence of degenerative or inflammatory changes in the presacral nerve have been described but their existence is very doubtful. The function of the ovarian hormones in causing spasmodic dysmenorrhoea is also not clear. For the first 2 or 3 years of anovular menstruation the periods do not as a rule cause pain. But when ovulation begins, a corpus luteum is formed and progesterone secreted and the periods become painful. Inhibition of ovulation by the use of the contraceptive pill usually renders the periods painless in such cases unless there is a large psychogenic element. It is tempting to explain spasmodic dysmenorrhoea by saying it is due to an ovarian dysfunction but if this is so its nature is unknown. The psychogenic factor is also emphasized and said to be increased by a doting mother who herself suffered from severe dysmenorrhoea. Marriage and child-bearing may improve or cure spasmodic dysmenorrhoea but this does not prove its psychogenic origin in the first place. Nevertheless, a healthy attitude by the patient to the condition and an assurance that it does not signify disease helps her to put up with it.

2. Congestive cases

It is unnecessary to differentiate the congestive cases as tubal, ovarian or uterine because the underlying cause in all is pelvic congestion accompanying such lesions as are shown in the table above. Their differential diagnosis is made by careful consideration of the history, combined with bimanual examination of the pelvic organs, and if required, laparoscopy. Simple *retroversion and flexion* can be recognized on bimanual examination; the fundus will be felt posteriorly, the cervix looking directly down the vagina in a forward direction. Retroversion of the uterus by itself does not cause dysmenorrhoea and painful periods mean that either pelvic infection or endometriosis coexists. *Salpingo-oophoritis* in its typical chronic form gives rise to irregular tender swellings on either side and behind the uterus, sometimes forming definitely retort-shaped swellings, especially if pus is present in the tubes. Fixation of these swellings and of the uterus is a very definite sign of the disease; while the history of one or more attacks of acute illness, with pelvic pain, will assist to make the diagnosis certain. Small haemorrhagic cysts of the ovary, the contents of which may be 'tarry' or of chocolate-like consistence, are also important causes of premenstrual dysmenorrhoea; they are always fixed, and are of endometrial origin (*endometrioma of the ovary*). Adenomyosis may produce general enlargement of the uterus or there may be a localized adenomyoma in part of the uterus. Then an asymmetrical swelling can be felt in the uterus on bimanual vaginal examination, as in the case of a uterine fibroid.

Any psychogenic factor will naturally accentuate the pain. Often associated with this type of dysmenorrhoea is some constitutional disability, the result of anaemia, overwork, worry, anxiety or other conditions leading to a lowering of the pain threshold.

In nearly all cases of congestive dysmenorrhoea the underlying cause also produces other symptoms such as menorrhagia, dyspareunia, backache and vaginal discharge. It is unusual to find congestive dysmenorrhoea as a symptom by itself.

3. Membranous cases

A cast of uterine endometrium, complete or incomplete, may be passed in either spasmodic or congestive dysmenorrhoea. Its passage through the cervix is likely to cause spasmodic pain because of the colicky uterine contractions. The cast may have to be distinguished from a decidual cast passed following the rupture of an ectopic pregnancy or from the cast of an early miscarriage. In either of these conditions a careful review of the history should lead to the diagnosis but if there is doubt histology of the cast should settle it. In ectopic pregnancy the cast contains the decidua of pregnancy but no chorionic villi and in the case of an early miscarriage there are villi in the decidua.

Cases of dysmenorrhoea may be confused with those of abdominal pain due to other lesions unconnected with menstruation; and the differentiation of such cases may be a matter of considerable importance. It is conceivable that the following conditions may be mistaken for dysmenorrhoea:

Appendicitis
Colic: intestinal, renal or biliary
Ruptured tubal gestation
Torsion of an ovarian cyst pedicle
Haemorrhage from or into a Graafian follicle
Rupture of an ovarian cyst or pyosalpinx
Threatened or actual abortion
Endometriosis

Obviously, some of these lesions are dangerous to life, and therefore it is essential that they are not overlooked. The danger of this occurring is increased if any of these lesions start at or near the expected time of a menstrual period, and would hardly arise if a menstrual period had terminated recently, or was not expected for some days. It will be noted that all these lesions are accompanied by sudden abdominal pain, which might perhaps lead to a suspicion of spasmodic dysmenorrhoea, but hardly of congestive, owing to the character of the pain.

N. Patel

Dyspareunia

Dyspareunia, or painful coitus, may depend on a variety of local lesions, or it may occur when no local lesion can be found. It is associated closely with vaginismus, or painful spasm of the levator ani muscle on attempts at coitus, and the same lesions which cause simple dyspareunia may also give rise to vaginismus; vaginismus is particularly likely to develop if the simple dyspareunia remains untreated for any length of time. In some women a local lesion produces no pain upon attempts at coitus which in others will cause pain accompanied by violent spasm of the levator ani. In some cases pain arises because there is a difficulty of penetration of the vaginal orifice, while in others there is no difficulty, but pain is caused on deep penetration—'deep dyspareunia'. The following lesions commonly give rise to dyspareunia:

Congenital absence of the lower part of the vagina
Unruptured hymen
Inflamed hymeneal orifice
Vulvitis
Bartholinitis
Disparity in size
Vulval dystrophy
—hyperplastic (leucoplakia)
—hypoplastic (atrophic vulvitis)
Healed perineal lacerations giving rise to a narrow introitus
Urethral caruncle
Urethritis
Cystitis
Prolapsed tender ovaries with retroverted uterus
Salpingo-oophoritis
Anal fissure
Thrombosed piles
Endometriosis
Arthritis of the hips
'Functional' causes

The lesions fall into natural groups, according to whether the situation of the lesion is at the vulva, the uterus and ovaries, the urinary passages, or at the anus and rectum; it is necessary to carry out a detailed examination of any case of dyspareunia in order to find out whether any of these well-defined lesions are present. The commonest is *inflamed hymeneal remains*, sometimes gonorrhoeal, accompanied by redness and swelling of the orifice of the duct of Bartholin's gland. The lesion is evident on inspection, and the parts are acutely sensitive to the least touch. Hyperplastic vulval dystrophy is a lesion that is obvious from the white, sodden appearance of the labia, and causes pain on account of the sensitive cracks and fissures which accompany it. Hypoplastic vulval dystrophy causes actual contraction of the vaginal orifice, and consequently penetration is difficult and causes pain. The red projecting growth from the urinary meatus, *caruncle*, is self-evident and acutely tender, while *urethritis* is diagnosed by the issue of pus on squeezing

the urethra. *Cystitis* is diagnosed by the presence of pus and bacilli in the urine, accompanied by frequency of micturition, and it causes pain because the bladder is painful and intolerant of the disturbance caused by coitus. *Prolapsed, tender ovaries* and *backward displacements of the uterus* cause no pain on penetration and no difficulty, but coitus with deep penetration gives acute pain at the time or a dull pelvic ache later; the condition is recognized by a bimanual examination, as is also *salpingo-oophoritis*, in connection with which there is usually a history of some acute attack of pelvic peritonitis. Vaginitis due to a trichomonas infection, or a chronic endocervitis with or without erosion, may be responsible. Endometriosis in the pelvis is a common cause of deep dyspareunia. Ovarian and other neoplasms are hardly ever responsible; severe constipation is not an uncommon cause. Disproportion in size is rarely in itself of importance as the vagina is very distensile, but if in addition there is any local lesion the pain will be accentuated. *Anal fissure* and *thrombosed and inflamed piles* are recognized by careful examination of the anus and rectum by the finger or speculum. Arthritis of the hips or lumbar spine may cause dyspareunia.

In the cases which occur without local lesions the vaginal entrance will be found to be acutely hyperaesthetic and penetration difficult, and there is spasmodic vaginismus. Careful examination fails to demonstrate a lesion, and these cases are usually termed 'neurotic' or 'functional'; sexual desire is not necessarily absent; indeed many such patients are over-desirous of the consummation of marriage. Fear, arising from painful attempts at coitus, is often the cause of the condition. Enlarging the orifice by gradual dilatation, using vaginal dilators, or by a small plastic operation often leads to cure as the patient gains confidence. Child-bearing also cures a case of this nature. These cases must be distinguished from those in which the underlying factor is absence of sexual desire and actual dislike of the sexual act, when the dyspareunia is merely a defence mechanism built up by the woman to avoid coitus. Unhappy and unsuitable marriages or fear of pregnancy conduce to this state of affairs, and the patient is prone to complain of pain when dislike is really what is meant. There is no difficulty in penetration in such cases.

N. Patel

Dysphagia

Dysphagia means difficulty in swallowing. The difficulty may be in the initiation of swallowing, which is of course under voluntary control, or in the later involuntary stages of swallowing, in which no conscious sensation is associated with the normal passage of a swallowed bolus from pharynx to stomach. If this transit is impeded, however, there is a sensation that swallowed food does not progress normally through the oesophagus. The patients then perceive a hold-up to the swallowed food and will complain of 'food sticking'. Dysphagia should be distinguished from painful swallowing, sometimes termed odynophagia, and from the globus sensation—a feeling of a lump in the throat—which does not interfere with swallowing in any way.

Oropharyngeal dysphagia

Neuromuscular disorders which affect oropharyngeal function cause difficulty in swallowing which is associated with a tendency to aspirate swallowed material into the airway, and with nasopharyngeal reflux. Unilateral cerebral lesions, such as cerebrovascular accidents cause transient dysphagia of this type. Infarction of the brainstem, as in pseudo-bulbar palsy and the posteroinferior cerebellar artery syndrome causes oropharyngeal dysphagia, as will any cause of lower cranial nerve palsies including motor neurone disease, the Guillain-Barré syndrome and poliomyelitis affecting the brainstem. Dysphagia will also occur when the brainstem is affected by multiple sclerosis and with extrapyramidal disorders such as Parkinsonism. The oropharyngeal dysphagia which occurs in rabies, tetanus and botulism is likewise a consequence of neural dysfunction.

Myasthenia gravis and diseases affecting the pharyngeal musculature impair the ability to swallow normally. The inherited muscular dystrophies, including dystrophia myotonica, polymyositis and dermatomyositis may involve the pharynx.

Structural abnormality in the pharynx should be suspected when oropharyngeal dysphagia occurs in the absence of nasopharyngeal regurgitation or a tendency to aspirate into the airway. Pharyngeal carcinoma and lymphoma cause dysphagia of this type. Xerostomia may be responsible for a similar complaint, however, as grossly impaired salivary secretion may be recognized particularly by elderly patients only in terms of difficulty in initiating swallowing. Extrapharyngeal tumours causing pharyngeal compression can give rise to dysphagia, especially when they also invade the pharyngeal wall. Thyroid enlargement, however, seldom does so except when retrosternal extension of the gland compresses the proximal oesophagus.

Partial obstructions of the high oesophagus produce a clinical picture virtually indistinguishable from pharyngeal obstruction. An oesophageal web situated just below the cricopharyngeus and associated with iron-deficiency anaemia (the Plummer-Vinson or Paterson-Kelly syndrome) is now an uncommon cause

of high oesophageal obstruction; squamous carcinomas occasionally occur at this level.

Cricopharyngeal spasm is sometimes suggested when a prominent indentation produced by the cricopharyngeus muscle is seen on a radiograph of the barium-filled upper oesophagus. The existence of a relationship between this radiological sign and a complaint of dysphagia or abnormality of cricopharyngeal muscle function is far from certain.

A *pharyngeal diverticulum* (Zenker's diverticulum) (*Fig.* D.8) is a posterior herniation of the pharnyx giving rise to a pouch liable to fill with food and saliva. Dysphagia occurs in consequence of compression of the lower pharynx and upper oesophagus. Regurgitation of some of the diverticulum contents may occur long after they have been swallowed. There is a view that disordered contraction of the cricopharyngeus muscle contributes both to the dysphagia of this condition and to the development of the diverticulum itself.

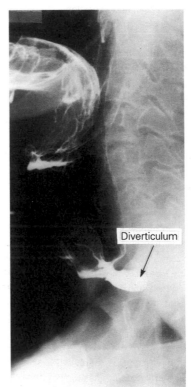
Diverticulum

Fig. D.8. Barium radiograph of cervical oesophagus, showing contrast in a pharyngeal diverticulum (See arrow).

Oesophageal dysphagia

A sensation that swallowed food is 'sticking' during its passage from the pharynx to the stomach is readily recognized and described by patients. Many will indicate the level at which the sticking sensation is felt, though this correlates imperfectly with the level at which obstruction actually occurs. Mechanical obstruction of the oesophagus characteristically manifests with dysphagia for solid foods such as meat, fish or bread whereas dysphagia due to disordered motility of the oesophagus is perceived to affect both solids and liquids.

MECHANICAL OBSTRUCTION OF THE OESOPHAGUS

Benign and malignant strictures of the oesophagus are the common causes of mechanical obstruction. *Benign (peptic) strictures* develop in consequence of long-standing gastro-oesophageal reflux and are encountered most commonly in the lower oesophagus, though they may develop at any level. Most, but not all patients with such strictures give a clear history of troublesome heartburn. Benign stricturing of the oesophagus may also develop as a consequence of swallowing corrosive substances. Accidental ingestion of such materials occurs particularly in young children. Epidermolysis bullosa affects the squamous epithelium of the oesophagus as well as the skin, and benign oesophageal strictures often develop in patients with this rare disease.

Malignant strictures of the oesophagus characteristically present with a short history of progressively worsening dysphagia, initially for solids but potentially evolving to cause complete oesophageal obstruction (*Fig.* D.9). Squamous carcinoma may develop at any level; adenocarcinomas are less common and usually occur at the lower end of the oesophagus but may develop at any level in an oesophagus lined with Barrett's epithelium. An adenocarcinoma of the gastric fundus is an important cause dysphagia if it invades or obstructs the lower oesophagus (*Fig.* D.10).

A Schatzki ring is a web which occasionally develops at the oesophago-gastric junction, usually in association with a hiatus hernia. Many of these rings cause no symptoms but the minority which narrow the lumen to 12 mm or less present a risk of oesophageal obstruction by impaction of a bolus of solid food.

Extraluminal compression of the oesophagus is an uncommon cause of dysphagia. Mediastinal tumours, however, particularly lymphoma and bronchial carcinoma may encircle and compress the oesophagus sufficiently to cause the symptom.

In older patients, a prominent indentation or even right lateral displacement of the oesophagus at the level of the aortic arch is frequently seen on barium radiographs. Dysphagia is rare, however, even when there is aneurysmal dilatation of the aorta. Enlargement of the left atrium, as in long-standing mitral stenosis, likewise rarely causes dysphagia even when oeso-

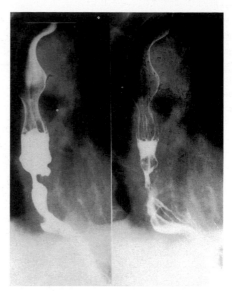

Fig. D.9. Oesophageal carcinoma.

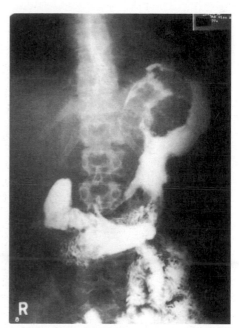

Fig. D.10. Barium meal of a female aged 60 with dysphagia. There is an extensive proliferative adenocarcinoma of the cardia extending into the gastric fundus.

phageal displacement is pronounced. In contrast, compression of the oesophagus by the aorta at the level of the diaphragm may give rise to significant obstruction and consequent dysphagia.

Dysphagia lusoria is a very rare condition in which the oesophagus is compressed by an anomalous right subclavian artery.

OESOPHAGEAL MOTILITY DISORDERS

Motility disorders of the oesophagus are well-recognized causes of dysphagia, but are uncommon. *Achalasia* is a disorder in which there is degeneration or functional failure of the oesophageal myenteric plexus, resulting in loss of all peristaltic contraction in the oesophageal body and failure of the lower oesophageal sphincter to relax in response to swallowing. (*Fig. D.11*). Food and fluid thus tend to accumulate in the oesophagus, although most food ingested at each meal does very gradually pass through to the stomach. The patient is aware that ingested food and fluid are 'held-up' and the consequent discomfort is sometimes relieved by self-induced regurgitation. Spasms of more severe retrosternal pain sometimes occur. Fluid retained in the achalasic oesophagus may regurgitate into the pharynx, particularly at night. Aspiration of this fluid into the airway may cause the patient to awaken with a bout of coughing; more commonly the fluid just dribbles from the mouth, resulting in a damp patch on the pillow each morning.

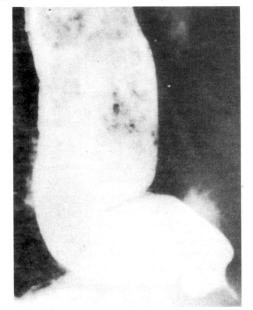

Fig. D.11. Achalasia, showing the 'bird-beak' appearance at the cardia. Many patients with achalasia present before significant oesophageal dilatation has developed, as in this example. (Dr RC Heading).

Chagas' disease is a degeneration of the oesophageal myenteric plexus caused by South American trypanosomal infection. The oesophageal manifestations are identical to those of achalasia.

Diffuse oesophageal spasm is even rarer than achalasia. Frequent non-peristaltic contractions of the oesophageal circular muscle cause dysphagia for solids and liquids and may be responsible for severe chest pain resembling that of myocardial infarction. Dys-

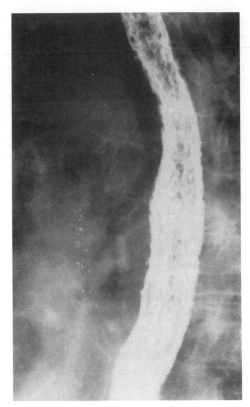

Fig. D.12. Extensive oesophageal candidiasis in a patient receiving chemotherapy for lymphoma.

phagia and pain can sometimes be provoked by drinking hot or ice cold fluids, and many patients avoid such drinks.

The endoscopic appearances of the oesophagus may be normal both in achalasia and in diffuse oesophageal spasm. Barium-swallow examination will establish the diagnosis in most cases of achalasia and in some cases of diffuse oesophageal spasm but oesophageal manometry provides a more secure foundation for either diagnosis.

Impaired or absent peristalsis in the distal oesophagus occurs in scleroderma, and in a minority of patients with gastro-oesophageal reflux. Intermittent dysphagia for solids, which is usually mild, may then occur.

Dysphagia associated with painful swallowing

Acute inflammatory conditions affecting the mouth, pharynx or oesophagus may cause swallowing to be painful (odynophagia) with a consequent difficulty in swallowing. The clinical history usually makes clear that painful swallowing is the dominant symptom. Ludwig's angina, acute laryngitis and the laryngeal element of angioneurotic oedema are rare causes of painful swallowing; candidiasis of the oesophagus is more often encountered. Patients who are debilitated or immunosuppressed are at particular risk of oesophageal candidiasis (*Fig.* D.12) but it is occasionally encountered in individuals who are otherwise healthy.

Acute inflammation and ulceration of the oesophagus may be caused by some drugs when an ingested tablet or capsule lodges for some hours in the oesophagus instead of passing promptly to the stomach. This is particularly likely with tablets which are taken last thing at night. Emepronium bromide and doxycycline have been notable for causing oesophageal ulceration in this way. Swallowing is then painful and there may also be an element of dysphagia.

R. C. Heading

Dyspnoea

Dyspnoea is the clinical word for breathlessness; although it is the ordinary Greek word for breathlessness, it is not an everyday term for English-speaking people. Thus, the word breathlessness, rather than dyspnoea, will be used throughout this section to emphasize that we are dealing with a sensation or symptom, not a physical sign. Most people intuitively know what is meant by breathlessness but would find it hard to describe in words. A useful definition is that offered by Comroe in 1966: 'difficult, laboured, uncomfortable breathing; it is an unpleasant type of breathing, though it is not painful in the usual sense of the word'. Most definitions of the term involve concepts of effort and awareness of a need to breathe.

Breathlessness may be a single sensation or, like pain, several related sensations. It is not clear to what extent the breathless sensation is the same in physiological circumstances (e.g. on vigorous exercise in normal subjects) and pathological circumstances, such as in respiratory disease; it is also not clear whether the breathlessness of different disease states is qualitatively the same. These issues, although intriguing, are rarely of practical importance in the clinical situation.

Conditions associated with breathlessness can be grouped into three main categories, which are not mutually exclusive. Breathlessness occurs in conditions where there is: an increased chemical or neurological drive to breathe; an increased work of breathing; or a decreased neuromuscular power. In all these situations, there is likely to be an increased drive to breathe, whether primary or secondary, and whether or not accompanied by an actual increase in ventilation. Recent experimental work on breathlessness, in both normal subjects and patients with respiratory disease has led to a general hypothesis for the genesis of the sensation. This suggests that breathlessness occurs when a drive to breathe exists that is abnormal, either qualitatively or quantitatively, and is translated in the medulla into a descending motor command to the respiratory muscles.

Table D.7 lists the important causes of breathlessness, in terms of the three categories described above. In practice, many of these conditions have their effects via more than one mechanism. There are some conditions associated with increased ventilation that are only rarely associated with breathlessness. When increased ventilation is voluntary, the descending path from the cortex to the respiratory anterior horn cells bypasses the medullary respiratory centre and breathlessness is much reduced or absent. This is evidence for the origin of the sensation in the region of the respiratory centre. In many forms of acidosis, if the respiratory apparatus is normal breathlessness is rare despite the increased ventilation.

Respiratory function tests

In most respiratory conditions severe enough to cause breathlessness, sophisticated tests of function are not necessary as the problem is obvious. However, respiratory function tests can be of use in determining patterns of impairment that can help in diagnosing the cause of the problem, and are particularly useful for monitoring changes in function over time or in response to treatment. Most respiratory function testing is done at rest, but important information about the cardiorespiratory system can also be obtained from measurements made during exercise.

The basic and most useful indices of lung function can be measured using a spirometer to record expired volume over time. Many machines are now available, with results produced either as flow-volume curves (*Fig.* D.13) or as volume-time curves (*Fig.* D.14). The major variables obtained from spirometry during forced expiration are the forced expiratory volume in one second (FEV_1), the forced vital capacity (FVC) and the peak expiratory flow rate (PEFR). Other variables that can be obtained from the same manoeuvre include flows at different points in the expiration such as at 50 per cent and 75 per cent of the vital capacity. The relaxed vital capacity can be measured using the same equipment but with a slow expiration. The PEFR can also be measured by simpler, cheaper peak flow meters; these are convenient when repeated estimates of PEFR are required, for example to diagnose variable airflow limitation in asthma.

To estimate other lung volumes it is necessary to use helium dilution to give an estimate of residual volume (RV—the volume remaining in the lungs at the end of a full expiration). Total lung capacity (TLC) is the sum of the RV and the VC. Another aspect of lung function is gas exchange between the alveoli and

Table D.7. Causes of breathlessness

Conditions associated with an increased chemical or neurological drive to breathe

Common causes	Uncommon causes
Pulmonary oedema	Acidosis
Pulmonary embolus	Pregnancy
Pneumothorax	Cyanotic congenital heart disease
Pneumonia	High altitude
Lobar collapse	Arteriovenous fistula
Pulmonary fibrosis	
Anaemia	

Conditions associated with an increased work of breathing

Obstructive ventilatory defects

Common causes	Uncommon causes
Chronic obstructive airways disease	Upper airways obstruction
Emphysema	
Asthma	
Bronchiectasis	
Cystic fibrosis	
Byssinosis	

Restrictive ventilatory defects

Common causes	Uncommon causes
Sarcoidosis	Large tumours
Fibrosing alveolitis	Large hiatus hernia
Extrinsic allergic alveolitis	Lymphangitis carcinomatosa
Pneumoconioses	Connective tissue diseases
Large pleural effusion	Aspiration pneumonitis
Extensive lung resection	Infections
Chest wall deformity	
Pulmonary oedema	
Left ventricular dysfunction	

Conditions associated with decreased neuromuscular power

Common causes	Uncommon causes
Myasthenia gravis	Poliomyelitis
Polyneuritis	Motor neurone disease
	Muscular dystrophies

(Conditions associated with decreased neuromuscular power are all relatively rare causes of breathlessness)

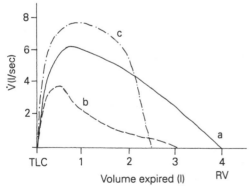

Fig. D.13. Superimposed expiratory flow-volume curves: a, normal; b, obstructive airways disease; c, restrictive lung disease.

the blood. This can be assessed by measuring the transfer factor for carbon monoxide. Of course, arterial oxygen tension is also a good indication of gas exchange and a fall during exercise is a sensitive means of detecting interstitial lung disease affecting gas exchange. Measurement of arterial blood gas tensions requires arterial puncture, which can be uncomfortable and even hazardous and, in the absence of an indwelling arterial line, difficult to repeat frequently.

It is also possible to measure arterial oxygen saturation non-invasively using oximeters. These function by shining different wavelengths of light through the tissue (usually the ear lobe); they can be left in place for several hours, for example during exercise testing or during sleep. Similarly it is now possible to measure arterial blood CO_2 tension (PCO_2) non-invasively, using a sensor strapped to the skin.

Exercise tests can assess the functioning of the cardiorespiratory system under stress. Commonly, exercise of progressively greater severity is performed on the treadmill or bicycle ergometer. Variables such as ventilation, heart rate, O_2 consumption and CO_2 production can be measured; it is also possible to obtain the subject's assessments of degree of breathlessness during the test. Such testing is mainly of research interest, but can sometimes elucidate the cause of breathlessness on exercise in someone with relatively normal results at rest (for example, an exercise induced cardiac dysrhythmia or a profound fall in arterial PO_2 due to a reversal of an arteriovenous shunt).

The pattern of lung function abnormality is particularly useful in deciding what type of disease is present. In airways obstruction, such as is found in chronic

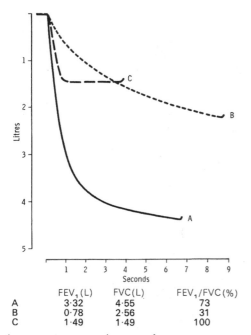

	FEV$_1$(L)	FVC(L)	FEV$_1$/FVC(%)
A	3·32	4·55	73
B	0·78	2·56	31
C	1·49	1·49	100

Fig. D.14. Superimposed tracings of expiratory spirograms in normal (A), obstructive airways disease (B) and restrictive lung disease (C). The measurements derived from these records are given below the graph.

obstructive airways disease, emphysema or asthma, spirometry typically shows a reduction in FEV$_1$ and in the FEV$_1$/FVC ratio. If a flow-volume curve is examined, the descending part of the curve tends to be concave due to reductions in flow at low lung volumes (*Fig. D.13*). In some cases, there is quite a marked reduction in FVC, due to air-trapping during the forced expiration. This is especially likely in emphysema and asthma. Spirometry alone in such cases cannot distinguish between obstruction with air-trapping and a mixed obstructive/restrictive defect. Restrictive lung conditions, such as diffuse pulmonary fibrosis, typically produce a reduction in FVC but have less effect on the FEV$_1$, so that the FEV$_1$/FVC ratio tends to be high. A typical flow-volume curve in restrictive lung disease is shown in *Fig D.14*.

Additional tests are not always necessary to distinguish between obstructive and restrictive conditions. Static lung volumes are uniformly reduced in restrictive conditions, with a normal RV/TLC ratio, and there is frequently a reduction in gas transfer factor. In obstructive conditions, it is common to find that the relaxed VC is greater than the FVC and that the RV/TLC ratio is increased, both due to air trapping. If emphysema is present, destruction of lung tissue often results in a reduction in gas transfer factor.

Blood gases can become abnormal in any severe lung disease. In respiratory failure secondary to chronic obstructive airways disease, the PO_2 is reduced and

there is a tendency for the PCO_2 to increase due to alveolar hypoventilation. In asthma a reduction in PO_2 is the main feature and the PCO_2 tends to be low due to hyperventilation in response to the hypoxaemia, only rising as a late event in life-threatening asthma. In restrictive lung conditions, a low PO_2 with a low PCO_2 is the usual pattern. In all these situations, including restrictive lung conditions, the hypoxaemia is mainly secondary to a mismatch between ventilation and perfusion of alveoli rather than to an actual diffusion defect.

The various conditions associated with breathlessness will be discussed under the headings used in *Table* D.7. Many of them produce breathlessness by several mechanisms but are classified according to the primary mechanism operating in most cases.

Conditions associated with an increased chemical or neurological drive to breathe

A characteristic of increased ventilation due to chemical or neurological stimulation is a high respiratory frequency and a low arterial PCO_2. Hypoxia and acidosis are the important chemical drives to breathe. Potential sources of neurological drives to breathe include pulmonary receptors, chest wall receptors and other skeletal muscle receptors. Neurological drives to breathe are probably important in parenchymal lung conditions associated with breathlessness, such as *pulmonary oedema* and *pulmonary infarction secondary to pulmonary embolus*. They may also be a mechanism for the breathlessness associated with *pneumonia* and *lobar collapse* (for example secondary to bronchial obstruction produced by *bronchogenic carcinoma*). It has been demonstrated that the increased ventilation associated with lobar collapse occurs even when the collapsed segment is small and there is little or no hypoxia. Breathlessness, due perhaps to stimulation of lung receptors, is a prominent early symptom of *Pneumocystis carinii pneumonia* associated with AIDS; the chest radiograph may be normal but arterial oxygen desaturation on exercise is usual. The breathlessness that accompanies a relatively small *spontaneous pneumothorax* is often quite marked, especially in the early stages, and cannot be explained by mechanical difficulties with ventilation. Again, it may be that stimulation of lung receptors plays a part.

Hypoxia from any cause can lead to breathlessness via stimulation of ventilation, for example in *cyanotic congenital heart disease, high altitude (mountaineers)* and *parenchymal lung disease* such as the various types of *pulmonary fibrosis*. It is not clear whether hypoxia can act as a direct stimulus to breathlessness, independent of its effects on ventilation; experiments have produced conflicting results.

In *cyanotic congenital heart disease*, such as Fallot's tetralogy, the mixed venous oxygen saturation falls on exercise due to increased extraction by the exercising muscles (this is a normal phenomenon); some of this venous blood passes into the aorta via the ventricular septal defect, causing a steep fall in arterial oxygen saturation. This stimulates ventilation and leads to severe breathlessness on exercise. Children with Fallot's tetralogy are often observed to squat. This produces some obstruction of venous return from the exercising muscles of the legs, reducing the fall in arterial oxygen saturation and the resultant increased ventilation and breathlessness.

Severe arterial hypoxaemia occurs in *respiratory distress syndrome of the newborn*. Due to lack of pulmonary surfactant, parts of the lung fail to expand and there is marked mismatching of ventilation and perfusion in the lungs. Perfusion of unventilated segments contributes to the arterial hypoxia. There is profound stimulation of ventilation, with respiratory rates of up to 100 per minute. It is, of course, only speculation to suggest that this is accompanied by breathlessness in these infants.

Hypoxia is a common feature of many types of *parenchymal lung disease*; it is more often due to mismatching of ventilation and perfusion than to an actual block to diffusion (*see above*). A more important cause of breathlessness in many of these conditions is the increased work of breathing, due to decreased compliance of the lung tissue, and they are discussed more fully below.

Anaemia is frequently accompanied by a complaint of breathlessness. The mechanism is probably inefficient oxygen delivery to exercising muscles, with a resultant increase in anaerobic metabolism and lactate production which drives ventilation. The breathlessness that sometimes accompanies *pregnancy* and *arteriovenous fistula* may in part be due to a similar mechanism, with changes in distribution of the cardiac output leaving some muscle groups relatively hypoxic. In late pregnancy mechanical difficulties with ventilation are likely to be more important. Other causes of acidosis also produce an increase in ventilation, such as *renal failure* and *diabetic keto-acidosis*. In practice, these conditions are rarely accompanied by breathlessness unless there is concomitant lung disease. In the case of keto-acidosis this may be because consciousness is obtunded, but it remains unclear why there is relatively little breathlessness associated with other causes of acidosis.

Isocapnic *voluntary hyperventilation* is not accompanied by breathlessness in the experimental situation as discussed above. Similarly, breathlessness is a relatively rare complaint in the *hyperventilation syndrome*; symptoms such as nausea, lightheadedness and paraesthesiae are much more common. Although it has been suggested that some people with lung disease have *disproportionate dyspnoea*, associated with various psychiatric symptoms, true *psychogenic dyspnoea* is a very rare phenomenon and should never be diagnosed without very thorough investigation, including exercise testing. It should be noted, however, that the sighing respiration of *cardiac neurosis* may be referred to by the patient as 'breathlessness'.

Conditions associated with an increased work of breathing

OBSTRUCTIVE VENTILATORY DEFECTS
The term *chronic obstructive airways disease* refers to the situation where there is chronic, more or less irreversible, obstruction of the airways, especially the smaller airways. It is sometimes referred to by other names, such as *chronic airflow limitation* or *chronic obstructive pulmonary (or lung) disease*. The most important association is with cigarette smoking, but general atmospheric pollution also plays a part and it is common in some dusty occupations. The old term 'chronic bronchitis' should probably no longer be used as it is unclear whether it refers to chronic mucous hypersecretion (it was often diagnosed on the basis of this) or to airways obstruction. There is now convincing epidemiological evidence that the two conditions are distinct, connected through cigarette smoking, and that it is only the airways obstruction that is related to increased mortality.

Chronic obstructive airways disease remains a very common condition and an important cause of breathlessness due to increased drive to breathe required to overcome the increased resistance to airflow. It is diagnosed by the finding of airflow limitation, not reversible by bronchodilators, usually with a history of cigarette smoking and productive cough. The main differential diagnosis is asthma (*see below*).

Emphysema is defined as an increase in size, due to destruction of the alveolar walls, of the air spaces distal to the terminal bronchioles. It commonly coexists with chronic obstructive airways disease; it is also related to smoking and to some occupational exposures, such as to cadmium and to coal dust. In advanced emphysema, the chest becomes chronically overinflated with an increased anteroposterior diameter—the so-called 'barrel chest'. The chest radiograph shows loss of normal lung markings, flattened domes of the diaphragm and sometimes the presence of bullae (*Fig. D.15*). The lung function defect is obstructive, with collapse of the airways during expiration due to lack of support from the surrounding lung tissue. Other common lung function findings are an increased RV, an increased TLC, an increased RV/TLC ratio, and a decreased transfer factor. Occasionally, large bullae may act as space-occupying lesions and add a restrictive component to the picture. There is debate about whether resection of the bullae relieves breathlessness in these cases. A particular type of emphysema is that related to inherited deficiency of α-1-proteinase inhibitor; the emphysema is panacinar rather than centrilobular and tends to affect the upper, rather than the lower, lobes (*Fig*. D.16).

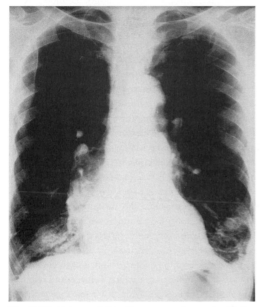

Fig. D.15. Male, aged 65, with severe emphysema and bullae in both upper and middle zones. The increased markings in the lower zones are due to compression of relatively normal lung tissue.

Breathlessness due to chronic irreversible obstructive airways disease presents as a major feature in a well-known clinical picture. Expiratory wheezes at the mouth and on auscultation are common but not invariable. Respiratory failure, with hypoxia and often hypercapnia, develops. Cor pulmonale, with peripheral oedema, develops in some cases. Two extremes have been described, depending on the degree to which the respiratory centre retains its sensitivity to carbon dioxide. Where sensitivity is lost, the $P\text{CO}_2$ rises, oedema is present and there is cyanosis due to hypoxia and sometimes secondary polycythaemia; this is the so-called 'blue bloater'. Where CO_2 sensitivity is retained, there tends to be a greater drive to breathe, with correspondingly more severe breathlessness, but relatively normal blood gases until a late stage of disease; this is described as the 'pink puffer'. In practice, there is considerable overlap between these two extremes.

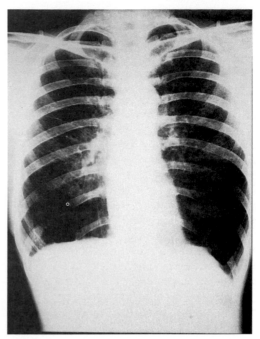

Fig. D.16. Female, aged 45, with emphysema secondary to α-1-proteinase deficiency. The lower lobes, unusually, are affected predominantly in this case.

Bronchiectasis is associated with breathlessness if there is appreciable airways obstruction present and if the lung destruction is extensive. The diagnosis is suggested by a history of production of copious purulent sputum, often with haemoptysis. Clubbing may be present with extensive disease. A bronchogram is the traditional way to confirm the diagnosis (*Fig*. D.17) but a more recent, non-invasive, alternative is computerized tomography. The lung disease of *cystic fibrosis* in children is similar to bronchiectasis of adults, with destruction of lung tissue and airways obstruction.

A common cause of breathlessness in all age groups is the episodic airways obstruction of *asthma*. The cardinal feature of asthma is the variable nature of the airways obstruction, with partial or complete reversal after bronchodilators. The typical history is of episodes of breathlessness, accompanied by wheezing, coughing or chest tightness, occurring especially at night and *after* exercise. During an attack, there is overinflation of the chest, wheezing and rapid ventilation. The breathlessness is made worse by the ventilatory stimulation from the accompanying hypoxia. Palpable 'paradox' of the arterial pulse is often present during a severe episode due to the large intrathoracic pressure swings. There are some particular causes of asthma that merit mention. *Bronchopulmonary aspergillosis* may provoke episodes of asthma or worsen pre-existing asthma. The chest radiograph may show transient pulmonary infiltrations and there is

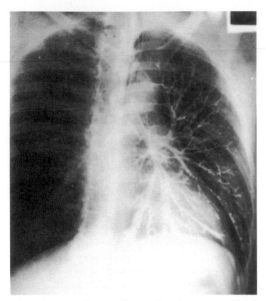

Fig. D.17. Bronchogram showing bronchiectasis in the left lower lobe. (*Dr Basil Strickland.*)

often an eosinophilia in the peripheral blood. A rare cause of asthma is *polyarteritis nodosa*, where it may be an early manifestation of this more general condition. *Occupational asthma* is being recognized with increasing frequency recently and should always be considered, especially when asthma fails to respond to usual treatments. A careful occupational history should be taken in all cases of asthma.

Airways obstruction is the main feature of *byssinosis*, a lung condition due to the inhalation of cotton and other vegetable dusts. The typical history is of breathlessness and chest tightness occurring on the first day back at work after a break, then gradually progressing so that it is constantly present. The late stages of byssinosis are indistinguishable from other causes of chronic obstructive airways disease.

Upper airways obstruction is an uncommon cause of breathlessness, but it is important to recognize because it can be rapidly fatal and can be rapidly relieved by intubation or tracheostomy. Obstruction at the level of the larynx may be due to severe *laryngitis*, which may still be secondary to *diphtheria*, or to *laryngeal oedema* as part of an allergic reaction. Severe *laryngotracheobronchitis* as occurs in *croup* can rapidly produce life-threatening respiratory obstruction and breathlessness and respiratory embarrassment can occur with severe *tonsillitis*. Obstruction can also be due to an impacted *foreign body* or to problems with the vocal cords themselves, as in *bilateral abductor paralysis*. Obstruction at the level of the trachea can be produced by intrinsic *carcinoma of the trachea* or by external compression from *carcinoma of the*

thyroid, *haemorrhage into a thyroid cyst, neoplastic glands* in the neck or mediastinum, *aortic aneurysm* or *dermoid tumour* of the mediastinum. Obstruction of the upper airways may be accompanied by inspiratory stridor and the flow-volume loop shows a characteristic truncation of the inspiratory part of the loop.

Restrictive ventilatory defects

The most obvious form of restrictive ventilatory defect is when there has been actual loss of lung tissue, following *surgical resection* of a lung or lobe. Breathlessness following pneumonectomy is more likely when there is disease of the remaining lung, such as obstructive lung disease in a smoker who has had a pneumonectomy for lung cancer. Space-occupying lesions can produce a similar effect. Examples are a large *pleural effusion* or *spontaneous pneumothorax*. Part of the breathlessness associated with these conditions is probably due to a neurological drive to breathe, but they also produce a restriction of lung tissue when large. A pleural effusion has to be very large before it produces noticeable breathlessness in young, healthy adults, but even a small effusion can lead to a worsening of breathlessness when it occurs in association with left ventricular failure, when there may already be pulmonary hypertension and oedema. Common features of a spontaneous pneumothorax are chest pain, often pleuritic in nature, and moderate breathlessness. A tension pneumothorax, actively increasing in size and compressing lung tissue, produces extreme breathlessness and often cardiovascular collapse and requires urgent relief through insertion of a cannula (*Fig.* D.18). Physical signs of a large pneumthorax are of reduced movement and reduced or absent breath sounds on the affected side. Large *tumours* can behave as space-occupying lesions, a particularly unpleasant example being a *mesothelioma* secondary to asbestos exposure. At post-mortem, the tumour is often seen to have replaced most of the original lung volume (*Fig.* D.19). A large *hiatus hernia* can occasionally cause breathlessness by acting as a space-occupying lesion within the chest.

Lung restriction can result from conditions of the chest wall. Deformity of the thoracic cage, such as occurs in severe *kyphoscoliosis, ankylosing spondylitis* or after a *thoracoplasty*, reduces the inspiratory volume that can be achieved, and may be associated with breathlessness as a result. Extensive pleural fibrosis or calcification can similarly produce a restrictive ventilatory defect; this may be found following *tuberculosis* or secondary to *asbestos exposure*. In severe cases, the lungs become encased in a rigid shell of pleura, sometimes called a cuirass. Restrictive ventilatory defects due to conditions outside the lung itself are

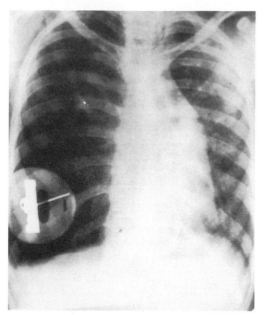

Fig. D.18. Male, aged 20, with pulmonary tuberculosis. Tension pneumothorax on right. Note the displacement of the heart to the left and an aspirating cannula *in situ*. (*Dr Basil Strickland.*)

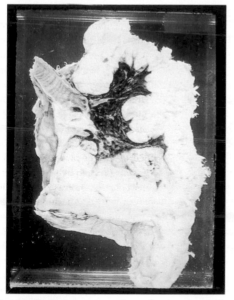

Fig. D.19. Post-mortem specimen showing mesothelioma replacing virtually all the lung tissue. The remaining lung is seen in the centre of the tumour.

characterized by reduced lung volumes but a normal or even increased transfer factor for carbon monoxide. This is because the lung tissue itself is normal, though compressed, and there may be a higher blood flow in the smaller volume of tissue causing the increase in transfer factor.

The largest group of conditions producing restrictive ventilatory defects are those involving the lung parenchyma itself. *Fibrosing alveolitis* is a generalized condition of the lung parenchyma, beginning as an inflammatory process and frequently progressing to established fibrosis. There are a number of variants of this condition, differing in their rate of progression and response to treatment with corticosteroids or immunosuppressants. The most acute form, sometimes known as the Hamman–Rich syndrome, progresses to severe disability and death within weeks or months. Other forms can be present for years before causing severe symptoms. Common features are breathlessness on exertion, dry cough, clubbing of the fingers (and toes) and inspiratory crackles especially at the lung bases. The chest radiograph shows reticulo-nodular shadowing, usually more marked in the lower zones.

In most cases of fibrosing alveolitis the cause is unknown. A somewhat similar clinical picture can develop in some cases of *extrinsic allergic alveolitis* which develops in response to inhaled organic dusts. The major mechanism is a type III allergy, with IgG antibodies against the allergen present in the blood. The best-known example of typical extrinsic allergic alveolitis (EAA) is farmer's lung. Acute episodes follow heavy exposure to the allergen, in this case spores of fungi such as *Micropolyspora faeni* contaminating damp hay. There is fever, breathlessness, cough, sometimes cyanosis, and crackles audible in the chest. Hypoxia and a restrictive ventilatory defect are present and there are scattered small, nodular shadows on the chest radiograph. Such acute episodes are often difficult to distinguish from atypical pneumonia, although the presence of precipitating antibodies can help. If exposure to the responsible agent continues, chronic disease develops. This is characterized by persistent breathlessness and dry cough, sometimes with clubbing and cyanosis. Airways obstruction can develop in addition to the restrictive defect and there may be emphysema as well as fibrosis in the lungs. The diagnosis is helped if there is a history of preceding acute episodes. In some types of extrinsic allergic alveolitis these are rare; in budgerigar fancier's lung an insidious development of fibrosis is common, probably because of the continuous low level exposure in this case. There are numerous other causes of EAA including: fungal spores, involved in bagassosis of sugar cane workers, in suberosis of cork workers, in sequoiosis of redwood sawyers, in lung disease of mushroom workers, malt-workers, maple-bark strippers and cheese makers; animal proteins in pigeon fancier's lung; and bacterial or amoebal proteins in humidifier fever (as distinct from legionnaires disease where lung infection is involved).

Extrinsic allergic alveolitis has some clinical and pathological features in common with *sarcoidosis*, although in the latter no causative agent has been identified. Acute, subacute and chronic forms of sarcoidosis are described. The acute form may have little in the way of respiratory symptoms and is characterized by bilateral hilar lymphadenopathy, often with fever, erythema nodosum and arthralgia. In the subacute and chronic forms there is a granulomatous infiltration in the lungs with increasing breathlessness. The chest radiograph shows pulmonary infiltration, said to be characteristically peri-hilar but often more generalized (*Fig.* D.20). Sarcoidosis is a systemic condition and many organs apart from the lungs can be affected, including the eyes (iridocyclitis), the lacrimal and salivary glands, the lymph nodes, the liver, the skin and the central and peripheral nervous system. The Kveim test is positive in acute disease but may be negative in the chronic form. A useful diagnostic feature of sarcoidosis, and EAA, is the presence of a large number of lymphocytes in the bronchoalveolar lavage fluid. In idiopathic fibrosing alveolitis, on the other hand, the fluid contains increased numbers of neutrophils.

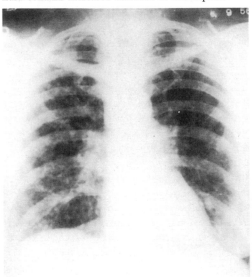

Fig. D.20. Pulmonary sarcoidosis in a middle-aged female complaining of breathlessness. Note the coarse nodular changes. The diagnosis has been confirmed by liver biopsy. (Dr Basil Strickland.)

Pneumoconiosis is a general term for lung disease due to dust inhalation but it is used mainly to describe the conditions associated with inhaling inorganic dusts where allergy is not an important mechanism. Symptoms and signs of lung disease tend to develop after exposure over many months or years. *Silicosis* is still an important disease world-wide. Breathlessness develops gradually and the restrictive pattern of deficit is frequently complicated by airways obstruction due to airways disease and lung distortion by fibrotic masses. The fibrosis of silicosis is nodular rather than

diffuse, and the chest radiograph shows distinct nodules which tend to coalesce to form large masses. In *coalworker's pneumoconiosis*, the chest radiograph shows a background of small nodular opacities, with large masses as the disease progresses (*Fig.* D.21). Disability is due mainly to the associated emphysema which may be severe. *Asbestosis* describes the lung fibrosis associated with asbestos exposure, which is diffuse and affects especially the lower lobes. It is frequently accompanied by pleural thickening or plaques which may calcify. An important complication is lung cancer, or more rarely mesothelioma. The restrictive lung function deficit and breathlessness of asbestosis is only poorly related to the severity of the radiographic changes. A number of other dusts can produce forms of pneumoconiosis. *Berylliosis*, due to exposure to beryllium, has many features in common with sarcoidosis and sometimes responds to treatment with corticosteroids.

Carcinoma of the lung rarely causes breathlessness as an early feature but breathlessness in more advanced disease may be due to a lobar collapse (as discussed above), to multiple metastases in the lungs or to lymphatic involvement producing lymphangitis carcinomatosa. This may also be due to the spread of extrapulmonary tumours and is associated with very severe breathlessness.

Most of the generalized *connective tissue diseases* can affect the lungs. Systemic lupus erythematosus frequently involves the pleura, with recurrent episodes of pleurisy, but can also lead to lung fibrosis. Systemic sclerosis (scleroderma) produces a diffuse interstitial pulmonary fibrosis, which can go on to produce cor pulmonale. A further cause of lung damage in this condition is recurrent aspiration if the oesophagus is also affected. Pulmonary involvement in rheumatoid disease is rare but diffuse fibrosis or rheumatoid nodules in the lung can occasionally occur. Caplan's syndrome is a type of coalworker's pneumoconiosis that occurs in men who have the rheumatoid diathesis. Multiple rounded opacities occur on a background of scanty small nodules; calcification and cavitation are quite common (*Fig* D.22). The lung condition can occur without overt arthritis but rheumatoid factor is nevertheless present in the serum.

Lung destruction as a result of infections can produce breathlessness secondary to a restrictive defect. *Tuberculosis*, with extensive cavitation, is often associated with breathlessness before adequate treatment; the breathlessness may persist after bacteriological cure due to the loss of lung tissue. *Klebsiella* pneumonia frequently destroys lung tissue and severe cases may be left with breathlessness after recovery from the infection.

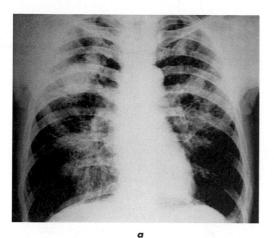 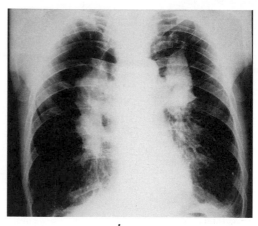

a   b

Fig. D.21. Coalworkers' pneumoconiosis with progressive massive fibrosis. a, In 1967, showing background small opacities and formation of large masses. (b), In 1980, showing enlargement of the massive lesions and reduction of opacities in the remaining lung due to increasing emphysema.

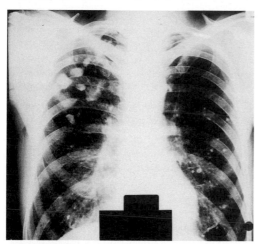

Fig. D.22. Caplan's syndrome in a coalworker. Rheumatoid factor was present in the serum. Note the large calcified opacities in both upper zones.

Other conditions of the lung parenchyma that can produce a restrictive ventilatory defect include *schistosomiasis*, fungal infections such as *blastomycosis* and *coccidioidomycosis*, and *alveolar proteinosis*. Poisoning with the weed-killer *paraquat* leads to severe breathlessness due to an obliterative bronchiolitis.

An important group of conditions in which breathlessness occurs at least partially due to a restrictive ventilatory defect is that causing *pulmonary oedema*. Cardiac causes of pulmonary oedema include valvular lesions, such as *mitral stenosis*, and *left ventricular failure*. The most common cause of left ventricular failure is ischaemic heart disease; other causes are hypertensive heart disease and non-ischaemic cardiomyopathies. As the pulmonary venous and capillary pressures rise, the lungs become stiffer; the accumulation of fluid in the interstitial tissue and in the alveoli increases the lung stiffness. Thus the work of ventilation is increased. In addition, gas transfer is impaired leading to increasingly severe arterial hypoxaemia which further drives ventilation. Breathlessness on exertion is accompanied by orthopnoea and bouts of nocturnal breathlessness (so-called paroxysmal nocturnal dyspnoea). The breathlessness that is frequently the symptom that limits exercise in heart disease with left ventricular dysfunction is not fully understood. The mechanism just outlined operates in some cases but other mechanisms, perhaps involving neurological drives to breathe, may also be important.

Acute pulmonary oedema, as every house officer knows, is a dramatic condition, with severe breathlessness developing rapidly, accompanied by a cough productive of frothy, pink sputum. There are widespread crackles in the chest and wheezing is often a prominent feature due to oedema of the bronchial walls. It can sometimes be difficult to differentiate between acute asthma and pulmonary oedema; radiographic appearances and the finding of mitral stenosis or a cause of left ventricular failure can be helpful. It is always worth remembering that an elderly patient with severe breathlessness might be suffering from acute asthma rather than pulmonary oedema secondary to cardiac disease. The radiographic features of pulmonary venous hypertension include engorgement of the upper lobe veins and septal lymphatic lines (*Fig.* D.23). In acute pulmonary oedema there is enlargement of the hilar shadows and fan-shaped mid-zone opacities (*Fig.* D.24).

Pulmonary oedema can be precipitated by infusion of saline. This is unlikely to occur with a normal heart and adequate renal function but it can readily occur in oliguric renal failure. Other non-cardiac causes

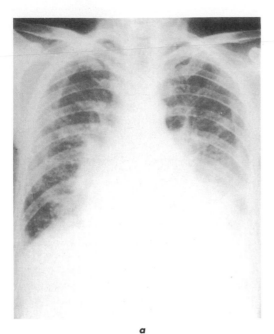
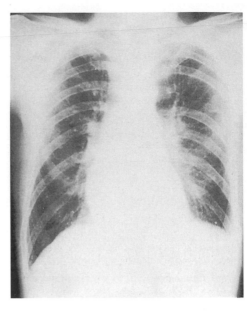

a

b

Fig. D.23. Male, aged 58, with mitral stenosis. In *a*, gross pulmonary congestion is present and ossific nodules are seen at the lung bases. In *b*, after mitral valvotomy, all the congestive changes have cleared and the ossific nodules are more clearly visible.

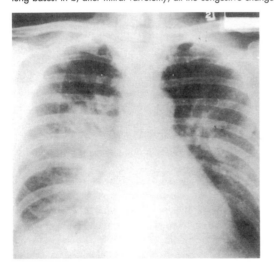

Fig. D.24. Acute pulmonary oedema following myocardial infarction. The changes are more marked on the right where the fan-shaped opacity spreading from the hilum is clearly seen.

of pulmonary oedema include cerebral vascular accidents, salicylate poisoning, hypersensitivity to radiographic contrast media, and adult respiratory distress syndrome when the pulmonary vasculature becomes abnormally 'leaky'. Pulmonary oedema can be caused by inhalation of smoke or other irritant gases, such as chlorine. *Aspiration pneumonitis* (Mendelson's syndrome) is similar to pulmonary oedema. It is due to the aspiration of gastric acid and the symptoms are virtually the same as for acute pulmonary oedema.

Conditions associated with decreased neuromuscular power

In these conditions an increased drive to the functioning respiratory muscles is required in order to attempt to maintain ventilation. *Weakness of the respiratory muscles* may be due to primary muscle disorders or to neurological disease. Examples include: myasthenia gravis, polyneuritis, poliomyelitis, motor neurone disease and muscular dystrophies. Despite the drive to breathe, hypoventilation is a feature of these conditions. It is also a feature of the respiratory failure associated with end-stage chronic obstructive airways disease, in particular. The hypoventilation associated with rare lesions of the respiratory centre itself is not usually associated with breathlessness, nor is the hypoventilation found in some cases of obesity (the so-called Pickwickian syndrome).

Differential diagnosis of acute breathlessness

Acute severe breathlessness is a common medical emergency, alarming for the patient and medical attendant alike. The urgency of the situation may be such that no time is available for radiographic or other investigation and the initial diagnosis must be made on the basis of clinical examination. The differential diagnosis will be discussed in terms of the physical signs which may be elicited in such an examination.

Simple inspection can be informative. If the patient is deeply cyanosed with engorged cervical veins, struggling for breath with violent movements of the larynx, *laryngeal or upper tracheal obstruction* should be considered. The stridor of upper airways obstruction is heard during both inspiration and expiration and should be distinguished from the expiratory wheeze of ordinary bronchial obstruction. The possible causes of upper airways obstruction are discussed above. The mucosal pallor of severe *anaemia* as a cause of breathlessness may also be noted on inspection.

Examination of the arterial pulse may reveal uncontrolled *atrial fibrillation* or other dysrhythmias, which can lead to sudden breathlessness especially if there is valvular or other cardiac disease. *Cardiac tamponade* is associated with marked 'paradox' of the arterial pulse and elevation of the jugular venous pressure, with a paradoxical rise in pressure during inspiration. It may be secondary to intrapericardial haemorrhage from malignant metastases; in association with cardiac rupture from a mycardial infarction it is usually rapidly fatal. The venous pressure is also markedly elevated following a massive *pulmonary embolus*, another cause of acute severe breathlessness.

Mediastinal displacement, as indicated by lateral displacement of the trachea, can be a valuable physical sign in acute breathlessness. In *massive collapse* of a lung, for example postoperatively, the trachea is displaced towards the affected side. The trachea is deviated away from the side of the lesion in *pleural effusion* and *tension pneumothorax*. The most likely fluid to accumulate rapidly enough in the pleural space to cause acute breathlessness is blood; *haemothorax* may follow chest trauma or even occur after pleural aspiration.

In acute *pulmonary oedema*, the venous pressure is usually also elevated and there may be signs on examination of the heart, such as a murmur of *mitral stenosis* or a gallop rhythm in *left ventricular failure*. Auscultation of the lungs usually reveals widespread crackles in pulmonary oedema and expiratory wheezes in *acute asthma*; in very severe asthma the wheeze can disappear because of gross reduction of air movement. If acute breathlessness is due to severe pulmonary infection, features such as pyrexia, purulent sputum and signs of consolidation in the lungs can be helpful diagnostically.

Anne Cockcroft

Dysuria

Dysuria is pain felt during the act of micturition. It is a urethral pain and relates to irritation of the urethral mucosa. It may, therefore, be experienced by an otherwise normal individual when concentrated or acid urine is passed, for example, when the patient is dehydrated from the excessive fluid loss associated with exercise or hot climate, or from an inability to drink enough fluid, for example during an intercontinental flight. Dysuria under these circumstances is rarely severe, and felt more as a tingling or slight stinging as urine is passed. The symptom is short-lived and corrected as soon as the relative dehydration resolves.

True dysuria is associated with a urinary tract infection. This may have arisen in the upper tract as pyelitis, in which case the bladder is invariably infected secondarily. It may be due to primary cystitis, or due to acute urethritis. True dysuria in women may also be found in the 'urethral syndrome', otherwise known as 'acute abacterial cystitis'. The feeling exactly mimicks a true cystitis but no microbiological evidence of infection can be found. This condition is noted elsewhere under URINE, RETENTION OF.

Pain felt in the bladder area is not true dysuria but may also be present during an acute episode of cystitis. Bladder pain can also be experienced in the presence of a bladder stone, when the stone bounces up and down on the trigone during the act of micturition. The trigone is a particularly sensitive area of the bladder and can therefore cause pain when involved by bladder or prostatic carcinoma and in acute and chronic prostatitis. Prostatitis is a difficult condition to diagnose—acute prostatitis renders digital examination of the prostate per rectum virtually impossible, as the gland is exquisitely tender; the diagnosis of chronic prostatitis is rarely satisfactory although the presence of threads on post-massage urine examination is usually taken as sufficient evidence of the condition. Positive cultures are rarely obtained from cases of 'chronic prostatitis' even when tissue cores of prostate are subject to bacteriological examination. Tuberculous cystitis may not be particularly symptomatic but bladder pain and true dysuria may both occur. When diagnosed, often after prolonged searching for positive cultures of early morning urines, it should be considered as a disease of the whole urinary tract.

Perineal pain during micturition is often indicative of prostatic disease, usually inflammatory. Prostatic carcinoma occasionally presents in this manner.

Acute urethral pain during micturition, associated with sudden cessation of a stream, implies the impaction of a calculus, a retained 'chip' following transurethral resection of the prostate or a dislodged portion of bladder tumour, along the urethra. As the narrowest portion of the urethra is the meatus, examination of the patient under these circumstances may reveal the object responsible protruding in part through the orifice. A stone impacted at the ureteric meatus provokes an intense oedematous reaction around the uretero-vesical junction and this may also cause a severe pain radiated to the distal end of the urethra.

In children, acute cystitis often presents in a non-specific way, the child having a sequence of screaming attacks which are obviously related to pain, the cause of which is not immediately apparent. Meatal ulceration and acute balanitis, both in the male infant, may provoke similar screaming attacks as the affected areas are, in effect, burnt by the ammonia in the urine each time micturition occurs.

Lynn Edwards

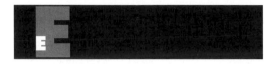

Earache

Earache (otalgia) may be due to a considerable number of diseases of the auricle or pinna, the external auditory meatus or middle ear. It may also be caused, most importantly, by referred pain from structures which share a common nerve supply. It is one of the common symptoms of childhood and may be one of the most deep-seated and unpleasant pains to bear. The causes of earache are listed in *Table* E.1

Local causes of otalgia

Auricle—causes in the auricle are usually obvious and include direct trauma, haematoma, furuncles and otitis externa which cause pain because of the swelling of the skin which is firmly attached to the underlying cartilage. Perichondritis may occur following infection. 'Chondrodermatitis nodularis chronicis helicis' is the name given to a very painful nodular lesion of the pinna thought to be due to vasoconstriction following exposure to cold. Malignant disease may be painful; rodent ulcers and squamous carcinomas are usually only markedly so during the later stages.

Meatus—the external auditory meatus is the site of many painful conditions; local infection of the skin and small furuncles may be extremely painful, the amount of pain bearing little relationship to the size of the furuncle which may be only the size of a pin's head.

In many cases of diffuse otitis externa there is great swelling of the meatal skin and it may not be possible to see the drum. There is pain on moving the pinna and this is a valuable sign to differentiate the condition from mastoiditis. Fungal infection (oto-mycosis) is often especially painful (*Fig.* E.1.)

Table E.1. Causes of earache

Local
Auricle
  Trauma
    Direct
    Haematoma
  Furuncle
  Boils
  Otitis externa (*see Fig.* E.1.)
  Perichondritis
  Chondrodermatitis nodularis
  Malignant disease
External auditory meatus
  Diffuse otitis externa
    Infective
      Bacterial
      Fungal
      Viral
    Reactive
      Eczematous
      Seborrhoeic dermatitis
      Neurodermatitis
  Malignant otitis externa
  Necrotizing osteitis
  Wax
  Keratosis obturans
  Foreign body—impacted
  Trauma
  Malignant disease
Middle ear
  Acute otitis media
  Chronic otitis media
    Tubotympanic otitis media
    Attic disease
  Serous otitis (rarely)
  Mastoiditis
  Malignant disease

Referred
Dental
  Caries
  Abscess
  Impacted molar
  Costen's syndrome
Pharynx
  Tonsillitis
  Pharyngitis
  Postoperative pain
  Quinsy
  Foreign bodies
  Malignant disease
Cervical spine
  Osteoarthritis
  Spondylosis

Neurological
Herpes zoster
Glossopharyngeal neuralgia
Trigeminal neuralgia (occasional)

In addition to the above, a condition called by Chandler (1968) 'malignant' otitis externa is found usually in diabetics where advancing infection leads to osteomyelitis and mastoiditis. The organism is always *B. pyocyaneus*.

Otitis externa haemorrhagica is described but it is best known as 'bullous myringitis' and is an infection of the middle layers of the tympanic membrane, usually caused by infection by *H. influenzae*. There is considerable pain when the layers of the drum are separated

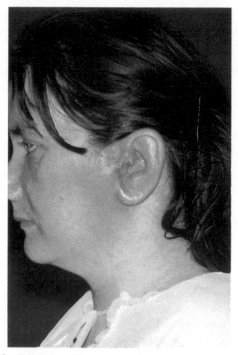

Fig. E.1. Severe otitis externa.

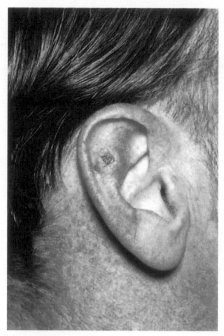

Fig. E.2. Epithelioma of the pinna.

by fluid which causes a bleb within the drum, which must be carefully differentiated from the bulging drum of otitis media. The pain ceases if the bleb discharges its serosanguineous contents.

Finally, among the infections, necrotizing osteitis of the tympanic ring is a chronic condition with low grade aching in the ear. A small ulcer with bare bone exposed at the base may be seen in the deep meatus and this may rarely go on to extensive necrosis around the tympanic plate. The aetiology is obscure.

Impacted wax may cause considerable pain and discomfort especially following swimming and ineffective attempts at removal by syringeing. Water may cause swelling of the wax and sudden deafness follows complete occlusion of the meatus. A more severe condition is keratosis obturans, where abnormal desquamation of the epithelium comes to lie in layers together with the wax and is most difficult to move. Pressure of this mass may cause bony necrosis and enlargement of the meatus. There is an association with chronic bronchitis and bronchiectasis, perhaps due to stimulation of the vagus and consequent reflex secretion of wax.

Foreign bodies may cause pain, usually after ineffective and incompetent attempts at removal. Insects are not infrequently found in tropical lands. Trauma, often self-inflicted in attempts to relieve irritation or remove wax, may cause scratches, ulcers or even perforations of the drum.

Malignant disease of the external meatus (*Fig. E.2*) is usually squamous-cell carcinoma. It often follows prolonged suppuration and is locally invasive, causing severe pain in the later stages. Rodent ulcers, common on the pinna, are rare in the meatus.

Middle ear. Acute otitis media is one of the commonest infections in childhood—hardly a child escapes one or more attacks. The infection follows an upper respiratory infection or cold and the pain may come on with great rapidity usually becomes worse in the evening. It often ceases abruptly as the drum ruptures and the child falls asleep, the discharge not being noticed by the mother till the following morning. It must be remembered that young children do not localize pain accurately and earache may not be a complaint. Unresolved acute otitis media may go on to acute mastoiditis where there is severe pain and tenderness behind and above the ear centred over the mastoid antrum. Swelling behind the ear may follow and a subperiosteal abscess may push the pinna forwards. Differentiation from otitis externa is most important. In otitis media and mastoiditis deafness is invariable, while good hearing and pain on moving the pinna indicate otitis externa.

Chronic otitis media (*Fig. E.3*) is not often accompanied by pain though exacerbations of infection in both tubotympanic otitis media and in attic disease causing earache are often of serious import. The intracranial complications of otogenic disease—subperiosteal abscess, extradural abscess and brain abscess—are all accompanied by headache and when this occurs

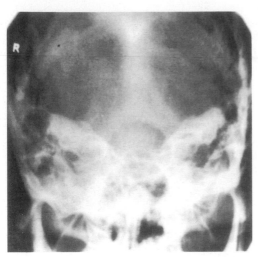

Fig. E.3. Chronic suppurative otitis media with a large choleste-atoma of the right temporal bone. (*Dr Lorna Davison.*)

together with pyrexia and vertigo in a patient with chronic otitis media great care should be taken.

Trauma may be direct due to perforation of the drum by foreign bodies (a matchstick used in an ear is a most dangerous weapon) or by water or air pressure changes, diving or a blow on the ear. Otitic barotrauma is not so common now that aircraft are pressurized but it may still occur on descent if the air pressure is increased suddenly or if the patient is suffering from Eustachian tubal dysfunction at the time of the flight.

Secretory otitis media, so common in children, is usually characterized by a symptomless deafness. Dull aching pain or, rarely, stabs of acute pain may be a symptom.

Malignant disease, again usually squamous-cell carcinoma, occurring in chronically infected ears, rare tumours such as the glomus tumour, myelomas and secondary malignant disease all cause pain. Diagnosis is by observation, X-ray studies and biopsy.

Referred pain

Referred pain affecting the ear is very common. Pain is referred through the 5th, 7th, 9th and 10th cranial nerves, the upper cervical nerves and possibly the sympathetic nerve supply. Despite careful examination no abnormality is found in the ear. It has always been taught that 'a swelling in the neck and cottonwool in the ear' is a sign of malignant disease of pharynx or nasopharynx, one of the most important causes of referred otalgia.

Dental causes—caries, dental abscess and impacted lower molars are all common causes of earache. Malocclusion may give rise to dysfunction of the temporo-mandibular joint (Costen's syndrome). These patients often have a history of dental extractions or

a badly fitting denture and tenderness will be found over the joint especially on movement, which may be restricted.

Pharynx. Tonsillitis, pharyngitis and even the initial stages of the common cold are all accompanied by earache which may vary from a mild stinging pain to very severe pain. The postoperative period after tonsillectomy is very consistently a time of quite unpleasant earache. This can be relieved by aspirin which has both a general and local action. Other simple pharyngeal causes are a quinsy, impacted foreign bodies or scratches due to trauma from bones and sharp objects that have been swallowed.

The most important group from a diagnostic point of view are malignant lesions of the nasopharynx, pharynx, laryngopharynx and larynx. Earache is found very consistently in these conditions and careful examination is always necessary if there is any doubt about a possible local cause.

Cervical spine. Cervical osteoarthritis or cervical spondylosis causing pain in the C2 and C3 regions may lead to referred pain around the ear in the middle-aged or elderly people who may have a history of trauma, such as 'whiplash injury'.

Neurological causes

A number of conditions come under this heading.

Herpes zoster oticus. Herpes zoster of the geniculate ganglion gives rise to lesions of the meatus, pinna and sometimes the palate and fauces. If facial palsy occurs (Ramsay–Hunt syndrome) this coincides with the vesicles and follows some days of severe otalgia which may precede all other signs. Sometimes there is tinnitus and vertigo.

Other cranial and upper cervical nerves are also affected by herpes.

Glossopharyngeal neuralgia. Very severe pain radiating from the throat to the tongue and ear is a rare condition sometimes associated with an elongated styloid process. There is often a trigger area in the throat in the same way as a trigger area may initiate trigeminal neuralgia or *tic doloreux* which, though usually involving the face, may also largely affect the ear.

A. G. D. Maran

Eating, disorders of

Disturbances of eating remain inadequately understood and often difficult to diagnose because the behaviour is frequently secretive and does not come to medical attention unless a complication develops or the condition is severe. Consequently the prevalence of these disorders is uncertain although there is mounting evidence that clinically significant conditions are the tip of an iceberg with transient, mild or partial disturbances occurring frequently and an overconcern with weight or shape which has no behavioural dimension being extremely common. Such attitudes can be identified in prepubertal schoolgirls, becoming accentuated as adolescence develops and sociocultural pressures exert their influence upon the equation of thinness with attractiveness.

The boundary between normal and abnormal concerns, eating habits and weight loss has posed major difficulties in the classification of eating disorders. This is well exemplified in the recently revised, standard American diagnostic system, DSM IIIR, where the amount of weight loss required to diagnose anorexia nervosa has been reduced from 25 per cent to 15 per cent; obesity continues to be classified as a physical disorder in spite of many patients' obesity being obviously psychologically based and behaviourally maintained; and a category of atypical eating disorders has been developed to classify a pot-pourri of partial syndromes and single symptoms. In short, the classification of eating disorders is unsatisfactory and the non-specialist should be more concerned with the recognition of an eating disorder rather than the intricacies of diagnostic classification (*Table* E.2).

Table E.2. Causes of disorders

Commonest
Transient disturbance or fad
Stress reaction

Common
Anorexia nervosa
Bulimia nervosa

Rare
a. Unexplained severe wasting
Hypopituitarism
Diabetes mellitus
Thyrotoxicosis
Malignant disease
Tuberculosis
Malabsorption syndrome

b. Bingeing
Cerebral damage
Cerebral tumour
Kleine–Levin syndrome
Kluver–Bucy syndrome

c. Self-induced vomiting
Pyloric stenosis
Postgastrectomy
Habit disorder

d. Psychiatric disorders
Depression
Schizophrenia
Obsessive-compulsive disorder

The only worthwhile distinction in practice is between *anorexia nervosa* and *bulimia nervosa*, with significant degrees of weight loss and amenorrhoea being confined to anorexia nervosa and loss of control over eating characteristic of bulimia nervosa. Bingeing, self-induced vomiting and purgation, disturbance of body image (p. 66) and a crucially persistent, morbid fear of becoming fat are shared features.

A notable difference between these conditions is the mode of presentation. In bulimia nervosa the patient usually seeks help for herself, expressing open distress about the loss of control over her eating behaviour; she tends not to deny or minimize symptoms. On the other hand patients with anorexia nervosa are usually highly secretive and misleading, failing to disclose important information. This has two effects in clinical practice—first the patient may present with a complication of their disorder as the primary complaint; second their inanition may present unexplained. Both these types of presentation are less common than the patient who is brought to medical attention by concerned relatives, but more common than the anorectic who presents with open concern about her own eating pattern.

The best-known somatic presentation of anorexia nervosa is amenorrhoea, usually secondary, and sometimes disguised by taking oral contraceptives. Gastrointestinal presentations include abdominal pain, constipation and diarrhoea caused by laxative abuse. Complications of repeated self-induced vomiting such as cardiac arrhythmias, impaired renal function, tetany, painless swelling of the parotid glands, erosion of dental enamel and chronic hoarseness, are unusual but potentially fatal, particularly when metabolic disturbances (especially hypokalaemia) and dehydration develop. This may result in a dramatic medical emergency presentation with profound cardiovascular collapse, although faints, blackouts and convulsions are more common sudden presentations.

Of course the commonest presentation of anorexia nervosa is a young female with unexplained weight loss, less than 10 per cent of cases being male. On examination the severe anorectic has marked wasting, lanugo hair, slow pulse, low blood pressure and cold extremities. Pubic and axillary hair are retained differentiating anorexia nervosa from hypopituitarism, where the patient also tends to be less emaciated. Other readily excluded causes of severe wasting are diabetes mellitus and thyrotoxicosis, but more difficulty may occur in distinguishing a malignancy (especially a reticulosis or cerebral tumour), occult tuberculosis and malabsorption syndromes.

Associated behaviours also have their own differential diagnoses. *Bingeing* may occur in hypothalmic damage or tumour, Kleine–Levin syndrome and Kluver–Bucy syndrome, all of which are very rare. *Self-induced vomiting* can develop in patients who have pyloric stenosis or following partial/total gastrectomy, while some individuals practise vomiting either to relieve stress (with no intention of controlling weight), or to titillate or disgust observers. *Purging* by laxative abuse is a common phenomenon, especially in older obsessional or hypochondriacal patients who require regulated bowels to lead a regulated life.

Psychiatric disorders enter the differential diagnosis, particularly depression, which also develops frequently in patients with eating disorders. The distinction can sometimes be difficult with marked weight loss, amenorrhoea, loss of energy, interests and concentration, sleep disturbance, obsessional ruminations and even suicidal ideation and overeating being potentially shared features. However there are differences— appetite is typically diminished in depression but normal or increased in eating disorders; more importantly preoccupation with food and its caloric content, disturbance of body image and a phobia of normal weight are not features of a primary depressive illness. Similarly these features distinguish an eating disorder from schizophrenia and obsessive compulsive disorder which may occasionally present with superficial resemblances through bizarre eating habits or food/weight-related rituals and overvalued ideas.

Indeed the distinction between an eating disorder and all the physical and psychiatric conditions that enter the differential diagnosis rests not with weight loss, dieting or any particular form of eating abuse, but with the constellation of fears, urges and attitudes that always form the psychological backdrop in both male and female patients. There is a cardinal *morbid fear of becoming fat* which persists even when grossly underweight or losing weight. Any weight gain or eating provokes anxiety that is relieved only by losing weight either by not eating or by elimination through vomiting, purgation or exercise. Food becomes an enemy, calories an obsession; life becomes dominated by the need to control this aspect of living.

However there may be great difficulty encountered in penetrating the patient's resistance to elicit the information that is necessary to confirm the diagnosis. Failure to establish this psychological driving force after careful, repeated assessment should alert the physician to the possibility of one of the rare, cryptic presentations in the differential diagnosis.

George Masterton

ELBOW
See JOINTS, AFFECTIONS OF.

Encopresis

(*See also* FAECES, INCONTINENCE OF)

Encopresis is often defined as the passage of faeces into socially unacceptable places, however it is more accurate to restrict this term to the passage of normal stools in this way. Encopresis is therefore one of the forms of faecal incontinence in children, others being overflow soiling in association with a faecally-loaded rectum (seen in children with non-Hirschsprung's megarectum) or the incontinence associated with diarrhoea (especially if the stools are persistently loose as in Toddler diarrhoea).

Encopresis is normal in the first 3 years of life. Persistence of encopresis occurs with developmental delay, chaotic training or neglect, or neurogenic rectum (spina bifida, sacral agenesis, spinal tumours or idiopathic). Secondary encopresis (occurring after bowel control has been acquired) is most frequently a response to emotional stress especially associated with anxiety or suppressed anger. Child physical or sexual abuse may present in this way. The development of a neurogenic rectum due to spinal tumours, cord damage from trauma or infection will lead to secondary encopresis.

G. S. Clayden

Enophthalmos (or retraction of the eyeball)

This may occur in: (1) fractures of the orbital floor (fractures of the orbital floor and necrosis of incarcerated orbital fat, results in progressive enophthalmos); (2) wasting diseases; (3) paralysis of the cervical sympathetic; (4) various congenital affections; (5) phthisis bulbi (shrinkage of the eyeball from prolonged endophthalmitis).

The enophthalmos in *wasting diseases* is due to the absorption of the orbital fat, and the diagnosis as regards the eye presents no difficulty.

Enophthalmos due to *paralysis of the cervical sympathetic* is never very gross, and is always associated with the other well-defined symptoms of this lesion, namely, diminution in the size of the palpebral aperture, constriction of the pupil, absence of sweating and blushing on the paralysed side. Occasionally it may be noticed that the hair over the affected side of the head is behaving differently from that on the sound side—it may lie flatter, or may lack lustre to a degree that the patient observes. The pupil is constricted owing to the paralysis of the dilator fibres.

In certain *congenital cases* there is well-marked retraction, associated with defective or irregular movements of the affected eyeball. Rarely, the condition is simulated by a maldevelopment of the globe, which has remained small and is usually extremely hypermetropic and poor-sighted.

W. M. Haining

Enuresis

(*See also* URINE, INCONTINENCE OF)

Enuresis means incontinence of urine in children and can be diurnal, nocturnal or both. Children vary in the age at which they become reliably continent of urine. The majority of children are continent during the day by age two-and-a-half years and by night by three-and-a-half years. The prevalence of wetting diminishes with age and is approximately 20 per cent of 4 year olds, 10 per cent of 5 year olds, 7 per cent of 7 year olds and 1.4 per cent of 14 year olds.

The commonest organic disease to lead to enuresis is urinary tract infection especially in girls; enuretic girls have a four-fold increased likelihood of having a urinary tract infection compared to non-enuretics. Dribbling urinary incontinence may be the presenting sign of an ectopic ureter draining below the sphincter or overflow from an obstructed bladder. Secondary enuresis (having previously been reliably continent) should be considered suspicious of a urinary tract infection especially when associated with other symptoms such as urinary frequency, abdominal pain, dysuria and wetting in the daytime. Secondary enuresis can be caused by neurological problems such as neurogenic bladder (associated with spina bifida or other cord lesions such as tumours). Polyuria often leads to enuresis in children and so diseases such as diabetes mellitus or insipidus, or chronic renal failure must be considered. Emotional problems can lead to enuresis which compounds the psychological difficulties because of parental reaction (similar to encopresis). Secondary enuresis is common following family break-up or bereavement. Child sexual abuse may present in this way.

G. S. Clayden

EPILEPSY
See CONVULSIONS AND FITS.

Epiphora

Epiphora is the overflow of tears on to the cheek and may be due either to increased production of tears or inadequate drainage of tears.

Increased production. Psychic lacrimation is normally associated with pain or emotional upset. Reflex stimulation of lacrimation causing epiphora is commonly associated with irritative conditions or corneal disease. Corneal injury, a blast of air or foreign body on the surface of the eye causes irritation of the trigeminal nerve that excites lacrimation. Even strong light, yawning, vomiting and laughing are associated with reflex lacrimation.

Inadequate drainage of tears. This may be due to malposition of the lacrimal puncta which should normally be closely applied to the eye in order to attract tears by capillary action. Such malposition may occur in ectropion associated with laxity of the lids

which may occur with age, or paralysis of the eyelid muscles which are responsible for blinking in facial palsy or cicatricial lid disease with scarring, which pulls the punctum out of its correct position. Obstruction of the lacrimal drainage apparatus (common canaliculus and nasolacrimal duct) will also cause epiphora.

S. T. D. Roxburgh

Epistaxis

It is important to realize that epistaxis is a sign not a disease. The causes of the condition are shown in (*Table* E.3.)

Table E.3. Causes of epistaxis

A. Local causes
Trauma to Little's area
Dryness of nasal mucosa, e.g. sex, drugs
Abnormal anatomy, e.g. septal deviations
Ulceration and excoriation
Nasal fracture
Nasal infections
Tumours of the nose and sinuses
Septal granulomas and perforations
Foreign bodies

B. Systemic causes
Coagulopathy—haemophilia, Christmas disease, von
  Willebrand's disease, purpura, leukaemia
Hypertension
Drugs, anticoagulants, aspirin, cytotoxic drugs
Atherosclerosis
Hereditary haemorrhagic telangiectasis
Vitamin deficiency—vitamin C, vitamin K
Renal dialysis

Epistaxis usually occurs from the anterior part of the nasal septum, an area known as Little's area. The feeding vessels are the greater palatine artery, the facial artery, the anterior ethmoidal artery and the sphenopalatine artery. At the junction of these vessels the area is very vascular and is easily traumatized, since it is at the front of the most prominent feature of the face.

Bleeding higher up the nose usually comes from the sphenopalatine arteries or the anterior ethmoidal arteries. It is important to try to identify the site as accurately as possible because, in the event of persistent epistaxis where packing has failed, a vessel may need to be tied. Different approaches are needed for the anterior ethmoidal artery, a branch of the internal carotid, and the maxillary artery as the terminal branch of the external carotid and so as accurate identification as possible is required.

The management of epistaxis is the management of the cause. If the nose has been traumatized then it is possible that a spicule of ethmoid bone has penetrated the anterior ethmoid artery and an open reduction may be required. Neoplasms of the nose and sinus need to be identified and treated accordingly (*Fig.* E.4).

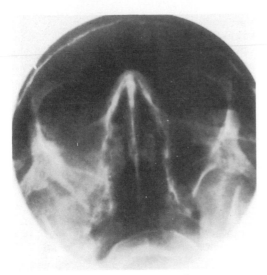

Fig. E.4. Carcinoma of the antrum. Note the opaque antrum and dehiscent orbital floor. (*Dr Lorna Davison.*)

Coagulopathies require the appropriate medical therapy and if the patient is on anticoagulants or aspirin then the effects of these need to be reversed. Many patients are hypertensive and a period of bed-rest and adequate sedation is helpful. Patients with hereditary telangiectasis may require skin grafting of the septum.

The most usual cause in children is bleeding from Little's area. In this instance the blood vessels are easily identified if the nose is packed for a short time with cocaine and adrenalin. Once the vessels are identified they can be easily cauterized either with electro-cautery, silver nitrate or trichloracetic acid.

Bleeding that comes from areas other than Little's area often requires admission to hospital. The first thing to do is to replace the blood volume, put the patient to bed and adequately sedate him. The nose is packed with ½-inch ribbon gauze impregnated with an antiseptic such as BIPP or an antibiotic such as terracortril. It is left in place for 48 hours and then removed. If the epistaxis recurs then the nose is packed again. If there is a further recurrence then either the anterior ethmoidal artery or the maxillary artery is ligated. The access to the maxillary artery is through the maxillary sinus.

A. G. D. Maran

Erythema

Erythema is a reddening of the skin due to persistent vasodilatation of the superficial vessels. It can result from a wide variety of causes and may be localized or generalized (*Table* E.4).

Table E.4. Erythema

A. Localized erythema
Internal
  Boil, herpes simplex, herpes zoster, impetigo,
  erysipelas, gout, thrombophlebitis, lymphangitis
External
  Irritant (thermal, caustic, traumatic)
  Allergic (allergic contact dermatitis)
  Fixed drug eruption

B. Localized patterns of erythema
Rosacea
Palmar erythema
Erythema ab igne
Livedo reticularis
Erythema annulare centrifugum (Lyme disease)
Erythema induratum (Bazin's disease)

C. Generalized erythema
Toxic erythema
Exanthems
  Measles, rubella, scarlet fever, erythema infectiosum,
  HIV infection
Erythema multiforme
Erythema nodosum
Lupus erythematosus
Dermatomyositis

A. Local erythema

A localized patch of cutaneous erythema can be of internal or external origin. Internal causes are most often local inflammatory processes where the diagnosis, if not at first obvious, soon becomes so, e.g. boil or carbuncle, herpes simplex or zoster, impetigo, erysipelas, gout, thrombophlebitis or lymphangitis. External causes may be irritant (e.g. thermal, caustic or traumatic) or allergic (e.g. allergic contact dermatitis). (*Fig.* E.5). A fixed drug eruption (e.g. to phenolph-thalein, codeine or sulpha drugs) gives a violent local erythema (*Fig.* B.45) which rapidly darkens to a magenta colour, and usually blisters. It recurs at the same skin sites at each drug exposure.

B. Localized patterns of erythema

1. ROSACEA

Erythema is a characteristic feature of rosacea (*Fig.* E.6). It may occur alone or in conjunction with telangiectasia, papules and pustules. The erythema is initially transient, like a prominent flush, but later persists for long periods. It is most characteristically seen over the cheeks and nose and may also affect the forehead and upper part of the neck.

2. PALMAR ERYTHEMA (*Fig.* E.7)

As an isolated phenomenon, this is best known in pregnancy, but is also seen in liver disease, thyrotoxicosis, rheumatoid arthritis and high output cardiac states and can also occur as a familial trait.

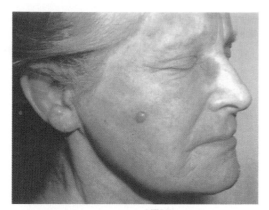

Fig. E.5. Contact dermatitis to chrysanthemum. (*Dr Paul August.*)

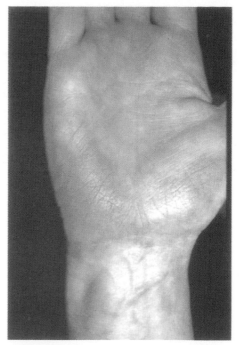

Fig. E.7. Palmar erythema. (*Dr Paul August.*)

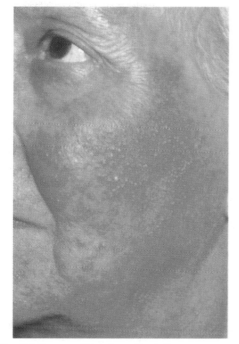

Fig. E.6. Rosacea. (*Westminster Hospital.*)

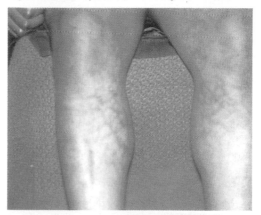

Fig. E.8. Erythema ab igne in a young West Indian girl. (*Dr Richard Staughton.*)

3. ERYTHEMA AB IGNE (*Fig.* E.8)

This is a reticulate erythema which progresses to persistent haemosiderin pigmentation due to long continued exposure to heat (infrared radiation). It is most common on the legs of elderly women.

4. LIVEDO RETICULARIS

This is a similarly patterned erythema, seen usually on the lower limbs, which may be due to polyarteritis nodosa, rheumatoid arthritis, lupus erythematosus and dermatomyositis. A physiological form called *cutis marmorata* is a reaction to cold and seen especially in children. There are a number of other rarer erythematous conditions in which patches of erythema appear on the trunk (*Fig.* E9), often in circular or gyrate patterns.

5. ERYTHEMA ANNULARE CENTRIFUGUM (LYME DISEASE)

This was known as a gradually spreading circle of cutaneous erythema responsive to penicillin for many years before the causative spirochaete *Borrelia burgdorferi* was discovered (from a epidemic of patients around the town of Lyme, New Hampshire—hence the alternative name—*Lyme disease*). The natural reservoir of infection is the red deer and it is only transferred to humans bitten by an infected deer tick, *Ixodes ricinus*. Patients either live in or have visited

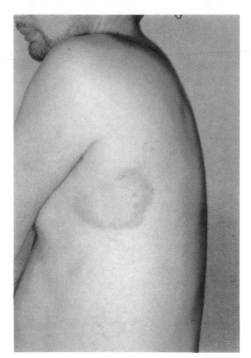

Fig. E.9. Annular erythema. (*Westminster Hospital.*)

forested areas in the weeks before the erythema begins. A rising specific IgA titre aids clinical diagnosis. Adequate treatment with penicillin or tetracycline is very important as a proportion of untreated patients progress to serious CNS infection, sometimes *after* the erythema has resolved.

Some very rare migratory erythemas can be cutaneous markers of underlying neoplasia, e.g. necrolytic migratory erythema (glucagon secreting pancreatic tumour), erythema gyratum repens (carcinoma or lymphoma).

6. ERYTHEMA INDURATUM (BAZIN'S DISEASE)

This is a rare manifestation of tuberculosis seen in middle-aged women. The site affected is the posterior aspect of the legs and the condition begins as a symmetrical eruption of deep-seated painless red nodules. The surface becomes purple and deep cold ulcers with undermined borders form. The patients show extreme sensitivity to tuberculin on skin testing.

C. Generalized erythema

1. TOXIC ERYTHEMA

This is a widespread symmetrical blotchy erythema tending to affect the trunk more than the extremities (*Fig.* E.10), and often accompanied by malaise, fever and lymphadenopathy. This cutaneous reaction pattern

may be provoked by many causes, e.g. viral infections, especially glandular fever, and also drug hypersensitivity, especially to ampicillin, amoxycillin, sulphonamides and non-steroid anti-inflammatory drugs. Often no cause is found. Spontaneous resolution, which usually occurs within 10–15 days, is often followed by desquamation.

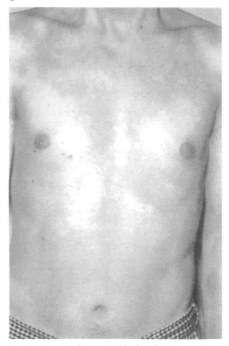

Fig. E.10. Toxic erythema. (*Addenbrooke's Hospital.*)

2. EXANTHEMS

In *measles*, the rash usually develops on the fourth day behind the ears. It spreads to the face and downwards to the trunk and extremities on the fifth to seventh days. The eruption is usually preceded by 1–7 days of prodromal coryza, nasal discharge and conjunctival injection, on the second or third day of which Koplik's spots appear, as white specks surrounded by redness, on the buccal mucosa opposite the molar teeth. Koplik's spots may be lentil-sized and few in number or salt grain-sized and very numerous. The fever, which may have been high during the prodromal stage, persists while the rash appears and usually decreases as it fades. Cough, facial puffiness and photophobia are also diagnostic pointers.

Rubella usually affects an older child or young adult and is typically accompanied by posterior cervical and postauricular lymph-node enlargement. The rash, which also begins on the face and spreads downwards to trunk and extremities, is composed of faint pink macules, and fades in 3 days. Constitutional symptoms are mild but joint pain may be prominent in adults.

Scarlet fever usually affects children under 10 years of age, who become acutely ill with high fever and vomiting. The throat is red and oedematous and there is characteristically a 'strawberry tongue'. The rash is lobster-red with punctate deeper red lesions (likened to small spots of red ink on red blotting paper) and appears on the second and third day behind the ears, spreading rapidly to the face, upper chest and flexor surfaces of the limbs. Purpura may develop in the skin creases. The fever persists with the rash from 2 to 5 days and is followed by desquamation in large flakes from palms and soles.

Erythema infectiosum (fifth disease) affects children between 2 and 10 years of age. It begins with a 'slapped-face' erythema on the cheeks in an otherwise well child. Over the next few days a maculopapular eruption spreads, sometimes in gyrate pattern over the limbs and trunk. The illness is due to a parvovirus and heals in 1–2 weeks, though successive bouts may occur.

Sero-conversion rash of HIV. A macular erythematous rash accompanies the seroconversion illness of primary infection with Human Immunodeficiency Virus in some 50 per cent of patients. Between 10 and 14 days after exposure, fever, systemic toxicity and lymphadenopathy may occur. From 5 to 8 days later oval macular erythematous lesions may appear on the trunk and limbs, extending beyond the usual T-shirt distribution of pityriasis rosea onto the palms and soles. The oral mucosa can be affected with superficial erosions. The whole illness most closely resembles secondary syphilis or glandular fever with rash. Lymphopenia and thrombocytopenia may occur. HIV seroconversion occurs at 4–8 weeks.

3. ERYTHEMA MULTIFORME (*SEE* P. 89)

This is a dramatic symmetrical eruption manifested by violaceous red macules and discs, 1–2 cm in diameter, the centres of which become cyanotic, forming the characteristic target (or iris) lesions (*Fig.* E.11). A blister may form in the centre. Lesions chiefly appear on extensor surfaces, particularly dorsa of hands and feet, knees and elbows. The mucous membranes are often involved, and there is accompanying fever, lymphadenopathy and leucocytosis. The severe bullous form that involves the mucous membranes is referred to as the *Stevens–Johnson syndrome*. No cause is discovered in half of the patients, but erythema multiforme may be precipitated by viruses (herpes simplex, vaccinia), bacteria (streptococcal infection), deep mycotic or protozoan infections, drugs (sulphonamides, salicylates, tetracyclines, antirheumatics), radiotherapy or collagen diseases (e.g. systemic lupus erythematosus).

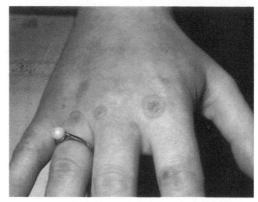

Fig. E.11. Erythema multiforme. (*Dr Richard Staughton.*)

Recurrent erythema multiforme is almost always due to recurrent herpes simplex infections.

4. ERYTHEMA NODOSUM

This is largely a condition of women between the ages of 15 and 30. Erythematous nodules begin suddenly, sometimes in crops, usually over the extensor aspects of the legs, but thighs, buttocks and extensor surfaces of the arms may be involved. Nodules are hard, deep and tender, with shiny red overlying skin. Gradually they soften and the colour changes to violet and finally yellow, but they never suppurate or ulcerate. An accompanying arthralgia is common and there may be fever and malaise whatever the underlying cause. The commonest cause in Britain, amongst women, is *sarcoidosis*, but *streptococci* are still an important cause in men.

In Irish or Asian patients *tuberculosis* should be suspected but, world-wide, *leprosy* is still the most common cause. Penicillin, sulphonamides and barbiturates are the most commonly implicated drugs. Rarer causes include ulcerative colitis, Crohn's disease, histoplasmosis, coccidioidomycosis, blastomycosis, chlamydial infections and Behçet's syndrome.

5. LUPUS ERYTHEMATOSUS

This is an important cause of erythema. It is more common in women than men and usually classified into two varieties: systemic and discoid. The systemic form affects joints, kidneys, haemopoietic, cardiovascular, respiratory and central nervous systems as well as the skin, and occurs in a younger age-group than the discoid form, which is a dermatological disorder. In the skin both types of lupus erythematosus cause perifollicular inflammation which is followed by scarring. The classic lesion of lupus erythematosus is an atrophic red scaly plaque with follicular plugging. The histopathology is characteristic showing epidermal thinning and basal cell liquefaction. Direct immunofluorescence microscopy demonstrates linear staining at the basement membrane in the lesions of both types.

Systemic lupus erythematosus (SLE) should be suspected in young women presenting with weakness, fever, weight loss, arthralgia and proteinuria, as well as a persistent erythematous rash on the face or areas exposed to sunlight. Though typical lupus erythematosus plaques may be found, particularly over the dorsa of the hands and fingers (*Fig.* E.12), they are less common than other erythematous rashes seen in SLE, such as: urticaria, urticated plaques, livedo reticularis and nailfold erythema. A diffuse telogen effluvium (*see* p. 18) is not infrequent. Established cases often have tell-tale signs on the hands; as well as nailfold erythema and telangiectasia, there may be infarcts of the cuticles, finger nodules and pulp atrophy. Between 80 and 90 per cent of such patients will have circulating antinuclear antibodies in high titre and raised DNA-binding proteins. Different varieties of antinuclear antibodies exist and relate to differing clinical presentations, a subject of current clinical research. The antinuclear antibodies can often be demonstrated throughout the skin, e.g. by taking a biopsy of non-light-exposed normal skin. This test is negative in the discoid variety. A systemic pattern, but without renal mortality, can be induced by certain drugs, e.g. hydralazine, procaine amide, griseofulvin and phenytoin.

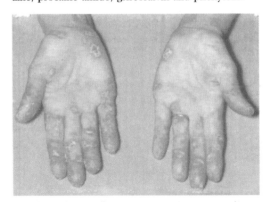

Fig. E.12. Lupus erythematosus. (*Westminster Hospital.*)

Chronic discoid lupus erythematosus (CDLE) lesions largely occur on sun-exposed sites, e.g. cheeks, forehead, nose and perioral skin, although the scalp is not infrequently affected. Lesions persist for many months extending slowly and leaving depigmented, central atrophic and hairless scars. Close examination of the erythematous active edge shows telangiectasia and follicular plugging (which can be demonstrated by detaching an adherent scale and observing downward-projecting 'tin-tack' plugs). Although the direct immunofluorescent test of such lesions will be positive, in 80 per cent of patients no circulating antinuclear anti-

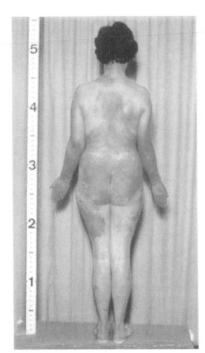

Fig. E.13. Dermatomyositis (carcinoma of breast). (*Westminster Hospital.*)

bodies are found. Less than 5 per cent of patients progress to the systemic form.

6. DERMATOMYOSITIS

The principal cutaneous signs of dermatomyositis are erythema and oedema. The proximal myopathy is described in detail elsewhere (*see* p. 346). The dermatological hallmark is a particular periorbital bluish-red oedema ('heliotrope' erythema): periungual changes identical to SLE (*see above*) may be seen, often with papules over the dorsa of the fingers (Gottron's papules). A diffuse scaling erythema of sun-exposed areas can occur, as well as psoriasiform lesions over elbows and knees (*Fig.* E.13). In common with SLE, there is histological basal cell liquefaction and follicular plugging. A patient over 40 years of age with dermatomyositis should be investigated for underlying neoplasia. Childhood dermatomyositis is almost never associated with malignancy, but can be responsible for considerable and disabling soft tissue calcification.

Richard Staughton

Euphoria

Euphoria describes an elevation of a person's mood. It is frequently the presenting symptom of manic-depressive (bipolar) illness or schizophrenia but these diagnoses should not be made before drug-induced

Table E.5. Euphoria

Common causes
Alcohol
Mania (bipolar illness)
Schizophrenia and schizoaffective illness
Cyclothymic personality
Early dementia (Alzheimer's type dementia, multi-infarct)
Frontal lobe syndrome
Frontal tumours (meningioma)
Head injury
Therapeutic drugs
    Corticosteroids
    L-dopa
    Bromocriptine
    Benzhexol
    Procyclidine
    Antidepressants (e.g. tricyclics and MAOIs)
Substance abuse:
    Amphetamines and other sympathomimetics
    Cannabis
    Cocaine
    Hallucinogens (e.g. LSD, psilocybins, mescaline)
    Phencyclidine and related compounds
    Opioids (heroin, morphine, codeine etc.)
    Inhalants (many solvents and spray can propellants)
    Sedatives, hypnotics, anxiolytics (benzodiazepines, barbiturates)

Less common causes
Temporal lobe epilepsy
Multiple sclerosis
Hyperthyroidism
Pick's disease
Neurosyphilis
Mild hypoxia (e.g. high altitudes)

---

mania and organic mood syndromes have been ruled out. The causes of euphoria are listed in (*Table* E.5). Mania is one of the commonest and most clearly identified causes of euphoria but the diagnosis is frequently missed or delayed until the patient and their family has come to harm through a combination of grandiosity and poor judgement. Diagnosis is based on the presence of either elated or irritable mood associated with some or all of the following features: overactivity; increased flow of speech; racing thoughts or flight of ideas; distractability; grandiose ideas which may be delusional; decreased sleep; increased appetite; behaviour which indicates poor judgement. The patient may become sexually disinhibited, spend too much money or drive recklessly endangering life. The mood can have the quality of infectious good humour but irritability is also common and at interview euphoria may be quickly and dramatically replaced by tearfulness, feelings of depression and remorse lasting for a few minutes before euphoria once again dominates the picture (labile mood).

In *bipolar illness* bouts of euphoria lasting more than a week or so may be preceded or followed by periods of depression. *Cyclothymia* describes a milder chronic form of bipolar illness in which the subject is prone to constant swings between mood elevation and depression with only brief stretches of normality. In such cases a moderate level of euphoria persisting for weeks or even months serves the subject well by increasing drive and enthusiasm, leading to increased sociability and greater involvement in sexual, political, religious or occupational activities. When a patient's mood is significantly elevated it can be a difficult judgement for the clinician to decide when to try to intervene. Mania sometimes presents for the first time in the puerperium and in some depressed patients it is precipitated by the use of treatments including monoamine oxidase inhibitors, tricyclic antidepressants or electroconvulsant therapy (ECT). The acute phase of a severe manic illness may be impossible to distinguish from schizophrenia and the diagnosis will only be clarified by follow-up. The relationship between manic illness and schizophrenia is controversial but there is little doubt that an episode of mania may precede or follow sometimes by several years, the development of a classically schizophrenic illness. In schizophrenia itself states of excitement with increased activity and euphoria are quite common although often there is a bizarre quality to the thoughts and incongruity of affect that distinguishes the schizophrenic states from manic illness. *Schizoaffective disorder* describes those conditions which have features both of schizophrenia and depression or mania.

Many organic conditions may present with an elevated mood resembling a manic episode and these include causes of *delirium* (*see* p. 114) where there will be impairment of consciousness. Hyperthyroidism may produce a manic syndrome, and the use of corticosteroids, L-dopa, bromocriptine, and the anticholinergic drugs procyclidine and benzhexol may cause euphoria.

Damage to the frontal lobes is sometimes associated with mild euphoria out of keeping with the patient's situation. The mood is often facile or facetious and accompanied by changes in personality including disinhibition, deteriorating social behaviour and a loss of spontaneity and volition. Slow growing frontal tumours (e.g. meningiomas), multiple sclerosis and dementia (Alzheimer's and Pick's disease) may cause a *frontal lobe syndrome*. *Temporal lobe epilepsy* may be associated with a psychosis resembling manic illness. Rarely neurosyphilis and porphyria can cause euphoric or grandiose states.

Many drugs are taken because of their ability to cause euphoria the commonest being alcohol. The list of compounds used to obtain a high include sympathomimetics (amphetamine, dextroamphetamine, methamphetamine, methylphenadate and appetite suppressants); cannabis; cocaine; hallucinogens, e.g. LSD, mescaline, magic mushrooms; inhalants including the aliphatic and aromatic hydrocarbons found in petrol, glue, paint, typewriter correction fluid; spray can propellants; anaesthetic gases, e.g. nitrous oxide and ether; short-acting vasodilators such as amyl or butyl nitrite; opioids (heroin, morphine), many compounds prescribed as analgesics, anaesthetics or cough suppressants, e.g. codeine, methadone); sedatives, hypnotics and anxiolytics, e.g. benzodiazepines and barbiturates. The diagnosis of a drug-induced euphoric state is made from the history and circumstances of the admission and by urine and blood drug screening for substances. Typically, the altered mood state is relatively brief. Diagnostic difficulties can arise in patients with a history of prolonged drug abuse, for example, with cocaine which may trigger a psychosis indistinguishable from mania or schizophrenia. The picture is further complicated because patients with manic depressive illness or schizophrenia may be heavy drinkers or drug abusers and may experience an exacerbation of their underlying condition through the drugs they are using.

D. Blackwood

Exophthalmos (or proptosis)

This may be bilateral or unilateral.

Bilateral exophthalmos

The commonest cause of this condition is *Graves' disease*, in which the exophthalmos is associated with thyroid gland swelling, with other general symptoms such as tachycardia, fine tremors and general nervousness. The degree of prominence of the eyes is variable, in some cases being so great that there is inadequate lid coverage of the cornea on attempted eye closure. A protrusion causes the upper lid to be unusually raised and the eyes look wide open, giving the patient an expression of alarm or astonishment (Stellwag's sign). When the eyes are lowered, the upper lids lag behind the downward excursion of the eye, leaving a broad portion of the sclera visible above the cornea (von Graefe's sign). The extent of exophthalmos may be asymmetrical with minimal involvement of the fellow eye. The condition sometimes appears to be unilateral. Increasing oedema of the lids along with inflammation of the conjunctiva and dilatation of the vessels over the insertion, particularly of the lateral rectus, are significant findings. The myopathy of Graves' disease most frequently involves the vertically acting muscles with limitation of upward eye movement. Other uncommon causes of bilateral exophthalmos are septic thrombosis of the cavernous sinus historically associated with skin infection at the inner angle of the eye or ethmoidal sinus suppuration,

bilateral lymphomatous deposits or pseudotumour and in children the craniodysostoses or other rare causes.

Unilateral exophthalmos

Unilateral exophthalmos may be due to:

Orbital cellulitis
Cavernous sinus thrombosis
Pseudotumour
Lymphoma
Cavernous haemangioma
Lacrimal gland tumour
Peripheral nerve tumour
Meningioma
Mucocele
Metastatic and secondary tumours

Orbital cellulitis can begin as a primary inflammatory process in front of the orbital septum, thereafter extending backwards or rising from direct orbital extension of paranasal sinus infection. The dire complication of further progression is septic cavernous sinus thrombosis. The general signs and symptoms of cavernous sinus thrombosis are more grave than in uncomplicated orbital cellulitis. Headache, nausea, vomiting and altered consciousness are early signs. Venous congestion produces gross chemosis and proptosis with a bluish discoloration of the eyelids. There is early onset of pan-ocular motor paresis. Bilateral involvement is virtually diagnostic of cavernous sinus thrombosis. Pseudotumour involvement of the orbit usually first appears above, but may also be found in the inferior retrobulbar tissues. Another involvement is at the apex of the orbit, visual loss may be of early onset. A pseudotumour along the superior orbital fissure causes a painful external ophthalmoplegia (Tolosa–Hunt syndrome).

Capillary haemangioma is the commonest cause of unilateral proptosis in childhood, the adult cavernous haemangioma causes a slowly progressive exophthalmos.

Orbital lymphomas usually occur in the anterior orbit involving the conjunctiva and lids. However posterior orbital involvement may occur and it is important to exclude a primary systemic lymphoma. Lacrimal gland tumours occur characteristically at the upper lateral portion of the orbit, causing painless downward and medial displacement of the globe and irregular enlargement of the lacrimal fossa.

Dermoid cysts specifically appear in childhood at the upper lateral quadrant of the orbit. Superior and medial swellings are more suggestive of mucocoeles of the frontal or ethmoidal sinus. Teratomas may occur congenitally or in very early life. Rhabdomyosarcoma is the commonest intraorbital malignant tumour of childhood presenting within the first decade. Development of proptosis is rapid, occurring within 1–3 weeks.

The rapidity of progression is more or less pathognomonic of this tumour.

Optic nerve gliomas usually manifest before the age of 5, resulting in a downwards nasal and forward proptosis. Meningiomas usually occur in older women, but can occur in childhood and their course is much more rapid. Ultrasound scan, CT, MRI and biopsy are all useful in assessing cases of exophthalmos.

Orbital haemorrhage may arise from trauma or sudden extreme physical effort causing bleeding from orbital varices leading to alarming, progressive orbital swelling. Arteriovenous fistula can occur following fracture of the base of the skull, with rupture of the internal carotid artery as it passes through the cavernous sinus. The caroticocavernous fistula causes a pulsatile proptosis of the eyeball associated with a bruit which is synchronous with the pulse. Gross dilatation of the conjunctival vessels is visible with arterialization of the conjunctival veins. Compression of the ipsilateral internal carotid diminishes the pulsation and audible bruit. Intermittent unilateral exophthalmos in children following coughing or crying is nearly always associated with a deep cavernous haemangioma.

S. T. D. Roxburgh

Eye, blindness of

See also VISION, DISORDERS OF

The World Health Organization defines blindness as a central visual acuity of less than 3/60 (1/20) or a visual field of less than 10 degrees. An alternative functional definition is loss of vision sufficient to prevent one from being self-supporting in an occupation, making the individual dependent on other persons, agencies and devices in order to live.

Colour blindness is a genetically determined disorder which is a minor handicap and is not true blindness.

The causes and prevalence of blindness through the world vary from country to country. It is estimated that 75 per cent of blindness in the world is avoidable.

The leading causes of blindness are trachoma, leprosy, onchocerciasis, xerophthalmia and cataract. In western countries age-related macular degeneration, diabetic retinopathy and glaucoma are the most common problems.

Different categories of the blind have different needs and the agencies for the blind access the individual blind person's requirements and provide a variety of services, including mobility training, visual magnifying aids, talking books, training of Braille, educational assessment, job rehabilitation and psychological counselling.

S. T. D. Roxburgh

Eye, inflammation of (red eye)

Inflammation of the eye may involve the conjunctiva (as a *conjunctivitis*), the cornea (*keratitis*—usually in the form of a *corneal ulcer*), and less commonly the uvea (*uveitis*) and sclera (*scleritis*). Localized patches of *episcleritis* may superficially resemble conjunctivitis, and the dusky circumcorneal congestion in an *acute glaucoma* may stimulate that from an acute anterior uveitis. The character of the inflammation varies with the type of the disease, but certain symptoms, such as *pain, photophobia* and *lacrimation*, are common to all inflammatory conditions, and are by themselves of little value in the differential diagnosis.

Conjunctivitis

In conjunctivitis the conjunctival vessels are dilated; they are freely movable over the subjacent sclera, and the conjunctival injection is most evident at a little distance from the corneal margin; the circumcorneal portion of the conjunctiva, owing to its firmer attachment to the sclera in this region, being relatively less injected. If the condition is purely conjunctival the cornea is clear and bright, the anterior chamber and iris are normal in appearance, the pupil is black with normal reactions. Purulent discharge may occur and there is often a feeling of grittiness as of sand or dust in the eye. Hyperaemia of the conjunctiva may be secondary to a foreign body on the cornea or on the conjunctiva itself, particularly underneath the upper lid.

Inturning of the eyelid (entropion) allows the eyelashes to rub against the cornea and conjunctiva (trichiasis) producing conjunctival hyperaemia and predisposing to conjunctivitis.

The use of topical drugs may produce an allergic conjunctivitis which is often associated with signs of allergy of the skin of the lids. Strong ultraviolet irradiation damages the conjunctival corneal epithelium, when using a sun-lamp or arc-welder without eye protection, producing conjunctival hyperaemia with considerable irritation or pain.

Conjunctivitis may be associated with a *mucopurulent* ocular discharge (*Fig. E.14*). The lids may be stuck together after sleep, the pain is generally slight, and allayed by closing the eyes. Mucopurulent conjunctivitis is characterized by more profuse discharge and is frequently due to infection by the staphylococcus or streptococcus and haemophilus species.

Some particular forms of conjunctivitis deserve special mention. In *ophthalmia neonatorum* (acute conjunctivitis of the newborn), caused by infection from the birth canal (chlamydia, staphylococcus or gonococcus), there is often profuse mucopurulent discharge; the condition is differentiated from imperfect

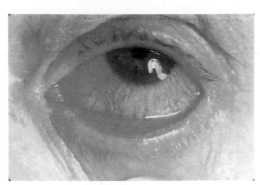

Fig. E.14. Acute conjunctivitis.

canalization of the nasolacrimal ducts by the fact that in the latter the discharge is present without the accompanying inflammation. Untreated cases are at grave risk of secondary corneal ulceration and require identification and early antibiotic therapy.

In *trachoma* (*Fig.* E.15), a chlamydial infection, endemic in the Middle East, but rate in the UK, the conjunctiva is studded with enlarged follicles, particularly on the under-surface of the upper lid and in the upper conjunctival fornix. The follicular enlargement is associated with thickening and oedema of the tissues of the upper lid causing partial ptosis, with excess lacrimation, and, in the later stages, vascular infiltrate (pannus) of the upper part of the cornea. In the later stages of trachoma the infiltration is followed by scarring which may buckle the tarsal plate, leading to cicatricial entropion and trichiasis.

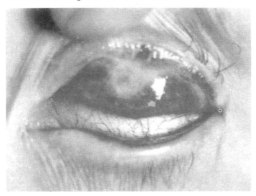

Fig. E.15. Trachomatous scarring of everted upper lid. (*Institute of Ophthalmology.*)

Conjunctival *allergies* are characterized particularly by oedema of the conjunctiva (conjunctival chemosis) and of the skin of the lids, epiphora and itch. They include non-specific responses to a wide miscellany of drugs, cosmetics and other irritants, and three specific clinical forms are recognized: (1) *Hayfever*, from exogenous pollens, etc.; (2) *Phlyctenular conjunctivitis* (due to an allergic reaction, e.g. to staphylococcus organism), featuring marked photophobia and one or

more round yellowish raised masses at the corneoscleral junction surrounded by a localized area of vascular conjunctiva. In some cases the phlycten encroach on the corneal surface, being followed by a trail or leash of conjunctival vessels; (3) *Spring catarrh*, exists in a palpebral and a bulbar form, the former showing polygonal flat-topped conjunctival nodules resembling cobblestones, the latter showing focal gelatinous limbal thickening.

Keratitis

Corneal ulcers produce greyish or white opacities of the corneal stroma with loss of the corneal epithelium. In more serious untreated cases infiltrations of the cornea may lead to loss of corneal tissue and progress to perforation of the cornea. In severe cases there may be pus in the anterior chamber—hypopyon (*see Fig.* C.39). The diagnosis presents no difficulty; the ulcers are obvious if the cornea is examined carefully, and stained with fluorescein.

Iritis

In iritis or 'anterior uveitis' the eye is congested and painful (in contrast to a 'posterior uveitis', or choroiditis, which simply blurs the vision). This vasodilatation differs from that in a conjunctivitis in that it is most evident in the circumcorneal region, with the tarsal conjunctiva remaining unaffected and that the colour of the injection is brick-red rather than pink. The cornea retains its clarity, but the aqueous may be turbid due to the presence of cells and protein, and there may be punctate deposits of leucocytes on the posterior surface of the cornea (*keratic precipitates*), or rarely a hypopyon or pus level within the anterior chamber (*see Fig.* C.39). Owing to the increased vascularity of the iris, and to the exudation into iris substance, its volume is increased and its mobility impaired; hence the pupil becomes small and sluggish. The presence of blood and exudate in the substance of the iris also changes its colour—a blue iris becomes greenish, and the fine detail of the iris structure is blurred and obliterated. Adhesions are apt to occur between the iris and the lens at the point of their immediate contact, the edge of the pupil; in the constricted state of the pupil these may not be seen, but on dilatation with cyclopentolate or atropine these adhesions or *posterior synechiae* prevent the enlargement of the pupil at certain points, and it therefore becomes irregular in shape (*Fig.* E.16). Small masses of iris pigment may also be seen on the anterior surface of the lens where the mydriatic may have broken down some of the weaker adhesions. An exudate into the pupillary aperture may form a fibrinous membrane completely or partially blocking the pupil.

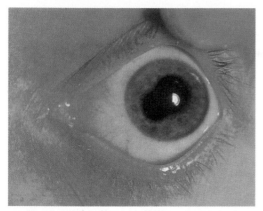

Fig. E.16. Iridocyclitis synechiae. (*Institute of Ophthalmology.*)

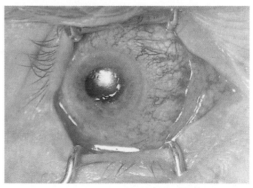

Fig. E.17. Acute glaucoma. (*Institute of Ophthalmology.*)

An important form of iritis (or, more properly, of 'uveitis', since the ciliary body and choroid are also involved), may occur in the second eye following a perforating injury in the first—'sympathetic ophthalmitis'. This possibility must always be borne in mind in cases of previous perforation of the globe, as it relentlessly leads to blindness unless suppressed by steroid treatment at an early stage.

Glaucoma

Acute angle closure glaucoma is a disease of the later years of life, and of hypermetropes rather than myopes. It is precipitated by any of the factors that may provoke dilatation of the pupil.

At first the chief complaint in subacute attacks is of temporary obscuring of vision and the appearance of haloes or rainbows around light sources; there is often a feeling of tension in the eye and a dull frontal headache in addition to the loss of vision. In acute attacks the pain is severe radiating from the eye to the head, the ears and teeth, and is associated with nausea, a symptom that *may* lead to the mistaken diagnosis of migraine. The lids may be oedematous and the conjunctiva injected (*Fig.* E.17). The cornea is hazy due to oedema, the anterior chamber shallow, the iris discolored, and the pupil mid-dilated and fixed. The eye is hard to the touch and very tender. Vision fails rapidly, even down to bare perception of light, within a few hours.

The distinction between subacute or acute glaucoma, as just described, and chronic simple glaucoma is easily made. Chronic simple glaucoma is an asymptomatic disease, and is usually discovered in the course

Table E.6.   A summary of the points of distinction between conjunctivitis, iritis and acute glaucoma and keratitis

	Conjunctivitis	Iritis	Acute glaucoma	Keratitis
Conjunctiva	Conjunctival vessels bright red and injected; movable over subjacent sclera; injection most marked away from corneoscleral margin; colour fades on pressure	Ciliary vessels injected, deep-red; most marked at corneoscleral margin; colour does not fade on pressure	Both conjunctival and ciliary vessels injected but dusky in colour	Conjunctival vessels red and injected. Injection most marked near the corneoscleral margin
Cornea	Clear, sensitive	Clear, sensitive	Steamy, hazy, insensitive	Irregular reflex, corneal opacity
Anterior chamber	Clear; normal depth	Aqueous may be turbid	Very shallow	Normal, hypopyon
Iris	Normal	Swollen, adherent to lens and muddy-coloured	Injected	Normal
Pupil	Black, active (normal)	Small and fixed, later festooned after adhesions form to lens	Mid-dilated, fixed, oval	Black active (normal)
Intraocular tension	Normal	Normal	Raised	Normal

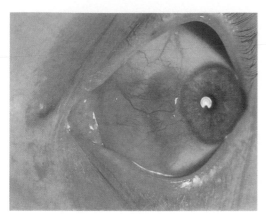

Fig. E.18. Episcleritis.

of routine examination. No pain, blurring of vision, haloes or feeling of tension are complained of; and the visual field loss which characterizes this disease is rarely noticed by the patient in the early stages.

The importance of discriminating between iritis and acute angle closure glaucoma cannot be overemphasized; the use of atropine or some similar mydriatic is a basic treatment of iritis, while in acute glaucoma it is disastrous (*Table* E.6).

Acute inflammation of the eye may be seen in *episcleritis* and *scleritis* (*Fig.* E.18). Episcleritis may be simple or nodular producing localized injection of the episcleral vessels. In either type the condition is normally idiopathic and asymptomatic with the patient merely complaining of redness of the eye. Scleritis is a more serious condition, often associated with the connective-tissue disorders. In contrast to episcleritis, the eye is painful and tender with a deep-seated bluish injection. Recurrent episodes of inflammation of the sclera may produce progressive scleral thinning. Early treatment with systemic anti-inflammatory drugs or corticosteroids is mandatory.

S. T. D. Roxburgh

Eye, pain in

Pain in the eye is not by itself pathognomonic of any particular lesion; but it may occur in a variety of circumstances, grouped as follows:

1. Pain associated with visible inflammatory changes

Due to:

Foreign body
Entropion or ingrowing lashes
Conjunctivitis
Keratitis
Iritis
Acute glaucoma

The differential diagnosis between these is discussed in the section on EYE, INFLAMMATION OF

2. Pain without visible changes in the eyeball, with loss of sight

Loss of vision in retrobulbar neuritis is usually unilateral and progresses during the first week sometimes to perception of light only.

The pain is generally referred to the back (retrobulbar) rather than to the front of the eye, and is exacerbated by ocular movement. The diagnosis is suggested if considerable loss of sight occurs in an eye, which, on examination, proves not to be affected by intraocular haemorrhage, detachment of the retina or any other visible lesion. After days or weeks, the pain may disappear and sight return to normal. On the other hand, in more severe cases, the inflammation in the optic nerve may extend forward to the back of the eyeball and become visible as a papillitis. The cause of the optic neuritis may be difficult to determine. Most commonly it is due to multiple sclerosis; often it remains obscure; sometimes it is traced successfully to some acute viral illness such as influenza.

3. Pain without inflammation and without impaired sight

An indefinite discomfort, sometimes (erroneously) labelled 'eyestrain', with a feeling of fatigue and congestion in the eyes, usually occurs in the evenings after prolonged close work which may be enhanced by difficulty in focusing (inadequate presbyopic correction), or an unclear image from incorrect glasses. If the refractive error is largely to blame, this is usually because of over-correction, as absence of glasses rarely causes eyestrain. Much more commonly the primary troubles are inadequate (or excessive) illumination, infrequent blinking, and especially a mild chronic blepharitis. The sensitivity of patients to such errors of refraction is variable, and is largely conditioned by the neurotic tendencies of the individual, for the errors to which eyestrain is attributed are usually of very small degree. It should be emphasized that myopia does not cause eyestrain, but simply a blurring of distance vision, that presbyopes normally complain of having to hold the book too far away, and that before the general availability of astigmatic lenses, a few decades ago, eyestrain was rarely mentioned—even among close workers, in poor illumination. A further occasional cause of eyestrain is an error of muscle balance, notably convergence insufficiency, which commonly responds to orthoptic exercises.

4. Pain in the eyes due to febrile or other constitutional causes

The most familiar example in this category is *influenza*. The pain is generally referred to the backs of the eyeballs rather than to the eyes themselves, but the complaint is one of pain in the eyes. The trouble occurs both at an early stage of the disease and as a sequel when the fever has subsided. The diagnosis is made from the course of the pyrexia and the general symptoms. There may be coryza as well as pain, for instance in the early stages of measles. In other conditions, such as meningitis, there is photophobia rather than pain in the eyes.

5. Pain in the eyes due to inflammation in ethmoid, sphenoid or frontal air sinuses

Sinusitis is probably the commonest cause of pain referred to the eye. It may be influenced by posture, and is commonest on waking (after prolonged recumbency).

W. M. Haining

Eyelids, disorders of

Apart from those conditions considered under EYE, INFLAMMATION OF, there are various others of which the patient may complain that deserve mention.

Blepharitis, or inflammation of the lid margin, is normally a sequel to seborrhoea with an allergic aggravation; and, if secondary infected with staphylococci, may become ulcerative. The margins are red, scales or crusts are found between the lashes, which are often small, distorted or destroyed. Entropion or trichiasis (ingrowing of the eyelashes) may result. The symptoms can normally be allayed by steroid/antibiotic applications.

External stye is a suppurative inflammation of an eyelash follicle. The condition is common and easily recognized; it is nearly always secondary to blepharitis, and is provoked by impairment of the general health.

A *Meibomian cyst or internal stye* is a similar infection of a Meibomian gland (in the posterior half of the eyelid margin). It may clear spontaneously, or the inflammatory signs and symptoms may recede, leaving a pea-sized swelling (which may also develop without antecedent inflammatory signs) called a 'chalazion'.

Entropion, or rolling inwards of the lid margin, may be *spastic* or *cicatricial*. *Trichiasis*, or rubbing of the lashes on the eye, with consequent discomfort and inflammation, is a frequent result. The opposite condition of *ectropion* may also be *spastic* or *cicatricial*, but it also occurs as a *senile* and *paralytic* phenomenon.

Symblepharon, or adhesion of the conjunctival surface of the lids to the globe, usually results from caustic burns. *Ankyloblepharon* is the term applied to adhesion of the two lids to each other, and may be due to similar causes, or may be congenital.

Xanthelasma is a slightly raised plaque, yellowish in colour, found in the skin at the inner end of either lid, often symmetrical and multiple. It may occur spontaneously or in association with hypercholesterolaemia. It should be removed if sufficiently disfiguring. A small clear cyst situated among the lashes is due to retention of secretion in a *gland of Moll*. Removal of the anterior wall results in its disappearance.

Molluscum contagiosum often occurs on the lids. The nodules are small, white, umbilicated and characterized by the ease with which contact with another portion of skin (not infrequently during removal) may allow the virus to provoke the appearance of further nodules.

Naevi or *moles* may occur on the lid, especially the margin, and involve the conjunctiva as well. They are usually pigmented. *Haemangiomata* may be similarly sited, as may *papillomata*. The commonest malignant tumour of the lid is a *basal cell carcinoma* or *rodent ulcer*. Congenital lesions of the lid already mentioned include ptosis, symblepharon, ankyloblepharon, ectropion, entropion and trichiasis. *Coloboma* occurs as a notch in the lid margin, usually towards the nasal end in the upper lid. A double row of lashes (*distichiasis*) may be found as a congenital malformation, possibly causing trichiasis. A frequent site for a *dermoid cyst* is near the outer canthus; there is often a corresponding bony defect, and the condition needs careful distinction from *meningocele* before exploration. *Epicanthus* is a disfiguring semilunar fold of skin across the inner canthus, usually disappearing as the nose develops. Though not primarily diseases of the lids, inflammatory conditions of the lacrimal gland or sac cause swelling and oedema in this region. *Dacryo-adenitis* is rare; it causes a painful swelling in the outer end of the upper lid; a similarly situated, though painless, swelling is caused by tumours of the lacrimal gland, histologically resembling the mixed parotid tumours. In *Mikulicz's disease* there is enlargement of both lacrimal and salivary glands, probably lymphomatous in nature. *Acute dacryocystitis* causes a painful red swelling at the inner end of the lower lid; it should be treated as an abscess, and no attempt made to relieve the underlying condition surgically (dacryocystrhinostomy) until the inflammation has subsided. The abscess may rupture through the skin, or require incision. It is frequently preceded by chronic dacryocystitis and EPIPHORA.

A disturbing symptom sometimes complained of, especially by elderly people, is 'flickering' of the lid—

a periodic clonic spasm of the orbicularis muscle. It may respond to general sedatives, though obstinate cases may call for blockage of the peripheral branches of the facial nerve by injecting botulinum toxin.

It is important to note that swelling and oedema of the lids, and oedema of the conjunctiva (*chemosis*) may be so intense as to suggest a far more serious state of affairs than the local inflammatory lesion which is its usual cause. Chemosis may occur from acute conjunctivitis, ocular inflammations or orbital cellulitis, obstruction to the lymph-flow from an orbital tumour may be the cause; or general disorders, such as anaemia or angioneurotic oedema.

W. M. Haining

Face, abnormalities of appearance and movement

The patient's features, expression and facial movements can in many cases suggest an instant diagnosis. While such 'spot' diagnoses may often be wildly inaccurate, in many cases they prove more telling than many investigative procedures done later to prove or disprove a diagnosis. Experience alone can teach the student to detect all that is to be learned from the patient's facies. The more subtle abnormalities of expression, the play of the emotions and the response of the features to questioning and intellectual and emotional challenge are transient and fleeting and cannot be recorded or reproduced and are sometimes so intangible as to defy any attempt to describe them. The passive vacant aspect of a chronic alcoholic, the tremor of his mouth when he opens it to protest his temperance, are clinical observations which cannot be reproduced visually, except by a television camera. The shifty eyes of the drug addict, the fatuous placidity of the patient with advanced multiple sclerosis, the anxious look of those within a few days of death, the explosive suddenness with which the victim of multiple sclerosis or brain damage bursts into laughter or tears, the vacant stare of the mentally defective child, the unsmiling sad appearance of the melancholic, the distant removed look of the schizoid personality, the excessive vivaciousness of the hypomanic—these are a few of the many familiar and striking lessons of the face which must be seen in real life if they are to be learned and utilized. It is upon the appearance of the face that people most rely for the judgement of general health and well-being, for this is the only part

of the body which everybody is habitually accustomed to see—plumpness or wasting, the complexion, the expression, the carriage of the head, the way the eyes, brows, cheeks and mouth move, for example, may all suggest certain disorders. Appearances may be deceptive however (*Fig.* F.1). Pallor is by no means the same thing as anaemia; a ruddy complexion is not necessarily a sign of rude health; it is often far from easy to distinguish the appearance of illness from the expression of unhappiness; it is all too easy to mistake for aggression what is really shyness.

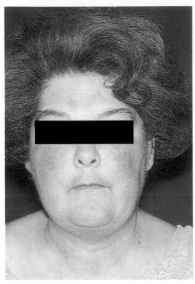

Fig. F.1. Red moon face in an anaemic woman on large doses of corticosteroids. Note the increased hair growth on the upper lip.

CRETINOID FACIES

Compared with the general stunted growth of the rest of the body the head of the child hypothyroid from birth is relatively large. The expression is dull or stolid. The face is broad, and remarkable for thick eyelids, broad flat nose, thick lips and widely spaced eyes (*Fig.* F.2). The mouth is usually open, the tongue may be more or less constantly protruded, and the chin is poorly developed. The hair is scanty and brittle, the skin coarse, dry or muddy, and often almost yellow.

MYXOEDEMATOUS FACIES

The dulled intelligence of the patient is betrayed by the apathetic physiognomy (*Fig.* F.3). The skin of the myxoedematous face is coarse, dry, sallow, pale and waxy, with occasionally a tinted rose-purple flush over each cheek. The puffiness of the eyelids may suggest acute glomerulonephritis, but the subcutaneous tissue everywhere is of firm consistence, and doughy rather than oedematous. The tongue is enlarged. The nose

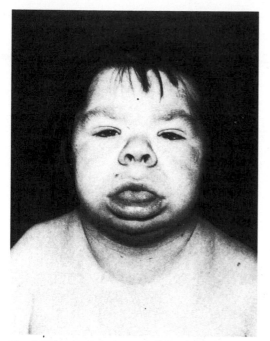

Fig. F.2. Female cretin, showing half closed eyes, thick nose, tongue and lips, fat chin and squat neck (*Dr R.G. Ollerenshaw, Manchester Royal Infirmary.*)

is broadened, the ears are thickened and the lips swollen. The hair is scanty, receding from the forehead, the eyebrows are thin and sparse (although the scantiness of the outer half often regarded as a diagnostic feature occurs too frequently in normal subjects for this to be reliable), the nails brittle and striated. Masses of fatty tissue may be found in the neck and trunk. The slow, husky speech, the expressionless face, and the general attitude of the patient may superficially suggest Parkinsonism, but the diagnosis may be made by paying attention to other clinical features. In hypopituitarism, the eyelids and nose, in contrast to myxoedema, are unaffected, and show no undue thickening. Another point of differentiation is that in pituitary disease complete loss of axillary and pubic hair is common, a feature that does not always occur in myxoedema. In hypopituitarism the face is hairless in males or females (*Fig. F.4*) and unduly wrinkled. The features are those of a middle-aged Peter (or Pauline) Pan. In contrast the patient with myxoedema looks like a wax doll who has been left in a sunlit shop window too long. In hypopituitarism the skin is soft and smooth and the hair of soft texture, whilst in myxoedema hairs and skin are of coarser quality. The voice in myxoedema is a husky croak, in hypopituitarism normal.

CONGENITAL SYPHILITIC FACIES

The victims of congenital syphilis, now an extreme rarity, after 10 or 12 years of age, may present a facies which is unmistakable—an overhanging forehead, perhaps frontal bosses, a depressed nasal bridge (*Fig.* F.5), striated scars radiating from the corners and other parts of the lips, with a sallow, earthy complexion. Closer observation of the eyes and teeth may detect the opacities of old keratitis and the changes in the upper incisors which were stated by Jonathan Hutchinson to be pathognomonic (*Fig.* F.6). These teeth are wide-gapped, irregular, and so deficient in enamel over the anterior and median parts of their cutting edges that the resulting crescentic notch imparts a striking appearance.

MYOPATHIC FACIES

Many cases of myopathy show no characteristic facies; in *facioscapulohumeral dystrophy* the face is always involved, the muscles around the mouth being affected most with a loose pout of the lips at rest and 'transverse' smile (*rire en travers*). These features are due to defective facial musculature, particularly to weakness of the orbicularis oris. Paresis of the orbiculares palpebrarum is only evident when an attempt is made to close the eyes, although it may sometimes lead to prominent and perhaps staring eyeballs. Inability of the patient to whistle or to blow out his cheek demonstrates the weakness of the orbicularis oris which is often rendered obvious by the large amount of labial mucous membrane exposed while the mouth is at rest.

In *dystrophia myotonica (myotonia atrophica, Steinert's disease)*, ptosis, facial weakness and dysarthria occur. There is a characteristic weakness and diminution in the size of the sternomastoids and the masticatory muscles are poorly developed or waste early, giving a long lean facial appearance. In males, frontal baldness is common. In the rare *ocular myopathy* there is progressive ptosis of the eyelids and immobility of the eyes.

MYASTHENIC FACIES

In patients suffering from myasthenia gravis there are two types of facies. The first is the patient whose lids lag with fatigue (*Fig.* F7). The second depends on the characteristic myasthenic smile, almost a sneer. This unfortunate and misleading facial expression is the result of deficient action on the part of the zygomatic and risorius muscles and exemplifies the curious way in which in this disease some muscles are affected and others escape, even when they derive their innervation from the same source. In patients with this disorder facial weakness is worsened by repeated movement but responds rapidly but transiently to anticholinesterase drugs such as intravenous edrophonium which acts more rapidly than neostigmine. In ocular myasthenia only the extra-ocular muscles are involved.

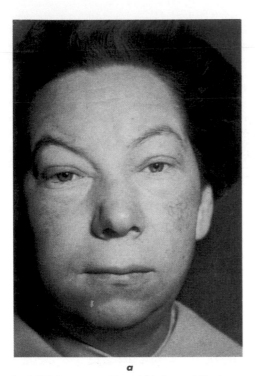 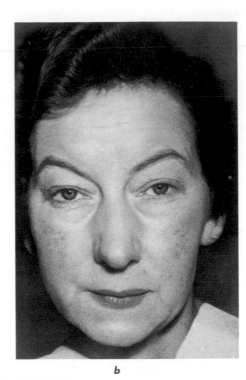

a b

Fig. F.3. Facies in myxoedema (a) before and (b) after treatment. (*Dr P. M. F. Bishop.*)

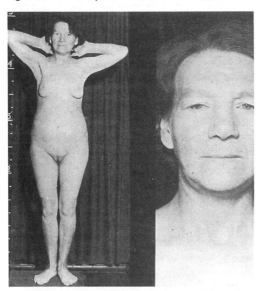

Fig. F.4. Sheehan's syndrome (hypopituitarism following hae-morrhage at childbirth) here gives a very different picture from that of primary hypothyroidism (myxoedema).

HYPERTHYROIDISM

The *facies of hyperthyroidism* depends chiefly upon the 'stare' (*see Fig.* T.8). Surprise or terror is suggested by the prominence of the eyeballs and the retraction of the eyelids. The degree of exophthalmos varies greatly and it may be completely absent; it is sometimes unilateral. The sclera is visible between the edge of the iris and the eyelids; the usual harmony of movement between the eyeball and the eyelid is lacking; normal blinking is much diminished or entirely in abeyance. The surface of the conjunctiva may be abnormally bright and glistening, and the secretion of tears may be excessive. In contrast with the white of the eyeballs, there is often considerable dark pigmentation of the eyelids which may also be the site of some oedema. The size of the pupils varies, undue dilatation occurring only in exceptional cases. The upper eyelid lags as the eye follows the examiner's finger downwards. Eye movements are often diminished in range due to intrinsic muscle weakness and the muscles of the brow are wasted, giving diminished wrinkling on raising the eyebrows (Joffroy's sign). A moist skin and a readiness to flush may often be remarked in the face.

THE FACIES OF PARKINSONISM

In this disease a cardinal symptom is muscular rigidity which affects the skeletal muscles generally as well as those of the face (*Fig.* F.8). The ocular muscles, however, escape and, as a consequence, while the face as a whole is expressionless or 'mask-like', the eyes appear to move with natural or even abnormal rapidity; for instance, they will turn in the direction to which the patient desires to look before the head has assumed a corresponding position. The face has often a staring

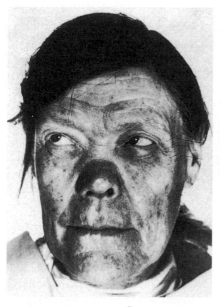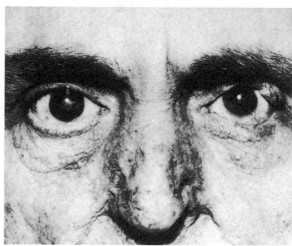

a   *b*

Fig. F.5. *a*, Congenital syphilis, showing depressed nasal bridge and rhagades (*Dr J.C. Houston*) *b*, Interstitial keratitis and nasal scarring in congenital syphilis (*Mr Rex Lawrie.*)

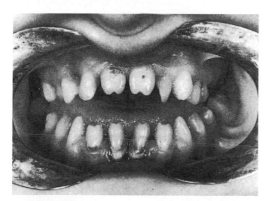

Fig. F.6. Hutchinson's teeth in congenital syphilis. Note the upper central incisors which are peg shaped and notched (*Professor W.E. Herbert.*)

expression, the eyelids being retracted by the tonic spasm of the orbiculares palpebrarum. An absence of normal blinking has been ascribed to the same cause. In contrast with the slow development of facial expression, under the influence of emotion there may be marked want of control over the fully developed emotional movement, and the patient protests that the exuberance of his laughter or tears is entirely out of proportion to his feelings of merriment or sorrow. The poverty of facial and general movement may falsely suggest a lack of intelligence and mental activity.

Parkinsonism may occur in patients who are suffering or have suffered from an attack of *encephalitis*. This syndrome, which is now very rare, may often be distinguished from primary Parkinson's disease by the presence of disturbances in pupillary and other reflexes, tics, localized spasms and the so-called 'oculogyric crises' in which the eyes are suddenly deviated upwards, downwards or sideways so that only the white of the eye is visible to the observer. These crises, highly unpleasant for the patient, usually last for several minutes and occasionally for hours. The facies of Parkinsonism may also be caused by certain drugs, which interfere with the action of dopamine within the basal ganglia; these include chlorpromazine, phenothiazines, butyrophenones and reserpine in large doses. In most cases, the abnormalities disappear after stopping the drug except for tardive dyskinesia which may become permanent. This serious variety of drug-induced extrapyramidal disease consists of involuntary 'mouthing' movements of the lips, lip-smacking and protrusion of the tongue. Neuroleptic drugs with the least anticholinergic activity, such as haloperidol, produce the larger number of cases of drug-induced Parkinsonism. Thioridazine has potent anticholinergic activity and does not have this side-effect. Less common causes of Parkinsonism include carbon monoxide and manganese poisoning.

TABETIC FACIES

In a considerable number of the few remaining cases of tabes dorsalis the appearance of the face is sufficiently striking to afford a clue to diagnosis. The small size or the inequality of the pupils reacting to accommodation but not to light (Argyll Robertson pupils) may first attract attention. The drooping of the upper eyelids,

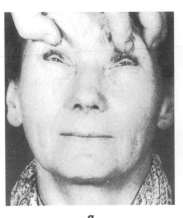
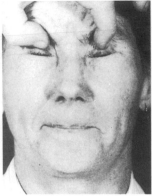
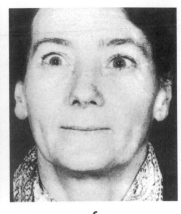

a   b   c

Fig. F.7. Myasthenia gravis showing: *a*, Inability to keep eyes closed against light traction on upper eyelid; *b*, Effective resistance after neostigmine—note the return of power to the orbicularis oris; *c*, Normal facies under the influence of neostigmine. (*Dr R.G. Ollerenshaw, Manchester Royal Infirmary.*)

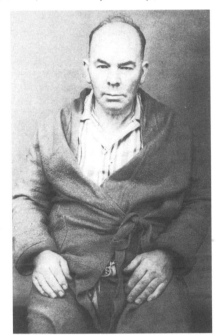

Fig. F.8. Paralysis agitans (Parkinson's disease) showing expressionless gaze and typical rigid immobility. (*Dr R.G. Ollerenshaw, Manchester Royal Infirmary.*)

combined with some wrinkling of the forehead produced by a compensating effort on the part of the frontalis muscle, imparts a sad expression. This drooping of the eyelid is not due to any paresis of the levator palpebrae superioris, as may be shown by the raising of the lid when the patient is looking upwards, but depends on the fact that this muscle, like most of the muscles of the body, is in a condition of hypotonia so that under the influence of gravity the lid hangs like a half-raised curtain in front of the eyeball. In other respects the face may be normal, but the majority of tabetics have a sallow complexion and very little subcutaneous fat, two conditions which contribute to their generally unhealthy appearance. Many victims of this disease exhibit a deficiency of the emotional reflex movements of the facial muscles; during conversation the play of the features appropriate to the subject of their talk is not so noticeable as in the case of healthy individuals.

FACIES OF ACROMEGALY (*Fig.* F.9)

In acromegaly changes in appearance frequently take place to such a degree that the patient becomes

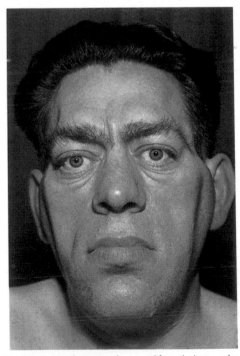

Fig. F.9. A case of acromegaly, exemplifying the heavy enlargement of the front of the lower jaw.

unrecognizable to friends, who have known him or her only before the onset of the disease. These are the result of abnormal growth of the bony and subcutaneous tissues especially in the skull and extremities. The characteristic facies is brought about by osseous hyperplasia of the frontal ridges, the mastoid, zygomatic, malar and nasal processes, while the lower jaw is usually enlarged in all directions. The prominent, arched brows, with retreating and wrinkled forehead, the massive nose, the long, thick upper lip and the heavy chin (*Fig.* F.9) form the most conspicuous features. The lower teeth are unduly wide apart and may project some distance in front of the upper. The tongue may be so enlarged as to keep the mouth open and to display many fissures and indentations as the result of its pressure against the teeth. In some cases the lower jaw is not affected, and the face may be described as abnormally square (*type carrée*).

DOWN'S SYNDROME

This facies is so distinctive that the diagnosis may usually be made at a glance. The head is brachycephalic; the palpebral fissures slant obliquely inwards and downwards towards a broad flat nose, rendered even broader by the presence of epicanthus; the eyelids show signs of chronic blepharitis; the ears are large and pitcher-shaped; the lips are fissured and often left open to allow a coarse tongue to protrude; the forehead is downy, and the hair of the scalp scanty, wiry and frequently mouse-coloured; the complexion is florid and mottled. The almond-shaped eyes, the presence of epicanthus, the florid complexion and the absence of fatty masses serve to distinguish Down's syndrome from cretinism.

THE ADENOID FACIES

This used to be described in the child sufferer with wide open mouth resulting in the oral breathing demanded by nasal obstruction, and the overslung lower jaw and dental occlusion with consequent incomplete musculature of the mouth and receding cheeks.

FACIES OF HEPATOLENTICULAR DEGENERATION (WILSON'S DISEASE)

The characteristic facies of this disease is seen only in advanced cases, and may be described as one of 'fixed emotion'. The slightest attempt to engage in conversation may evoke a sustained expression of exaggerated mirth, which is quite unlike that seen in other diseases of the nervous system. There is also a tendency to fall to one side when in the sitting position. The malady is associated with bilateral degenerative changes in the lenticular nuclei together with cirrhosis of the liver, due to the excessive amounts of copper in the tissues. The most remarkable feature of the disease is the Kayser–Fleischer ring, present in about 50 per cent of patients; this is a ring of rusty-brown pigment at the periphery of the cornea (*Fig.* F.10). Radiating brownish spokes of copper carbonate on the anterior or posterior lens capsule less often cause the characteristic 'sunflower' cataract.

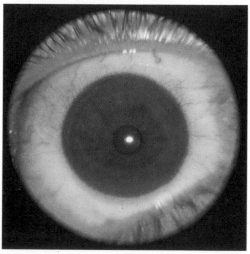

Fig. F.10. Kayser–Fleischer ring in a patient with Wilson's disease, due to deposition of copper-containing pigment in the cornea. (*Courtesy of Dr R. Guiloff.*)

FACIES OF MITRAL STENOSIS

It is occasionally possible to suspect mitral stenosis at sight, on account of the remarkable malar hyperaemia and dark-crimson lips contrasting with the yellowish pallor of the forehead, peri-oral and perinasal skin. If one covers the malar regions and the lips the face looks sallow, yet the malar flush and the dark-crimson lips give a look almost of plethora (*Fig.* F.11). When cardiac failure occurs and the liver becomes engorged, an element of icterus may be added.

FACIES OF PRIMARY POLYCYTHAEMIA

The coloration of the nose, lips, ears and palpebral conjunctiva is the chief feature of the facies in this malady, presenting an appearance which may be described as a combination of exposure to weather, of plethora and of cyanosis. The diagnosis depends on discovering pronounced polycythaemia, and generally a large, firm spleen. Polycythaemia may also be secondary to other conditions, cardiac, pulmonary or malignant disease (*Fig.* F.12).

FACIES OF CIRRHOSIS OF THE LIVER

There is nothing characteristic in the facies when cirrhosis of the liver is in an early stage. Nor can one

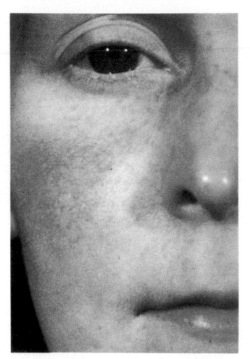

Fig. F.11. The facies in mitral stenosis, showing the malar flush (*Dr R.G. Ollerenshaw, Manchester Royal Infirmary.*)

FACIES OF ADDISONIAN PERNICIOUS ANAEMIA

Though today rarely seen, the facies in untreated Addisonian pernicious anaemia may be absolutely characteristic in the later stages. There is no emaciation, but the color is remarkable. Often described as 'lemon-yellow', it is more often a pale primrose yellow, with a peculiar delicacy in the yellowish tint that is unmistakable when it is fully developed.

FACIES OF ACUTE GLOMERULONEPHRITIS

The generally swollen half-bloated look, the partial closing up of the eyes by oedema, are usually unmistakable, but a somewhat similar appearance may be presented by the effects of insect bites, of angioneurotic oedema, or after the administration of aspirin or other drugs to which the patient is allergic. In the nephrotic syndrome, kwashiorkor and many other conditions with extensive oedema this may extend to involve the face but not usually in cardiac or starvation oedema which affects the dependent parts. In leprosy a similar puffy appearance of the face, particularly around the eyes, may be seen; a variety of skin lesions may occur with nodules, plaques and thickening of the skin. The ear lobes may enlarge and the lines of the face may coarsen and become deeper, giving the so-called 'leonine facies'. Patches of depigmentation may occur

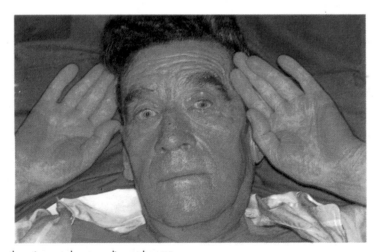

Fig. F.12. Polycythaemia secondary to malignant hepatoma.

diagnose the existence of cirrhosis with certainty even when the facies is that of chronic alcoholism, with its telangiectases over the cheeks, coarsening of the tissues, especially on and around the nose and mouth, with purplish reddening in general. But in the later stages of cirrhosis the sallow, dull, diffusely pigmented facies is often distinctive, though the actual peculiarities are not easily described.

or bronzed hyperpigmentation. Eyebrows and eyelashes may fall out and lips swell. Nasal blockage may occur and a saddle-nose deformity develop.

FACIES OF ARTHRITIS AND CONNECTIVE TISSUE DISORDERS

In *dermatomyositis* the most characteristic rash consists of a dusky red eruption on the face, over nose and cheeks, periorbital regions, occasionally on the forehead and on the neck, shoulders, front and back of the chest and on the arms. The erythema may be mottled or diffuse and either intensely red or cyanotic or a mixture of both. Sometimes on the upper eyelids a dusky lilac hue is seen, the so-called heliotrope rash said to be typical of dermatomyositis. Telangiectasia may be present as it may in systemic lupus erythematosus and scleroderma.

A common skin lesion of *lupus erythematosus* has a 'butterfly' distribution over the bridge of the nose and the cheeks (*Fig.* F.13). The facial skin lesion of *sarcoidosis* may have the same distribution but the eyelids and ears may be infiltrated with brownish nodules.

of the pigmentation only, without any suggestion at the time that there is malignant disease anywhere. It is probably an extreme degree of the liability to diffuse pigmentation of the skin that malignant disease in general tends to produce. It may precede malignant disease or follow it but usually appears at the same time. It may also occur in Cushing's syndrome, acromegaly, the Stein–Leventhal syndrome, adrenal insufficiency, pituitary or hypothalamic tumours or other lesions at the base of the brain. When associated with a malignant process these tend to be aggressive and rapidly fatal. Neither clinically nor histologically can acanthosis nigricans associated with a malignant process be differentiated from the disease without this association.

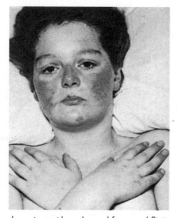 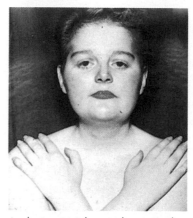

Fig. F.13. Female patient with prolonged fever and flitting joint pains due to systemic lupus erythematosus. The contrast is striking between the red butterfly rash of the disorder and the Cushingoid appearance on full steroid therapy 1 month later.

In *scleroderma* the parchment-like skin may be so tightly drawn over the underlying muscles that the face becomes completely expressionless (*Fig.* F.14) and the mouth cannot open widely.

In *giant cell (temporal) arteritis*, the inflamed temporal arteries are tender to touch and become thrombosed. Vision may be affected if the retinal arteries become involved. Tophi in the ears (*Fig.* F.15) indicate the presence of *gout*.

FACIES OF ACANTHOSIS NIGRICANS

The outstanding feature of this disease is the extreme pigmentation which develops in various parts of the body, as in the axillae, groin, nipples and umbilicus, but also in the neck or face; the degree may be described as what would, more or less, result if a collier's hands were stroked over the skin, producing massive darkening, almost blackening, in the areas affected. Although rarely generalized it is usually bilateral and symmetrical, blending into adjacent normal skin. Although the disease usually indicates abdominal carcinoma, especially carcinoma of the stomach, the patient may present himself for treatment on account

Other colorations of diagnostic significance are those of *haemochromatosis* where over 90 per cent of patients show bronzing of the skin from melanin deposition, about half having haemosiderin deposition also causing a slate-grey colour. The bluish tinge of the cartilage of the ears and sclerae in *ochronosis* appears usually between the age of 20 and 30. The cartilages of the ears may be slate-blue or grey and are often thickened and irregular. Pigmentation of the sclera is usually localized to a small area half way between the cornea and the inner or outer canthus. The skin over the malar areas and nose is often darker than usual. Other abnormal colours which may be seen in the face include the patchy pigmentation of the chloasma of pregnancy or that of vitiligo or albinism, and that resulting from prolonged administration of arsenic.

FACIES OF ADDISON'S DISEASE

Generalized darkening of the skin of the face may be the first thing to attract attention in a case of Addison's disease, but the distinctive character of the pigmentation is that it occurs in the mucous membranes within

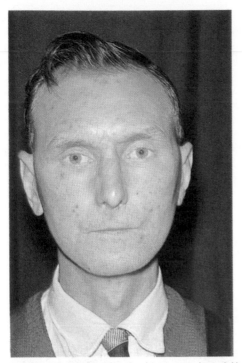

Fig. F.14. Scleroderma, showing the pigmented, mask-like smooth expressionless face.

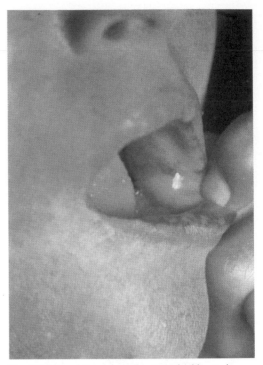

Fig. F.16. Buccal pigmentation in untreated Addison's disease. Under treatment with cortisone all pigmentation disappeared within a few weeks.

FACIES IN CUSHING'S SYNDROME

The red 'moon face' and hirsutism (q.v.) are characteristic and often seen as the result of corticosteroid therapy (*Fig.* F.17). Although the features look plethoric there is no true polycythaemia. This is one point of differentiation from the features of simple obesity, others being the presence of bruising (ecchymoses), muscle weakness, wide purple red striae (those in simple obesity being more narrow and pink) and hypertension. In Cushing's syndrome the cheeks may become so chubby that seen full-face they obscure the ears.

FACIES OF ARGYRIA

This condition is rare nowadays. It may still be met with amongst workers in silver. The coloration is even and uniform; it has a blue-grey appearance which persists when pressure is applied to the skin, and does not blanch as does a cyanotic skin. It is a subcutaneous rather than a dermal pigmentation.

The features in *pachydermoperiostosis*, a rare familial condition associated with pseudohypertrophic osteoarthropathy (with finger clubbing), are typical with thickening and furrowing of the face, with deep nasolabial folds, greasy skin of face and scalp and often excessive sweating. It appears to be transmitted by an autosomal dominant gene with variable expression.

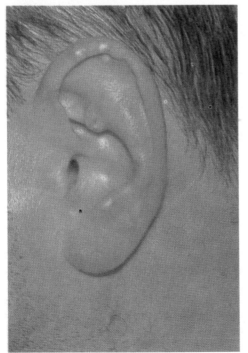

Fig. F.15. Typical tophi in the ear. They are opaque to transillumination.

the mouth (*Fig.* F.16), where it tends to be grey, as well as on the skin of the face and other parts of the body, where it is dark brown.

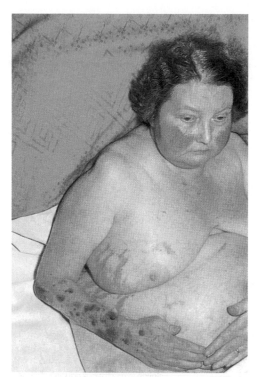

Fig. F.17. The Cushingoid picture of corticosteroid therapy. Note also the striae and subcutaneous haemorrhages.

FACIES OF ACUTE ILLNESS

Erysipelas, measles, scarlatina and mumps often permit an immediate facial diagnosis. Cellulitis, also, is self-evident (*Fig.* F.18). In lobar pneumonia the bright eyes, flushed cheeks, active alae nasi and labial herpes constitute what may fairly be termed a typical picture. Respiratory distress advertises itself by expression of anxiety and fear in pulmonary and cardiac disease, although alterations in colour due to cyanosis contribute to the appearance. Labial herpes (herpes febrilis) may also accompany many other febrile diseases, even a simple coryza, and may be due to sun sensitivity. Herpes zoster may affect the face and the periorbital region (*Fig.* F.19) and, when the nasociliary nerve is involved, lesions appear on the end of the nose and on the cornea.

ALTERATIONS IN CONTOUR

Slight facial asymmetry is very common. Marked asymmetry occurs in patients with lipodystrophy, hemiatrophy or hemihypertrophy, or congenital absence of the condyle of the mandible. Lack of teeth or bad dentures may contribute to asymmetry as may swelling of the parotid or other salivary glands or of the lymph nodes. Some rarer conditions may be mentioned as generally identifiable at sight. In osteitis deformans (Paget's disease) the face has the shape of an inverted

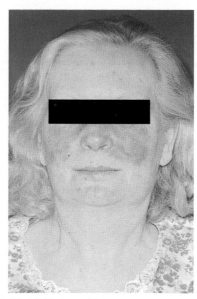

Fig. F.18. Cellulitis in an elderly woman.

triangle and, in consequence of the prominence of the forehead, appears to be toppling forwards (*Fig.* F.20). In leontiasis ossea there is progressive irregular enlargement of the bones of the cranium and face, with consequent asymmetry; the superior maxilla is particularly prominent. The rare condition of oxycephaly ('steeple head') need to be seen only once to be subsequently recognizable.

THE EYES

The eyes alone often provide diagnostic evidence of general as well as local disease. Pigmentation, oedema of the lids and exophthalmos have been mentioned. A squint may demand a detailed consideration of the central nervous system, as will spontaneous nystagmus. Icterus of the conjunctiva may be evidence of hepatic disease and the comparatively rare but striking appearance of blue sclerotics points to fragilitas ossium. 'Bags under the eyes' are generally devoid of any baleful significance but may possibly point to lack of sleep or overindulgence in alcohol.

VOLUNTARY MOVEMENTS

Weakness of the facial muscles is discussed in FACE, PARALYSIS OF.

Abnormal movement of the jaw may be due to any painful condition of the temporomandibular joint.

INVOLUNTARY MOVEMENTS

Besides the tremor of the head of old age and Parkinsonism, tremor may be due to alcohol, tobacco or other drugs. There is also a familial tremor of the hands, face and/or head affecting several members of

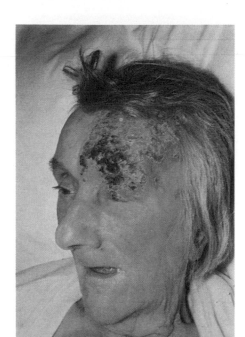

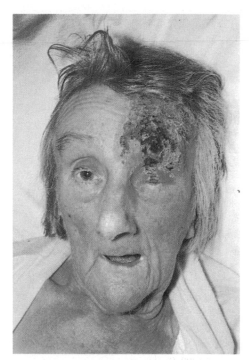

Fig. F.19. Severe herpes zoster affecting the brow and sclera. Not only may scarring interfere with vision subsequently, but at this age post-herpetic neuralgia is common, causing persistent pain in the area subsequently.

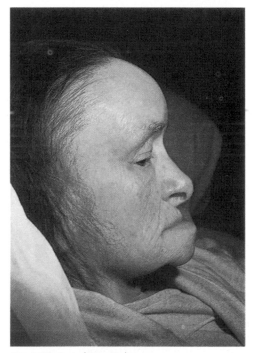

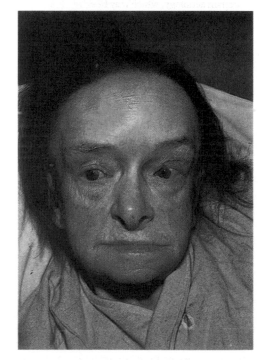

Fig. F.20. Typical Paget's disease.

the same family, usually commencing before the age of 25 years. The head-nodding of children may be mentioned in this connection. Other involuntary movements point to chorea, which may be hereditary (Huntington's), rheumatic or, rarely, senile, to habit spasms, or to tics (see p. 667). In aortic regurgitation there may be a constant jerking of the head synchronous with the heart beat (De Musset's sign). Facial paralysis and the peculiar condition of facial hemiatrophy or hemi-hypertrophy are sometimes obvious, sometimes evident only on careful examination.

EXPRESSION

The patient's expression, at interview, may give an indication of his attitude not only to his illness but also to his physician and what he expects of him or her. Differentiation of the emotional from the physical factors may be very difficult. There may be an expression of melancholy or depression, of anxiety, nervous tension, or querulousness. In some cases depression hangs over the patient like a black cloud, the face being dull, without hope for the future, expressionless, and uninterested in what is going on around.

F. Dudley Hart

Face, pain in

Pain in the face may be due to: (1) local disease of the eyes, sinuses, facial bones, nose, temporomandibular joint, teeth or tongue; (2) disease affecting the intracranial portion of the trigeminal nerve and its root; (3) tic douloureux, an easily recognized condition of uncertain aetiology, which may be more or less closely simulated by the conditions falling under (1) and (2) above; (4) migraine.

Trigeminal neuralgia

Trigeminal neuralgia (tic douloureux) is a distinct clinical entity, but its pathology is unknown in the majority of cases. Beginning usually over 50 years of age it is a paroxysmal facial pain tending in the early stages to occur in bouts lasting days or weeks. The pain then recurs and as time goes on the periods of pain become longer and the periods of remission become shorter so that eventually, although still intermittent, the pain will occur at some time on most days. The pain is intense and usually described as 'shooting' or 'stabbing' and each series of stabs lasts a few seconds or a few minutes. It usually starts in the maxillary or mandibular division, rarely in the ophthalmic division to which it may later spread, and is provoked by touching the face as in washing or blowing the nose, or by a draught or by talking or eating. The severity of the pain often causes the patient to screw up the affected side of the face, hence the name *tic douloureux*. On examination there are no abnormal signs in the nervous system but the tongue may be furred on the affected side.

The pain may be relieved in more than half the patients by carbamazepine (Tegretol), but in those in whom the treatment is ineffective and in those who relapse *tic douloureux* can be relieved by numbing the face over the area where provoking factors cause pain. This can be done most simply by alcoholic injection of the maxillary or mandibular branches and the pain will be relieved as long as sensory loss persists. Although sensation will return within a few months pain will not necessarily reappear at the same time and this treatment may well be adequate in elderly patients. Other treatments are by alcoholic injection in the Gasserian ganglion, which will permanently destroy the nerve cells, or by complete or partial section of the posterior root. With these procedures the cornea is rendered insensitive and thus becomes exposed to damage and possible ulceration so that glasses with a protective side-piece must be worn. In order to obviate this and the discomfort arising from numbness (touch loss) over the face, the procedure of medullary tractomy was devised in which the spinothalamic tract (carrying only pain and temperature fibres) is divided in the medulla. This carries, however, a certain morbidity. More recently injection around the Gasserian ganglion with phenol rather than alcohol has been tried and this certainly reduces the numbness but carries with it a higher relapse rate.

Symptomatic trigeminal neuralgia

This is the name given to pain similar to tic douloureux but caused by disease of the sinuses, teeth, temporomandibular joint and central nervous system. Although the quality and distribution of the pain may simulate the 'idiopathic' type, symptoms do not run the prolonged and intermittent course found in tic douloureux. This fact is clearly of no value in the diagnosis of a first attack, and identification of the source of the pain requires thorough clinical and radiological examination. In general, however, the evidence of disease is unequivocal in this symptomatic group, and it is a mistake to embark on extensive dental extractions or sinus operations unless the indications are clear. Active infection of the *frontal and maxillary sinuses, apical abscesses of the teeth, glaucoma* and *iritis*, and *malignant disease of the tongue* may simulate the pain of tic douloureux. The same is true of *multiple sclerosis, gummatous meningitis, neuromas* and *meningiomas* in the posterior fossa, *nasopharyngeal carcinomas, posterior fossa angioma* and *tabes* (lightning pains). The neuralgia which follows *herpes zoster* of the Gasserian ganglion in elderly subjects is unlikely to cause confusion unless the history of herpetic eruption is missed.

Periodic migrainous neuralgia

This is a particular variety of paroxysmal headache and differs from migraine in that the headaches occur in bouts and are of greater frequency and shorter duration. The headache is sharply localized to one or other supraorbital region but may spread into the temple, eye or cheek. Typically it wakens the patient from sleep every night an hour or two after he has gone to bed and it is very intense. It lasts from 30 to 90 minutes and may be accompanied by watering of the eye and blocking of the nose on that side. There may also be a partial ptosis and smaller pupil on the affected side.

Such a headache may also occur irregularly, not necessarily at night or every day but sometimes two or three times in 24 hours. A bout of such headaches usually lasts for several weeks when there is spontaneous remission. There is, however, a tendency for the headache to recur, usually after an interval of months or years, sometimes with a seasonal incidence. It is commoner in men and may occur at any time in adult life. Its cause is unknown.

Treatment is preventive by subcutaneous injections of ergotamine tartrate 0·25 or 0·5 mg or suppository containing 2 mg. If the attacks are occurring exclusively at night, this is given at bedtime. If, as usually happens, this brings freedom from attacks, the dose must be withheld every seventh night in order to see whether the bout has come to an end. If the attacks are irregular or more frequent, it will be necessary to give such medication two or three times in 24 hours in order to ensure control of the headache. At the same time the patient may benefit from regular sedation.

Frontal pain can be due to *upper cervical spondylosis* and also to *temporal arteritis*. Internal derangements of the temporomandibular joint, resulting as a rule from malocclusion of the teeth, can cause severe pain in the face and tongue on one side. The pain occurs only when the jaws are moved, as in speaking or in chewing, and its stabbing quality may lead to confusion with tic douloureux. Temporomandibular pain of this type is one of the components of *Costen's syndrome*, which includes tinnitus and Eustachian deafness in its rather confused symptomatology.

Ian Mackenzie

Face, paralysis of

Facial paralysis is seen in three clinical forms: (1) upper motor neurone paralysis, in which the lower half of the face is affected, and the upper half spared; (2) lower motor neurone paralysis, in which there is loss of movement in all the muscles on the affected side; (3) myopathy.

Upper motor neurone paralysis

This is due to a lesion of the corticopontine fibres of the pyramidal tract anywhere between the cortex and the middle of the pons. The eye can be closed and the forehead wrinkled, but the teeth cannot be bared on the affected side and there is weakness of the lips and buccinator muscles. In some cases involuntary emotional movements remain normal despite loss of purposive movements. In bilateral pyramidal lesions the upper part of the face is paralysed as well as the lower, and emotional movements are also involved. Rarely, emotional movements are lost and voluntary movements retained; this is occasionally seen in tumours or other lesions of the temporal lobe and premotor cortex.

Upper motor neurone facial paralysis occurs in many conditions—vascular accidents, neoplasms, cerebral contusion, degenerative cerebral disease and so on. It is usually associated with hemiparesis, or with weakness of the upper limb owing to the condensation of fibres which occurs in the pyramidal tract in the internal capsule and below, and in cortical and subcortical lesions it may occur independently.

Lower motor neurone paralysis

This occurs as a result of a lesion of the 7th nucleus or of the nerve itself. The upper and lower halves of the face are affected equally, and there is none of the dissociation of emotional and voluntary movements which may occur in upper motor neurone paralysis. If there is no recovery contractures may occur, the corners of the mouth being drawn to the affected side, thereby giving a false impression of weakness on the normal side. Fasciculation may be seen. Twitching movements are not uncommon in irritative lesions of the 7th nerve.

By far the most common form of peripheral facial palsy is *Bell's palsy*, which appears to be due to an inflammatory lesion in the facial canal of the temporal bone near the stylomastoid foramen. The onset is rapid, the patient often waking up in the morning to find the face paralysed on one side; in other cases the condition takes a day or two to reach its climax. There is often slight pain just below the mastoid at the onset. The eye cannot be closed and is liable to injury by dust; slight ectropion of the lower lid leads to epiphora. Taste in the anterior two-thirds of the affected side of the tongue may be perverted or lost if the disease has spread up the Fallopian canal. At a still higher level, paralysis of the nerve to the stapedius may cause hyperacusis.

Other causes of facial paralysis are less common than Bell's palsy. *Trauma* stands relatively high on the list, whether it be due to stab wounds, gunshot wounds, surgical attacks on the parotid gland and mastoid, or fracture of the petrous portion of the temporal bone. Paralysis usually occurs immediately in the fracture cases, but may appear for the first time a week or more after the injury, in which the event the prognosis for recovery is good. Among infective causes are *poliomyelitis, infectious mononucleosis, polyneuritis cranialis, polyneuritis of Guillain Barré type, gummatous or other form of meningitis* and *leprosy*. The swelling of the parotid gland which occurs in *uveoparotid polyneuritis*, a form of sarcoidosis, is often associated with a bilateral facial paralysis. *Geniculate herpes*, in which herpes of the tonsil, soft palate, auditory meatus and pinna is associated with facial paralysis, is so named from the belief that it is due to a zoster infection of the geniculate ganglion as suggested by Ramsey Hunt.

Neurofibroma of the 8th cranial nerve stretches the adjacent facial nerve and so adds facial palsy to the deafness, vertigo and tinnitus which occur early in the condition. As the tumour grows it encroaches upon the trigeminal nerve above, with loss of the corneal reflex and sensory loss in the face, and causes cerebellar symptoms by posterolateral pressure on the cerebellum. A glioma of the pons may have a somewhat similar symptomatology, but if the nucleus of the facial nerve is involved by the growth the adjacent 6th nucleus is likely to be affected too. Primary and secondary *tumours of the petrous bone* are a rare cause of facial paralysis.

Congenital bilateral facial paralysis is due to absence of the facial nerves. The upper part of the face is sometimes affected alone, or the entire face may be affected. The condition is always bilateral and is then easy to distinguish from facial palsy due to birth injury.

Diseases of muscle

Myopathy may cause facial weakness. This occurs in the heredofamilial dystrophies and myotonic dystrophy, but in these conditions the affection is not limited to the face, the weakness is bilateral, and confusion is unlikely to occur. *Myathenia gravis*, with its ptosis, diplopia, characteristic aggravation by exercise and ready response to edrophonium chloride (Tensilon), is usually easy to recognize. *Facial hemi-atrophy* may, superficially, resemble unilateral facial paralysis, but it is differentiated by the fact that the weakness is associated with an atrophy of all the tissues—skin, muscle, bone, nasal cartilage and even the eye.

Ian Mackenzie

Face, swelling of

In this article are included only swellings of the skin and subcutaneous tissues. Malignant and other diseases of the facial bones, etc., are considered under JAW, SWELLING OF; BONE, SWELLING OF and SALIVARY GLANDS, SWELLING OF. It is necessary therefore to determine the anatomical site of the lesion before considering the pathology. Swelling of the parotid gland will lie below and in front of the ear, or in the anterior prolongation of the gland, lying on the outer surface of the masseter. Swelling of the lingual gland will be seen in the floor of the mouth close to the fraenum, while lateral to this will be felt the submandibular gland, which is also palpable from outside in the submandibular fossa.

Occasionally a patient may present himself with painless symmetrical *oedema of the face*, commonly of the eyelids where the tissues are loosest. This will almost certainly be of renal origin, cardiac oedema causing oedema primarily in the dependent parts. Another form of oedema which may involve the whole face, but chiefly the eyelids and lips, is angioneurotic oedema. The recurrent attacks, each of sudden onset, the familial history, the associated symptoms of burning and irritation and the presence of similar areas of other parts of the body should clinch the diagnosis.

Swelling of the face and neck is seen in Cushing's syndrome (p. 200) whether primary or secondary to corticosteroid therapy, and when there is obstruction to the venous return to the heart from the head and neck, as is seen with mediastinal and bronchial neoplasms. In trichiniasis oedema of the eyelids is common, though more diffuse oedema of the face may occur.

A well-defined *cystic swelling* on the face is most commonly a *sebaceous cyst*, a structure freely movable on the deeper tissues but attached to skin. *Dermoid cyst* is much rarer and occurs only at lines of suture, the commonest site being above the outer canthus of the eye (*external angular dermoid*). A cyst in this situation is strongly suggestive of dermoid origin, and the diagnosis is confirmed if there is attachment to bone but not to skin, and particularly if depression of the bone has occurred, as it does in long-standing cases, the edge of the depressed area being palpable. *Meningocele* may occur occasionally as a translucent swelling at the root of the nose. It will be present at birth and will exhibit an impulse on coughing or straining. *Haemangiomas* are frequently found on the face and may appear cystic on palpation, but their dusky colour and surrounding dilated vessels will give the clue to their identity; they empty on pressure. Pigmented naevi will be recognized on sight.

Solid tumours of the face are *lipomas* and *fibromas*. The latter are fairly common and include an important variety, the neurofibromas. These tumours vary in size from being quite minute to an inch or more in diameter, and may be hard or soft. Other stigmas of von Recklinghausen's disease such as pigmentation, either diffuse or in multiple café-au-lait spots, or a profusion of soft, fleshy neurofibromas in other parts of the body, chiefly the trunk, help in the diagnosis. The condition sometimes runs in families.

Rodent ulcer is particularly common on the face and eyelids; it is the exception to find it elsewhere. It starts as a small nodule, often with a 'pearly' appearance, but soon breaks down to form the characteristic indurated ulcer with hard rolled edges (*Fig.* F.21). *Epithelioma*, with its raised everted margin and indurated base, and possibly secondary enlargement of regional nodes, is another malignant condition found on the face, particularly the lips (*Fig.* F.22). Confusion may arise in distinguishing epithelioma from the innocent condition *molluscum sebaceum*. However, molluscum runs a short course and the centre sloughs leaving an unsightly scar. Biopsy must be done early in any suspicious lesion.

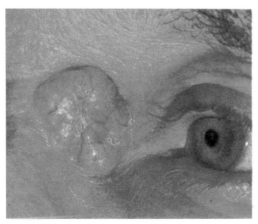

Fig. F.21. Rodent ulcer.

Various inflammatory swellings are found on the face, of which the following are some of the most important:

Boils and carbuncles are common, particularly around the lips. They have the same character as elsewhere, except that oedema is more marked.

Erysipelas is prone to occur on the face. It is marked by a vivid red oedematous swelling associated with fever. The redness tends to spread, the edges being raised and well defined from the healthy skin. The oedema may be continuous, or it may disappear in one place and reappear in another. In very severe cases the fever is high, rigors occur, the cuticle may be raised in blebs, and sloughing may ensue.

Alveolar abscess and *dental caries* are fertile sources of facial swelling, as is abscess in the nasal sinuses. (*See* JAW, SWELLING OF).

Anthrax chiefly affects operatives in wool and horse-hair factories and workers of raw hides. The

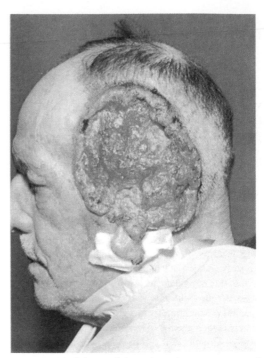

Fig. F.22. Epithelioma of the scalp and pinna (*Courtesy of the Gordon Museum, Guy's Hospital.*)

disease is characterized by the formation of a vesicle, which bursts, forms a scab, and then becomes surrounded by a ring of vesicles around which is an area of oedema. The diagnosis is confirmed by discovering anthrax bacilli in the discharge; a fluid prepared from a drop of fluid from one of the vesicles contains long chains of large, square-ended, Gram-staining bacilli, which have a characteristic growth on culture media.

Vaccinia. An accidental infection about the face may be mistaken for an anthrax pustule. If inquiry into the attendant circumstances is not sufficient to exclude the graver disorder, a bacteriological examination should be made.

Primary syphilitic sore, if found on the face, is generally situated on the upper lip, though it may also occur upon an eyelid, the nose or elsewhere. It is not so indurated as when on the glans penis, but the surrounding oedema is more marked, and the neighbouring lymphatic nodes become enlarged. The condition is often missed because it is not expected. An absolute diagnosis can be made by finding the spirochaetes in the serum discharged from the ulcer, and by serological tests, though the latter may not yet be positive if the facial chancre is of recent date.

Insect bites or stings—from mosquitoes, gnats, bees, etc.—often cause large, lumpy, irritating swellings. The only difficulty in diagnosis is when the original bite or sting has become indistinguishable owing to infection with pyogenic organisms.

The various skin diseases which may be associated with swelling of the face are considered under VESICLES.

Harold Ellis

Face, ulceration of

Most ulcers of the face have a serious cause (*see Table F.1*). If in doubt any persistent ulcer on the face should be subjected to biopsy. The more benign causes include neurotic excoriations of the face—so-called *acne excoriée des jeunes filles*—and ulceration due to accidental thermal or chemical burns. Such traumatic ulceration can, of course, be non-accidental—*dermatitis artefacta* (*see* Fig. F.23). *Anaesthetic* skin is soon traumatized and often prevented from healing by recurrent excoriation, and this can lead to extensive ulceration, as seen following surgery to the Gasserian ganglion for trigeminal neuralgia (*Fig.* F.24). Other causes of facial anaesthesia include posterior inferior cerebellar artery thrombosis and syringobulbia.

Table F.1. Causes of face ulceration

Benign
Excoriation
Trauma
Artefacta (*Fig.* F.23)
Anaesthetic areas (*Fig.* F.24)

Tumours
Basal-cell carcinoma (*Figs* F.21, F.25)
Squamous-cell carcinoma (*Fig.* F.22, see Fig. L.18)
Keratoacanthoma (*Fig.* S.31)
Malignant melanoma (*Fig.* S.27)
Lentigo maligna

Infection
Syphilitic chancre
Gumma
Yaws
Leishmaniasis
Lupus vulgaris (*Fig.* F.26)
Swimming pool granuloma (*See* p. 461)
Buruli ulcer

Other
Pyoderma gangrenosum
Cancrum oris (*Fig.* F.27)
Dental sinus (*Fig.* F.28)

Facial ulceration always raises the possibility of malignancy. Perhaps the best-known malignant ulcer on the face is the *rodent ulcer* (basal-cell carcinoma) (*Figs.* F.21, F.25) seen chiefly on exposed white skin. There is usually a background of solar skin damage (*see* p. 206). The hallmark of a rodent ulcer is its edge, which is raised and rolled with a pearly colour and crossed by multiple telangiectatic capillaries; usually there is central ulceration but some lesions remain nodular or cystic for many months before ulcerating. Rodent ulcers can be deeply pigmented making the true diagnosis less obvious, with simulation of a banal seborrhoeic wart, or malignant melanoma. *Squamous-cell carcinoma* is also common on sun-damaged skin

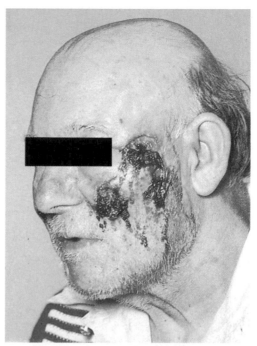

Fig. F.23. Dermatitis artefacta. (*Westminster Hospital.*)

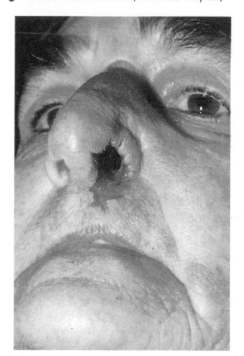

Fig. F.24. Ulceration of anaesthetic skin. (*Dr Paul August.*)

(*see Fig.* L.18), especially the lower lip, and may ulcerate. Lesions begin as firm fleshy tumours, and grow slowly and asymmetrically. A *keratoacanthoma* is also a fleshy papular tumour on sun-damaged skin, but the lesion is too symmetrical and grows too rapidly

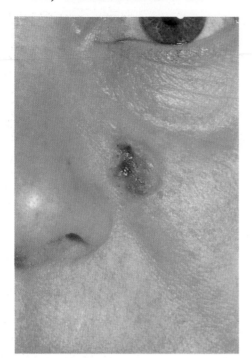

Fig. F.25. Basal-cell carcinoma. (*Westminster Hospital.*)

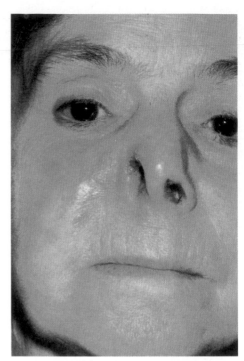

Fig. F.26. Lupus vulgaris. (*Westminster Hospital.*)

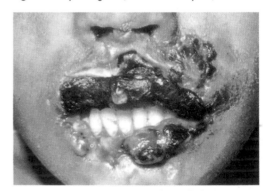

Fig. F.27. Cancrum oris. Herpes simplex in a leukaemic patient. (*Dr Richard Staughton.*)

to be a malignancy. There is a central keratin plug which may extrude, the whole lesion then having an ulcerated appearance. If not surgically removed, such lesions involve spontaneously within 3 months, leaving depressed scars. Ulcerating *malignant melanoma*, both melanotic and amelanotic, are also seen on the face. *Lentigo maligna* (Hutchinson's freckle) is an indolent black patch on elderly exposed skin. Pigmentation within the patch is variegate and histology shows stage I malignant change of melanocytes. Later fleshy pink nodules and/or ulceration indicate change to a more aggressive and vertical growth phase; despite this, lethal distant spread is unusual.

Infectious causes of facial ulceration are also usually serious. A primary *syphilitic* chancre may occur anywhere on the face, but especially on the lips. It develops rapidly from a small nodule to an indurated, painless ulcer with associated marked lymphadenopathy. Its rapid growth should distinguish it from neoplasms, save keratoacanthoma, and *Treponema pallidum* can be found in large numbers on dark field examination of the serous exudate. Serological tests will be positive 10–14 days from the onset of the chancre. A tertiary *syphilitic gumma* tends to ulcerate rapidly, extending at the margins, healing centrally. A primary *yaws* ulcer is rare on the face; in the secondary phase there are exudative nodules around the mouth, but tertiary gummatous ulcers can cause facial ulcers as well as destruction of the nasal septum or palate, as seen in syphilis. Cutaneous *leishmaniasis* may also

cause a facial ulcer. The lesion begins at the site of a sand fly (phlebotomus) bite, usually on a visit to South America or the Mediterranean littoral. Within a few weeks a livid papule develops and grows to 1–2 cm in size before ulcerating. The smear at this stage will be positive for Leishman–Donovan bodies. Untreated most such ulcers heal with scaring in 12–18 months. In *lupus vulgaris*, which is now very rare, the ulceration is chronic. It begins with deep-seated nodules, which after a time break down to form a granulomatous ulcer, covered with crusts. Around the edge the characteristic 'apple-jelly' nodules may be seen. Necrosis of cartilage of the nose and pinna is not uncommon (*Fig. F.26*), but bone is never attacked (in contrast to syphilis and malignancy). Lupus vulgaris usually begins in child-

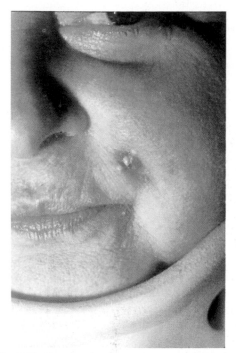

Fig. F.28. Ulcerating dental sinu:. (*Westminster Hospital.*)

hood. Other mycobacteria can produce granulomatous ulcers on the face, e.g. *swimming pool granuloma* and *Buruli ulcer* e.q.: in Uganda (*Mycobacterium ulcerans*). Rare causes of facial ulceration include *pyoderma gangrenosum, cancrum oris* (*see Fig.* F.27) and *ulcerating dental sinus* (*Fig.* F.28).

Richard Staughton

Factitious disorders

Factitious or artefactual disorders are conditions in which *illnesses are simulated or induced*, with *deliberate deceit* but with no *obvious motive or goal*. Their prevalence is uncertain but likely to be seriously underestimated as recognition is difficult unless the presentation is characteristic, persistent, repeated or closely observed—and suspected.

Broadly there are three types of presentation: (1) the fabrication of symptoms or signs of illness; (2) self-inflicted injuries to induce or simulate illness; and (3) the aggravation or elaboration of established disease.

Any physical or psychiatric condition can be feigned, even cases of artefactual AIDS were reported within a year or two of its emergence. There seems to be no limitation to the ingenuity or self-inflicted suffering of some patients, and particularly among people with a medical background or training, the application of drugs, medical equipment or pathology samples to devise illness can be scarcely credible.

The first and greatest problem facing the doctor

is to recognize that the presentation is not a bona fide illness. There are usually clues in the history which may be dramatic but is more frequently vague, inconsistent and 'hollow', while pressing for better information can provoke resentment or anger. Detailed medical knowledge or excessive interest in the investigations or treatment may be evident. The rapid development of 'complications' or fresh, unrelated symptoms as the investigations undertaken begin to report negative results is most characteristic.

There are few readily identifiable presentations but dermatitis artefacta is both common and may have a classically geometrical pattern to the lesions with sharply demarcated edges; the surgical wound or ulcer that repeatedly breaks down is another suspicious scenario, with tampering sometimes apparent. Fever is frequently simulated usually by interference with the thermometer, but has been induced by injecting pyrogenic material. Bleeding from any orifice can be especially dramatic although sometimes identifiable as self-inflicted upon careful examination—surreptitious anticoagulant ingestion or the addition of blood to samples can prove harder to identify, while occasionally the patient may induce anaemia before presenting. Gastrointestinal and endocrine disturbances are well documented, often involving drugs. Psychosis, bereavement and parasuicide are commonly feigned psychological presentations.

The diagnosis becomes even more difficult when the factitious behaviour is superimposed upon a genuine illness or abnormal test result, such as chest pain in the setting of ECG evidence of an old infarct, or when the patient accepts treatment knowing he should not have the treatment, such as with an established anaphylactic response to penicillin.

Finally manufacturing factitious disorders in others is a rare but recognized phenomenon occurring very occasionally with health staff fabricating abnormalities in patients and more often in parents inducing or simulating illness in their child or children. This form of the disorder, *Munchausen's syndrome by proxy*, is associated with factitious illness or somatization disorder in the mother and differs from typical child abuse in that the parents usually make no attempt to disguise their children's disorders nor give patently inadequate explanations: thus the spectre of non-accidental injury is rarely raised first by the parents' behaviour and attitudes. When a factitious condition is uncovered in an adult it is always worthwhile reviewing the medical histories of any children (*Table* F.2).

The differential diagnosis of factitious disorder is relatively straightforward compared with the problems usually encountered in establishing the nature of the

Table F.2. Differential diagnosis of factitious disorder

	Behaviour is evident and admitted	Behaviour is under voluntary control	Behaviour is directed towards an obvious goal
Factitious disorder	No	Yes	No
Deliberate self-harm	Usually	Yes	Sometimes
Hysteria	No	No	Yes
Malingering	No	Yes	Yes

condition (*Table* F.3). *Deliberate self-harm/parasuicide* is also self-injurious behaviour but is overt and does not entail deception in the sense of intentionally mimicking other diseases. *Hysteria* involves functional complaints and signs but these are not under conscious control and have identifiable gain. *Malingering* is self-induced and consciously operated—but is directed towards an understandable goal which, once achieved, ends the behaviour. In effect a factitious disorder is malingering without a sensible purpose: the presentation resolves nothing.

Table F.3. Causes of factitious disorder

Commonest
Personality disorder
  Antisocial
  Inadequate/dependent
Adjustment reaction to illness
Stress reaction

Less common
Depression
Anxiety
Mental impairment
Brain damage

Rare
Schizophrenia
Schizoaffective disorder
Anorexia nervosa

The classical presentation of factitious disorder is *Munchausen's syndrome*. Typically the patient is a young or middle-aged male, has repeated presentations and must wander. Their bizarre and multiple presentations, disruptive demanding behaviour, maladjusted unstable background and rootless existence are all hallmarks of severe personality disorder. It is because they are caricatures of the disorder that they are readily recognized and their importance, numerically and in the literature, has undoubtedly become exaggerated.

In fact the patient with factitious disorder is more likely to be female than male, to be undramatic, not to be admitted to hospital and to behave in a compliant manner. She tends to be a young adult, socially conforming, in employment and with an apparently stable family background. Pre-existing disease, ready access to drugs, medical knowledge gained from training or working in health care or having a close relative in the health profession are all surprisingly common. The personality is characterized as passive, dependent,

sensitive, introverted, obsessional, immature and with low self-esteem; sexual difficulties are common.

The condition sometimes represents a means of coping with an illness, a stress or relationship problem in an individual who cannot articulate or assert, or be the expression of an underlying depressive illness. In acute cases the outcome is favourable given appropriate management of the presentation and resolution of the primary problem. For those patients in whom the behaviour is repeated and arises in a more fundamental disorder of personality, themes of masochism and self-destruction figure persistently and prominently, self-injury is compelling and suicide or assisted death a not uncommon outcome.

Finally the doctor who establishes his patient is simulating illness is invariably faced with a key question—to confront or not to confront? The answer is almost always *to confront* but to approach the denouement gently, dispassionately, gradually and as part of a management plan, not in a hot-tempered accusatory way. When confronted, the Munchausen will get up, go and materialize elsewhere; but the remainder, the majority, will usually either respond positively to the suggestion of psychological help or will desist from their behaviour even if hotly denying the problem was self-induced. It helps if this is carried out by the physician who assessed the patient and has made the diagnosis after careful evaluation: the psychiatrist is also freed from implication in the detection process and can be seen as a helper after the event. Revealment can come as considerable relief for some patients who dislike their dishonesty as much as their doctor does, but not matter how skilfully and sensitively handled, these cases seldom prove satisfying and very rarely conclude with the doctor–patient relationship unscathed.

George Masterton

Faeces, abnormal consistency and shape

Sometimes abnormal consistency and unusual shape of stools may give some indication as to the underlying diagnosis.

Large bulky stools are characteristic of malabsorption and steatorrhoea. Classically the stools are pale brown, yellow or white. Small hard stools may be associated with motility problems secondary to tumours in the colon or irritable bowel syndrome. Narrow ribbon-shaped stools may indicate the presence of anal stenosis. This condition, usually in children, is associated with straining at defaecation and may lead to the development of fulminating enterocolitis.

Watery stools containing large quantities of fluid may be a feature of acute exacerbations of inflammatory bowel disease, especially Crohn's disease, or coeliac disease. They may also be characteristic of cholerheic diarrhoea associated with bile acid malabsorption and increased faecal excretion of bile acids leading to a secretory state with excess amount of water and electrolytes in the faeces. Cholerheic diarrhoea may occur in severe ileo-caecal Crohn's disease or after resection of the terminal ileum for Crohn's disease or caecal tumour. Watery diarrhoea of similar type is also a characteristic of severe infection such as cholera and more common infections such as dysentery.

R. I. Russell

Faeces, abnormal contents

Abnormal contents of faeces include blood, mucus, pus, bacteria and viruses and worms.

Blood

Red blood in the stools suggests a bleeding lesion at or near the anal margin but the source may be anywhere in the colon. This may be due to ulcerative colitis or, more rarely, Crohn's disease, haemorrhoids, fissures, tumours (benign or malignant), dysenteric infections, diverticular disease of the colon, or angiodysplasia of the colon. Patients with bleeding haemorrhoids usually complain of the passage of blood following defaecation. Bleeding anal fissures are intensely painful. Intussusception is classically associated with red-current stools due to engorgement and ischaemia of the bowel; pain and abdominal distension are usually also present.

Melaena stools are black in colour, containing altered blood which is due to bleeding from a lesion in the upper gastrointestinal tract proximal to the ileocaecal junction such as gastric or duodenal ulcer or tumour or a small bowel lesion (*see* MELAENA). Rarely a lesion in the low ascending colon may manifest as melaena.

Investigations into the presence of blood in the stools include digital rectal examination, sigmoidoscopy, colonoscopy and radiology (plain X-ray of abdomen and barium enema contrast examination).

Mucus

The presence of mucus in the stool may indicate an inflammatory process and is characteristic of acute exacerbations of ulcerative colitis, sometimes Crohn's disease, or infective lesions. This is particularly so if blood and pus are present. However, mucus may be a normal constituent of the stool without indicating any disease process. Patients occasionally mistake mucus strands for worms. Mucus with or without altered bowel habit may occur in the irritable bowel syndrome.

Bacteria and viruses

Infection with bacteria or viruses generally leads to diarrhoea, often with watery stools. Bacterial infections range widely from common pathogenic organisms, dysentery, pseudomembranous colitis and other infections due to a wide range of viruses associated, particularly in children, with watery diarrhoea. These include rotaviruses, enteroviruses, reoviruses, adenoviruses, Norwalk, astrovirus, coronoviruses and others.

Bacteria can generally be isolated from stool culture but viruses are rarely grown. They may be identified by electronmicroscopy.

Worms

Occasionally worms may be found in faeces.

TAPEWORMS

A common indication of tapeworm infestation is the passage per rectum of detached segments in either long or short tape-like strips. Close examination reveals the regular segmentation of a tapeworm and examination with a lens reveals the glandular structure of the uterus in tapeworm segments.

Patients may be symptomless or may complain of abdominal discomfort or diarrhoea; anaemia and eosinophilia may be present. The four forms of tapeworm which occur in the human intestine are *Taenia solium* (pork tapeworm), *T. saginata* (beef tapeworm), *Hymenolepis nana* (dwarf tapeworm) and *Diphyllobothrium latum* (fish tapeworm). *T. saginata* is the commonest tapeworm found in Britain. Microscopic examination of the faeces will show the characteristic eggs. Identification of the species is generally possible by the gravid proglottides. Tapeworms may also be seen on a straight X-ray film of the abdomen, or occasionally on barium meal examination.

ROUNDWORMS

The only roundworm which infests man in Britain is *Ascaris lumbricoides*. Symptoms of intestinal colic or biliary obstruction, particularly in children, may occur together with pneumonitis, urticaria and eosinophilia. There may be no symptoms until a worm is found in the stool; typical ova may be discovered in faeces. They are of relatively large size and of oval shape.

THREADWORMS

Oxyuris vermicularis, if present, generally occurs in large numbers. They can be detected by naked eye examination of the faeces. Each parasite is 3–10 mm in length and is colourless. They may be associated with frequency of micturition, pruritus ani, irritability and restlessness.

Other worm infections include hookworm (*Ankylostoma duodenale* and *Necator americanus*). The ova are oval with a clear transparent shell detected on a direct faecal film or a slide mounted in saline or iodine solution, commonly associated with iron deficiency anaemia. *Trichuris trichuria* (whipworm) is very common worldwide and presents with nocturnal pruritus ani. The worm is visible to the naked eye in the stool or perianal area.

Pus

The presence of pus in the stools indicates an infective lesion such as an abscess most commonly at or near the anal margin or in the distal colon. It may also be associated with conditions such as Crohn's disease, ulcerative colitis, tumours, diverticular disease, fistula or appendicular abscess.

The diagnosis may be made by digital rectal examination, contrast radiology or isotope scanning. Pus in the stools in large quantities indicates the rupture of an abscess into the gastrointestinal tract. The less the pus is mixed with other intestinal contents, the nearer to the anus is the site of rupture. A complete clinical history is essential and a vaginal examination may be required. Other abscesses leading to pus in the stools include pericolic, pelvic, prostatic, perirectal and pyosalpinx.

Microscopical amounts of pus in the stools may be due to any of the above lesions but is most commonly associated with ulcerative colitis, Crohn's disease, dysenteric infections, cholera, dengue fever, tumours, tuberculosis, typhoidal or venereal ulceration of the bowel.

Pus cells are generally identified under the microscope; digital rectal examination, sigmoidoscopy, barium enema, X-ray and isotope scanning using labelled white cells may be helpful in making the diagnosis.

Undigested food

The presence of undigested foodstuff in the faeces suggests a malabsorption/maldigestion problem such as severe coeliac disease, Crohn's disease or more likely pancreatic insufficiency. Tests of small intestinal and pancreatic function will provide the diagnosis.

Another cause is an intestinal fistula between stomach and colon or distal small bowel.

R. I. Russell

Faeces, colour

Change in colour of the faeces can sometimes be helpful in suggesting a diagnosis. However, severe changes generally require to be present before significant alterations in colour of the faeces are present.

Yellow or white stools

The presence of excess amounts of fat in the faeces characteristically gives yellow or white stools, known as steatorrhoea. It is associated with maldigestion and/or malabsorption states, but is most marked when maldigestion is present. It may be found in chronic pancreatic insufficiency, cystic fibrosis, pancreatic tumours or postgastrectomy conditions; it occurs more rarely in malabsorption states such as coeliac disease, tropical malabsorption, Crohn's disease, intestinal lymphangiectasia, bacterial overgrowth, ischaemia, chronic liver disease, endocrine abnormalities, lymphoma and Whipple's disease.

The presence of steatorrhoea can be confirmed by collecting stools over 3 or 5 days and measuring the amount of fat present together with the daily weight of stools. Steatorrhoea is defined as a fat content greater than 20 mmol per day. Daily weight of stools should be not more than 200 g and is often increased in the presence of steatorrhoea.

The range of causes of maldigestion and malabsorption should be systematically considered in the patient found to have steatorrhoea (*Table* F.4).

Clear-coloured stools

Clear-coloured or pure white stools are a characteristic feature of biliary obstruction or biliary atresia. In the newborn this is generally regarded as an inflammatory process, a progressively sclerosing cholangitis affecting both the extrahepatic and intrahepatic biliary tree. It may be of viral origin in some cases, and the progression from hepatitis to ductal hypoplasia or obliteration being observed. It may also be a congenital abnormality in some infants.

It is associated with liver damage and the clinical features are persistent jaundice, hepatomegaly and clear-coloured faeces. The diagnosis can be suggested by ultrasound or sometimes percutaneous liver biopsy although laparotomy may often be required in infants. Complete obstruction in the adult extrahepatic biliary tree may occur: bile duct or pancreatic cancers, sclerosing cholangitis, gallstones, following surgical trauma or occlusion due to round worms.

Table F.4. The causes of maldigestion and malabsorption

Gastric
Resection
Gastroenterostomy
Vagotomy
Gastrinoma

Pancreatic
Cancer
Chronic pancreatitis
Resection
Cystic fibrosis
Hypoplasia (Schwachman's syndrome)
Congenital enzyme defects

Hepatic
Cholestatic liver disease
　Drugs
　Primary biliary cirrhosis
　Viral
　Pregnancy
　Alcohol
　Biliary tract obstruction

Small intestinal causes
Infections and infestations
Resection
Bacterial overgrowth
Coeliac disease
Tropical sprue
Crohn's disease
Eosinophilic enteritis
Whipple's disease
Vasculitis
Vascular insufficiency
Lymphoma
Lymphangiectasia
Abetalipoproteinaemia
Drugs
Systemic sclerosis
Visceral myopathy
Autonomic neuropathy
Ulcerative ileojejunitis
Immunodeficiency
Graft versus host disease

Red or reddish-brown or deep brown stools

Red stools may indicate the presence of blood and suggest a bleeding lesion fairly near the anal margin. This may be due to ulcerative colitis, or, more rarely, Crohn's disease (in which there is rectal bleeding, diarrhoea, mucus and abdominal pain), fissure haemorrhoids, tumours (benign or malignant), dysenteric infections, angiodysplasia of the colon or diverticulitis.

Investigations include digital rectal examination, stool culture, sigmoidoscopy and radiology if necessary.

Red-current stools are a classical feature of intussusception, commonly in infants. The engorged and ischaemic intussusception bleeds, resulting in red-current stools; pain and distension are also present. Occasionally the intussusception is palpable per rectum. Straight X-ray of the abdomen or contrast radiology may be helpful in confirming the diagnosis.

Deep-brown stools may also occur due to excess urobilinogen associated with haemolytic jaundice. Urobilinogen can be measured in stools to confirm its presence.

Dark red or reddish-brown faeces may be a feature of porphyria. It may also be associated with deep-red or reddish-brown colour in the urine. The presence of porphyrins and porphobilinogen are tested for by taking a small piece of faeces which is shaken hard in 2 ml of solvent. A red fluorescence under an ultraviolet light confined to the upper (solvent) layer suggests the presence of porphyrins in urine or in faeces chlorophyll. Further extraction of the fluorescing solvent layer from faeces with 1·5 N HCl will remove porphyrins but not chlorophyll. Ingestion of large quantities of beetroot colour the stools red; large amounts of liquorice turn the stools a reddish-black colour.

R. I. Russell

Faeces, incontinence of

The individual affected by the inadvertent voiding of rectal contents per anum exists in a state of social alienation and professional isolation. Contrary to popular belief, of those who seek treatment, the disorder is most frequently seen in women of middle age. The overall estimated community prevalence for women is 1·7 per 1000 aged 15–64 and 13·3 per 1000 aged 65 or more. The latter figures suggest that many elderly patients are failing to attend for treatment, partly because of embarrassment and partly because many medical practitioners mistakenly adopt a defeatist attitude to functional problems in this age group.

Anorectal control is maintained under normal conditions by a combination of several factors the most important of which include: (*a*) the internal anal sphincter; (*b*) the external anal sphincter; (*c*) the puborectalis muscle; and (*d*) anorectal sensation. The role of the internal anal sphincter appears to be largely one of support providing a 'fine-tuning' mechanism. Weakness of this muscle (e.g. following manual dilation of the anus or sphincterotomy) leads to incontinence of flatus and soiling in the presence of diarrhoea but not to major functional disturbance. The external anal sphincter can contract vigorously for approximately 60 seconds before fatiguing. This is probably a mechanism to prevent soiling (for a short period) should the anal sphincters become 'threatened' by the presence of loose stool in the rectum. A major contribution to anorectal control is provided by the contraction of the puborectalis muscle which creates an angle between the lower rectum and upper anal canal (the anorectal angle). Sharp angulation permits a flap-valve mechanism to operate such that increases in intra-abdominal pressure cause the anterior rectal wall to close over the top of the anal canal excluding it from rectal contents. The sensation of a full rectum is probably caused by tension on pressure receptors situated in the pelvic floor rather than within the rectum itself. The discrimination of the nature of rectal contents is achieved by a simple locally mediated reflex whereby rectal distension (from flatus or faeces) initiates internal anal sphincter relaxation. A sample of rectal contents thereby intrudes into the anal canal and makes contact with the sensory rich anoderm at the dentate line where it is perceived.

Table F.5. Classification of the causes of faecal incontinence

Normal sphincters and pelvic floor
Faecal impaction
Causes of diarrhoea (e.g. infection, inflammatory
  bowel disease)
Faecal fistula/colostomy

Abnormal sphincters and/or pelvic floor

Minor incontinence
Internal sphincter deficiency
  Previous surgery (e.g. anal dilatation,
    sphincterotomy)
  Rectal prolapse
  Third degree haemorrhoids
  Idiopathic
Minor denervation of external sphincter and pelvic floor

Major incontinence
Congenital anomalies of the anorectum
Trauma
  Iatrogenic
  Obstetric
  Fractures of the pelvis
  Impalement
Denervation
  Obstetric
  Rectal prolapse
  Peripheral neuropathy (e.g. diabetes mellitus)
  Cauda equina lesion (tumour or trauma)
  Tabes dorsalis
  Lumbar meningomyelocoele (spina bifida)
Upper motor neurone lesion
  Cerebral
    Multiple stroke
    Metastases and other tumours
    Trauma
    Dementia and other degenerative disorders
  Spinal
    Multiple sclerosis
    Metastases and other tumours
    Degenerative diseases (e.g. B_{12} deficiency)
Rectal carcinoma
Anorectal infection (e.g. lymphogranuloma)
Drug intoxication (particularly in the elderly)

A complete classification of the causes of faecal incontinence is provided in *Table* F.5. At the outset it is of importance to establish the degree of disability since clearly the management of the patient with partial soiling secondary to a prolapsed haemorrhoid will differ from that in a patient with frequent and incapacitating incontinence of formed stool. In all patients a full clinical examination with special reference to the anorectum should be carried out. Digital examination

of the anorectum will provide a subjective assessment of anorectal function which ought to be supported, wherever possible: by (*a*) proctography; (*b*) anal canal manometry; and (*c*) electromyography of the external anal sphincter and puborectalis muscles.

Faecal incontinence in the presence of normal anal sphincters and pelvic floor

It is important to stress that the symptom of faecal incontinence need not necessarily imply deficiency of the anal sphincters or pelvic floor. Hence, any patient experiencing severe diarrhoea will frequently develop soiling of varying degree. The commonest cause of faecal incontinence therefore is probably *gastroenteritis*. Patients with severe *inflammatory bowel disease* frequently state that the urgency and frank faecal incontinence is the most distressing aspect of the disease and this, rather than the bleeding, may militate towards a surgical approach to management. Elderly patients and those who have *depressed cortical awareness* of rectal filling (e.g. following CVA or spinal cord section) may develop faecal impaction. Incontinence in these patients probably results from overactivation of a visceral reflex whereby the internal sphincter relaxes in response to rectal distension. A wide open internal sphincter then permits the leakage of stool of looser consistency.

Minor faecal incontinence

This is defined as the inadvertent loss of flatus or liquid stool per anum and is usually the consequence of a weak internal anal sphincter. This situation may arise secondary to some *surgical procedures* (e.g. manual dilatation of the anus) or be caused by a stretch effect in patients with a full thickness *rectal prolapse* or with third degree *haemorrhoids*. In some patients internal sphincter dysfunction is observed *without any underlying cause* apparent; in these patients there may be disease affecting the autonomic supply to this muscle. Finally, minor degrees of incontinence may result from *denervation* and other *injuries* affecting the external anal sphincter and pelvic floor; these are discussed below.

Major faecal incontinence

This is defined as the inadvertent and frequent loss of fully formed stool per anum and, as such, represents the most severe degree of functional impairment of the anorectum. *Congenital abnormalities* of the lower gut may be associated with anorectal incontinence particularly in some forms of rectal atresia where there has been total failure of development of the pelvic floor musculature. *Traumatic damage* may be inflicted on the external sphincter during vaginal delivery in which case the damage sustained is usually confined to the anterior section of the sphincter (third degree perineal tear) or by the surgeon during treatment of anal fistula when perhaps the puborectalis muscle or too much external sphincter muscle has been inappropriately divided. The pelvic floor can be damaged by 'shearing' forces when there has been complete disruption of the bony pelvis following compression injury to the pelvis. Rarely, impalement injuries to the anal sphincters and pelvic floor can lead to severe functional loss.

The greatest number of patients presenting for treatment of major faecal incontinence are found to have *denervation of the striated component of the anal sphincter musculature*. The source of nerve damage seems to be local (i.e. pudendal) in the majority and a major factor would appear to be traumatic childbirth where the nerves are subjected to undue compression and stretching forces. Damage may also be sustained in patients who strain excessively with defaecation and less commonly in patients with peripheral neuropathies, particularly diabetes mellitus. Finally, very rarely, lower motor neurone lesions can be the consequence of cauda equina tumours. If there is a history of severe perineal pain and the history of incontinence is brief this diagnosis should be considered and a myelogram or spinal MRI obtained.

Upper motor neurone lesions cause faecal incontinence for imprecise reasons. There is little doubt that interruption of suprasegmental control causes incontinence partly as a consequence of a motor deficit and partly because of sensory loss which in turn leads to impaction.

Rarely *rectal carcinoma and infection* (specifically by lymphogranuloma venereum) can give rise to extensive destruction of the pelvic floor such that faecal incontinence might be the presenting symptom.

M. M. Henry

Faints

(*See also* CONVULSIONS AND FITS; DIZZINESS; VERTIGO). Attacks of transient loss of consciousness are common and the causes range from simple vasovagal attacks to epilepsy. Furthermore, a complaint of 'fainting' may not always imply actual loss of consciousness; some patients may mean no more than a feeling of unsteadiness or 'light-headedness'. It is important, as always, to obtain from the patient and, whenever possible, from a witness a precise description of the nature of the attacks. The term 'syncope' has a more exact connotation and can be defined as 'transient loss of consciousness due to a reduction in the cerebral blood flow'. It is this condition with which this discussion will be mainly concerned.

The common causes of syncope are summarized in *Table* F.6.

Table F.6. Causes of syncope

1. **Vasomotor**
   Vasovagal attacks
   Postural hypotension
   Carotid sinus syncope

2. **Cardiac syncope**
   Stokes–Adams attacks in atrioventricular block
   Paroxysmal dysrhythmias
   Central circulatory obstruction, e.g. aortic stenosis
   Cyanotic attacks in congenital heart disease

3. **Cerebrovascular disease**

4. **Miscellaneous**
   Cough syncope
   Micturition syncope
   Breath-holding attacks

1. Vasomotor syncope

This rather imprecise term will be taken to include the large group of conditions in which the cardiac output and blood pressure fall as a result of a sudden fall in peripheral resistance and in the central venous pressure.

Vasovagal Attacks These are extremely common and are almost always of no serious significance. Many predisposing factors are known including emotion, fatigue, prolonged standing and chronic illness of almost any kind. There are other, more serious, conditions of which an apparently simple faint may be a manifestation. Haemorrhage causes syncope as a direct result of the fall in central venous pressure; if the bleeding is external no diagnostic difficulty arises, but, with internal bleeding as, for example, into the gastrointestinal tract, syncope may occur before there is any direct evidence such as haematemesis or melaena. The mechanism whereby haemorrhage causes syncope can also operate in a few patients with very large varicose veins or angiomatous malformations in the legs in which the blood accumulates in the upright posture. Severe pain can also cause syncope as in dissecting aneurysm or myocardial infarction although, in the latter condition, there may also be a fall in cardiac output sufficient on its own to cause syncope. In elderly patients especially, syncope is quite commonly the presenting symptom of myocardial infarction; on recovering consciousness the patient may not complain of chest pain, being perhaps more preoccupied with any trauma he may have suffered in his fall.

The clinical picture is well known, not least to the many medical students who have fainted at their first operation. The patient is nearly always in the upright position; indeed, a 'faint' occurring in the recumbent position is good evidence of some cause other than a vasovagal attack. A minor exception to this rule is the syncope experienced by some pregnant women while lying on their backs; this is probably due to pressure by the uterus on the inferior vena cava producing a fall in venous return. Prodromal symptoms include a feeling of weakness, nausea, sweating and epigastric discomfort; within a few seconds or minutes the patient falls unconscious. The pulse is of small volume and slow and the blood pressure very low; the face is pale and the skin cold and sweating. Incontinence of urine and muscular twitching are rare but can occur in transient loss of consciousness from any cause and do not necessarily imply that the attack is epileptic. Recovery is rapid as the cerebral blood flow increases in the recumbent posture unless the patient is prevented from falling as in a crowd or by well-meaning bystanders. Weakness and nausea may persist for some time after recovery of consciousness.

The term 'vasovagal', which has been used to denote this type of vasomotor syncope, is now widely accepted. However, in the past, it was used, originally by Sir William Gowers, to describe curious 'seizures' which resembled the attacks described above in most respects. They differed only in that loss of consciousness was rare and, usually, no precipitating cause could be found. A theory that they represented a specific entity and were possibly epileptic in nature has now been discredited and it seems certain that these attacks were no more than a mild form of vasomotor syncope occurring in unusually susceptible subjects. All practising physicians have seen patients who faint not only from venepuncture but from a tourniquet or sphygmomanometer cuff being put around an arm.

Postural Hypotension This condition overlaps with vasovagal syncope which, as has been said, almost always occurs when the patient is upright. It is, however, worth distinguishing a group of patients who have a steep fall in blood pressure whenever they stand upright. In some of these patients a neurological cause for the failure of vasoconstriction and other compensatory mechanisms can be identified; to others the label 'idiopathic' has been applied but, in many of these, it is probable that detailed investigation would localize a neurological lesion.

Many drugs can cause a marked postural fall in blood pressure. Among these are hypotensive agents such as guanethidine and bethanidine; nitrites, phenothiazine derivatives, monoamine-oxidase inhibitors, imipramine, barbiturates, amitriptyline and other psychotherapeutic agents have also been incriminated. The hypotensive agent prazosin seems to be unusually liable to cause sudden loss of consciousness for periods of time ranging up to 1 hour. It is not known whether this is always due to postural hypotension and it may be a specific side-effect of this drug. Lesions of peripheral nervous pathways can produce a similar effect by interruption of the afferent or efferent pathways of reflex arcs. Thus postural hypotension is well known in tabes, diabetes and acute polyneuritis, and has been described in alcoholic and carcinomatous neuropathy and in porphyria. Lesions of the central pathways are less easy to demonstrate but degeneration of the intermediolateral column in the spinal cord, vascular lesions of the brainstem and craniopharyngioma, and other parasellar tumours, possibly involving the hypothalamus, have been demonstrated in some cases. Many of these neurological conditions have in common an abnormal response to the Valsalva manoeuvre in that the blood pressure continues to fall throughout the period of strain and no overshoot or reflex bradycardia occurs.

Carotid-Sinus Syncope In many subjects massage of a carotid sinus can cause bradycardia with some fall in blood pressure. In some, mostly elderly patients, these changes may be more marked and this increased sensitivity of the carotid-sinus reflex can be produced by neoplastic or inflammatory lesions in the neck or by digitalis intoxication. In a few patients the haemodynamic changes may be so profound and the reflexes so easily elicited, as by a tight collar, shaving or turning the head, that recurrent syncope occurs. Various types of carotid-sinus syncope have been described with or without bradycardia in addition to the hypotension but the distinction is largely of academic interest. The carotid sinus is innervated by the glossopharyngeal nerve, and a rare condition which may be related to carotid-sinus syncope is the fainting sometimes associated with glossopharyngeal neuralgia, a condition similar to trigeminal neuralgia but causing pain in the tongue, pharynx and ear.

2. Cardiac syncope

In this group of conditions the cardiac output falls as a result of a primary cardiac lesion. It differs from vasomotor syncope in that attacks are much less closely related to the upright posture.

Stokes-Adams Attacks These are due to cardiac arrest usually in asystole but occasionally in ventricular fibrillation on a basis of atrioventricular block. Loss of consciousness can occur in any posture and is abrupt. The patient is pale and pulseless; respiration continues. After about 15–20 seconds twitching may begin due to cerebral anoxia. The attack usually lasts for about 30 seconds but may last longer and death may result. On recovery the patient becomes flushed; this is due to well-oxygenated blood which has been in the pulmonary capillaries during the period of circulatory arrest being flung into systemic capillaries which are widely dilated as a result of the accumulation of vasodilator metabolites. Occasionally, if the attacks occur when the patient is asleep, the only complaint may be of waking with the face feeling hot and flushed.

Paroxysmal Dysrhythmias A paroxysm of tachycardia with a heart rate much in excess of 200 per minute may cause syncope as diastolic filling of the heart is markedly reduced at these heart rates.

Central Circulatory Obstruction Syncope on effort and, more seriously, at rest is a well-recognized feature of aortic stenosis. The mechanism is not clear as this valve lesion is not associated with a low cardiac output unless failure has occurred. It may be that baroceptors within the left ventricular wall, stimulated by the very high pressure, are in some way responsible. Effort syncope is also not uncommon in other obstructive lesions such as pulmonary stenosis and severe pulmonary hypertension, but it is rare in mitral stenosis. The acute circulatory obstruction produced by massive pulmonary embolism or by the impaction of a left atrial thrombus or myxoma in the mitral orifice may also cause syncope. Obstruction to cardiac filling due to cardiac tamponade and constrictive pericarditis can have the same effect.

Cyanotic Attacks Syncope in Fallot's tetralogy and other types of cyanotic congenital heart disease is due not so much to a fall in cardiac output as to a sudden increase in the veno-arterial shunt. This can be due to a fall in systemic resistance or to an increase in the severity of a muscular infundibular stenosis. There is little change in blood pressure, but the patient becomes deeply cyanosed and the murmur of pulmonary stenosis becomes much softer as the greater part of the systemic venous return is shunted into the aorta via the ventricular septal defect.

Ischaemic Heart Disease Syncope due to acute myocardial infarction has already been discussed under 'vasomotor syncope' *above*.

3. Syncope due to cerebral vascular disease

Fainting is rare as a symptom of disease of the carotid arteries and their branches but is more common with stenosis or occlusion of the vertebral arterial system. Atherosclerosis of the vertebral or basilar arteries and external compression of the vertebral arteries by cervical spondylosis or in the Klippel–Feil syndrome can be responsible for syncopal attacks which may be induced by sudden rotatory movements of the neck.

4. Miscellaneous

There is a group of conditions in which syncope is associated with a rise in intrathoracic and intra-abdominal pressure. This includes *cough syncope* in which loss of consciousness occurs at the end of a violent paroxysm of coughing. A series of coughs produces the same circulatory effects as a Valsalva manoeuvre and a marked fall in cardiac output and blood pressure, probably combined with some degree of arterial hypoxaemia, is the mechanism of the syncope. The *breath-holding attacks* of early childhood producing syncope and cyanosis probably have a similar mechanism. The mechanism of *micturition syncope* is not fully understood. It occurs typically when, after heavy beer-drinking, the subject rises in the middle of the night to pass urine. The sudden assumption of the upright posture and the vasodilatory action of alcohol are certainly relevant factors and this condition may be nothing more than a vasomotor syncope. However, it is possible that afferent impulses from the bladder may play some part.

Differential diagnosis. The most important condition from which syncope must be distinguished is *epilepsy*. This can be very difficult but a careful history will usually resolve the problem. Epileptic attacks are characteristically stereotyped in their nature and duration and often occur without warning. Even if there is an aura it bears little resemblance to the prodromal symptoms of syncope except, possibly, in the case of complex partial seizures. Most varieties of syncope, with the notable exception of cardiac syncope, occur almost exclusively in the upright posture whereas the onset of an epileptic fit is unrelated to posture. The typical tonic and clonic phases of major epilepsy should not be confused with the minor twitches which may occur in syncope if a history can be obtained from a reliable eye-witness. Urinary incontinence, a very common feature of epilepsy, is not a major differentiating factor as it can occur in severe or prolonged syncope. Electro-encephalography is certainly of value in some cases but, even with this aid, some doubt may remain.

Consciousness is not loss in *vertigo* so that a history from the patient himself should elicit an account of the typical sensation of rotation. However, the use by the patient of such terms as 'giddiness' to describe the premonitory symptoms of vasomotor syncope together with the nausea which is common to both conditions may confuse the unwary.

Hysterical attacks are nearly always described by the patients as 'faints' but the gracefully dramatic fall into a convenient armchair bears no resemblance to syncope in which the patient collapses like a house of cards. Swoons are out of fashion unless one includes the hysterical faints of teenage girls at 'pop' sessions. It is possible that the so-called 'Toronto blessing' experienced in some charismatic church services is of the same nature.

Hyperventilation is usually a hysterical phenomenon and the feeling of light-headedness induced may be described as faintness. Here, as always, a careful history will resolve the issue but it is worth recalling that hyperventilation followed by a Valsalva manoeuvre will infallibly cause loss of consciousness. This is known variously as the 'mess trick' or the 'fainting lark'.

Peter R. Fleming

Fasciculation

Fasciculation is one of the classical features of a lower motor neurone lesion. It is observed clinically as an intermittent twitching movement under the skin and it is due to the contraction of groups of muscle fibres. The term fibrillation is applied to the contraction of single muscle fibres. It too occurs in lesions of the lower motor neurone but it is a phenomenon that is recorded electrically rather than observed clinically.

Whilst fasciculation can occur with inflammatory or compressive lesions of peripheral nerves, it is in chronic degeneration of anterior horn cells that it is most conspicuous. It is thus a common and an important diagnostic feature of motor neurone disease. Intermittent flickering movements, often around the shoulder girdle or in the thenar muscles, and sometimes felt by the patient, may be an early sign of the disease. Inspection over 2 or 3 minutes may be necessary before the tell-tale movement is detected. Sometimes it can be provoked by a light tap over the muscles.

It is important to note that fasciculation can also be benign. Transitory twitching of facial muscles, particularly the orbicularis oculi, is common experience in normal people; so too is fasciculation in calf muscles, sometimes after unaccustomed exercise. Such benign fasciculation, particularly when it is prolonged or extensive as it occasionally is, can be a cause of major anxiety in doctors and others familiar with the features of motor neurone disease.

D. A. Shaw

Fatigue

Fatigue is a normal reaction to exertion but may be produced excessively by minor exertion in any condition of ill-health, whether it be organic, psychogenic or both. It may be caused by malignant disease, infections and their sequelae, anaemia and states of low cardiac output, endocrine and metabolic disorders and malnutrition. It may be due to lack of sleep, boredom or overwork. The so-called 'combat fatigue' seen in the troops in the Second World War resulted more from the mental than the physical stress of active service. Fatigue on waking in the morning is more commonly due to mental rather than physical factors but it may be due to either or both. Depending on the cause, fatigue may be constant or episodic and in some cases, as in myasthenia gravis, may be anticipated, physical effort being avoided to prevent the later onset of fatigue.

Fatigue is at least as often psychological in origin as due to organic disease but many cases are multifactorial in origin. The following list, although inevitably incomplete, includes most of the common causes.

1. EMOTIONAL AND PSYCHOLOGICAL CAUSES

These include continued unhappiness, boredom, disappointment, overwork, lack of sleep, anxiety and depression. Neurasthenia, a nineteenth-century diagnosis, is undergoing something of a revival.

2. MALIGNANT DISEASE

Any neoplastic disease can be associated with fatigue, which may be a very early symptom—sometimes earlier than loss of weight.

3. CHRONIC INFECTION

Tuberculosis, brucellosis, infective endocarditis and toxoplasmosis are examples of conditions of which the most obvious manifestation may be fatigue.

4. POSTVIRAL FATIGUE SYNDROME

Many viral infections, of which infectious mononucleosis is the best-known example, may be followed, sometimes for many months, by profound fatigue; this may be curiously episodic. The status of myalgic encephalomyelitis (ME) as a specific entity is unclear. Some believe that it is a severe variety of the postviral syndrome. Others maintain that it is a different condition; in particular, it has been suggested that graded exercise, usually beneficial in most cases of the postviral syndrome, causes deterioration in ME.

5. TISSUE HYPOXIA

Anaemia of any type is a common cause of fatigue as are conditions in which the cardiac output is chronically low. These include severe pulmonary hypertension, mitral and tricuspid regurgitation, Addison's disease and excessive diuretic therapy.

6. CONNECTIVE TISSUE DISEASES

These include rheumatoid arthritis, systemic lupus erythematosus, polyarteritis nodosa, polymyalgia rheumatica, giant-cell arteritis and polymyositis.

7. ENDOCRINE AND METABOLIC DISORDERS

Apart from Addison's disease, which has already been mentioned, many conditions in this category, such as hyperthyroidism, renal or hepatic failure and diabetes mellitus, can present with fatigue.

8. MALNUTRITION

Whether this is due to dietary deficiency or to conditions associated with chronic diarrhoea such as ulcerative colitis or Crohn's disease, fatigue is likely to be present.

9. CHRONIC PAIN

Fatigue can be due to persistent chronic pain causing discomfort by day, as in osteoarthritis, or lack of sleep at night, as in some cases of Paget's disease or metastatic disease of bone.

10. MUSCULAR WEAKNESS

Chronic neurological disorders, such as multiple sclerosis, motor neurone disease and, especially, myasthenia gravis and the myopathies are typically associated with excessive fatiguability.

11. CHRONIC DRUG INTOXICATION

The long-term administration of beta-adrenergic blocking agents is an important cause of fatigue; alcohol abuse and the chronic administration of benzodiazepines have a similar but less specific effect.

12. DRUG WITHDRAWAL SYNDROMES

Fatigue may be a consequence of the withdrawal of addictive drugs such as morphine and diamorphine. It can also occur after the withdrawal of corticosteroids, benzodiazepines, alcohol, antidepressants and non-steroidal anti-inflammatory or analgesic agents on which the patient has become reliant.

F. Dudley Hart

FEVER

See PYREXIA.

Fingers, clubbed

The four features of finger clubbing are loss of nail bed angle, increased nail curvature (*Fig.* F.29), fluctuation of the nail bed and drumstick-like swelling of the terminal phalanx. Identification is easy when all four features are present, but dispute is common when only some occur. The first two criteria must be present for finger clubbing to be diagnosed; thus nail bed fluctuation on its own does not constitute clubbing. The first two criteria combine to increase the hypony-chial angle, subtended at the nail base by the skin crease at the dorsum of the distal interphalangeal joint and the skin immediately below the free edge of the nail (*Fig.* F.30). This angle, which is best measured from a shadowgram, is usually less than 190 degrees in normal subjects but exceeds 195 degrees in individuals with clubbing. Clubbing may affect the toes as well as the fingers, but is usually more obvious in the hands. Clubbing is usually bilateral but occasionally may be unilateral in the presence of local vascular abnormalities, such as a subclavian aneurysm, an arteriovenous fistula or disruption of the cervical sympathetic nerves. The pathophysiology of finger clubbing is not understood.

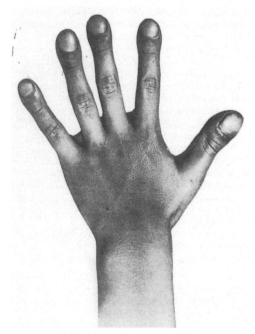

Fig. F.29. Clubbed fingers from a case of bronchiectasis.

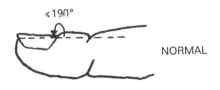

Fig. F.30. Measurement of the hyponychial angle.

Clubbing is an important physical sign and may be the first and only sign of serious organic disease.

The relative frequencies of causes will vary between countries but in Britain the rank may be:

COMMON CAUSE
Bronchial carcinoma
LESS COMMON CAUSES
Cardiac
Cyanotic congenital heart disease
Infective endocarditis
Pulmonary
Bronchiectasis
Cystic fibrosis
Empyema
Mesothelioma
Idiopathic pulmonary fibrosis
Extra-thoracic
Idiopathic/familial/congenital
Cirrhosis of liver
Coeliac disease
Crohn's disease
Ulcerative colitis
Thyrotoxicosis

UNCOMMON CAUSES
Cardiac
Atrial myxoma
Pulmonary
Lung abscess
Fibrotic tuberculosis
Pleural fibroma
Arteriovenous malformation
Metastatic deposits
Mediastinal
Lymphoma
Thymoma
Chronic granulocytic leukaemia
Oesophageal carcinoma
Oesophageal leiomyoma
Peptic oesophagitis
Achalasia of oesophagus
Extra thoracic
Nasopharygeal carcinoma
Thyroid carcinoma
Purgative abuse
Repeated pregnancies
Pachydermoperiostosis

Among pulmonary diseases, lung carcinoma is the commonest cause of finger clubbing and it is wise always to consider this diagnosis. Other intrathoracic malignancies including mesothelioma, lymphomas, and rarely secondary carcinomas or sarcomas can cause finger clubbing. Intrathoracic sepsis is associated with clubbing although this is now an unusual cause in Britain. Chronic bronchitis and emphysema do not cause clubbing. Diffuse pulmonary fibrosis may be associated with clubbing but different causes vary markedly in the frequency of this association. Clubbing is common in idiopathic pulmonary fibrosis, but rare in extrinsic allergic alveolitis and sarcoidosis. Pulmonary asbestosis is the only pneumoconiosis directly associated with clubbing.

Among diseases of the cardiovascular system,

cyanotic congenital heart disease is almost always associated with finger clubbing in those surviving beyond infancy. However, clubbing does not occur in non-cyanotic congenital heart disease such as uncomplicated atrial or ventricular septal defects or persistent ductus arteriosus. Clubbing is a well-recognized, but rather uncommon, feature of infective endocarditis; its absence must not be regarded as important evidence against the diagnosis. It usually appears 6 weeks or more after the onset of the illness but can occasionally develop within a month. Mild finger clubbing develops late in some cases of cirrhosis of the liver, especially in biliary cirrhosis, in coeliac disease, and, rarely, in ulcerative colitis and Crohn's disease.

Clubbing due to any cause may progress to hypertrophic pulmonary osteoarthropathy although this is almost always due to lung carcinoma. Periosteal new bone formation will then be evident especially at the distal ends of long bones at the affected joints.

Familial forms of clubbing and of hypertrophic osteoarthropathy are rare. The presence in family members and the absence of associated disease provide clues to the diagnosis. Heredity osteoarthropathy is associated with thickening of the skin of the hands and face, the latter giving rise to a characteristic appearance of large features with coarse deeply creased skin. This rare familial condition is called 'pachydermoperiostosis'.

Patients are rarely aware of their clubbed fingers. Thus, statements that there has been no recent change in their fingers should not be taken to indicate congenital clubbing.

Neil J. Douglas

Fingers, dead (white, cold)

Primary Raynaud's phenomenon

The digital arteries of the fingers serve two purposes: (a) to supply blood for nutrition of the finger and (b) by controlling blood flow through the skin of the fingers, they vary the heat loss and assist in regulating the core temperature of the body. Thus, on exposure of the body to cold they normally constrict, reducing blood flow through, and heat loss from, the fingers. In some people this reflex appears to be excessive and the digital arteries close completely and the finger becomes 'dead' white and numb. With rewarming the arteries open up again and blood flushes vigorously through the fingers often causing throbbing discomfort ('rewarming pain'). This condition of primary Raynaud's phenomenon probably occurs in about 5 per cent of healthy young females in Britain. It is sometimes seen in males. A family history is common indicating a constitutional basis for the condition. It virtually always begins between the ages of 10 and 30, and does not progress beyond this stage. The fingers remain healthy and normal in appearance and do not develop ulcers or gangrene.

Secondary Raynaud's phenomenon

Much less common is Raynaud's phenomenon secondary to some underlying disease. In these patients the phenomenon usually appears later in life, often middle age, though it can occur in younger patients and men are affected more often than in primary Raynaud's phenomenon. From the beginning the digital ischaemia tends to be more severe and is often at first asymmetrical. The white colour phase is often followed by a blue colour phase persisting for a long time and, in cold weather, the fingers may be permanently blue and cold. Within a short time, and usually within a year or two, the fingers begin to change in appearance becoming shrunken with tight skin and loss of subcutaneous tissue. Ulcers commonly appear under the fingernails (*Fig*. F.31) and, when healed, leave puckered scars (*Fig*. F.32). Repeated attacks lead to loss of tissue of the terminal phalanx with resorption of the phalanx and curved overhanging nails (*Fig*. F.33).

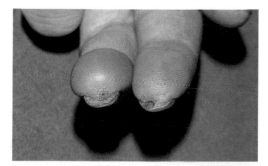

Fig. F.31. Subungal ulcers in secondary Raynauds' phenomenon.

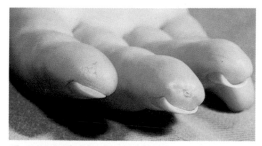

Fig. F.32. Healed ulcers in secondary Raynauds' phenomenon.

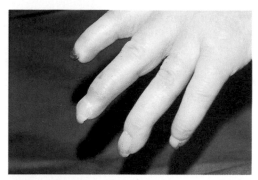

Fig. F.33. Loss of tissue and overhanging nails in secondary Raynauds' phenomenon.

The causes of secondary Raynaud's phenomenon may be listed as follows:

A. THE MORE COMMON CAUSES
    Scleroderma (CRST syndrome)
    Systemic lupus erythematosus
    Rheumatoid arthritis
    Vibration injury

B. THE LESS COMMON CAUSES
    Beta-blocking drugs
    Chronic ergot administration
    Thrombo-angiitis obliterans (Buerger's disease)
    Cold agglutinins

Scleroderma is the commonest cause of secondary Raynaud's phenomenon. It is usually the variety of scleroderma known as the CRST syndrome (Calcinosis, Raynaud's phenomenon, Sclerodactyly, Telangiectases). At first only one or two of these four components of the syndrome will be present, usually the Raynaud's and the telangiectases. The telangiectases are first seen on the nail bed but later larger ones appear on the fingers and face. Subcutaneous calcification eventually appears, which at first is felt as tender nodules under the skin of the fingers but eventually extrude through the skin (*Fig*. F.34). Although severe involvement of the fingers often leads to loss of digits it does not usually affect vital organs and does not usually shorten life-expectancy. Progressive systemic sclerosis with widespread skin involvement and involvement of vital organs is a rare cause of Raynaud's phenomenon and ulceration and gangrene of digits is unusual.

Systemic lupus erythematosus (SLE) may cause severe digital arteritis with Raynaud's phenomenon and repeated attacks of digital gangrene causing extensive loss of digits (*Fig*. F.35). *Rheumatoid arthritis* can similarly affect the fingers with digital gangrene.

Vibration injury, e.g. in foundry workers using pneumatic powered hand-held buffers and grinders, caulkers and welders in the shipbuilding industry and forestry workers using hand-held power driven saws, can cause severe Raynaud's phenomenon. The disorder

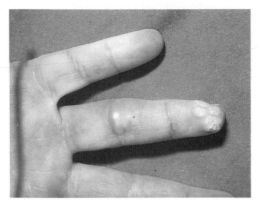

Fig. F.34. Subcutaneous calcification in scleroderma (CRST syndrome).

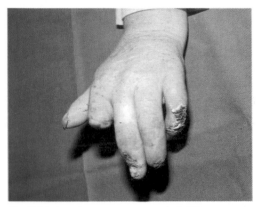

Fig. F.35. Digital gangrene in patient with SLE.

may appear within a few months in foundry workers but takes longer to appear in shipyard and forestry workers. In addition to the white fingers these patients develop numbness and tingling of the fingers. Although the Raynaud's phenomenon can be very severe and a considerable nuisance during cold weather, ulcers and gangrene generally do not occur.

Beta-blocking drugs used in the treatment of angina and hypertension, commonly cause cold hands but do not seem to induce classic Raynaud's pheno-menon, i.e. digital vasoconstriction, in patients who would not otherwise have Raynaud's but may make Raynaud's worse in those already suffering from the condition.

Persistent digital ischaemia

Sudden onset of ischaemia of one or more digits pers-isting for days, weeks or months (persistent digital ischaemia) is not uncommon in the middle aged and elderly. On examination the finger is usually blue and cold (*Fig.* F.36) but capillary circulation is present and the finger usually survives. In younger patients this condition is usually due to some form of arteritis, e.g. *SLE* or *Rheumatoid disease* but in older patients

investigation usually fails to reveal any abnormality except the presence of atheroma and in these patients the ischaemia is due to rupture of an atheromatous plaque higher in the arterial tree with cholesterol debris embolizing the digit.

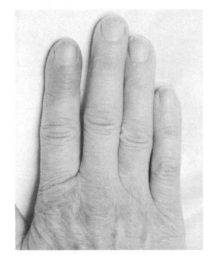

Fig. F.36. Persistent digital ischaemia.

Frostbite

Prolonged exposure of the fingers to cold, e.g. in hill walkers or outdoor workers in winter, may result in the patient complaining of cold, dead, numb fingers. This is due to freezing of the superficial layers of the skin. in the early stages there are white and dead patches of skin on the fingers (*Fig.* F.37) but later and in more severe cases, gangrene of the skin appears and may envelop the whole digit (*Fig.* F.38). Although it appears alarming at first, the gangrene is limited in most causes to the superficial layers of the skin and the skin will eventually peel off leaving a normal digit beneath.

E. Housley

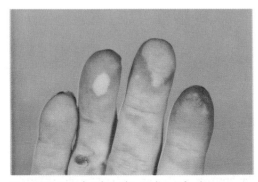

Fig. F.37. Limited early (within 12 hours) frostbite.

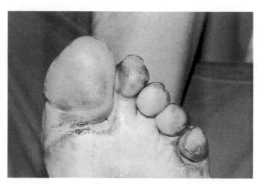

Fig. F.38. Frostbite of toes at 10 days.

Fingers, skin affections of

The skin of the fingers is particularly prone to those dermatoses that are precipitated by exposure to sunlight, climatic change and handled substances (e.g. irritants and chemicals). The fingers are often the site of inoculation of infectious skin conditions. (*Table* F.7) gives a comprehensive list of conditions that can be seen on fingers, divided into morphological types. (*Table* F.8) lists conditions by anatomical site.

Table F.8. Anatomical sites of skin affections

Finger webs
Irritant dermatitis
Contact dermatitis
Scabies
Candidiasis
Dermatophytosis

Peri-ungual
Whitlow
Warts
Mucous cysts
Herpetic whitlow (*Fig.* F.39)
Chronic paronychia
Fibroma (tuberous sclerosis) (*Fig.* P.4)
Chancre

eventually become colonized with moisture-loving organisms such as *Candida albicans, Pseudomonas* or *Staphylococcus aureus*. When this occurs an *acute paronychia* develops with swelling and considerable pain. Either side of any nail may be affected and the condition is difficult to eliminate unless the hands are kept scrupulously dry long enough for the natural seal to re-form. Acute paronychia can also be caused by *herpes simplex* (herpetic whitlow) (*Fig.* F.39), and the

Table F.7. Skin affections of the fingers

Erythematous	*Ulcers*	*Vesico-bullous*
Chilblains	Chilblains	Contact dermatitis
Actinic dermatitis	Frost-bite	Actinic dermatitis
Erythema multiforme (*See Fig.* E.11)	Lupus erythematosus	Erythema multiforme (*See Fig.* E.11)
Urticaria	Scleroderma (*See Fig.* S.21)	Pompholyx (*See Figs.* B.44, V.6)
Lupus erythematosus (*See Fig.* E.12)	Leprosy (*Fig.* F.40)	Scabies (*See Fig.* V.5)
Dermatomyositis (*See Fig.* E.13)	Syphilitic chancre/gumma	Epidermolysis bullosa
Frost-bite	Chrome ulcer	Pemphigoid
Erysipeloid	Trophic ulcer	Herpes simplex (*Fig.* F.39)
	Basal-cell carcinoma	
Papular/nodular	Squamous-cell carcinoma	
Warts	Lupus vulgaris	*Scaly*
Cellular naevi		Atopic eczema
Actinic dermatitis		Chronic dermatitis
Chilblains	*Macular*	Dermatophytosis
Granuloma annulare	Lentigo	Psoriasis
Keratoacanthoma	Junctional naevi	Ichthyosis
Basal-cell carcinoma	Telangiectases	
Squamous-cell carcinoma	Scleroderma	
Lichen planus	Liver disease	
Papular syphilide	Hereditary	
Mucous cyst	Vitiligo (*See Fig.* M.5)	
Fish tank granuloma (*See Fig.* N.48)		
Periungual fibroma (*See Fig.* P.5)		
Pustular		
Scabies		
Boils		
Whitlow (*Fig.* F.39)		
Impetigo		

A condition peculiar to the finger is a paronychia. The most important precipitating factor is the loss of the 'seal' at the nail quick; age, wear and tear, abrasive jobs such as gardening, irritant and penetrating chemicals such as solvents and detergents and skin conditions such as dermatitis or psoriasis may contribute to the breakage of this seal. After this has occurred a pocket tends to form between nail and skin which

presence of a painless ulcer at the lateral margin of the nailfold, frequently of the index finger, should arouse suspicion of a *syphilitic chancre*. Positive serological tests after the 10th to 14th day or the development of a secondary rash after from 2 to 3 weeks will clinch the diagnosis.

Richard Staughton

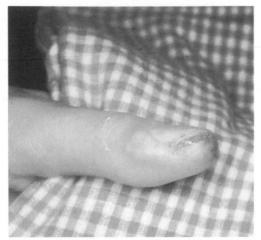

Fig. F.39. Whitlow due to herpes simplex. (*Dr Richard Staughton.*)

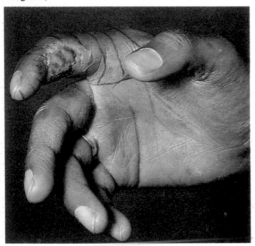

Fig. F.40.. Trophic ulcer in leprosy. (Westminster Hospital.)

Flatulence

Excess gas in the abdomen, wind, or flatulence is one of the most common complaints encountered in medical practice and yet it is seldom possible to offer a rational or convincing explanation, and therapy is often unrewarding. While it is widely believed that excessive gas in the gut is a frequent cause of abdominal discomfort there is objective evidence to suggest many of the patients who complain of bloating, pain, and gas are suffering from a disorder of intestinal motility rather than any increased production of intestinal gas.

Nitrogen, oxygen, hydrogen, carbon dioxide and methane make up more than 99 per cent of intestinal gas; the most important quantitatively are carbon dioxide, hydrogen and methane. Hydrogen and methane are not produced by human metabolic processes but are the consequence of the action of bacterial flora in the gastrointestinal tract. Carbon dioxide arises from bacterial metabolism and from the interaction of bicarbonate and hydrogen ion.

There are three ways in which patients with flatulence may present; with excessive belching, intestinal distension or meteorism, and the passage of excess flatus.

Belching

Air that is belched has always been swallowed and intraluminal production plays only a minor role. Because carbon dioxide, hydrogen, methane and swallowed air (nitrogen and oxygen) are odourless, it is normal for eructation not to have any odour. All healthy subjects may produce methane but only when production reaches a threshold does it appear in the breath. Excessive bacterial action in an oesophagus or stomach that is obstructed may produce gas which is unpleasant in odour. Bacterial gases may become detectable when the extrapulmonary route of removal is defective as in fetor hepaticus which results from the failure of the liver to clear volatile bacterial metabolites such as mercaptans from the blood. Patients with excessive gastric air may complain either of excessive or troublesome eructation of gas, or when the gas is unable to be belched, a discomfort in the left upper quadrant, the so-called *gas bloat* syndrome.

Hypersalivation or chewing gum may give rise to flatulence but sucking sweets, smoking or loose dentures are implicated on less secure grounds.

Intestinal distension and excess flatus

It is convenient to consider these two complaints together. Excess gas in the intestine usually arises from fermentation although aerophagy may contribute. The patient complains of distension, bloating, borborygmi which may be audible, discomfort, cramping abdominal pain and the passage of excessive volumes of flatus. Many patients are socially embarrassed and some admit to a fear of cancer. Gas accumulating in the splenic flexure may give rise to pain in the left upper quadrant, a condition which has been called the *splenic flexure syndrome* and which may possibly be a variant of the irritable bowel syndrome. Most patients who complain of excessive flatus are producing intestinal gas (hydrogen, carbon dioxide and methane) in the colon rather than the swallowing of excessive air (oxygen and nitrogen).

It is a common experience that certain types of food regularly cause flatulence and excessive flatus in normal individuals. The storage carbohydrates of vegetable material are resistant to the digestive enzymes and become available as substrate for bacterial enzymes. Those most commonly implicated include nuts, beans, raisins, onions, cabbage, brussels sprouts, prunes and apples. Patients who have carbohydrate malabsorption such as lactose or starch will produce excessive gas from the breakdown of unabsorbed oligosaccharides. The production of hydrogen following the ingestion of carbohydrates is utilized in the breath hydrogen test which can be used as a test for malabsorption of carbohydrate or bacterial overgrowth in the gut. Methane differs from hydrogen in that about two-thirds of the population produce very little of this gas. Increased quantities of methane are produced in the presence of carcinoma of the colon but this gas is not thought to play any role in the pathogenesis of the malignancy.

There is a group of young or middle-aged women who complain bitterly of abdominal distension prior to the menses or at the time of menopause and for whom no cause can be identified. These patients complain that they cannot fasten or comfortably wear clothing about the abdomen and they often maintain that they feel socially embarrassed although physical examination usually fails to reveal any abdominal swelling. This syndrome is probably a variation of the irritable bowel syndrome and should not be regarded as a syndrome involving excess intestinal gas.

The quantity of flatus which is passed varies between 200 and 2000 ml per day with a mean of about 600 ml daily in normal persons. Flatus varies from being odourless to unpleasantly odiferous. There is little information about the nature of the odiferous gases. Carbon dioxide, hydrogen, methane and swallowed air are odourless. Gases which can be detected by the human nose in concentrations of small amounts include ammonia, hydrogen sulphide, skatol, indole, volatile amines and short fatty acids. The ingestion of certain foods such as French green cheeses may also be a factor in creating foul-smelling flatus.

The flatus frequently contains quantities of hydrogen and methane which are within the explosive range and a dramatic, though rare event, is gas explosion during electrocautery of the colon.

Ian A. D. Bouchier

Flushing

Flushing is a slowly spreading erythema of the skin due to a temporary dilatation of the capillaries and is conventionally differentiated from emotional blushing only by severity, duration and extent. Flushing may be caused by many conditions and is often accompanied by light-headedness, a sense of suffocation, tremors, tinnitus and sometimes nausea and vomiting. The skin of the face, neck and upper anterior chest may be involved. In general flushing is more common in women than in men.

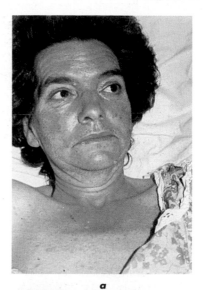

a

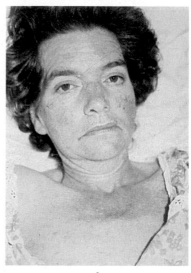

b

Fig. F.41. Before and after carcinoid flush. (Dr Richard Staughton.)

Menopausal flushing ('hot flushes') is extremely common at and just after the menopause, but may occur earlier following bilateral oophorectomy. The flushes, which can last 15 minutes, may be accompanied by sweating and develop spontaneously, sometimes even during sleep. The mechanism is still unknown though presumably neurohormonal.

Alcohol-induced flushing can be related to quantity or variety of drink consumed. Large amounts of histamine are found in sherry and some red wines though none in distilled spirits. Histamine causes flushing, and certain drugs and food may release enough from mast cells to cause a blush. Some diabetics on chlorpropamide flush with alcohol as do those taking disulfiram, metronidazole, and after percut-aneous absorption of the anti-scabetic Tetmosol (mono-sulfiram). Flushing is the commonest clinical feature of the *carcinoid* syndrome (*Fig.* F.41), also comprising diarrhoea, dyspnoea and right-sided heart lesions. In this condition, as in recurrent flushing of any cause, persistent cheek telangiectasis eventually occurs. In *systemic mastocytosis* severe flushing attacks, often accompanied by headache, may occur spontaneously or after trauma to skin lesions. Episodes of flushing and diarrhoea may accompany the *Zollinger–Ellison syndrome*, and fainting with flushing can occur with an adrenaline-secreting *phaeochromocytoma*. It may also occur in insulin-dependent *diabetics* with both hypo- and hyperglycaemia. It may be part of an *epileptic* aura.

Postprandial flushing of the face, especially the muzzle area, is a characteristic of *rosacea*. In this disease reddening later becomes permanent with telangiectasia, as well as papules and pustules (*see Fig.* E.6).

A flushed facial appearance is seen in patients with Cushing's syndrome, polycythemia rubra vera and ACTH secreting bronchogenic tumour (*see Fig.* S.24).

Richard Staughton

Foot and toes, deformities of

A deformity of the foot and ankle is described as a 'talipes' and this is the generic term commonly used for foot deformities of congenital origin. The primary deformities of the foot are *varus* (the heel is inverted), *valgus* (the heel is everted), *equinus* (the foot is plantar flexed) and *calcaneus* (the foot is dorsiflexed). A *cavus* foot is one with a high arch and a combination of deformities may occur so that a cavo-equino-varus foot may be seen.

Talipes equino-varus or club foot

The term 'club foot' is routinely restricted to a talipes equino-varus and it may be congenital or acquired (*Fig.* F.42).

CONGENITAL CLUB FOOT

The incidence is approximately 5 per 1000 live births in the United Kingdom and approximately 2 per 1000 live births are severe. The factors involved are partly genetic and partly environmental with the latter features acting upon the fetus in utero. There is a familial incidence with a greater incidence among the male offspring of a female patient. The male is predominant but there is no recognizable pattern of inheritance. The very moulded baby in utero with an oligohydramnios may present with a club foot. Congenital contractures in arthrogryphosis multiplex congenita or in spina bifida may produce a congenital club foot.

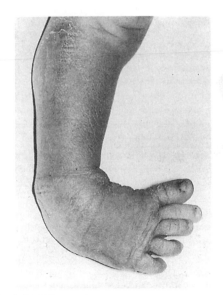

Fig. F.42. Talipes equino-varus.

The club foot is one in which the foot and ankle are in equinus and the forefoot is moulded into varus. The heel is in marked varus and there may be some minor cavus deformity associated.

CLINICAL FEATURES

There is a great variation in the degrees of talipes equino-varus from a mild deformity to one in which the sole and the toes touch the medial side of the lower leg. In the severe deformity there is an associated incidence of congenital dislocation of the hip, and the spine must be carefully examined for neurological abnormality.

Talipes varus

A minor varus deformity of the foot is frequently seen after intra-uterine moulding. Manual stretching will produce easy correction and spontaneous resolution is expected.

Talipes calcaneo-valgus

This is a common position of the foot of the newborn and is considered due to intra-uterine moulding (*Fig.* F.43). It is a benign condition and simple stretching will rapidly correct this position. The eventual prognosis is one of normality.

Congenital metatarsus varus

Adduction of the forefoot is again a common deformity in the baby and toddler. The constant face-lying of the baby tends to aggravate the position and alteration of the sleeping posture should be encouraged. Spontaneous resolution occurs in the vast majority without

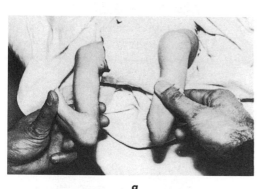

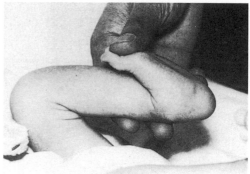

a b

Fig. F.43. a. Calcaneo-valgus feet in the neonate. b. The dorsum of the foot easily reaches the anterior shin.

treatment and only very rarely is surgical correction required.

Pes valgus (*Fig.* F.44)

A flat foot is one in which the heel is in some valgus and is common. The structure of the skeleton of this

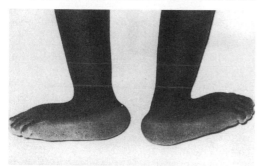

Fig. F.44. Valgus feet in spina bifida paralysis.

foot is normal and there may be associated ligament laxity. A painless flat foot should be considered normal, but if the foot is in spasm and painful the possibility of an abnormal tarsal coalition should be considered (peroneal spastic flat foot).

Pes cavus

Pes cavus is a fixed deformity of the foot with a very high arch in which there is an equinus deformity of the forefoot on the hindfoot (*Fig.* F.45). There is associated clawing of the toes and the term 'claw foot' is sometimes used to describe this extremity. The cavus deformity of the foot is usually associated with some underlying neurological abnormality. There may be associated muscular dystrophy, Charcot–Marie–Tooth or peroneal muscular atrophy causing the peripheral muscular imbalance. Poliomyelitis and Friedreich's ataxia are also causes. Spastic hemiplegia may also cause a rigid pes cavus. In those feet in which a neurological deficit cannot be demonstrated, the term 'idiopathic pes cavus' is used.

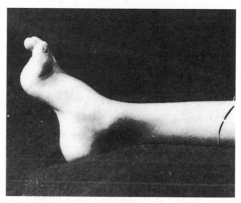

Fig. F.45. Pes cavus with claw toes.

Acquired talipes: paralytic causes

It is possible for any paralytic condition of neurological or muscular origin to produce deformities of the foot: (*a*) spastic paralysis due to upper motor neurone lesions; (*b*) flaccid paralyses due to lower motor neurone lesions; (*c*) cerebellar ataxias; (*d*) muscular dystrophies.

a. Lesions of the upper motor neurone (*Figs* F.46, F.47)

Cerebral palsy is usually due to a birth injury and produces a spastic paresis. Acquired lesions such as meningeal infections or cerebrovascular accidents may cause similar spastic weakness. The cord may be affected by injury, haemorrhage, thrombosis and tumour. Spinal dysraphism, a malformation arising from abnormal splitting of the notochord, may produce cord lesions and a diastematomyelia or congenital splitting in the upper part of the spine may affect the cord with a bony or fibrous bar obstructing the spinal canal.

b. Lesions of the lower motor neurone

Spina bifida affecting the cauda equina, poliomyelitis, peroneal muscular atrophy (Charcot–Marie–Tooth

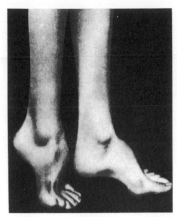

Fig. F.46. Infantile hemiplegia causing extreme talipes equinus of the right foot.

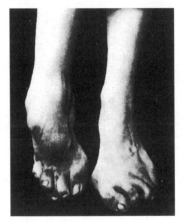

Fig. F.47. Bilateral talipes equinus from congenital spastic paraplegia.

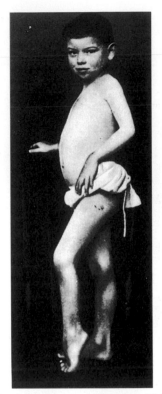

Fig. F.48. Talipes equino-varus due to spina bifida.

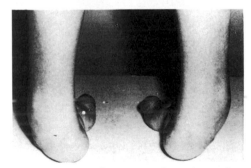

Fig. F.49. Cavo-varus feet in peroneal muscular atrophy.

disease), progressive muscular atrophy and amyotrophic lateral sclerosis may all cause a foot deformity (*Figs.* F.48, F.49). The nerves of the cauda equina or lumbar and sacral plexuses may be compressed by tumours, by untreated disc prolapse and by congenital bone abnormalities and in particular the bony abnormality associated with diastematomyelia.

c. Lesions of the cerebellum

Friedreich's ataxia may produce a talipes equino-varus.

d. Primary muscular disease

Pseudo-hypertrophic muscular paralysis (Duchenne disease) produces an equino-varus deformity. The family history, the enlargement of the calves and the way in which the patient raises himself from the supine position is characteristic. Amyotonia congenita is a similar condition with similar effects.

Foot deformities may develop in a variety of other rarer conditions such as Volkmann's ischaemic contracture with peripheral lower limb ischaemic

changes analogous to that occurring in the forearm. Acute flat foot may be due to inflammatory softening of the plantar ligaments as is seen in acute arthritis (Reiter's disease). Contracting scars following injuries or burns may cause deformity and the hysteric may produce what appears to be a fixed deformity but which in the early stages may be corrected during sleep or under anaesthesia.

Hallux valgus

The hallux is deviated into valgus at the metatarsophalangeal joint. There is a genetic predisposition and the female is more commonly affected. The commencement of the deformity may occur in adolescence and it may be exacerbated by the use of overtight and pointed shoes.

A bunion develops in associated with hallux valgus. The apex of the angle between the toe and the metatarsal may be pressurized in the patient's shoe. Reactive new bone produces a metatarsal head exostosis and the adventitial bursa medial to it becomes enlarged, inflamed and sometimes infected (*Fig*. F.50), the so-called 'bunion'.

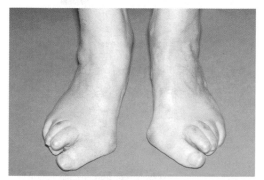

Fig. F.50. Gross bilateral hallux valgus with associated bunions.

Hammer toe

The constant lateral pressure of the hallux against the other digits may produce a hammer toe. The proximal interphalangeal joint flexes and becomes contracted with a painful and tender dorsal callosity (*Fig*. F.51).

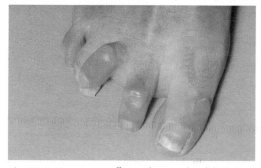

Fig. F.51. Hammer toes affecting the second and third digits.

The distal joint hyperextends. The same hammer deformity may occur if the second digit is extremely long.

Claw toes

Clawing of the toes may occur if there is a neurological imbalance with partial paralysis of the foot intrinsic muscles. This is seen in poliomyelitis and peroneal muscle atrophy. A pes cavus may be found in association (*Fig*. F.45). This deformity is also seen in Volkmann's contracture involving the lower limb.

Paul Aichroth

Foot, ulceration of

Perforating ulcers of the foot usually occur under the ball of the great toe, but may affect any pressure area.

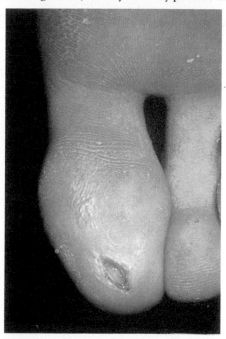

Fig. F.52. Ischaemic ulcer. (Addenbrooke's Hospital.)

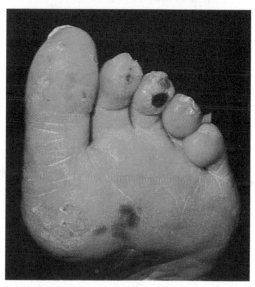

Fig. F.53. Cryoproteinaemia. (Westminster Hospital.)

Ulcers can form under hard *callouses*. Anaesthesia appears to be the most important factor and such lesions are seen in patients with *sensory neuropathy* of any cause, e.g. *diabetes, leprosy, alcoholism*, etc. Pressure ulcers are also seen in paraplegics of any cause. Chronic ulceration of the sole can be the presentation of *ischaemia* (*Fig*. F.52), and occurs in those

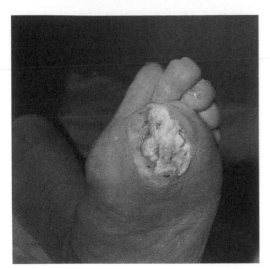

Fig. F.54. Squamous cell carcinoma. (*Dr Richard Staughton.*)

with *arteriosclerosis, heavy smokers* and patients with *familial hyperlipidaemia*. Ulceration of the feet can be the presenting feature of *cryoproteinaemia* (*Fig.* F.53). Deep fungal infections can cause foot ulceration, e.g. *blastomycosis, sporotrichosis* and *maduromycosis*. Rare causes include *syphilitic gumma* and neoplasms, e.g. *carcinoma cunniculatum* and *squamouscell carcinoma* (*Fig.* F.54).

Richard Staughton

Frigidity (anorgasmia)

Frigidity, or *anorgasmia* (a less pejorative term), like impotence (*see* p. 306), is due to a wide variety of causes, by far the most important of which are psychogenic. However, severe physical malformations of the genital tract whether congenital or acquired can, of course, interfere with sexual intercourse or lead to a failure to achieve orgasm. The same may also be an outcome of *dyspareunia*, due also to some physical lesion.

Quite a substantial proportion of women appear to be *constitutionally anorgasmic*. This implies that there seems to be no good physical or psychological reason for their inability to achieve orgasm, however hard or long they try. This may, however, be more apparent than real and, in the case of many women, be related to lack of knowledge of what is to be expected from sexual intercourse. However, with increasing sophistication, in part the outcome of better sex education, the level of expectation among women appears to be rising, which in turn may have led to a fall in the number of those who might once have been regarded as constitutionally anorgasmic. None the less, there remains an unknown number of women who, while they insist, on superficial questioning, that

their sex lives are satisfactory, may, when pressed, reveal that they have never actually obtained full sexual satisfaction. Such women have often been brought up to believe that sexual intercourse is something to be endured rather than enjoyed.

Before considering what may be pathological, two other relevant factors need consideration. One is that the achievement of sexual satisfaction by women appears to be more closely bound up with an affectionate or loving relationship than is the case with men, to whom mere physical attraction may be sufficient. The second is that women are slower to arouse sexually than are men. This means that if the male partner lacks technique, hurries the proceedings unduly, or, being partially impotent, suffers from premature ejaculation, with loss of tumescence, the woman concerned may not have sufficient time in which to achieve orgasm. If she is herself inexperienced and does not understand the reason for this, she may come to regard herself as frigid.

This type of difficulty may be regarded as *pseudofrigidity*, a state in which potential ability to achieve orgasm is present but, owing to unpropitious circumstances, may not be realized. Other circumstances which may likewise lead to failure of orgasm may be *fear of pregnancy*—some women deliberately suppress orgasm in the belief that this may prevent pregnancy occurring—sleeping in the same house as parents or in-laws, or sharing a bedroom with children, etc. *Alcoholism* in the marital partner may also be a source of difficulty, the inconsideration of a partly intoxicated spouse tending in due course to bring about an intense revulsion for sexual intercourse.

Like impotence, anorgasmia may arise out of *inexperience* or be due to *simple anxiety*. It may also be an outcome of *emotional immaturity*, a state often reflected by the inability of a young bride to live a separate existence independent of her parents. This is a common affliction among neurotic women who are either over-attached to their fathers or have a poor relationship with their parents which may be the outcome of cruelty in marriage, alcoholism, etc. *Sexual interference* in childhood or adolescence by a male relative or some other person may also later impair a normal capacity for satisfactory intercourse.

The other main sexual problem leading to anorgasmia is *vaginismus*. This is an intense spasm of the muscles surrounding the introitus, leading to it remaining tightly shut and thereby interfering with penetration by the male penis. Once such spasm occurs further attempts at penetration are painful enough to reinforce reflex closure of the introitus, creating thereby a vicious cycle. Vaginismus may be severe enough to lead to non-consummation of marriage, although in milder cases initial introital pain and spasm which may be largely the outcome of inexperience and apprehension may lessen as intercourse proceeds. Many instances of *dyspareunia* are in fact cases of vaginismus. However, in all cases of female sexual dysfunction gynaecological causes must be excluded. It may be necessary to carry out an examination under anaesthesia to exclude this.

In the case of *female homosexuals (lesbians)*, frigidity in a heterosexual relationship is common though not apparently invariable. Some basically homosexual women marry and make a success of it sometimes by arranging a *ménage à trois*. Many professional *prostitutes* are said to be frigid and many are probably homosexual also. The same, paradoxically, applies to *nymphomania* in which state, although there is an apparently intense desire for sexual relationships, sometimes with any available male partner, satisfaction is never achieved. It has also been suggested that nymphomania represents an attempt by the female to denigrate male sexuality.

Certain matters pertaining to childbirth may be important. In some women an *abortion* may occasionally give rise to frigidity, though the vast majority remain unaffected by this event. Fear of pregnancy has already been mentioned, but, even in the absence of this and where satisfactory contraceptive methods are employed, some women tend to become anorgasmic after the birth of a second or third child when no more children are desired, which may be a reflection of the more intimate relationship between childbearing and sex which exists in women as opposed to their husbands. Likewise, and sometimes surprisingly, a loss of libido quite often appears to follow sterilization—for whatever reason. Loss of sexual desire is not necessarily a sequel to the menopause; indeed, a capacity to enjoy sexual relationships may persist in some women to a relatively advanced age, although there is naturally a wide variation.

As in the case of the male, loss of libido may occur in women due to a *depressive illness*. Following treatment and satisfactory resolution of the illness sexual function may be restored once again to normal.

N. Patel

Gait, abnormalities of

Gait may be disturbed by: (1) mechanical defects in the lower limbs and pelvis; (2) pain in the legs, pelvis and lower lumbar spine; (3) disease of muscles; (4) disease of the nervous system: (a) increased tone, either striatal or pyramidal; (b) weakness, either pyramidal or peripheral; (c) ataxia, either sensory or cerebellar; (5) disease of the vestibular apparatus; (6) hysteria.

1. Mechanical defects

Inequality in the length of the legs, congenital dislocation of the hips, ankylosis of the knee or hip joints and deformities of the feet give rise to a characteristic bold, painless limp, the source of which is readily found on examination of the limbs.

Coxa vara and coxa valga may lead to characteristic gaits. Painless ankylosis of both hips leads to all movements being made at knees, ankles and feet, giving a short-stepping smooth gait, almost as if the patient were on roller-skates. This is seen, for instance, in some cases of ankylosing spondylitis.

2. Painful limp

Painful limp, due to pain in the pelvis or lower limb, is easily recognized by the manner in which the patient puts the weight on the sound leg and hurries off the affected one. The source of the pain may be in the limb itself, or it may be referred from disease in the pelvis, lumbar spine or cauda equina. Localized pain usually means localized disease at that site, referred pain tending to have a more diffuse and linear distribution, but many exceptions occur. The pain referred from a diseased hip may be felt only in the knee—an important feature in children with tuberculosis of the hip, and occasionally a root pain is limited to a small area in the foot (S1) or the lateral border of the leg (L5). Local tenderness at the site of the pain often indicates local disease, but it may equally well be present in referred pain. On the other hand, local deformity or swelling always means disease at that point. The more important causes of a painful limp are enumerated in the following list:

THE JOINTS
Injuries
Arthritis or arthrosis of lumbar spine, or of hip, knee, ankle
  and/or foot on one or both sides
THE BONES
Injuries
Neoplastic, congenital or metabolic disease
Inflammatory and/or infective disease
THE MUSCLES
Injury

Wasting and weakness
THE BLOOD VESSELS
Intermittent claudication from arterial disease or embolism
Phlebitis
THE LUMBOSACRAL ROOTS
Prolapse of intervertebral disc
Lesions of cauda equina
Lesions of lumbar vertebrae
Pelvic masses
OTHER TISSUES
Foreign body in foot (children)
Bursitis (gluteal, patellar and tendo Achillis)
Corns and bunions
Flat feet
Chilblains

3. Diseases of muscles

Diseases of muscles, although rare, can cause character-istic disturbances of gait. In the heredofamilial *my-opathies*, usually seen in early life, the gait is waddling, the muscles weak and either hypertrophied or atro-phied, and sensation is normal. In *myotonia congenita*, members of affected families experience from birth a peculiar difficulty in relaxing muscles after voluntary contraction. Thus on attempting to walk, the muscles go into a tonic spasm, but this can be worked off by continued exercise. Diagnosis is made on the family history, the presence of prolonged contraction after voluntary effort, the production of a persistent local-ized contraction on percussion of the affected muscles, and high-frequency discharges in the electromyogram, likened on the loudspeaker to the noise of a div-ebomber. A similar myotonia is seen in *dystrophia myotonica*, a familial disease usually of adult life but occurring also in children; the gait is disturbed by myotonia, but weakness and atrophy of the quadriceps and of the dorsiflexors of the feet are a further embar-rassment to walking. The presence of wasting and myotonia in the face, sternomastoids and forearm, and the frequent presence of premature baldness, cataracts and testicular atrophy, indicate the correct diagnosis. In *myasthenia gravis*, the legs, in common with the rest of the musculature, may fatigue rapidly: the gait is normal after rest, but as fatigue supervenes it becomes shuffling, unsteady and weak. The weakness and extreme hypotonia of the muscles in *amyotonia cong-enita* interfere with gait in those children who survive the first critical years of infancy. They learn to walk later, and they then present the unsteadiness of weak-ness, but even this incapacity may be outgrown.

4. Disease of the nervous system

a. Spasticity due to bilateral pyramidal disease will affect both legs, as in congenital spastic diplegia, spinal cord compression, multiple sclerosis, subacute com-bined degeneration of the cord in the early stages,

intramedullary tumours, syringomyelia, etc. Tone is increased in the extensors and adductors, so that the limb is held in extension, with plantar flexion of the foot, and some degree of adduction. Gait is stiff, the toes scrape the ground, and if the adduction and spasticity are severe, there is a 'scissors gait'. Weakness increases the disability. A unilateral pyramidal lesion gives rise to a similar stiff, extended limb, which is dragged around its normal fellow by tilting the pelvis, thus overcoming the adduction and allowing the flexed foot to clear the ground.

The rigidity of *extrapyramidal disease* affects extensors and flexors equally, but the legs are held slightly flexed at the hip and knee because the flexors are more powerful than the extensors. Steps are short and shuffling. The patient tends to walk faster and faster, as if chasing his centre of gravity. If pushed backwards, he tends to run backwards with short hasty steps. Fixity of expression, flexion of the neck and trunk, adduction of the arm with flexion of the elbows and the characteristic rhythmic tremor of the forearms, hands and fingers afford diagnostic assistance when the extrapyramidal lesions are due to Parkinson's disease, one of the earliest signs being a failure to swing the arm on walking. A similar gait results from extrapyramidal lesions due to encephalitis lethargica, arteriopathic cerebral degeneration, carbon monoxide poisoning, hepatolenticular degeneration, and (rarely) after severe head injuries.

b. Weakness plays a part in pyramidal lesions, but it is often difficult to distinguish the relative import-ance of this weakness and the associated spasticity in the disturbances of gait which are described above. On the other hand, weakness due to disease of the anterior horn cells or of the peripheral nerves to the legs gives rise to abnormal gaits, the features of which depend on the distribution of the weak or paralysed muscles. Where there is foot-drop, as in any form of polyneuritis, injuries to the common peroneal nerve, poliomyelitis or a lesion of the cauda equina, there is a high-stepping gait, in which the foot is lifted high and then slapped down on the ground. If the calf muscles are paralysed, as in a lesion of the posterior tibial nerve, the gait loses its natural spring. Further-more, disease affecting the motor fibres often attacks the sensory fibres too; proprioceptive sensory loss then adds a sensory ataxic element to the gait, which becomes clumsy, unsteady, irregular and broad based as in tabes, many types of polyneuritis and gross disease of the cauda equina. When sensory ataxia thus com-plicates muscular weakness, balance is worse in the dark or when the eyes are shut.

c. Sensory *ataxia* has been mentioned as a factor in the clumsy, incoordinated, noisy, wide-based gait of polyneuritis, tabes, lesions of the cauda equina and some cases of subacute combined degeneration of the cord. A second form of ataxic gait is seen as a result of disease or injury of the cerebellum or its connections. The gait is wide-based and clumsy, but it is little aggravated by darkness or by closing the eyes. There is a tendency to deviate towards the side of the lesion, but overcompensation may occur, with consequent deviation to both sides in an irregular, staggering and drunken manner. The normal 'swing' of the arm on the affected side may be diminished or lost, but this feature is often absent. 'Cerebellar' ataxia is seen in multiple sclerosis, the heredofamilial ataxias, occasional cases of tabes without proprioceptive sensory loss, and in inflammatory, neoplastic, degenerative, traumatic and vascular lesions of the cerebellum.

5. Vestibular ataxia

Disease of the labyrinth, the vestibular nerve or the vestibular nucleus in the pons can give rise to disturbances of gait. Vertigo makes the patient feel disorientated; the gait is unsteady and there is a tendency to deviate to the affected side. This occurs in acute phases of Menière's disease, acute labyrinthitis and vascular lesions of the pons.

6. Hysteria

Hysteria is sometimes responsible for abnormal gaits. There is no set pattern, but, however bizarre hysterical gaits may be, they have in common a certain improbability and flamboyance; a tendency to subside gracefully and safely on the floor, and to stagger in the direction of objects upon which to lean. 'Astasia abasia' is a term which was formerly used for inability to stand or walk despite normal movements of the limbs when recumbent, but it is desirable to recall that in hereditary spinocerebellar ataxia, and in affections of the flocculonodular lobe and the vermis of the cerebellum, a gross ataxia of gait may be found despite good performance in all tests of coordination when in bed. This is due to the fact that these functions, of balance and co-ordination, are subserved by different regions of the cerebellum which can be involved separately in disease processes, coordination depending on the integrity of the lateral lobes of the cerebellum and balance on the midline structures. Hysterical gaits are recognized by their inconsistencies, and by a quality which can best be described as insincerity; confirmation is to be found in the presence of psychoneurosis and the absence of organic disease. Unlike organic disorders of gait, they can sometimes be cured by suggestion.

Ian Mackenzie

Gallbladder, palpable

Physical signs

On occasions a grossly distended gallbladder in a thin subject may be visible as a distinct globular swelling in the right upper abdomen. However, palpation is the physical method of examination in detecting enlargement of the gallbladder. One may feel an oval, smooth swelling moving downwards close behind the anterior abdominal wall when the patient inspires, descending either from beneath the right costal margin near the tip of the 9th rib, or attached to the undersurface of a palpable liver in the right nipple line. As it enlarges, the tumour generally extends inwards as well as downwards so that it may ultimately cross the midline below the level of the umbilicus. It may be large enough to be palpable bimanually in a thin patient but it does not fill out the loin in a way that a renal tumour may do. It may or may not be tender, depending on whether the cause of the enlargement is or is not associated with inflammation. It feels firm and tense rather than hard. An impaired but not quite dull note is obtained on percussion.

Diagnosis from other swellings

It has to be distinguished particularly from four groups of conditions: (1) from *carcinoma* arising in the bile ducts or gallbladder itself; (2) from *tumours* in or attached to the liver in the neighbourhood of the gallbladder—secondary new growth, primary hepatoma or more rarely gumma, abscess or hydatid cyst; (3) from *mobile kidney, hydronephrosis* or *renal tumour*; (4) from *tumours in the neighbouring organs*, such as carcinoma of the pyloric antrum or the right suprarenal.

Clinical features, as described below, will often enable an accurate diagnosis to be made. These may be supplemented by appropriate radiological studies and by ultrasound or computerized tomography imaging—if necessary with fine needle aspiration.

1. CARCINOMA OF THE GALLBLADDER

It is often difficult to decide whether a tumour is merely an enlarged gallbladder or a growth infiltrating and replacing it, since in either case there may be a history extending over years of gallstones, with biliary colic, pyrexia and even jaundice, and primary new growth of the gallbladder is often associated with gallstones. The rapidity of the enlargement in the absence of any definite cause will suggest growth, particularly in a person of the cancer age; careful palpation may show that the mass is not smooth as in the case of most simple gallbladder enlargements, but more or less nodulated or covered with bosses or irregularities, which in themselves suggest new growth. In some cases there may be secondary deposits in the liver, ascites, and sometimes the enlargement of the left supraclavicular lymph nodes points to malignant disease with metastasis. Notwithstanding these points, however, the differential diagnosis may be so difficult that laparotomy will be necessary for decision.

2. TUMOURS ATTACHED TO OR IN THE LIVER

Those most likely to be mistaken for enlargement of the gallbladder are Riedel's lobe, secondary carcinoma of the liver and, much more rarely, hepatoma, gumma, abscess or hydatid cyst. It may, by physical examination, be impossible to distinguish a *Riedel's lobe* from an enlarged gallbladder or from a mobile kidney. Speaking generally, a Riedel's lobe usually descends from the liver farther to the right than does a gallbladder, and it is more apt to simulate an enlarged or a mobile kidney.

Metastatic deposits in the liver nearly always cause considerable and sometimes enormous enlargement and great hardness of the organ, not infrequently associated with jaundice. The diagnosis depends, first, upon the discovery of a primary growth, which in the case of carcinoma is likely to be in the stomach, pancreas, colon or rectum, or, in the case of melanoma, the eye, and secondly, on the discovery in the liver of several separate nodules, some of which may be felt to be umbilicated, that is to say depressed in their central part and raised around the edges.

Hepatoma, although rare in Great Britain, occasionally occurs in cirrhotics and may be multifocal. In the Far East and in eastern Africa it is far more common and, in patients from those areas, is an important condition to consider in differential diagnosis.

Gumma of the liver is rarely encountered nowadays, and when it occurs is usually mistaken for new growth unless there is a convincing history of syphilis or the effects of tertiary lesions are visible elsewhere, especially gummatous lesions of the skin or leucoplakia of the tongue. The diagnosis may be confirmed by obtaining a positive serological reaction, or by the beneficial effects of antisyphilitic treatment, though this does not always lead to rapid disappearance of a gumma of the liver. Even when the liver is inspected at laparotomy the diagnosis between gumma and new growth is not always easy.

Abscess of the liver, if it is to simulate an enlargement of the gallbladder, is likely to be a single large one which, if it has not arisen in some pre-existent mass, such as a gumma, new growth or hydatid cyst, is almost certain to have been acquired in a tropical country where the patient has suffered from amoebic dysentery. The diagnosis may not be evident until laparotomy is undertaken or the mass is punctured with an exploring needle.

Hydatid cyst of the liver is seldom situated in such a position as to cause difficulty of diagnosis for gallbladder enlargement; more usually the cyst is embedded in the liver substance, or projects from its upper surface. The diagnosis might be entertained if the patient were known to have hydatid cysts elsewhere or came from an area where this disease is endemic; but in most cases it is suggested by ultrasonography or CT of the liver and sometimes determined only when laparotomy has been performed. It might have been suggested by the discovery of eosinophilia, and also by the specific hydatid serum reaction if the hydatid cyst is alive and active. But latent or calcified hydatid cysts cause no symptoms, do not produce an eosinophilia and are not associated with a positive hydatid blood-serum reaction. Their walls, if calcified, can be seen on radiographs of the region.

3. THE DISTINCTION BETWEEN AN ENLARGED GALLBLADDER AND A MOBILE KIDNEY OR HYDRONEPHROSIS

There may be no jaundice to suggest gallbladder trouble, nor need there be any urinary changes to suggest kidney, so that the diagnosis may have to be made chiefly by palpation. Facts to stress are that a gallbladder is more easily felt anteriorly than posteriorly, whilst the reverse is the case with the kidney; that the kidney is, as a rule, the more freely movable of the two; that it is seldom possible to demarcate the upper pole of an enlarged gallbladder in the way that the top of a movable kidney can sometimes be defined; that with kidney tumour the loin is dull, whilst with gallbladder enlargement it is resonant; and that, on rather firm bimanual palpation, the patient may experience a peculiar sickening sensation which is characteristic of kidney. In cases of doubt, an intravenous pyelogram will demonstrate whether or not the right kidney is normal. (*See also* KIDNEY, PALPABLE.)

4. TUMOURS OF OTHER ORGANS SIMULATING ENLARGEMENT OF THE GALLBLADDER

These may be distinguished to some extent by the fact that new growths of the pylorus, transverse colon or suprarenal big enough to simulate an enlargement of the gallbladder seldom have the smooth oval outline that the gallbladder nearly always possesses. In addition, there may have been symptoms attributable to the primary growth, such as dilatation of the stomach, coffee-ground vomit, or evidence of secondary deposits in the liver, in the left supraclavicular lymph nodes, or elsewhere, to indicate the diagnosis.

Modern imaging techniques (ultrasound and computerized axial tomography) can usually give anatomical delineation of an enlarged gallbladder and differentiate the other masses enumerated above. Nevertheless in some of these cases it is impossible to exclude enlargement of the gallbladder without resorting to laparotomy.

The causes of enlargement of the gallbladder

Empyema of the gallbladder
Chronic pancreatitis.
Carcinoma of the head of the pancreas.
Cholecystitis from: (1) gallstones; (2) new growth.
Typhoid fever.
Obstruction of the common bile duct by a gallstone.
Obstruction of the cystic duct by a gallstone.
Simple mucocele.

It is noteworthy that *gallstones* comparatively seldom lead to enlargement of the gallbladder. If the associated inflammation does not progress to empyema, the gallbladder usually becomes thick-walled, contracted and embedded in dense adhesions which prevent it from dilating even when the cystic or common bile ducts become obstructed by a stone. Indeed, in a middle-aged patient in whom there has not been any very definite attack of biliary colic, the occurrence of progressive and considerable enlargement of the gallbladder, associated with a deepening jaundice and without ascites, arouses serious suspicion of a *lesion of the head of the pancreas* which has extended along the pancreatic duct so as gradually to occlude the common bile duct, the commonest cause of these symptoms being either *chronic pancreatitis* or *carcinoma* of the head of the pancreas or of the ampulla of Vater. In obstruction of the common bile duct due to gallstones, the gallbladder is as a rule not palpable; in obstruction due to carcinoma of the head of the pancreas it is usually distended and is palpable in about 50 per cent of patients (Courvoisier's law, *Fig.* G.1). Painless progressive jaundice suggests a carcinoma arising at the ampulla of Vater and, if this ulcerates, the stools may be positive for occult blood. Jaundice preceded by epigastric or upper lumbar pain is more likely to be due to carcinoma or chronic pancreatitis of the body of the pancreas. Sometimes sloughing of part of the tumour allows the pent-up bile to escape into the duodenum with puzzling temporary remission or even disappearance of the jaundice. In cases in which gallstones are the cause of the enlargement there is nearly always tenderness over the gallbladder and pain when it is palpated firmly, associ-

ated with a rise of temperature, possibly with rigors, especially if the inflammation has spread to the bile ducts (infective or suppurative cholangitis). Leucocytosis, with a relative increase in the polymorphonuclear cells, would indicate that in addition to gallstones there is *empyema of the gallbladder* demanding urgent surgical treatment.

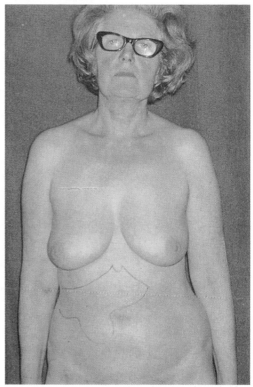

Fig. G.1. Courvoisier's law. Obstructive jaundice due to a carcinoma of the head of the pancreas. The liver is smoothly enlarged due to biliary obstruction. The gallbladder forms a globular palpable mass at its lower border.

Another cause of empyema of the gallbladder, albeit rare, is *typhoid fever*. The diagnosis is not difficult as a rule, for in most of the cases there will be no question of new growth or of gallstones and the patient will have been suffering from a prolonged asthenic fever already diagnosed serologically. In some typhoid patients bacillary infection of the gallbladder causes it to enlarge rapidly even to the extent of rupturing spontaneously and causing general peritonitis. In less severe cases, the inflammatory products discharge themselves naturally by the bile passages.

Simple mucocele of the gallbladder is a relatively unusual event which results from impaction of a gallstone at the outlet of the gallbladder when it happens to be empty. The walls of this organ continue to secrete mucus so that it becomes greatly distended with perfectly colourless mucoid liquid, free from bile pigment though sometimes containing crystals of cholesterol. The fluid is sterile. There are usually no symptoms. Such a mucocele may be mistaken for a mobile kidney. Usually the differential diagnosis can be established by radiological examination (cholecystography or intravenous urography) or by ultrasound or computerized tomography. However, the diagnosis of the nature of the mass is sometimes obscure until revealed by operation.

Harold Ellis

Gangrene

Gangrene means death of a part of the body from deprivation of its blood supply with superadded bacterial infection of the dead tissues. Ischaemia without infection results in a sterile infarction. This obstruction to the blood vessels may be mechanical, infective, degenerative, spasmodic or neoplastic.

Common causes of gangrene

TRAUMA

Division of the main artery to a limb, or pressure by splints or plaster-of-Paris. The effect of extreme heat or cold—frostbite, etc.

DISEASES OF THE BLOOD VESSELS

Embolism, thrombosis, Buerger's disease (thromboangiitis obliterans), Raynaud's disease, arteriosclerosis, venous gangrene.

INFECTION

Carbuncle, 'gas gangrene', etc. (Both arteriosclerotic and infective gangrene are common in diabetes mellitus.)

Less common causes

TRAUMA

Electric shock, chemical burns.

INFECTION

Septic wounds, erysipelas, anthrax, cancrum oris.

Complicating the following diseases and due to slight trauma

The typhoids, typhus, measles, marasmus, cholera, plague, yellow fever, malaria, poisoning by snake venom, leukaemias.

Neuropathic

Peripheral neuritis, syringomyelia, tabes dorsalis, leprosy, myelitis, meningomyelitis, lesions of the medulla spinalis.

Circulatory

Rheumatoid arteritis, syphilitic endarteritis, ergotism, erythromelalgia, carbolic dressings, aneurysm, polyarteritis nodosa, systemic lupus erythematosus, intraarterial injection of barbiturates and other drugs, obstruction by new growth, following carbonmonoxide poisoning.

The clinical picture of gangrene is exemplified best in the extremities. Here the failing blood supply is often first manifest by cramps in the muscles on exercise (intermittent claudication), and cyanosis of the toes or fingers, which may be colder than normal. Later, in the case of the legs, there is pain at rest, especially in bed at night when the warm environment raises the metabolic requirements of the part beyond that with which the inadequate circulation is able to cope. Finally some minor trauma, such as friction from a tight shoe or irritation from a protruding nail in the shoe, enables ingress of bacteria and gangrene supervenes. The toes, heel and malleoli are especial sites for trauma and hence for commencement of the gangrenous process.

Adjacent to the dead area there is a zone of inflammatory hyperaemia (*Fig.* G.2.) distal to which a definite line of demarcation eventually develops. This classic picture is modified in different sites, and dependent upon the presence and degree of infection, so that it will be necessary now to examine the individual causes of gangrene and see how these may be differentiated according to the clinical picture presented.

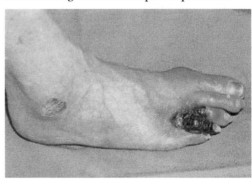

Fig. G.2. Gangrene of the foot, due to arteriosclerotic arterial obliteration.

It is of paramount importance to confirm or exclude the diagnosis of associated diabetes mellitus in all cases of gangrene (*Fig.* G.3.).

Trauma

The diagnosis of the pathology of traumatic gangrene can rarely give rise to any difficulty in that the history will betray the cause. Nevertheless, it may be important to ascertain *where* the vascular obstruction has occurred, and, although there are exceptions, it may

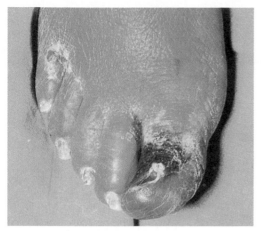

Fig. G.3. Diabetic gangrene.

be stated that where the distal half of the foot becomes gangrenous the obstruction is probably in the region of the popliteal artery; when the gangrene affects the lower half of the leg, the obstruction is at about the level of the bifurcation of the common femoral artery, observations which hold good whatever may have been the cause of the obstruction.

Diseases of the blood vessels

EMBOLUS

Gangrene due to embolism will be sudden in its inception and rapid in its onset. The embolus is commonly from vegetations on cardiac valves from a thrombus within the left atrium associated with mitral stenosis and atrial fibrillation, and occasionally from thrombi forming on the wall of the left ventricle after a coronary thrombosis, or from atheromatous plaques detached from large-bore vessels proximal to the site of the obstruction. The condition must be differentiated from acute thrombosis. Both may require urgent surgery, but an embolus is treated by balloon embolectomy whereas acute thrombosis may necessitate urgent end-arterectomy or a by-pass procedure.

If, in a case of acute onset, the heart is known to be diseased and the valves known to have vegetations, while the peripheral vascular system is normal, the diagnosis of embolism may be made with confidence and the only problem of diagnosis is to ascertain precisely where the embolus has lodged. If, on the other hand, the patient is known, or can be shown, to have atheromatous disease of the peripheral vessels then the case may be one of embolism or acute thrombosis, and arteriography is necessary to differentiate between the two, the filling defect in an embolism showing a smooth, rounded outline like a cigar butt, that of acute thrombosis being irregular and merging indefinitely with the jagged outline of the locally diseased vessels.

The diagnosis as to *where* the embolism has lodged depends partly on clinical signs and symptoms, but in the last analysis upon arteriography which, if the limb is to be saved, should be performed upon these cases of acute vascular obstruction, in the first place to exclude acute thrombosis, and in the second to localize the obstruction with precision. Nevertheless, the level of the developing gangrene (*see below*) will be of some help, particularly if it be remembered that emboli commonly ride astride a vessel at its point of bifurcation. The site of the initial pain may be misleading and attempts should always be made, by palpating along the course of a vessel, to find at what point the pulse is lost.

THROMBOSIS

Gangrene from this cause is usually of slow onset and always accompanies localized arterial disease, which latter may of itself have already obstructed the blood supply to a considerable extent; in fact the final occlusion, whatever the underlying pathology, is almost invariably due to thrombosis. Cases of acute thrombosis can only be diagnosed from embolism by arteriography (*see above*).

Venous gangrene is rare but is seen occasionally in the foot in severe cases of iliofemoral venous thrombosis (*Fig.* G.4).

BUERGER'S DISEASE (THROMBO-ANGIITIS OBLITERANS)

This disease affects the medium-sized arteries, chiefly of the lower extremity, and usually in men under the age of 45. Heavy smoking is invariable and the condition is more common in Eastern Europeans than in other population groups. The first symptom of vascular insufficiency is generally intermittent claudication and later rest pain at night in bed. There are often minor attacks of superficial thrombophlebitis. Examination of the affected leg may show absence of pulsations in the line of the dorsalis pedis and posterior tibial arteries. In advanced cases the popliteal pulse is also absent, but femoral pulsations usually persist indefinitely. The affected foot and toes are at first blue and cold; later gangrene of one or more toes ensues.

Buerger's disease usually affects both legs eventually, although, one being slightly worse than the other, the intermittent claudication in the more advanced leg brings the patient to a halt and masks the symptoms which would otherwise soon develop on the other side. In very advanced cases the upper limbs are also affected and very occasionally the upper limbs may

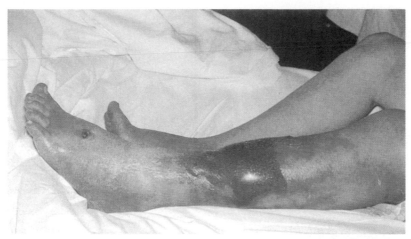

Fig. G.4. Gangrene secondary to iliofemoral venous thrombosis.

be the first to suffer. Smoking is absolutely forbidden in these cases as nicotine aggravates the condition.

RAYNAUD'S PHENOMENON

This may be primary Raynaud's disease, almost invariably in young females, or Raynaud's phenomenon, secondary to some other lesion, e.g. scleroderma (*see below*), polyarteritis nodosa or other collagen diseases; it may occur in patients with cryoglobulinaemia, or it can result in men working with vibrating tools. It is important to exclude other causes of cold, cyanosed hands, for instance pressure on the subclavian artery from a cervical rib or main vessel occlusion from arteriosclerosis or Buerger's disease.

As a result of exposure to cold, the fingers become white and later slate-blue. As they are 'thawed out' they change from a livid purple to deep red, this cycle being readily precipitated by plunging the hands into a basin of cold water. Because the disease affects only the terminal vessels, the radial pulse is normal and, in those cases where the toes are affected, the dorsalis pedis and posterior tibial pulsations are not lost. The disease, as might be expected, is subject to exacerbations in the winter and remissions in the summer, but at least for some years is gradually progressive so that, in a severe case, the tips of the fingers become gangrenous (*Fig*. G.5). Raynaud's phenomenon is commonly associated with *scleroderma*, in which the skin over the fingers becomes thickened and stiff so that they are held immobile in a position of semiflexion; and microstomia, a similar condition affecting the skin of the face and causing, as the name implies, a contraction of the mouth with radiating creases at the corners, together with pinching of the nostrils. Disappearance of the distal half of the distal phalanges causes shortening of the fingers and this effect is well demonstrated

radiologically. In addition there may be calcinosis, or the deposit of calcium salts in the subcutaneous tissues.

ARTERIOSCLEROSIS

This term is used here to cover the degenerative process which affect the arteries with age. In a proportion of cases the arterial deprivation is sufficiently severe to produce gangrene (almost invariably in heavy smokers), and in this event it is usually the lower limb which is affected, and the stages of intermittent claudication and rest pain are passed through just as in Buerger's disease. In fact the condition mimics Buerger's disease very closely apart from the age of onset, which is usually over 50, the presence of calcification in the arteries which may be shown-up by radiographs, and other evidences of vascular degeneration as revealed by palpation of the brachial artery or by retinoscopy. Just as in Buerger's disease, too, the peripheral pulsations are lost progressively in the leg, but the femoral pulses are usually retained. Sooner or later an embolus or more often thrombus (*see above*) may completely occlude the already constricted vessel and gangrene will rapidly ensue. Diagnosis can be confirmed by femoral arteriography, which will also enable the surgeon to decide if vascular reconstruction is possible surgically (by endarterectomy, balloon angioplasty or by-pass graft).

Infective gangrene

The inclusion of carbuncle, cancrum oris and 'gas-gangrene' together with the causes of gangrene hitherto described is such a well-established convention that no account of this syndrome is held to be complete without mentioning them. Nevertheless, carbuncle, cancrum oris, 'gas-gangrene' and other acute infections with thrombosis of the surrounding vessels

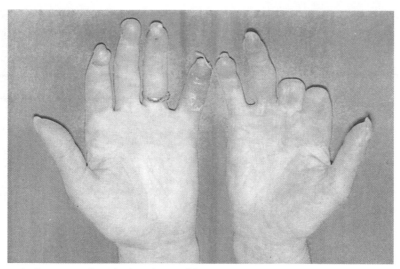

Fig. G.5. Raynaud's disease. Note loss of pulp and parts of fingers.

are distinct clinical entities and are hardly likely to be confused with other types of gangrene.

Listed above, under the heading 'Less Common Causes' are mostly those conditions in which gangrene is an incidental complication of a clinical picture otherwise coloured by the primary condition; or, on the other hand, local causes, such as carbolic acid dressings and the accidental injection of pentothal sodium into an artery, where the diagnosis is clear cut. Finally, it may be explained that a degree of trauma, which under normal conditions would produce little in the way of tissue damage, may, where the body is wearied by infection or racked by the torments of an unsuitable environment, lead to widespread gangrene. In this connection one may recall the fate of the slight injury to the finger of Evans on Captain Scott's second polar expedition, or the high incidence of *sphacelatio* which complicated the epidemics (? typhoid, ? typhus) ravaging the armies of Rome in their North African campaigns against the Numidians, or later, the similar fate which befell the invading French Armies of 1848, when the conditions in Algeria so decimated their ranks and gangrene was so common that the whole venture ended in catastrophe.

Ergotism

This now rare cause of gangrene arises from frequent ingestion of rye bread made from infected grain attacked by *Claviceps purpura*. The fingers are affected more frequently than the toes. Nowadays this phenomenon, once called 'St Anthony's fire', is more likely to be seen following excessive use of ergotamine for migraine.

Harold Ellis

GRIMACE
See FACE, ABNORMALITIES OF APPEARANCE AND MOVEMENT.

Grip, disturbances of

Man's privileged position in the animal kingdom is attributable to his prehensile upper limbs as well as to his superior brain. Our capacity to grip enables us to lift, carry, climb and handle tools. In terms of functional anatomy, grip depends primarily on the long flexor muscles of the fingers and the opposition of the thumb to the other digits. The latter movement is possible because the metacarpal bone of the thumb lies in a plane at right angles to that of the other metacarpals and because the carpo-metacarpal joint of the thumb has such a wide range of movement. Flexion thus carries the thumb medially across the palm in opposition to the other fingers.

Grip is impaired by any lesion affecting the motor supply of muscles of the forearm and hand. Thus upper motor neurone lesions in corticospinal pathways, radicular lesions affecting C7, C8 and T1 roots, and peripheral nerve lesions, may all result in weakness of grip (*see* MONOPLEGIA). As regards single peripheral nerve lesions, it is noteworthy that whilst median or ulnar nerve palsies can affect grip, the greatest disability results from an isolated radial nerve palsy. This is because without fixation of the wrist in extension, the grip becomes ineffectual.

Apart from purely motor lesions, grip can obviously be impaired also by severe incoordination, dystonia, involuntary movement or sensory deprivation. It may also be affected by disease of joints or muscles although, in general, muscle disease tends to be of proximal rather than distal distribution.

D. A. Shaw

Groin, swellings in

The general surgical clinic would seem incomplete without a number of patients with swellings in the groin whose diagnosis depends almost entirely on history and physical examination. As many of the patients are not urgent they become ideal subjects for both undergraduate and postgraduate examinations, particularly as they demonstrate the need for careful classification of the likely pathologies.

Anatomy

The groin is a region not easily defined anatomically but which may be divided into the inguinal and femoral regions by the inguinal ligament (not the groin crease). Swellings above the medial part of the inguinal ligament might be described as *inguinal* with those below the ligament *femoral*. The femoral triangle is more easily described as it is bounded by the inguinal ligament above, the medial border of the sartorius laterally and the medial border of adductor longus medially. These boundaries are not apparent in obese patients but the anterior-superior iliac spine and the pubic tubercle, representing the two ends of the inguinal ligament, allow most groin swellings to be appropriately classified. The mid-point of the inguinal ligament, above which lies the internal inguinal ring, can easily be identified and should not be confused with the *mid-inguinal point* which bisects the line drawn between the anterior-superior iliac spine and the pubic symphysis. Deep to this latter point, the external iliac artery passes beneath the inguinal ligament to become the common femoral artery (*Fig.* G.6.) These anatomical points should always be used as the groin skin crease may vary considerably, sometimes by as much as 5 cm in obese patients.

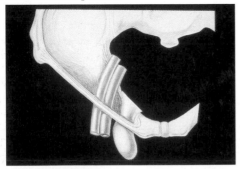

Fig. G.6. Anatomy of the groin.

Classification

As there are many potential causes, it is logical to classify groin swellings by the structures from which

they may arise. Within the various structures the potential pathologies may also be classified as congenital, acquired, traumatic, inflammatory or neoplastic in the usual way (*Table* G.1).

Table G.1. Classification of groin swellings according to tissues of origin

1. Skin and subcutaneous tissue
Sebaceous cyst
Lipoma
Neurofibroma

2. Lymphadenopathy
Reactive or inflammatory
Metastatic abscess
Metastatic tumour
Lymphoma

3. Body wall
Simple inguinal bulge
Inguinal hernia
Femoral hernia

4. Arteries and veins
Femoral aneurysm
Saphena varix

5. Miscellaneous
Abscess
Low appendix mass pelvic/inguinal fossa tumours
Hip pathology

A classification such as this enables a considered and complete assessment of any groin swelling. In practice by far the most common are inguinal or femoral hernias, lymphadenopathy and saphena varices whose features will be described in more detail.

SKIN AND SUBCUTANEOUS TISSUES

Sebaceous cysts are considerably less common in the groin than they are on the scrotum. Benign skin polyps, papillomas and pendunculated lipomas are all frequent in this region and may be easily diagnosed by their typical features. Other skin pathology may occur, as anywhere in the body, but are infrequent. Lipomas represent by far the most frequent swellings arising from the subcutaneous tissue and may also be found in the inguinal canal, although these may merely represent herniating extraperitoneal fat. Occasionally a minor injury may result in fat necrosis where a firm lump of saponified fat may initially be tender with features of inflammation that may be confused with either an inflamed and irreducible hernia or an abscess. This should be resolved by a careful history and examination but where a firm tender lump is related to the inguinal or femoral canal, exploration may be the safer option.

LYMPHATICS

There are three groups of lymph nodes in the groin. The inguinal nodes lie in the subcutaneous tissue just below and occasionally anterior to the inguinal ligament and drain the external genitals, the perineum and anus, the lower abdomen, buttock and upper third of thigh. The femoral nodes are around and below the sapheno-femoral junction and drain the lower two-thirds of the lower limb. The iliac nodes lie above and deep to the inguinal ligament and follow the iliac artery. They drain from the femoral and inguinal nodes but also may become enlarged secondary to intra-abdominal or pelvic pathology.

Groin lymphadenopathy is usually multiple but a large single node near the femoral canal may be confused with a femoral hernia. Essentially the causes of lymphadenopathy may be classified as either inflammatory or neoplastic and by custom non-specific inflammatory lymphadenopathy is described as *reactive* (Table G.2.)

Table G.2. Common causes of lymphadenopathy

A. Inflammatory

Non-specific (reactive)
Mechanical irritation
Septic foci in the feet, legs, genitalia or perineum
Part of generalized lymphadenopathy (e.g. viral)

Specific
Tuberculosis lymphogranuloma inguinalae
Cat scratch fever
Syphilis

B. Neoplasms

Primary non-Hodgkin lymphoma
Low, intermediate or high grade

Hodgkin's lymphoma
Lymphocyte predominant
Nodular sclerosing
Mixed cellular
Lymphocyte depleted

Metstatic carcinoma
Malignant melanoma
Squamous cell carcinoma
  Penis
  Scrotum
  Anal canal
  Lower limb skin

Inflammatory lymphadenopathy

There is usually a history of an inflammatory lesion involving the tissue drained by the relevant lymph nodes. This may appear trivial and the lymphadenopathy may continue for up to 3-4 weeks following resolution of the initial cause. In the early phase the node may feel indurated and tender, following which it becomes firm and softens as it resolves. Reactive lymphadenopathy may be single or multiple but the nodes usually feel discrete. Should resolution fail to occur over 3-4 weeks then biopsy becomes important to identify specific infections or malignancy.

SPECIFIC INFECTIONS

Tuberculous lymphadenopathy is now uncommon in the groin but may be associated with a chronic sore on the foot or leg which had not been recognized as tuberculous. The nodes are indurated but with little signs of inflammation in the overlying skin. They tend to become hard and usually do not suppurate or ulcerate for months. Ultimately chronic discharging sinuses will form.

Syphilitic nodes are hard and, like lymphogranuloma inguinale and other venereal infections, extremely uncommon in this country. On histology *Spirochaeta pallida* may be identified but serology may occasionally be negative. Frei's serological test is positive in lymphogranuloma inguinale.

GENERALIZED LYMPHADENOPATHY

A range of viral infections will cause generalized lymphadenopathy but when sustained over weeks with ill-health and malaise the Paul Bunnell antibody reaction may be requested where infectious mononucleosis is suspected. In modern practice toxoplasmosis and other causes of lymphadenopathy related to AIDS should be considered. In these cases the appearance and feel of the lymph nodes are similar to that with other reactive lymphadenopathies, but in AIDS lymphadenopathy is more common in the neck and axillae. Where generalized lymphadenopathy fails to settle within 2-3 weeks and serology is negative for both infectious mononucleosis and AIDS then biopsy may be indicated. Histology is more reliable if a node is taken from the neck or axilla.

Neoplastic lymphadenopathy

Relentlessly progressive lymphadenopathy requires urgent biopsy as neoplastic disease is very much more common than specific infections.

LYMPHOMA

The clinical features of both Hodgkin's and non-Hodgkin's lymphomas are similar but in non-Hodgkin's lymphoma the nodes may be hard and more closely resembling those of metastatic carcinoma. In Hodgkin's lymphoma the nodes often have a typical rubbery feel and may be matted together such that a clinical diagnosis can be quite confident. The diagnosis is confirmed by biopsy which should include an intact node taken, if possible, from a region other than the groin. Once the diagnosis has been confirmed then the extent of the disease should be fully identified (staging) by further investigations which include chest X-ray and CT scanning of chest and abdomen.

Metastatic carcinoma

Firm, hard nodes that grow into a confluent fixed mass as the disease progresses are typical of metastatic carcinoma which may be confirmed by either biopsy or needle aspiration cytology. If the primary has not been identified then a careful search must be performed for primary lesions in the territory drained by the relevant lymphatics. This includes rectal examination with proctoscopy and sigmoidoscopy, careful examination of the perineum and scrotum and a thorough search of the legs, feet and between the toes. Occasionally in melanoma the primary lesion may resolve despite rapidly progressive metastatic melanoma in the regional lymph nodes.

Body wall

Groin hernias are the most frequent type of hernia and may give rise to a number of acute complications. They are distinguished by simple clinical features readily identified on examination.

Inguinal hernia

The inguinal hernia is by far the most common variety of hernia. Approximately 3–5 per cent of the population have some variety of hernia with 70–75 per cent of these being inguinal. Inguinal hernias are very much more common in men and represent over 90 per cent of all hernias in men. In women, inguinal hernias are also nearly twice as common as femoral hernias although there is a misconception that as femoral hernias commonly occur in women they are also more common than inguinal hernias.

Most groin hernias present as a soft lump in the groin that may be associated with local pain or discomfort on standing, lifting or after heavy work. The clinical features of an inguinal hernia are of a lump arising just superior to the lower one third of the inguinal ligament. Most hernias are reducible, in which case there will be an impulse on coughing. In small hernias the sensation of reduction is perhaps the most reliable clinical sign confirming the presence of a hernia. This sensation of reduction helps to distinguish a genuine hernia from the bulge throughout the inguinal canal which is so often seen in thin men (Malgaigne's bulges) and which has little significance.

ANATOMY

The inguinal canal is formed by the descent of the testis from the posterior abdominal wall during early development and passes obliquely through the anterior abdominal wall extending from the internal inguinal ring at the mid-point of the inguinal ligament to the external inguinal ring just above the pubic tubercle. The anterior wall is formed by the external oblique aponeurosis and incorporates the lower-most fibres of the internal oblique at the internal ring. Inferiorly there is the inguinal ligament and posteriorly the transversalis fascia reinforced medially by the fibres of the conjoint tendon. The internal oblique and transversus muscles arch over the canal superiorly. Indirect inguinal herniae arise through the internal ring passing into what is probably a congenital sac consisting of a persistent or patent processus vaginalis. Direct inguinal herniae occur as a result of weakness in the posterior wall of the inguinal canal medial to the inferior epigastric artery which passes in the medial border of the internal ring.

CLINICAL FEATURES

The vast majority of patients notice a lump in the groin which may be asymptomatic or cause an aching or dragging sensation (*Fig.* G.7.) Occasionally the presenting symptoms are those of small-bowel obstruction when bowel herniates and then becomes stuck in the sac with oedema and obstruction at the hernia ring. A local, irreducible and acutely inflamed lump suggests either inflammation in an irreducible hernia or strangulation of the hernial contents which may be extraperitoneal fat, omentum or intestine.

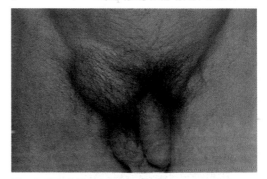

Fig. G.7. Right inguinal hernia.

Inguinal herniae in infants and children

These are almost invariably indirect with 90 per cent in boys. The lump may be noticed by the mother while bathing the child or when the child is straining, coughing or upset, or may be detected either during the postnatal examination or as the child first starts to walk. It is frequently difficult to demonstrate the hernia in the clinic but a clear history from the mother is sufficient to make a confident diagnosis. As there is a definite risk of obstruction and strangulation the surgeon should not refrain from exploring the affected side where an appropriate and reliable history can be obtained. The differential diagnosis consists of a hydrocele, encysted hydrocele of the cord, undescended testis or torsion of the testis.

Inguinal hernia in adults

Essentially adults may have either indirect or direct inguinal hernias with sliding hernias representing a variety, usually indirect, in which an adjacent partly peritonealized organ herniates as part of the hernia sac wall. This usually involves the caecum, the sigmoid colon or the bladder.

INDIRECT HERNIAS

These arise from the internal ring lateral to the inferior epigastric vessels and pass down the inguinal canal within the cord. Frequently they pass down into the scrotum and may reach substantial size (*Fig. G.8.*) This variety of hernia is ten times more frequent in men than women and is more common than the direct variety. It is identified by an impulse passing obliquely from lateral to medial as the hernia is produced on coughing and by the sensation of reduction in the line of the inguinal canal on gentle pressure. Once the hernia is reduced it can be controlled by digital pressure over the internal ring even with the patient standing or coughing. A finger gently introduced from the upper scrotum into the neck of the inguinal canal at the external ring may identify filling from above and laterally rather than from posteriorly.

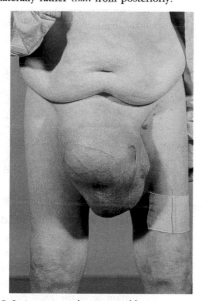

Fig. G.8. A massive indirect inguinal hernia.

DIRECT INGUINAL HERNIA

This variety of hernia is extremely rare under the age of 40 and typically presents in the elderly. A bulge is identified over the most medial part of the inguinal ligament which may reach sizeable proportions but rarely descends into the scrotum (*Fig.* G.7.) It is uncommon for direct hernias to obstruct and they usually have an obvious and prominent cough impulse which appears to come directly out through the body wall rather than obliquely in the line of the inguinal canal.

The differential diagnosis of inguinal herniae include encysted hydroceles of the cord, herniated extraperitoneal fat or lipomas of the cord, inguinal lymphadenopathy, ectopic testis and femoral hernias. The inguinal hernia is best distinguished from the femoral hernia by carefully identifying the pubic tubercle where the insertion of the inguinal ligament can usually be felt. The inguinal hernia arises above the inguinal ligament, passing over this point towards the medial side. The femoral hernia, which may appear to fold over the inguinal ligament, can be felt to arise in its deeper part from the femoral canal below and lateral to a finger on the pubic tubercle.

Femoral hernia

Although relatively common as a cause of small-bowel obstruction, femoral hernias are less common than inguinal, incisional and paraumbilical hernias, representing only 3–5 per cent of all hernias. They are two to three times more common in women than men so that femoral hernias do represent over 20 per cent of all hernias in women. They more frequently occur on the right side and over 30 per cent present with a complication such as obstruction or strangulation.

ANATOMY

The femoral hernia descends through the femoral canal bordered medially by the lacunar ligament, posteriorly by the iliopectineal band and anteriorly by the inguinal ligament. As these three rigid walls limit femoral canal expansion, which can only occur by displacing the femoral vein laterally, there is a definite risk that the hernia will become irreducible, obstructed or strangulate. The sac then descends to the saphena-femoral junction where least resistance turns the hernia forwards and upwards to lie anterior and sometimes even extends above the inguinal ligament (*Fig.* G.9.).

CLINICAL FEATURES

Femoral herniation is rare before late adult life. It may present as a firm or even rubbery lump in the groin which often represents no more than herniated extraperitoneal fat together with the tissue accumulated around the sac as it descends through the femoral canal and up through the cribriform fascia. As a result, the hernial sac can almost invariably be palpated in the upper medial femoral triangle even when the contents are reduced. It is unusual to feel a cough impulse in a femoral hernia unless it contains omentum or gut which is freely reducible. An irreducible hernia,

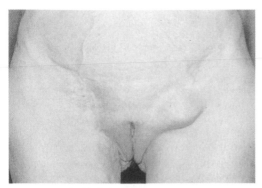

Fig. G.9. Irreducible femoral hernia.

particularly in the presence of obstruction or strangulation will be tender, tense, often inflamed and will not have a cough impulse. On careful palpation of the pubic tubercle the neck of the sac may be felt below and lateral as it passes under the inguinal ligament.

Vascular swellings

Vascular swellings in the groin should be easily recognized and yet the saphena varix is often mistaken for a femoral hernia. Aneurysms of the common femoral artery are relatively rare and most frequently seen following previous arterial surgery as a pseudoaneurysm (*Fig.* G.10.) Occasionally an inflamed pseudoaneurysm or mycotic aneurysm may present in a drug addict who has used the femoral artery for vascular access. The diagnostic importance of this is that it may be mistaken for an abscess with catastrophic results when drainage is attempted.

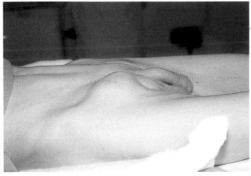

Fig. G.10. Pseudoaneurysm in the right groin 8 years following aorto-bifemoral bypass using a Dacron graft.

Saphena varix

ANATOMY

The saphena varix develops when there is incompetence of the saphena femoral junction and long saphenous system. The proximal part of the long saphenous becomes dilated where reflux of turbulent

blood impinges on the anterior wall of the vein. It lies in the upper femoral triangle just below the usual location for a femoral hernia and just medial to the femoral pulse.

CLINICAL FEATURES

A saphena varix is only visible or palpable when the patient stands and disappears on lying. A cough impulse is pronounced and is usually associated with a fluid thrill which clearly feels different from the impulse in a hernia. On compression the swelling collapses completely and reappears immediately the finger is withdrawn. Almost invariably there are varicose veins in the distribution of the long saphenous vein from which a tap impulse may be transmitted into the saphena varix.

Femoral aneurysm

Aneurysms of the femoral artery are not common but usually involve the common femoral just above its bifurcation. Atherosclerotic aneurysms rarely cause symptoms but occasionally thrombose spontaneously with resulting acute ischaemia or claudication. More worrying are pseudoaneurysms following bypass to the groin using prosthetic grafts such as Dacron which may expand rapidly and rupture. Needle puncture (often iatrogenic during arteriography) may result in pseudoaneurysm formation or, in drug addicts, mycotic aneurysm.

ANATOMY

The common femoral artery lies immediately below and medial to the mid-point of the inguinal ligament. Aneurysms rarely extend into the profunda or superficial femoral artery and resulting bleeding tends to involve the groin tissues, spreading up and down in the line of the inguinal canal promoting swelling and bruising of the scrotum or labia.

CLINICAL FEATURES

In the absence of inflammation the diagnosis is obvious with easily palpated pulsation. A rapidly expanding pseudoaneurysm or more particularly mycotic aneurysm may be mistaken for an abscess. Gentle palpation through the induration will always reveal substantial and abnormal pulsation. Occasionally there may be swelling of the distal limb due to compression of the vein or lymphatics.

Miscellaneous

ABSCESS

Groin abscesses are not infrequent and may arise primarily from skin or subcutaneous infection, by metastasis to the regional lymph nodes or by extension from the hip, sacroiliac joint or lumbar spine in chronic abscesses.

In achieving a diagnosis a careful search must be made for a primary source of infection either from the toes, foot or leg or from the scrotal or perineal skin including the perianal region.

CHRONIC ABSCESS

Abscesses from the retroperitoneum, either arising from skeletal structures or occasionally from appendicitis or regional enteritis may track down the psoas sheath to point just below the inguinal ligament. An abscess such as this must be distinguished from a femoral hernia as incision into an irreducible or strangulating femoral hernia will almost certainly result in fistula formation. Aspiration may aid in the diagnosis, remembering that occasionally tuberculosis infection of the spine or fallopian tubes may present in this way as may actinomycosis of the appendix, which is now extremely rare.

A number of rarer lumps may develop in the groin including all the usual soft tissue or mesenchymal tumours that may occur in any other part of the body such as a neurofibroma or neurolemmoma. These are rare in the groin and more usually extend from pelvic tumours. An ectopic testis may be felt in the region of the external inguinal ring where they occasionally lie superficial to the inguinal ligament, in the upper femoral triangle or just above and lateral to the scrotum. This diagnosis may be suspected when the testis is absent in the scrotum and is usually obvious as the patient recognizes the sensation on gentle compression.

C. McCollum

Gums, bleeding

Bleeding from the gums is a common complaint and the predominant underlying local cause is infection, both bacterial and viral, as the induced inflammatory response renders the mucosa very susceptible to minor trauma. The coexistence of systemic disease can exacerbate this gingival inflammation or may even initiate it through a reduced resistance to infection or a defect in blood coagulation.

Dental diseases

Periodontal disease is almost endemic within the human race. The most significant factor is poor oral hygiene, leading to the accumulation of food debris and bacteria in the supporting tissues, which subsequently becomes organized into dental plaque and calculus. Bacterial toxins cause destruction of the periodontal ligament supporting the teeth; pockets form, where further bacteria may accumulate. Slow progressive destruction and infection of the supporting tissues follow. The gingival mucosa becomes swollen and hyperaemic, leading to a reluctance to clean the teeth which aids further infection. Any minor trauma to this swollen and inflamed mucosa, such as mastication or toothbrushing, causes bleeding. There may also be a purulent discharge from the necks of the teeth and the breath smells unpleasant (*Fig.* G.11.)

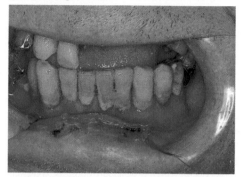

Fig. G.11. Gingival erythema due to chronic periodontal disease.

Dental caries, when present, may be obvious to the naked eye, or, less conspicuously between the teeth or beneath the gingival mucosa. This also allows an accumulation of bacteria leading to localized infection and, again, gingival hyperaemia and haemorrhage.

If both these conditions are left untreated then eventually abscess formation will occur which is discussed in the section JAW, SWELLING OF.

Blood dyscrasias

Abnormal or defective bone marrow activity as in aplastic anaemia, or neoplastic infiltration, will cause bleeding of the gums due to a reduced resistance to infection and a reduction in the number of circulating platelets. The gingival mucosa becomes acutely inflamed, swollen and bleeds readily. In acute leukaemia the swelling is also due to the local accumulation of leukaemic cells in the gingival tissues. Thrombocytopenia also occurs as part of marrow disorders any of which may give rise to purpura in the oral cavity. Purpuric spots may best be seen in the hard and soft palates and haemorrhage from the gums occurs readily. In the mucosal tissues of the cheeks and lips, where the surface epithelium is not so tightly bound down to the underlying supporting connective tissue, large ecchymoses may be found.

The coagulation defect in haemophilia and von Willebrand's disease may cause spontaneous haemorrhage within the oral tissues and may be particularly troublesome after dental extraction unless appropriate measures are taken.

Disorders of blood vessels

Scurvy can be conveniently discussed under this heading, as the main defect is of abnormal collagen production causing capillary fragility. There is also a general lack of tissue resistance which, in the gingival mucosa, may lead to superimposed infection. It is probably this latter aspect which produces the majority of the gingival enlargement characteristic of the disease, as in the presence of good oral hygiene the swelling is far less marked. Whilst scurvy in the developed world is now an uncommon disease, it can still be found amongst old and neglected people with a restricted diet and, in people who for dietary reasons reduce their input of food containing ascorbic acid. It may also be found in alcoholics and patients with peptic ulceration existing on a milk diet.

Hereditary haemorrhagic telangiectasia (*Fig.* G.12.) is caused by a capillary abnormality and the head and neck region is a common site. In the mouth these abnormal vessels are visible through the mucous membrane and minor trauma may produce a persistent haemorrhage, which is difficult to control. Von Willebrand's disease and Henoch-Schölein purpura both may occur in the oral cavity but are not a predominant feature of the disease.

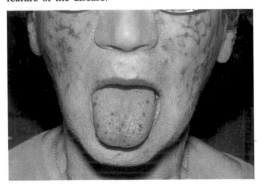

Fig. G.12. Hereditary haemorrhagic telangiectasia.

Chemical poisoning

Mercury was previously used in the treatment of syphilis and frequently produced a severe acute stomatitis with profuse salivation, halitosis and painful swellings of the lips, gums, tongue and cheeks. The patient suffered a metallic taste and the regional lymph nodes could be involved. This method of treatment has long been discontinued but poisoning can still occasionally occur from industrial exposure. The gums become hyperaemic and tend to bleed which, as always, is aggravated by poor oral hygiene. Eventually necrosis of the gingival mucosa may occur.

Phosphorus was at one time responsible for severe stomatitis, going on to necrosis of the jaw— 'phossy jaw'—not infrequently ending in death as the result of fatty degeneration of the liver and heart. Since restrictions are now laid upon the use of crude yellow phosphorus in the manufacture of matches it is now almost unknown. Apart from occupation, the patient may, with suicidal intent, have been taking a rat paste or other vermin-killer containing phosphorus.

Arsenic and *lead* are rare causes of gingival bleeding and usually arise from industrial contamination. The gingivae are again inflamed, swollen and bleed easily and, in the case of lead, there is a characteristic blue line at the gingival margin known as the Burtonian line. Other signs of poisoning may be present, particularly pigmentation of the skin, vomiting, diarrhoea, hyperkeratosis of the soles of the feet and the palms of the hands. Generalized peripheral neuritis may be found in the case of arsenic and the symptoms given under anaemia in the case of lead. Arsenic may be found in excess in the hair, or lead may be detected in the faeces, or in the urine.

Pregnancy

The hormonal changes which take place during pregnancy may have the effect of exacerbating a pre-existing gingivitis. Generalized swelling of the gingival mucosa may occur, or it may be confined to one papilla, giving rise to a pregnancy tumour (*Fig.* G.13). Histologically this tissue consists of immature granulation tissue and is extremely vascular. Haemorrhage readily occurs and, provided the diagnosis is certain, all that is necessary are oral hygiene measures, as once the pregnancy is completed, the vascular tissue will recede. Isolated lesions which, however, remain should be excised.

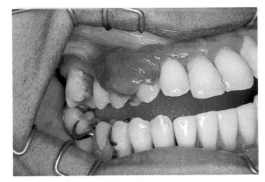

Fig. G.13. 'Pregnancy tumour'.

Malabsorption

Patients with malabsorption may show signs of anaemia in the mouth with a red and swollen tongue and pallor of the mucosa. In addition to this, the gingival mucosa may haemorrhage readily.

Iatrogenic

Overdose with the drug Warfarin may produce spontaneous bleeding of the oral mucosa and will require vitamin K preparations or transfusion of fresh frozen plasma to arrest the haemorrhage. In the mouth with pre-existing gingivitis, the drug phenytoin, used in the control of epilepsy, may produce hypertrophy of the gingival mucosa, predominantly involving the interdental papillae. Regular maintenance of good oral hygiene becomes very difficult and further secondary infection supervenes. At this stage, the gingival mucosa becomes inflamed and is associated with local haemorrhage. Treatment is through scaling and polishing of the teeth and the maintenance of good oral hygiene but, in some cases it may be necessary to withdraw the drug or excise the hyperplastic tissue.

Radiotherapy

Radiation to the oral cavity in the management of malignant tumours induces a severe mucositis of the oral mucosa, which is characterized by erythema, superficial ulceration and pain. Good oral hygiene is difficult to maintain and supra-infection, especially with candida may ensue. Spontaneous haemorrhage of the mucosa during mastication and tooth cleaning is not uncommon.

Chemotherapy

Because of their toxic effect on the bone marrow, cytotoxic agents may produce changes in the oral cavity similar to those which are seen with the blood dyscrasias.

Infection

The oral cavity is commonly involved in bacterial infection due to dental causes. However, generalized infection of the oral mucous membrane due to bacteria is rare, the majority being caused by viruses.

BACTERIAL

The most important example of the former is acute ulcerative gingivitis, which is characterized by a proliferation of Vincent's organisms, *Treponema vincentii* and *Fusiformis fusiformis*. The predominant features are bleeding of the gums, soreness and halitosis. There is a characteristic ulceration and blunting of the interdental papillae and there is considerable debris and slough in the gingival crevice. There may be an associated fever, malaise and regional lymphadenitis.

Infection may be associated with pre-existing poor oral hygiene and stress has also been implicated. It may also be a feature of patients with a reduced resistance to infection as in acute leukaemia, agranulocytosis and those undergoing cytotoxic chemotherapy.

In the African continent, the association with measles and the suppression of the immune system by malnutrition leading to cancrum oris is well described. Here, small areas of dark necrosis occur in the cheeks or lips, which rapidly progress to produce widespread necrosis and destruction of the circum-oral and oral structures.

VIRAL

Acute inflammation of the oral cavity occurs with viral infections, the most common being herpes simplex and herpes varicella-zoster. The primary infection with herpes simplex may often be subclinical, but if not then acute herpetic gingivostomatitis is encountered. This is characterized by severe inflammation and vesicle formation, leading to ulceration of the entire oral mucous membrane with constitutional symptoms of fever, malaise and enlargement of the regional lymph nodes.

The gingivae are acutely inflamed, swollen and bleed easily. The disease is usually self-limiting after a few days and only symptomatic relief is required and the maintenance of oral hygiene. Secondary infection of the vesicles may be prevented by chlorhexadine or tetracycline mouthwashes.

The reactivation of the herpes zoster virus (shingles) in the distribution of the trigeminal nerve may cause severe erythema, ulceration and haemorrhage of the oral mucosa in the exact distribution of the branch involved, usually the maxillary branch. The condition is again self-limiting and the intraoral lesions require only symptomatic relief, although one of the new antiviral agents may be valuable in the protracted case.

The Epstein–Barr virus (infectious mononucleosis) may cause a gingivostomatitis where the gingivae are characteristically red, swollen and haemorrhagic, similar to the appearance found in acute leukaemia or scurvy. Acute bacterial ulcerative gingivitis may follow. A high proportion of patients show petechiae in the soft palate, which, because it is so characteristic, is of diagnostic importance.

Autoimmune disease

The oral mucous membrane is frequently involved by autoimmune conditions whereby the mucosa undergoes superficial bullous formation followed by ulceration. This is invariably associated with inflammation, a degree of secondary infection and haemorrhage. The commonest is aphthous ulceration of the minor and major type, but the mouth is also not infrequently involved by systemic lupus erythematosus, pemphigus, mucous membrane pemphigoid, bullous erythema multiforme and epidermolysis bullosa. The auto-immune skin condition lichen planus frequently involves the mouth and the erosive type is associated with widespread ulceration and haemorrhage.

Neoplastic disease

The commonest malignant tumour of the oral cavity is the squamous cell carcinoma, which is liable to undergo central necrosis, producing ulceration and secondary infection. This may produce intermittent haemorrhage, especially if the tumour erodes one of the adjacent blood vessels.

Developmental lesions

The oral cavity may be involved by capillary or cavernous haemangiomas and on occasions lymphangiomas. All these lesions are liable to bleed with trauma and are particularly hazardous following dental extractions, should they involve the bone of the mandible or the maxilla.

Inflammation

The fibrous epulis, denture granuloma, pyogenic granuloma and the giant-cell epulis have a similar clinical and histological appearance. These soft-tissue swellings arise within the oral or gingival mucosa and consist of a fibrous tissue stroma which may be vascular and covered by squamous epithelium. These swellings when subjected to trauma will be a source of haemorrhage within the oral cavity.

P. T. Blenkinsopp

Gums, hypertrophy of

True hypertrophy of the gingival mucosa is relatively rare, accordingly, enlargement can conveniently be classified into that caused by predominantly *fibrous tissue* and that caused by a *cellular infiltration*. It should be remembered that the commonest cause of gingival enlargement is infection associated with the dental structures, and this is discussed in the sections on BLEEDING GUMS and JAW, SWELLING OF.

Fibrous infiltration

Hereditary gingival fibromatosis is a rare autosomal dominant condition in which all the gingival tissues become enlarged to such an extent that the teeth may become almost buried, and in the child will interfere with their eruption. Mucosal inflammation is not always a feature and treatment is by surgical reduction and the maintenance of good oral hygiene. There may, in addition, be hirsutism and thickening of the facial features, associated epilepsy and mental retardation.

A high proportion of patients taking the anticonvulsant drug phenytoin over a long period of time will develop fibrous hyperplasia of the gingival tissues but

this predominantly affects the interdental papillae (*Fig.* G.14.) Again, the enlargement may be such as partially to obscure the teeth from view and is made worse by the presence of chronic infection. In severe cases, it may be necessary to consider substituting a different drug; local measures consist of improving the oral hygiene and gingivectomy.

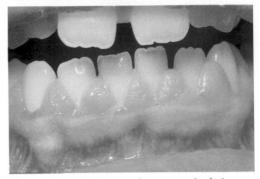

Fig. G.14. Gingival hypertrophy as a result of phenytoin therapy.

Vascular or inflammatory enlargement

Pregnancy gingivitis, acute leukaemia and scurvy have been discussed under GUMS, BLEEDING. Wegener's granulomatosis is a disease of focal necrotizing vasculitis affecting the upper and lower respiratory tracts (*See* p. 443). Occasionally, a proliferative gingivitis may occur which arises interdentally and spreads mainly along the buccal gingivae. Extensive periodontal destruction may occur and the diagnosis can only be obtained by biopsy.

Infiltration of the gingivae by angiomatous tissue occurs as part of a haemangioma (*see* JAW, SWELLING OF) and should be distinguished from a localized proliferation of capillaries due to chronic irritation, such as that which is caused by a carious tooth or a retained dental root. The latter will resolve with removal of the irritant stimulus, while the former is usually part of a more extensive proliferation involving adjacent structures.

P. T. Blenkinsopp

Gums, retraction of

Retraction of the gingival mucosa is mostly associated with chronic periodontal disease (*Fig.* G.15.) Accumulation of dental plaque causes progressive destruction of the alveolar bone supporting the teeth and the mucous membrane, if not swollen by inflammation, recedes with the bone. So common is this process with age, it is often referred to as 'getting long in the tooth'. Vigorous attention to the periodontal tissues will limit the rate of bone loss but in some patients it is progressive with little evidence of infection.

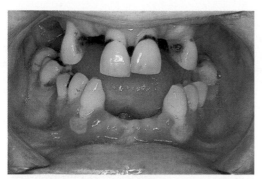

Fig. G.15. Gingival recession due to chronic periodontal disease.

Retraction of the gingivae may also be associated with intraoral scarring as occurs in epidermolysis bullosa, submucous fibrosis and various connective tissue disorders. Occasionally high muscle attachments will cause localized recession due to recurrent traction during function.

P. T. Blenkinsopp

Gynaecomastia

Gynaecomastia is enlargement of the male breast due to an increase in the duct tissue and in the periductal stroma. If the condition lasts for longer than a year the stroma becomes fibrous and the gynaecomastia tends to persist. The condition should not be confused with fat in the mammary region; in this case no glandular tissue is palpable behind the areola. Other conditions which cause swelling in the breast should be excluded, such as carcinoma, lipoma or neurofibroma.

Gynaecomastia is common in neonates and at puberty. When it occurs in older age-groups a pathological cause is more likely, though in the elderly it may be a physiological accompaniment of declining testicular function.

The pathophysiology of gynaecomastia is poorly understood. In some cases there has been shown to be a decreased ratio of free androgens to free oestrogens. In other cases the cause may be an undue sensitivity of breast tissue to normal circulating hormones; sometimes the enlargement is unilateral. The causes of gynaecomastia are set out in *Table* G.3.

Table G.3. Causes of gynaecomastia

Physiological
Neonatal
Pubertal
Senescent
Familial
Endocrine pathology
Hypogonadism
  Prepubertal testicular failure
    Agenesis
    Bilateral torsion of the testes

    Klinefelter's syndrome
    Reifenstein's syndrome
    Noonan's syndrome
    Cryptorchidism
  Destructive lesions of the testes
    Trauma
    Castration
    Mumps orchitis
    Tuberculous orchitis
    Leprous orchitis
    External radiation
  Defects in testosterone synthesis

Testicular tumours
Leydig-cell tumour
Sertoli-cell tumour
Chorion carcinoma
Teratoma
Seminoma

Other tumours
Bronchogenic carcinoma

Thyroid
Hyperthyroidism
Hypothyroidism

Adrenal
Adrenocortical carcinoma or adenoma

Pituitary
Acromegaly
Chromophobe adenoma

Hypothalamic lesions
Disorders of sex differentiation
Male pseudohermaphroditism
True hermaphroditism

Liver dysfunction
Hepatitis
Cirrhosis
Haemochromatosis
Hepatic carcinoma

Neurological disorders
Traumatic paraplegia
Dystrophia myotonica
Friedreich's ataxia
Syringomyelia

Respiratory disorders
Carcinoma of the bronchus
Chronic suppurative lung disease

Renal disorders
Chronic renal failure
During maintenance haemodialysis
Hypernephroma

Gastrointestinal disorders
Chronic ulcerative colitis
Following extensive gut surgery

Polyostolic fibrous dysplasia
  (McCune–Albright syndrome)

Renutrition following starvation and malnutrition

Drugs
Hormones
  Oestrogens
  Human chorionic gonadotrophin
  Methyl testosterone
  Desoxycorticosterone

Androgen antagonists
  Spironolactone
  Progestogens
  Cyproterone
  Cannabis

Cimetidine
Griseofulvin
Digitalis glycosides
Flutamide

Other drugs
Amphetamines
Tricyclic antidepressants
Methadone
Amphetamines
Diethylpropion
Isoniazid

Neonatal gynaecomastia

Seventy per cent of male neonates have some breast enlargement. In just over half of these fluid ('witch's milk') can be expressed on squeezing. The breast enlargement is probably due to the effect of placental oestrogens and human chorionic gonadotrophin stimulating the Leydig cells of the baby's testes to produce oestrogen. The witch's milk may possibly be the result of maternal prolactin. Histological examination shows the typical features of a lactating breast.

Pubertal gynaecomastia

The vast majority of boys develop a minor degree of gynaecomastia at the time of puberty (*Fig.* G.16a). Before the gynaecomastia appears there is a rise in plasma oestradiol which anticipates the expected pubertal rise in plasma testosterone. Along with the increased oestradiol there is an increase in prolactin, but the levels fall as the gynaecomastia develops. In boys in whom pubertal gynaecomastia does not occur, this sequence of hormonal events does not take place. In some boys the gynaecomastia is more marked and may even approximate to the normal female breast (*Fig.* G.16b). Often the condition arises in one breast only, or develops on one side some weeks or months before it appears in the other. Occasionally fluid can be expressed. In an appreciable number of cases there is a history of neonatal gynaecomastia, or even a family history, suggesting that there may be a constitutional sensitivity to oestrogen secreted by the Leydig cells of the testis. This sensitivity could possibly be mediated by increased numbers of oestrogen receptors in breast tissue.

Mild, early gynaecomastia usually regresses, but moderate to marked degrees of it tend to persist. Although anti-oestrogens such as tamoxifen should theoretically be of value, they seem to have little effect on anything but mild gynaecomastia. The patient is best referred early for plastic surgery. A peri-areolar incision should leave a virtually invisible scar.

It is important to consider other causes of gynaecomastia in a pubertal boy, such as drug ingestion, and to examine the testicles carefully for the presence of a tumour. If one testis appears to be normal and the

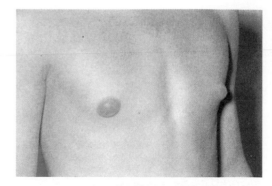

a

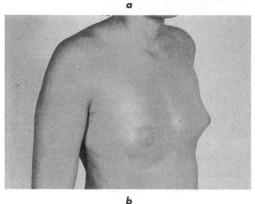

b

Fig. G.16. Gynaecomastia in boys at puberty.

other one is small, the 'normal' testis may be harbouring a tumour. The oestrogens produced by the tumour may have suppressed pituitary gonadotrophins and caused failure of development of the contralateral testis. Testicular ultrasonography is a useful way of detecting small tumours.

Senescent gynaecomastia

Occasionally patients in the sixth or later decades of life may develop gynaecomastia (*Fig.* G.17.) There may be associated loss of libido and occasionally hot flushes. The plasma testosterone is reduced. Plasma oestradiol levels remain normal, but plasma oestrone rises due to increased conversion from androstenedione. Sex hormone binding globulin levels rise with a consequent increase in the binding of testosterone. The result is a further reduction in free testosterone and an imbalance in the ratio of free testosterone to free oestrogens. The serum gonadotrophins are raised. It is important, however, in this age group to consider other causes of gynaecomastia, such as bronchogenic carcinoma, drug ingestion, liver disease, etc.

Testicular disorders

HYPOGONADISM

Gynaecomastia is usually due to testicular agenesis or to Klinefelter's syndrome (*see* p. 632). In cryptorchidism,

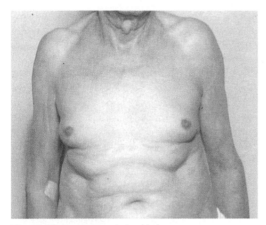

Fig. G.17. Gynaecomastia in elderly man.

while sterility is the rule, Leydig-cell function is usually normal, so gynaecomastia is not a common feature. It should be noted that gynaecomastia is not usually a feature of hypogonadism secondary to pituitary or hypothalamic disease.

Destructive lesions of the testes such as castration, trauma and mumps orchitis are relatively commonly associated with gynaecomastia.

Rare defects in testosterone synthesis due to enzyme deficiency have been associated with gynaecomastia.

TESTICULAR TUMOURS

Testicular tumours such as those of the Leydig cell produce gynaecomastia because of increased oestrogen secretion. Others, e.g. chorion carcinoma, do so because human chorionic gonadotrophin (hCG), produced by the tumour, stimulates testicular tissue to secrete oestrogens. In the early stages chorion carcinoma of the testis may be impalpable, so estimations of serum hCG are important in the investigation of gynaecomastia, particularly since chorion carcinoma is the commonest testicular tumour to cause it.

Leydig-cell tumours are rare before puberty but should be considered as a cause of gynaecomastia in adult males. Seminomas rarely may cause gynaecomastia. The rarest testicular tumour of all, the Sertoli-cell tumour, frequently presents with gynaecomastia and loss of libido.

Thyroid disorders

Five per cent of male thyrotoxics have gynaecomastia. There is an increased conversion of androgen to oestrogen in the liver. Increased oestrogen levels and excess thyroid hormones both lead to a rise in sex hormone binding globulin (SHBG) levels, so that more testosterone is bound and the free testosterone to free oestradiol ratio falls.

Rare patients with hypothyroidism have been noted to have gynaecomastia; the mechanism is uncertain.

Adrenal tumours

Adrenocortical carcinoma and, more rarely, adenoma may produce oestrogens and lead to the development of gynaecomastia. Plasma or urinary oestrogens may be raised and gonadotrophin levels may be suppressed. Urinary 17-oxo-steroids can be increased or normal. The testes are small and aspermia is present. Testicular biopsy may show hypoplasia of Leydig cells. Localization by computer-assisted tomography should be carried out.

Pituitary tumours

Acidophil or chromophobe tumours of the pituitary causing acromegaly or chromophobe tumours not producing excess growth hormone not infrequently secrete large amounts of prolactin. This occurs particularly when associated with secondary hypogonadism and an alteration in the free testosterone: free oestradiol ratio may lead to gynaecomastia. Some pituitary tumours have caused gynaecomastia because of the secretion of luteinizing hormone.

Hypothalamic disorders

Lesions in the hypothalamus may give rise to precocious puberty and gynaecomastia.

Disorders of sex differentiation

Male pseudohermaphroditism is a term used to describe individuals who have testes and an XY chromosomal constitution but ambiguous external genitalia. There are two main varieties. The first is due to abnormal testicular function, usually deficient testosterone production. This may be caused by certain enzyme deficiencies occurring in congenital adrenal hyperplasia (20, 22-desmolase deficiency, 3-β-hydroxysteroid dehydrogenase deficiency and 17-α-hydroxylase deficiency), to failure of conversion of testosterone to dihydrotestosterone because of 5-α-reductase deficiency or to failure of testosterone production because of 17-β-hydroxysteroid dehydrogenase deficiency. The clinical manifestations vary widely from hypospadias only to grossly abnormal appearances with a small penis exhibiting chordee, a bifid scrotum, a persistent urogenital sinus and a vagina opening into the posterior urethra. A rudimentary uterus and Fallopian tubes may be present. The testes are undescended or present in the labio-scrotal folds. Gynaecomastia may appear at puberty.

In the other variety of male pseudohermaphroditism (*testicular feminization syndrome*) there is end-organ resistance to the action of androgens due to lack of androgen receptors (*Fig.* G.18.) The appearance is female, there is absent pubic and axillary hair, the external genitalia look like those of a normal female, but there is a blind vagina. Testes are usually intra-abdominal, but may lie in the inguinal canal or in the labia majora. The breasts are those of a normal female except that the nipples and areolae are often small.

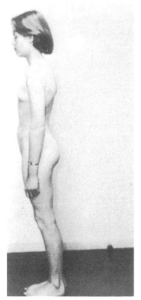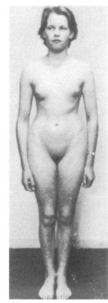

Fig. G.18. Testicular feminization. Normal female configuration. Note absence of pubic hair. (*Courtesy of the Gordon Photographic Museum, Guy's Hospital.*)

Liver dysfunction

In chronic liver disease there is a decline in testosterone production and an increased conversion of androgens to oestrogens. The sex hormone binding globulin goes up and reduces further the level of free testosterone. During recovery from liver diseases such as hepatitis the gynaecomastia may be due to an improvement in nutrition.

Neurological disorders

About 20 per cent of patients with *traumatic para-plegia* develop gynaecomastia. In the cases in which testicular histology has been studied the findings are similar to those found in Klinefelter's syndrome. Traumatic paraplegia is followed by a period of catabolism with marked loss of protein. It is possible that this is responsible for the testicular changes.

Patients with *dystrophia myotonica* very rarely develop gynaecomastia and then it is usually accompanied by extreme physical debility. The same applies to patients with *syringomyelia* and *Friedreich's*

ataxia. In all of them the histological appearances in the testis are similar to those of Klinefelter's syndrome.

Respiratory disorders

Carcinoma of the bronchus may secrete human chorionic gonadotrophin (hCG), which by stimulating the testes may lead to increased oestrogen production. In most cases where bronchial carcinoma has caused gynaecomastia there has been associated hypertrophic pulmonary osteoarthropathy. In patients recovering from chronic suppurative lung disease the gynaecomastia is probably due to improved nutrition.

Gynaecomastia may occur in any chronic debilitating disease such as renal failure, neoplasia, congestive cardiac failure, tuberculosis, cirrhosis and diabetes, particularly during a recovery phase. It has been especially noted during maintenance dialysis. The mechanism is probably similar to that noted in starving ex-prisoners of war when re-fed. In them gonadotrophin levels which were depressed during the period of starvation rise following the receipt of food. The testes become stimulated again and the individual goes through what is, in effect, a second puberty. However, in renal failure there are low levels of testosterone and evidence of testicular resistance to gonadotrophin action.

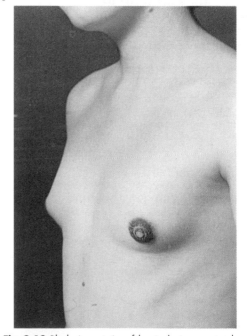

Fig. G.19. Black pigmentation of the nipples in a man to whom stilboestrol has been administered. (*Courtesy of the Gordon Photographic Museum, Guy's Hospital.*)

Drugs

Drugs are an important cause of gynaecomastia, especially in adults. Oestrogen therapy invariably produces gynaecomastia and when stilboestrol is used a deep brown pigmentation of the nipple and areola develops (*Fig.* G.19.) Gynaecomastia has been described in workers in the pharmaceutical industry who were involved in the manufacture of oestrogens. Human chorionic gonadotrophin administration may cause gynaecomastia when used for the treatment of undescended testicles. Methyl testosterone can occasionally lead to breast enlargement, possibly because of peripheral conversion to oestrogens. Any drug which is an androgen antagonist (*see* Table G.3) may cause gynaecomastia by allowing the unopposed action of oestrogens on breast tissue. However, the major reason for the association of digitalis glycosides with gynaecomastia may be because they are used for the treatment of heart failure and it may be that the improvement in the individual's health and nutrition is the important factor.

A few other drugs have been reported as causing gynaecomastia (*see* Table G.3). It is possible that with isoniazid, used for the treatment of tuberculosis, the most important factor in the causation of gynaecomastia is the recovery from a chronic disease.

Ian D. Ramsay

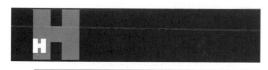

Haematemesis

Causes of haematemesis

Gastrointestinal haemorrhage commonly presents as vomiting of blood or blood-stained gastric content; this is defined as haematemesis.

1. Swallowed blood

Epistaxis
Haemoptysis
Bleeding from mouth or throat
Spurious

2. Diseases of the oesophagus

Hiatus hernia and reflux oesophagitis
Oesophageal varices
Mallory–Weiss syndrome
Oesophageal ulcer
Mediastinal tumour perforating oesophagus and aorta
Foreign body perforating oesophagus and aorta

3. Diseases of the stomach

Gastric ulcer
Acute gastritis and haemorrhagic erosions
Tumours, carcinoma, haemangioma, leiomyosarcoma

Pseudoxanthoma elasticum
Hereditary haemorrhagic telangiectasia (Osler-Rendu–Weber syndrome)

4. Diseases of the duodenum

Duodenal ulcer
Diverticula
Tumours, primary or invasion from pancreas
Gallstones ulcerating into duodenum

5. Portal obstruction

Hepatic cirrhosis
Portal vein thrombosis

6. Disordered haemostasis

Thrombocytopenia
Polycythaemia
Purpura
Leukaemia and related disorders
Aplastic anaemia
Haemophilia and related disorders
Von Willebrand's diseases
Scurvy
Chronic liver disease

7. Drugs

Anticoagulant therapy
Non-steroidal anti-inflammatory drugs (NSAIDs), aspirin, phenylbutazone; indomethacin and many others

8. Miscellaneous

Adbominal aneurysm opening into stomach or duodenum
Uraemia
Abdominal surgery, trauma or burns (Curling's ulcer)
Polyarteritis nodosa, systemic lupus erythematosus
Malignant hypertension
Acute febrile disorders, variola, scarlet fever, measles, malaria, yellow fever, Dengue, infective endocarditis

The commonest causes of profuse haematemesis are acute gastric erosions, gastric ulcer, duodenal ulcer and cirrhosis of the liver. A long history of typical peptic ulcer symptoms may be present in patients bleeding from gastric or duodenal ulcer but this may not always be present. Acute erosions are particularly common in patients taking aspirin or other non-steroidal anti-inflammatory drugs or may follow acute alcohol ingestion. A history of alcoholism may point to cirrhosis of the liver and may be accompanied by jaundice, palmar erythema, spider naevi and ascites; the liver may be enlarged and the spleen may also be palpable. Absence of these features does not exclude the diagnosis. Endoscopic examination of oesophagus, stomach and duodenum is essential in all cases of significant haematemesis.

1. Swallowed blood

EPISTAXIS

Bleeding from the nose may be followed by haematemesis when blood has been swallowed and then vomited; this may occur at night when blood has been swallowed during sleep.

HAEMOPTYSIS

Blood coming from the lungs may be swallowed, especially if haemorrhage occurs during sleep. The patient may cough up blood which is subsequently swallowed.

BLEEDING FROM THE MOUTH AND THROAT

Bleeding may occur from the gums, tongue and fauces, and blood from these sources may be swallowed and subsequently vomited. Bleeding from the gums may occur in scurvy or mercurial stomatitis.

SPURIOUS

Some patients suffering from a variant of the Munchausen syndrome may swallow blood in secret and subsequently vomit this with an intent to deceive.

2. Diseases of the oesophagus

HIATUS HERNIA AND REFLUX OESOPHAGITIS

Hiatus hernia is common but is mostly associated with the symptoms of acid reflux and oesophagitis than with gastrointestinal bleeding. Blood loss in oesophagitis and hiatus hernia is usually chronic, presenting as iron-deficiency anaemia, but occasionally haematemesis does occur. This most commonly occurs from the gastric side of the oesophago-gastric junction and is more common with a paraoesophageal rather than a sliding hiatus hernia. Haematemesis may be associated with Barrett's syndrome, in which ulceration of gastric mucosa may occur in the lower oesophagus.

OESOPHAGEAL VARICES

Varices developing at the lower end of the oesophagus or the upper end of the stomach as a result of portal hypertension are generally associated with cirrhosis of the liver and may be the cause of profuse haematemesis if rupture occurs. Stigmata of chronic liver disease may be present such as jaundice, ascites, palmar erythema or spider naevi. The absence of these features does not exclude the presence of portal hypertension and varices.

MALLORY–WEISS SYNDROME

Rupture of the gastric mucosa at the oesophago-gastric junction may result in haematemesis. This may follow vomiting and is particularly common in alcoholics. Such tears are generally linear, at or just below the mucosal junction, and may extend into a submucosal plexus of thin-walled vessels. The characteristic clinical picture of retching and vomiting followed by haemorrhage is not the only way the Mallory–Weiss syndrome presents, as early endoscopy in patients has shown this to be a relatively common cause of haematemesis.

OESOPHAGEAL ULCER

Such ulcers may be benign or malignant and may be associated with hiatus hernia and reflux oesophagitis. Although a relatively uncommon cause of haematemesis, significant bleeding may occur, the diagnosis being confirmed by endoscopy with biopsy.

MEDIASTINAL TUMOUR PERFORATING OESOPHAGUS AND AORTA

This is an infrequent complication of such tumours but may occur if the tumour erodes into the oesophagus. It may be associated with compression and invasion of large veins leading to oedema of the neck and extremities, cyanosis and dilated superficial veins.

FOREIGN BODY PERFORATING OESOPHAGUS AND AORTA

This rare cause of haematemesis may be induced by a fish bone, pin or dental plate perforating both oesophagus and a large vessel or aorta. A history of a foreign body being swallowed, followed by a feeling of discomfort in the oesophagus, suggests the condition which is generally confirmed by radiology or endoscopy.

3. Diseases of the stomach

GASTRIC ULCER

Haematemesis may occur in acute or chronic gastric ulcer. Gradual loss of blood may allow sufficient time for acid gastric juice to convert haemoglobin into haematin which gives the vomit a dark brown or 'coffee-ground' appearance. Severe bleeding may occur if a medium-sized or large vessel is eroded. Profuse haemorrhage causes a feeling of faintness, restlessness, syncope and a rapid feeble pulse. There may be abdominal pain, nausea, vomiting and associated melaena. The pain is generally epigastric, but many haematemeses from ulcers are associated with no abdominal discomfort.

Endoscopy is the most important investigation in determining gastric ulcer as a cause of haematemesis; the site of the ulcer can be positively identified, the severity of the bleeding assessed and biopsy obtained to determine if the ulcer is benign or malignant. Usually a biopsy is not taken from bleeding ulcers, the endoscopy being repeated in a few days for the purpose of obtaining suitable biopsies.

ACUTE GASTRITIS AND HAEMORRHAGIC EROSIONS

In acute gastritis the mucosa is congested and small haemorrhages and erosions are identified at endoscopy. Generally slight haemorrhage occurs although it may be occasionally profuse. Haemorrhagic erosions are small or minute ulcers, the differences between these and multiple small gastric ulcers being that of degree rather than of kind.

Acute gastritis and haemorrhagic erosions may be associated with the ingestion of irritating foods, alcohol, or corrosive and irritant poisons. There may be a feeling of discomfort and tenderness in the epigastrium, nausea and vomiting.

Non-steroidal anti-inflammatory drugs are now perhaps the commonest cause of bleeding from erosive gastritis.

Other causes of bleeding from such lesions are very severe acute infections such as variola, infective endocarditis, yellow fever, black water fever and Dengue fever.

Gastritis and haematemesis may also be due to corrosive poisons, strong acids or alkalis destroying the surface membranes of mouth, throat, oesophagus or stomach, causing intense pain, dysphagia, retrosternal discomfort, abdominal distension, collapse and haematemesis. In arsenic poisoning the mucous membrane of the stomach is red, inflamed, partly detached and covered with blood-stained mucus. The principal symptoms are nausea, severe sickness, burning epigastric pain and diarrhoea. The vomitus is usually brown, turbid fluid mixed with mucus and streaked with blood in which arsenic may be detected by appropriate tests; severe diarrhoea may come later.

TUMOURS

Severe haematemesis is relatively rare in *carcinoma of the stomach*, accounting for less than 5 per cent of all haematemeses. The patient may have epigastric discomfort, nausea, vomiting, anorexia and weight loss. Pyrexia, anaemia, cachexia and an abdominal mass may also be present. Sometimes no preceding symptoms occur and the patient presents with haematemesis. Pain is variable but when present is generally central, sometimes being referred to the back. If nar-

rowing at the pyloric area has occurred, the patient may have regular vomiting streaked with blood of 'coffee-ground' appearance. If the tumour is at the cardia, regurgitation of food may occur rather than true vomiting, and may occur a few minutes after eating. Troisier's sign—enlargement of the left supraclavicular lymph node—is a rare finding but if present strongly suggests malignant disease.

Gastric tumours are best diagnosed by endoscopy through which adequate biopsies under direct vision can be obtained.

Other tumours of the stomach may rarely occur; these include haemangioma—a benign tumour comprising newly formed blood vessels—and leiomyoma—a sarcoma containing large spindle cells of unstriped muscle. These are rare tumours but are likely to ulcerate and bleed.

PSEUDOXANTHOMA ELASTICUM (GRÖNDBLAD–STRANDBERG SYNDROME)

This is a hereditary disease characterized by widespread abiotrophy of elastic tissue throughout the body. Disintegration of submucosal artery elastica leads to severe haemorrhage from the stomach. Characteristic appearances of the skin of head, neck and body may suggest the diagnosis.

HEREDITARY HAEMORRHAGIC TELANGIECTASIA (OSLER–RENDU–WEBER SYNDROME)

This is caused by dilatation of normal vascular structure following congenital thinning of arterial muscle coat and absent elastin in arteriolar wells. There are multiple telangiectasia which are commonly found on the lips and mucous membranes of the mouth and throughout the gastrointestinal tract. There may also be an arteriovenous fistulae in the lungs and liver. The condition is inherited as an autosomal dominant. The most common presentations are gastrointestinal tract bleeding, often haematemesis, sometimes melaena, or epistaxis. Endoscopic examination of the stomach generally identifies such lesions, but milder bleeding distal to the stomach is often difficult to diagnose.

4. Diseases of the duodenum

DUODENAL ULCER

Haematemesis occurs when a duodenal ulcer erodes a blood vessel, some of the blood regurgitating through the pylorus into the stomach to be vomited, the rest passing down the gastrointestinal tract to cause melaena. If bleeding is severe, red blood may be passed per rectum. It is common for duodenal ulcer and haematemesis to have little pain. If pain is present it is central, upper abdominal and possibly radiating to the back. There may be a dyspeptic history with pain occurring some hours after food, often at night, with symptoms showing periodicity. Generally endoscopy can rapidly identify the presence and site of a bleeding duodenal ulcer.

DIVERTICULA

Duodenal diverticula are fairly commonly seen on radiological examination, but are generally asymptomatic. If inflammation occurs within a diverticulum the symptoms may resemble those of duodenal ulcer although there is generally not the classical regular food relationship. A coexisting ulcer may be present. Haematemesis is rare in association with duodenal diverticula.

TUMOURS

Duodenal tumours are rare, mostly arising from the ampulla of Vater, being associated with jaundice and pale or silvery stools. Occasionally, invasion of the duodenum occurs from tumour in the head of the pancreas resulting in haematemesis.

GALLSTONES ULCERATING INTO THE DUODENUM

This is a rare cause of haematemesis and is generally associated with previous attacks of colicky abdominal pain, classically under the right costal margin, and sometimes associated with jaundice. The diagnosis is generally confirmed by plain abdominal X-ray showing air in the biliary tree, ultrasound examination, or the passage of stone in the faeces, or endoscopy.

5. Portal hypertension

CHRONIC LIVER DISEASE

Chronic liver disease may be associated with disordered haemostasis in the form of thrombocytopenia associated with portal hypertension, or coagulation abnormalities. Thus any other cause of bleeding such as peptic ulceration or oesophageal varices may lead to a major haematemesis because of the abnormal haemostatic mechanisms.

PORTAL VEIN OBSTRUCTION

Extrahepatic portal vein thrombosis usually occurs in infants and early childhood. The cause is usually unknown and infection is rare. The patients present with haematemesis from oesophageal varices, or splenomegaly. There is rarely evidence of liver dysfunction clinically or biochemically. The outlook is good. Surgery should be avoided, but if bleeding is a problem some form of portal systemic shunt surgery is required.

In adults, portal vein thrombosis is usually due to thrombosis, trauma or neoplastic invasion.

6. Disordered haemostasis

A large number of conditions may be associated with disordered haemostasis. These may cause gastrointestinal haemorrhage with haematemesis. Often another lesion in the stomach or duodenum, such as a small erosion or ulcer, may start to bleed but the bleeding may become significant in the presence of conditions leading to abnormal haemostasis. There may be a small erosion or ulcer in either stomach or duodenum which may start to bleed, the bleeding becoming significant due to the abnormal haemostasis which may be present.

THROMBOCYTOPENIA

A number of conditions may be associated with thrombocytopenia, including hepatic cirrhosis with portal hypertension, side-effects of drugs or reticuloses. Any of these conditions may be associated with bleeding, becoming significant and leading to haematemesis.

POLYCYTHAEMIA

Patients with polycythaemia rubra vera may develop thrombotic episodes leading to ulceration and followed by bleeding from the stomach or duodenum.

PURPURA

Purpuric conditions may be associated with haemorrhage from any mucous membranes, anywhere in the gastrointestinal tract. The underlying cause of the purpura should be investigated.

LEUKAEMIA AND RELATED DISORDERS

Leukaemia and other associated conditions such as Hodgkin's disease, lymphomas and other reticuloses may develop haemorrhages from any part of the gastrointestinal tract, leading to haematemesis. Enlargement of the spleen may indicate the underlying condition. The diagnosis is established by blood or bone-marrow examination.

APLASTIC ANAEMIA

Aplastic anaemias may be related to a range of conditions including viral infection and the side-effects of drugs. They may rarely be associated with gastrointestinal haemorrhage and haematemesis. The diagnosis is again established by blood or bone-marrow examination.

HAEMOPHILIA AND RELATED DISORDERS

Excessive bleeding from many sites may be associated with haemophilia and other disorders of coagulation.

Gastrointestinal bleeding presenting as haematemesis is relatively common in these conditions; the diagnosis has generally been made before such bleeding occurs. Haemorrhage into joints may be present.

VON WILLEBRAND'S DISEASE

Deficiency of Von Willebrand factor leads to ineffective platelet adhesion. Bleeding may result, although the defect is generally mild. Sometimes there may be an associated haematemesis.

SCURVY

Haematemesis may occur in severe cases of scurvy. The patient may also have swollen spongy gums, anaemia, cutaneous haemorrhages and subcutaneous indurations. The patient may give a history of a diet deficient in fresh vegetables or there may be underlying conditions such as Crohn's disease or coeliac disease leading to malabsorption and malnutrition. Measurement of ascorbic acid levels in blood and in tissues will give the diagnosis.

7. Drugs

A number of drugs may be associated with haematemesis, the cause being suspected by an accurate and detailed drug history from the patient or the presence of a disorder such as arthopathy, suggesting that the patient may be having, or have had, drugs, such as non-steroidal anti-inflammatory agents, which may lead to gastrointestinal haemorrhage.

ANTICOAGULANT THERAPY

Anticoagulants may be indicated in various conditions including deep venous thrombosis or pulmonary thromboembolism, and patients on long-term anticoagulant therapy may have significant gastrointestinal haemorrhage from relatively minor lesions in the stomach or duodenum such as small ulcers or erosions. An accurate drug history should provide a guide to the cause.

NON-STEROIDAL ANTI-INFLAMMATORY DRUGS (NSAIDS)

These drugs are widely used in all forms of arthropathy and may lead to the development of haemorrhagic erosions or erosive gastritis in the stomach or duodenum, with haematemesis. They are being more widely used especially in elderly patients. An accurate drug history should provide the clue to the cause but endoscopy will localize the site and assess the severity of the lesion.

8. Miscellaneous

A number of rarer conditions may be associated with gastrointestinal haemorrhage and haematemesis. These include severe bleeding from an abdominal aneurysm opening into the stomach or duodenum, uraemia associated with chronic nephritis (in which the presence of high blood pressure, cardiac hypertrophy, retinopathy, polyuria and urine of low specific gravity with albumin or blood present may point to the diagnosis); abdominal surgery; trauma or burns (Curling's ulcer); autoimmune disorders such as polyarteritis nodosa or systemic lupus erythematosus. Gastrointestinal bleeding may be associated rarely with malignant hypertension and acute febrile disorders.

R. I. Russell

Haematuria

Haematuria means the presence of red blood cells in the urine and, although free haemoglobin may be present in the urine as a result of lysis of cells in the urinary tract, it should not be confused with haemoglobinuria in which the pigment alone is filtered through the glomeruli. In clinical practice there are two main ways in which haematuria may pose a diagnostic problem. Macroscopic haematuria may be a presenting feature, with or without other symptoms, or blood may be found in the urine only by 'dipstick' testing or microscopy. In the former case the remainder of the history and examination together with special investigations will be aimed directly at finding the site and cause of the bleeding. In the latter, the finding of microscopic haematuria will either support a diagnosis already made or suspected or will prompt specific investigations; the only reason for ignoring this finding, temporarily, is when blood is found on routine urine testing in a menstruating woman.

In a patient complaining of frank haematuria, with no other symptoms, enquiry should be directed to the details of the symptom itself. The colour of the blood may be of some slight significance as, if it is bright red, it is more likely to have come from the bladder or urethra. The opposite does not apply as dark-coloured blood is of no diagnostic significance. The time at which the blood appears *during* micturition is rather more helpful. Thus, if the blood appears only during the final expulsive efforts or the terminal urine is more deeply blood-stained than the rest, the bleeding is almost certainly from the bladder; if it is the first urine passed which is most blood-stained, the urethra or prostate are the likely source. Even distribution of the blood throughout micturition suggests either that the source of bleeding is in the kidneys or ureters or that the bleeding is profuse from any site above the urethra. The amount of blood present is also of diagnostic importance; in the absence of trauma, a large quantity of blood is suggestive of a tumour of the urinary tract although profuse bleeding is quite common in several other conditions, for example benign prostatic hypertrophy.

The history should, naturally, include the patient's past and family history together with details of his or her occupation and of any drugs being taken. All other symptoms are relevant until proved otherwise and, specifically, symptoms related to the urinary tract should be enquired about. Thus unilateral lumbar pain, passing forward into the groin, with occasional attacks of colic, would suggest a renal lesion while increased frequency of micturition or penile pain immediately after micturition would suggest vesical disease. Sacral pain would suggest malignant disease in the bladder or prostate. The site of associated symptoms may, however, be misleading. For example, a tumour in the bladder might, by occluding a ureteric orifice, cause unilateral hydronephrosis with lumbar pain and tuberculosis of the kidney and ureter can cause increased frequency of micturition in the absence of vesical infection.

Physical examination must be thorough as there is virtually no abnormal physical sign which may not be associated with one of the numerous causes of haematuria. The kidneys should be palpated to determine their size, if possible, and to elicit any tenderness. Suprapubic palpation will detect a distended bladder and may cause pain in the presence of cystitis but it is by rectal and vaginal examination that the pelvic viscera are most easily palpated. On rectal examination the uniform, elastic and movable prostate affected by benign hypertrophy can be distinguished from the hard, nodular, often immovable gland without a median groove characteristic of carcinoma. Thickening of the lower end of the ureter is suggestive of tuberculosis and infiltration at the base of the bladder may be present with a vesical carcinoma. Lymphatic spread from a carcinoma of the bladder or prostate may be palpable as thickening in the lateral pelvic space. Vaginal examination will also allow palpation of the bladder base and lateral pelvic space as well as of the other pelvic organs; in the fornices the lower end of each ureter can sometimes be felt if it is diseased or contains a calculus. The testes should be examined, particularly for evidence of tuberculosis of the epididymis.

The urine itself should be examined. Macroscopic inspection may reveal clots, which can be studied by floating them in the urine diluted with water in a flat tray. Their shape may suggest the source of bleeding; thus, clots formed in a renal pelvis may be triangular in shape while those formed in a ureter are likely to

be thin and 'worm-like'. Microscopy of the urine is more revealing but it must be carried out on a fresh specimen. The presence of red-cell casts is pathognomonic of glomerular bleeding. Large numbers of oxalate crystals may indicate a tendency to oxalate stone formation; the much rarer crystals of cystine are diagnostic of cystinuria, with its strong tendency to the formation of calculi. The finding of clumps of transitional epithelial cells (*Fig.* H.1) is suggestive of carcinoma or papilloma of the bladder and is an indication for formal cytological examination of the urine. Rarely fragments of renal papillae may be seen, sometimes with the naked eye, in papillary necrosis associated with chronic interstitial nephritis. The presence of leucocytes is not very helpful as they are likely to be found not only in bacterial infections but also in tuberculosis, tumours and benign prostatic hypertrophy.

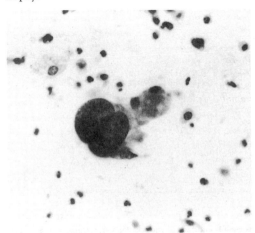

Fig. H.1. Clumps of transitional carcinoma cells in the urine in a case of carcinoma of the bladder. (Dr J.O.W. Beilby, Middlesex Hospital.)

Further investigation of haematuria should usually include plain X-rays of the abdomen, ultrasound scanning of the urinary tract and, in many cases, intravenous and retrograde urography; cystoscopy can rarely be omitted unless there is strong evidence of a glomerular lesion causing the bleeding. The latter investigation will reveal not only tumours and other lesions of the bladder but, even if the bladder is normal, may help to locate the site of bleeding if blood-stained urine is seem issuing from one ureteric orifice.

The main causes of haematuria are summarized in *Table* H.1.

Renal causes of haematuria

Haematuria can follow *trauma* of any degree of severity. A history of an accident or a blow or kick to the lumbar region suggests damage to the kidneys. Even slight injury to the loin, of which there may be

Table H.1. Causes of haematuria

Renal
Trauma
Tumours
Calculus
Glomerulonephritis
Polycystic kidneys
Tuberculosis
Pyelonephritis
Infarction
Polyarteritis nodosa
Chronic interstitial nephritis
Hydronephrosis
Irradiation nephritis
Hydatid disease
Medullary sponge kidney
Relief of tension

Ureteric
Calculus
Tumours

Vesical
Trauma
Tumours
Prostatic enlargement
Tuberculosis
Calculus
Cystitis
Foreign body
Disease of adjacent organs

Urethral
Urethritis
Calculus
Tumours
Foreign body
Caruncle

General
Drugs
Bleeding disorders

no recollection or external sign, can cause haematuria, especially if there is a pre-existing renal lesion. The kidney may be palpable but this must be distinguished from an extravasation of blood in the perinephric tissues. In any case of haematuria following trauma it is essential to distinguish an injury to the kidney from one to the urethra or bladder. With urethral injury the canal may be merely contused or partially or completely ruptured. Blood may be found at the meatus or may be present only in the first portion of urine passed; complete rupture will produce signs of extravasation of urine with an inability to micturate. Evidence of extravasation of urine or of fluid in the peritoneal cavity causing peritoneal irritation may accompany haematuria following injury to the bladder. Evidence, including radiographic, should be sought of fracture of the bony pelvis which may have caused the vesical or urethral injury.

Renal tumours are important causes of haematuria. The commonest presenting symptom in *carcinoma of the kidney* ('hypernephroma') (*Fig.* H.2) is profuse intermittent haematuria. A mass may be felt in the loin and there may be pain in that region resulting from increasing tension or colic from the passage of clots. Occasionally the initial symptom is unexplained fever and polycythaemia or hypercalcaemia may also be found; hypertension is present in about 30 per cent of cases. An intravenous urogram will show deformity of the renal pelvis or calyces but the most useful investigations are CT scanning and renal arteriography; the latter will show a characteristic pattern of vessels in the tumour. In children with *nephroblastoma* (Wilms tumour) the presenting feature is commonly abdominal distension and a mass is almost always palpable; haematuria occurs later. An *adenoma* of the kidney or an *angioma* at or near the apex of a papilla can cause profuse haematuria. Both are rare and can usually be diagnosed only at surgery or post-mortem, although angiography may sometimes show a tumour 'blush'. *Papilloma* or *papillary carcinoma* of the renal pelvis is uncommon; either may cause profuse haematuria and enlargement of the kidney due to hydronephrosis. Pyelography may show a filling defect in the renal pelvis. Clinically the benign and malignant lesions are indistinguishable although the older the patient the more likely is the tumour to be malignant. *Squamous-cell carcinoma* of the renal pelvis is a very rare cause of slight or moderate haematuria.

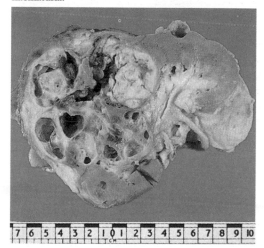

Fig. H.2. Carcinoma of the kidney.

Renal calculus seldom causes profuse bleeding but haematuria, and often pyuria, may occur, especially after exercise or the jolting of a journey. An aching pain in the loin is common while the stone remains in the kidney and may be followed by renal colic if the stone begins to descend down the ureter. This typical very severe pain passes from the loin downwards and forwards to the groin, upper part of the thigh and testicle and is accompanied by a frequent desire to micturate. The previous passage of a small calculus per urethram following an attack of renal colic is an important diagnostic feature. The radiographic diagnosis of ureteric calculus is discussed below (p. 262). A renal calculus may become too large to pass into the ureter and may then cause hydronephrosis or pyonephrosis with corresponding symptoms including haematuria (*Fig.* H.3).

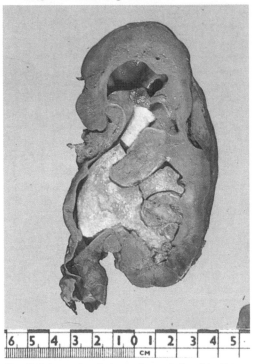

Fig. H.3. Large phosphatic stag-horn calculus of the kidney.

Glomerular disease is a common and important cause of haematuria, macroscopic or microscopic. *Post-streptococcal glomerulonephritis* is now rare in the Western world but is still common in developing countries where it often follows streptococcal skin infections. The characteristic features are haematuria, producing the typical 'smoky' appearance, and proteinuria, generalized oedema and hypertension. A similar lesion is a common complication of *infective endocarditis*, in which the glomerular changes are focal and segmental. Careful examination of a fresh specimen of urine will show red cells in a majority of cases of endocarditis and thus is an important diagnostic procedure. In both these conditions the glomerulitis is due to deposition of immune complexes as it is in *shunt nephritis* associated with infection of shunts used to drain hydrocephalus and in the nephritis occasionally associated with *chronic sepsis. Rapidly progressive glomerulonephritis* is a cause of macroscopic haematuria with loin pain; it causes rapid deterioration and can lead to acute renal failure within a few days. It can occur in Henoch-Schönlein syndrome, cryoglobulinaemia, microscopic polyarteritis, Wegener's granulomatosis and the nephritis associated with the development of antibodies to glomerular basement membrane (*anti-GBM nephritis*). The latter is often associated with pulmonary haemorrhage (*Goodpasture's syndrome*). Another cause of recurrent macroscopic or microscopic haematuria is *Berger's nephritis* (*IgA disease*). The aetiology is unknown but the episodes of haematuria commonly follow upper respiratory tract infections; the characteristic histological feature is the deposition of IgA in the glomeruli. It predominantly affects children and young adults; when it was first described, the prognosis was thought to be good but it is now known to account for a significant number of cases of chronic renal failure. Nephritis is also a common feature of *Henoch–Schönlein syndrome* which, although occasionally severe (*see above*), is more often a relatively benign condition characterized by haematuria with typical purpuric and oedematous skin lesions, arthritis and abdominal pain with intestinal bleeding. A number of hereditary varieties of nephritis can also cause haematuria; of these the most common is *Alport's syndrome* in which a renal lesion, often severe but less so in females, is associated with nerve deafness; the differential diagnosis, which can be made by renal biopsy, includes *familial benign haematuria* in which proteinuria and deafness do not occur and intermittent or persistent microscopic haematuria continues for many years without any deterioration in renal function. Nephritis with haematuria is also a feature of several systemic diseases of which the most important is *systemic lupus erythematosus* (SLE); of the numerous manifestations of this disease, arthritis, cutaneous lesions and hypertension are those most often associated with nephritis. Haematuria is not one of the typical features of the nephrotic syndrome but some of the causes of the latter, including SLE, produce sufficient glomerular inflammation to cause haemorrhage. Apart from this, *renal vein thrombosis* which is a recognized complication of the nephrotic syndrome, causes sudden deterioration in renal function together with haematuria, which is often macroscopic. *Postural proteinuria*, i.e. proteinuria occurring *only* in the erect position, is occasionally associated with slight haematuria which does not affect the generally good prognosis; also haematuria may occur with the proteinuria associated with *vigorous exercise*—so-called 'jogger's nephritis'.

Adult polycystic disease of the kidneys is frequently associated with haematuria, either painless or with clot colic; it can be precipitated by mild trauma. Both kidneys are usually palpable and hypertension is common (*Fig.* H.4). The differential diagnosis includes bilateral hydronephrosis; in the latter haematuria is less common and there will usually be evidence of a lesion of the bladder, prostate or urethra causing obstruction. The pyelographic appearances are quite different; in polycystic disease the calyces are narrow and elongated, quite unlike the dilated pelvis in hydronephrosis.

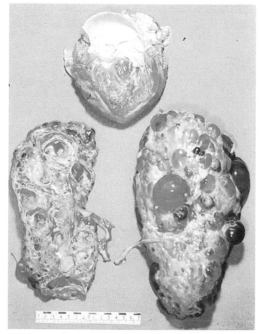

Fig. H.4. Bilateral grossly enlarged polycystic kidneys. Note the associated hypertensive cardiomegaly.

Haematuria in *renal tuberculosis* is usually slight and is associated with pyuria; occasionally an episode of gross haematuria is the presenting feature. The patients affected are usually young adults who may complain of a dull ache in one loin with occasional exacerbations resembling renal colic. Once the tuberculous focus has ruptured into the renal pelvis the characteristic symptom is increased frequency of micturition both by day and by night even without any involvement of the bladder. The bleeding is rarely increased by exertion, unlike with renal calculus. The thickened lower end of the ureter may be palpable on rectal or vaginal examination and, in males, nodules may be felt in the prostate or seminal vesicles. The cystoscopic appearance of the ureteric orifice may be distinctive. Hydronephrosis may develop in the affected kidney and intravenous urography will reveal characteristic changes (*Fig.* H.5). The diagnosis can be confirmed by culture of early morning specimens of urine. Other infections of the kidney, such as *acute pyelonephritis*, occasionally cause haematuria.

Vascular lesions of the kidneys can cause haematuria. *Infarction* is usually due to an embolus arising, for example, from a fibrillating left atrium, mural thrombus following myocardial infarction, a large vegetation in

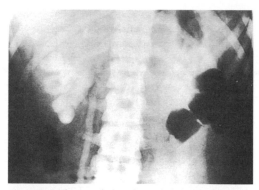

Fig. H.5. Pyelogram of tuberculous right kidney. Note the fine scattered calcification in the upper pole. The calices are dilated and clubbed.

infective endocarditis or, very rarely, left atrial myxoma. Infarction can also occur in *macroscopic polyarteritis nodosa*; the diagnosis can be confirmed by arteriography. *Sickle-cell disease* may cause haematuria as a consequence of vascular damage and *aneurysm of the renal artery* and *intrarenal arteriovenous fistula* are also rare causes of haematuria. Accelerated ('malignant') hypertension can cause haematuria, usually microscopic but occasionally macroscopic.

Less common causes of haematuria include *chronic interstitial nephritis* due commonly to the ingestion of analgesics; bleeding may be profuse when there has been recent papillary necrosis. Recurrent bleeding in such a case should, however, prompt a search for transitional-cell carcinoma of the renal pelvis which is a recognized complication of this condition. In *hydronephrosis* likewise haematuria is more likely to be due to an obstructive lesion than to the hydronephrosis itself. *Irradiation nephritis* is a rare cause of haematuria with modern radiotherapeutic techniques as is, in Britain, *hydatid disease*. *Medullary sponge kidney* is usually symptomless but haematuria and renal colic may occur as a result of calculus formation. *Relief of tension* by the sudden emptying of the bladder in a case of chronic urinary retention may cause bleeding, commonly from the bladder but sometimes from the kidney.

Ureteric causes of haematuria

Ureteric calculus may cause haematuria, either during the descent of the stone or when it becomes arrested without causing complete obstruction to the flow of urine. The diagnosis is usually easy from the history and the character of the pain, accompanied by the increased desire to micturate; but, in some cases, a calculus on the right side may be mistaken for appendicitis. A previous history of the passage of a calculus or of symptoms of renal stone may be elicited. A calculus may become impacted in any part of the ureter, though most commonly in the pelvic portion. Cystoscopy may show swelling and ecchymosis of the ureteric orifice if the stone is near the bladder or occasionally it may be seen projecting from the orifice. Radiographic examination may show an opacity in the line of the ureter, but this should always be confirmed by a stereoscopic radiograph taken with an opaque bougie passed into the ureter or by intravenous urography. Shadows very similar to calculi may be caused by phleboliths or calcified nodes; these are frequently multiple and calcified nodes show variations in density with indistinct outlines but, if single and apparently in the line of the ureter, may cause diagnostic confusion unless investigations are carried out as described above.

Papilloma of the ureter may cause haematuria, even after the removal of the primary disease in the renal pelvis by nephrectomy. For this reason it is usual to carry out complete ureterectomy at the same time as the nephrectomy, if this cause of haematuria is suspected.

Carcinoma of the ureter is rare (*Fig.* H.6); it can be diagnosed by the filling defect in the ureter with dilatation above on ureterography, and by the brisk bleeding which occurs when a ureteric catheter is passed. The differential diagnosis of the negative shadow produced by a tumour in the ureterogram includes a non-opaque calculus and an air bubble.

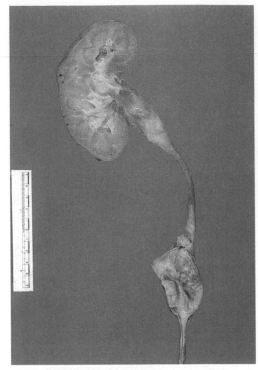

Fig. H.6. Carcinoma of the ureter producing hydronephrosis and treated by nephro-ureterectomy.

Vesical causes of haematuria

Intermittent profuse painless haematuria is characteristic of *papilloma* or *papillary carcinoma* of the bladder. Other symptoms which may be present include an urgent desire to micturate or retention of urine due to clot formation in the bladder or, with carcinoma, increased frequency of micturition. Bimanual pelvic examination under general anaesthesia may provide evidence of carcinomatous infiltration of the base of the bladder or of the pelvic lymphatics but an innocent tumour can rarely be felt per rectum. Cystoscopy is the essential diagnostic procedure and a malignant tumour will most commonly be seen at the base of the bladder above and lateral to a ureteric orifice. This orifice may be occluded causing hydronephrosis so that a bladder carcinoma may cause renal pain and swelling and, initially, be confused with a renal tumour. A papilloma of the bladder may occur at any age but is rare below the age of 25; a papillary carcinoma is uncommon before the age of 45. Papillomas may be multiple, either from direct implantation or as a result of an inherent tendency of some vesical mucosae to produce multicentric lesions.

Nodular and *ulcerative carcinomas* occur in elderly patients and cause slight but fairly constant haematuria. Other symptoms are commonly present;

these include increased frequency of micturition by day and by night and penile pain following micturition. Pyuria is also common. The blood often appears as a few drops at the end of the stream or may be present throughout micturition. Usually the tumour is seen at cystoscopy at the base of the bladder but there is a rare form of adenocarcinoma, derived from the urachus, which occurs at the dome of the bladder.

Sarcoma of the bladder is rare. It occurs in children and, occasionally, in adults and forms a rapidly growing mass, sometimes resembling a bunch of grapes (sarcoma botryoides). *Haemangioma* may occur as a flat lesion or as a solid tumour of considerable size.

Profuse haematuria is common in patients with *prostatic enlargement*, either benign or due to carcinoma. It is, surprisingly, more common with the former. The patient is usually over the age of 50 and there is typically a history of gradually increasing frequency of micturition. The enlarged prostate can be felt on rectal examination and, at cystoscopy, dilated veins ('prostatic varices') can be seen over the surface of the gland.

Vesical tuberculosis occurs most commonly in young adults. Persistent frequency, slight haematuria and pus in a urine sterile on normal culture are very suggestive features although, as indicated above, such symptoms can occur in renal tuberculosis before bladder infection has occurred. Evidence of tuberculosis elsewhere, in the lungs or the genital organs, may be found. Cystoscopy may reveal evidence of vesical infection.

Vesical calculus also causes slight haematuria, usually as a few drops in the terminal urine. In the absence of cystitis, increased frequency of micturition by day but not by night is typical. There may be pain of a pricking character in the glans penis after micturition and sometimes a history of sudden stoppage of the urinary stream. The patients are usually male and there may be a history of previous renal or vesical calculi. Stones are often visible in radiographs, except for urate calculi which contain little calcium and are, therefore, not very radio-opaque. Haematuria is more likely to be associated with the spiky oxalate calculi than with the smooth urate and phosphate calculi.

Acute cystitis is often accompanied by haematuria; the diagnosis will usually be obvious on other grounds. There is, however, a form of haemorrhagic cystitis in which bleeding predominates over other symptoms; a similar form of haemorrhagic cystitis is a complication of treatment with cyclophosphamide.

Simple ulcer of the bladder may occur as a result of severe localized inflammation in acute cystitis.

Chronic interstitial cystitis (Hunner's ulcer) in the female is often associated with painful haematuria and increased frequency of micturition from a small contracted bladder.

Radiation cystitis is characterized by multiple telangiectases in the vesical mucosa which may bleed severely. Vesical *schistosomiasis* causes slight haematuria and other symptoms similar to those of vesical tuberculosis. There is likely to be a history of residence in an endemic area such as Iraq and the neighbouring countries, Egypt and much of Africa. The typical ova of schistosoma haematobium may be found in the urine and at cystoscopy so-called 'sandy patches' may be seen; these consist of numerous ova without any inflammatory reaction. *Foreign bodies* may be introduced into the bladder by accident or design and cause bleeding; their presence will be revealed by cystoscopy or radiography.

Haematuria may occur as a result of spread of *disease of neighbouring viscera* to the bladder. Carcinoma of the uterus, vagina, rectum or pelvic colon can all invade the bladder, usually at a late stage of the disease. Of more clinical importance is the haematuria which may result from contact of an acutely inflamed appendix with the bladder wall and consequent localized cystitis; this is obviously a possible source of diagnostic confusion but the other symptoms of acute appendicitis are likely to be present and rectal examination will reveal the inflammatory process in the right side of the pelvis. More rarely, acute salpingitis or pelvic abscess can cause haematuria by a similar mechanism. Haematuria can also be caused by direct spread of inflammation from tuberculous or dysenteric ulceration of the intestines or from diverticulitis of the colon; the latter is particularly likely to lead to a vesicocolic fistula with pneumaturia as well as haematuria.

Urethral causes of haematuria

Lesions of the urethra can cause blood to appear spontaneously at the meatus as well as haematuria. Such conditions include *acute urethritis, calculus* (Fig. H.7), *papilloma* (Fig. H.8). and *carcinoma. Angiomas* are rare but can bleed heavily; there may be other similar lesions elsewhere in the body. *Foreign bodies* may be introduced into the urethra as a form of sexual excitement and, in females, a *caruncle* at the urethral orifice may cause haematuria which is inexplicable unless a thorough physical examination is carried out.

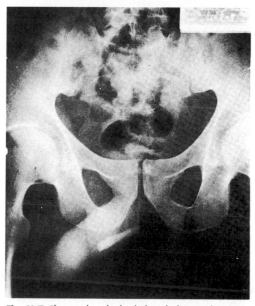

Fig. H.7. Elongated urethral calculus which caused retention of urine.

General causes of haematuria

Several drugs have been implicated as causes of haematuria but *anticoagulants* are the only ones of practical importance. Haematuria is common if control is poor but it must be remembered that, in such a patient, the fact that he or she is on anticoagulants does not exclude other causes of haematuria; bleeding apparently induced by anticoagulant therapy can be the first sign of renal carcinoma. Finally *thrombocytopenia* and disorders of platelet function can cause haematuria as can *haemophilia, Christmas disease* and, occasionally,

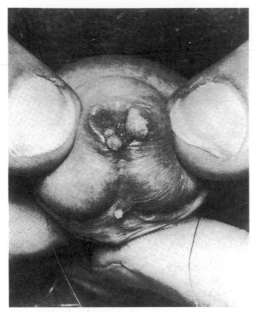

Fig. H.8. Papillomas of the urethra projecting from the external urinary meatus.

scurvy. In these conditions the diagnosis will usually be clear on other grounds.

Peter R. Fleming

Haemoptysis

The coughing up of blood is defined as haemoptysis, a term generally accepted to refer specifically to expectoration of blood resulting from bleeding in the lungs or bronchi. The amount of expectorated blood may vary widely from slight streaking of the sputum to massive exsanguinating haemorrhage. Blood, either alone or mixed with sputum, is nearly always produced by coughing, but rarely may trickle past the larynx to 'well up in the throat'. For this reason some patients with *true haemoptysis* present to an otolaryngologist. Blood from the nasopharynx or larynx may lead to spitting of blood or blood-stained secretions. This is sometimes called *spurious haemoptysis* since the blood does not in the strict sense arise from the lungs.

In the assessment of haemoptysis it is important to establish whether the bleeding has arisen from the chest, from the nasopharynx or upper gastrointestinal tract. Although examination of the nasopharynx should never be omitted it is unusual to find bleeding lesions in the upper respiratory tract. Bleeding of oesophageal, gastric or duodenal origin can usually be differentiated from haemoptysis by the presence of gastrointestinal symptoms, such as nausea or vomiting, or a history of oesophageal varices or peptic ulcer disease. Prompt upper-gastrointestinal endoscopy will settle the issue in doubtful cases. *Table* H.2 lists distinguishing features

that might help differentiate between haemoptysis and haematemesis.

Patients usually regard the presence of blood in the sputum as a sinister sign of serious lung disease. Haemoptysis may be a single event and of little prognostic importance if a slight blood-staining of the sputum follows a repeated violent bout of coughing. An effortless haemoptysis of 1 or 2 ml of blood is much more likely to be of importance, especially if it is followed by the production of further blood-stained sputum. The history and physical examination, with special attention to the respiratory and cardiovascular systems including the leg veins and to the nasopharynx, may provide clues to the underlying cause of haemoptysis but are seldom diagnostic. A technically satisfactory chest radiograph is mandatory and may reveal evidence of old or new inflammatory lesions, probable malignancies, or vascular abnormalities. Routine laboratory tests should include a full blood count and tests to exclude a bleeding diathesis. Virtually every patient with significant haemoptysis should undergo bronchoscopy to determine the site of bleeding and its cause, but the timing of the procedure is controversial. While it is desirable to determine the site of bleeding this can be difficult if all the airways contain fresh blood. Sputum cytology may be of value. If routine investigations are normal but haemoptysis persists further imaging of the chest by CT scanning may be helpful to exclude the possibility of localized bronchiectasis and to assist in identifying the presence of arteriovenous fistulae.

Haemoptysis, especially isolated instances of blood-staining of sputum, often remains unexplained even after extensive investigations. Up to one fifth of patients are in this category and it is conventional to follow them with further chest radiographs after an interval of about 2 months with the view also to obtaining the results of culture for mycobacteria and repeating investigations as necessary. *Table* H.3 lists the causes of haemoptysis according to the appearances of the chest radiograph.

SPURIOUS HAEMOPTYSIS

Bleeding from the upper respiratory tract usually presents as obvious bleeding from the gums or from the nose (*See* EPISTAXIS). As noted above it may give rise to 'haemoptysis', because blood can be aspirated into the lungs during sleep and subsequently expectorated on awakening, possibly mixed with bronchial secretions. The nasopharynx should be examined in all cases of haemoptysis.

TRUE HAEMOPTYSIS

The patient's age and environment are of importance. Where tuberculosis is a common disease haemoptysis

Table H.2. Haemoptysis and haematemesis: distinguishing features

Suggesting haemoptysis	Suggesting haematemesis
Respiratory symptoms	Dyspepsia
Tickle or gurgle in the throat; cough	Faintness; abdominal pain; nausea
Blood produced by repeated acts of coughing; may be mixed with sputum; blood-stained sputum may be produced for several days	Blood produced by isolated acts of vomiting; may be mixed with food debris
Usually bright red; may be frothy; reaction on alkaline side	Usually dark in colour; may resemble coffee-grounds; usually acid in reaction
Rapid bleeding either from lung or from upper alimentary tract produces only slightly altered blood, with or without clots	
Stools usually normal in appearance; may contain occult blood	Stools often dark and tarry (melaena) and always give positive test for occult blood

Table H.3. Causes of haemoptysis

Radiological abnormality which is readily diagnosed
Pulmonary tuberculosis
Tumours of the lung—carcinoma, adenoma, etc.
Pneumonia
Pulmonary infarction
Aspergilloma
Contused lung due to trauma
Mitral stenosis
Large arteriovenous malformation

Radiological abnormality, the nature of which is not immediately obvious
Pulmonary infarction
Pulmonary haemosiderosis
  Childhood haemosiderosis
  Adult haemosiderosis
Goodpasture's syndrome
Associated with systemic lupus erythematosus
Associated with pulmonary vasculitis

With no gross radiological abnormality
Mitral stenosis
Pulmonary embolism
Essential hypertension
Bronchitis and/or bronchiectasis
Tumours of the larynx, trachea or larger bronchi not yet blocking the lumen
Hereditary haemorrhagic telangiectasia and other pulmonary arteriovenous malformations

Bleeding diathesis
The primary disease is virtually always obvious from its other manifestations. Puzzling haemoptysis is rarely due to an unrecognized bleeding disorder

Iatrogenic
Needle lung biopsy
Transbronchial lung biopsy

must always give rise to a suspicion of pulmonary tuberculosis, especially in younger patients. Bronchial carcinoma is a frequent cause of haemoptysis in middle-aged or older patients who smoke cigarettes. With either of these diseases there may be a history of ill-health with non-specific respiratory symptoms preceding haemoptysis by a few weeks or months; but the haemoptysis is often the first event to alert the patient to seek medical advice.

Pulmonary tuberculosis

Haemoptysis is often an early symptom of pulmonary tuberculosis. At this stage physical examination is seldom abnormal but radiographic changes are to be expected with localized mottled shadowing or consolidation, possibly with cavitation. Rarely, haemoptysis may arise from radiographically obscure disease with localized shadowing concealed by the overlying skeleton, hilar or mediastinal shadows. Lateral, apical, tomographic or CT scanning views may then be required for diagnosis. Haemoptysis in patients with active tuberculosis varies in severity from streaky staining of the sputum to profuse life-threatening bleeding. Severe haemoptysis may arise in chronic cavitated disease from rupture of aneurysmal dilatation of an artery, exceptionally remaining patent in a strand of tissue traversing a cavity—the so-called 'aneurysm of Rasmussen'. Old calcified tuberculous lesions may also be sufficient cause for haemoptysis simply due to local bronchiectasis, though reactivation of tuberculosis must be considered. Investigation of all cases in which there is radiological evidence suggesting active or inactive tuberculosis must include examination of the sputum for tubercle bacilli.

Fungal infections

When commoner diseases such as tuberculosis have been excluded, *histoplasmosis*, *coccidioidomycosis* and *blastomycosis* must be considered in the differential diagnosis of haemoptysis associated with abnormal appearances in the lung, especially in areas where these diseases are prevalent. Diagnosis depends upon isolation of the causal organism and may be aided by serological tests. Other rare infections that must be similarly considered when tuberculosis has been excluded include *actinomycosis*, *nocardiosis* and *cryptococcosis*; diagnosis of these depends upon isolation of the causal organism.

Bronchial carcinoma

Haemoptysis, an early symptom of bronchial carcinoma, usually takes the form of blood-streaking of sputum and possibly small free haemoptysis, often repeated over days or weeks. Later more severe bleeding may occur from erosion of larger vessels either by the tumour or by the suppuration which often results from bacterial infection beyond it. Bronchial carcinoma must be suspected especially in cigarette smokers at or past middle-age, but may occur in younger individuals. There is usually an obvious abnormality on the chest radiograph; the more common findings are of two sorts. The first is associated with tumours originating in large bronchi and consists of air-absorption collapse or consolidation of a segment, a lobe (*Fig.* H.9) or even a whole lung beyond a complete obstruction, or patchy inflammatory consolidation beyond a partial obstruction. The second consists of localized, usually rounded shadows in the lung fields, produced by tumours originating more peripherally. In some cases of squamous-cell carcinoma, a rounded shadow of this sort may show a central transradiant area, due to necrosis of the central part of the tumour. Such appearances must lead to a provisional diagnosis of bronchial carcinoma. In occasional cases, a bronchial carcinoma arising in a large bronchus causes haemoptysis before it has obstructed the bronchus and before there is any abnormality on the ordinary chest radiograph taken in full inspiration. In such patients there is likely to be a wheeze that may be mistaken for an asthmatic or bronchitic wheeze of expiratory airflow obstruction. Wheezes due to partial obstruction of larger airways differ in two respects. First, they may be localized and 'fixed', i.e. do not clear on coughing. Secondly, they are as apparent in inspiration as in expiration, a fact that can be confirmed on spirometry; inspiratory flow rates are decreased as much as expiratory flow rates, resulting in characteristic changes in the volume flow loops. Another way of recognizing partial obstruction of one of the lobar or main bronchi is to take a chest radiograph on full expiration. This may result in air trapping in the affected lobe or lung.

In all cases of suspected bronchial carcinoma at least three specimens of sputum should be examined for malignant cells. These will yield about 70 per cent true positive and 30 per cent false negative results on patients who have bronchial carcinoma. The tumour cell type can be predicted as accurately by sputum cytology as by a specimen obtained at bronchoscopy, so, if sputum cytology is positive, bronchoscopy is unnecessary in patients who are clearly inoperable by reason of general frailty or the spread of the tumour.

When sputum cytology yields negative results

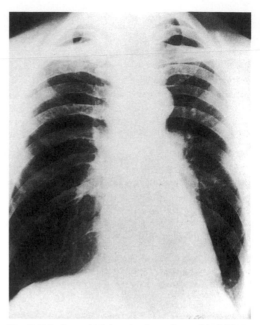

Fig. H.9. Radiograph of chest showing collapse of the left lower lobe due to carcinoma of the bronchus. Note the displacement of the heart to the left, the slight raising of the diaphragm, and slight narrowing of the spaces between the left lower ribs; the displaced heart almost hides the characteristic triangular shadow of the collapsed lung itself.

fibreoptic bronchoscopy is indicated to obtain histological specimens by brush biopsy, forceps biopsy and bronchial washings. In the case of peripheral tumours that cannot be reached by fibreoptic bronchoscopy, even under fluoroscopic control, transthoracic biopsy with a thin needle may be indicated. As transthoracic needle biopsy is a 'rule in' test—i.e. while a positive result is diagnostic, a negative result does not rule out carcinoma—patients should not be unnecessarily exposed to the risks of this when thoracotomy will be indicated whatever the result.

Bronchial adenoma

Haemoptysis is an important symptom in *bronchial adenoma*; these tumours may be very vascular. Episodes of haemoptysis may occur over several years, and there may also be a history of recurrent attacks of pneumonia always involving the same lobe. There may be clinical and radiological evidence of lobar collapse or consolidation, possibly with abscess formation; an adenoma in a central bronchus may present with the manifestations of partial obstruction of a large airway described above for bronchial carcinoma. Since most of the tumours arise in large bronchi, bronchoscopic diagnosis is easy.

Pneumonia

Bacterial pneumonias usually present as an acute illness with chest pain, dyspnoea, cough, fever and even rigors. *Table* H.4 shows the characteristic clinical features and the results of the blood count and direct examination of the Gram-stained smear of sputum that indicate the likely organism (for initiation of therapy) before the results of sputum cultures become available. Haemoptysis rarely amounts to more than blood-staining; the rusty sputum associated especially with *pneumococcal pneumonia* usually does not appear until several days after the beginning of the illness. If the sputum is or becomes frankly purulent, the possibility of a *suppurative pneumonia* or *lung abscess* must be considered. Haemoptysis associated with lung abscess may be secondary to bronchial obstruction, e.g. by carcinoma, especially in middle-aged or older smokers, more rarely by an adenoma in younger adults or a foreign body in children.

of pelvic or leg vein thrombosis do not become clinically manifest until days or weeks after an episode of pulmonary embolism, and sometimes never at all. *Table* H.5 lists the disorders known to increase the risk of venous thromboembolism, which, if present, should raise the diagnostic suspicion of *pulmonary infarction* as the cause of haemoptysis.

Bronchiectasis

Haemoptysis in a patient with a long history of cough and persistently or intermittently purulent sputum, possibly with episodes of increased volume and purulence associated with fever, suggests *bronchiectasis*. Localized crackles may be found persistently over the affected part of the lung, and clubbing of the fingers may be present, particularly in those with long-standing persistently purulent infection. Bleeding probably arises from the large pulmonary-systemic arterial anastomoses that develop in long-standing cases; it may

Table H.4. Acute pneumonia in previously healthy adults and children

Causes of pneumonia	Initial clinical features	Age	Blood count	Gram-stained sputum smear
Streptococcus pneumoniae Staphylococcus aureus	Sudden onset with fever, cough and pleuritic chest pain	All ages especially adults	Leucocytosis >12 000/mm³	Smear shows bacteria and large numbers of leucocytes
Haemophilus influenzae		Children		
Legionella pneumophila	Onset with 'flu'-like symptoms and chest pain, confusion, diarrhoea and abdominal pain	Middle aged or elderly males	Leucocytosis <15 000/mm³ Lymphocytopenia <1000/mm³	
Mycoplasma pneumoniae	More gradual onset with general symptoms of malaise, body pains and headache, with symptoms of upper respiratory tract infection	Young adults and children		Sputum mucoid Few leucocytes No significant pathogens seen
Chlamydia psittaci		Adults		
Coxiella burnetti Influenza viruses		Adults All ages	Normal or a leucopenia	
Adenovirus		Young adults and children		
RS virus		Children 3–5 years old		
Measles	Rash, etc.	Children		
Varicella	Rash, etc.	Adults		

Pulmonary infarction

This diagnosis is simple if haemoptysis is preceded or accompanied by pleuritic pain of sudden onset, and possibly by slight fever with or without dyspnoea, in a patient with heart disease, especially if there is atrial fibrillation, or the patient has present evidence of deep leg vein thrombosis providing an obvious origin for a *pulmonary embolus*. However, in many patients, signs

be the principal symptom and may be severe, even with bronchiectasis of limited extent. Computer tomography scanning of the thorax may help to establish the diagnosis. Bronchography may be performed prior to surgical resection of bronchiectasis but is seldom required for diagnosis.

Chronic bronchitis

Patients with chronic bronchitis not uncommonly cough up blood-streaked sputum especially during an

Table H.5. Factors predisposing to increased risk of venous thromboembolism

Disease process	General
Surgery—especially pelvic	Increasing age
Myocardial infarction	Previous thrombo-embolism
Congestive cardiac failure	Varicose veins
Trauma	Obesity
Stroke	Pregnancy
Malignant disease—especially pancreatic	Oral contraceptive use
Lower limb fracture—especially the hip	Immobility
	Bed rest
	Air and bus travel

exacerbation of their condition; expectoration of pure blood is much less common. In either case some explanation for the haemoptysis, other than chronic bronchitis, should always be considered. Chronic bronchitics are nearly always cigarette-smokers and they are also candidates for carcinoma of the lung. The recognition of chronic bronchitis is discussed on page 166.

Aspergilloma

The fungus *Aspergillus fumigatus* particularly colonizes open healed tuberculous cavities, but also any previously damaged lung tissue, such as occurs in bronchiectasis, sarcoidosis and pneumoconiosis, diffuse fibrosis and localized fibrosis of the lung such as that associated with ankylosing spondylitis. The mycelia grow into a ball that almost fills the cavity but leaves a crescent of air above the opacity. This results in the characteristic radiological appearances.

Aspergillomas are usually discovered on a routine chest radiograph but recurrent haemoptysis is a characteristic feature and may herald a massive pulmonary haemorrhage.

Sputum examination for aspergilli is unhelpful because they may be present in healthy persons and are, in any case, not often identified in the sputum of patients with aspergilloma. There is a useful precipitin test which is almost always strongly positive but the aspergillin skin test is positive only in about 20 per cent of cases.

Foreign bodies in the tracheobronchial tree

These can give rise to haemoptysis in two ways. Soon after lodgement, a hard foreign body with sharp edges may lacerate the mucosa and cause local ulceration and lead to bleeding, usually slight with no more than blood-streaked sputum. Later, infection beyond a foreign body obstructing a bronchus can cause pneumonia, abscess formation and, if neglected, eventually bronchiectasis, all of which are possible causes of haemoptysis. If it is not radio-opaque or if it is lodged centrally where it may be hidden in the mediastinal shadow, a foreign body will be radiologically inapparent, and cause no radiological evidence of its presence until the secondary changes arising from bronchial obstruction appear. A non-occluding foreign body of metal, bone or plastic material often produces no immediate irritative symptoms, and haemoptysis may be the first symptom to draw attention to its presence. The diagnosis will be made or confirmed at bronchoscopy.

Hydatid cyst

Infection with *Echinococcus granulosus* is particularly prevalent in the Middle East, Mediterranean coastal countries, South America, South Africa and Australia. Haemoptysis is the most common single symptom of an intact hydatid cyst and is possibly due to the size of the cyst causing congestion and blood vessel erosion; it often precedes rupture of a cyst. When a cyst has ruptured, infection often complicates the picture, with all the possible consequences of pulmonary suppuration, including severe haemoptysis. The diagnosis will be suggested by the chest radiograph, which will show one or more rounded shadows; rupture of cysts and added infection will, of course, affect the appearances. Complement fixation and Casoni skin tests may be helpful in diagnosis.

Paragonimiasis

Haemoptysis is a leading feature of infection with the lung fluke, *Paragonimus westermani*. This occurs endemically in Japan, China, Korea and Taiwan; it occurs in Africa, particularly in the Cameroons. In addition to haemoptysis, cough and chest pain occur. The chest radiograph shows characteristic air-containing cysts, usually 1–2 mm^3 in diameter with a thickened base, scattered throughout the lungs; these cysts may be mistaken for tuberculous cavities, particularly if the changes are limited to the subclavicular zones as frequently happens. The diagnosis finally depends upon the finding of ova in sputum or stool.

Other parasitic infestations

Haemoptysis may occur either as parasites pass through or when they finally settle in the lungs. Most of them have fairly well-defined geographic distributions and are only likely to affect those who are or have been resident in endemic areas. Among parasites which may cause haemoptysis by their passage through the lungs are: *Ascaris lumbricoides*, which has a worldwide distribution; *Schistosoma*, of which various species have different, mainly tropical, distributions, and which may cause haemoptysis during the passage of larvae through the lungs, but of which the principal pulmonary manifestation, obliterative arteriolitis with granuloma formation, arises later and is not especially associated with haemoptysis; and *Dirofilaria immitis*, the heart-worm of dogs in Australia, which may cause haemoptysis and radiologically detectable lesions in the lungs of man.

Pulmonary haemosiderosis

Pulmonary haemosiderosis is a condition, characterized by episodic bleeding into the lungs, which results in deposition of haemosiderin in intra-alveolar macrophages and in interstitial histiocytes, together with a variable degree of alveolar wall fibrosis in the more chronic forms of the disease. The disorder presents in different ways at different ages.

In *childhood haemosiderosis* acute episodes of pulmonary haemorrhage with fever, cough, haemoptysis and breathlessness occur and the child is found to be anaemic. The individual episodes are often self-limiting and clear rapidly but can be life-threatening. The sputum characteristically contains iron-laden macrophages between the episodes of haemorrhage. Physical signs in the chest are unimpressive; crackles are sometimes heard. The chest radiograph shows large bilateral confluent lesions which appear and disappear rapidly. Antibasement membrane (ABM) antibodies are not found.

In *adult idiopathic haemosiderosis* gradually increasing breathlessness accompanied by small 'fleck' haemoptyses occurs, repeatedly over a prolonged period. The chest radiograph shows widespread fine stippling, often of pinhead size, and most densely distributed at the bases. Areas of acute confluent shadowing are rarely seen. The appearances may remain unaltered over many years. Physical examination of the chest usually reveals little in the way of abnormal signs unless alveolar wall fibrosis is marked, when finger clubbing may develop. The diagnosis is made by finding haemosiderin-laden macrophages in the sputum between episodes of haemoptysis. If there is no sputum for examination, macrophages can be obtained by bronchoalveolar lavage using the fibreoptic bronchoscope. Large numbers of these iron-laden cells are obtained, sometimes rendering the lavage fluid almost black. Some patients have air-flow obstruction as well as a restrictive defect; the explanation for this is not known but the finding does not negate the diagnosis.

Goodpasture's syndrome occurs most frequently but not exclusively in young male cigarette smokers (6:1 male/female ratio). The pulmonary lesions usually develop first; there is episodic haemoptysis sometimes severe enough to be life-threatening and the chest radiograph shows confluent or widespread fine shadows related to the severity of the bleeding. Within about a year renal impairment develops with fairly rapid progression to renal failure and death.

The features that distinguish this form of pulmonary haemosiderosis from the other is the presence in the serum of antibasement membrane (ABM) antibodies. Such antibodies are believed to cross-react with the basement membranes of both the lungs and the kidneys. Renal and lung biopsies demonstrate a pattern of linear fluorescence both in the glomeruli and along the capillaries in the alveolar walls. Typically the disorder affects cigarette smokers who present with cough, dyspnoea and haemoptysis which may be streaky and intermittent or sometimes severe enough to be life-threatening. The lungs are usually spared in non-smokers.

Systemic lupus erythematosus (SLE) may be associated with recurrent haemoptyses. The chest radiograph usually shows widespread confluent patchy shadows and the patient has other clinical features of SLE; immunological tests confirm this diagnosis. The lesion in the lung is believed to be due to a pulmonary vasculitis. In contrast to some other types of haemosiderosis, resolution with corticosteroids is often dramatic.

Diffuse lymphangioleiomyomatosis

This exceedingly rare condition is diagnosed by histological examination of a lung biopsy from patients who present with a diffuse lung disorder, haemoptysis and slowly increasing breathlessness. Obstructive distortion of the pulmonary veins by hypertrophic muscle leads to capillary haemorrhage and resulting siderosis. Other clinical features are recurrent pneumothoraces and chylothorax. The aetiology has not been established but the condition is probably a hamartomatous malformation of lymphatic and perilymphatic tissue.

Systemic vasculitides

In the rare cases of *polyarteritis nodosa* in which the pulmonary arteries are involved with consequent small infarctions of the lung, haemoptysis may occur. Suspicion of the diagnosis depends on the other systemic features of polyarteritis nodosa. Confirmation of the diagnosis may be by tissue biopsy or the demonstration of multiple intraparenchymal aneurysms on visceral angiography.

In the *Churg–Strauss syndrome (eosinophilic granulomatosis, allergic angiitis and granulomatosis)* there is usually a long history of asthma with eosinophilia and eventually the patient develops other manifestations of generalized vasculitis. Haemoptysis, though not a particular feature, may occur; the chest radiograph may be normal or show transient or 'fixed infiltrations' or nodules.

Haemoptysis is more likely to be a clinical symptom in *Wegener's granulomatosis*. This condition is characterized by necrotizing granulomas in the respiratory tract including the nose and sinuses. There is also widespread vasculitis usually affecting the kidney. The chest radiograph shows multiple, usually bilateral nodular shadows which may vary in size from time to time and may cavitate; when they do so the cavities often have thick irregular walls. Diagnosis is made by biopsy of a lesion in the nose, sinuses or lung.

Arteriovenous fistula of the lung

This usually causes symptoms and signs arising from shunting of mixed venous blood directly from pulmonary artery into pulmonary vein, effectively a 'right-to-left' shunt. Haemoptysis occurs in only a minority of cases. About half are associated with *hereditary haemorrhagic telangiectasia* of which epistaxis is a frequent symptom.

Trauma

Haemoptysis occurs not only when the lung is directly penetrated, or lacerated by fractured ribs, but also in non-penetrating injuries. These may be associated with contusion of the lung, even without rib fractures. Exposure to blast from explosions may cause haemorrhagic consolidation of the lung (*blast injury*) with haemoptysis.

Mitral stenosis

The heart should be carefully auscultated for signs of mitral stenosis in all cases of haemoptysis. Rheumatic heart disease is less often encountered in Western countries. The cause of the haemoptysis may be the high pulmonary venous pressure or pulmonary embolism and infarction, particularly in patients with atrial fibrillation and/or cardiac failure. Pulmonary embolism leading to infarcts, especially in patients with atrial fibrillation, is a frequent cause. Less severe bleeding leading to blood-stained sputum may be associated with the high pulmonary venous pressure.

Left ventricular failure

The thin frothy sputum produced in pulmonary oedema is frequently tinged pink with blood. Diagnosis depends upon the recognition of the underlying cardiac disease.

Aortic aneurysm

An aortic aneurysm may erode into a bronchus, leading to rapidly fatal haemorrhage with massive haemoptysis. Most aneurysms of the thoracic aorta seen now arise as a result of traumatic dissection following a road traffic accident. The classic syphilitic aortic aneurysm has become a rarity.

Bleeding diathesis

In disease associated with disturbances of haemostasis and clotting, such as *thrombocytopenia, Henoch–Schönlein purpura, scurvy, leukaemias* and *aplastic anaemia*, haemoptysis may occur, but as a minor feature of a generalized bleeding tendency in which epistaxis and bleeding from the gums are more prominent. These may be accompanied by bleeding from the alimentary or urinary tracts, or by purpura, leading to appropriate haematological investigations. Haemoptysis is virtually never the sole clinically evident presenting feature of these diseases.

Factitious 'haemoptysis'

When a patient presents with a history of haemoptysis as the sole symptom, and investigation has shown no evidence of its source, nor of any organic disease, it must be remembered that single episodes of unexplained haemoptysis are not uncommon. Moreover, the patient may have come for investigation because he wanted reassurance; for instance, he may have a friend who has been found to be suffering from tuberculosis or bronchial carcinoma with haemoptysis as an initial symptom, and becomes alarmed lest the streaks of blood he notices after cleaning his teeth are the first sign of the same thing in himself. Very occasionally, a patient returns with recurrent complaints of haemoptyses, the blood being deliberately produced by various forms of trauma in the mouth or pharynx.

P. R. Studdy

Hallucinations

A patient's perception may be distorted by a variety of causes including an active imagination; stimulant and hallucinogenic drugs such as amphetamine, cocaine and LSD; the functional psychoses; specific intracranial pathology in particular that is associated with temporal lobe epilepsy (*Table H.6*).

Table H.6.   Causes of hallucinations

Sleep and sensory deprivation
Extreme fatigue
Bereavement
Narcolepsy
Delirium
Alcoholic hallucinosis
Drugs
   Amphetamine
   Cocaine
   LSD, mescaline, magic mushrooms,
     dimethyltryptamine, anticholinergics,
     bromocriptine, inhaled solvents
Schizophrenia
Mania
Depression
Postconcussional states
Temporal lobe epilepsy
Intracranial space-occupying lesions

During the aura of epilepsy, distortions in the form of objects (*micropsia* and *macropsia*) or in the quality or intensity of sounds or colours are frequently described. *Illusions* are sensory deceptions which typically occur when a person is apprehensive and distressed. For example a fearful person walking alone on a dark night might misidentify the branch of a tree for a crouching assailant. *Hallucinations* however have a very different quality distinct from illusions and are described as sensory perceptions which occur without any external stimulus. *A functional hallucination* is a hallucination only heard in the midst of some background noise such as traffic or a running tap. It has no particular diagnostic relevance and may merely reflect a diminution of the severity of the symptom. It should always be borne in mind that what is described as a hallucination is, for the patient, a very real, normal and often troublesome sensory experience and the patient may be puzzled why others cannot share the experience and, for example, hear for themselves the voices persecuting him. Hallucinations occur in normal people, following sleep or sensory deprivation and in states of extreme physical tiredness. Auditory and visual hallucinations of the departed spouse are particularly common during *bereavement*. In many normal people vivid visual hallucinations occur during the process of falling asleep (*hypnagogic hallucinations*) or when awaking from sleep (*hypnopompic hallucinations*). These sleep-related experiences are also common in *narcolepsy*. During *delirious states* patients may experience quite bizarre visual, auditory and tactile hallucinations.

Auditory hallucinations are often of considerable diagnostic significance although many patients may be reluctant to describe them unless asked because they may feel that 'hearing voices' is synonymous with madness. Auditory hallucinations are most commonly found in *schizophrenia*, and are also features of *depres-*

sive psychosis, *mania* and *chronic alcoholic hallucinosis*. The patient may hear simple sounds such as tapping, whistling or rattling noises and not uncommonly musical experiences. When voices are heard these may be uttering single words such as the patient's name or single expletives. Of greater diagnostic significance are auditory hallucinations consisting of whole sentences since certain characteristic features are strongly indicative of schizophrenia although not completely unknown in manic-depressive illness. Voices which say the patient's own thoughts out loud, which give a running commentary on the patient's actions, or voices which argue or discuss the patient amongst themselves referring to the patient in the third person are usually a symptom of schizophrenia when in the absence of a marked mood change. In acute schizophrenia these voices are often abusive and unpleasant and cause great distress to the patient. As the disease progresses however the content of the auditory hallucinations may become more neutral or even supportive and the person's response is less distressed. In *depressive psychosis* auditory hallucinations may be equally clear to the patient and the content will be congruent with depressed mood often containing accusations of sinful deeds or threats of impending disaster. On the contrary, in *mania* auditory hallucinations are more likely to be congruent with an elated mood and grandiose delusions. In affective psychosis the hallucinations disappear as the mood state recovers.

Visual hallucinations are much less common in schizophrenia and affective psychoses and characteristically occur in organic states or as an effect of drugs. *Space-occupying lesions* involving the visual areas of the occipital lobe or the association areas in the temporal and parietal lobes cause visual distortions and hallucinations which may be accompanied by varying degrees of loss of visual field, dyslexia or cortical blindness. Bizarre visual hallucinations and delusions occur in *delirium*, the *post concussional state*, *temporal lobe epilepsy* and *metabolic disturbances*, such as hepatic failure. *Amphetamine, cocaine, phencyclidine* and *solvents* may all cause visual experiences which may be hallucinations, illusions or sensory distortions. *Alcohol withdrawal (delirium tremens)* is characterized by dramatic perceptual changes which may be quite bizarre and cause terror in the sufferer.

Drugs taken orally specifically for their hallucinogenic properties include those related to 5-hydroxytryptamine such as LSD and dimethyltryptamine (DMT) and some related to catecholamines such as mescaline.

Within an hour or so of ingestion of a sufficient dose of LSD the subject begins to develop perceptual changes in a state of full wakefulness. These include the intensification of colours and sounds and synesthesias (senses become mixed up so that a colour is seen when a sound is heard). Hallucinations and illusions are usually visual consisting of geometrical forms, persons or objects. The mood is usually euphoric accompanied by intense mystical feelings, though anxiety may predominate in some, depending on the setting. Physical symptoms include sweating, tachycardia, tremor and incoordination. The abnormal perceptions may persist for up to 12 hours but flashback recurrent hallucinations sometimes cause distress.

Tactile hallucinations which include the feeling that 'ant-like' insects are crawling in the skin (formication) are found in alcohol withdrawal and cocaine abuse. Bizarre somatic hallucinations are frequently experienced by schizophrenics and may be elaborated into fantastic delusions (feeling that a radio-transmitter implanted in the spine is controlling movements), or sexual delusions (a somatic hallucination involving the sexual organs may lead to the delusion in a female patient that she has been raped). *Olfactory hallucinations* are common in schizophrenia but also occur in the aura of *temporal lobe epilepsy*. The hallucination of a smell is usually unpleasant and often described as a smell of faeces, of burning or of escaping gas. In schizophrenia such experiences may develop into delusional beliefs of persecution. In temporal lobe epilepsy, brief olfactory hallucinations during the aura will immediately precede other manifestations of a seizure and the diagnosis will not be in doubt.

D. Blackwood

HAND, DEFORMITY OF
See JOINTS, AFFECTION OF.

Head, retraction of

Usually the result of severe meningitis, this can also occur in children as the result of asphyxia. Intermittent spasms of retraction occur in tetanus, strychnine poisoning, rabies, torsion spasm and spasmodic torticollis. Stiffness of the neck, short of actual retraction, will also be considered in this section; it can be due to meningism, meningitis, subarachnoid haemorrhage, meningeal carcinomatosis, and pressure cones resulting from increased intracranial pressure. Stiffness due to disease of the cervical spine and paraspinal tissues is dealt with separately on page 609.

Causes of retraction of the head (including stiffness of the neck)

1. MENINGISM
2. MENINGITIS
   a. Bacterial
   b. Viral
   c. Spirochaetal
   d. Fungal
   e. Carcinomatous
   f. Sarcoid
3. SUBARACHNOID HAEMORRHAGE
4. PRESSURE CONES
5. ASPHYXIA
6. INTERMITTENT RETRACTION
   a. Spasmodic torticollis
   b. Torsion spasm
   c. Tetanus
   d. Rabies
   e. Strychnine poisoning
7. SPINAL AND PARASPINAL DISEASE

The term *meningism* is applied to the headache, photophobia and stiff neck which occur, as a rule, in children, in the course of general infections such as tonsillitis, pneumonia and pyelitis. The pressure of the spinal fluid is raised, but its contents are normal.

Meningitis causes resistance to forward flexion of the neck, but this may be absent in very mild cases and also in fulminating infections. Actual retraction of the head is best seen in tuberculous meningitis and in meningococcal meningitis; it has become rare since the introduction of antibiotics. Inflammation of the leptomeninges is caused by many organisms—bacteria, viruses, spirochaetes and yeasts—and a low-grade 'meningitis' can occur when the meninges are invaded by secondary carcinomatosis and sarcoidosis. It is sometimes possible to guess the identity of the agent from a consideration of the clinical features of the case, but examination of the spinal fluid is always essential for confirmation.

Features common to most cases of meningitis are headache, photophobia, vomiting, giddiness and fever. There may be a rigor, or a convulsion, at the onset of the more virulent types, especially in children. There is stiffness of the neck, spinal muscles and hamstrings. Thus, forward flexion of the neck is resisted, and it may evoke flexion of the hips and knees (Brudzinski's sign). There is resistance to extension of the knee on the flexed thigh (Kernig's sign), because this movement pulls on the roots of the cauda equina. There may or may not be evidence of focal damage to the brain and cranial nerves. The latter are involved as they traverse the subarachnoid space, and the brain itself can be damaged by spread of the infection along the meningeal sheaths which cover the vessels as they penetrate the surface of the brain. Moreover, thrombosis both of arteries and of veins can occur, with infarction, oedema or brain abscess as a result.

Thrombosis of the dural sinuses is a serious occurrence, the results of which depend on which sinus is involved. It is especially likely to occur as a complication of infection in the middle ear, the mastoid and the paranasal sinuses. Thrombosis of the superior longitudinal sinus interferes with the venous return from the cerebral veins and with the absorption of cerebrospinal fluid, so leading to cerebral oedema and a rise of intracranial pressure. A similar train of events follows the spread of a thrombus from the lateral sinus to the torcula. If the sigmoid sinus thromboses, clot will spread thence to the internal jugular vein. There are two further factors which can raise intracranial pressure in meningitis: the presence of inflammatory exudate itself, and hydrocephalus caused by interference with the free passage of spinal fluid from the fourth ventricle to the convexity of the brain, where it is absorbed. Finally, intracranial pressure may be raised by the presence of subdural collections of fluid (subdural hygroma), which are not infrequent after meningococcal meningitis in young children.

Infection can gain access to the meninges by several routes. In most cases it is blood-borne, and in an important minority it spreads from local infections in the ear, accessory nasal sinuses, face and scalp. The existence of this second group emphasizes the need to seek for evidence in the history and on physical examination as to the possibility of local infection in every case. Points to be looked for are the presence of otitis, mastoiditis or sinusitis. Moreover, a history of head injury, whether recent or remote, may mean that there is a fracture and a dural tear leading into an air sinus, thereby providing a path for the entry of micro-organisms. In such cases, meningitis is apt to be associated with an abscess, whether extradural, intradural or intracerebral, along the track of entry. Sepsis in the face or scalp, such as furunculosis, erysipelas, infected scalp wounds or herpes, can lead to meningitis in debilitated persons. Infection may also enter via a meningocele, or a congenital dermal sinus at the base of the spine, and these must be looked for in unexplained meningitis in infants. Yet another manner of infection is following lumbar puncture or spinal anaesthesia, fortunately rare; in such cases lowgrade infection is usual, e.g. by *Bacillus pyocyaneus*

Meningococcal meningitis (syn. spotted fever, cerebrospinal fever) usually occurs in epidemics which are initiated by droplet infection from healthy carriers. A bacteraemia precedes the meningitis by hours, days or even weeks. Occasionally there is a *chronic meningococcal septicaemia* with fever, purpura and transient pain, and swelling in the joints, and a proportion of such cases will end up with meningitis. In another small group, the patient is overwhelmed by a fulminating septicaemia within a few hours of the onset; some pass rapidly into coma, without a significant fall of blood pressure, while others remain clear in mind but suffer a drastic fall of pressure due to circulatory collapse, and these cases usually present a diffuse

purpuric rash on the skin (the *Waterhouse-Friderichsen syndrome*, which is also seen in other severe infections). In the usual type of meningococcal meningitis, however, there is fever, meningeal irritation, severe headache and sometimes a purpuric or macular rash. Convulsions may occur at the onset. Transient cranial nerve palsies and papilloedema may be found, and delirium is common. Tendon reflexes are reduced, and extensor plantar responses are common in the more severe cases. The condition is one of meningo-encephalitis, and this explains the intellectual and emotional changes which may be present in survivors. These symptoms are not unlike those which may follow cerebral contusion, and they may be complicated by an anxiety state in persons who find themselves unable to cope with life as a result of the mental incapacity caused by the meningo-encephalitis. The spinal fluid in meningitis usually contains a polymorph pleocytosis, with a rise of protein and a fall of glucose. Both intra- and extra-cellular diplococci are found.

In some cases of *meningococcal meningitis*, the exudate is largely confined to the base of the brain, thereby leading to an obstructive hydrocephalus. There is mild fever, vomiting, papilloedema and head retraction. In infants—the usual victims—the head enlarges, and there is a slow downward course with emaciation, vomiting and increasing stupor. In the first few days of the illness the changes in the spinal fluid are the same as in the ordinary type of meningococcal meningitis, but thereafter the meningococci disappear and there is merely a lymphocytic pleocytosis, a rise of protein, and rather a low sugar content. In such cases ventricular tap may produce the diplococcus.

Further sequels of meningococcal meningitis are the subdural hygroma referred to above, cranial nerve palsies, and disabilities arising from the formation of scar tissue around the spinal cord. These include a lower-motor neurone paralysis of muscles in the limbs, and occasionally an incomplete transverse lesion of the cord with paraplegia, sensory impairment and sphincter disturbances.

Other forms of pyogenic meningitis are sporadic rather than epidemic in incidence, do not as a rule produce a rash, and are usually derived from a more or less obvious source of infection. Thus *pneumococcal cases* commonly arise from infection in the ears or sinuses, or from pneumococcal pneumonia. *Streptococcal meningitis* is rarer than the pneumococcal form but occurs in similar circumstances; in a proportion of cases, however, there is a cerebral abscess in addition to the meningitis, and this must always be looked for, if necessary by CT scan. *H. influenzae*— (Pfeiffer)—is an important cause of meningitis in infants, and may cause the disease in adults; it may or may not be preceded by upper respiratory infection or by pneumonia. The signs of meningeal irritation may be slight. Other bacterial causes of meningitis are relatively rare and they will be identified by culture of the spinal fluid.

Meningitis with a predominantly lymphocytic response in the cerebrospinal fluid occurs in infection by tuberculosis, viruses, yeasts and spirochaetes. Of these, tuberculosis is the most important. The meningitis is secondary to tuberculosis elsewhere, although the source may not be clinically apparent. It rarely occurs before the age of 6 months and is most common in children and young adults. The onset is commonly insidious, with malaise and occasional headaches which may precede the signs of meningitis for days, weeks or even months. The meningeal phase includes headaches, signs of meningeal irritation and retraction of the head. Epileptic attacks—whether focal or general—and sudden hemi- or monoplegia, aphasia or cranial nerve palsies, mental changes, and papilloedema with visual loss, are common; hydrocephalus tends to increase, leading in untreated cases to stupor, incontinence, a rise in pulse and medullary failure. Choroidal tubercles may be found on examination of the retina, and the Mantoux test is positive in the majority of cases. The spinal fluid is under increased pressure, and may be either clear or opalescent; a fibrin clot forms on standing for some hours. There is an excess of lymphocytes and there may be a few polymorphs. The protein is raised, and the chloride is reduced *in the later stages of the disease*; the sugar content falls at an early stage. The definitive test is the demonstration of the organism in the fluid, whether by direct smear, culture or guinea-pig inoculation; if the evidence in favour of the disease is good, treatment should not be withheld until the organism is found. In the early stages of the disease the conditions which may cause difficulty in diagnosis are acute lymphocytic choriomeningitis and other virus infections of the meninges in which, however, the sugar and chloride content of the cerebrospinal fluid are normal, and the clinical course quite different, with rapid recovery in most cases. In acute syphilitic meningitis the VDRL reaction is positive, while in meningitis associated with aural and sinus infections there may be both lymphocytes and polymorphs present, with negative culture and a normal sugar content in some cases (*aseptic meningitis*).

Meningitis can complicate *Weil's disease* (*spirochaetosis icterohaemorrhagica*), but an acute and predominantly lymphocytic meningitis can also occur without jaundice, renal damage or haemorrhagic symptoms, and this is called *meningitis leptospirosa*.

It occurs in persons who have been in contact with rats, e.g. canal bathers, sewage workers, etc., and the spinal fluid is sterile if ordinary culture media are used. Sugar and chloride contents are normal. A benign meningitis can also be caused by *L. canicola*, which is carried by dogs. There may be conjunctival suffusion, and a rash which may resemble erythema nodosum. The spinal fluid contains an excess of lymphocytes, while the chloride and sugar content are normal, and the fluid is sterile in ordinary culture media. Diagnosis is confirmed, as in Weil's disease, by guinea-pig inoculation and by the detection of antibodies in the blood.

Lymphocytic meningitis may also occur with *tick-borne relapsing fever* (*T. recurrentis*), either during the first attack of fever, or more often in subsequent bouts. There is severe headache, neck stiffness and slight papilloedema. Cranial nerve palsies, notably the 7th, are not uncommon. There is increase of protein and lymphocytes in the spinal fluid, and the organism can be identified by dark ground illumination, or by inoculation of the spinal fluid into a suitable animal.

A well-marked lymphocytic meningitis can be caused by the viruses of acute choriomeningitis, mumps and glandular fever, whereas the meningeal reaction of poliomyelitis, zoster and arthropod-borne encephalitis is usually less obtrusive. A specific virus is responsible for acute *lymphocytic choriomeningitis*, a benign disease characterized by a prodromal period of malaise, headaches, muscle pains, pyrexia and upper respiratory catarrh; this is followed after a week or two by severe headache, photophobia, neck stiffness and a positive Kernig sign. In a minority of cases transverse myelitis, facial palsy or temporary mental and emotional changes may occur. In the cerebrospinal fluid the protein is raised, and there may be from 50 to 3000 cells, of which at least 95 per cent are usually lymphocytes. Chlorides and sugar are normal, and the virus can sometimes be got from the fluid. *Mumps meningitis* usually starts on the 5th to the 10th day of the illness, but meningeal symptoms may precede the parotitis, or they may occur with orchitis but without parotitis. The meningitis may be accompanied by encephalitis with disturbances of consciousness and, rarely, focal cerebral and cerebellar signs. Cranial nerve palsies and myelitis have been described. Sudden permanent deafness, in one or both ears, with or without vertigo and vomiting, may occur in mumps without evidence of meningo-encephalitis. In *glandular fever* there may be a well-marked lymphocytic meningitis of sudden onset, with enlargement of glands, increase of the mononuclears in the blood, and an increasing titre in the Paul–Bunnell test. Acute polyneuritis may complicate the disease, or may occur in glandular fever without meningitis. Of the *arthropod-borne forms of virus encephalitis, Louping-ill* is an epidemic disease of sheep, found in the northern parts of the British Isles, which is sometimes transmitted to sheep farmers and laboratory workers. It is carried by a tick. A phase of malaise and headache for a few days is followed by apparent recovery, and then illness characterized by fever, meningeal irritation, drowsiness, and cerebellar or other focal signs. There is a lymphocytosis in the cerebrospinal fluid. The prognosis is good. *Japanese B. encephalitis* occurs in Japan and China, and a celebrated outbreak occurred in Okinawa. The virus is spread by mosquitoes. There are meningeal signs, drowsiness, stupor, signs of diffuse cerebral involvement, convulsions and tremors. There is a lymphocytosis in the spinal fluid, the sugar remaining normal. The mortality in this disease can be over 50 per cent. Moreover, both mental impairment and change of personality may occur in the survivors. *St Louis encephalitis* occurs in the USA and is transmitted by mosquitoes. It is a summer disease, with fever, headache, meningeal signs, tremor, ataxia and difficulty in speech, and these are sometimes preceded by pain in the muscles, sore throat and malaise. There is usually a lymphocytosis and increase of protein in the spinal fluid, but no fall in the sugar content. *Equine encephalomyelitis* is a disease of horses in North and South America, but has been transmitted to humans, probably by mosquitoes. It is a feverish illness with meningeal signs and convulsions. In the early stages the cerebrospinal fluid may contain 1000 or more cells per cubic millimetre, polymorphs predominating at first. Cases of lymphocytic meningitis have occasionally appeared during *epidemics* of *pleurodynia* (Bornholm disease), but there is no good evidence that the meningitis in such cases is caused by a Coxsackie virus.

Infection by yeasts has been uncommon in the past, but it appears to be on the increase since the advent of antibiotics. *Cryptococcosis (Torula histolytica)* involves the subcutaneous tissues, the lungs, and the central nervous system, alone, or in combination, or in series. Subcutaneous granulomas break down to form abscesses and ulcers. Pulmonary lesions may mimic either chronic tuberculosis or carcinoma. The cerebral type usually starts insidiously with headaches, dizziness and stiffness of the neck, but it may commence suddenly. There is little or no fever, but gradually the cerebrospinal pressure rises producing papilloedema, and there may be cranial nerve palsies, hemiparesis or ataxia. Large granulomas may, in fact, cause symptoms of a cerebral tumour. The patient eventually sinks into coma. There is a marked mononuclear pleocytosis in the spinal fluid, and the protein is raised. The glucose content is reduced, and cryptococci—

which are readily mistaken for erythrocytes or lymphocytes—can be found in small numbers in the fluid.

Sarcoidosis, which causes uveoparotid polyneuritis, can also give rise to a low-grade meningitis with headaches, slight stiffness of the neck, and a rise of lymphocytes and protein in the spinal fluid. It can pass on to cause an obstructive hydrocephalus, with papilloedema and optic atrophy. Cranial nerve palsies and diabetes insipidus have been described. The diagnosis can only be inferred by the presence of typical lesions in other areas, e.g. skin, liver, lungs and eyes.

Subarachnoid haemorrhage is usually due to rupture of a saccular aneurysm, or of an atheromatous aneurysm. Less common causes are hypertension, angiomatous malformations, mycotic and syphilitic aneurysms, and purpura. An abrupt onset, early loss of consciousness in most cases, and the presence of blood in the spinal fluid distinguish the average case from meningitis. When the leak is slow, however, the severe headache, stiffness of the neck, slight pyrexia, ocular palsies and positive Kernig sign may simulate meningitis, and it is only the blood in the spinal fluid which clinches the diagnosis. If the lumbar puncture is delayed for a day or two, the fluid may be found to be yellowish in colour (xanthochromia), and not bloodstained. Rarely, pain starts in the lumbar region and gradually spreads down the back of the legs and up to the neck. Another unusual form presents as sudden coma, and there may, in such a case, be a history of former attacks of unexplained coma with neck stiffness.

Pressure cones at the tentorial hiatus and at the foramen magnum can cause stiffness of the neck. They occur as a result of space-occupying lesions and, occasionally, from cerebral oedema. The local rise of pressure from an expanding mass in the head, or from hydrocephalus, dislocates and displaces brain substance. Thus a mass in the middle fossa, e.g. tumour or extradural haematoma, can dislocate part of the temporal lobe into the posterior fossa, with the result that the mid-brain and the displaced tissue are tightly wedged in the dural ring. This may obstruct the aqueduct, thus aggravating the situation by causing internal hydrocephalus. In posterior fossa tumours, the reverse is seen: oedematous brainstem and cerebellar tissue is displaced upwards through the tentorial notch. Downward herniation of the medulla and cerebellar tonsils through the foramen also occurs, and will also give rise to rigidity of the neck.

Pressure cones can arise as the result of intracranial space-occupying lesions: tumour, abscess, haematoma, internal hydrocephalus and occasionally from cerebral oedema due to vascular lesions. All these conditions may therefore cause stiffness of the neck.

It is important to recognize the presence of a pressure cone, because the removal of even a small quantity of spinal fluid by lumbar puncture may cause collapse and death.

Asphyxia can cause retraction of the head, or stiffness of the neck. The more striking examples are usually seen in children with bronchopneumonia, bronchiolitis, or foreign body in the larynx. It has also sometimes been noted in retropharyngeal abscess. Even in adults with severe bronchopneumonia there may be stiffness of the neck, though retraction is rare. That asphyxia without cerebral oedema can cause retraction of the head is well illustrated by the retraction which is seen during the administration of pure nitrous oxide, e.g. for the extraction of teeth, but this may not be the whole explanation in the diseases mentioned.

Ian Mackenzie

Headache

Headache is of minor significance in the majority of cases but it may be the first, indeed the only, symptom of grave disease. Symptomatic treatment of a headache should never precede careful examination, and possibly investigation, with the object either of excluding or of recognizing one or other of its more serious causes.

The explanation of the mode of production of the pain known as *headache* is not easy. It is generally agreed that the principal pain structures of the head are extracranial, especially the arteries, though some intracranial structures, such as the venous sinuses, parts of the dura mater at the base of the brain, the dural arteries, the cerebral arteries at the base, the 5th, 7th, 9th and 10th cranial and upper three cervical nerves may play a part in some cases. To arrive at the diagnosis of the cause in a particular case, attention should be paid to the character, situation and time of occurrence of the pain, to its constancy, intermissions or paroxysmal exacerbations, to circumstances which alleviate or aggravate it, and also to accompanying symptoms.

Character. Diagnostic assistance may be afforded by such descriptions as throbbing, paroxysmal, or as being affected by movement or alterations of position.

Situation. This may be frontal, vertical, occipital or unilateral, and in cases of organic disease of the cerebrum may occasionally aid in localizing the situation of the lesion. It may be unilateral in migraine, tumour, abscess, middle-ear disease, or occipital in cerebellar disease. Occipital headache spreading to the vertex and even to the forehead may be produced by cervical spondylosis, although a similar headache may occur in basal subarachnoid haemorrhage, in some cases of tumour in the posterior fossa, and in meningitis. Purely frontal headache is suggestive of frontal sinusitis. Headaches over the vertex associated with other bizarre symptoms, such as a sensation of the skull closing and opening, are usually manifestations of psychoneurosis.

Time of occurrence. Headache associated with organic disease of the brain or its meninges often persists or becomes worse at night. It may wake the patient from sleep, being usually more severe in the morning, whereas headache due to toxic and functional causes is relieved by rest in a horizontal position. Grave suspicion should be entertained of an organic nature of the headache which disturbs the patient's sleep at night. A headache experienced on rising in the morning may also, however, be due to a stuffy ill-ventilated room, to excessive smoking or consumption of alcohol the previous evening, or to cervical spondylosis. In antritis and sinusitis, frontal and facial headache may come on after breakfast, persist most unpleasantly through the day, and pass off in the late afternoon. Evening headaches are often due to mental stress or eyestrain. Even a normal eye can suffer strain if work is excessive, the light bad, or the general health poor. True ocular headache is, however, relatively infrequent, apart from that associated with glaucoma and acute inflammatory states of the eye. It is more common with hypermetropia and astigmatism than myopia.

For the purposes of classification it is convenient to divide the causes of headache into three main groups: (A) Headaches of extracranial origin; (B) Headaches of intracranial origin; (C) Headaches originating elsewhere: miscellaneous.

A. Headaches of extracranial origin

1. Vascular headaches
    a. Migraine: classical and atypical
    b. Cluster headaches (migrainous neuralgia)
    c. Non-migrainous headaches (post-traumatic, hypertensive)
    d. Extracranial arteritis (e.g. giant-cell arteritis)
2. Muscle-contraction headaches (tension or 'nervous' headaches)
3. Anterior headaches (arising from nose and paranasal structures) (sinus headache)
4. Ocular headaches
5. Aural headaches
6. Dental headaches
7. Cranial neuritides
8. Cervical headaches

B. Headaches of intracranial origin

1. Traction on intracranial structures, mostly vascular, by—
    a. Primary or metastatic tumours involving vessels, meninges or brain
    b. Abscess (epi- or subdural or parenchymal)

c. Haematoma (epi- or subdural or parenchymal)
d. Subarachnoid haemorrhage
e. Post-lumbar puncture
f. Increased brain swelling (pseudotumor cerebri)
2. Headaches from congestion or inflammation of intracranial structures.

C. Miscellaneous

Emotional, psychiatric
Drugs, gases, poisons
Toxic states, renal failure
Heat-stroke

A. Headaches of extracranial origin

1. **Vascular.** These headaches are very common, and are in general due to painful dilatation and distension of an extracranial branch (or branches) of the external carotid artery, and possibly intracranial dural branches also, with surrounding oedema. In *migraine*, frontal supraorbital and superficial temporal arteries are associated with pains in temple or forehead on one or both sides, but posterior headaches may be due to similar dilatation and distension of occipital and/or postauricular arteries. Similar pains of vascular origin occur in the lower half of the head, the face and upper jaw around the back teeth. Classical migraine is usually unilateral but may spread to become bilateral or generalized; attacks are episodic, lasting from a few minutes to several hours or even days, and may be mild or extremely severe. Nausea is common, sometimes with vomiting. Preceding the headache a variety of visual sensations may occur due to constriction of retinal arteries: flashing lights or other spectra, visual field defects such as unilateral or homonymous hemianopia and rarely transient hemiplegia from transient constriction of cerebral arteries. After these initial vasoconstrictive symptoms the throbbing headache of vasodilatation begins either as the initial symptoms fade or a short time later. Pressure on the common carotid or affected superficial artery may temporarily reduce the headache.

In the closely related *cluster headaches* which are more common in middle-aged men, attacks come on suddenly, high in one nostril, the intense throbbing pain spreading behind the eye on that side and sometimes into the forehead. The attacks last up to 2 hours and during this time the nose and eyes water, the skin reddens and a Horner's syndrome may develop on the same side with ptosis and contraction of the pupil. The attacks may come once or several times in the day for several weeks, then abruptly cease only to recur in a new 'cluster' of attacks some weeks or months later. During these cluster periods, but not between, alcohol is likely to provoke attacks.

These cluster headaches may be extremely severe and prostrating and may occur at night. They seldom coexist with migraine. *Non-migrainous vascular headaches* may follow head injuries, with attacks of throbbing and aching but a variety of headaches may follow head injuries from a number of different causative factors. Although arterial hypertension is usually *not* accompanied by headaches, about 10 per cent of patients do complain on occasion of severe headaches, particularly in the early morning, only sometimes being associated with unduly high pressure readings. The headaches associated with *giant-cell arteritis* occur in the elderly of either sex, usually over one temporal artery, severe and throbbing, the affected artery being tender to the touch and thickened and nodular but sometimes occluded and pulseless. The onset may be sudden, sometimes accompanied by fever. Depending which areas are affected, pain may be in the jaw, face, occipital area of the side of the neck, and combing the hair or touching the scalp may be very unpleasant. A biopsy may confirm the diagnosis, but therapy with corticosteroids should not be delayed as involvement of branches of the ophthalmic artery may cause partial or complete loss of vision. The erythrocyte sedimentation rate is usually, but not invariably, elevated above 50 mm in one hour.

2. **Muscle contraction** (tension or 'nervous' headaches) are non-pulsatile, persistent, unilateral or bilateral aches, sometimes felt as tight or band-like feelings in temporal, frontal, occipital or parietal regions. Emotional tension is usually present; sometimes anxiety and/or depressive states. Prolonged mental concentration may cause a similar headache.

3. **Anterior headaches** arise from acute sinusitis, dull and aching but sometimes severe and aggravated by sudden movement of the head, with tenderness over the affected sinuses, frontal or maxillary. The turbinates are usually engorged and inflamed. Chronic suppurative disease in frontal, ethmoid, sphenoidal sinuses or maxillary antra may cause recurring persistent anterior headaches.

4. **Ocular headaches** usually start around and over the eyes, being due to uncorrected errors of refraction, disturbances of ocular muscle balance and glaucoma (*see* EYE, PAIN IN). The pain of increased intraocular pressure (acute angle-closure glaucoma), at first localized to the eye itself, may spread

throughout much of the area supplied by the ophthalmic division of the trigeminal nerve; it may be severe and prostrating and accompanied by nausea and vomiting. The eyeball is usually tender to digital pressure. Acute angle-closure glaucoma is an ophthalmic emergency as vision is at risk. It is a rare event compared with the much more common chronic primary open-angle glaucoma of insidious onset which is usually symptomless until some loss of vision has occurred. Headaches associated with various ocular disturbances are usually considered secondary to maintained contraction of intra-ocular muscles due to excessive effort of accommodation or of extraocular muscles in an effort to get a clear retinal image. Simple myopia does *not* produce headaches.

5. **Aural headaches.** Trauma, new growth or inflammation may be a source of headache in the region of the ear, but the 5th, 7th, 9th and 10th cranial nerves may convey pains from pharynx, larynx and jaws. Primary ear disease as a cause of headache is uncommon but important as it usually denotes destructive or inflammatory disease.

6. **Dental headaches.** Afferent fibres may convey painful sensations from dental disease or after dental extractions via the third division of the 5th cranial nerve.

7. **Cranial neuritides.** Herpes zoster of the 5th and 7th and, rarely, the 9th cranial nerves may cause pains around the ear.

8. **Cervical headaches** referred over the occiput and back of the head from degenerative and traumatic changes in the cervical spine are common. Cervical spondylosis is probably the commonest cause of headaches in the back of the head. Such headaches may extend over the head to temples, vertex and frontal regions. The neck movements are restricted and usually painful, pain often running also into one or both shoulders or arms.

B. Headaches of intracranial origin

Although headache is the presenting symptom in a high proportion of patients with tumours of the posterior fossa, it occurs in only about 33 per cent of supratentorial tumours. Headache from intracranial sources is due to traction and displacement of venous sinuses, middle meningeal arteries, large arteries at the base of the brain, and dilatation and distension of intracranial arteries. Inflammation or pressure on pain-sensitive structures may cause headaches.

Time of occurrence. Organic cerebral disease should be suspected when there is a history of recurrent nocturnal or morning headaches.

Severity. The pain is often intense and sometimes paroxysmal in character, but seldom interferes with sleep. In cases of brain tumour rarely is it as bad as a severe migraine, but it tends to be a dull steady deep ache, not throbbing. Even if a tumour exerts considerable traction or displacement of cranial nerves there may be little or no headache in some cases, but if a tumour intermittently obstructs the cerebral ventricles there may be a transient but very severe generalized headache lasting up to 30 minutes, then disappearing as rapidly as it appeared.

Situation. This may give some clue to the existence and localization of an organic lesion. In cases of cerebral tumour the pain may be unilateral or frontal; with a cerebellar lesion it is more often occipital. About one-third of all headaches roughly overlie the tumour, about two-thirds if there is no raised intracranial pressure. In middle-ear and mastoid disease headache is unilateral with localized tenderness. Occipital headache may be one of the earliest symptoms of meningitis.

Associated signs and symptoms. One or more of the following signs and symptoms may present themselves at an early period in cases of headache due to organic cerebral disease, so that their prompt recognition is important:

Vomiting of the 'cerebral type' (*see* VOMITING): usually bears no relation to food. There is usually no preceding nausea; it may occur unexpectedly and in projectile form.
Inequality of the pupils
Squint
Papilloedema
Drowsiness
Twitchings
Convulsions

Tapping the skull over the site of the pain may reveal local tenderness.

The presence of any of these signs associated with headache would point to the existence of one or other of the organic lesions enumerated above. If lumbar puncture and investigation of the cerebrospinal fluid is performed the development of a pressure cone is a very real danger in cases with increased intracranial pressure and fresh symptoms may be precipitated by this investigation. It should therefore be avoided.

Cerebral haemorrhage, thrombosis and *embolism* are often followed by headache of varying severity. With embolic or arteriosclerotic infarction the headache, thought to be due to vasodilatation of nearby unoccluded vessels, is usually mild and localized to the side of the lesion. Headaches are more common when vessels near the base of the brain are occluded. The headache of cerebral haemorrhage may be severe. It commonly occurs in hypertensive subjects with abrupt onset of neurological physical signs. The bleeding is usually from microaneurysms situated on striatal arteries.

In *subarachnoid haemorrhage*, usually from rupture of a berry aneurysm or arteriovenous fistula, headache is sudden in onset, often very severe and accompanied by neck stiffness and photophobia.

In *meningitis*, the character of the headache is significant. It is intense, occipital, and even at an early stage attended by stiffness of the neck and retraction of the head. It may be throbbing in nature.

Lumbar puncture may be followed by severe headache which is usually relieved by absolute rest in the recumbent position without pillows. It is usually occipital and throbbing, usually dull but sometimes severe. It is probably due to leakage of cerebrospinal fluid through tears in the dura mater. The headache usually appears within 12-24 hours of the puncture, coming on usually when the patient is erect. The use of narrow bore needles, slow withdrawal of fluid and accurate siting are important preventive measures. In *pseudotumor cerebri*, or benign intracranial hypertension, the intracranial pressure is raised in the absence of a space-occupying lesion. The headache is often mild, often worse on waking, is aggravated by coughing or sneezing and may be accompanied by visual blurring or some other visual defect and occasionally temporary loss of vision. Ophthalmological examination may reveal slight or marked papilloedema, sometimes with retinal haemorrhages, but the more common visual findings are enlargement of the blind spots and sometimes central or paracentral scotomas and/or constriction of the peripheral fields. The intracranial pressure, normally 50-180 mm of water, as measured by lumbar puncture with the patient lying on his side, may rise to 300-600 mm. There are many causes, intracranial venous sinus thrombosis, as after mastoiditis or head injury, being among the more common. It may occur also rarely in pregnancy, in obesity with menstrual irregularities, in children on corticosteroid therapy, after consumption of excessive amounts of vitamin A, in severe iron deficiency anaemia and obstructive pulmonary disease, and in many other conditions. In some cases there is no obvious cause. Radiological studies have shown smaller than normal ventricles, suggesting that the cause is not due to diminished cerebrospinal fluid absorption but to cerebral swelling from oedema.

Headaches from congestion or inflammation of intracranial structures include those occurring with febrile states, hypoxia, carbon-monoxide inhalation, asphyxia, the taking of nitrites, probably post-epileptic and 'hangover' states, in hypertensive episodes occurring with phaeochromocytoma, in acute hypertensive encephalopathy and other causes of rapid rises in arterial blood pressure. Paget's disease of the skull may be accompanied by severe headaches.

C.   Miscellaneous

Emotional and fatigue states may be accompanied by headaches. In tension (anxiety) states extracranial muscle contraction is probably a major factor but not the only one. Headaches are not an uncommon complaint when no medical condition is present, being an excuse for evading certain situations. Some people have such a remarkable susceptibility to headache that the slightest provocation can produce it. This is particularly true of migrainous subjects, but headaches may also be used by the patient for a variety of social and other reasons. Headaches occur not only during heat-stroke but sometimes afterwards, and after head injuries headaches may persist for many weeks or months, particularly in compensation cases or other situations awaiting the results of legal or medico-legal decisions. A large number of poisons or drugs, inhaled or swallowed, may cause headaches, for instance lead and carbon-monoxide poisoning. Nitrites or mono-sodium glutamate (in soy sauce) may cause headaches, as may excessive vitamin A intake. Chronic 'toxic' or infective states, for example chronic renal failure are often accompanied by recurrent or chronic headaches. Lack of sleep is yet another not uncommon cause; so too the deprivation of a drug to which the patient is attached and on which he is dependent.

There are, therefore, almost as many causes for headache in medicine as there are disorders. The most common are tension and anxiety states, sinusitis, migraine, cervical spondylosis, eyestrain and states of fatigue. Advanced imaging techniques, such as computed tomography and magnetic resonance imaging are of great value in the differential diagnosis of disorders of the central nervous system. Nevertheless, in the large majority of cases, the cause of a headache can be established satisfactorily on a carefully taken history and clinical examination.

F. Dudley Hart

Heart, enlargement of

Cardiac enlargement may be detected or suspected on the basis of clinical examination (*see* HEART IMPULSE, DISPLACED), a chest radiograph or an electrocardiogram. Full assessment usually requires the combination of these three forms of investigation, plus echocardiography. When considering a patient with apparent cardiac enlargement, it is necessary to decide: (1) whether the enlargement is genuine or spurious; (2) if genuine, whether it is physiological or pathological; and (3) if pathological, whether it is due primarily to a myocardial disorder or a haemodynamic lesion.

The identification of genuine cardiac enlargement

The clinical diagnosis of cardiac enlargement is usually made because of displacement of the cardiac impulse. With left ventricular hypertrophy due to hypertension, aortic stenosis or hypertrophic cardiomyopathy the apex may not be displaced, but has a heaving, sustained character quite different from the normal. *Radiographic* cardiac enlargement is diagnosed when the cardiothoracic ratio is greater than 0·5 in a posteroanterior chest radiograph with a tube-to-film distance of at least 2 m, taken in full inspiration. The cardiothoracic ratio is the ratio of the widest part of the cardiac shadow to the widest part of the lung fields. A spurious impression of cardiomegaly is caused by antero-posterior projections, portable apparatus with a reduced tube–film distance, and a poor inspiratory effort. In pectus excavation (funnel chest) a false impression of cardiac enlargement may be obtained from a posteroanterior film but a lateral film will clarify the issue.

Radiological enlargement of the cardiac shadow may be due to a pericardial effusion. This is more likely if the enlargement is rapid (and previous films are available for comparison). Clinically there will usually be elevation of the jugular venous pressure, there may be a pericardial friction rub, and an increased area of cardiac dullness. The ECG usually shows low voltages and there may be electrical alternans (alternating large and small QRS complexes in the same lead). Echocardiography is diagnostic (*Fig.* H.10).

An electrocardiographic diagnosis of cardiac enlargement is usually based on large QRS voltages. By convention, a sum of the S wave in lead V2 and the R wave in V5 of greater than 4·5 mv is one of the criteria for left ventricular hypertrophy. However this criterion is sometimes met in fit muscular young men with thin chest walls, and in this circumstance other criteria such as a QRS duration of more than 0·1 second or T wave changes should be sought before making a firm diagnosis.

The identification of a pathological process

Athletes tend to have enlarged hearts, a slow resting pulse rate, and often a soft ejection systolic murmur related to a large resting stroke volume. In 'duration'

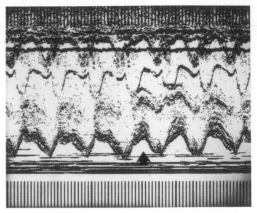

Fig. H.10. M-mode echocardiogram from a patient with pericardial effusion. The echo-free space between chest wall and the front of the right ventricle is arrowed.

sports such as running or swimming there is chamber enlargement without disproportionate hypertrophy of the ventricular walls. In 'power' sports such as weightlifting there may also be ventricular hypertrophy. If left ventricular hypertrophy is marked on electrocardiography or echocardiography it is worth asking about, and warning against, abuse of anabolic steroids.

Cardiac enlargement is sometimes found in patients with congenital heart block, as an adaptive response to a slow pulse rate. It is usually present in acromegaly—sometimes as part of a general process of soft tissue hypertrophy, but sometimes as a feature of acromegalic heart muscle disease.

The distinction between myocardial and haemodynamic disorders

Cardiac enlargement, without a murmur but with an added third or fourth heart sound, is more likely to be due to a myocardial disorder and, with a murmur, to a haemodynamic lesion; the distinction is not absolute, however. The best diagnostic tool is duplex ultrasound (echocardiography plus Doppler cardiography) which gives information both about valve performance and about ventricular function.

MYOCARDIAL PROBLEMS

The principal heart muscle problems (in order of frequency in 'Western' practice) are ischaemic heart disease, dilated cardiomyopathy, hypertrophic cardiomyopathy and the 'specific heart muscle diseases' which mimic dilated cardiomyopathy.

Ischaemic heart disease

Myocardial infarction can lead to left ventricular aneurysm formation. This is more frequent after anterior infarction. The cardiac impulse is displaced and has a diffuse 'dyskinetic' feel. The ECG shows evidence of old infarction, sometimes with persistent ST segment elevation. The chest radiograph usually shows cardiomegaly, occasionally with calcification in the aneurysm. Echocardiography is diagnostic. Ischaemic heart disease can also cause global left ventricular dilatation indistinguishable clinically from a dilated cardiomyopathy, though symptoms of angina or a history of myocardial infarction may provide clues.

Dilated cardiomyopathy

Dilated cardiomyopathy is the consequence of diffuse damage to cardiac muscle. By definition, the cause of 'cardiomyopathy' is unknown, but a similar clinical pattern is found in acute myocarditis and in association with a number of 'specific heart muscle diseases' (*Table H.7*). The heart is clinically and radiologically enlarged and there are usually features of cardiac failure. There is a tachycardia and often a gallop rhythm with a loud third heart sound. The apex is displaced, and there may be soft systolic murmurs from functional mitral or tricuspid regurgitation. The electrocardiogram is usually abnormal, but the changes are non-specific. Echocardiography shows a characteristic pattern with dilatation of all four cardiac chambers and very poor ventricular contraction. Myocardial biopsy has a limited role, largely in excluding myocarditis or a specific cause. The prognosis is best when there is a remediable cause such as alcohol abuse, or where acute myocarditis is followed by spontaneous recovery.

Acute myocarditis is probably the commonest cause of a dilated cardiomyopathy pattern in younger adults. There is often a preceding acute febrile illness or respiratory tract infection. Many viruses have been implicated, but the most consistent link is with the Coxsackie B group. The vast majority of cases of myocarditis probably goes unrecognized, but the prognosis in cases which present with cardiac failure is poor.

Alcoholic heart disease is probably the most common of the specific heart muscle diseases in middle-aged Western males, and there is some evidence that it may be reversible. Amyloid heart disease is unusual, among the specific heart muscle diseases, in that ventricular dilatation is not a prominent feature, although ventricular function is impaired.

Hypertrophic cardiomyopathy

Hypertrophic cardiomyopathy is characterized by abnormal hypertrophy of all or part of the ventricular muscle in the absence of an obvious stimulus. One form, usually inherited as an autosomal dominant trait, tends to present in childhood or adolescence and may cause sudden death, usually after physical exertion. Another form, whose genetic status is less clear, presents in the fifth or sixth decade and has a more benign course.

Table H.7. Specific heart muscle diseases

This is not an exhaustive list of specific heart muscle diseases, but emphasizes those which may present with cardiac enlargement.

Connective tissue diseases
Sarcoidosis
Systemic lupus erythematosus
Polyarteritis nodosa
Rheumatoid arthritis (+ pericardial effusion)

Infections
Chagas disease
Viral myocarditis
Rickettsial myocarditis

Neurological/neuromuscular disorders
Duchenne's progressive muscular dystrophy
Friedreich's ataxia (mimics hypertrophic
  cardiomyopathy)
Dystrophia myotonica (+ heart block)
X-linked humeroperoneal neuromuscular disease
  (mainly heart block)

Neoplastic disease (primary or metastatic)
Leukaemia, lymphomas

Metabolic disease
Amyloidosis
Haemochromatosis
Cardiac glycogenosis
Polysaccharide storage disease
Tay–Sachs disease
Fabry's disease
Gout
Oxalosis
Mucopolysaccharidoses (Hurler's syndrome)
Refsum's disease

Endocrine
Diabetes (+ ischaemic heart disease)
Phaeochromocytoma
Thyrotoxicosis
Myxoedema (+ pericardial effusion)
Acromegaly
Cushing's syndrome (+ hypertension)

Nutritional
Beri-beri
Kwashiorkhor

Toxic chemical and drug effects
Alcohol
Cobalt
Emetine and chloroquine
Daunorubicin and doxorubicin

There is usually clinical cardiac enlargement. The apex is displaced and often has 'double beat' character from a palpable atrial impulse, as well as the sustained lift of ventricular hypertrophy. There is usually a systolic murmur, which gets louder during a Valsalva manoeuvre. There may be reversed splitting of the second heart sound, and the peripheral pulses are 'jerky'. The electrocardiogram is abnormal, sometimes showing left ventricular hypertrophy with marked T wave changes, sometimes mimicking an inferior infarct. Echocardiography is diagnostic. Patients with the hereditary neurological disorder, Friedreich's ataxia, frequently have cardiac lesions similar to those of hypertrophic cardiomyopathy.

HAEMODYNAMIC PROBLEMS

Haemodynamic problems causing cardiac enlargement can be divided into those causing a *volume load* and those causing a *pressure load*. The initial response to a volume load is an increase in stroke volume, with enlargement of the cardiac chambers concerned but preservation of vigorous contraction. The response to a pressure load is hypertrophy, without dilatation, of the chambers involved. If either a volume or a pressure load persists beyond the capacity of the heart to compensate, then the chambers will dilate and contraction will become impaired. Chronic failure of the 'left side' of the heart, from mitral valve disease, or left ventricular impairment, may be accompanied by reactive pulmonary vasoconstriction and secondary pulmonary hypertension, with ensuing dilatation of the right heart chambers as well.

Causes of pressure load
Left-sided
   Common
   Systemic hypertension
   Aortic stenosis
   Less common
   Coarctation of the aorta
   Rare
   Phaeochromocytoma
Right-sided
   Common
   Cor pulmonale
   Reactive pulmonary hypertension from left-sided problem
   Less common
   Chronic thromboembolic pulmonary hypertension
   Pulmonary stenosis
   Eisenmenger's syndrome
   Rare
   Primary pulmonary hypertension
   Carcinoid syndrome
   Appetite suppressants

Systemic hypertension is by far the commonest 'pressure load' cause of cardiac enlargement. Most cases are due to 'essential' hypertension, but renal and endocrine causes should be remembered. Aortic coarctation causes delayed femoral pulses, and there is often a systolic murmur. A phaeochromocytoma can cause severe, but intermittent, hypertension. Murmurs should lead to the diagnosis of aortic or pulmonary stenosis. Aortic stenosis is frequently severe even when there is little or no radiological cardiac enlargement, but the presence of poststenotic dilatation of the ascending aorta may give a clue (*Fig.* H.11). The diagnosis of pulmonary hypertension is often missed. The circumstances may be suggestive, and clinically the combination of a pronounced right parasternal impulse with changes of right ventricular hypertrophy in the electrocardiogram should lead it to be suspected.

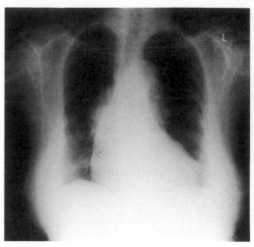

Fig. H.11. Chest radiograph from a patient with severe aortic stenosis. There is little ventricular dilatation, but there is poststenotic dilatation of the ascending aorta.

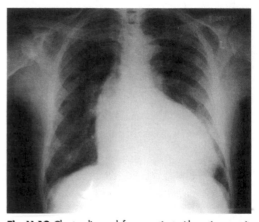

Fig. H.12. Chest radiograph from a patient with aortic regurgitation and previous hypertension. There is predominantly left ventricular enlargement, with, in addition, some dilatation of the ascending aorta ('sitting duck' profile). This combination is frequently seen in patients with aortic regurgitation or mixed aortic valve disease.

Causes of volume load
Left-sided
   Common
   Mitral regurgitation
   Aortic regurgitation
   Less common
   Systemic arteriovenous fistula
   Severe anaemia
   Congenital heart disease: persistent ductus arteriosus, ventricular septal defect
   Rare
   Paget's disease of bone
   Erythroderma (in both cases via arteriovenous shunts)
Right-sided
   Atrial septal defect
   Other complex congenital heart disease
   Tricuspid regurgitation

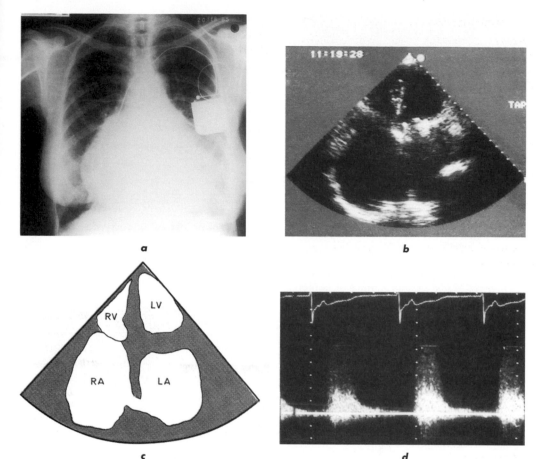

Fig. H.13. *a,* Chest radiograph showing massive cardiac enlargement in a patient with mitral and aortic valve disease and a cardiac pacemaker. The radiographic appearances do not permit easy identification of the specific chambers involved, but echocardiography *(b,c)* from the apex shows that most of the enlargement is due to atrial dilatation. *d,* Doppler cardiography showed that in fact the predominant lesion was aortic stenosis. This case emphasizes the need to combine different diagnostic techniques in solving complex problems.

Mitral and aortic regurgitation are detected through their distinctive murmurs. Selective enlargement of the different cardiac chambers may give a characteristic radiographic appearance (*Fig.* H.12), but in some cases the radiographic appearance is nonspecific and further aid must be sought from ultrasound scanning (*Fig.* H.13). 'Extracardiac' causes of an increased volume load are often difficult to detect, and require careful clinical assessment, possibly backed by objective measurement of cardiac output at rest by echocardiography, dye dilution or radionuclide techniques.

D. De Bono

Heart impulse, displaced

The position of the cardiac apex is defined as the furthest outward and downward point at which a cardiac impulse can be felt in the supine unrotated patient. This point usually lies in the 5th or 6th left intercostal space in the midclavicular line.

Displacement of the apex may be due to a congenitally abnormal position of the heart, to cardiac enlargement, or to cardiac displacement resulting from chest wall or intrathoracic abnormalities.

Congenital dextrocardia may involve simple mirror-image inversion of the heart and other viscera (situs inversus) or may be associated with a variety of complex congenital cardiac defects (*Fig.* H.14). In adults, simple dextrocardia without associated defects is more common, and is benign.

Displacement of the cardiac apex resulting from *cardiac enlargement* can usually be suspected on the basis of the patient's symptoms of heart disease, or the presence of murmurs or abnormal heart sounds. Confirmation can be made by chest radiography, ECG and echocardiography, and the differential diagnosis is discussed more fully in HEART, ENLARGEMENT OF.

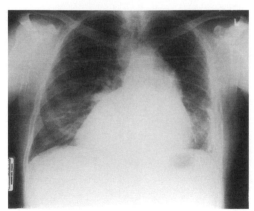

Fig. H.14. Dextrocardia in an adult patient with complex cyanotic congenital heart disease. The abdominal viscera were not inverted—note the position of the gastric air bubble.

Displacement of the cardiac apex from *abnormalities of the chest wall* is usually apparent on inspection of the patient; these abnormalities include pectus excavatum (funnel chest), pectus carinatum (pigeon chest), kyphoscoliosis and thoracoplasty.

An exception is sometimes a 'compensated' thoracic kyphoscoliosis, which may be more easily appreciated on a chest radiograph. Conversely, pectus excavatum is obvious clinically, but is sometimes missed on cursory inspection of a postero-anterior chest radiograph (*Fig.* H.15).

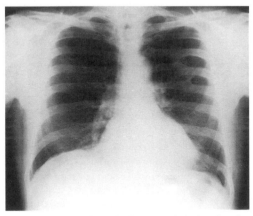

Fig. H.15. Chest radiograph of patient with displaced cardiac apex resulting from pectus excavatum. The ribs appear more horizontal than usual (fractured ribs also seen on left).

Displacements of the cardiac apex as a result of intrathoracic abnormalities are listed below according to the organ or tissue involved. Pulmonary or diaphragmatic causes are common, the rest rare.

LUNG AND PLEURA

Pleural effusion
Pneumonectomy
Tension pneumothorax

DIAPHRAGM

Congenital diaphragmatic hernia
Hiatus hernia

PERICARDIUM

Clearwater cyst of pericardium
Pericardial tumour

OESOPHAGUS

Achalasia of the cardia/megaoesophagus
Foregut duplication cyst

AORTA

Aneurysm of descending aorta

Lymphoid tissue and thymus

Enlargement of thoracic lymph nodes is common, but seldom causes cardiac displacement. Rarely, enlargement of para-aortic nodes or aberrant thymus tissues may do so.

The differential diagnosis can often be clarified by radiography in the postero-anterior and lateral projections, with the help of a barium swallow to outline the oesophagus. In more difficult cases CT scanning and echocardiography—particularly transoesophageal echocardiography—are useful.

D. De Bono

Heart, murmurs in

A heart murmur is the audible sign of turbulent blood flow within the heart. The site of maximum intensity of the murmur should be noted together with the direction in which it radiates—as a rule this is the direction in which the turbulent blood is flowing. Other clues such as cardiac enlargement or abnormal pulsation in the precordium or neck vessels should also be sought. A thrill is a palpable vibration and, for practical purposes, thrills can be regarded as 'palpable' murmurs. High-pitched vibration is usually more easily heard than felt and the significance of a thrill is simply that of a loud murmur. With low-frequency vibrations, some observers claim to find a thrill easier to feel than a low-pitched murmur is to hear.

Heart murmurs can be classified as *systolic* or *diastolic* (the continuous murmur of persistent ductus arteriosus is, strictly speaking, exocardiac), though a single lesion can sometimes cause both. Systolic murmurs accompany the upstroke of the carotid pulse, diastolic murmurs precede or follow it.

Systolic murmurs

These are further classified as *ejection systolic murmurs*, which increase to a crescendo in midsystole and then die away before the second sound, and *pansystolic murmurs*, which remain at a more or less constant amplitude throughout systole. Late systolic murmurs are a variant of the latter, appearing in mid or late systole and continuing to the second sound (*Fig.* H.16).

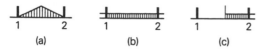

1	2	1	2	1	2
(a)		(b)		(c)	

Fig. H.16. Diagrammatic representation of ejection systolic (*a*), pansystolic (*b*) and late systolic murmurs (*c*).

Ejection systolic murmurs

The causes of these are listed in *Table* H.8.

Table H.8. Causes of ejection systolic murmurs

Most common
Innocent murmur
Flow murmur of high cardiac output
Mild aortic stenosis; bicuspid aortic valve
Mild pulmonary stenosis

Common
More severe aortic stenosis
Flow murmur of aortic regurgitation
Pulmonary stenosis
Pulmonary flow murmur of atrial septal defect
Hypertrophic cardiomyopathy

Uncommon
Supra- or subvalvar aortic stenosis
Severe hypercholesterolaemia

INNOCENT SYSTOLIC MURMURS

An ejection systolic murmur is commonly heard in fit children or young adults, particularly after exercise or vasodilatation, for example during pregnancy. Characteristically, the murmur is soft, best heard in the second left intercostal space and gets louder on inspiration; the second sound is normally split (*see* HEART SOUNDS) and there are no other abnormal signs. Further investigation of these patients is almost always negative and the long-term prognosis is excellent.

AORTIC AND PULMONARY STENOSIS

The murmurs of mild aortic or pulmonary stenosis differ from innocent murmurs principally in that they tend to be louder and the murmur is often preceded by an ejection click. Most patients with mild congenital aortic stenosis have bicuspid valves. Eventually the abnormal valve tends to calcify and a mild stenosis may become severe. In elderly patients a soft ejection systolic murmur is usually due to calcific infiltration of the aortic valve and an ejection click is absent. The murmur of aortic stenosis can usually be heard all over the precordium and tends to radiate to the upper right sternal edge and the neck. The murmur of pulmonary stenosis is loudest at the left sternal edge and may radiate to the back. In aortic coarctation, an ejection

murmur may be heard beneath the left scapula; other signs such as delayed femoral pulses are also present.

In young patients, the murmurs of severe pulmonary or aortic stenosis tend to be loud and harsh, but loudness is a poor guide to the severity of aortic stenosis in the elderly or when the cardiac output is low. Other features of severe aortic stenosis include clinical evidence of left ventricular hypertrophy and a slow-rising carotid pulse. In severe pulmonary stenosis the second sound is widely split. Duplex ultrasound scanning (two-dimensional echocardiography plus Doppler studies) is the most useful investigation. A Doppler record from a patient with aortic stenosis is shown in (*Fig.* H.17).

FLOW MURMURS

Ejection systolic murmurs may be due to turbulence caused by a normal blood flow through a stenotic valve orifice, as in aortic stenosis, or by an increased blood flow through a non-stenotic valve. The latter mechanism accounts for most innocent murmurs and, also, for the pulmonary ejection systolic murmur of atrial septal defect, in which the flow through the pulmonary valve orifice may be increased two or three-fold above normal. These patients have an 'active' feel to the precordium, there is fixed splitting of the second sound and there may be a tricuspid diastolic flow murmur. Similarly, patients with marked aortic regurgitation may have a systolic murmur despite the absence of anatomical stenosis.

HYPERTROPHIC CARDIOMYOPATHY

Patients with this condition usually have an ejection systolic murmur, clinical evidence of left ventricular hypertrophy and often a characteristic 'jerky' pulse. In these patients, the murmur paradoxically tends to get softer in inspiration and louder during expiration or a Valsalva manoeuvre. Echocardiography is usually diagnostic.

Pansystolic murmurs

The causes of such murmurs are listed in *Table* H.9.

MITRAL REGURGITATION

The murmur of mitral regurgitation is usually loudest at the apex and radiates to the axilla. Loudness is some indication of severity, but there are exceptions. Torrential mitral regurgitation from papillary muscle rupture may be almost silent, while some patients with mitral valve prolapse and haemodynamically mild regurgitation may occasionally emit exceedingly loud 'honks' or 'whoops' audible across the room. The severity can be assessed from the patient's general condition, cardiac enlargement, the presence of cardiac

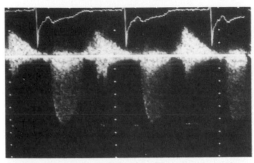
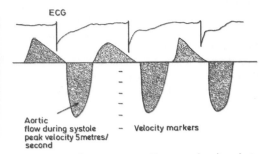

Fig. H.17. Doppler cardiographic trace from the cardiac apex in a patient with aortic stenosis. The trace plots the velocity against time profile of blood ejected through the aortic valve. The maximum velocity is 5 metres per second, corresponding to a peak instantaneous gradient of approximately $4 \times 5^2 = 100$ mmHg.

Table H.9. Causes of pansystolic murmurs

Most common
Mitral regurgitation (in adults)
   Rheumatic
   Mitral valve prolapse
   Ischaemic
   Due to endocarditis
   Secondary to dilatation of mitral annulus
Ventricular septal defect (in children)

Common
Tricuspid regurgitation
   Secondary
   Rheumatic
   Due to endocarditis
Postinfarction ventricular septal defect

Uncommon
Pneumomediastinum 'pseudomurmur' or 'pericardial
   crunch'

failure and the radiographic appearances as well as from the murmur. The term 'mitral valve prolapse' is used, confusingly, to describe either a diverse group of causes of non-rheumatic mitral regurgitation which have in common excessive elongation of the chordae tendineae, or a clinical syndrome which includes both the consequences of mitral regurgitation and also other features such as a predisposition to dysrhythmias and, possibly, sudden death. Echocardiography is sometimes able to distinguish patients who simply have thin, stretched chordae tendineae (pellucid valve syndrome) from those with thickened, redundant, myxomatous valve tissue. It is in the latter group that most of the 'extra-valvar' events occur.

Clinically, patients with mitral valve prolapse are sometimes indistinguishable from those with other causes of regurgitation. The murmur of prolapse tends, however, to be mid- or late-systolic rather than pansystolic, at least in the early stages, and there may be one or more mid-systolic 'clicks' which are due to tensing of the chordae.

CONGENITAL VENTRICULAR SEPTAL DEFECT

This is the commonest cause of a pansystolic murmur in children and young adults. Large ventricular septal

defects can cause cardiac failure within the first 3 months of life and, if untreated, sometimes induce reactive pulmonary hypertension with diminution, and eventual reversal, of shunt blood flow, cyanosis and disappearance of the murmur. Most pansystolic murmurs in older children are due to small defects with a loud murmur but a small shunt (maladie de Roger). The murmur is heard all over the precordium but maximally at the upper left sternal edge. Duplex ultrasound scanning is the investigation of choice. Accurate knowledge of the size and position of a defect helps predict whether it is likely to close spontaneously.

ACQUIRED VENTRICULAR SEPTAL DEFECT

In adults, this may follow stab wounds or, more commonly, acute myocardial infarction. Clinical distinction between postinfarction septal defect and mitral regurgitation is difficult but ultrasound is diagnostic.

TRICUSPID REGURGITATION

This may be primary, from rheumatic heart disease or endocarditis, or secondary to right ventricular dilatation in response to pulmonary hypertension. The murmur is loudest at the lower left sternal edge and is accompanied by pathognomonic 'v' waves in the jugular venous pulse. This lesion is seen much more often in conjunction with other cardiac lesions than on its own.

PERICARDIAL 'CRUNCH'

Patients with acute rupture of the oesophagus may develop a noise in the chest, synchronous with the heart beat, which is virtually indistinguishable from a loud pansystolic murmur. It is presumably a consequence of surgical emphysema in the mediastinum being 'crunched' with each systole.

Diastolic murmurs

These can be divided into early diastolic and mid-diastolic. Early diastolic murmurs are usually soft, decrescendo, high-pitched—'like the letter R whispered', and best heard with the diaphragm of the stethoscope. They immediately follow the second heart sound, or the downstroke of the carotid pulse, and tend to be best heard at the left (sometimes right) sternal border with the patient sitting up, leaning forward and breathing out. Mid-diastolic murmurs are usually low-pitched, rumbling and best heard with the stethoscope bell (*Fig.* H.18).

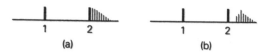

Fig. H.18. Diagrammatic representation of early diastolic (*a*) and mid-diastolic (*b*) murmurs.

Early diastolic murmurs

There are only two important causes of such murmurs, *aortic* and *pulmonary regurgitation*. The causes of these lesions are listed in *Table* H.10.

Table H.10. Causes of early diastolic murmurs

Aortic regurgitation due to	
Most common	Bicuspid aortic valve Chronic rheumatic heart disease
Common	Chronic hypertension Dissecting aneurysm of aorta Infective endocarditis Failing aortic prosthesis
Uncommon	Acute rheumatic fever Rheumatoid heart disease Ankylosing spondylitis Reiter's syndrome Chronic renal failure
Pulmonary regurgitation due to	
Common	Secondary pulmonary hypertension, e.g. in mitral valve disease Following pulmonary valvotomy or valvuloplasty
Uncommon	Primary pulmonary hypertension Thromboembolic pulmonary hypertension Eisenmenger's syndrome

AORTIC REGURGITATION

Unless this lesion is mild, it is usually accompanied by a wide pulse pressure and a collapsing arterial pulse. Features such as exaggerated carotid pulsation (Corrigan's sign), 'pistol shot' femoral bruits and capillary pulsation (Quincke's sign) are 'makeweights' to be sought when the diagnosis is already firm. The murmur of *acute* aortic regurgitation, as in acute endocarditis, is similar in timing to the more usual early diastolic murmur but may be quite different in quality,

being loud and harsh and apt to be confused with a systolic murmur unless it is timed against the pulse.

PULMONARY REGURGITATION

This is usually secondary to pulmonary hypertension; the murmur of pulmonary regurgitation secondary to chronic rheumatic mitral stenosis was described by Graham Steell. Pulmonary regurgitation may also be due to a damaged pulmonary valve resulting from a previous valvotomy or balloon valvuloplasty; in the absence of pulmonary hypertension pulmonary regurgitation seems to be very well tolerated. Distinction from aortic regurgitation is usually easy from the clinical circumstances and the absence of other features of aortic regurgitation. Confirmation is possible by Doppler cardiography.

Mid-diastolic murmurs

The causes of these murmurs are listed in *Table* H.11.

Table H.11. Causes of mid-diastolic murmurs

Common
Rheumatic mitral stenosis
Uncommon
Austin Flint murmur in aortic regurgitation Tricuspid flow murmur in atrial septal defect Tricuspid stenosis Carey Coombs murmur in acute rheumatic fever Left or right atrial myxoma Mitral flow murmur in ventricular septal defect or persistent ductus arteriosus with large shunt

MITRAL STENOSIS

This is by far the most common cause of a mid-diastolic murmur, which is best heard at the cardiac apex. There is often an audible or palpable opening snap in addition (*Fig.* H.19). The murmur of mitral stenosis is often accentuated just before the first sound (presystolic accentuation). This is most often recognized in sinus rhythm and attributed to an increased flow during atrial systole but it is sometimes heard in atrial fibrillation.

CAREY COOMBS MURMUR

A soft low-pitched mid-diastolic murmur is sometimes heard in acute rheumatic fever, called after the physician who first described it. It is not due to mitral stenosis but probably represents turbulence from minute vegetations on the mitral valve surface and from stiffening of the valve itself.

AUSTIN FLINT MURMUR

This murmur is due to fluttering of the anterior leaflet of the mitral valve, as a result of turbulence caused by aortic regurgitation. There is invariably an early

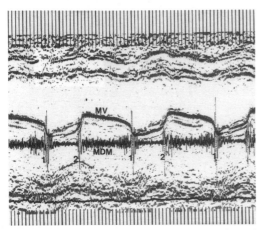

Fig. H.19. Echophonocardiogram from a patient with mitral stenosis showing the relationship of the mid-diastolic murmur (MDM) to the opening of the mitral valve (MV).

diastolic murmur of aortic regurgitation and the opening snap of mitral stenosis is absent. Echocardiography is diagnostic.

MID-DIASTOLIC FLOW MURMURS

The mid-diastolic murmur of increased tricuspid flow in atrial septal defect is usually heard only in children and adolescents. It tends to be higher pitched than the murmur of mitral stenosis and is best heard at the lower left sternal edge. A similar murmur may be heard at the apex in patients with a large ventricular septal defect or persistent ductus arteriosus.

TRICUSPID STENOSIS

The murmurs of tricuspid stenosis are similar to those of mitral stenosis, but the condition is much less common. The jugular venous pressure is elevated and the venous pulse has a characteristic waveform (*see* NECK, ENGORGED VEINS IN).

ATRIAL MYXOMA

Left atrial myxomas are commoner than right though both are rare. They may cause murmurs mimicking mitral stenosis but, often, the murmurs vary with posture as the myxoma prolapses in or out of the valve orifice. The first sound is loud and there may be an extra sound, called a 'tumour plop', from movement of the myxoma.

D. De Bono

Heart sounds

Tradition describes four heart sounds. The first and second are almost always audible, the third and fourth occur only in specific circumstances. There is also a medley of *added sounds*, mainly described as 'clicks',

'snaps' or 'plops', which can be heard in patients with particular conditions—these are distinguished from murmurs and rubs (*see* HEART, MURMURS IN and RUB, PERICARDIAL) by their short duration.

First sound

The first heart sound is due to the closure of the mitral and tricuspid valves. Closure is normally simultaneous, but occasionally one valve closes slightly before the other, causing splitting of the first sound. This may be associated with right bundle branch block, but is seldom of clinical importance.

The first sound is usually readily recognized as the 'lub' in the traditional 'lub-dup' cadence of heart sounds. It is the sound which immediately precedes the upstroke of the carotid pulse. A *loud* first heart sound is most commonly associated with a hyperdynamic circulation (e.g. in pregnancy, febrile illness, thyrotoxicosis). Echocardiography has shown that the mitral cusps are still wide apart at the onset of systole as a consequence of the atrial augmentation of ventricular filling, and it is this together with the increased rate of rise of ventricular pressure (dp/dt) as a result of sympathetic stimulation and a low peripheral resistance which increase the force of valve closure. A loud first sound is not a feature of paroxysmal tachycardia, where ventricular stroke volume is reduced and the synchrony of atrial and ventricular contraction may be disturbed. *Mitral stenosis* is the other common cause of an abnormally loud first sound. In rheumatic mitral stenosis the mitral cusps are fused together laterally to form a diaphragm which bulges into the left ventricle during diastole, and is propelled sharply back towards the left atrium in systole. The latter movement produces a loud, ringing first sound, often palpable as well as audible. A loud first sound is best heard in patients with a stenosed but still mobile valve in sinus rhythm. Progressive calcification restricts valve movement, and the sound gets quieter. A loud first sound alone does not make the diagnosis of mitral stenosis, but should prompt a careful search for a mid-diastolic murmur. A much rarer cause of a loud first heart sound is left atrial myxoma. Tricuspid stenosis may also cause a loud first sound, but this is rare. Apparently increased loudness of the first heart sound may simply be due to a relative lack of soft tissue between heart and stethoscope, as in fit thin young subjects or patients who have had a mastectomy. Conversely, obesity or emphysema may muffle the heart sounds.

Varying intensity of the first sound occurs in three common conditions—atrial fibrillation, extrasystoles, and complete heart block. In atrial fibrillation the varying length of diastole causes the mitral cusps to be in varying positions at the onset of systole, and ventricular stroke volume also varies with the length of diastole. To some extent these effects cancel out, so the variation in first sound intensity may be less than in complete heart block, where stroke volume is relatively constant but where the varying relationship of atrial to ventricular systole causes the position of the mitral cusps to vary from beat to beat at the onset of systole. With extrasystoles, the first sound of the premature beat is invariably softer. Coupled extrasystoles cause a characteristic cadence of loud first, normal second sound, soft first and second sound, pause. This is often misinterpreted because the premature beat gives no palpable pulse and all the sounds are ascribed to a single cardiac cycle.

An abnormally quiet first heart sound, unless an artefact of obesity or emphysema, is usually due to a reduced cardiac output. In left ventricular failure a small increase in left ventricular volume during diastole causes a large rise in pressure, and echocardiography shows that the mitral cusps have virtually drifted together before the onset of systole. In these circumstances a quiet first heart sound frequently accompanies a third or fourth sound, as described below.

A sudden diminution in the intensity of the first sound may occur in acute mitral regurgitation, when it will be associated with the appearance of a pansystolic murmur. Even more rarely, an endocarditic vegetation or an atrial myxoma (*see below*) may interfere with mitral valve closure and cause a sudden reduction in the first sound.

The changes in intensity of the first heart sound can be summarised as follows:

LOUD
Thin chest wall
Hyperdynamic circulation
Mitral stenosis
Atrial myxoma

SOFT
Obesity/emphysema
Cardiac failure
Acute mitral regurgitation
Endocarditis/myxoma

VARIABLE
Atrial fibrillation
Extrasystoles
Complete heart block
Atrial myxoma

Second sound

The second heart sound is due to closure of the aortic and pulmonary valves. In expiration their closure is normally synchronous, but in inspiration there is a tendency for the aortic valve to close slightly earlier, the negative intrathoracic pressure causing blood to pool in the pulmonary veins, and the pulmonary valve slightly later, as venous return to the right side of the heart is increased. *Inspiratory splitting of the second heart sound* is the result—a normal finding in children and in some adults. It is best appreciated with the stethoscope diaphragm applied at the left of the sternum in the second or third intercostal space.

Fixed splitting of the second heart sound is virtually pathognomonic of atrial septal defect. The second sound is split because of the increased volume load on the right ventricle, and the split is fixed because the septal defect equalizes right and left atrial pressure throughout the cardiac cycle. Fixed splitting is not a feature of ventricular septal defect or persistent ductus arteriosus.

Fixed splitting has to be distinguished from *wide splitting* of the second sound where the split is audible in both inspiration and expiration but wider in inspiration. This occurs in right bundle branch block and in pulmonary stenosis. There is a direct relationship between the width of the expiratory split and the pulmonary gradient. In severe pulmonary stenosis or Fallot's tetralogy the pulmonary component of the second sound may be so quiet as to be inaudible. Wide splitting of the second sound is not usually found in pulmonary hypertension.

Reversed splitting of the second sound occurs when left ventricular ejection is prolonged or delayed so that pulmonary closure precedes aortic valve closure. Inspiration now causes the sounds to move together, so wider splitting is heard in expiration. In practice, reversed splitting is uncommon, and is mainly associated with left bundle branch block, hypertrophic obstructive cardiomyopathy and some cases of congenital aortic stenosis. In most adult cases of aortic stenosis the valve cusps are so rigid that the aortic second sound is inaudible.

An abnormally loud second heart sound is most commonly due to systemic hypertension. The second sound may also be loud in patients with a dilated or aneurysmal ascending aorta. Because the pulmonary artery lies closer to the surface than the ascending aorta, pulmonary hypertension can cause a very loud second heart sound which may be palpable as well as audible. In patients with transposition of the aorta and pulmonary arteries a loud second sound is heard for the same reason.

The characteristics of the second heart sound in various conditions can be summarised as follows:

LOUD

Thin chest wall
Hyperdynamic circulation
Pulmonary hypertension
Transposition of great arteries

SOFT

Obesity
Low cardiac output
Severe aortic or pulmonary stenosis

NORMAL SPLIT

Healthy children, some adults

WIDE SPLIT

Pulmonary stenosis
Right bundle branch block

FIXED SPLIT

Atrial septal defect

REVERSED SPLIT

Hypertrophic cardiomyopathy
Left bundle branch block

Third sound

The third heart sound is a low-pitched sound, like a thump or a thud, which occurs in mid-diastole. It is 'physiological' in athletes, some children, and in association with a hyperdynamic circulation, e.g. during pregnancy. In other patients it is associated with a dilated, poorly contracting left ventricle with a high end-diastolic pressure. The precise mechanism of the third heart sound is controversial. Its timing has been shown to coincide with the end of the phase of rapid diastolic ventricular filling.

A third sound in a fit patient with a resting bradycardia is nearly always physiological. Likewise, when there is evidence of a hyperdynamic circulation such as loud first and second heart sounds, peripheral vasodilatation and a good pulse volume, a third sound is little cause for worry. A third sound is also often heard in severe mitral regurgitation, even in the absence of heart failure.

A pathological third sound is usually part of a characteristic cadence described as a gallop rhythm. There is a tachycardia, a soft first heart sound quickly followed by a soft second sound, and then a loud third sound: da-da-*dum*, da-da-*dum*. The patient often looks ill, the cardiac apex is displaced and has a diffuse or dyskinetic feel. A chest radiograph will confirm cardiac enlargement, and the best way to confirm impaired ventricular function is by echocardiography.

Fourth sound

The fourth heart sound is associated with a hypertrophied atrium emptying into a rather stiff left ventricle. It is only heard in sinus rhythm, and precedes the first sound by about 0·15 seconds: da-lub-dup, da-lub-dup. It is characteristically heard in hypertension and in hypertrophic cardiomyopathy, and occasionally in patients with ischaemic heart disease, especially soon after myocardial infarction, or aortic stenosis. In severe hypertension or hypertrophic cardiomyopathy there is often a separate palpable and visible component to the apex beat which coincides with the fourth heart sound. A fourth sound is not a feature of mitral stenosis (where the stenosed valve prevents rapid atrial emptying) or of mitral regurgitation where the atrium is too distended to contract forcefully. Some authorities describe patients with a fourth sound as having a 'presystolic gallop rhythm'.

Added or extra sounds

The *opening snap* is a feature of mitral (more rarely tricuspid) stenosis. It coincides with the bulging of the mitral valve 'diaphragm' into the ventricle in early diastole. It is a sharp, high-pitched sound best heard with the stethoscope diaphragm in the third or fourth left intercostal space about 3 cm from the left sternal edge, and apt to be confused with a widely split second sound. The presence of an opening snap indicates that the valve, though stenosed, is still mobile. The interval between the second sound and opening snap reflects left atrial pressure—a high pressure, and thus severe stenosis, causing an early opening snap.

An *ejection click* is a short, loud, ringing sound immediately following the first heart sound ('as the l follows c in click'). It is a feature of valvar aortic stenosis with a mobile aortic valve, bicuspid aortic valve, or valvar pulmonary stenosis, and it is usually followed by an ejection systolic murmur. It is best heard in the aortic or pulmonary 'areas' depending on its cause. The mechanism is thought to be tensing of the aortic or pulmonary cusps just prior to ejection. An ejection click without a murmur sometimes occurs in idiopathic dilatation of the pulmonary artery.

Midsystolic clicks are usually associated with mitral valve prolapse (*see* HEART, MURMURS IN, p. 284) and are due to sudden tensing of parts of the mitral valve apparatus during systole (*Fig.* H.20). There may or may not be an associated systolic murmur. Both clicks and murmur may vary with posture and phase of respiration.

Clicking pneumothorax occurs when a small left pneumothorax causes a clicking sound, often loud and audible to the patient, in phase with the cardiac cycle. It is benign and self-limiting, but may recur.

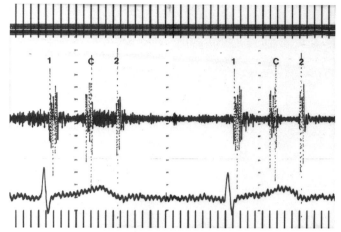

Fig. H.20. Phonocardiogram from a patient with mitral valve prolapse showing first and second heart sounds (1,2) and a midsystolic click (C).

Prosthetic valve sounds are heard in patients who have undergone valve replacement with mechanical prostheses (e.g. Starr–Edwards, Bjork–Shiley or St Jude valves). Each valve has an opening sound (analogous to the opening snap or ejection click) and a closing sound analogous to the first or second heart sound. The closing sound is usually much the louder—if it accompanies the first sound the patient has had a mitral valve replacement and conversely for aortic valve replacement. The sound and cadence of the clicks are fairly constant for an individual patient, and sudden muffling of one or other prosthetic sound usually indicates prosthetic malfunction, perhaps due to thrombosis.

D. De Bono

Heartburn

Heartburn is a burning restrosternal discomfort, sometimes amounting to pain, which is usually perceived to originate in the high epigastrium and radiate towards the neck. Many who suffer from it find difficulty in describing the quality of the sensation, for which adjectives such as burning, hot, sharp, rough or acid are not wholly satisfactory but most sufferers will readily identify the discomfort as being felt up and down the midline anterior chest. The location of the discomfort may therefore be of greater value than descriptions of its quality in distinguishing heartburn from other varieties of chest pain.

Heartburn characteristically develops after meals and may be brought on by changes in posture such as stooping or lying down. Relief follows sitting or standing up, and may be derived from antacids and by drinking water, milk, tea or any other non-acid fluid.

The sensation of heartburn originates in the lower oesophagus and is produced by gastro-oesophageal reflux. Sensitivity of the oesophageal mucosa to acid appears to be at the root of the sensation, although the sensory mechanisms are ill-defined. Oesophagitis—inflammation and erosion of the oesophageal mucosa—is often present, but not invariably so and it is important to appreciate that many patients with troublesome heartburn have no detectable abnormality of the oesophageal mucosa.

Gastro-oesophageal reflux occurs to some degree in most healthy individuals. Excessive gastro-oesophageal reflux, which is likely to produce troublesome heartburn, arises most commonly from malfunction of the lower oesophageal sphincter. Loss of the normal anatomical relationships of the gastro-oesophageal junction, as occurs in hiatus hernia, impairs sphincter function to some extent but in most individuals with excessive gastro-oesophageal reflux there is an intrinsic failure of the sphincter to remain tightly closed and relax only in response to swallowing.

The term gastro-oesophageal reflux disease is currently fashionable to embrace all clinical manifestations and pathological consequences of excessive gastro-oesophageal reflux. Heartburn is its principal and classical symptom. It is clear, however, that many healthy individuals suffer occasional heartburn which they can sometimes relate to dietary indiscretions or overindulgence in alcohol or tobacco. Heartburn is also extremely common during pregnancy. Gastro-oesophageal reflux, and thus heartburn, may also occur in association with gastric and duodenal disorders such as peptic ulceration and acute gastritis, and as an element in the 'dyspepsia' provoked by drugs such as non-steroidal anti-inflammatory agents. The possibility of gastric or duodenal disease should be given particular consideration when upper abdominal discomfort and heartburn coexist.

R. C. Heading

Hemianopia

Hemianopia means inability to see objects in one-half of the visual field. An understanding of the different types of hemianopia requires an understanding of the anatomy of the visual pathways (*Fig.* H.21).

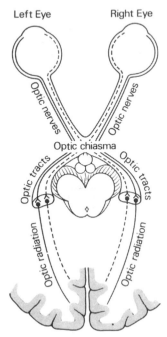

Fig. H.21. Diagram illustrating the connections of the optic nerves and tracts, and the occipital cortex. The left occipital cortex sees objects in the right half of the field of vision. The right occipital cortex sees objects in the left half of the field of vision.

Monocular hemianopia

Loss of half of the visual field of one eye usually indicates optic nerve pathology but may occasionally result from retinal damage. Monocular hemianopia may be either temporal or nasal depending on which fibres in the optic nerve have been damaged. A monocular quadrantanopia indicates loss of one-quarter of one field.

Compression of the optic nerve from a tumour may result in a monocular hemianopia but optic neuritis, such as frequently occurs in multiple sclerosis, more commonly produces a central field defect in the form of a scotoma. The commonest cause of monocular hemianopia is ischaemic damage to the optic nerve.

Bitemporal hemianopia

This most commonly results from damage to the optic chiasma, usually from a pituitary tumour. Less common causes are suprasellar cysts, aneurysms, meningiomas of the tuberculum sellae or craniopharyngiomas.

When the pressure upon the chiasma begins from below the visual field defect typically begins in the upper part of the temporal fields leading initially to a bitemporal quandrantanopia. Pressure from above the chiasma produces initially a lower bitemporal defect. By the time all the crossing fibres in the optic chiasma are compromised, a complete bitemporal hemianopia will have developed.

Skull X-rays will usually show an enlarged pituitary fossa when a bitemporal hemianopia has resulted from a pituitary tumour (*Figs.* H.22, H.23). When due to other causes, the skull X-ray may be normal. The investigation of choice is CT scan or MRI.

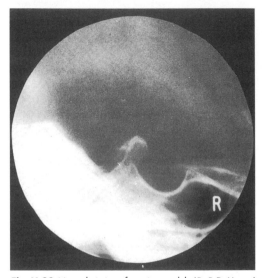

Fig. H.22. Normal pituitary fossa in an adult. (*Dr R.D. Hoare.*)

Homonymous hemianopia

In homonymous hemianopia the visual loss affects the right or left half of each visual field and usually results from damage to the optic radiation or visual cortex. Optic tract damage or damage to the lateral geniculate body may produce a homonymous hemianopia but such cases are rare. Homonymous hemianopia may be congruous or incongruous. Congruous defects are those that are identical in shape and degree in each field; incongruous defects are asymmetrical.

In the optic tracts the intermingling of fibres from the homonymous halves of the two retinae is not as complete as in the optic radiation. Consequently, a lesion of the tract tends to lead to an incongruous homonymous hemianopia whereas a lesion of the optic radiation is more likely to produce a congruous field defect.

Damage to the visual cortex may spare the area responsible for macular vision resulting in homonymous hemianopia with macular sparing. Lesions of the

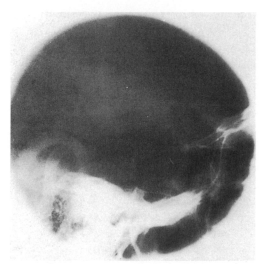

Fig. H.23. Pituitary fossa enlarged by tumour. Note erosion of posterior clinoid processes. (*Dr R.D. Hoare.*)

Table H.12. Brainstem syndromes which involve cranial nerves

Eponym	Signs
Weber's syndrome	Oculomotor palsy with crossed hemiplegia
Benedikt's syndrome	Oculomotor palsy with contralateral cerebellar ataxia, tremor and corticospinal signs
Millard–Gubler syndrome and Raymond–Foville syndrome	Facial and abducens palsy and contralateral hemiplegia; sometimes gaze palsy to side of lesion

Table H.13. The causes of hemiplegia

1. **Congenital**
   Porencephaly, cerebral agenesis, cerebral angioma, Sturge–Weber syndrome (cerebral palsy)
2. **Head injury**
   Birth injury, cerebral contusion, traumatic cerebral haemorrhage, subdural haematoma, extradural haematoma
3. **Vascular accidents**
   Cerebral thrombosis, hypertensive encephalopathy, cerebral haemorrhage (Fig. H.26), subarachnoid haemorrhage, cerebral embolism
4. **Neoplasms**
   Primary neoplasms (Figs H.24, H.25), secondary neoplasms
5. **Infection**
   Meningitis (various), cerebral abscess, cortical thrombophlebitis, encephalitis, hydatid cyst
6. **Demyelinating conditions**
   Multiple sclerosis, Schilder's disease, acute disseminated encephalomyelitis
7. **Degenerative conditions**
   Motor neurone disease
8. **Miscellaneous conditions**
   Pick's disease, epiloia
9. **Hysteria**

parietal lobe typically produce a hemianopia which begins with loss of vision in the lower parts of the field whereas a temporal lobe lesion characteristically affects the upper parts of the visual field (homonymous quandrantanopias). Associated signs may assist in localization.

The visual field defect, when plotted using the Bjerrum screen, may be the same for different size objects and is then said to have sharp edges. A visual field defect which varies depending on the size of the object presented, is said to have sloping edges. The former is more typical of a vascular cause whereas the latter is said to be more often encountered when the optic pathway is compressed by tumour.

In testing the visual fields clinically, it is customary to present an object, usually a finger or coloured pinhead, first to the temporal field of one eye and then to that of the other. It is also useful to present a wagging finger to both temporal fields simultaneously. Occasionally there is failure in this test to pick up the finger in one field although it is perceived when presented singly. This is the phenomenon of visual inattention (or extinction) and it is encountered in some parietal lobe lesions.

N. E. F. Cartlidge

Hemiplegia

Hemiplegia means paralysis of one side of the body affecting both arm and leg. Strictly speaking hemiparesis means partial paralysis, but the two terms are often regarded as interchangeable.

The terms are usually applied in cases in which the paralysis is of upper motor neurone type, although it is possible to see unilateral weakness affecting both arm and leg in lower motor neurone disorders, such as poliomyelitis, motor neurone disease or combined cervical and lumbar radiculopathy. Hemiplegia is most commonly seen in damage to the upper motor neurone above the level of the foramen magnum. A discrete lesion of the spinal cord in the upper cervical region may produce a hemiplegia but this is rare.

Localization of hemiplegia

A lesion of the motor cortex may produce a hemiplegia if extensive enough to involve the cortical areas for arm and leg. There will usually be associated facial weakness.

Damage to the converging fibres descending from the cortex into the internal capsule produces a dense hemiplegia and this is one of the commonest sites of pathology resulting from cerebrovascular disease. The

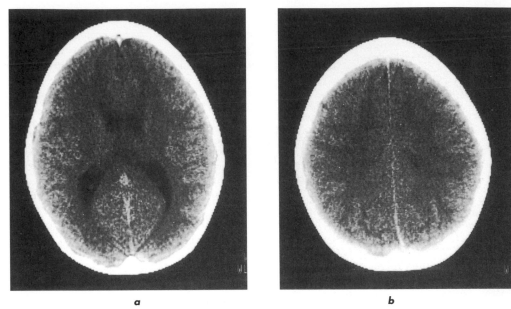

a   *b*

Fig. H.24. Normal CT scan. *a*, At the level of the lateral ventricles. *b*, Above the lateral ventricles showing the corona radiata and the cortex.

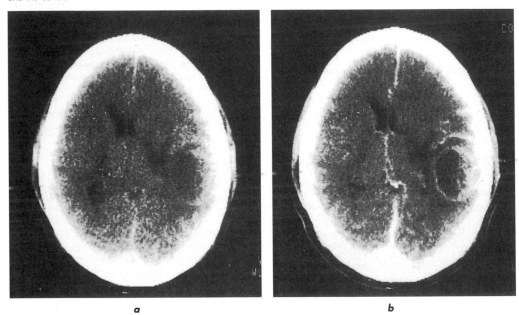

a   *b*

Fig. H.25. CT scan of a left parietal malignant glioma showing a mass effect. *a*, Before injection of contrast. *b*, After injection of contrast showing rim enhancement around necrotic tissues.

weakness typically affects the lower part of the face and the arm and leg in similar degree, although in some instances the hand may be more severely paretic than the proximal muscles of the arm. Typically the so-called 'physiological' flexors are weaker than the extensors. This results in more profound weakness of shoulder abduction, elbow extension, wrist extension, finger extension and finger abduction in the arm, and hip flexion, knee flexion and ankle dorsiflexion in the

leg. The opposing muscles tend to be those which are associated with spasticity resulting in the typical hemiplegic posture of an abducted flexed arm and an extended leg. Loss of all the descending motor axons from damage in one internal capsule is never associated with complete hemiplegia because of the uncrossed fibres from the opposite motor cortex. In dense hemiplegia there may be some weakness of the respiratory muscles and of the trunk. The upper part of the face

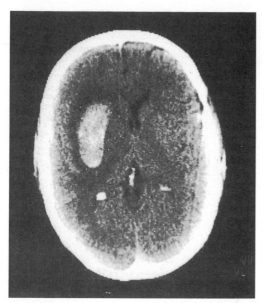

Fig. H.26. CT scan showing intracerebral haemorrhage.

is preserved and the pharyngeal and laryngeal muscles are similarly not greatly affected because of bilateral cortical representation. There may, however, be slight tongue weakness.

Associated signs include those of increased tendon reflexes, extensor plantar responses and ankle and knee clonus. The abdominal and cremasteric reflexes are lost on the side of the hemiplegia. In cases of chronic hemiplegia there may be some slight loss of muscle bulk and contractures may become prominent. Paralysis occurring in childhood before bone growth ceases may be associated with hemiatrophy.

Topographical localization

Damage to the motor cortex rarely produces complete hemiplegia unless the lesion is very extensive. The weakness is often localized to one limb or part of the limb.

In damage to the internal capsule the hemiplegia is often associated with sensory loss and visual field defect. Damage to the descending motor pathway in the brainstem rarely produces isolated hemiplegia because of the other important structures close to the corticospinal tract. One well-known combination resulting from a brainstem lesion is Weber's syndrome where there is an ipsilateral third nerve palsy and a contralateral hemiplegia. Other brainstem syndromes associated with hemiplegia are listed in *Table* H.12. The pathological causes of hemiplegia are listed in *Table* H.13.

N. E. F. Cartlidge

Hiccup

Hiccup is very common and is only significant if persistent. It is caused by sudden involuntary contraction of both the diaphragm and external intercostal muscles in association with rapid glottic closure. Hiccups may be induced by stimulating a variety of sensory nerves, particularly the vagus and phrenic. Hiccups usually occur with a frequency of between 4 and 60 per minute.

The commonest cause of hiccup is gastric distension after rapid ingestion of food, alcohol or air. Other common causes include excitement and a sudden change in temperature either of the environment or of the stomach induced by a hot or very cold meal. However, in persistent cases, the following causes should be considered:

1. Intrathoracic

A. MEDIASTINAL

Irritation of a phrenic nerve may cause recurrent attacks of intractable hiccup. In an adult this may be due to malignant lymphadenopathy due to tumours of the lung or oesophagus or to a lymphoma. An aortic aneurysm may rarely cause hiccup. Hiccup may also follow mediastinal surgery or mediastinitis.

B. DIAPHRAGMATIC

Hiccup may occur in pneumonia and empyema due to diaphragmatic pleurisy, and may also occur in myocardial infarction and pericarditis.

2. Intra-abdominal disease

Hiccup of intra-abdominal cause often results from diaphragmatic irritation due, for example, to diaphragmatic hernia, subphrenic abscess, peritonitis, pancreatitis, liver metastases, liver abscess, splenic infarct and carcinoma of the stomach. However, other conditions such as carcinoma of the sigmoid colon and carcinoma of the uterus have been associated with hiccup even without any obvious diaphragmatic involvement. Hiccup may occur after abdominal or pelvic operations and is seen in association with acute postoperative dilatation of the stomach and with intestinal obstruction.

3. Central

A. EPIDEMIC ENCEPHALITIS

This rare cause of hiccup was probably a variety of encephalitis lethargica in which there was inflammation affecting the third and fourth segments of the cervical cord, those from which the phrenic nerve originates. Hiccup may also follow lesions of the medulla.

B. INTRACRANIAL

Hiccup may rarely result from intracranial tumours, intracranial haemorrhage, brain abscess or meningitis, especially when the brainstem or basal meninges are involved.

C. TOXIC

Uraemic hiccups are uncommon but may be persistent. Acute severe fevers including typhoid, malaria and cholera may also be accompanied by hiccups.

D. HYSTERICAL HICCUP

This occasional cause of hiccup usually affects young women who may hiccup persistently during wakefulness. However, the hiccup stops during sleep.

E. DRUGS

Benzodiazepines and short-acting barbiturates can also cause hiccup.

Neil J. Douglas

HIP
See JOINTS, AFFECTIONS OF.

Hirsutism

Hirsutism is said to be present when a female has an amount of hair on her face, body or limbs which is inappropriate for the race she belongs to or the culture in which she lives. A problem posed by immigration is that individuals originally from places such as Cyprus, Southern Italy or Sicily, where women have more marked hair growth, compare themselves with women of Northern European extraction, who are less hairy, and come to the conclusion that they are abnormal.

Many doctors who encounter a patient with hirsutism worry about the presence of some serious pathology, such as an adrenal or ovarian tumour. In fact these causes are rare. The majority of patients are suffering from the polycystic ovary syndrome. However, it is worth while looking for evidence of virilization, which makes a pathological cause much more likely. A few relatively simple tests can be done to confirm or exclude serious pathology.

Types of hair growth

LANUGO

This is the very fine, silky, but sometimes quite long hair which covers the entire skin surface of the fetus; it is usually shed by the 7th or 8th month of intra-uterine life.

VELLUS

Males and females are born with the same number of hair follicles. In childhood the follicles produce vellus hair which is fine and non-pigmented. This type of hair persists into adult life in the areas of skin which are not producing terminal hair (*see below*). Occasionally a woman may notice vellus hair, particularly on the face, when looking into a mirror with the sun or light behind her head. She may then look for them elsewhere and be horrified to find them on her chest, arms and legs. This, of course, is not hirsutism but 'pseudohirsutism'. Non-androgenic causes of hirsutism usually result in increased vellus hair formation.

INTERMEDIATE HAIR

This hair is soft and silky but may grow long and become pigmented. It then becomes a source of embarrassment. A combination of vellus and intermediate hair over the face and shoulders is characteristic of Cushing's syndrome.

TERMINAL HAIR

Terminal hair is coarse and pigmented and is of three types:

Non-sexual hair which is present on the scalp, eyebrows, arms and legs.

Ambosexual hair which is initiated by low levels of androgens and is present in the axillae, lower pubic triangle and limbs.

Sexual hair which is produced by male levels of androgens and is present in the upper pubic triangle as the 'male escutcheon', on the face, nose, ears, trunk and limbs, where it is present in more profusion than ambosexual hair. When this type of sexual hair is present in a woman she is deemed to be suffering from 'hirsutism'. However, it is important to realize that there is an overlap between what can be considered to be normal and that which is regarded as 'hirsute'. In a study of 400 consecutive Welsh and English women students at the University of Wales, 26 per cent had terminal hair on the face, 17 per cent on the chest or breasts, 35 per cent on the lower abdomen (mainly linea alba) and 84 per cent on the lower arm and leg. Of these latter 84 per cent, nearly three-quarters, also had terminal hair on the thighs and upper arms. As mentioned before, Mediterranean (and some Indian) women tend to grow more terminal hair than Nordic women, whereas women of the Mongolian races (Japanese, Chinese, American Indians, etc.) grow much less. These racial factors must therefore be taken into account when assessing hirsutism. The presence of oligomenorrhoea, amenorrhoea, seborrhoea and acne in a hirsute woman are factors indicating the necessity for investigation.

Hirsutism and virilism

Virilism may accompany hirsutism and is characterized by clitoral enlargement, breast atrophy, temporal hair recession, frontal baldness and loss of normal female contours due to increased muscularity. Deepening of the voice often occurs and there is usually amenorrhoea. The presence of virilization should draw attention to the possibility of one of the conditions which are marked by an asterisk in *Table* H.14.

Table H.14. Causes of hirsutism (in order of frequency)

* Polycystic ovary syndrome
  Idiopathic (often familial)
  Menopause

Drugs
  Menopausal preparations (containing methyltestosterone)
* Androgens
* Anabolic steroids
  Synthetic 17-nor-progestogens
  ACTH
† Phenytoin
† Diazoxide
† Minoxidil
† Glucocorticoids

Metabolic disorders
† Anorexia nervosa
† Porphyria cutanea tarda

Miscellaneous disorders
† Cornelia de Lange syndrome
† Hypertrichosis lanuginosa

Endocrine disorders
  Acromegaly
*† Cushing's syndrome
† Congenital and juvenile hypothyroidism
* Congenital adrenal hyperplasia
* Adrenal carcinoma or adenoma
* Ovarian tumours
    Arrhenoblastoma
    Hilus cell tumour (and hyperplasia)
    Luteoma

---

* May be associated also with virilization.
† Associated with vellus rather than with terminal hair production.

Polycystic ovary syndrome

This is the commonest cause of hirsutism in clinical practice. The classic features originally described by Stein and Leventhal are hirsutism, obesity, oligo-menorrhoea or amenorrhoea, and enlarged cystic ovaries with thickened capsules. On microscopical examination numerous small atretic follicles are found, surrounded by hyperplastic theca interna. In most cases the menstrual disturbance starts shortly after puberty and tends to get progressively worse. Anovulation is invariable. Hirsutism is present in about 50 per cent of cases (*Fig.* H.27) and occasionally virilization is seen. The ovary produces excess androstenedione which is converted into testosterone. In addition, the androstenedione undergoes conversion to oestrone in

fatty tissue. Thus there is not only androgenization but also continuous oestrogen production. The result is continuous high LH production by the pituitary which tends to perpetuate the situation. FSH levels are low normal. 17-oxo- or keto-steroids are usually in the high normal range.

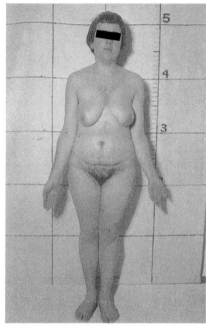

Fig. H.27. Polycystic syndrome with hirsutism.

The classic syndrome may not always be present. Obesity may be absent, hirsutism is not a feature in 50 per cent of patients and some patients may have normal-sized ovaries with a solitary atretic follicle.

Idiopathic hirsutism

This is the second commonest type of hirsutism, but the diagnosis should only be reached after excluding all the other possible causes listed above. If there is a history of hirsutism in other close female relatives or a history of baldness in father or brothers the diagnosis of idiopathic hirsutism is more certain. Although the condition is called 'idiopathic', minor hormonal abnormalities are frequently found. In normal women small amounts of the pro-androgens androstenedione and dehydroepiandrosterone are secreted mainly by the adrenal gland. These are then converted into testosterone and its derivative, the more powerful hormone dihydrotestosterone. In women with hirsutism there may be an increased production of androstenedione by the ovary as well as the adrenal and this leads to increased conversion to testosterone and dihydrotestosterone. The rise in active androgens lowers the concentration of sex hormone binding globulin (SHBG); the net effect is to decrease the amount of bound androgen and to increase the amount of free androgen, thus amplifying its biological action. In idiopathic hirsutism the usual finding is either a slightly raised or a normal plasma testosterone. If the SHBG is reduced then the free testosterone may be elevated. Urinary 17-keto- or oxosteroids are usually normal because they are only increased when very large amounts of androstenedione and dehydroepiandrosterone are being produced.

Menopause

At the time of the menopause there tends to be an increase in the growth of terminal hair in the moustache and beard areas, whereas, paradoxically, body hair gradually becomes less.

Drugs

Menopausal preparations containing methyltestosterone, androgens in general, anabolic steroids, the synthetic 17-nor-progestogens and ACTH may all cause an increased growth of terminal hair. Androgens and anabolic steroids may even cause some degree of virilization.

Other drugs (phenytoin, diazoxide, minoxidil and glucocorticoids) cause stimulation of vellus hair growth.

Metabolic and miscellaneous disorders

Vellus hair growth is seen as a feature of anorexia nervosa and porphyria cutanea tarda. In the condition known as 'hypertrichosis lanuginosa' the lanugo hair which was shed in utero at the 7th or 8th month suddenly regrows and completely covers the face so that the features become unrecognizable. In the Cornelia de Lange syndrome (*see* p. 629), which is associated with short stature ('Amsterdam dwarfism'), the scalp hair reaches down to the bushy and confluent eyebrows and there is also generalized hirsutism of a mixed vellus and intermediate type (*Fig.* H.28).

Endocrine disorders

ACROMEGALY

The incidence of this disease is about three newly diagnosed cases per million of the population each year, whereas the prevalence of previously diagnosed cases is approximately 40 per million of the population. Just over half the women with acromegaly complain of hirsutism and in them urinary 17-oxosteroids may be slightly raised. The mechanism for the increase in 17-oxosteroids is unknown. The hair is of the terminal type.

CUSHING'S SYNDROME

Apart from iatrogenic disease caused by the administration of glucocorticoids, Cushing's syndrome is rare, occurring in only one to two per million of the population each year. The condition is relatively more common in women, when it is usually associated with hirsutism. There is conspicuous hair growth in the beard and moustache areas but the characteristic feature is a rather widespread, vellus hirsutism on the face and over the shoulders. The plethoric moon-shaped face, buffalo hump, supraclavicular puffiness, livid cutaneous striae, central obesity, thin limbs and subcutaneous bruising of the *classic* case make the diagnosis easy. However, mild or early cases of Cushing's syndrome may not be easy to recognize and it is a diagnosis always worth bearing in mind in a woman with hirsutism. The best screening tests to use are a 24-hour urine collection for free cortisol or a 9 a.m. plasma cortisol following 1 mg of oral dexamethasone taken the previous night before retiring. A normal urinary free cortisol and a suppressed 9 a.m. plasma cortisol will exclude the diagnosis.

CONGENITAL AND JUVENILE HYPOTHYROIDISM

Congenital hypothyroidism occurs in approximately one per 5000 births in the United Kingdom. With the increasing use of neonatal TSH screening most cases should be diagnosed shortly after birth and treatment initiated. In cases diagnosed later on, the babies may develop a coat of vellus or intermediate hair over the back and extensor surfaces of the skin. A similar picture is sometimes seen in patients with juvenile hypothyroidism (*Fig.* H.29).

CONGENITAL ADRENAL HYPERPLASIA

Congenital adrenal hyperplasia results from excessive ACTH stimulation. This is caused by an inherited deficiency of an enzyme necessary for the synthesis of cortisol. Five different types of enzyme lack have been recognized, but 21-hydroxylase deficiency is by far the most common. This occurs with a frequency of 1 per 5000 live births. In the female the condition is usually recognized at birth because of genital abnormalities such as enlargement of the clitoris and fusion of the labia. In girls with less severe enzyme defects 21-hydroxylase may present at a later age with premature false puberty (*see* p. 524) and hirsutism. Occasionally the condition becomes apparent after puberty; in addition to hirsutism there may be clitoromegaly and either oligomenorrhoea or amenorrhoea.

The increase in adrenal androgens is caused by an ACTH-stimulated build-up of precursors of cortisol. They can be measured as 17-oxosteroids in the urine.

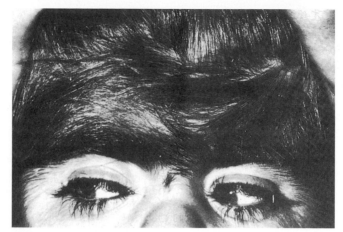

Fig. H.28. Cornelia de Lange syndrome. (*Dr D. M. MacDonald and the British Journal of Dermatology.*)

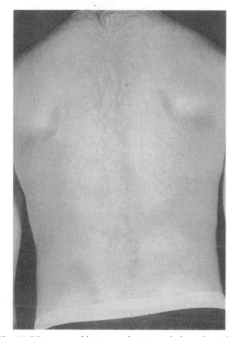

Fig. H.29. Increased hair growth in juvenile hypothyroidism.

In 21-hydroxylase defect, raised levels of 17-hydroxyprogesterone are found in the blood and its metabolite, pregnanetriol, is increased in the urine.

A few women with hirsutism are carriers for 21-hydroxylase deficiency and show marked rises in 17-hydroxyprogesterone when given ACTH.

ADRENAL CARCINOMA OR ADENOMA

Adrenal tumours producing hirsutism and virilization are rare. There are usually very high levels of urinary 17-oxosteroids which cannot be suppressed to 50 per cent of the original levels by 0·5 mg of dexamethasone 6-hourly for 3 days. Forty per cent of carcinomas are palpable. Adenomas may be very small. Calcification

in a carcinoma may sometimes be seen on X-ray. CT scanning is usually informative, but, if not, isotope scanning or selective venous sampling for adrenal androgens may localize the tumour.

OVARIAN TUMOURS

These are exceedingly rare as a cause of hirsutism and virilism. They usually give rise to extreme degrees of virilism because the androgen which they produce, testosterone, is very potent. Levels of testosterone are high in the blood, but urinary 17-oxosteroids, which only measure 25 per cent of all testosterone secreted, may be within the normal range. The tumour may be palpable on pelvic examination and the enlargement can be confirmed by ultrasound.

Ian D. Ramsay

Hyperventilation

Hyperventilation is overbreathing or ventilation in excess of metabolic requirements, with symptoms arising from respiratory alkalosis and hypocapnia (*Table* H.15).

A. Acute

Acute hyperventilation is easily recognized because overbreathing is apparent. The characteristic patient is a young 'hysterical' woman and the presentation has a readily identified precipitant which may have aroused anxiety, fear, distress, excitement, adulation or other powerful feelings. Occasionally the respiratory alkalosis is compensation for a metabolic acidosis, and especially in the young, diabetic ketoacidosis and salicylate poisoning can present occultly and ought to be excluded. Asthma, which has been identified as both a cause and a consequence of hyperventilation, may also present as stress-induced dyspnoea, although it is usually distinguishable by evident expiratory dif-

Table H.15. Causes of acute hyperventilation

Commonest
Stress reaction
Anxiety
Phobia
Panic

Less common
Acidotic disorders
  Diabetic ketoacidosis
  Salicylate poisoning
  Renal failure
Pulmonary disorders
  Asthma
  Pulmonary oedema
  Pulmonary embolism
  Pleural effusion
  Spontaneous pneumothorax
Vasovagal attacks
Following childbirth or abdominal surgery

Rare
Acidotic disorders
  Biguanide intolerance
  Intestinal fistula
  Surgical relocation of ureters in ileum or colon
Psychiatric disorders
  Hysteria
  Malingering
Others
  Epilepsy
  Acute porphyria
  Phaeochromocytoma
  Hepatic cirrhosis
  Pyloric stenosis

ficulty. In hospital, acute hyperventilation is not uncommonly precipitated by abdominal surgery or childbirth, when anxiety is accompanied by an avoidance of abdominal breathing as a protective mechanism against pain or fear of re-opening the wound. The differential diagnosis of acute breathlessness in these circumstances is pulmonary embolism, which may also provoke as well as mimic acute hyperventilation.

B. Chronic

Chronic hyperventilation syndrome is much more difficult to recognize because, once established, the disorder can be maintained by occasional deep breaths or sighs. Chronic hyperventilation accounts for 6–10 per cent of medical referrals, but is frequently unconsidered with the patient's multiple unexplained somatic and psychological complaints leading all too readily to a label of 'functional disorder'.

Even when chronic hyperventilation syndrome is contemplated the clinician faces difficulty establishing the disorder's presence because there is no satisfactorily reliable sign or test. The diagnosis rests upon a combination of typical symptoms and signs, clinical tests and investigations of respiratory function. The central symptom is breathlessness, an air hunger which is associated with gasping, sighing and a feeling of suffocating. Breathlessness tends to be worse at rest, following exercise or on awakening and it may be associated with a particular setting, such as shops or buses, or be triggered by emotions. Common physical symptoms include fatigue, dizziness, faintness, headaches, tremors, sweating, palpitations, chest pain, dysphagia, nausea, heartburn, diarrhoea, flatulence, while common psychological symptoms are anxiety, depression, poor concentration and memory, depersonalization: any of these may be the presenting complaint, but it is the sheer number and range of symptoms that give the clue. A more characteristic pointer is paraesthesiae in the hands, fingers and around the mouth, while tetany is strong but rare evidence. In susceptible individuals hyperventilation may present with fits.

At interview, gasping, sighing and a rapid, uneven respiratory pattern may be noted. The frequent interruption of speech by the need to breathe can be an important sign. Excessive thoracic movement during breathing is characteristic while forced, voluntary overbreathing may rapidly provoke the re-experience of presenting symptoms and rebreathing into a paper bag may abolish them. Assessment of respiratory function helps to establish the diagnosis (*Table* H.16).

Table H.16. Causes of chronic hyperventilation

Commonest
Anxiety

Less common
Pulmonary disorders
  Asthma
  Pulmonary embolism
  Bronchial neoplasm
  Diffuse pulmonary fibrosis
Renal failure
Psychiatric disorders
  Phobia
  Panic
  Depression
  Briquet's syndrome (somatization disorder)
  Hypochondriasis
Primary habit disorder

Rare
Neurological disorders
  Damage to respiratory pathways
  Raised intracranial pressure
Metabolic disorders
  Congestive cardiac failure
  Persistent hypoxaemia
  Liver failure
Psychiatric disorders
  Schizophrenia
  Malingering

It cannot be assumed that chronic hyperventilation invariably arises from a disturbed emotional state. *Physical causes* include disorders of ventilation-perfusion: asthma, pulmonary embolism, parenchymatous lung disease, and, rarely, neurological damage to the respiratory pathways, usually in the brainstem. However the commonest causes are *psychological disorders*, especially anxiety, phobias and panic disorder. Paradoxically it is now evident that chronic overbreathing may induce these conditions as well as result from them. This interaction is complex and best understood as a feedback loop (*Fig.* H.30), but the implication is that treatment can be focused upon either the breathing abnormality or the emotional disorder with the expectation of ameliorating both aspects.

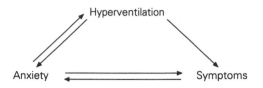

Fig. H.30. The relationship between hyperventilation and anxiety.

Finally, a substantial minority have no evidence of underlying physical or psychological disorder. In these patients chronic hyperventilation syndrome is probably a *primary habit disorder*, although the predisposing biological and psychosocial mechanisms are still unknown. All habits tend to be exaggerated when under pressure, so it should be anticipated that such individuals become symptomatic on stressful occasions: without considering this, it is easy to mislabel these patients as pathologically anxious.

George Masterton

Hypochondriasis

The 'worried well' account for 10–15 per cent of medical attendances, most of which are considered to be hypochondriacal complaints.

The characteristics of hypochondriasis are: (1) Concern with health or disease in oneself, present most of the time; (2) Preoccupation not justified by the amount of organic pathology; (3) Does not respond adequately to reassurance, given after a careful physical assessment.

When faced with a hypochondriacal patient, the first and most essential step is to defer reaching this conclusion until physical conditions are excluded. Suspicions that the presentation is not hypochondriacal are raised if: (*a*) the presentation is acute; (*b*) there is no past history of unexplained disorders; (*c*) there are no stressors evident; (*d*) there is no psychological disturbance beyond the anxiety/apprehension appropriate in the circumstances (*Table* H.17).

Table H.17. Causes of hypochondriasis

Commonest
Stress reaction
Adjustment reaction (especially to illness)
Anxiety
Depression (neurotic)
Early or otherwise undetected physical illness

Less common
Panic
Phobia
Obsessive—compulsive disorder
Depression (psychotic)
Schizophrenia
Primary hypochondriasis

Rare
Dementia
Mental impairment
Schizoaffective disorder
Monosymptomatic hypochondriacal psychosis
Post-traumatic stress disorder
Hysteria
Briquet's syndrome (somatization disorder)

Hypochondriacal presentations are usefully divided into *primary* and *secondary*, the distinction made more important by the poor prognosis found in primary hypochondriasis contrasting with the favourable outcome generally attained when hypochondriasis is in the setting of another psychological disorder.

Transient hypochondriacal *reactions* are common, usually responding well to explanation and reassurance but occasionally developing and persisting. Any stress or situation may be the trigger in a vulnerable individual, but there are some common circumstances in which personal vulnerability is less crucial. Recovering from serious illness may precipitate this response as part of an adjustment reaction; similarly serious illness in a close friend or relative may lead to concerns about having the same disease, the mental mechanism being identification with the loved one and sharing their suffering, or as part of a grief reaction when death has occurred. Hypochondriacal reactions are more common in the elderly particularly if the patient has an established painful condition, and in this group the loss of work, outside interests and friends may conspire to focus attention and interest on the functioning of the 'inner world'.

Hypochondriacal *delusions* are uncommon and may take easily recognizable, bizarre forms in schizophrenia, dementia and monosymptomatic hypochondriacal psychosis (a rare condition in which the delusions are not accompanied by features which would permit classification as a primary organic or functional psychosis). Among the commoner presentations are beliefs of infestation, emitting odours and changes in size, shape or function of organs. In major depression the delusions may be more subtle and difficult to detect, although detection is the more important because these phenomena are associated with a substantial risk of suicide. Generally, depressive hypochondriacal delusions are understandable in the context of other depressive changes—for instance delusions of venereal disease arise from depressive guilt and sometimes impotence, while delusions of cancer can be the outcome of morbid, pessimistic thinking accompanied by constipation, impaired appetite and weight loss.

Hypochondriacal *preoccupations, worries and fears* occur commonly in the setting of neurotic disorders. In anxiety, agoraphobia, panic disorder and depressive neurosis hypochondriacal features can usually be easily established as one element in a constellation of symptoms and signs that typify the underlying disorder. Physical symptoms may be the presenting feature of any of these conditions and may be perceived with enhanced alarm or dread by a patient who has an abnormal mood state. The presenting complaint is usually a typical feature of anxiety or depression, such as musculoskeletal pain, cardiovascular, gastrointestinal or neurological symptoms, which basically becomes magnified and misinterpreted.

Primary hypochondriasis is rare but its existence as an entity is now widely accepted. It is essentially a diagnosis by exclusion of the causes already outlined, but the condition has some characteristic features: (*a*) first and foremost—persistent complaining; (*b*) detailed accounts: 'the organ recital'; (*c*) matter-of-fact presentation; (*d*) less interest in the response than in the narrating. Such patients are usually obsessional and often anxiety prone. These characteristics of style and personality aid in distinguishing primary hypochondriasis from somatization disorder (Briquet's syndrome) where patients have persistent unexplained physical complaints but tend to be inarticulate, poor historians who give highly dramatic accounts of events but sketchy information about their symptoms with the emphasis upon extraordinariness rather than detail.

Finally it should be borne in mind that patients with primary hypochondriasis are not immune to physical illnesses and are indeed vulnerable to mental disorders: exaggeration in hypochondriacal complaining may indicate a superimposed depressive illness or anxiety state. On the other hand repeated specialist referrals and investigations reinforce this behaviour! Hence the doctor has a delicate balance to strike over when to investigate and treat, and unfortunately his decision-making is frequently hindered by the antipathy and alienation that tends to develop in the doctor–patient relationship. The hypochondriacal patient's compulsion to self-absorb and report understandably stresses all relationships, but usually the rewards evidently outweigh these considerations, for such patients are rarely interested in attempting to change their behaviour.

George Masterton

Hypothermia

Hypothermia is defined as a deep body or 'core' temperature of below 35°C (95°F). Normally protected parts, such as the abdomen, are cold to the touch. When hypothermia is suspected, deep rectal temperature should be measured with a thermocouple or special low-reading thermometer.

Mild hypothermia down to 32°C (90°F) may be characterized by confusion, slow responses, slurred husky speech, ataxia and involuntary movements resembling cerebellar incoordination. Skin pallor, shivering and some degree of tachycardia and mild hypertension are often noted.

Moderate–severe hypothermia is characterized by drowsiness, stupor or overt coma. Some patients may be comatose at 31°C, others may still be conscious at 27°C. The pupils are usually constricted and unresponsive to light (mimicking opium poisoning) but the low body temperature is against a diagnosis of pontine haemorrhage. Occasionally fixed dilated pupils are noted in those with severe, protracted hypothermia and then may mimic severe, closed head injury. The skin may show cyanotic or pink blotches, and sometimes purpuric lesions, skin haemorrhages or pressure lesions (*Fig.* H.31). Fluid shifts give it a typical puffy or oedematous consistency. At very low 'core' temperatures fine muscle tremors and muscle rigidity have replaced shivering. Tendon jerks, if still present, show slow contraction and relaxation phases; the knee jerk is the last to be lost. The plantar responses may be bilaterally extensor or absent; a unilateral extensor response usually indicates an underlying cerebrovascular catastrophe. Severe bradycardia or atrial fibrillation may be present; tachycardia is inappropriate in hypothermia and suggests internal haemorrhage, e.g. from severe gastric erosions. Any intra-abdominal catastrophe may not be detectable until after rewarming. Coarse pulmonary crepitations indicate oedematous and often infected lungs, but respiration may be too poor for these features to be recognized.

Severely hypothermic patients lack easily detectable vital signs, with imperceptible peripheral pulses, inaudible heart sounds, unrecordable BP and slow, shallow respiration; the pupils may sometimes be widely dilated and unresponsive. An ECG will exclude death, but even ventricular fibrillation may reverse with rewarming. If the diagnosis of hypothermia has been overlooked, the characteristic J waves in the ECG should remedy this oversight (*Fig.* H.32).

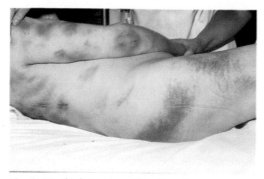

Fig. H.31. Skin lesions in accidental hypothermia.

2. Increased heat loss

Outdoors cold/wet exposure or cold water immersion
Ethanol
Vasoconstriction failure, e.g. elderly survivors of previous accidental hypothermia
Malnutrition, e.g. kwashiorkor
Erythroderma, e.g. generalized psoriasis, exfoliative dermatitis
Paget's disease of bone

3. Central thermoregulatory failure

Uraemia
Cerebrovascular injury or cerebral trauma
Drugs—including self-poisoning, e.g. phenothiazine tranquillizers, tricyclic antidepressants, barbiturates
Diabetic ketoacidosis

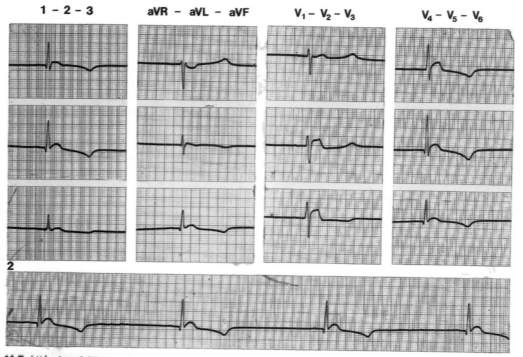

M.G. (♀) Aged 67 yrs. Myxoedema 18.12.76 25°C (rectal)

Fig. H.32. ECG showing characteristic J waves in a 67-year-old male with myxoedema (temperature 25°C rectal).

Many elderly hypothermic patients have complex physical signs, either because of complications of the hypothermia (e.g. pulmonary crepitations) or because the hypothermia is simply an epiphenomenon of serious underlying medical disorder.

The important causes of hypothermia are:

1. Decreased heat production

Inactivity and immobility, e.g. lying on floor after a stroke or fractured femur
Hypoglycaemia
Impaired shivering capacity (elderly)
Myxoedema
Starvation and malnutrition
Hypopituitarism

Wernicke's encephalopathy
CO poisoning/anoxic brain injury, e.g. after cardiac arrest
Organophosphate poisoning

4. Peripheral thermoregulatory failure

Spinal cord lesions, especially cervical

5. Mechanism(s) uncertain

Severe chronic or debilitating disease (preterminal), e.g. malignancy, hepatic cirrhosis
Overwhelming infection, e.g. severe bronchopneumonia, overwhelming TB, falciparum malaria
Severe congestive heart failure
Shock after multiple injury, major operation, severe coronary thrombosis or pulmonary embolism

Collapse due to severe dehydration, e.g. severe diarrhoea, including cholera

Pancreatitis

6. Cold weather

Irrespective of the above causes, hypothermia is more common during, but by no means confined to, the colder winter months

7. Rare forms

Intermittent hypothermia
Agenesis of the corpus callosum
Chronic hypothermia
Poikilothermia

Derek Maclean

Hysteria

The term *hysteria* has been dropped in ICD10 to be replaced by Dissociative (conversion) disorders. However *hysteria* will be used in this section.

Before describing hysterical presentations and their differential diagnosis the topic requires to be prefaced by some comments about related aspects that can lead to confusion. The terms 'hysteria' and 'hysterical' have different connotations when applied to behaviour and personality: hysterical *behaviour* refers to histrionic, attention-seeking behaviour while hysterical *personality* describes a shallow, flamboyant, self-absorbed, 'showbiz' individual—both terms tend to denote disapproval. Hysteria in its proper sense is a presentation of neurosis in which the stress or conflict and the anxiety this engenders are avoided through the defence mechanisms of conversion or dissociation. Although embracing these disorders under one umbrella has passed out of fashion in the United States where the term hysteria has largely been dropped, hysteria or hysterical neurosis remains an accepted unitary concept elsewhere.

The justification for delimiting hysteria lies in the features common to all presentations (*Table* H.18), and without all three characteristics being present the diagnosis is erroneous.

There are other features linked to hysterical symptoms none of which are invariable. The most important is *secondary gain(s)*, i.e. the spin-off benefits arising from being ill which may perpetuate the condition when the primary cause has been resolved. *Suggestibility* is a useful clinical sign (and a potent tool in therapy); this ability to influence site, characteristics and severity as well as inducing or removing symptoms altogether may sometimes be enhanced by hypnosis, or abreaction using diazepam or amytal, when the underlying conflict may also be explored if necessary. *La belle indifference* describes a bland lack of concern towards what is manifestly a serious condition—it is also frequently found in stoical, physically

Table H.18. Characteristics of hysteria

1. The presentation corresponds to an idea in the patient's mind of how the disorder should present, i.e. (*a*) physical or sensory changes do not obey anatomical and physiological rules; (*b*) psychological changes do not adhere to accepted psychological principles

2. The disability must be apparent and definable in terms of positive findings. Clinical examination usually reveals obvious inconsistencies or anomalies, particularly the preservation of functions that ought to be lost or the absence of abnormalities that ought to be present

3. Primary gain. The disorder resolves an emotional conflict or personal problem which is kept out of consciousness

ill patients and its presence in hysteria is usually confined to acute presentations as opposed to chronic states where high levels of anxiety are the rule. *Symbolism*, or what the symptom means is an important concept in psychoanalysis, sometimes being interpreted as a precise communication and representation of the nature of the underlying conflict—but in clinical practice this rarely seems relevant. Finally, failure to respond to conventional, physical interventions or drugs is characteristic, and should alert the doctor's suspicions before proceeding to more invasive techniques—while a sustained response to a physical treatment mitigates against a hysterical aetiology.

Perhaps surprisingly appreciable hysterical personality traits are found in only 15 per cent of cases. The breeding ground for hysteria is much more frequently a passive, dependent, inarticulate individual who is in a submissive role and cannot express themselves freely either through inability or fear of the consequences. Through illness hysteria generates control without confrontation, hence its links with other conditions in which sick role behaviour is prominent such as chronic pain and factitious disorder.

Hysteria divides easily into conversion disorders and dissociative states, with conversion (of the emotional disorder into a physical state) and dissociation (of emotions from thoughts and behaviour) being the principal mental defence mechanisms to be employed.

Conversion disorders can mimic any physical condition but by far the commonest presentations are neurological, involving mobility, sensory modalities (including pain and the special senses) and pseudoseizures, while less common presentations include vomiting, urinary retention and pseudocyesis. There are numerous signs and tests that aid in identifying a presentation as a conversion disorder, all of which are derived from the themes in the first and second requirements in *Table* H.18. The features of hysteria evolve and there is an impression that the more bizarre and obviously functional presentations such as glove and stocking anaesthesia are diminishing in frequency to be replaced by disorders that can be more difficult to distinguish clinically, hysterical epilepsy being a good example.

Similarly there seems to have been a change in the presentations of *dissociative states* from the trances, twilight states, automatisms and somnambulisms so common in the 'golden age of hysteria' a century ago, to amnesic states, fugues (journeys without memory—usually aimless wandering) and pseudodementia (*Table* H.19).

Table H.19. Causes of a hysterical presentation

Common
Hysteria—hysterical neurosis (Conversion disorder/ dissociative state)

Less common
Neurological disorders
Systemic disorders with CNS effects
Depression

Rare
Schizophrenia
Alcoholism

Before establishing the diagnosis of hysteria it is essential to exclude a primary physical or psychiatric explanation for the symptom *Neurological disorders* of all types and systemic diseases with CNS effects must be ruled out, by extensive investigation if necessary. Even if all investigations are negative and the presentation bears the unequivocal physical characteristics of a conversion disorder the diagnosis of hysteria must not be made unless the psychodynamic requirement is met, i.e primary gain is identified, because follow-up studies have demonstrated that such patients may proceed to develop neurological disorders such as tumour, multiple sclerosis and dementing processes. A conversion sign developing in a patient over 40 years of age with no psychological explanation and no past history of hysteria or other mental illness is a sinister occurrence which merits careful review. Indeed it was by maintaining an open mind in such circumstances that the physical basis has been established for conditions like globus hystericus, torticollis, paroxysmal hemicrania, thoracic outlet syndrome and the syndrome of painful legs and moving toes.

Hysterical presentations also occur in the setting of *psychiatric disorders*, particularly depression, but also dementia, schizophrenia and alcoholism (especially fugues). Occasionally the mental disorder only becomes apparent on follow-up after the hysterical presentation has resolved, but the possibility of an underlying depressive illness should be actively considered in older patients and those with a personal or family history of affective disorder (*Table* H.20).

Table H.20. Differential diagnosis of hysteria

Physical/mental illness
Hypochondriasis
Factitious disorder
Malingering

Differentiating hysteria from *factitious disorder* rarely presents problems because the former is, by definition, obviously produced to secure gain through the resolution of an emotional conflict while the gains obtained from factitious disorder are, at best, obscure. In practice neurological symptoms apart from epilepsy are rarely simulated in factitious conditions while in hysteria self-injury seldom occurs intentionally. An interesting distinction in presentation between the two conditions is that the hysteric knows and cares little about health issues while the patient with factitious disorder is often immersed in all aspects of illnesses and hospitals.

Differentiating hysteria from *malingering* is a much harder task because both conditions involve evident gains and the sole point of distinction is whether the patient's behaviour is consciously or unconsciously motivated. The only time when a definite diagnosis can be made with confidence is during the early stages of the first, acute presentation before the disorder has been elaborated by factors like suggestion and illness experiences. Here the nature of the primary gain frequently aids diagnosis, malingering being particularly linked to obvious environmental advantage such as compensation or avoiding military service. How important it is to make this distinction in the latter example has been given less consideration than cunning ways of catching out malingerers—for neither hysteria nor malingering seem likely to be conducive with good soldiering!

In almost all chronic cases, which includes all compensation cases, as well as in some acute cases, the distinction between hysteria and malingering is spurious, and irrelevant for clinical purposes. The problem is that insight is neither fixed nor dichotomous, it comes and it goes—hence the apposite maxim 'in time all malingerers become hysterics and all hysterics become malingerers'. It is also possible for both diagnoses to be present, for example pseudoseizures sometimes being used consciously for obvious gain while on other occasions being unconsciously motivated. This phenomenon is particularly evident in protracted compensation cases where many patients with functional disorders fail to improve even after a satisfactory financial settlement because secondary gains have superseded money as the basis for maintaining symptoms, having developed imperceptibly as part of the patient's and their family's adjustment. In these cases it is typical for there to be a number of gains understood with varying degrees of insight by the patient, and these gains and insights change as circumstances unfold. In such cases the application of a diagnosis of hysteria or malingering by a doctor frequently reveals more about his regard for the patient and his views upon human nature in general than the true state of affairs.

It is an understanding of the gains and the psychodynamics, what makes the patient tick and what are the circumstances including the nature and roles of close friends and relatives that matter in clinical practice. The malingering versus the hysteria debate is irrelevant in tipping the scales in the direction of shedding symptoms rather than maintaining them, or in encouraging the patient to get well through a combination of suggestion, problem solving and reward while avoiding reward and reinforcement of illness behaviour.

George Masterton

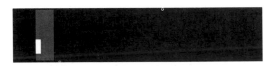

Impotence

This is defined as the inability to perform the sexual act. Erectile impotence is where this inability is caused by a lack of penile erection or deformity of the erect penis. Ejaculatory impotence is failure of ejaculation of semen into the vagina; this may be because of a lack of external ejaculation or premature ejaculation and may or may not be accompanied by lack of orgasm.

Erectile impotence

Impotence can be secondary to psychological problems (*psychogenic impotence*) or to disease affecting the endocrine mileau or the blood or nerve supply to the penis (*organic impotence*). The distinction between these two major categories of impotence can be difficult because inevitably men with organic impotence often develop a disturbed pysche because of their problem. If the man is married, whatever the cause of the impotence, it is usually better to involve his wife early on in the treatment.

IMPOTENCE SECONDARY TO PSYCHOLOGICAL PROBLEMS (PYSCHOGENIC IMPOTENCE)

In this situation the mechanisms of erection are intact but the libido is reduced or perverted. The commonest cause of reduced libido is depression but fortunately may resolve when the depression is treated. It should

be noted that tricyclic antidepressants may cause impotence in some patients. Abnormal sexual or homosexual inclination may also cause impotence. An example of abnormal sexual inclination is fetishism where erections may only be possible in response to some bizarre stimulus such as tight-fitting rubber garments, etc. Impotence may also be a symptom of marital disturbance and treatment should involve both husband and wife.

IMPOTENCE SECONDARY TO DISEASE (ORGANIC IMPOTENCE)

Any debilitating disease or excess of drugs including tobacco or alcohol may cause impotence. Endocrine disease associated with a lack of testosterone can also result in impotence but this is often not a problem to the patient because there is also a lack of sexual drive (e.g. some men with Klinefelter's syndrome). Impotence secondary to drugs or treatment may occur in two ways: first, drugs and treatments which interfere with testosterone production, e.g. castration for any reason, treatment of prostatic cancer with gonadotrophin analogues or oestrogens; second, drugs or treatments which interfere with neurological pathways such as the antihypertensive antiadrenergic drugs methyldopa and guanethidine or interuption of pelvic nerve pathways after surgery (e.g. abdominoperineal resection, postchemotherapy lymph node dissection for testicular tumours). Impotence and indeed ejaculatory failure may occur with many neurological disorders, e.g. diabetic autonomic neuropathy, spinal-cord compression and paraplegia, tabes dorsalis, multiple sclerosis, etc. Impotence secondary to vascular deficiency is usually a manifestation of a more generalized vascular disease and occurs in older men. Impotence associated with excessive cigarette smoking is vascular in origin.

IMPOTENCE IN THE ABSENCE OF ANY OVERT PSYCHIATRIC PROBLEM OR UNDERLYING DISEASE

This is the most common problem facing the clinician. In general, if the man is under the age of 45 and especially if the problem is longstanding then it is more likely to be psychogenic in origin. Assessment is by history and examination, when obvious factors may be discovered (*see above*). The mechanics of erection can be tested by monitoring sleep erections although the apparatus required for this is cumbersome and unreliable. Another more reliable test is by an intracorporeal injection of a vasoactive substance. This will cause the penis to become erect unless the blood supply is severely reduced. When the penis is erect the arterial pulses of the superficial and deep arteries can be assessed using Doppler examination. It is safest to start with a low dose of prostaglandin E1 e.g. 10 mcg. If this does not produce a response a higher dose can be tried but not for at least 24 hours (e.g. prostaglandin E1 20 mcg). An erection which is initially strong but rapidly fails may indicate excessive venous drainage. A prolonged and immediate erection after a low dose of prostaglandin may indicate neurological damage and if neurological problems are suspected it is very important to start with a low dose. If sleep erection testing and prostaglandin tests show a normal erection then efforts should be made to detect any hidden psychological problem.

The prostaglandin test should be used with care because there is a risk of prolonged painful erections which may require further medical attention. If painful priapism persists for more than about 8 hours the patient should report back to the doctor who gave the original injection. The problem may be solved by aspiration of 10 to 30 ml of blood from the corpora using a syringe and needle. If this dose does not work a slow intracorporeal injection of 10 mg phenylephrine in 10 ml saline may be given but care must be taken to monitor the blood pressure.

DEFORMITY OF THE ERECT PENIS AND PAINFUL ERECTION

This complaint is uncommon but when present is nearly always organic. Examination may reveal obvious factors such as a *phimosis* or *tight frenum* and these can be corrected by circumcision or division. The erect penis can be examined either after intracorporeal prostaglandin injections or by asking the man to take photographs of the erect penis at home using a polaroid camera. The extent of the deformity can be remarkable with minimal findings when the flaccid penis is examined. The two most common causes of deformity are those in relation to *hypospadias* either treated or untreated and *Peyronie's disease*. The former problem is present from birth and manifest as soon as the young man is concerned about his erections. Treatment is surgical correction. Peyronie's disease is a curious condition where plaques of scar tissue form in the wall of the corpora. The condition is usually painful and while the pain is present progressive. Treatment is conservative while pain is present (vitamin E may help) and surgical if the degree of deformity becomes so great as to interfere with intercourse. Other causes of penile deformity are congenital, fractured pelvis and unilateral thrombosis of the corpora.

Micropenis is rare and usually associated with marked obesity. A much more common problem is concern about penis size particularly amongst Indian and Arabic men. Almost always the penis is of normal size and after complete physical examination strong reassurance needs to be given.

Ejaculatory impotence

This condition is usually organic and is relatively common in *neurological disease* such as diabetic autonomic neuropathy, multiple sclerosis, etc. Paraplegia is another common cause. Psychogenic ejaculatory failure may occur but can usually be recognized because of the strange personality of the man. Sometimes this situation is seen in the infertility clinic where a child is very much wanted by the female partner but the husband is ambivalent. In the absence of any overt disorder the two main causes of failure of ejaculation are retrograde ejaculation and anejaculation. The former can be diagnosed by the finding of many sperm in the postcoital urine sample. The latter may be difficult to diagnose but there may be an absence of one or both vas deferens and an absent or very small prostrate.

A common problem is *premature ejaculation*. This may occur in younger men where the response to sexual stimuli may be very rapid. With reassurance from the doctor and familiarity with sexual stimuli the problem usually resolves. The problem can be particularly troublesome in men from countries where there is strict segregation of the sexes before marriage and strict taboos on masturbation or any sexual activity.

T. B. Hargreave

HEIGHT INCREASED
See STATURE, TALL.
HEIGHT REDUCED
See STATURE, SMALL.
HEMIANAESTHESIA
See SENSATION, ABNORMALITIES OF.

Indigestion

Indigestion is a very common symptom with a prevalence in the community approaching 30 per cent. *Dyspepsia* is synonomous with indigestion which may be defined as upper abdominal discomfort amounting even to pain, nausea, vomiting, heartburn and distension. Severe abdominal pain should not be regarded as either dyspepsia or indigestion. In the past dyspepsia was regarded as indicative of a chronic peptic ulcer. The advent of radiology soon revealed that the majority of patients with indigestion did not have an ulcer and the term 'X-ray negative' dyspepsia was introduced. This term has been superseded since the introduction of fibreoptic endoscopy and a better description for dyspepsia which is not of ulcer origin is 'non-ulcer dyspepsia'. Of all patients with dyspepsia, only 25 per cent have ulcers visible either on endoscopy or radiology. Of those with non-ulcer dyspepsia, about

15 per cent have no identifiable lesion in the gastro-intestinal tract. The cause of their dyspepsia is not always apparent and the term 'nervous dyspepsia' has been introduced but this must be used with caution and only in patients in whom a clearly disturbed emotional state can be defined. Indeed, recent work suggests that there is no clear psychological or psychiatric disturbance present in many patients who have no organic cause for their dyspepsia.

Indigestion frequently accompanies the symptoms of nausea and vomiting (p. 710). The causes of dyspepsia are listed in Table I.1. Under these circumstances the cause for dyspepsia readily becomes apparent. The discussion of indigestion in this section relates to abdominal discomfort which has been present for 1 month or more and is not precipitated by exertion or relieved by rest. The mechanism of dyspepsia is probably varied and can often be accounted for on the basis of a local lesion in the upper gastrointestinal tract, or some more generalized disturbance of gastroduodenal and small intestinal motility. In some circumstances, it is possible that gastric hyperacidity contributes. An attractive concept is that there is a functional disturbance of the upper gastrointestinal tract mediated by gastrointestinal peptide hormones. Although many hormones can be shown to have an influence on gastroduodenal motility, it has not been possible to identify any one particular pattern of hormone disturbance which correlates with indigestion. This interesting hypothesis remains to be proven.

Peptic ulcer dyspepsia

Both *duodenal* and *gastric ulcers* may present primarily with indigestion. The classical symptomatology of a *duodenal ulcer* includes intermittent pain felt in the epigastrium or to the left or right of the midline which is located precisely by the patient, and which is worse before meals and relieved by either taking food or antacids. Patients with a *gastric ulcer* tend to be older, and have relatively more pain; this occurs sooner after meals than in a duodenal ulcer and is less likely to be relieved by food or antacids. A characteristic feature of peptic ulcer disease is the periodicity with long periods when the patient is free of pain. Other features include flatulence, nausea and vomiting. One of the more reliable features of distinguishing a duodenal ulcer is the presence of pain which wakes the patient at night. Unfortunately, these characteristic features of gastric and duodenal ulcers are encountered in less than 50 per cent of patients. Not only are the symptoms of peptic ulcer disease non-specific and non-sensitive for the diagnosis of peptic ulcer as opposed to non-ulcer dyspepsia, but in addition it is not possible to distinguish reliably on history between a gastric and

Table I.1. Causes of dyspepsia

Common
Duodenal ulcer
Gastric ulcer
Gastritis
  Immune
  H. pylori
Gastric cancer
Hiatus hernia
Oesophageal reflux
Irritable bowel syndrome
Drugs
  Tobacco
  Alcohol
  Non-steroidal anti-inflammatory agents
  Theophylline
  Digoxin
  Iron preparations
  Cytotoxic agents
  Antibiotics
Gallstones
Psychiatric disorder
  Tension/anxiety
  Depression
Food intolerance
Aerophagy
Pregnancy

Less common
Other gastric tumours
  Lymphoma
  Leiomyosarcoma
Other gastric diseases
  Sarcoidosis
  Tuberculosis
  Eosinophilic granuloma
  Syphilis
Adult hypertrophic pyloric stenosis
Hypertrophic gastritis (Ménétrièr's disease)
Duodenitis
Other duodenal diseases
  Webs
  Polyps
  Cancer
  Lymphoma
Chronic pancreatitis
Pancreatic cancer
Crohn's disease
Colonic cancer
Metabolic diseases
  Diabetes mellitus
  Uraemia
  Suprarenal insufficiency
  Hyperthyroidism
  Hypothyroidism
  Hypercalcaemia
Coeliac disease
Tropical sprue
Chronic hepatitis
Pulmonary tuberculosis
Congestive cardiac failure
Autonomic neuropathy
Gastric and small intestinal motility disorders
Giardiasis
Strongyloidiasis

a duodenal ulcer. Furthermore, the physical examination is unreliable and there is much evidence to indicate that the physical sign of epigastric tenderness on light or deep palpation is insensitive, not specific, and has a low predictive value for peptic ulcer disease or indeed any other form of gastroduodenal disease. The only certain way of diagnosing either a gastric or duodenal ulcer is either by endoscopy or less reliably by a barium meal.

Non-ulcer dyspepsia

There are many causes for dyspepsia or indigestion which are not due to peptic ulcer disease. These include *gastritis* and *duodenitis, gastric carcinoma, drug dyspepsias, disease* of the *biliary tract, pancreatic disease* and a variety of other less common causes.

Gastritis can present in an identical way to peptic ulcer with indigestion, epigastric discomfort, flatulence, nausea and vomiting. There may or may not be epigastric tenderness. Two types of gastritis are recognized, fundal gastritis which is commonly associated with pernicious anaemia and antral gastritis. The latter form of gastritis appears in children and adults and there is a strong association with the organism *Helicobacter pylori*. Although a medical history is a poor discriminator between peptic ulcer and non-ulcer dyspepsia, upper abdominal pain which is not severe, is aggravated by food or milk, and in the absence of night pain, vomiting or weight loss is suggestive of gastritis.

Gastric cancer has become less common in the western world in the past decade. A short history of indigestion in a patient over the age of 55 which is accompanied by marked weight loss and persistent pain with no periodicity should raise the suspicion of a gastric cancer. All patients with indigestion which persists without remit for over a month should be investigated by gastroscopy or by a barium meal.

Indigestion is a poor guide to *cholelithiasis* and *cholecystitis*. The classic features of gallbladder disease include moderate to severe pain felt below the right costal margin or the epigastrium, passing round to the back on the right and occasionally felt in the scapular area. The pain is of variable intensity. If the stone impacts in the cystic duct the pain will be of a colicky nature. A stone impacted in the common bile duct gives rise to more persistent unremitting pain and will usually be accompanied by the presence of jaundice, dark urine and pale stools. A syndrome of intermittent jaundice, dark urine and pale stools with episodic fever and pain is a feature of stone in the common bile duct associated with infection. There is no characteristic gallbladder dyspepsia. Fatty food dyspepsia is a common symptom in clinical practice but has no relationship to gallbladder disease. Indeed, the mechanism of fatty food dyspepsia remains unclear.

Chronic pancreatitis is usually associated with more severe pain rather than indigestion. However, some patients do have a mild, continual discomfort in the upper abdomen which is accompanied by a bloated feeling and occasionally pain which is felt radiating through to the back. *Carcinoma of the pancreas* may present in a similar way with a much shorter history and the appearance of such symptomatology together with the onset of diabetes mellitus in an elderly person should raise the suspicion of a pancreatic cancer. One of the confusing ways in which *cancer of the colon* may present is with the symptomatology suggestive of an upper gastrointestinal disease and it must be borne in mind that should a patient who has presented with indigestion be shown to have no obvious upper gastrointestinal tract disease, a barium enema may well prove to be a fruitful investigation for revealing the cause of the illness.

Drug-induced dyspepsia is not uncommon, particularly with the widespread use of non-steroidal anti-inflammatory agents which is a well-recognized cause of indigestion and upper gastrointestinal discomfort. Other causes include antibiotic therapy, other analgesic agents, prednisolone, digitalis, and theophylline preparations.

Alcoholic gastritis is a well-recognized condition which usually presents with early morning nausea and vomiting but may be accompanied by epigastric discomfort or the latter may be the only feature of this illness. *Smoking* too is a cause of indigestion and may contribute to the dyspepsia of patients with alcohol abuse.

Indigestion is a well-known presenting feature of *pulmonary tuberculosis*. Although this is a less common disease in developed countries, it still occurs with sufficient frequency for a chest X-ray to be necessary in all patients who have dyspepsia which cannot be explained by obvious upper gastrointestinal disease. Two infections in the upper gastrointestinal tract are important causes of indigestion, *giardiasis* and *strongyloidiasis*. Giardiasis is a particularly important condition because it may present with upper abdominal discomfort, nausea and loss of appetite in the absence of diarrhoea or obvious malabsorption. The symptomatology may be quite irregular and misleading unless a specific search is made for giardia in the stool or in duodenal aspirates.

Patients with the *irritable bowel syndrome* frequently have a dyspeptic feature to their illness. Thus, although it is characteristic to have lower abdominal pain associated with a feeling of incomplete evacuation and flatulence with discomfort relieved by the passage of stools, indigestion and upper abdominal discomfort are now recognized with increasing frequency as a feature of this, as yet, unexplained syndrome.

Poor dentition or loss of teeth has been ascribed as the cause for indigestion; but the evidence is poor and it is likely that these are only uncommon causes of upper gastrointestinal discomfort. Similarly it remains controversial to what extent *stress* and other personal factors are responsible for indigestion. A number of well conducted studies suggest that stress is not a major factor in the genesis of dyspepsia and 'functional' dyspepsia is not a condition which can be diagnosed with any ease or certainty. Similarly, it is difficult to demonstrate convincingly a relationship between food and indigestion. Many patients will claim that certain *foods* cause indigestion but such studies that have been undertaken of these patients suggest that only a small number have verifiable specific food intolerance. It is also difficult to know whether the excessive consumption of tea or particularly coffee has a role in the genesis of indigestion. Dyspepsia, nausea and vomiting may be prominent in the early months of *pregnancy*.

Less common causes of dyspepsia include *Crohn's disease, tuberculosis* or *sarcoidosis* of the stomach, *adult hypertrophic pyloric stenosis, hypertrophic gastritis* (Ménétrièr's disease). Duodenal lesions which are rare but which may present with indigestion include an *annular pancreas, duodenal polyps or webs and cancer in the duodenum.*

Indigestion is a common and important symptom in clinical medicine. With careful history and a judicious use of investigations, it is possible to find a cause for many of the patients. However in an appreciable number of patients no clear cause can be identified. It is important that these people should not be falsely diagnosed as either having some psychiatric illness or food intolerance. Usually the dyspepsia subsides over a period of months or years with supportive therapy from the physicians and a judicious use of drugs acting on the upper gastrointestinal tract.

Ian A. D. Bouchier

Infertility

Involuntary infertility may be defined as a failure to conceive when regular intercourse has taken place over a reasonable length of time. After one year 80 per cent of women have managed to conceive and a further 5-10 per cent of pregnancies will have occurred at the end of the second year. The remainder 10-15 per cent of all marriages can be considered as barren requiring infertility investigations.

A precise diagnosis of the cause for infertility is often difficult, and although there are many well-defined conditions which give rise to it, there are a number of cases in which no definite cause can be found. In many patients the failure is due to a number of minor 'infertility factors' unimportant in themselves, but which in aggregate may result in inability to conceive.

In 20 per cent of patients a single cause for the infertile marriage will not be found; factors in the male or female alone may account for a further 30 per cent in each and in the rest both partners may have factors producing infertility. If the examination of a fresh ejaculate of semen shows it to be within normal limits with regard to volume >2 ml and number of spermatozoa (above 20 million per ml), 50 per cent showing motility, and in addition there are not more than 20 per cent of abnormal forms, the husband should not be regarded as subfertile. Repeated checks are not necessary if a fertile specimen has been produced, although the male counts vary much according to the stage of health. Any systemic illness of which fever is an example depresses spermatogenesis. The effect appears over the weeks after the start of fever and attains its maximum within 6 weeks. Spermatogenesis may not return to normal for several months. If live spermatozoa can be found in the cervical mucus after coitus about the time of ovulation the male can be excluded as the cause of the infertile marriage. Four active progressing spermatozoa to the high-power field is the average. Providing there are some spermatozoa in the ejaculate it is not possible to say that a man is infertile no matter how low the semen count. Pregnancies seem to occur in the face of very low counts.

The causes of male infertility are as follows:

1. Male factors

Impotence, oligospermia, necrospermia, aspermia, varicocele, premature ejaculation and failure to ejaculate during coitus.

Constitutional diseases associated with infertility are: tuberculosis, diabetes mellitus, anaemia, syphilis, alcoholism and dietetic deficiences. *Over-work* of a mental nature can affect sperm production. *Endocrine factors* such as hypothyroidism or hyperthyroidism. Hypopituitarism suggested by underdevelopment of the penis, and obesity. Drugs less commonly cause infertility but they include anti depressants and sulphasalazine.

Men suffering from the chromosomal anomaly, Klinefelter's syndrome (XXY), have undeveloped genitalia with small soft testes and are infertile. Between 3 and 5 per cent of men arc infertile because of autoimmunization with circulating antibodies to their own spermatozoa.

The commonest cause of complete sterility in the male is blockage of the epididymis due to gonorrhoea or other infection. Atrophy of the testes following orchitis as a complication of mumps (about 10 per cent of males contracting mumps develop orchitis) may be responsible. The male with both testes undescended is almost certainly sterile.

Failure of the male to ejaculate during coitus is a not infrequent cause when both partners are found to be normally fertile.

2. Female factors

LOCAL

a. *Gross pelvic lesions*
Absence of uterus, vagina, Fallopian tubes or ovaries
Closure of hymen, vagina or cervix
Fibroids, polyps, carcinoma
Tuberculosis of the endometrium
Endometriosis
b. *Cervical lesions*
Cervicitis
Abnormalities of cervical secretion
Stenosis of cervix
c. *Tubal lesions*
Inflammatory lesions
Tuberculosis
Rudimentary tubes
d. *Vaginal and vulval lesions*
Dyspareunia
Vaginismus
e. *Endocrine lesions*
Gross disorders:
Fröhlich's syndrome, myxoedema
Simmonds' disease
Adrenocortical tumours
Menstrual disorders:
Polysystic disease of the ovaries
Amenorrhoea, hypomenorrhoea
Metropathia
Anovular menstruation
Ovarian failure (primary or secondary)
f. *Chromosomal anomalies*
Turner's syndrome (XO)
Super-female (XXX)

GENERAL

Anxiety
Old age
Obesity
Anaemia
Nutritional: vitamin A, B deficiency
Occupational

3. Combined Male and Female factors present together

a. Subnormal sperm count with abnormal cervical secretion in the female
b. Incomplete penetration
c. Lack of seminal plasma
d. Defective germ plasma

The above lists shows that some causes of infertility are primary, others secondary. Thus absence of the uterus or infantile uterus means primary sterility, while failure to ovulate, salpingitis, etc. may occur in women who have had children, and only secondarily because sterile on account of these lesions.

Congenital lesions

Some of the congenital lesions are diagnosed easily, such as *imperforate hymen, absence of the vagina*, or *stenosis of the cervix*, while absence of the essential organs often requires an anaesthetic in order that a bimanual examination may be made satisfactorily or for a laparoscopic examination to be undertaken.

Patients with gonadal agenisis suffer from too short stature, sexual infantilism and primary amenorrhoea. Two-thirds have an XO chromosome complement and other features of Turner's syndrome. Laparoscopy reveals small elongated ovarian streaks of fibrous tissue in place of ovaries. Male pseudo-hermaphrodites with testicular feminization and a 46XY chromosome karyotype have the appearance of a female of normal height and often well-developed breasts. They have absent or scanty axillary and pubic hair, a short, blind vagina, absent uterus and tubes and suffer from primary amenorrhoea. Bilateral testes may be in the abdomen or in the inguinal canal. The cause is end-organ resistance to testosterone or androgen insensitivity. Other members of the family are liable to have the condition.

Acquired lesions

The differential diagnosis of acquired lesions can only be made by complete examination of the patient. This includes a clinical examination of the vulva, vagina, cervix and pelvic organs by inspection and bimanual vaginal examination; an assessment of the Fallopian tubes or salpingography or by injecting dye into the uterus and seeing if it spills out of the fimbrial ends into the pelvis; detection of ovulation by basal body temperatures or blood progesterone levels in the second half of the cycle or the finding of a secretory endometrium on biopsy; a study of the cervical mucus at ovulation time with special regard to the presence or absence of actively progressing sperms in it after intercourse.

Blockage of the Fallopian tubes

This occurs as the result of past salpingo-oophoritis. It can be demonstrated by insufflation of the tubes via the uterus with carbon dioxide (Rubin's test). It can also be demonstrated by injecting into the uterus and tubes a water-soluble substance that is radio-opaque. Radiographs are taken under a fluorescent screen and image intensifier. The tubes may appear to be blocked as the result of spasm (*Fig.* I.1). An alternative investigation and the method of choice is pelvic laparoscopy. This affords an opportunity to study the condition of all the pelvic organs, to see adhesions if they are present and to note if methylene blue dye injected

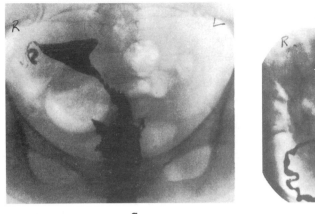
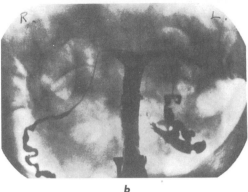

a   *b*

Fig. I.1. *a.* Radiograph of the uterus and Fallopian tubes after intrauterine injection of radio-opaque solution. The left tube is closed at the uterine end. The right tube is stenosed: *b.* Radiograph of the uterus and Fallopian tubes after intrauterine injection of radio-opaque solution. The left tube is patent. The right tube is closed at its outer end.

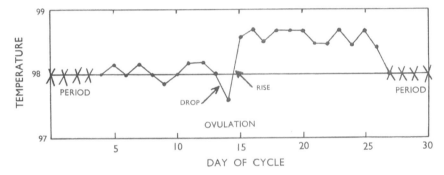

Fig I.2. A typical basal temperature chart

into the uterus comes out freely from the fimbrial ends of the tubes and spills into the pelvis.

When the man's sperm count is adequate and the woman's Fallopian tubes are patent, attention should be paid to the Simms–Hühner *post-coital test*. Mucus is aspirated from the cervical canal at the time of ovulation following intercourse the night before or the morning of the test. The mucus is placed on a slide, covered with a coverslip and examined under the high power of the microscope. There should be at least two, and normally five or more, motile sperms progressing in straight lines across the high power field. A negative postcoital test may be due to abnormal sperm production, inadequate intercourse, failure to ejaculate or hostile cervical mucus.

Endocrine causes of infertility

Endocrine causes are common. Pregnancy is not possible during periods of amenorrhoea because of failure to ovulate. Women who suffer from oligomenorrhoea have their fertility reduced. It is rare for women who menstruate regularly at monthly intervals not to ovulate although some of them do have a defective corpus

luteum and a poor or short luteal phase of the menstrual cycle. If an early menopause is suspected serum FSH will be more than 25 u/l and LH more than 25 u/l. The occurrence and timing of ovulation can be verified by taking the temperature by mouth first thing on waking before moving or getting out of bed. The basal temperature in the first half of the cycle is slightly lower than it is in the second half. A characteristic drop followed by a rise at mid-cycle indicates ovulation which, in most women, takes place about 14 days before the onset of the next period (*Fig* I.2). Ovulation is followed by the formation of a corpus luteum and this can be diagnosed by a raised serum level of progesterone (between 2·8 and 64 nmol/l) usually carried out on the 21st day of a normal cycle. Following ovulation the uterine endometrium undergoes the histological changes of the secretory (or progestational) phase which become more and more marked up to the time of the onset of menstruation. The stromal cells enlarge and the glands become tortuous with deep serrations in their walls and secretion in their lumina. A biopsy of the endometrium toward the end of the cycle will show these changes if ovulation has taken place. The finding in the cervix of the typical clear elastic mucus in mid-cycle is further proof that ovulation has taken place. Mid-cycle cervical mucus can be drawn into threads up to 10 cm in length. This is known as *spinnbarkeit* and is an indication of high oestrogen secretion by the ovary. 'Ferning' is another effect of high mid-cycle oestrogen. The mid-cycle cervical mucus is spread thickly on a glass slide, rinsed in distilled water and allowed to dry. A characteristic pattern resembling a fern leaf forms on the slide. Later in the cycle absence of spinnbarkeit and ferning indicate a progesterone effect and functioning corpus luteum.

Although serum levels of hormones are accurate measures of ovarian function, smears of vaginal cells in the hands of the expert cytologist also reflect the hormonal changes. The length and character of the luteal phase can be assessed by doing serial smears. A short luteal phase may prevent a fertilized ovum from embedding in the endometrium.

Other causes of infertility

Generalized endocrine disorders such as hypo- or hyperthyroidism, adrenocortical hypo- or hyperfunction and uncontrolled diabetes may result in infertility. Polycystic ovarian disease (Stein–Leventhal syndrome) is characterized by bilaterally enlarged polycystic ovaries, secondary amenorrhoea or oligomenorrhoea and infertility. About half the patients are hirsute and many are obese. Infertility is due to failure of ovulation. The enlarged ovaries can be felt on bimanual vaginal examination but are best diagnosed on ultrasonography or laparoscopy. Blood levels of LH are raised and there may be an increased excretion in urine of androstenedione or dehydroepiandrosterone.

N. Patel

Irritability

Irritability is a universally experienced feeling which becomes pathological when exaggerated in duration or degree. There have been disagreements over definition, in teasing irritability out from hostility, anger and aggression, but the core constituents appear to be: (1) reduced control over temper, often resulting in quarrelling or behavioural outbursts; (2) not initiated by the intention to harm or intimidate; and (3) unpleasant experiences which lack the purging effect of vindicated anger. The feeling may be brief or prolonged, and may have no overt manifestations; however destructive thoughts or actions emerge as extreme irritability shades into frank aggression (*Table* I.2.).

Table I.2. Causes of irritability

Commonest
Normal
Personality trait
Any debilitating/fatiguing condition

Less common
Drugs
  Alcohol
  Stimulants
  Benzodiazepines
Drug withdrawal
Endocrine disorders
  Thyroid dysfunction
  Hypoglycaemia
  Premenstrual tension syndrome
Neurological disorders
  Head injury
  Following neurosurgery
  Frontal lobe damage/disease
  Epilepsy
  Delirium
  Dementia
Psychiatric disorders
  Adjustment reaction
  Anxiety
  Depression
  Mania
  Paranoid disorder

Rare
Drugs
  Opiates
  Barbiturates
  Antihistamines
  Monoamine oxidase inhibitors
  Tricyclic antidepressants
Neurological disorders
  Temporal lobe disease/damage
  Multiple sclerosis
  Migraine
  Encephalitis
  Subdural haematoma
Endocrine disorders
  Parathyroid dysfunction
  Adrenal dysfunction
  Pituitary dysfunction
Psychiatric disorders
  Post-traumatic stress disorder
  Panic
  Schizophrenia
  Schizoaffective disorder
  Eating disorders
Other causes
  Postviral fatigue syndrome
  Infectious mononeucleosis
  Kleine-Levine syndrome
  Insomnia
  Sleep-wake schedule (night-shift syndrome)
  Pellagra
  Anaemia
  Hypercalcaemia

Irritability is a common complaint addressed to doctors, sometimes by the patient and sometimes by those who are the butt of this unwelcome irascibility. Like other emotions it varies constitutionally and some people are simply more bad-tempered and peevish than others while ill-health or tiredness are commonplace precipitants. Aspects of irritability also figure as a persistent trait in various types of *personality disorder*, including the psychopathic, paranoid, narcissistic and hysterical forms. However attention should be focused when this represents a distinct change, either as a new or exaggerated phenomenon.

Irritability can exist and present independently of other mood states, but there is no evidence suggesting it ever forms a primary disorder. The common underlying causes are *organic brain disease*, *drugs* and other *primary mood disorders*. Irritability occurs often following neurosurgery or head injury, even when the trauma is relatively minor. It is a rare accompaniment of temporal lobe disease, but is commonly and classically associated with frontal lobe disorders, with other features and signs usually being elicited. Irritable mood frequently develops in the early stages of dementia, especially multi-infarct dementia, when absurd irascibility can be a major source of distress among relatives: this 'improves'as the process advances.

Epilepsy and irritability is a well-known association, particularly the build up of touchiness that precedes a seizure and is relieved by it. However persistent irritability is an important interictal problem, especially in focal epilepsy (of any site) compared with primary generalized epilepsy. Phenobarbitone exacerbates irritability, and in some cases, switching anticonvulsant treatment to carbamazepine is helpful. In addition to barbiturates other drugs implicated in the generation of irritability are stimulants, benzodiazepines, antihistamines (rarely) and alcohol (commonly), while the abstinence syndrome induced by the withdrawal of any drug upon which the patient has become dependent is another potential cause. Other notable physical causes are endocrine disorders, the best-known association being with premenstrual tension syndrome where the mood changes are characteristically phasic and sometimes responsive to progestogens and/or pyridoxine.

Abnormal degrees of irritability are reported in around half of all patients with primary anxiety states, while post-traumatic stress disorder may present with touchiness or outbursts of temper that can progress to unprovoked aggression. In mania irritability is very common, indeed even more common than elation, as well as the source of much of the accompanying behavioural disturbance. However it is in depressive illness that the greatest diagnostic difficulties tend to occur. Depression presenting silently with irritability seems particularly common in the puerperium: there may be other persistent changes including emotional lability, constant fatigue and loss of libido, but without major depressive features or loss of love for the baby these changes can all too readily be ascribed to not sleeping, not coping or not adjusting. The condition normally resolves even if untreated but now and again

it may persist for years, causing major marital disruption and influencing important decisions like having further children, or even sterilization—decisions that can be regretted when effective treatment is initiated. The prescription of minor tranquillizers to such patients only serves to exacerbate the situation, and indeed it is important to remember that irrespective of cause or treatment, alcohol and benzodiazepines should be avoided in all cases where irritability is a major feature.

George Masterton

Jaundice

Types

Jaundice may be caused by a raised conjugated or unconjugated bilirubin. Unconjugated hyperbilirubinaemia may be due to excessive production of bilirubin (haemolysis), reduced uptake of bilirubin or a failure of conjugation by the liver. Conjugated hyperbilirubinaemia results from hepatocellular damage or obstruction of the bile ducts, either within the liver (intrahepatic cholestasis) or of a major bile duct (extrahepatic obstruction jaundice). Jaundice is also often classified into pre-hepatic (haemolysis), hepatic and extrahepatic types. Clues as to the cause of jaundice may be obtained from the history and physical examination (*Tables* J.1, J.2).

Investigations of jaundice

The simplest investigations are liver function tests and urine examinations; typical abnormalities are shown in (*Table* J.3). The liver enzymes, aspartate (AST) and alanine transaminase (ALT), are normally contained within the liver cells, and are released during hepatocellular necrosis whereas alkaline phosphatase is excreted into the biliary system and rises in obstructive jaundice.

There is no bilirubin present in the urine of patients with pre-hepatic (haemolytic) jaundice because unconjugated bilirubin is tightly bound to albumin and is not filtered at the glomerulus. On the other hand, conjugated bilirubin is water-soluble and stains the urine dark in hepatocellular and obstructive jaundice. Urobilinogen is produced by bacteria in the gut and is normally partially reabsorbed into the portal vein, taken up by hepatocytes and re-excreted in bile. When the liver is damaged hepatic extraction is less efficient and the concentration of urobilinogen in plasma, and hence in the urine, rises. The presence of urobilinogen in the urine is thus a test of liver

Table J.1. History of jaundice

Haemolytic	Hepatic		Obstructive
Family history	Flu symptoms		Abdominal
Racial origin	Rashes		pain
Drug history	Joint pains		Pale stools
Symptoms of anaemia	Contact with jaundice	Viral	Dark urine
	Blood transfusions		Itching
	Infections		
	Drug history		
	Alcoholic intake		
	Previous jaundice		

Table J.2. Physical signs associated with jaundice

Haemolytic	Hepatic		Obstructive
Splenomegaly, reduced stature	Dupuytren's contractures Parotid enlargement	} Alcohol	Scratch marks Mass in abdomen
	Spider naevi Gynaecomastia Testicular atrophy Loss of hair Red hands	} Endocrine	Gallbladder In a patient with obstructive jaundice if the gallbladder is palpable the cause is unlikely to be gallstones—Courvoisier's law
	White nails Ascites and oedema	} Hypoproteinaemia	
	Bruising	Prothrombin time prolonged	
	Splenomegaly Veins around umbilicus	} Portal hypertension	

Table J.3. Liver function tests and urinalysis in jaundice

	Unconjugated bilirubinaemia (haemolytic)	Hepatocellular jaundice	Obstructive jaundice
Liver function tests	Direct bilirubin ↑ AST ALT } normal ALK—P	Indirect bilirubin ↑ AST ↑↑ ALT ↑↑ ALK—P ↑	Indirect bilirubin ↑↑ AST ↑ ALT ↑ ALK—P ↑↑↑
Urine tests	Bilirubin 0 Urobilinogen Normally not raised	Bilirubin + Urobilinogen ++	Bilirubin +++ Urobilinogen →

function and one of the earliest signs of recovery from hepatocellular jaundice is the disappearance of urobilinogen from the urine as it is again removed by the liver. In complete obstructive jaundice, urobilinogen is absent from the urine as there is no bilirubin in the gut.

All patients presenting with cholestatic jaundice should undergo ultrasound examination of the liver (*Figs* J.1-J.3). This examination is cheap, without complication and in experienced hands accurate at determining whether or not there is obstruction to the biliary tree. If equivocal the ultrasound should be repeated as jaundice deepens and it may then be obvious that there is indeed an obstructive cause. In addition to demonstrating dilated ducts, expert ultrasonographers can often show the cause of obstruction

but this is unreliable and definitive cholangiography should be performed in all circumstances. The radiologist may also show dilatation of the gallbladder, cholelithiasis and secondary deposits within the liver. Furthermore the pancreas, portal and hepatic veins and the spleen can be visualized. Once the diagnosis of extra hepatic biliary obstruction has been made the bile ducts should be outlined by cholangiography. This is best done by endoscopic retrograde cholangiopancreatography (ERCP) in which a side-viewing endoscope is passed into the second part of the duodenum (*Fig.* J.4). The ampulla of Vater is first seen and ampullary tumours can be identified and biopsied. The bile duct and pancreas are cannulated and opacified using radiological contrast material. The procedure is successful in approximately 90 per cent of patients in expert hands and, as well as defining the cause of the obstruction, the endoscopist has the capacity to relieve obstruction by extracting calculi or placing stents within strictures. When the endoscopist fails to achieve a diagnosis the alternative approach to ERCP is to perform a percutaneous transhepatic cholangiogram (PTC) using a 'skinny' needle (*Fig.* J.5). This is a technically easier procedure in patients with a dilated biliary tract but is also successful in approximately 60 per cent of patients with non-dilated bile ducts.

A rational approach to the investigation of jaundice is illustrated in *Fig.* J.6. Liver biopsy confirms the presence of hepatocellular damage, but the differentiation of large duct obstruction from intrahepatic cholestasis may be difficult (*see later*) (*Fig.* J.7).

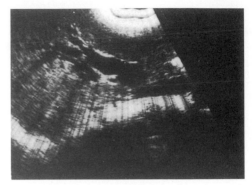

Fig J.3. Longitudinal ultrasound showing obstructive jaundice due to stone in common bile duct.

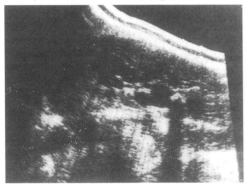

Fig. J.1. Longitudinal ultrasound showing dilated common bile duct and intrahepatic ducts.

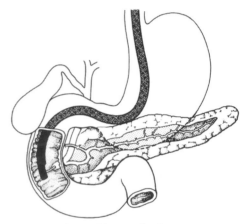

Fig.J.4. Cannulation of the ampulla of Vater.

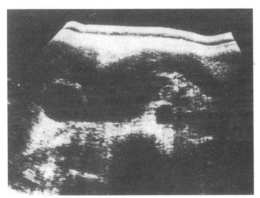

Fig J.2. Longitudinal ultrasound showing a carcinoma of the head of the pancreas as to a cause of obstructive jaundice.

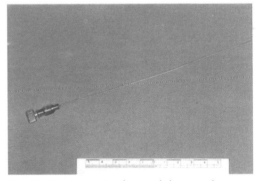

Fig. J.5. Percutaneous transhepatic cholangiography.

Unconjugated hyperbilirubinaemia

1. Increased production of bilirubin:
a. Inefficient marrow production
b. Increased breakdown (haemolysis)
    Haemoglobinopathies
    Antibody-mediated
    Drug-induced
2. Decreased uptake of bilirubin into the liver:
    Gilbert's disease
3. Decreased conjugation of bilirubin in the liver:
    Crigler–Najjar syndrome
    Neonatal jaundice
    Drugs
    Lucey–Driscoll syndrome

Increased production of bilirubin without haemolysis (shunt hyperbilirubinaemia)

Very rarely inefficient marrow production of haemoglobin results in increased amounts of unconjugated bilirubin being released into the circulation ('early

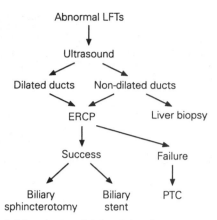

Abnormal LFTs

↓

Ultrasound

Dilated ducts   Non-dilated ducts

ERCP   Liver biopsy

Success   Failure

Biliary   Biliary   PTC
sphincterotomy   stent

Fig. J.6. Investigation of cholestatic jaundice.

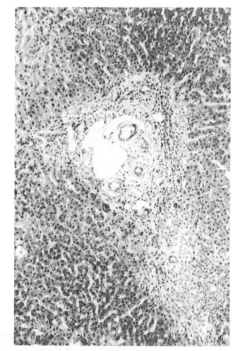

Fig. J.7. Liver histology of large duct obstruction showing expansion of portal tracts and proliferation of bile ducts.

label' bilirubin). The red cells manufactured, however, have a normal life span. This is a rare primary condition and also occurs in a number of other causes of inefficient erythropoiesis, for example anaemia.

Increased production of bilirubin due to haemolysis

Most commonly, unconjugated hyperbilirubinaemia results from haemolysis, either caused by an *intrinsic* abnormality of the red cells or due to the development of an abnormal mechanism of destruction (*extrinsic*). The general investigation of patients with a haemolytic anaemia is summarized below.

a. Evidence of intravascular haemolysis:

    Haptoglobins
    Haemoglobinaemia
    Haemoglobinuria
    Haemosiderinuria
    Methaemalbuminaemia

b. Evidence of increased marrow production:

    Reticulocytosis
    Skeletal changes
    Marrow hyperplasia

c. Evidence of red cell damage:

    Fragmented forms

d. Evidence of shortened red cell life:

    Radioactive labelling of red cells

A.   EVIDENCE OF INTRAVASCULAR HAEMOLYSIS

Haemoglobin released during intravascular haemolysis is normally attached to haptoglobin, the levels of which are usually reduced in chronic haemolytic states. However, levels may also be reduced by chronic liver disease and increased non-specifically in a number of connective tissue disorders. Haemoglobinaemia associated sometimes with methaemalbuminaemia, haemoglobinuria and haemosiderinuria, provide incontrovertible evidence of intravascular haemolysis, but are frequently absent in chronic haemolytic anaemias.

B.   EVIDENCE OF INCREASED MARROW PRODUCTION

In a compensated anaemia, reticulocytosis with a raised mean corpuscular volume (MCV) is common. Increased marrow activity results in skeletal changes which are frequent in thalassaemia and sickle-cell disease but rare in other conditions. The skull of such patients demonstrates a thickened vault and the diploe are widened. Bony trabeculae arising at right angles to the diploe may produce a 'hair-on-end' appearance (*Fig.* J.8). The bones of the limbs have a widened narrow cavity with a coarse trabecular pattern.

C.   EVIDENCE OF RED CELL DAMAGE

Fragmented forms may provide evidence of increased red cell destruction (*Fig.* J.9).

D.   EVIDENCE OF SHORT RED CELL LIFE SPAN

The standard clinical test to detect shortened red cell survival is to tag the patient's cells with a radioactive chromium and measure the decline in plasma radioactivity.

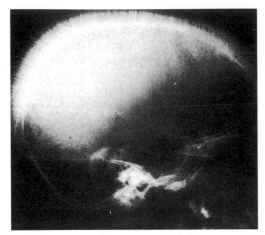

Fig. J.8. Hair-on-end appearance of skull in patient with thalassaemia.

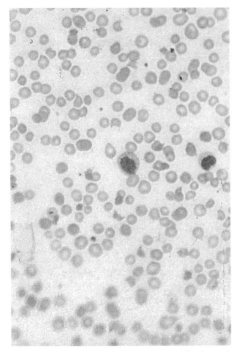

Fig. 9. Fragmented red cells seen in intravascular haemolysis.

Intrinsic defects of the red cells leading to increased haemolysis

a. Spherocytosis

b. Elliptocytosis

c. Enzyme defects

d. Haemoglobinopathies

  i. Sickle-cell disease

  ii. HbSC disease

  iii. Thalassaemia

e. Paroxysmal nocturnal haemoglobinuria

A.   CONGENITAL SPHEROCYTOSIS

This is a dominantly inherited defect which probably affects the red cell membrane, rendering it more permeable to sodium. The red cells are spherical rather than the usual biconcave shape and are more readily haemolysed in hypotonic saline (red cell fragility test). The patient usually presents in early childhood, even though jaundice may have been noticed in early childhood; often jaundice is first identified in the teens. Splenomegaly is common; bile pigment stones are frequently formed and patients occasionally present with obstructive jaundice. The disease is characterized by crises of worsening anaemia and jaundice caused by increased haemolysis due to infection. The diagnosis is usually straightforward with splenomegaly, a family history and a typical blood film, but it must be remembered that spherocytes may be a feature of a number of different types of haemolytic anaemia, and that occasional mild cases of congenital spherocytosis do not present until adulthood. Splenectomy is usually followed by long-term remission of symptoms.

B.   CONGENITAL ELLIPTOCYTOSIS

This is another Mendelian dominant disorder and it is usually asymptomatic, without haemolysis. Occasionally a compensated haemolytic anaemia occurs but anaemia sufficient to produce jaundice is extremely rare.

C.   ENZYME DEFECTS

A wide variety of enzyme defects in the red cells have been described which produce a haemolytic anaemia and jaundice. These are usually recessively inherited. Suspicion of this type of disorder is always aroused if haemoglobin electrophoresis and osmotic fragility are normal in a patient with haemolytic anaemia. Splenectomy in these patients is not beneficial. The commonest of these disorders is pyruvate kinase deficiency whose clinical features are more variable in severity, but similar to congenital spherocytosis.

D.   HAEMOGLOBINOPATHIES

The primary structure of haemoglobin is four polypeptide chains attached to a haem molecule. Normal adult haemoglobin has two identical alpha and two identical beta polypeptide chains attached to the haem. In the fetus the haemoglobin has two gamma chains replacing the beta chain (fetal haemoglobin) and a small proportion of adult haemoglobin has two delta chains instead of two beta chains (A2 haemoglobin).

A2 and fetal haemoglobins will increase in disease affecting the beta chains. There are two basic types of haemoglobinopathies. One involves qualitative defects affecting one of the polypeptide chains (usually a single amino acid substitution). The other is a quantitative defect affecting the production of the whole of one long chain.

Qualitative defects of haemoglobin

Single amino acid substitution in the polypeptide chain of haemoglobin commonly produces no disease. Occasionally an amino acid substitution produces a haemolytic anaemia and *sickle-cell anaemia* provides the model for such an illness. Patients who inherit one abnormal gene only (heterozygous or sickle-cell trait) are usually only mildly affected and do not become jaundiced. Patients who inherit two sickle-cell genes have sickle-cell disease. An amino acid substitution in the beta chain produces an unstable haemoglobin molecule which polymerizes into the reduced state into long chains which distort the red cells into a sickle shape. Sickle-cell disease affects Negroes predominantly and is characterized by jaundice, anaemia and skeletal changes. Although the clinical manifestations are variable, life for the patient is frequently punctuated by crises of spontaneous sickling in the circulation which produces severe abdominal and bone pain and a high fever. Although splenomegaly is common in children, repeated infarcts of the spleen usually lead to atrophy in adulthood. Gallstones are again common, which may produce obstructive jaundice. The prognosis is serious with many patients still dying either as children or in young adult life.

The diagnosis is made by haemoglobin electrophoresis which will show increased amounts of fetal and A2 haemoglobin, and by demonstrating *in vitro* sickling of cells by addition of a reducing agent to the blood (sickle-cell test).

Sickle-cell HbC disease

Although heterozygous sickle-cell disease is usually asymptomatic, if another abnormal haemoglobin (e.g. HbC) is inherited from the other parent haemolysis and jaundice may result, although the disease is usually milder than homozygous sickle-cell disease. Similar clinical symptoms may occur with the inheritance of one thalassaemia gene and one sickle-cell gene.

Qualitative defects of haemoglobin leading to increased haemolysis (thalassaemia)

The homozygous inheritance of defective production of alpha chains of haemoglobin is not compatible with life. The heterozygous inheritance of defective production of alpha or beta chains (alpha or beta thalassaemia minor) produces a mild abnormality rarely giving rise to jaundice. β-Thalassaemia major is the only homozygous thalassaemia syndrome which may occasionally result in jaundice. This condition is found most commonly in patients originating from the Mediterranean littoral, and anaemia dominates the clinical picture. Hepatosplenomegaly and marked skeletal changes may also occur. The blood picture is similar to that of iron deficiency anaemia and the diagnosis is made by an increased amount of circulating fetal haemoglobin on haemoglobin electrophoresis. For reasons that are unknown, A2 haemoglobin is not usually increased. There is often an *increased* resistance to haemolysis in hypotonic saline (osmotic fragility test).

E.   PAROXYSMAL NOCTURNAL HAEMOGLOBINURIA

Episodes of haemolysis may be accompanied by slight jaundice in this rare condition. Diagnosis can be made by the characteristic history of red urine, which contains haemoglobin, following sleeping. The abnormal haemolysis of the red cells can be demonstrated if the plasma is acidified (Ham's test).

Extrinsic factors leading to increased haemolysis

Autoimmune haemolytic anaemia
Cold haemoglobinuria
Drugs and chemicals
Glucose-6-phosphate dehydrogenase deficiency
Miscellaneous

A.   WARM ANTIBODY AUTOIMMUNE HAEMOLYTIC ANAEMIA

In this condition antibody coats the patient's red cells at 37°C resulting in increased extravascular destruction. The antibody is usually of the IgG class and incomplete (i.e. does not directly cause agglutination or haemolysis). This antibody can be detected by the direct Coombs' test where the addition of antibody to IgG in *in vitro* causes the red cells to agglutinate. Spherocytes are often present in the blood film, the white count may be raised and occasionally the platelets are low, producing purpura. In acute acquired haemolytic anaemia the patient is usually a child with a palpable spleen, jaundice, anaemia and the constitutional symptoms of fever, vomiting and prostration. In the chronic form the onset is insidious, usually in adults but again the patient is usually jaundiced (in 75 per cent of cases) and has a palpable spleen. In half the patients with acquired haemolytic anaemia no cause for the antibody formation is found, but in the rest it is secondary to a number of diseases, most importantly disseminated lupus erythematosus, but also recticuloendothelial malignancy, leukaemia and sarcoidosis. Resolution of the symptoms usually occurs following treatment with corticosteroids or, occasionally, splenectomy.

B. COLD ANTIBODY AUTOIMMUNE ANAEMIA

Occasionally antibody is produced which reacts with the patient's red cells at low temperatures. Depending on the thermal range of the antibody a continuous mild haemolytic anaemia may occur punctuated by paroxysms of intravenous haemolysis with abdominal pain, rigors, transient jaundice and splenomegaly, which may be provoked by exposure to the cold. Cold antibody haemolytic anaemia is frequently secondary to viral infections and malignancy.

C. DRUG AND CHEMICAL-INDUCED HAEMOLYSIS

Some chemicals (e.g. arsenic and naphthalene in moth balls) produce haemolysis and jaundice which is directly dose related. Haemolysis may occur with other drugs; this is unrelated to the dose and occurs in a few susceptible individuals only (*Table* J.4). The two important mechanisms for producing haemolysis in this situation are an associated deficiency of glucose-6-phosphate dehydrogenase in the red cell, or the production of auto-antibodies, often directed against the drug attached to the red cell membrane, which acts as a hapten. In this type of haemolysis the blood film often shows spherocytes and red cell inclusions (Heinz bodies).

Table J.4. Drugs occasionally causing haemolysis

a. In glucose-6-phosphate dehydrogenase deficient subjects

Antimalarials, e.g.	primaquine
	mepacrine
Antibacterials	chloramphenicol
	sulphonamides
Nitrofurans	nitrofurantoin
Quinines	quinidine

b. Auto-immune
Penicillin
Sulphonamides
Quinine and quinidine
Methyldopa
Mefenamic acid
Sulphasalazine
Para-aminosalicylic acid

Glucose-6-phosphate dehydrogenase deficiency is common in Negroes and inhabitants of the Mediterranean littoral. This enzyme helps to maintain the cell concentration of reduced glutathione which is turn stabilizes the haemoglobin molecule.

Favism is a disorder characterized by intravascular haemolysis and jaundice occurring when a glucose-6-phosphate dehydrogenase deficient patient, usually a child from the Mediterranean region, ingests fava beans or inhales the pollen.

Similar episodes occur when the patient is exposed to certain drugs (*see Table* J.4). Haemolysis ceases when the older population of red cells containing less of the enzyme is destroyed.

Autoimmune drug-induced haemolysis is particularly common with methyldopa where the direct Coombs' test is positive in 20 per cent of patients taking the drug, but haemolysis occurs in less than 1 per cent.

D. OTHER CONDITIONS CAUSING HAEMOLYSIS

Acute haemolysis with jaundice may occur with various infections, e.g. malaria and gangrene, and more mildly with viral pneumonia (usually due to cold agglutinins). It may also follow a mismatched blood transfusion or occur in a severely burned patient.

Excessive exercise, particularly on hard roads, may also lead to episodes of intravascular haemolysis (*march haemoglobinuria*).

Microangiopathic haemolytic anaemia is the name given to a group of conditions characterized by haemolysis in association with fragmentation of red cells as they pass through blood vessels damaged by clots. Evidence of disseminated intravascular coagulation is common. Such haemolytic anaemias are present in thrombotic thrombocytopaenic purpura, malignant hypertension, disseminated neoplasia and in association with uraemia in children (the haemolytic uraemic syndrome).

Unconjugated hyperbilirubinaemia caused by impaired uptake of bilirubin into the liver

GILBERT'S DISEASE

There is some debate as to whether this condition exists or whether it represents the upper range of a normal population distribution of unconjugated bilirubin. However, most would accept that it is a common familial condition in which there is a mild degree of unconjugated hyperbilirubinaemia. It is probably inherited as a Mendelian dominant with variable penetrance. The degree of jaundice varies and often increases following an infection or a period of fasting. Episodes of deepening jaundice may be associated with recurrent, vague abdominal pains. Mild decreases in red cell life span and the liver's ability to conjugate bilirubin are associated with a failure of transport of unconjugated bilirubin into the liver cell. The diagnosis is made by excluding liver disease. It may be confirmed by fasting the patient or by giving an intravenous injection of nicotinic acid. Both of these manoeuvres result in an increase in serum bilirubin concentrations.

They are rarely necessary since the diagnosis is usually obvious.

Unconjugated hyperbilirubinaemia caused by impaired conjugation in the liver

1. CRIGLER–NAJJAR SYNDROME

In this familial condition there is a deficiency of the liver enzyme, glucuronyl transferase, which conjugates bilirubin. In severely affected patients (Type 1) death occurs in the neonatal period. A partial enzyme defect with some conjugated bilirubin in the bile and a better prognosis (Type 2) also occurs.

2. NEONATAL JAUNDICE

Glucuronyl transferase matures shortly before birth and newborn babies, particularly if premature, will become mildly jaundiced. This may be severe in conditions increasing the bilirubin load (e.g. haemolysis) and kernicterus may result. Occasionally prolonged neonatal jaundice is thought to occur in breast-fed babies due to the presence of pregnandiol in the milk.

3. LUCEY–DRISCOLL SYNDROME

Unconjugated bilirubin has rarely been described in pregnancy due to hormonal inhibition of bilirubin conjugation.

Conjugated hyperbilirubinaemia

HEPATIC CAUSES

The hepatic causes of conjugated bilirubinaemia may be divided into acute hepatocellular damage, associated with considerable increases in hepatic enzymes and a short clinical course, and chronic damage where the course is protracted and there are lesser rises in liver enzymes.

a. *Acute liver damage*
   i. Viral hepatitis
   ii. Non-viral infections
   iii. Drug induced
   iv. Poisons
   v. Fatty liver of pregnancy
b. *Chronic liver damage*
   i. Cirrhosis
   ii. Tumours
      a. Primary
      b. Secondary
c. *Infiltrations*
   i. Reticuloendothelial tumours
   ii. Amyloidosis

Acute hepatic damage

Causes of acute hepatic damage may produce a mild clinical illness or a severe disease (fulminant hepatic failure) with encephalopathy and a high mortality, when cerebral oedema, renal failure and a bleeding diathesis are frequent causes of death.

VIRAL HEPATITIS

Although a large number of viruses occasionally cause hepatitis (including rubella, Coxsackie B, herpes simplex, yellow fever virus and cytomegalovirus) the four common ones are virus A, virus B, virus C and infectious mononucleosis. The recognition of serological markers for hepatitis A and B have revolutionized our understanding of viral hepatitis and it is now realized that many patients with these infections do not become jaundiced.

Virus A (infectious hepatitis)

This is an endemic infection with a short incubation period (15-20 days) causes by a 27 nm RNA virus. Outbreaks usually occur in conditions of poor hygiene or overcrowding. The usual transmission is faeco-oral. Patients present with malaise, anorexia, fever and a rapid onset of jaundice. There is often a vague ache in the right upper quadrant and the liver is enlarged and tender. The spleen may also be palpable. Complete recovery is usually within a few weeks, although relapses may occur. Occasionally patients develop deep jaundice due to intrahepatic cholestasis during the convalescent period. The diagnosis is confirmed by the demonstration of IgM antibody to the virus.

Virus B (serum hepatitis)

This infection has a longer incubation period and arthralgias and rashes may occur in the prodromal period. It is caused by a DNA virus which has an outer coat derived from the host cells and an inner core. Originally only blood transmission was recognized, e.g. blood transfusions, transfusions of blood products (haemophilic globulin), or by needles contaminated with blood in drug addicts and in tattooing. Outbreaks in renal dialysis units produced by blood contamination have caused great concern in the past. The disease is also venereally transmitted as the virus is present in semen. Hepatitis B is common in homosexuals, 10 per cent of whom have serological markers of past infection. Asymptomatic carriers of hepatitis B infection are very frequent in certain parts of the world, e.g. Africa, China and parts of the Mediterranean. These patients may transmit the infection vertically from mother to offspring. The diagnosis of virus B hepatitis is made by the detection of the presence of surface antigen (HbsAg) in the bloodstream. For the patient to be infectious whole virus (Dane) particles must be present in the bloodstream and the presence of e antigen is a marker for this.

The majority of patients develop an acute viral hepatitis and this is associated with formation of antibodies and clearance of the virus from the liver. Other individuals failed to clear the virus, become carriers and some of these develop chronic liver disease. Patients with persistent hepatitis B virus infection are at risk of developing primary hepatocellular carcinoma.

Patients with known chronic hepatitis B infection may suffer an acute exacerbation of hepatitis due to a coincident infection with the delta virus which secondarily infects only patients with chronic HB hepatitis.

Virus C (non-A non-B hepatitis)

Patients may present with a typical history of viral hepatitis but without evidence of infection with the usual hepatotrophic viruses. At least two types of non-A non-B are recognized. One has a short incubation period and is contracted by transfusion with blood or its products, Virus C. The other is sporadic, has a longer incubation period and is probably contracted by the orofaecal route, Virus E. It has a particularly bad prognosis in pregnant women.

Hepatitis C is characteristically a milder illness than HBV but leads to chronic liver disease in a high proportion of individuals.

Infectious mononucleosis

Up to 15 per cent of patients with glandular fever develop jaundice. The clinical picture is characteristic with malaise, sore throat, skin rashes, lymphadenopathy and splenomegaly. Atypical mononuclear cells are found in the peripheral blood and the test for heterophile antibody (Paul–Bunnell) is usually positive.

Yellow fever

This is a zoonosis and is transmitted to man from a primate pool by the mosquito in tropical Africa, the Caribbean and South America. The incubation period is short (3–4 days) with a sudden onset of rigors, jaundice and abdominal pain. Its course may be fulminant with renal failure and a bleeding diathesis.

NON-VIRAL INFECTIONS

Relapsing fever

This condition is caused by a spirochaete of the Borrelia group of bacteria and is characterized by jaundice and a fever of up to 40 °C which normally lasts for 4–5 days and then remits. The epidemic form of the disease is usually caused by lice and is common during periods of famine. An epidemic infection is usually transmitted by the tick and is common in the Far East, Africa and America.

Leptospirosis

The spirochaete *L. icterohaemorrhagica* infects a variety of small animals and man contracts the disease by bathing in water contaminated with infected urine. The disease is biphasic with an initial illness a few days after exposure, with a temperature, meningism and prominent myalgias and conjunctivitis. Recovery may occur, or after a week the patient may develop widespread bruising, jaundice and occasionally renal failure. *Leptospira icterohaemorrhagiae* is transmitted by rats' urine, mainly to agricultural and sewage workers, and produces a severe form of the disease where jaundice and renal failure are particularly likely to occur.

Other bacterial infections

Jaundice may complicate any septicaemic illness. Occasionally an infected thrombus in the portal vein may occur (portal pyaemia) following an acute infection in the area drained by the portal system, e.g. appendicitis. The signs of a portal pyaemia are severe prostration, a swinging pyrexia and jaundice.

DRUG-INDUCED ACUTE HEPATIC DAMAGE

Drugs either produce predictable dose-related hepatic necrosis, e.g. paracetamol, or more commonly, damage is produced unpredictably in only a few of the patients exposed to this drug and unrelated to its dosage. There are two basic patterns of liver damage, either acute hepatic cellular necrosis with features identical to viral hepatitis, or intrahepatic cholestasis. It is not possible to give an exhaustive list of drugs producing hepatocellular damage (*Table J.5*). and a high index of suspicion should exist in any jaundiced patient who is taking drugs.

Paracetamol

Paracetamol overdose is the commonest cause of fulminant hepatic failure in Britain. Hepatic damage is dose-related but death has been reported with amounts as low as 7·5 g. Following ingestion paracetamol is metabolized to a toxic intermediate which is scavenged by glutathione. When glutathione stores are exhausted the metabolite binds covalently to the membrane of hepatocytes causing cell death. Chronic alcoholics whose microsomal enzymes are reduced and whose glutathione stores tend to be depressed are at increased risk following the overdose. Nausea, vomiting and abdominal pain develop within 12–36 hours and jaundice develops 2–3 days later. In severe cases this leads to liver failure with coagulopathy and encephalopathy. A very characteristic feature of paracetamol poisoning is the development of renal failure.

Table J.5. Drug-induced hepatic damage

Those drugs in italics are the commonest causes of liver damage

	Acute hepatic necrosis	Cholestasis
Paracetamol	+	
Dextropropoxyphene	+	+
Halothane	+	
Tetracycline	+ (in pregnancy)	
Erythromycin estolate		+
Penicillin	+	
Sulphasalazine		+
Nitrofurantoin	+	
Pheniramine maleate	+	
Piperazine	+	
Isoniazid	+	
Rifampicin	+	
Para-aminosalicylic acid	+	+
Chlorpromazine		+
Monoamine-oxidase inhibitor	+	
Methyldopa	+ (? cirrhosis)	
Quinidine	+	
Perhexiline	+ (? cirrhosis)	
Chlorpropamide		+
Phenytoin	+	
Propylthiouracil	+	+
Oral contraceptives		+
Anabolic steroids		+

Halothane

Halothane is a very safe anaesthetic but there is an undoubted small incidence (0·003 per cent) of serious acute hepatic necrosis following the use of the drug, which may lead to fever, jaundice and death. Inadvertent repeated use in patients who were previously jaundiced following exposure to halothane results in recurrence of the patient's jaundice. Halothane hepatitis is more common after repeated exposures particularly in obese patients. Jaundice associated with pyrexia usually occurs 2 weeks after initial exposure but only 10 days after subsequent administration. Halothane should not be reused in patients who have suffered a febrile illness and abnormal liver function tests after a previous anaesthetic with this agent.

Oral contraceptives

The older oral contraceptives containing a relatively high concentration of oestrogen occasionally led to a mild cholestatic jaundice. These individuals are particularly prone to develop cholestasis in pregnancy. In addition the older contraceptives also had a tendency to cause the Budd–Chiari syndrome and a variety of tumours within the liver, in particular benign adenomas. The newer contraceptives which contain much lower concentrations of oestrogens are much safer and rarely cause these complications.

Anabolic steroids

The C17-alpha-alkalated-substituted testosterones, e.g. norethisterone and norethanandrolone, produce a dose-related cholestasis by a similar mechanism to the oral contraceptive.

Chlorpromazine

An unpredictable cholestatic jaundice may occur in 1 per cent of patients within a month of starting treatment with this drug. Eosinophilia and mitochondrial antibodies are frequently found in the bloodstream. The patient itches, has pale stools and dark urine. Three-quarters of patients recover on withdrawal of the drug but a few develop prolonged cholestasis resembling primary biliary cirrhosis (*see* later).

Antineoplastic drugs

A variety of such drugs cause jaundice and liver damage, e.g. methotrexate. However, the primary conditions for which these drugs are administered are often a cause for jaundice.

INDUSTRIAL TOXINS

These are only rarely a cause of jaundice in man. Most seem to act by inhibiting protein synthesis. *Carbon tetrachloride* and less commonly other volatile hydrocarbons produce acute hepatocellular necrosis and jaundice within 1-2 days of exposure. Renal failure, pancreatitis, pulmonary oedema and death may also occur. Dicophane (DDT) and trinitrotoluene (TNT) also occasionally produce hepatic necrosis.

A cholestatic jaundice has been described following accidental ingestion of flour contaminated by diaminodiphenyl methane (so-called 'Epping jaundice', after the place where the outbreak occurred).

Amanita

Ingestion of as little as three wild mushrooms of the Amanita species may be fatal. Abdominal pain and diarrhoea occur within 18 hours of ingestion followed 3 days later by the development of fulminant hepatic failure and jaundice.

ACUTE FATTY LIVER OF PREGNANCY

This condition occurs shortly before or after delivery and is frequently fatal. The cause is unknown but histology shows microvesicular fatty droplets in the liver cells.

Chronic liver damage—cirrhosis

Cirrhosis is defined as diffuse fibrosis with nodular regeneration of the liver which destroys the normal spatial relationship of the lobules. It is classified as micronodular, macronodular or mixed, depending on the size of the nodules. The condition may be suspected in cases of jaundice where the liver is firm and palpable, although sometimes it is shrunken and impalpable. The stigmata of chronic liver disease (*Table* J.2) are often present and the spleen may be enlarged because of portal hypertension. Oedema and ascites are caused by a combination of portal hypertension, sodium retention and hypoalbuminaemia. Hepatic encephalopathy may occur, with a sweet musty odour to the breath (caused by mercaptans originating from gut breakdown of methionine), a flapping tremor (asterixis), disorders of the sleep rhythm and then frank unconsciousness. A chronic form of encephalopathy with slowness and psychiatric changes may also occur. Jaundice is a relatively late complication of cirrhosis and many patients with compensated cirrhosis have relatively normal liver function tests.

Causes of cirrhosis

1. ALCOHOLIC LIVER DISEASE

2. INFECTIONS
a. Viral (HBV, HCV)
b. Bacterial (syphilis)
c. Protozoan (schistosomiasis)

3. CHRONIC ACTIVE HEPATITIS
a. Lupoid
b. HBV
c. Drugs

4. GENETIC DEFECTS
a. Haemochromatosis
b. Wilson's disease
c. Galactosaemia
d. Glycogen storage diseases
e. Alpha-1 antitrypsin deficiency

5. BILIARY DISEASE
a. Long-standing extrahepatic biliary obstruction
b. Primary biliary cirrhosis
c. Sclerosing cholangitis
d. Congenital hepatic fibrosis

6. VENOUS CONGESTION
a. Cardiac failure
b. Constrictive pericarditis
c. Budd–Chiari syndrome

7. JEJUNO-ILEAL BYPASS

1. ALCOHOLIC LIVER DISEASE

There is a strong relationship between the national figures for consumption of alcohol and death from cirrhosis. Women are more susceptible to the effects of alcohol than men, and drinking more than 20 g a day is associated with an increased risk of cirrhosis. In men, over 80 g a day is associated with an increased risk which rises to 25× normal if more than 100 g a day is consumed. Probably steady alcohol consumption for about 10 years is required rather than bouts of drinking. Individual susceptibility is also important as some patients never develop cirrhosis however much they drink. Three types of liver disease are associated with alcohol.

Fatty infiltration does not cause jaundice and does not lead to cirrhosis. *Alcoholic hepatitis* is a clinical syndrome which occurs after a bout of heavy drinking with fever, jaundice and multiple spider naevi. The aspartate transaminase is only mildly elevated but the patient may be deeply jaundiced. The white count is often markedly increased and the prothrombin time may be very prolonged. Such patients have a significant mortality and may later develop cirrhosis, even if they stop drinking completely. Histological changes consist of an acute inflammatory reaction at the portal tract and necrosis of liver cells, often with multiple protein inclusions (Mallory's alcoholic hyaline). These histological changes are seen quite frequently in patients who drink excessive alcohol and are not always associated with the full clinical syndrome of alcoholic hepatitis. In *Zieve's syndrome* alcoholic hepatitis is associated with haemolytic anaemia and hyperlipidaemia in addition to jaundice.

Cirrhosis. Alcohol produces a micronodular cirrhosis and the prognosis is undoubtedly worse if the patient continues to drink. It has been suggested that autoimmune mechanisms, particularly in alcoholic hepatitis, may be important. A combination of alcohol abuse and hepatitis B infection is particularly likely to lead to the development of cirrhosis and strongly predisposes to primary hepatic carcinoma.

2.   INFECTIONS

The discovery of markers for hepatitis B and C has demonstrated that these are both important causes of cirrhosis.

Congenital syphilis may produce a pericellular fibrosis but true cirrhosis is uncommon as regeneration nodules do not usually develop.

Schistosomiasis classically produces periportal fibrosis (pipesteam fibrosis) leading to portal hypertension, but cirrhosis may also develop and is thought to be due to associated conditions, e.g. hepatitis B infection which is also very common in these patients.

3.   CHRONIC ACTIVE HEPATITIS

Chronic active hepatitis is a consequence of a variety of diseases. The commonest cause worldwide is chronic infection with the hepatitis B virus. A history of drug abuse, homosexuality or exposure to blood products is often elucidated in patients presenting with hepatitis B in the Western hemisphere. Autoimmune chronic active hepatitis (lupoid hepatitis) is an auto-immune disease of women characterized by the presence of circulating smooth muscle antibodies, antinuclear factor and high titres of immunoglobulins (IgG). Chronic active hepatitis may also be due to ingestion of drugs including oxyphenacitin, methyldopa, antituberculous agents or anticonvulsants. Very similar appearances may also be seen in patients presenting with Wilson's disease and the appearances may be indistinguishable from conditions as apparently distinct as primary sclerosing cholangitis.

Chronic active hepatitis presents with malaise, jaundice and eventually with hepatic decompensation. The spleen is frequently enlarged and patients with the autoimmune type commonly have associated arthralgia.

The diagnosis is made by demonstrating abnormal liver function tests, particularly hypertransaminasaemia, which must persist for at least 6 months. There may be evidence of chronic hepatitis B infection, circulating smooth muscle antibodies or antinuclear factor. Liver biopsy reveals an inflammatory infiltrate radiating from the portal tracts and broaching the limiting plates. Fibrosis is almost invariable and may encircle groups of hepatocytes resulting in the formation of rosettes. Frank cirrhosis may be present at the time of diagnosis.

4.   GENETIC DEFECTS

a.   Haemochromatosis

This is an autosomal recessive disease characterized by increased intestinal iron absorption. The disease is rare in premenopausal women and most patients also abuse alcohol which further increases iron intake. Slate-grey pigmentation develops because of melanin and iron deposition in the skin. Cirrhosis occurs; the liver is invariably enlarged and there is evidence of portal hypertension and hepatic decomposition. Iron deposition in the pancreas causes diabetes mellitus ('bronze diabetes'). Accumulation in other endocrine glands leads to testicular atrophy, gynaecomastia and loss of body hair; hypopituitarism can occur. The diagnosis is suggested by a high serum ferritin concentration and confirmed by liver biopsy. Primary hepatocellular carcinoma is a relatively common complication and cause of death.

b.   Wilson's disease

Wilson's disease is a recessively inherited disease of impaired copper metabolism. Copper accumulates in the liver causing cirrhosis and in the basal ganglia of the brain causing an extrapyramidal neurological syndrome. Patients usually present between the age of 5 and 25 years with either or both liver and neurological disease. The hepatic presentation may be insidious with jaundice and ascites. The liver is usually small and fibrosed. The presentation may alternatively be acute with fulminant hepatic failure and severe haemolytic anaemia.

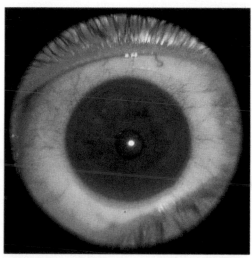

Fig. J.10. Kayser–Fleischer ring in a patient with Wilson's disease, due to deposition of copper-containing pigment in the cornea. (*Courtesy of Dr R. Guilloff.*)

The diagnosis is made by slit-lamp examination of the eyes when Kayser–Fleischer rings can be demonstrated (*Fig.* J.10). Urinary 24 hour copper excretion is increased and this increases further with penicillamine therapy. In addition serum copper concentrations are increased and caeruloplasmin levels are low. Liver biopsy shows cirrhosis. Copper stains are positive.

c. Other metabolic errors

All the other metabolic errors leading to cirrhosis and jaundice mentioned above are exceedingly rare. Of the glycogen storage disease, only type IV leads to cirrhosis and jaundice.

d. Alpha-1 antitrypsin deficiency

This autosomally recessively inherited disease may present as a severe neonatal hepatitis or as established cirrhosis in patients below the age of 20 years. There may be associated lung disease characteristically presenting as emphysema, pulmonary fibrosis and respiratory failure. Liver biopsy shows PAS-positive inclusion bodies within hepatocytes.

5. BILIARY DISEASE

Disease affecting the extrahepatic biliary tract, intrahepatic ductules or canaliculi can lead to cirrhosis. Extrahepatic biliary obstruction following trauma to the bile ducts can occasionally cause a secondary biliary cirrhosis; extrahepatic biliary obstruction is considered later. The most important causes of intrahepatic cholestasis are drugs and primary biliary cirrhosis.

Primary biliary cirrhosis predominantly affects middle-aged females and is due to destruction of bile ductules by a cell-mediated auto-immune process. The disease progresses extremely slowly in the majority of patients and usually presents with a cholestatic syndrome comprising itching, pale stools and dark urine. Hypercholesterolaemia is common and may lead to the development of xanthelasmas. The disease is associated with other auto-immune diseases including hypothyroidism, Addison's disease, systemic sclerosis, diabetes and renal tubular acidosis. Other patients present with bleeding oesophageal varices or ascites without a previous history of itching. Physical examination may reveal stigmata of chronic liver disease, jaundice, pigmentation and xanthelasmas. The liver is enlarged and firm; the spleen may be palpable and ascites develop because of portal hypertension.

Primary biliary cirrhosis should be considered in women presenting with cholestatic liver function tests. The mitochondrial antibody is positive in more than 98 per cent of patients. Serum IGM concentrations are increased. A liver biopsy shows chronic inflammatory infiltrate in the portal tract with destruction and paucity of bile ductules. Granulomas may be seen within portal tracts.

Sclerosing cholangitis

Secondary sclerosing cholangitis is a condition in which progressive fibrosis and narrowing of the intrahepatic and extrahepatic biliary tree occurs as a consequence of biliary sepsis. It follows bile duct injury. Primary sclerosing cholangitis is a disease strongly associated with ulcerative colitis. Many individuals are asymptomatic and merely have cholestatic liver function tests. Others present with fluctuating jaundice and in advanced disease this leads to secondary biliary cirrhosis. It is likely that the condition predisposes to the development of cholangiocarcinoma.

6. HEPATIC CONGESTION

True cirrhosis due to heart failure is very uncommon although jaundice may occur in association with heart failure

The Budd–Chiari syndrome

This syndrome is a rare condition in which the main hepatic veins are occluded. It is discussed in the chapter LIVER, ENLARGEMENT OF. The liver scan often shows a central area of uptake which is due to the enlargement of the caudate lobe of the liver whose veins drain separately into the inferior vena cava.

Chronic liver damage—infiltrations

AMYLOIDOSIS

The liver may be involved by infiltration with amyloid, both in the primary disease and where it is secondary to chronic suppuration, myelomatosis or rheumatoid arthritis. Amyloid is an antigen/antibody complex which stains metachromatically with crystal violet and shows birefringence with Congo red staining. The liver is enlarged and rubbery and the patient may show other features of amyloidosis such as nephrotic syndrome, cardiac failure and malabsorption. Hepatocellular failure, and hence jaundice, is rare in this condition, and the diagnosis may be made by liver or rectal biopsy.

Chronic liver damage—tumours

The liver may be affected both by benign and malignant tumours but only the latter will produce jaundice. Secondary deposits are 25 times more common than a primary malignant growth.

PRIMARY HEPATOCELLULAR CARCINOMA

Primary tumours of the liver are a frequent accompaniment of cirrhosis and are said to be found in between 50 and 60 per cent of postmortems in cirrhotic patients. Hepatocellular cancer is particularly common in certain parts of the world especially Africa and China where hepatitis B is the important aetiological agent. Aflatoxin, which is produced by a fungus growing on grain stored in humid conditions, and the now obsolete radiocontrast material Thorotrast (thorium dioxide), are often associated with the development of the tumour.

Primary hepatocellular carcinoma tumours may occur at any age, are five times more common in males than females and should be suspected in any patient with cirrhosis who deteriorates or who develops a lump in the liver. A friction sound is occasionally heard over the tumour and arterial murmurs may be present. The diagnosis is made by finding elevated alpha-feto protein concentrations, and by liver biopsy.

Primary sarcoma of the liver and malignant haemangiosarcoma

These are extremely rare tumours which may cause jaundice in their terminal stages. Malignant haemangiosarcoma is associated with exposure to Thorotrast and vinyl chloride.

SECONDARY TUMOURS

The liver is the most frequently site of blood-borne metastatic tumours, whether drained by systemic or portal veins. It is involved in about a third of all cancers, including half of those in the stomach, large bowel, breast and lung. The liver may be normal in size or grossly enlarged with palpable hard deposits. Jaundice may be absent and is usually mild. The serum alkaline phosphatase is often markedly raised.

Reticuloendothelial diseases in the liver

The reticuloendothelial cells of the liver may be involved by any malignant process involving this system. Jaundice is usually mild, and may occasionally be due to haemolysis.

Intrahepatic cholestasis

Drugs
Viral hepatitis
Cirrhosis (occasionally)
Dubin–Johnson syndrome
Pregnancy
Sclerosing cholangitis
Biliary atresia
Recurrent idiopathic cholestasis

In this group of conditions the patient presents with an obstructive jaundice, usually with pale stools, dark urine and itching, but investigations reveal no obstruction of the extrahepatic bile ducts.

DUBIN–JOHNSON AND ROTOR SYNDROMES

These are rare familial benign intermittent conditions producing jaundice with conjugated hyperbilirubinaemia. In the Dubin–Johnson type the liver is greenish black and contains brown pigment. Jaundice is rarely deep and the alkaline phosphatase remains normal. The diagnosis may be made by a bromsulphthalein retention test in which, after an initial fall, the serum level of BSP rises after 2 hours and remains detectable

for 48 hours. The condition is thought to be due to poor transport of conjugated bilirubin into the biliary canaliculi. The Rotor syndrome resembles Dubin–Johnson clinically and biochemically, the main difference being the absence of brown pigment in the liver.

PREGNANCY

Some women develop intrahepatic cholestasis in the last trimester of pregnancy associated with itching, pale stools or dark urine. The mechanism seems similar to that of oral contraceptive-induced cholestasis (*see* later).

Extrahepatic biliary obstruction

Extrahepatic biliary obstruction can be classified as being due to diseases within the lumen of the bile ducts, those affecting the wall of the ducts or diseases compressing the duct from outside (*Table* J.6).

Table J.6. Causes of obstruction to the bile ducts

Causes within the lumen of the bile ducts
Gallstones
Parasites

Causes affecting the wall of the ducts
Accidental division
Acute pancreatitis
Chronic pancreatitis
Carcinoma of the bile duct
Congenital obliteration of the bile duct

Causes compressing the bile duct or invading it from the outside
Tumours of the pancreas
Peritoneal adhesions
Enlarged portal lymph nodes
Aneurysm of the hepatic artery
Hydatid cysts
Retroperitoneal cysts
Duodenal diverticulum

Obstruction is usually followed by dilatation of the common bile duct although this may take some time to develop. The architecture of the liver is usually normal although biopsies show pigmentation, bile plugs and infarcts. Cirrhosis can rarely develop in extremely long-standing obstruction. The patient is clinically jaundiced and the degree of jaundice may be very deep resulting in a greenish tinge. The urine is dark because of an excess of bilirubin. The stools are pale, clay coloured and bulky because of increased fat content. Biochemical investigations reveal a raised serum alkaline phosphatase concentration, prolonged prothrombin time because of vitamin K malabsorption, hypocalcaemia because of vitamin D malabsorption. The serum albumin concentration is usually maintained until late stages.

The investigation of obstructive jaundice has already been alluded to. The steps involved are ultra-

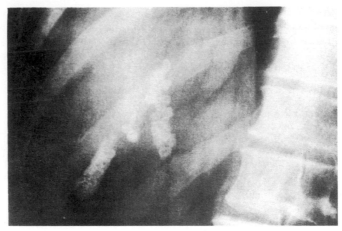

Fig. J.11. Multiple gallstones situated in the gallbladder and common bile duct. Patient presented with painless obstructive jaundice without any preceding history.

sound followed by either endoscopic, percutaneous cholangiography or liver biopsy.

Causes due to obstruction of the bile duct lumen

A. GALLSTONES

This is the commonest cause of extrahepatic biliary obstruction in the UK. The gallstones are mixed and usually originate from the gallbladder although it is likely that primary bile duct stones may also occur.

The patient presenting with choledocholithiasis and obstructive jaundice may or may not have had a previous cholecystectomy. Severe right upper quadrant pain radiating through to the back usually occurs. Fever associated with rigors is common. The jaundice fluctuates and may disappear completely, presumably because the calculus either passes into the duodenum, or disimpacts from the ampulla, and returns into the lumen of the duct. Another important consequence is gallstone pancreatitis. Occasional patients (usually elderly) present with painless progressive jaundice simulating a carcinoma of the pancreas. Some patients with bile duct calculi have no symptoms and present incidentally with abnormal liver function tests. Examination usually reveals mild jaundice. There may be tenderness of the liver and pyrexia. The gallbladder is usually impalpable.

Investigations reveal cholestatic liver function tests and leucocytosis. Calcified gallstones may be seen on plain abdominal X-ray in 20 per cent of patients with cholelithiasis (*Fig.* J.11). An ultrasound examination may or may not reveal a dilated biliary tree. Stones may be seen within the bile duct although they are often overlooked. Calculi may be identified within the gallbladder although this is uncommon in patients whose jaundice is not caused by choledocholithiasis.

Percutaneous transhepatic cholangiography (*Fig.* J.12.) and ERCP reveal filling defects within the common bile duct. Gallstones may also be demonstrated by computed tomography (*Fig.* J.13).

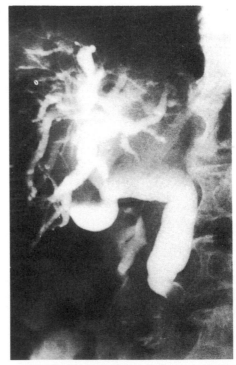

Fig. J.12. Percutaneous transhepatic cholangiogram (PTC) The bile ducts are dilated and the filling defect caused by a stone can be seen at the lower end of the common bile duct.

B. PARASITES

The most important of these is the worm *Ascaris lumbracoides* which is released from an ovum in the duodenum and migrates into the intestinal wall and

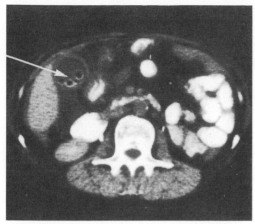

Fig. J.13. Occasionally gallstones may be demonstrated in the course of investigations for other conditions, as in this patient those CT scan clearly shows the presence of three gallstones situated within the gallbladder.

hence the portal circulation. Worms enter the liver, heart and lungs, migrate in the pharynx and are swallowed. Patients present with haemoptysis, bronchitis and pneumonia; occasionally a worm blocks the bile duct to cause jaundice or act as a nidus for the development of a calculus. Roundworm jaundice is a common cause of icterus in African children.

Causes affecting the wall of the bile duct

A. BILE DUCT TRAUMA

This is usually a consequence of division at operation and is more likely to occur if the surgeon is inexperienced, in patients who have had previous biliary operations or who have an inflammatory mass around the bile duct.

B. CHOLANGIOCARCINOMA

These are epithelial tumours of the bile duct and arise at any point within the biliary tree. Patients present with painless obstructive jaundice and it may be impossible to differentiate the lesion either clinically or by investigation from tumours of the pancreas. One important variant is a tumour arising at the bifurcation of the main left and right hepatic duct (Klatskin tumour). This is an extremely hard, fibrous, but slowly growing tumour and carries a better prognosis than tumours arising elsewhere in the biliary tree.

C. CARCINOMA OF THE AMPULLA

Tumours arising from the ampulla are uncommon and present with painless obstructive jaundice. They are more slowly growing than carcinoma of the pancreas and should be considered for Whipple's operation.

D. BILIARY ATRESIA

This presents as deepening obstructive jaundice within 2–3 days of birth. Liver failure develops by the age of 3–6 months. The diagnosis is made by HIDA scanning followed by cholangiography.

E. SCLEROSING CHOLANGITIS

Causes compressing the bile duct from outside

A. CARCINOMA OF THE PANCREAS

The most important cause is carcinoma of the pancreas which invades the common bile duct as it passes through the head of the gland. The patient presents with painless obstructive jaundice although others complain of progressive and continuous pain in the back due to invasion of the coeliac plexus and other retroperitoneal structures. Jaundice is progressive and associated with weight loss. Rigors are unusual.

Examination reveals cachexia, deep jaundice, hepatomegaly and a palpable gallbladder (*Fig.* J.14). There may be evidence of metastatic spread; in particular there may be supraclavicular lymphadenopathy or tumour nodules in the umbilicus (Sister Joseph's nodule).

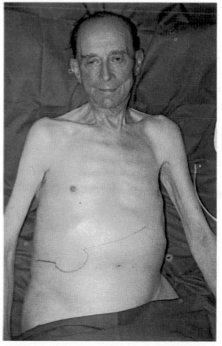

Fig. J.14. Jaundiced patient with enlarged gallbladder. Jaundice due to carcinoma of the pancreas.

Most tumours arise from ductular epithelium and carry a very poor prognosis. It is important however to remember that some tumours are more amenable to therapy; these include cystadenocarcinoma, a tumour of relatively young women, and apudomas.

Ultrasonography reveals dilated intrahepatic and extrahepatic bile ducts. It may also show a mass within the pancreatic head. Endoscopy may demonstrate invasion of the duodenum by tumour and the diagnosis can then be confirmed by biopsy. ERCP reveals a stricture within the lead of the pancreas corresponding to a low bile duct malignant stenosis (*Fig.* J.15.)

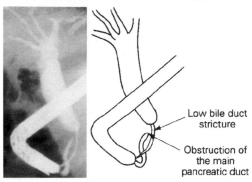

Low bile duct stricture

Obstruction of the main pancreatic duct

Fig. J.15. ERCP showing typical appearances of obstructive jaundice due to pancreatic carcinoma. A stricture in the head of the pancreas is associated with a corresponding stricture in the lower common bile duct.

Malignant obstruction of the extrahepatic bile duct may also be due to enlarged lymph nodes in the region of the porta hepatis and this is usually encountered in patients with breast carcinoma or secondary carcinoma from gastrointestinal origin. Occasionally true secondary deposits occur within the bile duct usually from melanoma or carcinoma of the breast.

B. MIRIZZI'S SYNDROME

This is a rare entity in which a stone impacts in Hartmann's pouch. It causes compression and obstruction of the common hepatic duct.

C. ANEURYSM OF THE HEPATIC ARTERY

This is a rare cause of obstructive jaundice diagnosed by arteriography.

D. CYSTS

Hydatid cyst is a rare cause of obstruction jaundice; far more commonly these are found incidentally by plain X-ray. Simple cysts or choledochal cysts may also cause obstructive jaundice.

K. R. Palmer

Jaw, deformity of

The jaws may become deformed by congenital or acquired disease and many of the latter are discussed under the heading JAW, SWELLING OF. The reader should

refer to this section for details of pathological conditions causing jaw deformity. Trauma to the jaws may cause deformity due to displacement and this will be maintained if inadequate treatment results in non-union or malunion of the fracture. The majority of conditions, however, to be considered here are of a developmental nature occurring before birth or during the growth period.

CONGENITAL

Cleft palate
Pierre Robin's syndrome
First arch syndrome
Treacher–Collins syndrome

ACQUIRED

Premature synostoses
Achondroplasia
Diseases of the temporomandibular joint
Acromegaly

Growth of the facial skeleton takes place by sutural growth, surface deposition and remodelling, and cartilagenous growth with secondary ossification. The main stimulus for growth of the maxilla is the growth of the brain, causing an increase in size of the cranial vault and the cranial base to which the maxilla is joined. The cranial base also increases in length by cartilagenous growth at the spheno-occipital synchrondrosis. Growth within the maxilla is stimulated by the development of the nasal capsule and the eyes.

The mandible forms *in utero* around a rod of cartilage known as Meckel's cartilage, which is replaced by the bone of the mandible, leaving only the condylar cartilage at the temporomandibular joint. Subsequent elongation of the mandible occurs by the growth of this cartilage with secondary ossification and development is completed by surface deposition and resorption.

There is an inherent genetic potential for growth of the facial skeleton, but this is aided by the eruption of the dentition and by the muscular forces placed upon it by the muscles of mastication. A defect in one or more of these mechanisms of growth will produce jaw deformity. However, the majority of cases of jaw deformity arise from a simple imbalance between the growth of the maxilla and the mandible to produce a dental malocclusion (*Fig.* J.16).

Congenital jaw deformity

CLEFT PALATE

Cleft palate occurs in approximately one in every two thousand live births and is due to a failure of growth and fusion of the palatal shelves in the embryo. Females are affected more than males and there may be an

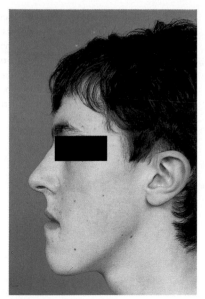

Fig. J.16. Patient exhibiting growth imbalance of the maxilla and mandible.

associated cleft of the lip (*Fig.* J.17). There is a genetic disposition to this deformity, but other exogenous factors have been implicated, such as drugs, e.g. phenytoin, or folic acid deficiency. Five per cent of cases of cleft lip and palate are associated with other congenital abnormalities.

palatal shelves. The syndrome is, therefore, characterized by a small mandible, cleft palate and protruding tongue. The baby may present with feeding and respiratory problems, which can be corrected by the construction of a small dental plate and nursing in the supine position.

FIRST ARCH SYNDROME

This syndrome characteristically exhibits a deformed or absent ear, macrostomia and an underdevelopment of the mandibular ramus and condyle. The masticatory muscles on that side are also deficient and there is hypoplasia of the orbit and zygoma on the ipsilateral side (*Fig.* J.18). Other associated abnormalities may be present, particularly of the vertebrae. According to Poswillo, haemorrhage of the stapedial artery in the region of the otic ganglion during uterine development is proposed as the cause.

TREACHER–COLLINS SYNDROME

This is an inherited autosomal dominant condition affecting the facial skeleton in a similar way to the first arch syndrome, but the abnormalities are bilateral and symmetrical. Due to the poor development of the zygomatic arches, prominent nose and small jaw, many of the patients have a fish-like appearance.

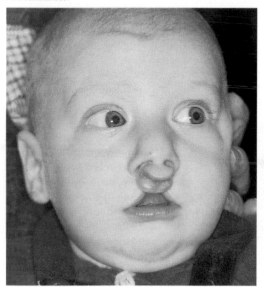
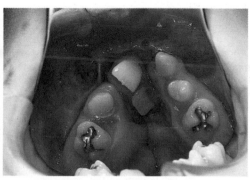

a *b*

Fig. J.17. a, b, Bilateral cleft lip and palate with rotation of the premaxilla.

PIERRE ROBIN'S SYNDROME

This syndrome is thought to be caused by hypoplasia of the mandible, preventing the normal descent of the tongue and thus preventing the fusion of the embryonic

Acquired jaw deformity

PREMATURE SYNOSTOSIS

Premature fusion of the cranial sutures are a feature of Cruzon's and Apert's syndrome, producing deformi-

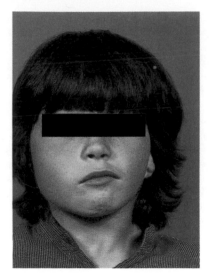

Fig. J.18. Patient with the first arch syndrome.

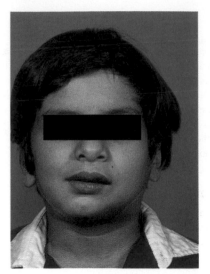

Fig J.19. Facial deformity due to ankylosis of the right temporomandibular joint.

ties of the cranial vault. Because of an associated lack of growth of the cranial base, patients also exhibit extreme underdevelopment of the mid-third of the face.

ACHONDROPLASIA

This rare condition usually represents a sporadic mutation; less than 20 per cent will be of a familial nature. The aetiology is not completely understood, but there is a defect of endochondrial ossification. Failure of growth at the spheno-occipital synchondrosis and lack of growth in the maxilla produces the characteristic underdevelopment of the mid-third of the face. Curiously, growth of the mandible is unaffected, leading to relative mandibular prognathism.

DISORDERS OF THE
TEMPOROMANDIBULAR JOINT

The mandibular condyle may be affected by trauma, infection from the middle ear or juvenile arthritis, all of which will damage the condylar growth centre. The result is under-development of one side of the mandible with compensatory growth on the contralateral side. This produces a facial asymmetry and underdevelopment of the ipsilateral side of the face in the vertical plane. Fractures of the temporomandibular joint may, on occasions, be followed by ankylosis and this, too, will prevent normal development of the affected side of the face (*Fig*. J.19). Treatment of all these conditions is by surgical correction.

In some patients there may be excessive growth of the condyle known as condylar hyperplasia, resulting in asymmetry of the facial skeleton with, overgrowth of the affected site. Asymmetry may also be caused by hemifacial hypertrophy or hemifacial atrophy. In the latter case there is slow progressive atrophy of the soft tissues of one side of the face with secondary deformity of the facial skeleton. Patients may also exhibit contralateral Jacksonian epilepsy and trigeminal neuralgia. This condition is thought to be due to an abnormality of the sympathetic system and is often associated with scleroderma.

ACROMEGALY

Acromegaly follows autonomous hypersecretion of growth hormone caused by hyperplasia or an adenoma of the pituitary acidophil cells. The face is invariably affected by this condition with overgrowth of the mandible to produce prognathism with malocclusion, enlargement of the tongue and deposition of bone at the supraorbital ridges and zygomas.

The facial skin also becomes thickened, as does the subcutaneous tissue, producing an accentuation of the normal skin folds. The nose becomes enlarged, especially at the tip, as do the lips. Treatment should be of the underlying pituitary problem and corrective jaw surgery should only be undertaken following stabilization of the condition. Many of these patients have cardiomyopathy and there may be serious complications during anaesthesia.

P. T. Blenkinsopp

Jaw, pain in

Pain in the jaw mostly arises from the dental structures and their supporting bone, the temporomandibular joint and the associated muscles of mastication. In the upper jaw, infections of the nose and paranasal sinuses may additionally cause pain in the maxilla. Disorders of the trigeminal nerve are a relatively rare cause of facial pain, but atypical facial pain which is part of a psychological illness (usually depression) is quite common.

Dental pain

Inflammation in the pulp chamber of a tooth caused by dental caries, inadequately insulated restorations or occlusal trauma characteristically causes pain with thermal stimulation or pressure. This then progresses to an ache which lasts for increasing periods of time or may be worse at night when the patient lies down.

As the inflammation progresses, the pain becomes very severe and constant until such time as remedial therapy is carried out, or gangrene of the pulp occurs. At this stage, the pain diminishes but is replaced by an ache within the alveolar bone should a dental alveolar abscess develop (*Fig.* J.20).

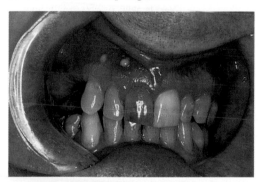

Fig. J.20. Upper right central incisor with gangrene of the dental pulp and pus discharging through the alveolar bone.

With increasing infection, the visible signs of inflammation become apparent and a swelling develops in the mucous membrane or associated soft tissues (*see* JAW, SWELLING OF). At any stage this pain may be worsened by occlusal trauma to the tooth during mastication or when the teeth are percussed. The pain associated with a periodontal abscess or pericoronal infection is similar to the pain associated with an alveolar abscess; that is, the pain is moderate to severe and throbbing in nature.

Any of the conditions developing within the jaw, e.g. dental cysts, ameloblastoma, etc. (*see* JAW, SWELLING OF) may become infected and again the pain is similar to abscess formation of dental origin. The diagnosis is usually readily apparent following a careful recording of the history followed by clinical and radiographical examination. Should the abscess formation involve the masticatory muscles, then trismus will also be present as well as signs of acute infection.

Acute post-extraction osteitis

This pain commences 2–3 days after the extraction of a tooth and is due to bacterial infection of the bone lining the tooth socket, should the normal healing blood clot break down. The pain is severe, dull, throbbing or gnawing in character. It is usually associated with a bad taste in the mouth and examination will demonstrate an empty tooth socket (dry socket) in which food has collected. Treatment is by local cleansing of the socket and installation of local antiseptic agents. Antibiotics are not normally required.

Acute maxillary sinusitis

Pain arising in the acutely infected maxillary sinus may be confused with pain of dental origin as the tooth roots of the upper teeth have a very close relationship to this structure. Maxillary sinusitis normally follows an upper respiratory tract infection, especially if the normal drainage of the antrum through the ostium is reduced, for example, by a deviated nasal septum. However, maxillary sinusitis can arise from dental infection should the abscess present in the maxillary antrum rather than in the oral cavity. Infection of the maxillary sinus may also follow the creation of an oro-antral fistula after dental extraction.

In maxillary sinusitis, the patient suffers from a throbbing pain in the cheek with radiation towards the eye, but there is never any swelling of the face. The teeth may be tender to percussion and the pain is aggravated by bending forward or lying down. Intranasal examination may demonstrate a mucopurulent discharge through the normal ostium. A reduction in translucency of one maxillary sinus compared with the other suggests that it contains fluid and this will be easily confirmed on an occipitomental X-ray (*Fig.* J.21).

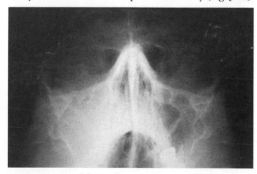

Fig. J.21. Acute left maxillary sinusitis.

A neoplastic process of the maxillary antrum should be considered if the pain does not respond to normal measures or if there is swelling of the face or oral cavity associated with bone destruction and displacement of the teeth. A tumour of the maxillary antrum may also cause epistaxis and sensory loss in the maxillary division of the trigeminal nerve. If this is suspected then a biopsy should be obtained either by antral puncture through the nose or via a Caldwell–Luc approach.

Temporomandibular joint

The temporomandibular joint may be affected by any of the conditions which afflict the other joints, e.g. rheumatoid arthritis, osteoarthritis and septic arthritis; in which case pain and swelling are exhibited in the preauricular region, in the acute phase, with limitation of jaw movements. An acute effusion, as a result of a blow to the jaw or a fracture involving the joint, may arise in the temporomandibular joint, also causing pain and swelling anterior to the ear.

However, the most common form of pain arising in the temporomandibular joint is associated with the temporomandibular joint pain dysfunction syndrome. This is an extremely common and much written about subject without there being a clear cut understanding of the mechanisms involved. The symptomatology is, however, well recorded and consists of pain arising in the region of the temporomandibular joint or ear which may be associated with a 'clicking' noise, and, is aggravated by wide opening of the mouth, as with yawning and chewing hard foods.

When masticatory muscle spasm is also present, which is common in this condition, the patient may have some limitation of jaw opening and complain of facial pain. This radiates across the face from the ear to the region of the eye, or down into the lower jaw on both lateral and medial aspects. Curiously, many patients also state that the face becomes swollen, which is probably a reflection of the shortening of the masseter muscle due to spasm. The alleged mechanisms are many, with minor trauma and associated stretching of the ligaments and displacement of the articular cartilage being currently accepted. However, severe dental malocclusion may be a factor and, without doubt, stress is a very important aetiological cause in many people. Patients under stress would appear to clench their teeth, bite their nails or, grind their teeth at night, all of which induces masticatory muscle spasm, ischaemia, and hence pain.

Primary neuralgias

Primary neuralgias may be defined as the disturbed function of a nerve without there being any recognized aetiological factor or pathological process acting at some point along the nerve pathway or its central connections. In the jaws the trigeminal nerve is affected and very occasionally the glossopharyngeal nerve. There is no associated signs and the diagnosis is made from the history.

The pain characteristically affects almost always only one branch of the trigeminal nerve initially, although later on in the disease it may spread to affect two or occasionally three divisions. The disease most commonly affects patients over 50 years old, and the incidence is twice as common in women as in men.

The pain is very severe. It is described as sharp, or similar to an electric shock. It is paroxysmal in nature, lasting only a few seconds with intervals of a few minutes or a few hours. The pain may be felt spontaneously or in response to stimulation within a trigger area on the face. This trigger area may be activated by a cold wind, shaving, washing, eating or cleaning the teeth. Natural remission is fairly common.

The main differential diagnosis is between causes of dental pain and these should be excluded before a diagnosis of trigeminal neuralgia is made. Treatment is with the specific drug carbamazepine but, as it occasionally causes agranulocytosis, regular monitoring of the white blood cell count is essential. Should medical treatment fail then a surgical approach should be considered. In every case, careful examination of the central nervous system should be made to exclude a neoplasm or, in the younger age group, the onset of multiple sclerosis, which can mimic trigeminal neuralgia in the early stages of the disease.

Secondary neuralgias

Here an identifiable pathological process is acting at some point along the trigeminal nerve or its central connections, producing pain at the periphery. The symptoms may be similar to trigeminal neuralgia or may be a duller more continuous pain. Neoplasms are the most significant cause, other examples being aneurysms or compression of the nerve in the bony canal in Paget's disease.

Exact testing of the function of the cranial nerves is essential followed by a full clinical and radiographical examination, including CT scans to establish the diagnosis.

Post-herpetic neuralgia

Involvement of one of the branches of the trigeminal nerve with the virus herpes zoster will produce pain and vesiculation in the anatomical distribution of that nerve. Once this attack has resolved, scarring of the involved nerve may leave the patient with post-herpetic neuralgia and possibly sensory disturbance. This pain can be severe and very resistent to treatment.

Migraine

Migraine and migrainous neuralgia may occasionally involve the maxilla, although the predominant features are manifested as headache. The diagnosis is normally made from the history when an intense pain is associated with visual disturbance, nausea and constitutional symptoms. In migrainous neuralgia, the pain is predominantly behind the eye and patients may also experience pain in the maxilla and temple regions. There may be watering of the eye and flushing of the facial skin (*see* pp. 42, 277).

Referred pain

The only important example of referred pain to the jaws is that of coronary artery insufficiency which may produce pain in the left side of the mandible.

Atypical facial pain

Large numbers of patients present with atypical facial pain which is symptomatic of a psychological illness. The pain is described as being very severe, but it does not produce any restriction upon the normal function of the jaws and oral cavity. It does not have an anatomical distribution, commonly involves both sides of the face and jaws and moves from one part of the facial skeleton to another. It does not respond to analgesics and usually there are many other associated symptoms such as a dry mouth, burning tongue, and other complaints throughout the body.

There can be some overlap between this condition, and temporomandibular joint dysfunction caused by stress but, in every case, it is essential to exclude pain due to any one of the other causes just described. Therefore, atypical facial pain is often a diagnosis of exclusion and once made, any underlying depression should be treated by medication or referral for psychiatric help. (*See also* FACIAL PAIN, p. 203.)

P. T. Blenkinsopp

Jaw, swelling of

Swellings of the jaw, once they have reached a certain size, will be obvious as a facial swelling or swelling in the submandibular region. The true nature will, however, only be ascertained by an intraoral examination and in many cases the taking of radiographs will also be required. Smaller swellings may only be visible on examination of the oral cavity or will have been discovered by the patient during normal oral function. Testing of the trigeminal cranial nerve should always be carried out as a change in sensation may have very significant consequences. Swellings of the jaws can, to the inexperienced clinician, be incorrectly diagnosed as swellings of the submandibular salivary gland, submandibular lymph nodes or swellings of the parotid gland.

Infection associated with the dental structures

Bacterial infection associated with the dental structures is by far the most common cause of swellings of the jaw. An alveolar abscess arises when gangrene of the dental pulp occurs following dental caries, extensive dental restorations or trauma (*Fig.* J.22). This infection then spreads to the alveolar bone to cause a localized osteitis but remarkably, in the majority of cases, does not cause osteomyelitis. Instead, the abscess as it enlarges becomes localized and perforates either the lateral or medial plate of the outer compact alveolar bone. It is at this stage that it presents as a swelling of the jaw which is tender and covered by inflamed mucosa. Occasionally an alveolar abscess is associated with sensory loss of the mandibular branch of the trigeminal nerve.

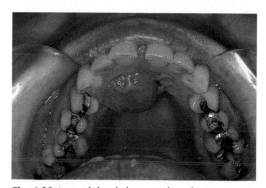

Fig. J.22. Intraoral dental abscess in the palate.

A periodontal abscess arises from bacterial infection within the periodontal membrane of the tooth, which is usually associated with previous chronic periodontal disease. A pericoronal abscess arises in the mucous membrane surrounding the crown of an erupting or impacted tooth; the majority being associated with wisdom teeth.

At this stage the swelling is largely confined to the region of the jaws and may discharge intraorally. However, should the bacteria gain access to the adjacent soft-tissue compartments, then facial cellulitis or soft-tissue abscess formation will follow. Depending upon the anatomical position of the infection, the submandibular area may become swollen, or the cheek (buccal space) or more posteriorly the submasseteric space, which may be misdiagnosed as a parotid swelling (*Fig.* J.23).

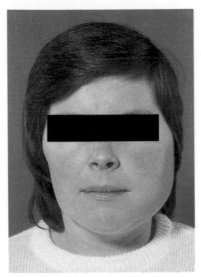

Fig. J.23. Facial swelling due to infection from an impacted wisdom tooth.

On the medial aspect of the jaw, swelling in the sublingual space may occur or more posteriorly in the pterygoid, lateral pharyngeal or peritonsillar space. Diagnosis of these latter space infections may be difficult and, if beneath a muscle compartment, are associated with severe trismus.

These medial swellings are potentially very serious as respiratory obstruction may follow unless the neck is decompressed in severe cases. Ludwig's angina is an acute emergency in which both sublingual and submandibular spaces are involved in acute infection. Again urgent surgical decompression of the neck is required to prevent respiratory obstruction.

Persistent recurrent infection causing chronic swelling and discharge may be due to an opportunistic infection with actinomycosis.

Osteomyelitis

True osteomyelitis of the jaws is now relatively rare following the improvement in general dental health and the use of antibiotics. However, when established, severe pain with loosening of the adjacent teeth is encountered and usually there is sensory loss of the mandibular branch of the trigeminal nerve. The overlying mucosa becomes swollen and hyperaemic and, indeed, sinuses may develop through which there is a discharge of pus and bony sequestra. In the acute phase, it is invariably associated with significant soft-tissue swelling. The radiographic changes take some time to develop, but show diffuse rarefaction and sequestrum formation. Subperiosteal woven bone may also be a feature and the infected bone may be subjected to a pathological fracture.

Management of all these infections is by antibi-

otics and drainage in the acute phase and then appropriate treatment of the causative dental structure, which may require extraction.

Trauma

Fractures of the mandible are relatively common and are associated with swelling caused by haematoma formation from the bleeding marrow space and periosteum. The swelling may be made worse by a protruding bone fragment or the presence of a foreign body. The injury may not be sufficient to cause a fracture but may nevertheless produce a haematoma in the soft tissue. This normally resolves without treatment but, occasionally, requires aspiration. The diagnosis of a fracture is normally easy to make from the history, the abnormal mobility of the fragments and the irregularity of the dental arches. In many fractures, a laceration of the oral mucosa is also present. The diagnosis is confirmed by radiographic examination.

Swellings associated with benign dental pathology

Unerupted teeth are a frequent cause of jaw swelling which, commonly, are the canine and premolar teeth in the palate and the premolars in the lower jaw. In the elderly, when the molar teeth have been lost, an erupting wisdom tooth may produce a swelling in the posterior area of the alveolus.

The follicle of unerupted teeth may undergo dentigerous cyst formation, which is an epithelial-lined sac embracing the crown of the tooth (*Fig.* J.24). This slowly enlarges and may cause displacement of the involved tooth or the adjacent teeth. As the expansion continues the alveolus enlarges and, just before perforation, exhibits the phenomenon of 'eggshell crackling'. Once perforated, the swelling is naturally fluctuant. The cyst may slowly enlarge or, should it become infected, acute swelling with inflammation occurs. Other cysts which have a similar clinical presentation are dental cysts, residual dental cysts and keratocysts. Keratocysts, however, tend to be multilocular and have a distinct tendency to recur after removal.

Odontomes, which are developmental abnormali-

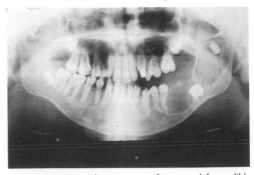

Fig. J.24. Extensive dentigerous cyst formation, left mandible.

ties of the dental lamina, may give rise to a swelling of the jaw and the diagnosis is confirmed by X-ray. Osteomas of the jaw present as hard, round, bony swellings which may be endosteal (central) or subperiosteal (peripheral). Multiple osteomas of the facial bones are found in Gardner's syndrome, the other main feature being polyps of the large intestine which have a tendency to become malignant. Radiologically osteomas may be composed of dense radio-opaque bone or may have a high cancellous component, in which case they are relatively radiolucent. Torus palatinus is a developmental abnormality of the midline of the hard palate characterized by a cylindrical enlargement in the region of the midline palatal suture (*Fig.* J.25). Torus mandibularis is a similar slowly enlarging developmental abnormality but it arises on the lingual aspect of the mandible in the premolar region. All these osteomas are simply removed if they prove troublesome as a result of trauma to the overlying mucosa.

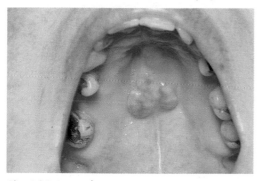

Fig. J.25. Torus palatinus.

Fibrous dysplasia

This condition of bone of unknown origin is characterized by replacement with fibrous tissue and enlargement in all three dimensions. At this stage the abnormal bone is very vascular but subsequently ossification occurs to produce an amorphous radio-opaque appearance on the radiograph. The process tends to cease at skeletal maturity. The jaws are frequently affected in monostotic fibrous dysplasia and may also be involved in polyostotic fibrous dysplasia and Albright's syndrome.

Ossifying fibroma

This is a benign fibro-osseous lesion which causes a well-circumscribed mass of fibrous tissue showing areas of speckled calcification. It normally arises within the substance of the bone and slowly expands in all directions to produce a sclerotic margin. With time, the lesion becomes more calcified and can cause loosening of the adjacent teeth. Treatment is by surgical excision.

Cementifying fibroma

This condition is similar in some ways to ossifying fibroma in that an area of bone is replaced by fibrous tissue, but subsequent calcification resembles dental cementum. Periapical cemental dysplasia is similar to cementifying fibroma but produces multiple sites of ossification with cementum. The diagnosis is usually easy to make from the radiographic appearances but may, in some patients, produce a bony hard irregularity of the dental alveolus.

Cherubism (familial fibrous dysplasia)

Symmetrical enlargement of the facial skeleton occurs in this inherited condition, which is usually apparent in early life and then arrests at puberty. Radiographs show symmetrical multilocular radiolucent areas of the jaws and, histologically, the bone is replaced by fibrous tissue with multinucleated giant cells as a predominant feature. The giant cells, in some cases, make the differential diagnosis difficult from giant-cell granuloma or hyperparathyroidism, the blood chemistry is, however, usually normal.

Paget's disease

This disease of bone of unknown aetiology found in patients in middle to late life may affect the mandible but, more commonly, the maxilla. According to some studies, approximately 15 per cent of cases show involvement of the facial skeleton. Enlargement of the facial bones may produce the characteristic 'leonine facies' and, intraorally, expansion of the dental alveolus occurs with displacement of the teeth. Pain may occur due to entrapment of the trigeminal nerve and the radiograph shows the typical areas of patchy sclerosis. Extraction of the teeth can be difficult due to hypercementosis and postextraction bleeding may be severe. In the active phase of the disease, the serum alkaline phosphatase is raised, which will aid the diagnosis of the condition. Sarcomatous change in longstanding Paget's disease occurs but is relatively rare.

Epulis

This term denotes a swelling arising from the gum of which the majority are either pyogenic granulomas, fibroepithelial polyps or peripheral giant-cell granulomas. They may be sessile or pedunculated in shape and covered by pink or red mucosa (*Fig.* J.26). Histologically they exhibit a core of granulation or fibrous tissue covered by epithelium.

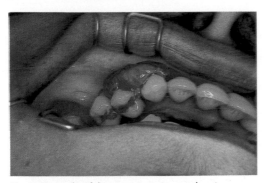

Fig. J.26. Epulis of the gum (pyogenic granuloma).

The pyogenic granuloma and fibroepithelial polyp represent an exaggerated soft-tissue response to minor trauma and are treated by simple excision and curettage. Pyogenic granulomas are common in pregnancy (*see* GUMS, BLEEDING).

Denture granulomas are histologically similar to the fibroepithelial polyp but arise from low-grade persistent denture trauma. Pseudofolds of mucous membrane with a fibrous tissue stroma are formed in the region of a traumatic denture flange. Treatment is again by excision, with attention to the prosthesis.

Papilloma

This benign tumour of epithelium is uncommon in the mouth and, when present, is usually found towards the back of the mouth in the soft palate or on the pillar of fauces. It is predunculated with an irregular surface of pale filiform projections. The lesion should be excised with its base.

Giant-cell granuloma

The aetiology of this lesion is again unknown. It arises in the young age group and is confined to the tooth-bearing areas of the jaws, with the mandible as the most frequent location. Radiographs show a radiolucent area, and histologically, the tissue is vascular fibrous tissue with multinucleated giant cells. The lesion can grow rapidly. The central giant-cell granuloma develops within the jaw, later perforating the alveolar bone to present in the mouth as a spherical purple swelling. Confusion can arise with the brown tumour of hyperparathyroidism but here the occurrence in the older age group with raised serum calcium and parathormone levels would indicate the diagnosis. Additionally, radiographs in hyperparathyroidism show multiple osteolytic lesions, osteitis fibrosa-cystica, on skeletal survey. The peripheral giant-cell granuloma is similar in every respect to the central, except that it arises from the gingival margin as a localized fleshy mass which bleeds easily. The treatment of both types is by surgical excision.

Ameloblastoma

Ameloblastoma is a tumour peculiar to the jaws and is a locally invasive neoplasm of odontogenic epithelium. Unless infection supervenes the tumour is quite painless as it slowly enlarges. In underdeveloped countries they may reach enormous proportions before assistance is sought. Radiographs usually show a multilocular radiolucency but, occasionally, unilocular variants may present. Spacing of the teeth may occur but sensory disturbance of the trigeminal nerve is not usually a feature. Treatment is by resection with a margin of healthy bone.

Eosinophilic granuloma

The solitary eosinophilic granuloma produces an area of bone loss in the jaw and there is an associated soft-tissue swelling with gingival ulceration. The condition may first come to be noticed because of loosening of the teeth, the failure of a tooth extraction site to heal or a pathological fracture. The jaws may also be affected by multifocal eosinophilic granuloma where, with loosening of the teeth, there is also generalized inflammation of the oral cavity and gingival enlargement.

Myxoma

Another benign tumour to affect the jaws and cause expansion is the myxoma, which is a rare benign neoplasm arising from odontogenic mesenchyme. It produces a multilocular radiolucent appearance with multiple criss-crossing septi in the defect.

Haemangioma

The endosteal haemangioma is more common in the mandible than the maxilla and, if truly endosteal, presents as a hard, non-tender, painless swelling. Haemorrhage may occur around the necks of the teeth, which may become loosened and severe haemorrhage follows dental extraction.

Minor salivary glands

The minor salivary glands are distributed widely throughout the oral mucosa but are found in abundance at the junction of the hard and soft palate. The important benign causes of enlargement are mucous extravasation cyst and pleomorphic adenoma (*Fig.* J.27).

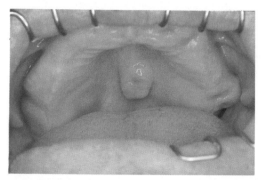

Fig. J.27. Pleomorphic adenoma arising from a minor salivary gland in the palate.

Malignant tumours

Sarcomas of the jaw are rare, with the mandible being affected more often than the maxilla. The tumour presents as a rapidly enlarging swelling with drifting and loosening of the teeth and sensory disturbance of the involved trigeminal nerve. Radiographs demonstrate irregular destruction of the jaw but in the osteogenic sarcoma there are, in addition, radiating trabeculae of new bone formation to give the characteristic 'sun ray' appearance. Treatment is by wide resection and blood borne metastases do not normally occur as rapidly as in osteosarcomas found elsewhere in the skeleton. More rarely a chondrosarcoma may involve the jaws with similar clinical signs to the osteosarcoma. Treatment is again by wide resection.

Intrabony squamous-cell carcinoma is rare but when present it causes a destructive lesion within the mandible on X-ray, sensory disturbance of the trigeminal nerve and expansion of the bone with loosening of the teeth. The more common squamous-cell carcinoma arising in the oral mucous membrane produces swelling of the soft tissue overlying the jaw, usually with central ulceration and underlying bone destruction (*Fig.* J.28).

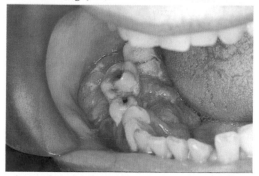

Fig. J.28. Squamous-cell carcinoma of the mandibular alveolus.

Carcinoma of the maxillary antrum and malignant tumours of the minor salivary glands contained within the mucosa of the palate, will eventually cause intraoral swelling of the upper jaw, leading to ulceration. A malignant lesion should be suspected if growth is rapid and is associated with bone destruction, loosening of the teeth, haemorrhage, and sensory disturbance of the trigeminal nerve. The diagnosis is confirmed by biopsy. The important malignant tumours affecting the upper jaw in addition to carcinoma of the antrum are adenocystic carcinoma, adenocarcinoma, malignant pleomorphic adenoma and lymphoma.

Metastatic tumours of the jaws

Secondary deposits of tumours rarely affect the jaws, with the mandible as the commoner site. Tumours of the bronchus, breast, kidney and thyroid produce osteolytic lesions while carcinoma of the prostate tends to form an osteosclerotic deposit. The clinical signs are similar to other intrabony malignant tumours with swelling, pain, loosening of the teeth and sensory disturbance. Eventually pathological facture occurs.

Secondary deposits may also develop in the overlying soft tissue of the jaws, especially at the gingival margin, and may be confused with a benign epulis. Rapid growth usually occurs to produce a fleshy mass, which may be friable and haemorrhagic. These lesions should be excised and all submitted for histological examination lest the diagnosis should be missed.

P. T. Blenkinsopp

Joints, affections of

Joint affections may be acute, as in rheumatic fever, gout or traumatic hydrarthrosis; acute relapsing becoming chronic, as in rheumatoid arthritis or Reiter's disease; chronic with acute onset, as in some cases of generalized osteoarthritis; or insidious and chronic as in most cases of osteoarthritis. The affection may be of one joint, a monarthritis, as may be seen in tuberculous arthritis; or it may be the start of a polyarthritis, as is seen not infrequently in psoriatic arthropathy, in which a number of joints are eventually affected. The pattern of joint involvement may be important: rheumatoid arthritis affects initially and chiefly peripheral joints; ankylosing spondylitis affects the sacroiliacs and spine; polymyalgia rheumatica affects the girdle joints, pelvis and shoulders. The terminal interphalangeal joints are affected commonly in osteoarthritis (Heberden's nodes) and psoriatic arthropathy, occasionally in adolescent rheumatoid arthritis, but rarely in adult rheumatoid arthritis. Interphalangeal involvement of the toes is rare in rheumatoid arthritis but more common in the arthritis associated with ulcerative colitis or Reiter's disease. Joint involvement may be in the form of a flitting and transient polyarthritis, as in rheumatic fever, some cases of systemic lupus erythematosus and in a number of other conditions or in a recurring or palindromic pattern subsiding completely between episodes, as in some cases of rheumatoid arthritis.

Joints may be swollen because of:

1. Bony enlargement, as in osteoarthritis or Charcot's joints in tabes dorsalis or syringomyelia
2. New periosteal bone deposition as in hypertrophic pulmonary osteoarthropathy or thyroid acropachy.
3. Synovial effusion. The joint fluid may be:
   clear and acellular in association with, e.g. serious injury; inflammatory and cellular as in rheumatoid arthritis; blood-stained as in traumatic haemarthrosis and bleeding disorders; purulent as in pyogenic infection or acute crystal synovitis; milky as in chylous arthritis associated with filiariasis.
4. Synovial proliferation as in rheumatoid arthritis.
5. Rarely because of malignant changes, as in sarcoma and secondary carcinoma.

Not infrequently joints are swollen from a combination of two or more of these factors. Swelling of synovial tendon sheaths or bursae alongside joints may also contribute greatly to the clinical picture, symmetrical involvement of extensor sheaths on the dorsum of the wrists being very typical of rheumatoid arthritis. Subacromial and semimembranosus bursal involvement may contribute much swelling when shoulders or knees are affected by an inflammatory arthritis. If there is doubt regarding the presence of infecting organisms aspiration should be performed. This will often contribute useful information in non-infective conditions such as gout, chondrocalcinosis, or haemarthrosis if diagnosis is in doubt.

Joints affected by any disease process may show a variable blend of five factors: swelling, pain, stiffness, tenderness and weakness. These five factors in variable combinations cause the dysfunction typical of the particular arthritic disease in question. In progressive systemic sclerosis (scleroderma) stiffness is the dominant. component; in gout swelling, tenderness and pain. The joints in rheumatoid arthritis vary and differ depending on activity and stage of the disease process; stiffness in early rheumatoid disease is largely due to joint swelling, in advanced disease to irreversible change, even in some patients, to the point of bony or fibrous ankylosis. In many instances chronic joint swelling produces excessive joint laxity allowing reversible deformity or subluxation. In other cases destruction of joint tissue in rheumatoid arthritis causes gross hypermobility, the so-called 'lorgnette' or 'telescopic fingers' being extreme examples of this.

Two of the cardinal signs of inflammation, heat and redness, are often absent in inflammatory arthritis, while in acute pyarthrosis the joint is hot and in gout hot and red. In most patients with rheumatoid arthritis the joints tend to be cold and moist without erythema,

though swollen, painful and tender. Palmar erythema is common in rheumatoid arthritis and in systemic lupus erythematosus, the palms and fingertips being often a bright pink. Inflammatory arthropathies usually cause most discomfort in the early morning, the tissues becoming 'gelled' with disuse in the night. This early morning increase in pain and stiffness of fingers, wrists and shoulders in particular is characteristic of rheumatoid and similar arthropathies; in ankylosing spondylitis a similar increase in stiffness and pain occurs in spine, hips and shoulders. Painful morning stiffness is also seen characteristically in polymyalgia rheumatica in shoulders and hips.

There are very many possible causes of joint involvement in systemic disease; these are listed below. Not all can be discussed and described; the following account deals only with the more common and distinctive.

A list of the arthropathies

1.   CONGENITAL

Achondroplasia and pseudoachondroplasia
Angiokeratoma corporis diffusum (Fabry's disease)
Arthrogryposis multiplex congenita
Camptodactyly
Chondrodysplasia punctata (Conradi's syndrome)
Congenital indifference to pain
Down's syndrome
Dysplasia epiphysalis multiplex
Ehlers–Danlos syndrome
Familial dysautonomia (Riley–Day syndrome)
Hereditary progressive arthro-ophthalmopathy
Hypermobility syndrome
Marfan's syndrome
Morquio–Brailsford syndrome
Osteodysplasty
Osteogenesis imperfecta
Spondyloepiphysial dysplasia

2.   DEGENERATIVE, TRAUMATIC AND OCCUPATIONAL

Ankylosing vertebral hyperostosis (Forrestier's disease, diffuse interstitial spinal hyperostosis (DISH))
Occupational syndromes, e.g. porter's neck, wicket-keeper's fingers
Osteoarthritis
Traumatic syndromes, e.g. traumatic haemarthrosis

3.   DIETETIC

Fluorosis
Kashin–Beck disease
Rickets
Scurvy

4.   ENDOCRINE

Acromegaly
Cretinous and myxoedematous arthropathy

Diabetic cheiroarthropathy
Hyperparathyroidism
Hypoparathyroidism
Thyroid acropachy

5. GUT-ASSOCIATED

Acute gastrointestinal bacterial infection
Antibiotic-induced (pseudomembranous) colitis
Crohn's disease
Jejuno-ileal bypass arthritis-dermatitis syndrome
Ulcerative colitis
Whipple's disease

6. IDIOPATHIC INFLAMMATORY

Acne fulminans arthritis
Behçet's syndrome
Erythema multiforme
Dermatomyositis and polymyositis
Dressler's syndrome
Erythema nodosum
Familial Mediterranean fever
Henoch–Schönlein syndrome (anaphylactoid purpura)
Intermittent hydrarthrosis
Juvenile chronic arthritis (Pauciarticular, Polyarticular, Systemic)
Mixed connective tissue disease
Palindromic rheumatism
Pigmented villonodular synovitis
Progressive systemic sclerosis (scleroderma)
Relapsing polychondritis
Rheumatoid arthritis, including Felty's syndrome, Caplan's syndrome
Sarcoidosis
Spondyloarthropathy, e.g. ankylosing spondylitis, Psoriatic arthritis, reactive arthritis, Reiter's syndrome, Enteropathic arthritis (Crohn's disease, Ulcerative arthritis)
SAPHO syndrome
Sjögren's syndrome
Systemic lupus erythematosus

7 IDIOPATHIC NON-INFLAMMATORY

Osteochondritis dissecans
Osteochondrosis

8. HAEMATOLOGICAL

Agammaglobulinaemia
Haemophilia and allied disorders
Leukaemia
Sickle-cell disease
Thalassaemia

9. INFECTIVE

Infections due to bacteria, spirochaetes and mycoplasma

Anthrax
Brucella abortus and *melitensis arthritis*
Cat-scratch fever

Clutton's joints
Diphtheria
Erysipelas
Glanders
Haverhill fever
Infective endocarditis
Jaccoud's arthropathy
Leprosy
Lyme arthritis
Lymphogranuloma venereum
Meningococcal fever
Mycoplasma pneumoniae
Poncet's disease
Pseudomonas pseudomallei (Melioidosis)
Pyogenic (staphylococcal, psittacosis, gonococcal, pneumococcal, etc.)
Rat-bite fever
Rheumatic fever
Secondary syphilis
Streptococcal reactive arthritis
Tuberculosis
Typhoid and paratyphoid fever
Weil's disease (*Leptospirosis icterohaemorrhagica*)
Yaws

Infections due to viruses

Chikungunya
Dengue
Echo virus infection
Glandular fever (infectious mononucleosis)
Influenza
Measles
Mumps
O'Nyong–Nyong fever
Parvovirus (human)
Poliomyelitis
Ross River virus arthritis
Rubella
Viral hepatitis (mainly 'B')

Infections due to fungi

Actinomycosis
Aspergillosis
Blastomycosis
Coccidioidomycosis
Cryptococcosis (torulosis)
Histoplasmosis
Madura foot (mycetoma pedis)
Sporotrichosis

Infections due to protozoa

Amoebiasis
Giardiasis

Infections due to worms

Chylous arthritis
Dracunculosis (Guinea-worm arthritis)
Filariasis
Trichiniasis
Schistosomiasis
Strongyloidiasis

10. METABOLIC

Amyloidosis
Biliary and alcoholic cirrhosis
Calcinosis circumscripta (pyrophosphate arthropathy)
Calcinosis uraemica
Chondrocalcinosis
Disseminated lipogranulomatosis (Farber's disease)
Familial hypercholesterolaemia
Familial lipochrome pigmentary arthritis
Gaucher's disease
Gout
Haemochromatosis
Hunter's syndrome
Hurler's syndrome (gargoylism)
Multicentric reticulohistiocytosis (lipoid dermato-arthritis)
Myositis ossificans
Ochronosis
Renal transplant and haemodialysis syndrome
Wilson's disease

11. VASCULAR

Avascular necrosis (fat emboli, caisson, etc.)
Polyarteritis nodosa
Polymyalgia arteritica (giant-cell arteritis and polymyalgia rheumatica)
Takayasu's (pulseless) disease
Wegener's granulomatosis

12. NEOPLASTIC

Chondrosarcoma
Haemangioma
Hypertrophic pulmonary osteoarthropathy
Left atrial myxoma
Lymphoma
Metastatic malignant disease
Multiple myeloma
Osteoid osteoma
Paget's sarcoma
Hypertrophic pulmonary osteoarthropathy
Synovioma

13. NEUROPATHIC

Algodystrophy (shoulder–hand syndrome, transient osteoporosis, Sudek's atrophy)
Charcot's joints, tabetic or syringomyelic
Diabetic arthopathy (neuropathic and infective)
Paraplegia syndrome
Ulcero-osteolytic neuropathy

14. DRUG-INDUCED

Anticoagulants
Barbiturates
Corticosteroid arthropathy
Hydralazine syndrome (procaine amide, oral contraceptives, etc.)
Isoniazid shoulder–hand syndrome
Quinidine
Serum sickness

15. MISCELLANEOUS

Acro-osteolysis syndrome
Dupuytren's contracture
Knuckle pads (Hale–White) (Garrod)
Paget's disease of bone
Periostitis deformans (Soriano)
Thorn synovitis
Septic focus syndrome
Subacute pancreatitis
Xiphoid syndrome

1. Congenital arthropathies

In classical *achondroplasia* bony growth is abnormal but epiphysial development is normal; premature osteoarthritis is not usual and spinal stenosis may occur. In *pseudoachondroplasia* and the various *spondyloepiphysial dysplasias* epiphyses are involved, rendering these subjects particularly prone to severe premature osteoarthritis in adult life. In *Conradi's syndrome* a widespread patchy calcification in articular and other cartilages is seen in infancy with shortening and asymmetry of the limbs; premature osteoarthritis follows in adult life as it does in *hereditary progressive arthro-ophthalmopathy* where progressive myopia is associated with multiple epiphysial dysplasia.

Arthrogryposis multiplex congenita is a rare congenital condition characterized by joint contractures, usually symmetrical and multiple, affecting lower limbs rather than upper and distal joints more than proximal ones. The subcutaneous tissues may be thick, doughy or gelatinous. While usually apparent at birth and readily recognized, if the patient is not seen until adult life the condition may be confused with advanced rheumatoid arthritis with joint contractures of fingers, knees, elbows and wrists. It is usually, but not always, painless, though secondary degenerative changes may occur later and cause considerable discomfort, particularly in the hips which may become dislocated. Other congenital abnormalities may be present, such as small or absent patellae, high palate, hypospadias and micrognathia. Clubbing of fingers and toes is common, mental deficiency rare.

Camptodactyly is an innocent congenital condition where the little fingers are flexed with thickening of the proximal interphalangeal joints. It is a relatively common condition and important only in that it may be confused with osteoarthritis. Other fingers are less often affected.

In *congenital indifference to pain* the patient traumatizes the joints and other tissues repeatedly and may develop secondary traumatic osteoarthritis or even neuropathic joints. Such patients are usually mentally and neurologically normal otherwise but are constantly suffering the effects of injury, fractures, bruises, dislocations, cuts and scratches, as they do not experience pain as do normal subjects. It is a rare condition.

Dysplasia epiphysalis multiplex is inherited as an autosomal dominant trait. The epiphyses of the long bones become deformed, the hips most commonly. Any or all of the epiphyses of the long bones may be affected, with resultant osteoarthritis, particularly of hips and knees, beginning in early life. The sufferers are often of short stature with short, squat digits. Such children presenting with pain, usually in the hip, are often misdiagnosed as cases of Perthe's disease.

The *Ehlers-Danlos syndrome* is a rare genetically determined disorder of connective tissue, characterized by hypermobile joints and hyperextensible skin which tends to split if mildly injured, with resulting gaping scars. There are probably seven entities included in this title; in one, in particular, the ecchymotic type IV, sudden death may occur from spontaneous arterial rupture or gastrointestinal perforation, though abnormalities in collagen biosynthesis occur also in three other types. Joint subluxations and dislocations occur if the joints are hypermobile and effusions into knees are common. Dislocations of clavicles, patellae, shoulders, radii and hips may occur and recur several times. Other developmental abnormalities are common, such as kyphoscoliosis, anterior wedging of vertebrae, spina bifida occulta, club-foot and genu recurvatum. Bleeding may occur in superficial tissues, or from vagina, rectum or mouth and haemarthrosis may occur. Children may be backward in walking and develop a tabetic-like gait. In the sixth to ninth months of pregnancy joints may become more lax and subluxable than previously. Premature osteoarthritis may occur in a few patients.

Familial dysautonomia (Riley-Day syndrome) is a congenital disorder almost completely confined to Ashkenazic Jews, transmitted as an autosomal recessive trait. Among many manifestations relative insensitivity to pain may lead to neuropathic joints in knee or shoulder in early adolescence.

Maldevelopment of axial and peripheral joints are features of the *mucopolysaccharidoses*. Features of these inherited disorders are due to accumulation of mucopolysaccharides (or glycosaminoglycans) in the tissues as a result of deficiency of lysosomal enzymes necessary for their degradation. In the commonest of these rare disorders, Hurler's syndrome (gargoylism), the onset is from 6 months to 2 years of age but the typical picture of gargoylism does not appear until 4 or 5 years later. The child develops coarse features with thick lips, large bulging head and flattened nose; the cervical spine is short with kyphosis of the lower dorsal and upper lumbar regions. Acetabula are shallow, epiphyses flattened, irregular and retarded in development. Limitation of joint movement is common, particularly abduction of shoulders and hips and extension of fingers, and contractures of hips and elbows may occur, the hands becoming clawed. The children are often intellectually impaired and rarely live beyond 20 years of age. Similar features are found in other mucopolysaccharidoses, the Hunter syndrome, the Sanfilippo syndrome, the Scheie syndrome and the Maroteaux-Lamy syndrome.

In the type IV *Morquio-Brailsford* mucopolysaccharidosis the children appear normal until 1-2 years of age when kyphosis is seen with protrusion of the sternum and prominence of the chin appearing a year later. Growth usually ceases at 10 years, the child showing a short trunk with kyphosis, knock knees, flat feet, waddling gait, muscle weakness and increased laxity of joints which is in sharp contrast with the contractures seen in the other mucopolysaccharidoses. In a severe case almost every joint may be affected, the spine, hips and knees most often, and cord compression may occur. Aortic regurgitation is common. Keratan sulphate excretion in the urine is increased and, though not invariably present, may be diagnostic. Mentally the children are normal.

Ganglioside storage diseases also result from inherited enzyme deficiencies. *Farber's disease* results from deposition of lipid with a vigorous granulomatous reaction (disseminated lipo-granulomatosis). Arthritis is an early feature with red swollen joints and periarticular pigmented swelling appearing in the first few months of life. It is a very rare condition. Death from respiratory infection is usual before the age of 2.

In the *hypermobility syndrome* generalized joint laxity occurs as an isolated finding, giving rise to recurrent joint pains and effusions, particularly after vigorous exercise. Symptoms, more common in females than in males, usually start from the age of 15. The knees are most commonly affected. Degenerative changes may begin early in the fourth decade. These children, who often consider themselves to be 'double-jointed', often suffer quite severe cramp-like pains in the legs after sporting activities. About 10 per cent of otherwise normal subjects have such hypermobility. Symptoms are related to the degree of hypermobility but often decrease with advancing age and crippling osteoarthritis is uncommon.

The picture of *Marfan's syndrome* is of a tall, thin loose-jointed youth or girl with long extremities, especially the fingers (arachnodactyly), dislocated lenses, tremulous irides and cardiovascular abnormalities, particularly dilatation of the ascending aorta and aortic regurgitation. Fifty per cent of these patients present with backache, pains in joints and/or effusions.

Joints may dislocate readily, hips or shoulders most commonly, but early development of osteoarthritis is unusual. Many other abnormalities may be present, pigeon chest or pectus excavatum particularly. The sexes are affected equally. The distance from pubis to sole exceeds that of pubis to vertex and arm span is greater than height. Distal bones are longer than proximal and subcutaneous fat is sparse.

Osteodysplasty (Melnick and Needles syndrome) is another inherited skeletal dysplasia, probably a congenital disorder of skeletal growth which leads to early degenerative changes in the large weight-bearing joints, including the spine. Radiographs show curvature of the long bones of the limbs with irregular cortex and widening and thinning of the metaphyses. These changes may roughly resemble those of rickets but ribs, clavicles and scapulae are also deformed.

The outstanding abnormality in *osteogenesis imperfecta* is the ease with which bones may be fractured. In addition joints are unduly mobile, thinness of the sclerae gives the eyes the typical pale blue appearance and there is atrophy of the skin with a tendency to subcutaneous haemorrhage. Joints dislocate readily and growth may be arrested by multiple small fractures in epiphyses. Spine and chest deformities may occur and deafness is not unusual. Ligaments are weakened and tendon ruptures may occur.

This list of congenital non-infective arthropathies is not complete and the different causes are not yet clear enough to classify them all accurately. Undue laxity, with recurrent subluxations or increased friability or fragility of tissues, leads to premature degenerative changes in the joints affected. Other coexistent congenital abnormalities are common.

2. Degenerative arthropathies

By *osteoarthritis* is meant the various painful syndromes arising primarily from degenerative changes in the joints (*Figs. J.29, J.33, J.34*). Age brings degenerative changes, but the pains experienced vary greatly depending on personality, degree of change and joints affected. Such changes are more likely to occur in any joint previously injured by fracture or dislocation or even mild subluxation or in any joint which is congenitally abnormal or, because of mechanical factors, working abnormally in the face of abnormal stresses. Repeated 'microtrauma' may also predispose to degenerative changes. Endocrine factors may play a part in some cases as in the so-called *generalized osteoarthritis* which usually affects women 1–5 years or more before or after the menopause. The most commonly affected joints are the terminal interphalangeal joints of the fingers (Heberden's nodes), the thumb bases (carpometacarpal and metacarpophalangeal

joints of the thumbs). cervical and lumbar spine, knees and hips and acromioclavicular joints. Less commonly affected are proximal interphalangeal and metacarpophalangeal joints of the fingers. Although essentially degenerative, Heberden's nodes may, in some cases, be tender, red and inflamed in the early stages; inflammation also occurs in osteoarthritis in other joints but does not dominate the scene as it does in rheumatoid arthritis. The hand in osteoarthritis differs from that in rheumatoid arthritis as shown in *Table* J.7.

In the knee, effusions may occur as a result of trauma and there may also be considerable synovial proliferation. It is not always easy to distinguish an osteoarthritic joint from a rheumatoid one but the pattern of the disease elsewhere in the body and the absence of systemic features in osteoarthritis usually suffice to distinguish the two. In any joint, the absence of inflammatory swelling, nodules and of enlarged lymph nodes favours osteoarthritis rather than inflammatory arthritis. Sedimentation rates are rarely elevated above 30 mm in the first hour (Westergren) in osteoarthritis and are usually normal as are haemoglobin and plasma proteins. Tests for rheumatoid factors are negative. In the cervical spine degenerative changes centre essentially around the lower 5th, 6th and 7th intervertebral discs, the pain often fanning up into the occiput, over the head and into the shoulders; neck movements are restricted and painful. In rheumatoid disease, particularly in childhood, involvement is more diffuse throughout the cervical spine though pain may be referred in a similar manner. Subluxation of the first on the second vertebra, which occurs in rheumatoid arthritis and ankylosing spondylitis, is not seen in osteoarthritis. A lateral radiograph of the cervical spine will readily distinguish the rough irregularity of disc degeneration from the straight, even intervertebral bridging of ankylosing spondylitis. The condition known as 'ankylosing hyperostosis' of the spine (Forrestier's disease) is a degenerative one occurring not infrequently in diabetics (*see* BACK PAIN IN), usually in the lower dorsal area.

3. Dietetic arthropathies

Kashin–Beck disease is a condition apparently resulting from fusarial infection of flour. In the valleys in eastern Siberia, northern China and North Korea, where it occurred, degenerative changes in joints and spine appeared in relatively young people as a result of cartilage destruction. It is now disappearing with the elimination of infected grain. *Rickets* is much less common than it was and for this reason may be more easily missed. Presenting symptoms may be pains and tenderness over bones, particularly the back, hips, thighs and legs generally. The pains are usually aggrav-

Table J.7. Differential diagnosis of osteoarthritic and rheumatoid joints

Osteoarthritis	Rheumatoid arthritis
Bony joint swelling	Spindle soft-tissue swellings of joints
Terminal interphalangeal joint involvement common (Heberden's nodes)	Terminal interphalangeal joint less commonly involved
Metacarpophalangeal and proximal interphalangeal joints less commonly involved	Metacarpophalangeal and proximal interphalangeal joints commonly involved
Wrists rarely affected	Wrists commonly affected
Tendon sheaths not involved	Swelling of tendon sheaths common
Affected joints not usually very tender	Affected joints usually tender
Gross deformity rare	
Joint effusions rare	Joint effusion common
Radiographs show:	
Juxta-articular bony sclerosis	Juxta-articular osteoporosis
Diffuse joint space loss	Bony erosions
Juxta-articular pseudocysts	Subluxation or deformity
Osteophytes	

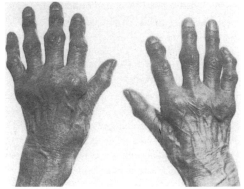

Fig. J.29. Typical osteoarthritic (Granny's) hands. The enlargement and distortion are essentially bony secondary to degenerative changes in the cartilages.

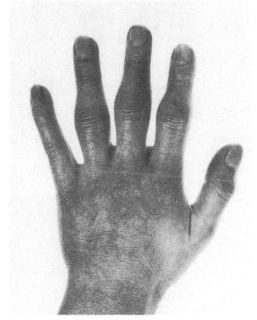

Fig. J.30. Typical spindling of proximal interphalangeal joints in rheumatoid arthritis. The swelling is due to inflammatory changes and increased fluid in these joints.

ated by rising from resting positions and by exercise. The dangers of missing the diagnosis lie in permanent bony deformities in the pelvis and lower extremities and in the thorax. Pelvic deformities, most serious in females, usually occur in the first year of life. In *scurvy* the child is listless and apathetic with poor appetite. Bones may be painful and tender from subperiosteal haemorrhages and tender swellings may be palpated. The disease is seldom seen in adults; when it occurs dietetic deficiencies are usually due to neglect, alcoholism or obsessional food fads, sometimes medically induced.

4. Endocrine arthropathies

In *acromegaly* recurrent pains in spine and limb joints may be mistaken for those occurring in rheumatoid or osteoarthritis. Effusions may occur in the knees and the carpal tunnel syndrome is not uncommon. The joints may be hypermobile in the early stages due to enlargement of the cartilages, and subluxations and traumatic effusions may occur as in the other hypermobility syndromes. Later bony overgrowth restricts movement, so that the picture resembles more that

of osteoarthritis, or, because of the fixed bent spine, that of advanced ankylosing spondylitis.

Diabetic cheiroarthropathy affects the hands of some patients with diabetes mellitus; the fingers may become stiff and partially flexed with thickening of the skin of the palms.

In the original description of *myxoedema*, in 1873 by Sir William Gull, muscular stiffness, joint swelling and broad spade-like hands were noted. In the early stages of the disease, before the classical features of myxoedema appear, the hands may be mistaken for those of early rheumatoid arthritis (*Fig. J.35*). The carpal tunnel syndrome occurs not infrequently and arthralgia is a common complaint. Signs of inflammation are absent but synovial thickening

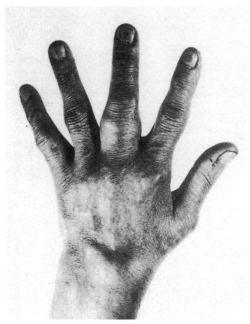

Fig. J.31. Swelling in a rheumatoid hand due to inflammatory changes in extensor tendon sheaths.

and, occasionally, effusions may occur, the knees and hands being most commonly affected. Traumatic lesions are not uncommon and hip pain may be due to a slipped femoral epiphysis.

roidism back pain and stiffness may cause a clinical picture similar to that of ankylosing spondylitis but, though ligamentous calcification is present, the sacro-iliac joints are normal. It is associated with hypocalcaemia, cataracts, fits, tetany and rashes. In *thyroid acropachy* subperiosteal thickening is seen in metacarpal and phalangeal bones of the hands in patients with hyperthyroidism who have in many cases been treated and rendered euthyroid. Exophthalmos is common and so-called 'pretibial myxoedema' may be present. The somewhat thickened hand resembles that seen in hypertrophic pulmonary osteoarthropathy, but the condition is milder and less extensive, being usually confined to the hands.

5. Gut-associated arthropathies

The more characteristic of these are considered in the next section under the spondyloarthropathies.

6. Idiopathic inflammatory arthropathies

In *dermatomyositis* and *polymyositis* minimal or moderate transitory arthralgia or arthritis occurs in about one-third of cases. Effusions are less common. Fingers and knees are most commonly affected. The skin and muscle manifestations point to the true diagnosis, muscles of the pelvic girdle and thighs and shoulder girdle becoming weak. The association of dermatomyositis

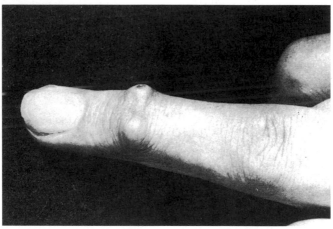

Fig. J.32. Rheumatoid nodules masquerading as Heberden's nodes. Note the necrotic (arteritic) centre in the upper one.

In *hyperparathyroidism*, as in some cases of osteomalacia, crush lesions may occur in juxta-articular bone with a traumatic type of synovitis, with effusions and impaired function of the affected joints. Calcification is not uncommon in synovial membrane and cartilage in these cases but it is rare in rheumatoid arthritis, a point of distinction between the two conditions. Not only may 'pseudorheumatoid arthritis' occur but also 'pseudo-gout' due to deposition of crystals of calcium pyrophosphate dihydrate. In idiopathic *hypoparathy-*

with malignant disease in adult cases should be kept in mind.

Dressler's syndrome following myocardial infarction or cardiac injury or surgery occurs around 2–4 weeks or more after the acute episode, with pericarditis, arthralgia and, rarely, arthritis.

The diagnosis *erythema multiforme* probably covers several different entities, some mild, some severe, the so-called 'Stevens–Johnson syndrome' being a severe variant. Arthritis or arthralgia may occur along

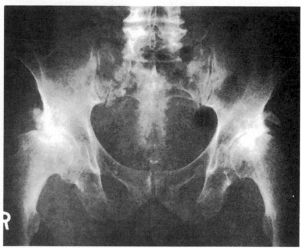

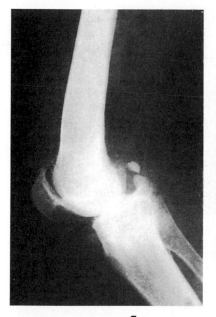

a   *b*

Fig. J.33. *a*, Osteoarthritis of the knee joint. *b*, Osteoarthritis of the hip joints. (*Dr T. A. Hills.*)

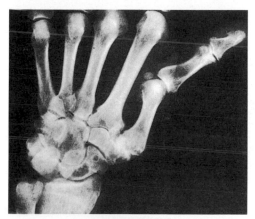

Fig. J.34. Severe osteoarthritis of the carpometacarpal joint of the thumb. (*Dr Keith Jefferson.*)

with other inflammatory reactions in skin, eye, mouth and elsewhere.

Familial Mediterranean fever is an ill-understood disorder characterized by recurrent and sometimes periodic attacks of arthralgia or arthritis. It occurs predominantly in people of Mediterranean origin, Armenians, Arabs and Sephardic Jews. Onset is in childhood or adolescence, episodes of fever recurring with polyserositis, abdominal pain, urticaria and other rashes, arthralgia and arthritis and, later, amyloidosis. Joint manifestations occur in one-third to one-half of the cases, usually arthralgia but sometimes mono- or oligoarthritis. The acute episodes last only a few days, rarely weeks, most cases showing no permanent

sequelae. Sacroiliac changes may occur late in the disease.

Henoch–Schönlein syndrome ('anaphylactoid purpura') is commonest in children under 12 years of age. The outstanding feature is a maculo-petechial and sometimes papular rash on the buttocks and extensor surfaces of the lower limbs particularly. Urticaria and purpura may occur. Pain, swelling and stiffness of joints, most commonly ankles and knees, is usually transient and lasts only a few days. Alimentary hae-morrhage and haematuria are not uncommon and about 10 per cent of cases develop renal failure.

Intermittent hydrarthrosis, usually in the knees, may resolve without sequelae but approximately 50 per cent of patients eventually develop rheumatoid arthritis or ankylosing spondylitis. Hydrarthrosis may, however, be a manifestation of infective systemic disease such as syphilis or brucellosis. There is usually complete or almost complete remission between attacks. It may also occur after trauma, in osteoarthritis and osteochondritis dissecans; in other words it is a physical sign and not a diagnosis. Some patients recover without showing signs of any other disorder.

Palindromic rheumatism is a name given to recurring episodes of arthritis due to many causes, the most common probably being the early phase of rheumatoid arthritis.

Pigmented villonodular synovitis presents as a persistent but usually relatively painless synovial proli-feration with blood-stained joint fluid. Brown nodular masses, possibly due to haemangiomas, form in the

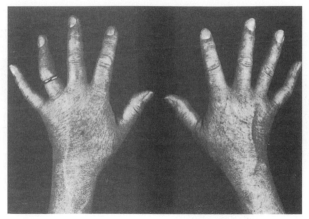

Fig. J.35. Typical swelling of hands in myxoedema.

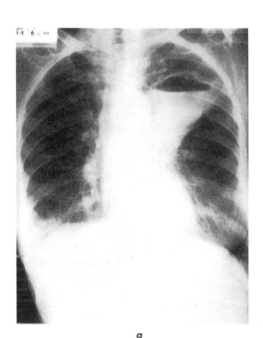

a

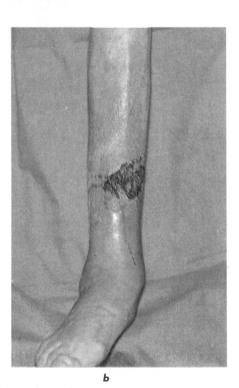

b

Fig. J.36. *a*, Lung abscess in neutropenic Felty's syndrome. *b*, Leg ulcer in Felty's syndrome.

synovia; these become traumatized, inflamed and hyperplastic, the hyperplastic synovial cells containing haemosiderin. The condition is usually monarticular, commonly of the knee, and occurs in young adults, males rather than females. The joint may lock repeatedly. The aspirated joint fluid is characteristically blood-stained or dark brown in colour.

In *progressive systemic sclerosis* (scleroderma) the skin is stretched tight over the underlying tissues (*Fig.* J.40), the joints being intact though initially showing changes resembling those of rheumatoid arthritis.

Relapsing (or atrophic) polychondritis is a rare disorder in which the cartilages of joints, ears, nose and trachea soften and collapse; this leads to arthritis, facial changes, dyspnoea or stridor and, occasionally, death.

Rheumatoid arthritis (*Figs.* J.30–32, 38) is sufficiently well known as to need no description. It is as well to remember that tendons and tendon sheaths and bursae are commonly involved by the inflammatory process and these add to the clinical picture. *Juvenile arthritis* is, in only a small minority of cases, an early form of rheumatoid arthritis. In a few cases, particularly

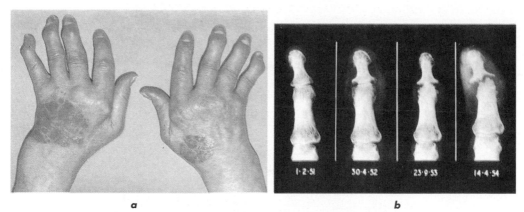

Fig. J.37. *a*, Psoriatic arthropathy, showing involvement of terminal interphalangeal joints. *b*, Advanced destructive changes in psoriatic arthropathy.

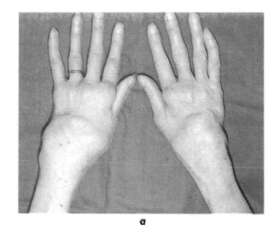

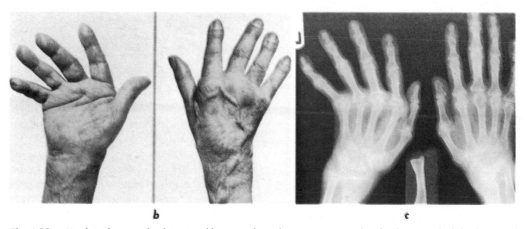

Fig. J.38. *a*, Hands in rheumatoid arthritis. In addition to arthritic changes extensor tendon sheaths are involved. *b*, Rheumatoid arthritis with ulnar deviation and palmar contraction (pseudo-Dupuytren). *c*, Unusual unilateral ulnar deviation with gross bilateral carpal rheumatoid changes. Changes in metacarpophalangeal joints are more marked in the left than the right hand.

in boys, it may be an early form of ankylosing spondylitis but it is usually a sero-negative chronic arthritis. It differs from adult polyarthritis in that splenomegaly and lymphadenopathy are more common, tests for rheumatoid factor usually negative, involvement of terminal interphalangeal joints of fingers and cervical spine more common (*Fig.* J.39), and skin rashes of maculopapular type more common. In the eye, iritis with band opacity in the cornea occurs, sometimes with secondary cataract formation; these are not seen

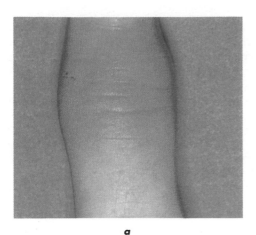 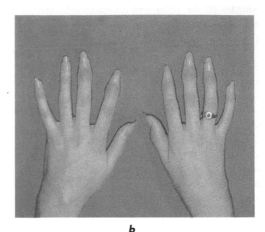

a   *b*

Fig. J.39. *a, b,* Involvement of terminal interphalangeal joints in juvenile chronic polyarthritis.

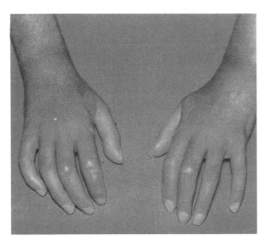

Fig. J.40. Scleroderma (progressive systemic sclerosis). Note the tight shiny skin over the flexed knuckles.

in rheumatoid arthritis in adults. Growth in general may be arrested if the disease is severe and premature fusion may occur in epiphyses adjacent to involved joints. Pericarditis is more common in juvenile arthritis than in adult rheumatoid arthritis.

In *Felty's syndrome* splenomegaly, enlargement of lymph nodes, neutropenia and sometimes pigmentation of the skin are superimposed on the usual picture of rheumatoid arthritis. The only reason for maintaining the title in what is merely a variant of rheumatoid arthritis is to emphasize the importance of the neutropenia, for intercurrent infections are the rule and splenectomy may be necessary. Leg ulcers are relatively common, the usual site being the lower shin anteriorly (*Fig.* J.36).

The arthropathy associated with *sarcoidosis* is often accompanied by erythema nodosum; a weak or negative tuberculin reaction is usual and the Kveim test may be positive. The arthropathy may be no

more than a migratory arthralgia or it may be a true polyarthritis with pain, fever, systemic upset and swelling of several joints, usually the larger ones. In the majority of cases polyarthritis subsides in a few weeks. Hilar node enlargement is common in chest radiographs, and lymph nodes may be palpable in the neck and axilla in some cases. Splenomegaly may be present. Histoplasmosis may also present with hilar lymphadenopathy and joint pains ('pseudosarcoidosis').

The term *spondyloarthropathy* is applied to a family of conditions whose key features are: involvement of the spine and sacroiliac joints; oligo-articular lower limb arthritis; an association with iritis, psoriasis and inflammatory bowel disease; a high prevalence of the HLA B27 antigen.

The principal members of this group are: ankylosing spondylitis; reactive arthritis; Reiter's disease; psoriatic arthropathy; enteropathic arthritis associated with ulcerative colitis and Crohn's disease.

Behçet's syndrome and the Stevens–Johnson syndrome share some features with this family though their inclusion within the group is contentious.

The classical picture of *ankylosing spondylitis* is that of a young male adult with stiff back and chest and often stiff neck and hips also. The sedimentation rate is elevated, anterior uveitis is present in 25 per cent of cases at some stage in the disease course, and radiographs show typical changes in sacroiliac joints and usually in the dorsolumbar spine.

Peripheral joint involvement may occur but is usually, though not always, transient. Knee effusions are not uncommon. The pattern of the disorder is essentially central, spine and girdle joints being predominantly affected, peripheral small joints rarely and transiently; this contrasts with rheumatoid arthritis.

Nodules do not occur and rheumatoid factor is not present in the serum. The histocompatibility antigen HLA-B27 is found in over 90 per cent of patients.

Reiter's disease comprises arthritis associated with genital-tract inflammation or recent gastrointestinal infection. The syndrome may be caused by either sexually transmitted infection or acute gastrointestinal infection and in either case urethritis or cervicitis may be present. Recognized causal pathogens include *Chlamydia trachomatis, Salmonella enteritidis* and *typhimurium, Shigella flexneri, Yersinia enterocolitica* and *pseudotuberculosis* and *Campylobacter jejuni*. Traditionally arthritis, urethritis and conjunctivitis comprise the classical triad; conjunctivitis is often transient or mild and genital tract symptoms may be mild, overlooked or denied. Diagnosis therefore requires a careful history and a genitourinary examination including microscopic examination of urethral and/or cervical smears. A variety of terms are used to describe this condition; commonly the relationship between infection in the genitourinary or gastrointestinal tract with aseptic arthritis is described by the term 'reactive arthritis'. Arthritic symptoms appear a few days or up to 3 weeks after the initial symptoms of the causative infection. The distribution of affected joints, ankles, heels and knees being principally affected, is characteristic and lesions of buccal mucosa, of the glans penis or prepuce (balanitis circinata), or of skin (keratoderma blenorrhagica) suggest the correct diagnosis. Later, sacroiliac changes may occur and sometimes a clinical picture similar to that seen in ankylosing spondylitis develops. Caucasian patients with Reiter's disease usually have the tissue antigen HLA-B27, those with the picture of ankylosing spondylitis almost 100 per cent. Rheumatoid factor is absent from the blood; nodules do not occur. When skin manifestations are present the condition may closely resemble that of psoriatic arthropathy. The interphalangeal joints of the toes, rarely involved in rheumatoid arthritis, may be affected in Reiter's disease. Iridocyclitis and iritis, rare in rheumatoid arthritis, are not uncommon in Reiter's disease.

In *psoriatic arthropathy (Fig. J.37)* the arthritis usually but not invariably follows the skin disorder by several years. The sero-negative, non-nodular polyarthritis tends to be more patchy and less evenly symmetrical than rheumatoid arthritis, and the terminal interphalangeal joints of the fingers are frequently affected, particularly if the nails are affected by the pitting, ridging and separation of psoriasis. When all the joints of a finger are affected by inflammatory arthritis the digit resembles a hot sausage, as was noted many years ago by French rheumatologists. In some cases the sacroiliac joints or the spine are affected, the clinical picture being that of ankylosing spondylitis.

In *Crohn's disease* and *ulcerative colitis* and, less commonly, in *Whipple's disease* (intestinal lipodystrophy) arthralgia or arthritis may occur in the spine or peripheral joints. In all of these, rheumatoid factor is absent from the blood and rheumatoid nodules are not seen. In the arthropathy of ulcerative colitis, the best documented of these three disorders, onset is usually between the ages of 15 and 45 years. It is usually symmetrical and often monarticular with short exacerbations and usually complete recovery, joint erosions being rare and minor in character. It affects both sexes equally and usually begins acutely, affecting one knee or ankle primarily, subsequent attacks being of similar pattern. The arthritis usually commences long after the onset of the colitis and may coincide with an exacerbation of the disease. In all three conditions, ulcerative colitis, Crohn's disease and Whipple's disease, a picture similar to that of ankylosing spondylitis may eventually appear after some years.

In *systemic lupus erythematosus* any or all systems of the body may be involved in addition to the joints, which are not invariably involved, though arthralgia is usually present at some stage in the course of the disease. The patient, usually a female, is more ill than arthritic in most cases, though joint involvement is present in about two-thirds of patients. The finding of numerous antibodies, including antinuclear antibody, in high titre, and DNA antibody in the blood is strong confirmatory diagnostic evidence. The joint involvement may be flitting, resembling rheumatic fever, or more constant, resembling rheumatoid arthritis. The coexistence of skin lesions and visceral manifestations suggests the correct diagnosis, the typical lupus butterfly rash over nose and cheeks being particularly characteristic. Neutropenia and anaemia are common, thrombocytopenia not uncommon. Asthma, proteinuria, neurological signs, splenomegaly, retinal exudates and a number of other coexistent findings in any arthritic should make one think of this disorder or a related connective tissue disease. Epileptiform fits occur in about 10 per cent of cases. Patients with neurological and renal involvement fare worst. Patients having a combination of clinical features of systemic lupus erythematosus, progressive systemic sclerosis and polymyositis with high titres of a circulating antinuclear antibody with specificity for a nuclear ribonucleoprotein are said to have *mixed connective tissue disease*.

7. Idiopathic non-inflammatory arthropathies

In *osteochondritis dissecans* flakes of articular cartilage, sometimes with a portion of the underlying bone, become detached without evident trauma, the condition manifesting itself as recurring attacks of arthritis. The commonest site (85 per cent) is the knee; the radial head is the next most common, hip and ankles being rarely involved. The condition may be bilateral and X-rays are usually diagnostic.

In *osteochondrosis* the diagnosis is also essentially a radiological one. It is essentially a disturbance of epiphysial ossification seen in childhood and early adult life, possibly ischaemic in origin. Early radiographs show dense fragments in the epiphysis and a broadening of the epiphysial line with, later, areas of rarefaction and condensation so that a core of dense bone is seen in a porotic matrix. The epiphyses are affected during the periods of their greatest activity, for instance the femoral head from 4-12 years (Legg–Calve–Perthes disease), the tibial tubercle from 10-16 years (Osgood–Schlatter disease).

8. Haematological arthropathies

It is wise to perform a full blood count, sedimentation rate and examination of plasma proteins in obscure cases of arthritis. Approximately 25 per cent of patients with *agammaglobulinaemia*, congenital or acquired, develop a non-suppurative arthritis not unlike rheumatoid arthritis, the joints showing effusions, pain, tenderness and stiffness. The condition is usually asymmetrical, is unaccompanied by radiological changes, and may be transient, subsiding in a few weeks without sequelae, or may persist for years but with little residual change. Biopsy of synovial tissue does not distinguish between the two conditions. The sedimentation rate is usually normal and tests for rheumatoid factor are negative. In some cases arthritis has been attributed to mycoplasma infection but recurrent infection with the usual pyogenic organisms is also common.

Haemarthrosis may occur in *haemophilia* (factor VIII deficiency) and allied disorders, such as *Christmas disease* (factor IX deficiency), and in patients on anticoagulant therapy but is rare in von Willebrand's disease. In *leukaemia* haemorrhages are common and flitting pains resembling rheumatic fever are not uncommon in acute leukaemia and this, taken in conjunction with a systolic cardiac murmur, may cause diagnostic confusion particularly in acute aleukaemic leukaemia. Pains in bones and joints occur not infrequently in acute leukaemia in childhood and in chronic leukaemia in adults, both myeloid and lymphatic. In children juvenile arthritis is often diagnosed in error.

In *sickle-cell anaemia* painful crises occur which are characteristic of the disorder, and these may occur not only in the abdomen but in bones and joints in children or adults. Although the most common symptoms are those of anaemia, some patients have no complaints except during crises. Aseptic necrosis of bone may occur, particularly in the head of the humerus or femur, radiographs showing subsequently areas of increased density and areas of necrosis. The course of the disease is that of a chronic haemolytic process punctuated by periodic painful crises. Chronic ulceration of the lower legs is relatively common and scars are commonly to be seen around the malleoli. Another striking complication of sickle-cell disease, particularly in children, is salmonella osteomyelitis, often multifocal. In *β-thalassaemia major* pains and swelling in ankles and feet may occur.

9. Infective arthropathies

In the infective arthropathies the infecting organism is present in locomotor tissues; in gonococcal arthritis, for instance, gonococci can be isolated from the infected joints or joint; the condition responds to appropriate antibiotics. Any of the infections due to bacteria, spirochaetes or mycoplasma may, if there is destruction of tissue, lead to chronic changes in bones and joints, but if the correct treatment is given early there may be little or no residual disability. In these days of extensive and rapid worldwide travel, conditions previously unknown in residents of one country can occur with resulting arthralgia or arthritis.

Viral arthropathies are common throughout the world but are usually mild and transient. Arbovirus infections including Chikungunya and O'Nyong-Nyong are common in some parts of Africa and South America. To a lesser extent arbovirus infections also occur in Scandinavia (Ockelbo, Pogosta) and Australia (Ross River virus arthritis). In Europe and the USA parvovirus arthritis is the commonest viral joint disease, also associated with a transient rash, upper respiratory infection and malaise (erythema infectiosum, fifth disease). Arthritis following natural rubella is uncommon because of widespread vaccination but may follow vaccination itself. If viral arthritis is suspected hepatitis B infection must also be excluded. Usually joint involvement is polyarticular and symmetrical and carpal tunnel syndrome may develop. Symptoms generally subside within 3 weeks. Postvaccination arthritis may affect a single joint only and persist or recur. Lyme arthritis, named after the part of East Connecticut in which it was first identified, comprises a variable multisystem disease combined with transient asymmetrical oligarthritis. The causative agent is a spirochaete *Borrelia burgdorferi* which is transmitted by tick bites. The disease is only acquired therefore in areas where ticks of the genus *Ixodes* are endemic. The disease responds to antibiotic treatment.

Rheumatic fever is seen much less often today than previously. It is as well to remember that many other arthropathies may present in similar form, joints being successively affected and remitting rapidly, the so-called 'flitting pains' rippling round the locomotor system. Not only may rheumatoid arthritis present in this way, but also systemic lupus erythematosus, ankylosing spondylitis, Hodgkin's lymphoma, leukaemia, brucellosis and a number of other disorders. The heart is rarely seriously involved if rheumatic fever first occurs over the age of 17 years.

Jaccoud's arthritis is an extremely rare disorder following repeated attacks of rheumatic fever, characterized by ulnar deviation of the fingers and hyperextension of the proximal interphalangeal joints without bone destruction.

tion occurs in many other disorders and is not in itself diagnostic. The presence of tophi in ears or elsewhere suggests the diagnosis although the symptoms and signs are usually diagnostic. The only absolute proof is the identification of urate crystals from the affected joint under the polarizing microscope.

In some cases, suggestive of gout, intra-articular crystals turn out to be not urate but calcium pyrophosphate, the condition being *chondrocalcinosis articularis* or 'pseudogout'. This condition affects knees most commonly but other joints are also affected, often in symmetrical fashion, with the appearance of calcification in the joint cartilages. Acute inflammatory episodes occur also in chronic *renal failure* with deposition of calcium salts in the soft tissues alongside, rather than in, joints. This may also be seen in patients following

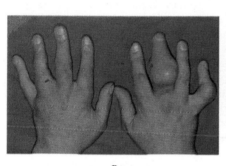
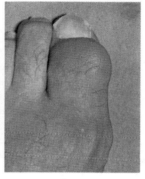
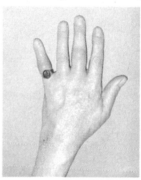

Fig. J.41. *a*, Severe tophaceous gout. *b*, Acute gout in big toe. *c*, Acute gout in middle and little fingers.

The arthropathy occurring after *prostatectomy*, and sometimes after gynaecological operations, affects hips particularly, the patient lying in great pain with hips partly flexed. On rising from his bed he may have to walk backwards as forward progression is too painful. The disorder is usually rapidly relieved by draining a pocket of fluid or infective material from behind the symphysis pubis; occasionally true osteitis pubis is present.

10. Metabolic arthropathies

The commonest of these is *gout*. This disorder is characterized by the sudden agonizing nature of the acute attack which is often so severe as to make the patient, almost always an adult male, feel he must have broken a bone in his foot, but for the fact that the disorder frequently starts in bed in the early morning about 5-6 a.m. There are usually clear signs of inflammation, the skin being tense, shiny, hot and red over the big toe metatarsophalangeal joint, ankle or hand, the first named being the commonest. Acute attacks may also occur in the knee (*Figs.* J.41–J.43). Although hyperuricaemia is usually present it is not invariably so, and an elevated plasma urate concentra-

renal transplantation from cadavers or living donors other than identical twins. Polyarthritis with effusions, often in the knees, may occur in these patients who may have rheumatoid factor in the blood.

In *calcinosis circumscripta*, calcium salts (carbonate and phosphate) may be deposited under the skin but they are again para-articular rather than in the joint tissues, which appear normal.

Amyloidosis may be secondary to rheumatoid arthritis, ankylosing spondylitis and (more rarely) Reiter's disease, but it may also occur in primary form associated with pains and swellings in joints and, when associated with multiple myeloma, may cause the carpal tunnel syndrome.

Joint symptoms and backache in particular occur in *ochronosis*. Here the diagnosis is made by examination of the urine for homogentisic acid and the cartilage of the ears for pigmentation. Radiographs of the spine are typical, heavy calcification occurring in the intervertebral cartilages (see p. 45).

Multicentric reticulohistiocytosis (lipoid dermato-arthritis) may be mistaken for rheumatoid arthritis in adults as changes in fingers and tenosynovitis occur, but the presence of yellow nodules on ears,

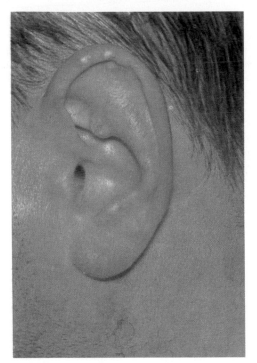

Fig. J.42. Typical tophi in ear. They are opaque on trans-illumination.

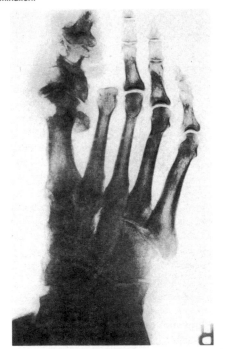

Fig. J.43. Severe destructive tophaceous gout. The second toe was even more severely affected and was removed.

forehead, neck, forearms and elsewhere, with groups of purple papules, suggests the true diagnosis which can be confirmed by biopsy. In advanced cases erosion of phalanges leads to shortening of the fingers.

In *Wilson's disease*, characterized by accumulation of copper in the tissues, arthritic changes, commonest in hands, wrists and knees, may start about the age of 30. Associated features are hepatic cirrhosis, psychiatric disease, and the Kayser–Fleischer green-brown ring around the cornea is diagnostic (*Fig*. J.10).

11. Vascular arthropathies

Avascular necrosis occurs in caisson disease (nitrogen or air embolism), from fat embolism, and occasionally in chronic alcoholism. The hips are often bilaterally involved with destruction of parts of the heads of the femurs but shoulders and one or both knees may also be affected.

Giant-cell arteritis and *polymyalgia rheumatica* are probably two facets of the same condition occurring in the elderly as, on existing evidence, both conditions are due to an arteritis of those vessels having an internal elastic lamina. Renal and cerebral vessels are therefore usually spared. The patients, usually over the age of 60, are of either sex, have marked morning stiffness, sedimentation rates up to 100 mm in the first hour (Westergren) and pains and stiffness of shoulder and hip girdles. When the temporal vessels are involved a splitting headache is often present, and the main danger is to vision if branches of the ophthalmic artery become affected. Pulses may disappear and murmurs be heard at the points of arterial narrowing. The sterno-clavicular joints may be affected, but the disorder, as far as the girdle joints in general are concerned, is one of pain and stiffness in hips and shoulders without progressive clinical or radiological change and eventually with full recovery. Diagnosis can be confirmed by arterial biopsy.

In *polyarteritis nodosa* arthralgia is much more common than actual arthritis, but any joint may be affected in any pattern, local or general, severe or mild, flitting or constant. The appearance of nodules clinches the diagnosis but these occur in only a minority of cases and many biopsies may have to be done before the diagnosis is confirmed. Eosinophilia occurs in about 15 per cent of cases. Bronchial spasm is among the more common manifestations elsewhere but it is the multisystem distribution of symptoms which may suggest the diagnosis. When asthma, allergic rhinitis and eosinophilia are present the term 'Churg–Strauss vasculitis' is used.

12. Neoplastic arthropathies

Metastatic malignant disease or *multiple myeloma* usually cause bony rather than joint changes. The serum alkaline phosphatase, often elevated in the former, is usually normal in the latter as there is no osteoblastic activity in myelomatosis. Joint changes

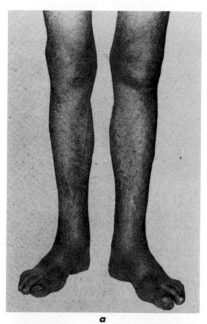

a

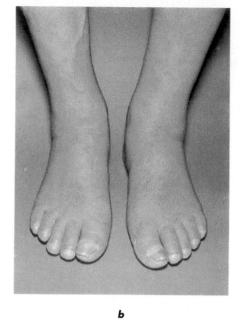

b

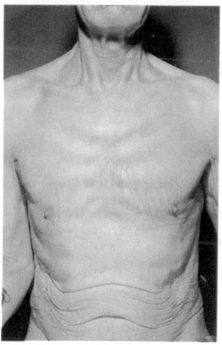

c

Fig. J.44. *a*, Hydrarthrosis of knees and swelling of ankles and feet due to bronchial carcinoma, causing pseudohypertrophic pulmonary osteoarthropathy. *b*, Swollen painful ankles in pseudohypertrophic pulmonary osteoarthropathy with *c*, wasting and loss of weight due to right basal bronchial carcinoma.

occur, however, in *hypertrophic pulmonary osteoarthropathy* (*Figs*. J.44, J.45), a condition mostly associated with a bronchial carcinoma, usually a peripheral one. Removal of the primary lesion leads to rapid resolution of the effusions and arthritic changes in the more commonly affected joints, the knees and ankles. Fingers and toes are clubbed and the extremities

show a thickening based on new subperiosteal bone deposition which can be seen in radiographs (*Fig*. J.46). Not all cases of hypertrophic osteoarthropathy are secondary to malignancy, however, some being due to cyanotic congenital heart disease, colonic and other conditions (*see* FINGERS, CLUBBED). In a familial primary form symptoms of *pachydermoperiostosis*

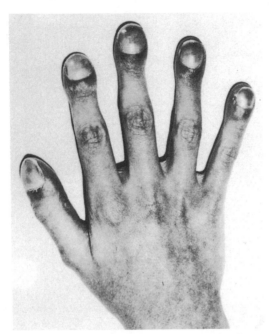
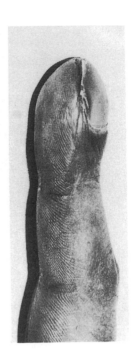

Fig. J.45. Pseudohypertrophic pulmonary osteoarthropathy, showing clubbed fingers.

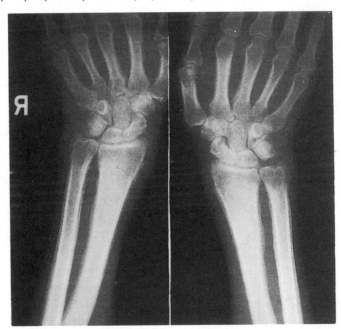

Fig. J.46. Pseudohypertrophic osteoarthropathy of the radius and ulna showing new periosteal bone deposition. (*Dr T. H. Hills.*)

start usually in adolescence, more commonly in males, the hands and feet enlarging with marked clubbing and cylindrical thickening of forearms and legs; recurrent joint effusions may occur. The patient's features thicken, giving a leonine appearance.

Osteoid osteoma is a benign disorder and, although not a disease of joints, it should be mentioned because of the pain it causes and the difficulties in

differential diagnosis. The pain is initially intermittent but becomes more persistent and severe and is often aggravated by movement. There are no physical signs. It affects adolescents and young adults and, although any bone except the skull may be affected, the commonest to be involved are femur and tibia, which account for half the cases. Radiographs show a characteristic central opacity surrounded by a translucent zone, surrounded in turn by a zone of sclerosis. It may affect the bones of the spine, where it is often very difficult to diagnose and is usually not suspected. The pains are sometimes worse at night than during the day.

loma and amyloidosis. There is also an idiopathic variety with no apparent cause. Characteristic symptoms are tingling and hot and cold electrical sensations up the arms, interfering with sleep.

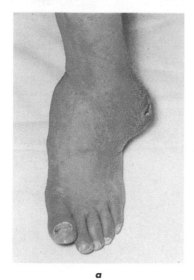
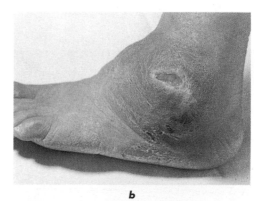

a

b

Fig. J.47. Charcot's disease of ankle showing disorganization of the joint (a) and gummatous ulcer (b). (Mr R. G. Beard.)

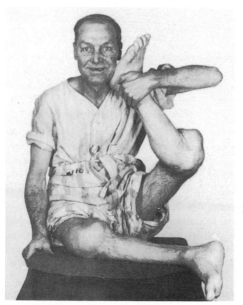

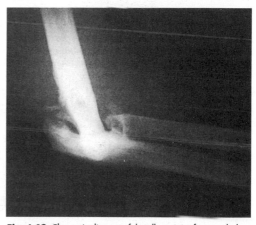

Fig. J.49. Charcot's disease of the elbow joint from pathological dislocation. (Dr T. H. Hills.)

Fig. J.48. Charcot's disease of the knee joints showing the extraordinary mobility arising from joint destruction. The absence of pain is evident from the facies. (Dr Ralph Kauntze.)

13. Neuropathic arthropathies

Although the *carpal tunnel syndrome* is not strictly a joint affection, it is so often a manifestation of rheumatoid arthritis that is should be mentioned. It is not infrequently the first sign of this disorder. Other causes are pregnancy, acromegaly, myxoedema, multiple mye-

Neuropathic joints (Figs. J.47–J.49). in the form of Charcot's joints in tabes dorsalis are characterized by their gross deformity, painlessness and florid X-ray appearances, where numbers of bone islands surround a grossly deformed or disorganized joint. Syringomyelia affects chiefly shoulder and elbow; knee, ankle, hip and spine are more commonly affected in tabes. Diabetic arthropathy is different in that clinical and radiological signs of infection are often present along with poor vascularization and signs of peripheral neuropathy; the condition is usually confined to the feet and toes.

Osborne's syndrome is due to ulnar nerve com-

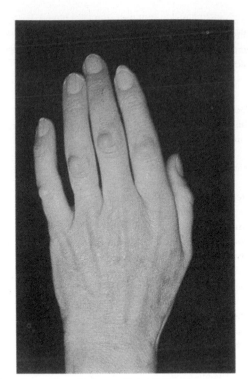

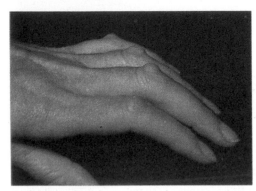

Fig. J.50. Extra-articular knuckle pads (Knobbly Knuckles, K.K. syndrome, Garrod's fatty or Hale White's nodes). They are fibrous, are not painful, and are only important in differential diagnosis from rheumatoid and osteoarthritic nodes.

pression beneath the arcuate ligament just below the elbow.

In the *shoulder–hand syndrome*, a reflex dystrophy, trophic changes follow soon after injury to the shoulder or weeks or months after myocardial infarction; a similar syndrome has been reported in patients on antituberculous therapy and in other pathological conditions. The shoulder is stiff and painful, the skin of the hand shiny and smooth and sometimes hyperaesthetic, the muscles atrophic. There is no joint swelling, though initially there may be considerable swelling of the whole hand and fingers. X-rays show initially osteoporosis of humeral head and wrist, later a more diffuse 'ground-glass' appearance. In many cases there is no apparent cause for the condition.

14. Drug-induced arthropathy

Alcoholics are especially likely to sustain injuries to bones and joints; they are also more prone to septic arthritis and avascular necrosis of bone. Prolonged *corticosteroid therapy* may also be associated with septic arthritis, osteoporosis, and fractures. Crush fractures of lumbar or dorsal vertebrae are not uncommon. A condition very similar to systemic lupus erythematosus with LE cells present in the blood can be due to a large range of drugs, the commonest being procaine amide; this is the so-called *hydralazine syndrome*.

Symptoms disappear on stopping the drug. It has also been reported with oral contraceptives, though such cases are very rare.

15. Miscellaneous arthropathies

The *knuckle pads* (Garrod's pads), seen not infrequently on the dorsal aspects of the proximal interphalangeal joints of the fingers (*Fig.* J.50), are usually not accompanied by any symptoms and are best disregarded. They are due to fibrous thickenings the size of small orange pips and are not part of the clinical picture of osteoarthritis or any other form of arthritis. They are not associated with any bony changes, though in some cases they occur with *Dupuytren's contracture* which, in turn, is occasionally associated with Peyronie's disease (induratio penis plastica). The palmar contractures occurring in rheumatoid arthritis may, on occasion, resemble Dupuytren's contracture (*see Fig.* J.38b). *Thorn synovitis* is an inflammatory condition due to a thorn or splinter of wood or a foreign body being knelt on by a child, who is hardly aware of it at the time. The *septic focus syndrome* is a rare disorder where diffuse aches and pains in and around joints are rapidly relieved by removal of a septic focus or drainage of an abscess. No residual changes are left in the tissues. Lastly, the *xiphoid syndrome* refers to pains which stem from a displaced or mobile xiphisternum, often the result of trauma. This simple condition is only noteworthy in that it may be mistaken for more serious disorders of stomach, duodenum, gall bladder or heart.

Joint disease in young children

The following conditions should be considered when children under 5 years of age present with joint symptoms.

In joint affections in early childhood under 5 years of age consider:

Septic arthritis: due to staphylococci, haemolytic streptococci, *H. influenzae*, tuberculosis).

Associated with or *following* infection: adenovirus, rubella, mumps, chickenpox, *Mycoplasma pneumoniae*, cytomegalovirus, rickettsia, Lyme arthritis, Kawasaki's syndrome.

Idiopathic: chronic juvenile arthritis (Still's disease), familial Mediterranean fever.

Vascular and haematological: Henoch–Schönlein syndrome, sickle-cell disease, leukaemia, haemophilia, haemangioma, hypogammaglobulinaemia.

Dietetic: rickets.

Miscellaneous: Farber's disease, the mucopolysaccharidoses (e.g. Hurler–Scheie syndrome), injuries (the battered child syndrome), neuroblastoma, thorn synovitis.

INFECTIVE (SEPTIC CONDITIONS)

Infection in infancy

Staphylococcal infection is common, but many organisms may be responsible. The infant is ill, often rejecting food, vomiting or convulsing, but sometimes only mildly ill with slight fever. The hip is the most common joint to be affected and is held flexed and adducted, oedema appearing around the adductors.

1-5 Years of age

Haemophilus influenzae infection is common in Great Britain. If several joints are affected suspect hypogammaglobulinaemia or some other immune abnormality. Staphylococcal, haemolytic streptococcal and, more rarely, tuberculous infection should be considered.

INFECTIONS

Other infections with adenoviruses often start with pharyngitis followed a few days later by fever, macular erythematous rash and a symmetrical arthritis which lasts up to 6 weeks. A similar transient arthropathy may occur with rubella, mumps and chickenpox. Infection with cytomegalovirus is often associated with abnormal tests of liver function and infection with *Mycoplasma pneumoniae* with erythema multiforme. Other infec-

tions not seen in the UK unless imported are rickettsial infections such as Rocky Mountain Spotted Fever or Lyme arthritis where a small red macule or papule enlarges to form a large erythematous ring followed by fever and arthritis, usually of only a few joints. In Japan and the East, Kawasaki's syndrome should be considered a possibility.

NON-INFECTIVE INFLAMMATORY CONDITIONS

Juvenile chronic arthritis often presents under 5 years of age (*see* p. 348). If of inflammatory onset it has to be distinguished from the infective conditions above.

Andrew Keat

Keloid

A keloid is a benign but uncontrolled fibrous overgrowth of the dermis in response to wounding. The tendency to form keloids is a personal trait, more common in blacks, young adults and in the stretched skin of neck and chest. Usually the antecedent damage is obvious, e.g. surgical incisions, pierced ear lobes (*Fig.* K.1), burns and chickenpox. Keloids may follow acne and folliculitis, chiefly on the chest (*Fig.* K.2)

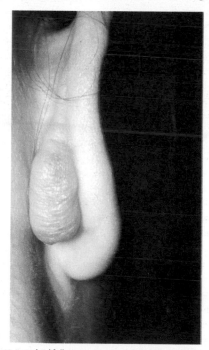

Fig. K.1. Keloid following ear piercing. (*Westminster Hospital.*)

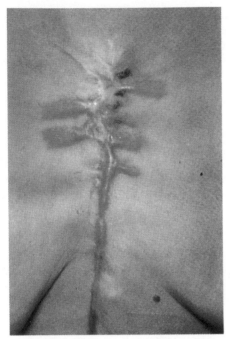

Fig. K.2. Keloid following cardiac surgery. (*Westminster Hospital.*)

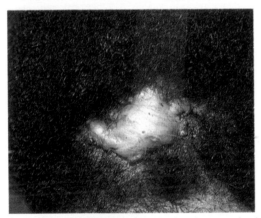

Fig. K.3. Keloid folliculitis on back of neck. (*Dr Richard Staughton.*)

and at the back of the neck (*Fig.* K.3), where ingrowing hairs may be a perpetuating factor. Keloids commonly recur following an excision unless intralesional steroids are injected at the time of operation or radiotherapy is administered during the postoperative period.

Richard Staughton

Kidney, palpable

A renal swelling may be so slight that it is only found upon clinical examination, or it may be large enough to attract the patient's attention. Hydronephrosis, pyonephrosis, renal tuberculosis or abscess, new growth or cysts (single or multiple) in the kidney have to be diagnosed not only from one another but also from other tumours simulating a renal swelling. The characteristic points of a renal tumour are:

1. The *intestine is in front of the tumour*. When either kidney is merely slightly enlarged, both large and small intestines will be in front of it; but when the organ is so enlarged as to reach the anterior abdominal wall the coils of small intestine are pushed aside. The anatomical relation of the large intestine to the kidney, and the absence of a mesentery, do not allow of the same mobility of the colon, which usually retains its position in front of the kidney, although it is sometimes pushed downwards by a tumour projecting forwards from the lower pole. Hence an area of resonance can usually be obtained in front of a renal swelling; if the colon is empty it can sometimes be felt in a thin subject and rolled by the fingers on the surface of the tumour. Bowel is almost never placed in front of a splenic tumour, and only rarely in front of a hepatic tumour.

2. The *area of dullness to percussion* is continuous from the lateral aspect of the swelling to the midline posteriorly—that is, there is no area of resonance between the mass and the vertebral spines, as with a splenic or ovarian tumour.

3. A renal tumour usually *retains the shape of the kidney*; it is rounded at its borders and poles, and does not possess any edge or sharp margin, as do splenic or hepatic swellings (*Fig.* K.4). The surface of the tumour may present rounded, smooth, raised bosses in cases of renal growths or in polycystic disease.

4. A *renal tumour* in the process of enlargement *projects forwards and downwards*. It may fill up the natural hollow of the loin, but seldom causes any prominence posteriorly. A perinephric abscess, which often simulates a renal swelling, may cause a distinct prominence in the loin.

5. A renal tumour may be movable downwards or inwards, unless it is fixed in the loin by preceding inflammation, or by the spread of carcinoma into the perirenal tissues; an enlarged kidney may be felt bimanually, and if grasped between the two hands *can be pushed into the loin*. A renal tumour rarely descends into the iliac fossa but it may be present there in congenital ectopia or in cases of excessive mobility.

6. When a renal tumour is large enough to reach the anterior abdominal wall it commonly comes in contact with it at the level of the umbilicus, at the same time bulging out the iliocostal space. There is usually a line of resonance between the upper margin of the tumour and the hepatic dullness.

7. A *varicocele* may be developed on the same side as the renal tumour due to obstruction of the

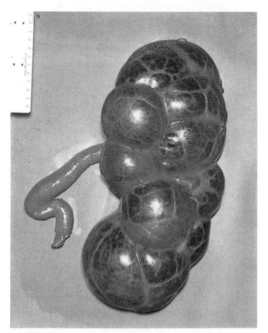

Fig. K.4. Enormous hydronephrosis due to small stone impacted in the distal ureter. The kidney was so large that it could readily be felt on rectal as well as abdominal examination, yet it has retained its reniform shape.

testicular vein as this drains into the renal vein on the left or the inferior vena cava on the right. This is especially significant on the right side, although it is a rare finding, and I have personally never seen a renal tumour associated with a rapidly developing varicocele due to involvement of the testicular vein.

8. With a renal tumour there may be *changes in the urine* pointing to renal disease; but on the other hand, the urine at any one time may be normal, free from blood or pus, from the fact that the ureter of the diseased side is blocked, or that the disease does not involve the renal pelvis.

9. In exceptional cases, a tumour of the right kidney may extend upwards towards the dome of the diaphragm, rotating the liver so that the anterior margin of the latter descends below the costal margin, and prevents satisfactory palpation of the renal areas.

Although, from the above physical characters, it would seem that a renal tumour should present little difficulty in diagnosis, yet it is by no means infrequent to find that a tumour possessing several of these characters may give rise to considerable doubt in the determination of the organ from which it arises. The following points will assist in the diagnosis of renal swellings from other tumours with which they are likely to be confused.

1. Enlargements of the gallbladder

These are placed immediately below the costal margin, so that no interval exists between the tumour and the

lower margin of the liver. They are usually oval in outline, with the long axis in the line between the 9th right costal cartilage and the umbilicus, are freely movable with the respiratory movements, and movable from side to side about an axis at the costal margin. There is dullness on percussion over them, and they cannot be felt in the loin or be grasped bimanually. With an enlarged gallbladder there may be attacks of colic, with or without jaundice. A good radiograph may show the outline of a distended gallbladder distinct from the shadow of the kidney, and gallstones may sometimes be seen, while a cholecystographic examination will show that no contrast medium enters the gallbladder. Ultrasonography is a particularly valuable non-invasive method of demonstrating the distended gallbladder and will also show up gallstones, which are highly echogenic.

2. Enlargements of the liver

These pass downwards from beneath the costal margin so that there is no line or resonance, or area in which the hand can be depressed, between the tumour and the costal margin. Hepatic tumours do not impair the normal resonance in the loin in the same manner as a renal tumour does. A tongue-shaped lobe of the liver (Riedel's lobe) may cause difficulty in diagnosis; but here the lower margin is seldom so rounded as is that of a renal tumour, nor will the mass be felt in the loin on bimanual examination. A tumour or cyst in the concave aspect, or of the left lobe, of the liver is especially liable to cause error in diagnosis, whereas, on the other hand, a tumour of the right kidney which projects upwards behind the liver may so rotate the latter that its anterior margin descends below the costal margin and completely obscures the kidney. In a case of a large carcinoma of the right kidney, the liver may in this way be so depressed as to render palpation of the kidney impossible. A pyelographic examination may reveal a normal renal picture or on the other hand may indicate a hydronephrosis or renal growth. Ultrasonography will readily differentiate between a hepatic and a renal swelling.

3. Enlargements of the spleen

These descend from beneath the left costal margin, and have no bowel in front of them, they are therefore dull to percussion. The edge of a splenic tumour is usually well defined and often notched and there is resonance between the posterior aspect of the tumour and the spinal column. A splenic tumour is more movable than is a left renal tumour. A blood count may help in deciding in favour of a splenic enlargement, and a pyelogram may show a normal kidney.

4. Perinephric effusions

Whether of blood, pus or urine, these may form a tumour in the loin which upon physical examination may be mistaken for a renal swelling. A perinephric effusion may arise from some suppurative condition of the kidney, so that the previous history and examination of the urine will not assist in differential; or it may be due to conditions entirely distinct from renal disease. An effusion of blood around the kidney is, in nearly all cases, caused by an injury to the loin, and will be accompanied by other signs of injury. It may, however, occur from the spontaneous growth and rupture of a renal neoplasm. A perinephric abscess forms a less well-defined tumour than that caused by a renal swelling, is more acute in its general symptoms, such as pain and temperature, and fills up the iliocostal space. The skin over it may be thickened or oedematous, and fluctuation may be felt to be more superficial than in a renal swelling. A perinephric abscess may result from suppuration about a carcinoma or diverticulum of the large bowel, from appendiceal inflammation, or from suppuration in a perinephric haematoma due to injury; it may be a sequel to a specific blow, or be due to a haematogenous infection. Bilateral palpation and comparison of the loins may detect a perinephric swelling by the way the loin is filled out and becomes even convex on the affected side. This is best seen by laying the patient prone and carefully inspecting both sides. A high leucocyte count in the blood with increased percentage of polymorphonuclear cells would be in favour of perinephric inflammation.

5. Tumours arising from the pelvic organs

Tumours arising from the pelvic organs, from the ovary or uterus, may in some cases simulate renal tumours. An ovarian cyst with a long pedicle occupying the loin may be mistaken for an enlarged or movable kidney, and any sudden attacks of pain occurring from torsion of the pedicle may be looked upon as due to renal colic. The usual ovarian cyst or uterine fibroid will seldom be confused with a renal swelling, for it is placed in the midline of the body, can be felt to come up from the pelvis, and can be felt on bimanual vaginal examination to be attached to the uterus or its appendages. These tumours give rise to dullness anteriorly, and do not alter the normal resonance in the loin. In cases of malignant ovarian tumours associated with ascites the lumbar resonance may be lost, but on turning the patient over on one side the previously dull note becomes replaced by resonance in the uppermost loin. In the case of an ovarian cyst with a long pedicle, or of a uterine fibroid of pedunculated,

subserous form, the position in the loin may sometimes suggest a renal tumour; it will be found, however, to occupy a more anterior position in the abdomen than a renal tumour, and to possess a much greater range of movement, and it does not slip back into the loin under the costal margin in the same manner as an enlarged kidney does; there is resonance posteriorly, the kidney may be actually palpated as well as the abdominal tumour, while a distinct connection with the pelvic organs can sometimes be traced from the tumour when the latter is drawn up.

In contradistinction to the above a very large cystic renal swelling may be mistaken for an ovarian cyst. It may occupy the greater part of the abdomen, and even be felt per vaginam to be encroaching upon the pelvis; but on careful examination of a renal tumour of this form there will be no line of resonance between the mass and the vertebral column posteriorly, the natural hollow of the loin will be filled up, and there is frequently a distinct bulging in the lower thoracic wall, together with an increased length of the iliocostal space on the affected side. Some assistance may be obtained from the history; a hydronephrosis may have been first noticed as a tumour starting under the costal margin and gradually increasing downwards towards the iliac fossa and inwards across the median line, whereas an ovarian tumour may have been noticed to increase upwards from the pelvis. With an ovarian or pelvic tumour, a pyelogram will show a normal renal pelvis. Ultrasonography usually enables accurate anatomical diagnosis of the pelvic mass.

6. Suprarenal tumours

Suprarenal tumours may occasionally be of sufficient size to form an abdominal tumour, presenting a rounded, movable swelling in the hypochondrium. It is sometimes possible to distinguish them from renal tumours by radiography after presacral insufflation of oxygen into the retroperitoneal tissue (*see* p. 368), or, more certainly and with far less disturbance to the patient, by computerized tomography.

7. Faecal accumulation in the colon, caecum or sigmoid flexure

These may give rise to a tumour and pain of a colicky nature in the loin; the tumour can sometimes be indented by the examining fingers. They will be distinguished from renal swellings by the general intestinal symptoms, flatulence and the changes in form consequent on the administration of large enemas. A patient with a collection of faeces in the colon may not complain of constipation, but may in fact have a small daily evacuation from the overloaded bowel.

8. Appendicular inflammatory mass

This will be diagnosed from renal tumours by the situation of the pain and by the swelling being in the iliac fossa rather than in the loin. In some cases, however, the pain may be referred to the lumbar region, or an appendiceal inflammatory mass may spread upwards. This is especially so when the appendix is retrocaecal in position. The onset of the trouble, the acute symptoms, and the febrile disturbance will usually distinguish these cases from renal lesions.

9. Malignant growth of the large intestine

Malignant growth of the large intestine, especially of the ascending or descending colon, may form a tumour in the loin which closely resembles a renal swelling. The mass formed by the growth may be grasped bimanually, is movable in the same directions as a renal tumour, and comes forward under the costal margin. The percussion note over the front of the lump is resonant, and there is usually an aching pain in the loin. If the growth has infiltrated through the wall of the bowel uncovered by peritoneum, the perirenal tissues may be thickened, or proteinuria may be produced by direct invasion of the kidney, when the case will even more resemble a renal lesion. Carcinoma of the large intestine should be suspected if there is any irregularity in the action of the bowels, mucus or blood in the motions, or any symptom of incipient obstruction in the intestine. The tumour may be irregular and nodular, whereas a renal tumour presents rounded margins. The occurrence of a tumour in either side, associated with discomfort or palpable distension of the caecum from the accumulation of faeces, would render a growth in the colon the more suspicious.

The diagnosis of a large bowel tumour can usually be established by a barium enema X-ray examination. Confirmation can be made by direct colonoscopic examination, at which, usually, biopsy material can be obtained for histological examination.

10. Tumours of the omentum, mesentery or pancreas

These tumours, either cystic or malignant, are more median in position, do not project into the loin and seldom resemble a renal tumour. Retroperitoneal and perirenal tumours may closely simulate renal tumours but can be distinguished on pyelography; they displace the ureter medially or laterally.

In many cases in which difficulty arises in the diagnosis of a swelling in the loin, great help may be obtained by excretion urography (p. 370) or by retrograde pyelography by the injection into the renal pelvis and calices of a medium opaque to X-rays, through a ureteric catheter. By these means the renal pelvis and calices may be outlined clearly in their normal position, and any change in position or shape may indicate that the swelling is of renal origin. The detailed anatomy of these masses can usually be demonstrated by computerized axial tomography.

THE DIFFERENTIAL DIAGNOSIS OF RADIOGRAPHIC SHADOWS IN THE ABDOMEN AND THE PELVIS

It is necessary for the true interpretation of radiographs that a clear conception should be held of the various conditions which may cast a shadow on an X-ray negative. In the diagnosis of cases of urinary disease much information may be gained by the use of X-rays, and not merely in the confirmation of the presence of calculi in some part of the urinary tract; in a good film the outline and the size of the kidney can be seen, while, by means of excretion urography or by the direct injection of the ureter and the pelvis of the kidney with a radio-opaque solution, the size, position and shape of either may be outlined accurately and compared with the normal (*Figs.* K.5, K.6). In a good film after efficient alimentary preparation the outline of a normal kidney should be visible, lying opposite the bodies of the 1st, 2nd and 3rd lumbar vertebrae (*Fig.* K.5), and having an excursion of from 4 to 5 cm in forced inspiration and expiration. A *renal calculus*

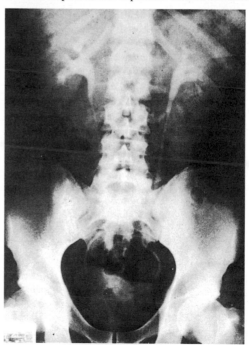

Fig. K.5. Normal excretion pyelogram, 30-minute film after removal of compression. The calices are cupped, the left ureter is filled completely and the right partially.

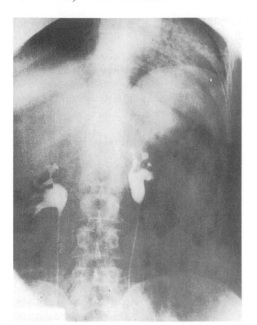

Fig. K.6. Retrograde pyelogram. The right kidney is normal. On the left the calices are clubbed and the pelvis dilated from the presence of a calculus, which is hidden by the contrast medium.

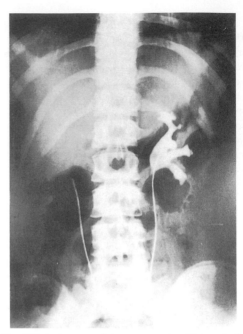

Fig. K.8. Pyelogram outlining a pure uric acid stone in the left kidney. It gave no shadow on the plain film.

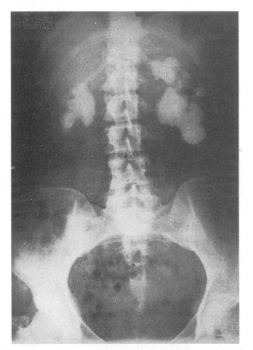

Fig. K.7. Radiograph showing bilateral renal calculi. On the left the dendritic stone forms a cast of the renal pelvis and calices.

(*Figs*. K.6, K.7) in a radiograph casts a shadow superimposed upon the renal shadow. If it is of triangular or branched outline, it is almost certainly a renal calculus; but others may give a shadow of even, uniform density, of sharp outline, yet clearly renal as shown by the

manner in which the opacity moves equally with the renal shadow in respiratory movements. In a film taken laterally through the transverse axis of the patient, a renal calculus should make a shadow superimposed upon the bodies of the upper lumbar vertebrae, usually the 2nd, unless the kidney is enlarged, when the shadow of a calculus may be displaced in front of the vertebral bodies. A stone composed of pure uric acid may give no shadow on a radiograph; one of calcium oxalate gives the most dense shadow; next in order of density is the phosphatic; those of urates, cystine and xanthine give a less definite shadow. A radiolucent stone may, however, be shown as a negative shadow in an excretion or retrograde pyelogram; it must be distinguished from a tumour of the renal pelvis, an air bubble or blood clot. In the case of a stone the contrast medium is more likely to surround the shadow completely (*Fig*. K.8) whilst a tumour will be attached at some point (*Fig*. K.9). Blood clot is irregular and an air bubble can be displaced in a second radiograph.

The shape of a shadow in the renal area will often indicate its position in the kidney and an excretion pyelogram will confirm it (*Fig*. K.10). There are, however, several other conditions which may cast a shadow in the renal area, and it is necessary to differentiate these from the shadow of a renal calculus. The following are the most frequent:

1. Intestinal contents
2. Calcification of mesenteric lymph nodes
3. Gallstones, on the right side
4. Calcification of the costal cartilages

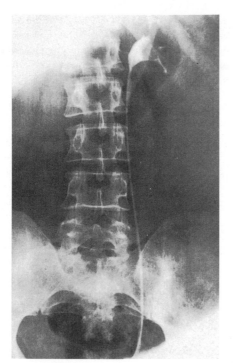

Fig. K.9. Pyelogram showing a benign tumour in the left renal pelvis.

5. Caseous masses in a tuberculous kidney
6. Areas of calcification in a renal growth
7. Foreign bodies

1. INTESTINAL CONTENTS may cast a shadow in the renal area owing to inefficient preparation of the patient or to the fact that he has recently taken as medicine bismuth, magnesium salts, etc. If any doubt exists a second examination should be made after further purgation. There may be some residue in the intestine from a recent barium-meal examination.

2. CALCIFICATION OF THE ABDOMINAL OR MESENTERIC LYMPH NODES may cause a shadow in any part of the abdominal cavity. Though they are most frequently seen near the lower lumbar vertebrae or about the sacroiliac joint, and therefore external to the renal shadow, they may be superimposed upon the latter and cause difficulty in diagnosis. The shadow of a calcified node is usually mottled in appearance, small areas in the shadow showing increased density owing to the irregular deposition of lime salts; calcareous nodes are frequently multiple, but their chief characteristic is their range of mobility. Thus if more than one negative is taken with varying degrees of compression the shadows of calcareous nodes may show a varying position with regard to the renal shadow, whilst in a lateral view a lymph node shadow is usually in front of the bodies of the vertebrae and not superimposed upon them. A calcified node may be placed immediately in front of the kidney and move equally with it, causing great difficulty in diagnosis; or there may be a calculus in one kidney and calcareous nodes imitating calculi on the other side.

A pyelogram will show the relation of a calculus to the renal pelvis (*Fig.* K.10).

3. GALLSTONES may give a shadow in the renal area on the right side. They are frequently multiple, and may be seen to be faceted in a fusiform collection

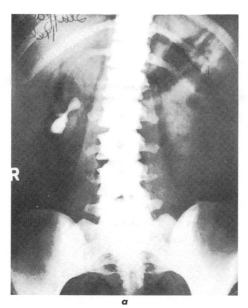

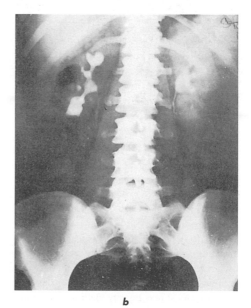

a *b*

Fig. K.10. *a.* Radiograph showing a dumb-bell shadow in the right renal area. *b.* The excretion pyelogram shows that the shadow is a stone occupying the lowest calix and pelvis of the right kidney.

presenting the shape of the distended gallbladder (*Fig.* K.11). A single gallstone superimposed on the renal shadow may cause difficulty; the shadow of a gallstone is less dense than is that of a renal stone, and is frequently more dense in the central than in the peripheral part. In a lateral view a stone in the gallbladder will occupy an anterior position in the abdomen, though one impacted in the common bile duct may be seen opposite the body of the 1st or 2nd lumbar vertebra; in this case there will probably be jaundice. In a cholecystographic examination a gallstone may cause a filling defect (negative shadow) in the area of the gallbladder occupied by the dye. The distribution of stones in a horseshoe kidney may cause confusion until a pyelogram is done (*Fig.* K.12).

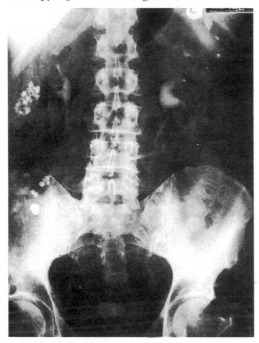

Fig. K.11. Intravenous pyelogram showing also a collection of faceted stones in the gallbladder, calcified mesenteric glands in the right iliac fossa and phleboliths in the pelvis.

4. CALCIFICATION OF THE COSTAL CARTILAGES may give a shadow in the renal area in an anteroposterior negative. The shadows are not dense, are hazy in outline, and tend to assume a horizontal or oblique axis. In a lateral view they will be placed immediately under the anterior abdominal wall.

5. CASEOUS MASSES IN A TUBERCULOUS KIDNEY. The shadow in this condition is rarely so defined as is that of a calculus, is of moderate density with blurred and indistinct margins, appearing as one or more blotches in the renal area; but occasionally, from the deposition of calcium salts, it may be very like the radiograph of a calculus (*see* Fig. H.5).

6. CALCAREOUS AREAS IN A RENAL CARCINOMA.

Rarely faint ill-defined areas may be present in a renal carcinoma. There will, however, be symptoms of growth, such as haematuria and renal tumour, whilst a pyelographic examination will show a deformity of the pelvis and renal calices.

7. A FOREIGN BODY, such as a shrapnel bullet, lying in front of or behind the kidney may mimic a calculus.

The line of the *normal ureter* lies anatomically along or just internal to the tips of the transverse processes of the 2nd to the 5th lumbar vertebrae, passes with a slight curve outwards in front of the sacro-iliac articulation, and then with a marked curve forwards and inwards to the base of the bladder. A shadow in this line may be due to a calculus in the ureter, but it must be differentiated carefully from other conditions. A calculus is usually small, rounded or oval, with a long axis in the line of the ureter. It may be found in any part of the course of the ureter, but it is seen most frequently in the lower end just before it enters the bladder. The conditions which may give a shadow that is likely to be mistaken for a ureteric calculus are:

1. Calcified lymph node
2. A concretion in the appendix or the intestinal contents
3. Phleboliths in the pelvis
4. A foreign body

1. CALCIFIED LYMPH NODES in the line of the ureter are placed most frequently in the angle between the last lumbar vertebra and the ala of the sacrum. They are usually multiple, forming a group in this situation in triangular form rather than in the longitudinal axis of the ureter; they are mottled in appearance, of irregular density, and are so movable that their position varies in successive radiographs. Should difficulty arise, the examination should be repeated after a radio-opaque catheter has been passed into the ureter by means of a cystoscope. In many cases a stereoscopic examination of the area with a catheter in the ureter or a radiograph by the 'double-shift' technique in which two exposures are made on the same film, the tube being moved laterally before the second exposure is made, will show that the suspicious shadow is some distance from the ureter. A catheter may often be passed up the ureter alongside and pass a calculus in the duct, but a stereoscopic examination will show that the two are actually in contact with each other.

2. A CONCRETION IN THE APPENDIX may occasionally give rise to a shadow in the line of the right ureter, suggesting a calculus with very similar clinical symptoms. Further examination with a radio-opaque catheter in the ureter will show that the shadow is extra-ureteric.

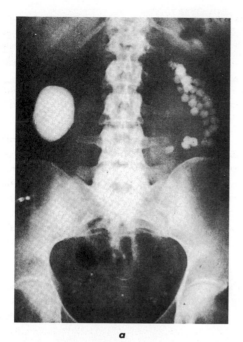

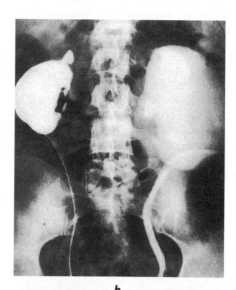

a

b

Fig. K.12. *a.* Large single dense shadow on the right and multiple small ones on the left. *b.* Pyelography shows that the shadows are enclosed in the dilated pelves of a horseshoe kidney. Note the inwardly pointing calices and the flower-vase pattern of the ureters.

3. PHLEBOLITHS IN THE PELVIS are liable to be mistaken for ureteric calculi, but they often have a characteristic ring-like appearance, which is quite diagnostic. They are usually multiple and are placed towards the peripheral areas of the pelvis, often about the level of the ischial spine. A stereoscopic examination with an opaque catheter in the ureter will differentiate them from calculi, though it may not be possible to distinguish them from calcified lymph nodes. It must not be forgotten that a calculus may be present in the ureter in addition to phleboliths, but the distinction can be made by excretion pyelography or radiography after the passage of a ureteric catheter. *Fig. K.13* shows that the shadow of the ureter does not impinge on any of the numerous phleboliths present in the pelvis.

4. FOREIGN BODIES, especially after periods of war, may occasionally lie near the line of the ureter. They are usually more dense than calculi.

A shadow may be present in a pelvic radiograph which must be differentiated from that of a vesical calculus. The latter is usually rounded or oval, occupies a fairly central position in the pelvis, and may show rings of varying density owing to the deposition of layers of urinary salts of different composition. Occasionally one or more vesical calculi may form a shadow in a more lateral position in successive negatives, when a suspicion of their presence in a diverticulum in the bladder will arise. The diagnosis of this condition is

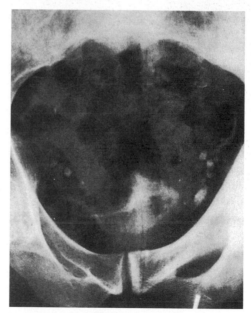

Fig. K.13. Excretion pyelogram showing numerous phleboliths in the pelvis; the left ureter is seen passing between them. Note the 'bite' defect in the bladder caused by a solid carcinoma.

discussed below. The following conditions may give rise to radiographic shadows in the pelvis.

1. Prostatic calculi
2. Calcification of a uterine fibroid
3. Opaque masses in a dermoid cyst of the ovary
4. Phosphatic encrustation upon a vesical growth

5. Foreign bodies in the bladder
6. Urethral calculi

1. PROSTATIC CALCULI may be single or multiple, but in the radiograph they occupy a position very low in the pelvis, often behind the shadow of the pubis (*Fig*. K.14). They would not be seen by a cystoscope, but might be felt during the passage of any instrument through the prostatic urethra. They are palpable in the gland per rectum, either as a hard, inelastic nodule embedded in the prostate, or by the grating of multiple calculi on each other on pressure.

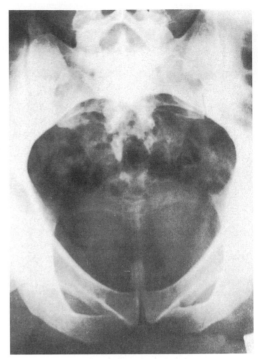

Fig. K.15. Radiograph showing a shadow due to a cystine calculus in the prostatic urethra.

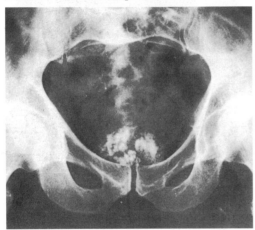

Fig. K.14. Radiograph showing shadows in the pelvis due to multiple prostatic calculi.

2. CALCIFICATION OF A FIBROID TUMOUR OF THE UTERUS gives a large, irregular shadow of varying degree of density. Bimanual palpation of a tumour moving with the uterus would point to the diagnosis.

3. OVARIAN DERMOIDS may give rise to irregular shadows in the pelvis due to the formation of bone or teeth in the cyst. They may be present in young adult life, and a tumour would be palpated on abdominal or pelvic examination.

4. PHOSPHATIC ENCRUSTATION UPON A VESICAL TUMOUR may occur in a case of growth in the presence of cystitis and give rise to faint ill-defined shadows in the pelvic radiograph. A cystoscopic examination will reveal the true nature of the lesion.

5. FOREIGN BODIES in the bladder may become so encrusted with urinary salts that a shadow like that of a calculus may be present. A variety of foreign bodies have been found in the bladder, either introduced by intent or by the accidental breaking off of a piece of catheter or the like. In some cases the shadow will show a central area of different density or even a metallic nucleus.

6. URETHRAL CALCULI may be retained in the canal behind a stricture and enlarge *in situ*. They form a shadow in a radiograph above or below the pubic arch (*Fig*. K.15).

Imaging techniques

Much assistance in the diagnosis of urinary disease apart from the presence of calculi may be afforded by means of imaging techniques (radiology, ultrasonography and computerized tomography), supplemented by methods used by the urologist. A good plain film taken in a thin subject may show the outline and size of the kidneys so plainly that one of them may be demonstrated to be enlarged, or the irregularity of outline may give rise to a suspicion of malignant growth. Methods have been devised by which more information may be gained—for example, by the injection of gas into the presacral tissues or by direct introduction into the renal pelvis, calices and ureter of radio-opaque solutions, or by the injection into the circulation of radio-opaque dye which is excreted by the kidneys, or by the injection of such substances into the aorta.

Presacral gas insufflation consists of distending the fatty tissue around the kidney with oxygen, CO_2 or air; by this method a more distinct outline of the kidney is obtained. The injection is made into the retroperitoneal tissues in the presacral hollow. The outline of the kidneys can usually be clearly demonstrated and sometimes that of the liver and spleen. The method is harmless and usually painless. Nowadays this technique has been almost entirely replaced by ultrasound scanning or computerized axial tomography, which, in turn, may be superseded by nuclear magnetic resonance scanning.

The injection of radio-opaque solutions into the renal pelvis and ureter, combined with radiography (*retrograde pyelography* and *ureterography*), has a wide application and renders more precise information than can be obtained by the perirenal insufflation method; the two investigations can be successfully combined. A dilute solution of 25 per cent sodium diatrizoate ('Hypaque') or 35 per cent meglumine iothalamate, the drug used for excretion urography, is used. For this method of pyelography (the 'ascending pyelogram') a ureteric catheter is passed by means of the cystoscope through the ureteric orifice; the solution is injected very slowly by means of a small syringe or allowed to run in by gravitation until the patient begins to feel discomfort in the loin, an accurate measure of the amount of fluid injected being recorded. The pelvis of the normal kidney will hold an average of 6 ml before pain is produced. A radiograph is taken immediately, when an exact outline of the renal pelvis and calices is displaced as a dense shadow (*Figs.* K.6, K.16). In cases of renal distension a much larger amount can be injected before pain is produced (*Figs.* K.17–K.19).

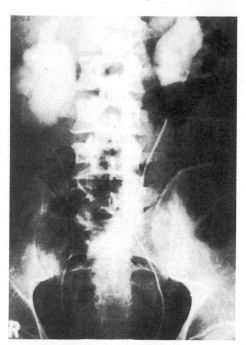

Fig. K.17. Retrograde pyelogram in a case of bilateral hydronephrosis associated with pelvi-ureteric obstruction.

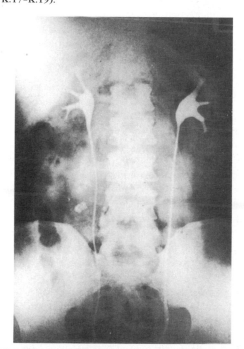

Fig. K.16. A normal bilateral retrograde pyelogram.

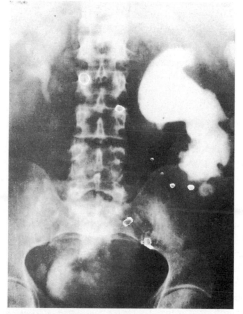

Fig. K.18. An excretion pyelogram showing a giant calculus in the left kidney. Note the filling defect in the bladder caused by a large papillary tumour.

The determination of a normal renal pelvis by radiography has also aided the diagnosis in many cases of doubtful abdominal tumours in which the clinical data have raised a suspicion of renal disease. There may be doubt as to whether a tumour palpable in the abdomen and causing pain in the loin is a renal tumour or whether it originates in the colon, gallbladder, pancreas or suprarenal gland. Examination by pyelography may demonstrate a normal renal pelvis which would in many cases exclude any disease of the kidney.

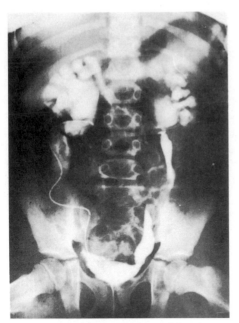

Fig. K.19. Retrograde pyelogram showing bilateral congenital hydro-ureter and hydronephrosis in a girl.

To obtain a radiograph of the ureter it is advisable to pass a ureteric catheter with an acorn tip only a short distance into the ureter before making the injection; in this way any dilatation or deviation from the normal line of the ureter is demonstrated, whereas the passage of the catheter along the whole length of the canal might straighten out the latter. In some cases the passage of the catheter may be obstructed in the ureter; in these the injection should be made with the catheter in situ, when the fluid may find its way past the obstruction and radiography may show a dilated or tortuous ureter (*Fig.* K.19) with dilatation of the pelvis of the kidney.

Occasionally a radiographic picture of the bladder is required to determine the size of a diverticulum, the vesical opening of which has been found on cystoscopy. For this purpose the same type and concentration of dye is used as in retrograde pyelography. Radiographs are then taken in both the anteroposterior and the oblique planes; it is also of advantage to repeat the exposures after the patient has voluntarily voided the vesical contents, when the diverticulum may be seen to remain filled with the solution.

Excretion urography is a method of pyelography consisting of the *intravenous injection* of non-toxic fluids of high iodine content and depends upon the excretion of the radio-opaque solution by the kidney. For this purpose 40–60 ml of 45 per cent sodium diatrizoate ('Hypaque') or meglumine iothalamate 60 per cent is injected into a vein after the patient has abstained from drinking any liquid for at least 6 hours.

Radiographs are then taken at intervals of 1, 5, 15 and 30 minutes after the injection. In cases in which the kidneys are of normal efficiency, a distinct shadow should be obtained of the renal pelvis and calices of each side in the first picture, increasing in definition in the second (*Fig.* K.5). The outlines of the ureters may be seen and in the later pictures the bladder is outlined in the pelvis. This test differs from the ascending method in being dependent upon the functional efficiency of the kidney; if this is impaired the test may fail to show any shadow owing to lack of excretion of the fluid, and therefore it may be used as a test of function as well as a radiographic test. The simplicity of the method has much to recommend it, but it must be said that the outlines of the renal pelvis and calices may be indistinct, and insufficient to rely upon for accurate diagnosis, in which case it has to be sometimes supplemented by the ascending method. In cases in which there is obstruction to the ureter, dilatation of the latter and of the renal pelvis may be distinctly seen. In cases of vesical tumour a distinct filling defect may be seen in the bladder in the later negatives (*Fig.* K.13). Compression of the lower ends of the ureters by a pneumatic belt and pads suitably placed after the first pictures have been taken improves the definition and filling even more.

Aortography is done by the translumbar route or by catheterization of the femoral artery (Seldinger's method). In the translumbar method 20–30 ml of 60 per cent meglumine iothalamate are injected directly into the upper part of the abdominal aorta in order to outline the renal vascular system. It is carried out under general or local anaesthesia with the patient in the prone position; a long needle, up to 10 in (25 cm) in length, is introduced from the left side of the body of the 1st lumbar vertebra below the last rib and passed forwards, inwards and upwards to enter the aorta above the origin of the renal arteries; 30 ml of solution are injected quickly and films are taken as soon as the injection starts and as rapidly as possible whilst it continues. The early ones show the arterial system and the later ones show the nephrographic phase when the whole of the renal substance is opacified; they may also show the veins and sometimes some filling of the pelvis. (*Fig.* K.20).

In the femoral approach by the Seldinger technique (now by far the more commonly used) a fine catheter is passed into the femoral artery and up the aorta as far as the renal vessels where the contrast medium is injected. A method of selective renal angiography has been developed in which the tip of the catheter can be turned to enter one or other renal artery; this gives the best demonstration of the renal vessels but it requires the use of an image-intensifier with a television monitor.

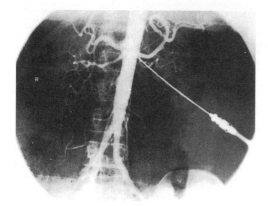

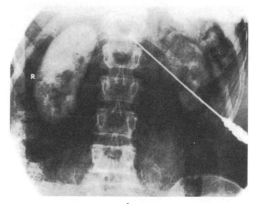

a *b*

Fig. K.20. *a.* Aortogram done by the translumbar method: arterial phase. The right renal artery, seen below the hepatic, is of normal size. The left, seen below the splenic, is small. *b.* Nephrographic phase in the same case. The left kidney is small and less densely opacified than the right, it contained a papillary carcinoma in the upper calix.

The investigation is of value in demonstrating new growths of the kidney, where pooling of the contrast occurs in the growth, and in detecting congenital abnormalities. It has been of use in verifying the existence of a solitary kidney. It can also differentiate tumours from cysts, which may also be aspirated under radiological control.

Nephrotomography. In this investigation 45 per cent sodium diatrizoate or 60 per cent meglumine iothalamate is injected rapidly into an antecubital vein, and a series of tomograms is taken at 1-cm levels through the whole thickness of the kidney. This investigation has its greatest value in distinguishing a renal tumour from a cyst; the tumour is irregularly and densely opacified; the cyst contains no vessels and remains radiolucent. (*Fig.* K.21).

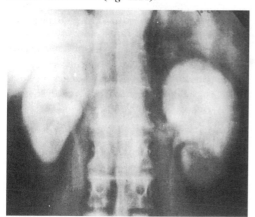

Fig. K.21. Nephrotomogram showing a solid tumour (carcinoma) in the upper pole of the left kidney. *Reproduced by courtesy of Dr John L. Emmett.*

Ultrasonography enables the skilled operator to differentiate between a solid and a cystic renal mass and also to detect a hydronephrosis. The simplicity

and non-invasiveness of this technique are especially advantageous.

Computerized tomography (CT scan) readily differentiates, again, between solid and cystic enlargements of the kidney and enables clear delineation of other masses in the region which may mimic a renal swelling.

CT enables the extent and local spread of a tumour of the kidney to be delineated and also allow lymph node and hepatic metastatic spread to be defined. Invasion of the vena cava by tumour can be shown if contrast is injected intravenously (*Figs.* K.22–K.24).

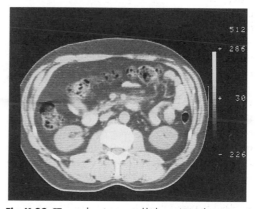

Fig. K.22. CT scan showing normal kidneys. (*Dr Adrian Dixon.*)

A kidney may be enlarged and yet not palpable from the fact that it is either wholly above the costal margin or obscured by the liver or the thick abdominal walls of the patient. On the other hand a kidney may be so diseased as to be functionless and shrunken, when it cannot be felt; but the remaining organ may be enlarged in a compensatory degree and may be distinctly palpable. One must remember the danger

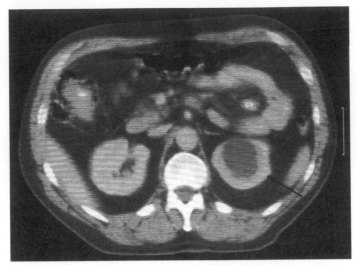

Fig. K.23. CT scan demonstrating a large left renal cyst (arrowed). (*Dr Adrian Dixon.*)

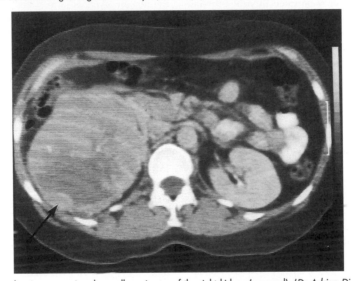

Fig. K.24. CT scan showing a massive clear cell carcinoma of the right kidney (arrowed). (*Dr Adrian Dixon.*)

of regarding an enlarged kidney as the diseased organ when it may in reality be the only functioning one. The kidney of normal size and position is not palpable from the abdomen, or on bimanual examination with one hand on the loin; but, in a thin subject, the lower pole of the right kidney may sometimes be felt to descend between the hands on the patient's taking a full inspiration; if, therefore, a kidney can be felt easily on bimanual examination, it is either unduly mobile, unduly low or enlarged. It is often difficult to say if a kidney that is movable is also enlarged to a slight degree; and a kidney which was thought clinically to be enlarged has often been found to be of normal size when exposed; this is in part due to the thick coverings of the abdominal wall, or to the amount of fatty tissue surrounding the organ.

Causes of kidney enlargement

If the kidney is definitely enlarged, it remains to determine the nature of the enlargement; in this one is guided, not only by the physical characters of the tumour present, but also by other symptoms that are associated with it, more especially, perhaps, by the altered characters of the urine. The kidney may be enlarged only slightly, as in tuberculosis, pyelonephritis, incipient hydronephrosis or carcinoma; or may be enlarged to a considerable degree in polycystic disease, hydro- or pyonephrosis, and in some forms of malignant growth. From the physical examination of the enlarged organ it is often possible to say that the swelling is fluid or solid in nature, but it is seldom that a true diagnosis of the lesion can be made from palpation of the kidney alone. In the following diseases, in which renal enlargement is usually present, the diagnosis must be arrived at by the consideration of associated symptoms.

In *renal tuberculosis* the disease occurs in a miliary or in a caseous form. Miliary tuberculosis occurs as part of a general tuberculosis, usually in children, is bilateral and causes no tumour. The caseous variety occurs most frequently in young adults who have had tuberculosis elsewhere in the body, as a disease in one kidney, in which one or several foci may be present. These enlarge and soften to form a tuberculous abscess, which invades the medullary tissues, to open eventually and discharge its contents into the renal pelvis. The kidney is slightly enlarged and tender, and there is persistent pyuria and haematuria in small amounts. The epithelial lining of the ureter is quickly invaded by the tuberculous process, becoming thickened and infiltrated, and at the same time shortened, so that cystoscopically the ureteric orifice is seen to be drawn upwards. An early symptom of renal tuberculosis is increased frequency of micturition, even before the bladder has become infected in the downward progress of the disease. The ureter may be felt to be thickened per rectum or per vaginam, or other tuberculous foci may be found in the prostate, vesiculae seminales or epididymes in the male. A thorough search should be made for tubercle bacilli in the urine by microscopy and specific culture. In cases in which caseous areas are present in the kidney, a radiograph may show blurred, indistinct shadows in the renal area, and a pyelographic examination will show a lack of definition of one or more renal calices and occasionally cavitation of the kidney. Intravenous pyelography may fail to show a shadow on the affected side owing to inefficient function of the kidney in the excretion of the contrast.

In *pyelonephritis* the kidney may be slightly enlarged, together with renal pain, pyuria and general malaise. Pyelonephritis is usually bilateral, and due to some infective or obstructive lesion in the lower urinary tract, symptoms of which are usually obvious (*see* PYURIA). Bacteriological examination by culture of a specimen of urine is essential to the diagnosis.

Malignant tumours of the kidney give rise either to an irregular nodular enlargement of the kidney, or to a general, uniform, solid tumour. There is usually aching pain in the loin, with intermittent attacks of profuse haematuria that occur when the growth has infiltrated the renal pelvis or sometimes sooner. The bleeding may be so profuse that clots are formed in the renal calices, pyramidal in shape, which in their passage down the ureter give rise to typical colic. Long worm-shaped clots from formation in the ureter may also be present. The common type of renal tumour

in the parenchyma of the kidney, the adenocarcinoma, arises in the renal tubular epithelium. It was formerly supposed to arise in small aberrant areas of suprarenal tissue which may be found in this situation and was known as a hypernephroma (Grawitz tumour). The malignant tumours arise in any part of the kidney, are often fairly well defined from the renal tissues, and are seen on macroscopical section to contain areas of yellow colour and areas of organizing blood clot from former interstitial haemorrhage. Microscopically, they show large polyhedral cells, with clear cytoplasm (clear cell carcinoma), arranged in an alveolar, tubular or papillary formation somewhat resembling the suprarenal cortical tissue; in some specimens granular cells predominate. They are now classified under the term 'adenocarcinoma'. Their rate of growth varies enormously, but the main symptoms are fairly constant. There is aching in the loin, and enlargement of the kidney may be found on examination (*Fig.* K.24), but at first the symptoms are slight. Haematuria occurs without any apparent exciting cause, and there may be renal colic from the passage of clots down the ureter; the tumour may be of fair size before any haematuria is noticed. Metastases to lungs, brain, liver and bones (skull, vertebrae, pelvis, ribs, upper humerus and upper femur) are common and, indeed, these manifestations may be the first evidence of the presence of the renal primary.

Another form of malignant tumour that occurs in the kidney is that which arises from embryonic tissues, and to which the name 'nephroblastoma' (Wilms' tumour) has been applied. These tumours are formed of mixed tissues, such as striated and non-striated muscle, cartilage or bone, and epithelial structures in tubular or glandular form. They grow in the renal tissues, expanding these to form a spurious capsule. They occur most frequently in children, and haematuria is infrequent. These tumours are of rapid growth, are exceedingly malignant, and the existence of a large tumour in the loin may be the earliest symptom.

Thus, the occurrence of a renal tumour, accompanied by intermittent attacks of haematuria, especially if profuse, should always give suspicion of renal growth in an adult. Renal tuberculosis and calculus may give rise to renal enlargement, but the haematuria is seldom profuse; with calculus, the haematuria is often brought on or increased by exertion, whereas with growth it may come on at any time, even during rest. At the same time it should be remembered that both profuse haematuria and renal enlargement may arise from a vesical tumour which obstructs the normal flow of urine from the ureteric orifice. In all cases, therefore, a full urological examination should be made before any operative measure is carried out. The rapid development of a *varicocele*, especially on the right side, is very rare but it is a point significant of renal growth. The pyelographic picture of a renal growth is usually distinctive. There is displacement or destruction of one or more calices and deformity of the renal pelvis, with frequently a filling defect in the latter (*Fig*. K.25). A filling defect in the pelvis alone, perhaps with dilatation of the calices, is more suggestive of a pelvic new growth of the papillary type.

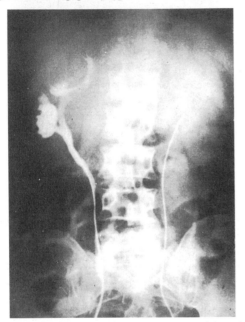

Fig. K.25. Pyelogram in a case of carcinoma of the right kidney. The crescentic filling defect is characteristic of a space-occupying lesion.

Hydronephrosis and *pyonephrosis* form definite enlargements of the kidney, which may attain a large size. The tumour is oval or rounded, smooth, and gives a sense of tenseness or elasticity, while occasionally distinct fluctuation may be obtained. Pyelography assists the diagnosis very materially (pp. 368 et seq. and *Fig*. K.25). A hydronephrosis occurs when there is a partial ureteric obstruction, or in cases of repeated attacks of temporarily complete obstruction to the ureter. Bilateral hydronephrosis may also arise from the back-pressure due to any obstruction of the normal passage of urine from the bladder. Hydronephrosis is often accompanied by renal pain, sometimes by renal colic, and occasionally by haematuria. The tumour may show marked changes in size, from the varying character of the lesion producing the obstruction; thus, if the ureter is wholly blocked, the tumour will increase in size and become more tense, whilst if the obstruction is partially relieved the tumour will diminish, synchronously with the passage of a larger quantity of urine of

low specific gravity. The presence of any obstruction to the normal flow of urine from the kidney predisposes to the onset of infection of the kidney by microorganisms, so that a hydronephrosis may become converted into a pyonephrosis, or the latter may arise from the obstruction of the ureter of a kidney already the seat of pyelitis. The physical examination of a kidney distended with urine or with pus shows practically no difference between them, but with pyonephrosis other indications are usually present to assist the diagnosis. Examination of the urine will reveal the presence of pus at some time, although, if the ureter is wholly obstructed at the time of examination, pus may be absent if the other kidney and the bladder are normal. If, however, the ureter is blocked only partially, pus will be found in the urine; in the intermittent form, pus may be present in large quantities at intervals coinciding with the decrease in the size of the renal tumour. With pyonephrosis, also, there will be the general evidence of suppuration, namely, raised temperature, sweating, pallor and often diarrhoea. The most frequent causation of pyonephrosis is renal calculus, so that a careful inquiry into the history of the case for symptoms of calculus may give important indications, and X-ray examination, etc., will be of service (pp. 368 et seq.) unless the stone has been passed. Very occasionally palpation of a kidney enlarged from calculus disease will give rise to distinct crepitation from the friction of one stone upon another. (*Fig*. K.26) illustrates recurrent bilateral calculi of the kidneys in a woman with raised serum calcium and lowered serum phosphate. After removal of the parathyroid tumour and pyelolithotomy there has been no more stone formation and the case also demonstrates the relationship between urinary calculi and the parathyroid glands, because of the influence of the latter upon the calcium metabolism of the body.

Cysts of the kidney

Hydatid cyst of the kidney may give rise to a tumour in the loin exactly resembling a hydronephrosis, and would usually be diagnosed as such. The discovery of hooklets or hydatid elements in the urine, or in the fluid aspirated from a renal cyst, will point to the nature of the disease.

Polycystic disease of the kidney may occur in children or in adults, and forms a tumour which is commonly bilateral, though that of one side may be larger than the other. In adults the disease causes practically no trouble, except the presence of the tumour, in the early stages, but later, symptoms of renal insufficiency develop, with thirst, drowsiness and vomiting. The tumour gives the usual physical signs of a renal enlargement, and may attain a great size on

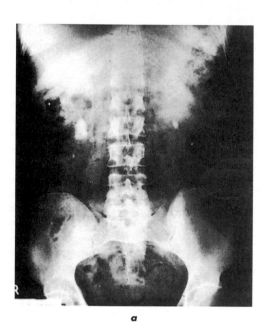

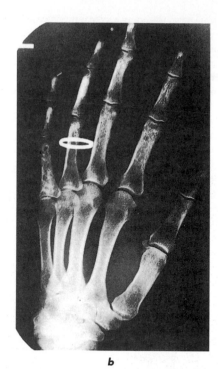

a   b

Fig. K.26. *a.* Recurrent bilateral calculi of the kidneys in a woman with a parathyroid adenoma. (Plain radiograph of abdomen.) *b.* The left hand of the same patient showing cystic changes in the 5th proximal phalanx.

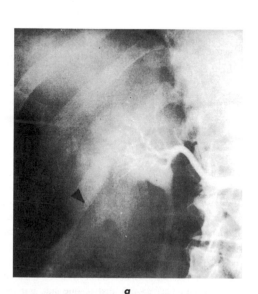

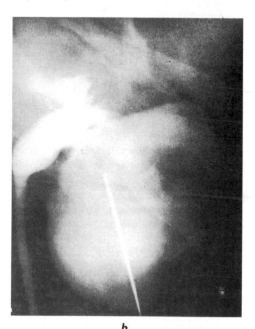

a   b

Fig. K.27. Arteriogram demonstrating a renal cyst. *a.* The avascular filling defect (anterior view). *b.* The cyst after aspiration and confirmation of the diagnosis by injection of contrast medium (posterior view).

both sides. In thin subjects rounded prominences may be felt on the surface of the tumour. There may be aching pain in the loins and, occasionally, marked haematuria. The urine is of low specific gravity, is increased in amount, and in the absence of blood often contains a small amount of protein. The disease is usually accompanied by arteriosclerosis and raised blood pressure. Indeed, death may result from hypertensive cardiac failure or a cerebrovascular accident. The character of the urine and the bilateral renal tumours are usually sufficient data upon which to form a diagnosis, but with a unilateral tumour, such as occasionally occurs, the diagnosis is very difficult. A hydronephrotic or pyonephrotic kidney may give evidence of fluctuation which will not be obtained with a polycystic kidney. The pyelographic picture of polycystic disease shows the calices to be considerably lengthened and drawn out by the disease, but shows no cavitation and rarely any pelvic dilatation as in a hydronephrosis.

A large *solitary cyst* of the kidney may produce a renal tumour and may cause aching in one loin. A pyelographic examination shows the calices to be displaced by the enlarging cyst, and in spite of the absence of haematuria, a diagnosis of renal growth is usually made and the true cause of the disease revealed by ultrasound or CT scanning and confirmed, if necessary, by aortography; the renal cyst is avascular in contrast to the marked tumour circulation seen in a renal carcinoma. The cyst can then be both confirmed and treated by aspiration under X-ray or ultrasound control (*Fig.* K.27).

Harold Ellis

KNEE
See JOINTS, AFFECTIONS OF.

Labour, difficult

Difficult labour is abnormally slow progress of labour. Once established, progressive labour is characterized by increasing dilatation of the cervix and descent of the presenting part. Abnormalities related to either the maternal or fetal factors, singly or jointly, may lead to difficult labour.

Uterine Dysfunction

Uterine contractions that are either not coordinated or are not of sufficient amplitude may lead to failure of cervical dilatation. The first stage of labour is divided into two stages; the early, latent phase and the later active phase of labour.

In the early phase the cervix becomes effaced and soft but only slightly dilated. The active phase is characterized by progressive dilatation of the cervix and descent of the presenting part. Assessment of labour using 'partograms' makes the temporal relationship of cervical dilatation and descent of the presenting

part easy to visualize. The two parameters are charted against time, and abnormalities of labour are more readily detectable. Two main types of uterine dysfunction are recognized. The hypertonic uterine inertia commonly occurs in the active phase of labour before, or at about, 4 cm dilatation of the cervix. The hypertonic uterine dysfunction is associated with elevation of the basal tone and the contractions are much more painful, usually occurring in the second half of the active phase. It is necessary to rule out pelvic contraction as a cause of dysfunctional labour prior to considering therapy with oxytocics. Pelvic contractions or fetal malposition is often the common cause but inappropriate and premature sedation in early labour may also be responsible for prolonging the latent phase. Prolongation of the latent phase is defined as labour lasting longer than 8–10 hours; prolonged active phase is defined as cervical dilatation of less than 1–1·5 cm per hour once labour is in the active phase.

Prolonged difficult labour increases perinatal morbidity and mortality, leads to maternal exhaustion and increases the risk of intrauterine infection.

N. Patel

Lacrimation

Lacrimation or tearing is a function of the lacrimal gland and the accessory lacrimal glands. Tears wet the surface of the cornea and conjunctivae protecting the surface epithelium. They inhibit growth of organisms, provide the cornea with nutrient substances and make the cornea a smooth optical surface by abolishing minute surface irregularities. Basal tear production provides enough tears for these purposes and reflex lacrimation occurs with irritative conditions or corneal disease (*see* EPIPHORA). Psychic lacrimation is normally associated with pain or emotional upset.

Tear production diminishes with age and dryness of the eyes is a common complaint of the elderly.

S. T. D. Roxburgh

Leg, oedema of

In the great majority of patients with generalized oedema, the legs, particularly the ankles, are likely to be affected (*see* OEDEMA, GENERALIZED). In most of these cases both legs will be involved but, occasionally and perhaps due to the patient's position in bed, the oedema may be somewhat asymmetrical. In most of the conditions discussed in this section, the oedema is strictly unilateral and there will, therefore, be little difficulty in distinguishing them from the causes of generalized oedema. The causes of oedema of the legs can be classified under the headings of *trauma, inflammation, venous obstruction* and *lymphatic obstruction*.

Trauma

The cause of the swelling associated with sprains and fractures, bites and stings, and burns and frostbite is likely to be obvious. There is, however, a late complication of trauma, of which oedema is a feature, which may present a diagnostic problem. This is *algodystrophy* or *Sudek's atrophy*. This rather rare condition usually follows trauma to a limb, which may be very mild, and, in the leg, most commonly affects the ankle. It is characterized by pain, which may be very severe, and the ankle is warm, red and oedematous, suggesting local inflammation; there is, however, no systemic evidence of inflammation. These changes subside after a few weeks and the skin around the joint becomes cold, cyanosed and, ultimately, atrophic. X-rays show local osteoporosis. Full recovery is usual but may not occur for many months. The aetiology is unknown but it has been suggested that abnormal autonomic reflexes may be responsible.

Inflammation

Oedema is one of the cardinal signs of inflammation. Local lesions, such as *boils* and *carbuncles*, are easily identified but more widespread inflammatory lesions may initially cause diagnostic confusion. The bright red areas with palpable raised margins of *erysipelas* are characteristic but oedema due to obstruction of cutaneous lymphatics may persist after the acute inflammation has subsided. *Cellulitis* causes more diffuse oedema as does *acute osteomyelitis*; lymphangitis and lymphadenitis are commoner in the former while, in the latter, the constitutional disturbance is greater. *Chronic osteomyelitis* can cause puzzling oedema but imaging will settle the diagnostic issue. *Acute arthritis* of any type is associated with local oedema. In most cases the swelling of the joint itself will make the diagnosis clear but *acute gout* can cause a swelling widespread enough to simulate cellulitis. *Acute rheumatoid arthritis* is less likely to cause confusion but it is worth remembering that, in this condition, more generalized oedema can occur; this is probably due to a combination of hypoalbuminaemia, stasis in an immobile patient and, perhaps, increased capillary permeability. The painful swelling of the calf with ankle oedema caused by a *ruptured Baker's cyst* is easily confused with deep venous thrombosis; a history of prior swelling of the joint, decreasing with the onset of the calf pain, is an important diagnostic feature.

Venous obstruction

Deep venous thrombosis in the calf muscles is an important cause of oedema of the ankle; the swelling will extend further up the leg if thrombus is also present in the femoral and iliac veins (*Fig*. L.1). Venous thrombosis is a common complication of major surgery and of prolonged recumbency for any reason; it can also often occur without any obvious cause. Long coach journeys by the elderly and, in women, the use of oestrogen-containing oral contraceptive agents increase the risk of deep venous thrombosis. In addition to the ankle oedema the calf is typically swollen and tender on pressure from behind and from side to side. Homan's sign (pain in the calf on dorsiflexion at the ankle) may be positive but is of no diagnostic value as it can be positive with any painful lesion of the calf. Very often, none of these signs are present; the first evidence of deep venous thrombosis may be a fatal pulmonary embolism.

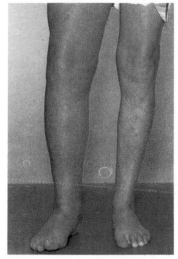

Fig. L.1. Iliofemoral venous thrombosis of the right leg with gross oedema.

Thrombus may spread upwards beyond the iliac veins to involve the *inferior vena cava* and, in that case, the other leg will become oedematous. With such a sequence of events, the diagnosis of inferior vena caval occlusion is clear. Primary occlusion of this vessel, however, will present with bilateral ankle and leg oedema, in which case the differential diagnosis includes all the causes of generalized oedema. Diagnostic assistance may be provided by investigations such as Doppler flow studies but the definitive diagnosis of venous occlusion can be made only by venography or CT scanning. In any patient in whom venous thrombosis has occurred without obvious cause, a thorough general examination, including rectal and vaginal examination, is essential to detect pelvic or abdominal tumours causing pressure on veins.

Varicose veins, with or without previous thrombosis, commonly cause ankle oedema, usually quite mild. Although, in the great majority of cases, it is the veins themselves which are the seat of the trouble, it is wise, at first presentation, to examine the patient with the possibility of external pressure on the large veins in mind, as in patients with acute venous occlusion.

Lymphatic obstruction

The oedema fluid in lymphatic obstruction contains

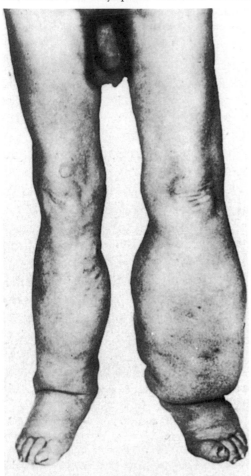

Fig. L.2. Milroy's disease in a man of 74. He had never been abroad. In this condition the lymphoedema may be symmetrical, may affect only one limb or, as in this case, may affect one limb more than the other.

much more protein than the fluid in other conditions causing oedema. Consequently, although, initially, the swelling 'pits' on pressure and disappears overnight, it later becomes firm and non-pitting ('brawny') and is present all the time. Later the skin becomes grossly thickened and, sometimes, ulcerated. The common causes of lymphatic obstruction in Western countries include *neoplastic infiltration* of the lymphatics and lymph nodes, and scarring from *trauma*, surgical or otherwise, and from *irradiation*; recurrent *streptococcal infection* can cause similar damage. In tropical countries, *filariasis* is a common cause of lymphatic obstruction and chronic oedema of the legs known as elephantiasis. The commonest form of filariasis is that due to *Wuchereria bancrofti*; this is widespread in the tropics and causes elephantiasis of the whole leg and also of the genitalia, especially in males. Another filaria, *Brugia malayi*, is found in the Far East, especially South-East Asia; the inguinal lymph nodes are affected, as in Bancroftian filariasis but, curiously, the oedema and elephantiasis are confined to the lower parts of the legs. There is also a *non-filarial elephantiasis* seen in parts of Africa and Central and South America; this is due to chronic lymphangitis apparently caused by microscopic particles of silica absorbed through the skin of the feet; it usually affects the feet and lower parts of the legs. *Lymphatic hypoplasia* is a rare cause of oedema. This occurs in two forms: a congenital variety presenting with oedema in early infancy and a familial form, sometimes known as Milroy's disease. In the latter there is an abrupt demarcation between the swollen and the normal tissue at the level of a joint—ankle, knee or hip (*Fig.* L.2). There is sometimes a history of attacks of pyrexia in association with the spread of the oedema which is typically episodic. Thus, the swelling, having been present at the ankle only for several years, may, rather suddenly, spread to reach the knee and, later, in a similar fashion, the hip.

Peter R. Fleming

Leg, pain in

This section deals specifically with the causes of pain referred into the limb or arising from local lesions rather than generalized diseases. The subdivision of the section is largely anatomical but nerve root compression (sciatica), ischaemia (intermittent claudication) and spinal stenosis (spinal claudication), which are responsible for a very large proportion of pain in the buttock and leg, are considered separately first.

Sciatica may affect the buttock, anterior or posterior thigh, calf or foot or the entire leg. Pain is affected by posture and is aggravated by sciatic and femoral nerve stretch tests; altered cutaneous sensation and motor weakness may or may not be present. Claudication pain occurs only during exercise, though the differentiation between arterial causes and spinal stenosis may be difficult. Most cases of sciatica in the elderly are due to spinal stenosis secondary to osteoarthritis of the apophyseal joints.

Sciatica

CAUSES

Intrathecal
Neurofibroma or other tumour
Irritation of the meninges by haemorrhage

Infection
Intrathecal injections
Hydatid cyst
Postherpetic neuralgia

Extradural
Prolapsed intervertebral disc
Spinal stenosis
Spinal abscess—tuberculous, brucella/osteomyelitis
Vertebral tumour—primary, secondary, myeloma
Fracture-dislocation
Spondylolisthesis

Extraspinal
Cysts and tumours of pelvic viscera
Fetal head during labour
Pelvic inflammatory disease
Neurofibroma of sciatic nerve
Penetrating injuries

Pain radiating from a lumbosacral nerve root into the leg is sciatica. In spite of the multitude of possible causes, in the vast majority of instances sciatica is due to a prolapsed intervertebral disc, apophyseal joint osteoarthritis (spondylosis) or spinal stenosis (especially in the elderly). These lesions do not always cause pain: central disc protrusions may induce cauda equina compression with urinary retention without any other symptoms.

Nerve root compression is characterized by complaints of well-localized pain with or without paraesthesiae, numbness, wasting and weakness. Paraesthesiae including numbness indicate direct involvement of sensory pathways and are not necessarily associated with referred pain. Nerve root pain may be aggravated by coughing and sneezing, straight-leg raising (Lasègue's sign) and by neck flexion. Aggravation of the pain or paraesthesiae by flexion of the hip (which stretches the cauda equina) is a reliable indicator of a root lesion. However, extraneural lesions may be associated with pain on coughing and Lasègue's sign; flexion of the neck may produce a surge of paraesthesiae down the trunk into the limbs (l'Hermitte's sign) in multiple sclerosis, subacute combined degeneration of the cord, cervical spondylosis or cervical cord tumour. A neural lesion is confirmed by the presence of muscular weakness, sensory loss and depression or loss of the knee or ankle jerk. Muscle wasting usually has the same significance but may be associated with extraneural disease or disuse. Nevertheless, radicular pain of recent onset may not be accompanied by any objective neurological signs.

Lesions of the cauda equina are uncommon. Tumours, notably slowly growing neurofibromas, may cause intermittent sciatic pain for months or even years before the diagnosis is established; neurological signs may be relatively late in appearing, but lumbar puncture will usually reveal a raised cerebrospinal fluid

protein level and there may be a partial or complete intrathecal block. Backward protrusion of the lower intervertebral lumbar discs or of the lumbosacral disc may compress the cauda equina with unilateral or bilateral sciatica. The spinal fluid may or may not show evidence of block and the protein level may be raised. Meningeal irritation from local meningitis, haemorrhage or intrathecal injections can give rise to severe bilateral sciatica, usually of short duration and obvious origin.

Posterolateral herniation of the nucleus pulposus of the intervertebral discs at L4/5 and L5/S1 spaces is the commonest cause of acute sciatica. There may be a history of an acute injury, which may be slight, or of preceding lumbago, but there may be no such history. Sciatica is usually unilateral, occasionally bilateral and rarely alternating. Examination reveals a stiff lumbar spine with tenderness at the level of the lesion. The lumbar lordosis may be lost and there may be a scoliosis which becomes more marked with forward flexion. Areas of reduced sensation to pinprick, weakness and reflex change associated with individual root lesions are summarized in *Fig.* L.3 and *Table* L.1.

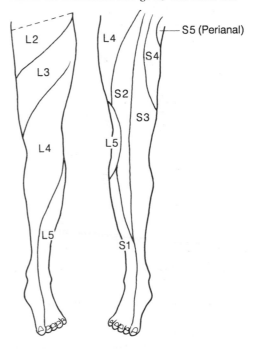

ANTERIOR   POSTERIOR

Fig. L.3. Areas of reduced sensation to pinprick in lumbosacral root lesion.

With an L5 root lesion weakness is most marked in extensor hallucis longus and with an S1 lesion calf wasting may be seen. After acute disc prolapse, the spinal fluid is often normal though there may be a slight rise in protein content. Radiographs of the

Table L.1. Signs associated with common nerve root lesions affecting the legs

Root	Paraesthesiae/numbness	Muscle weakness	Reflex change
L1	Groin	—	—
L2	Front of mid thigh	Quadriceps	—
L3	Front of lower thigh	Quadriceps	Knee ↓
L4	Front of lower thigh, knee and inner aspect of shin	Quadriceps and tibialis anterior	Knee ↓
L5	Back of thigh, lateral aspect of leg, dorsum of foot to big toe	Extensor hallucis longus	Ankle ↓
S1	Back of leg, lateral aspect of foot and sole	Calf wasting and weakness of plantar flexors	Ankle ↓

lumbar spine may show significant narrowing of the affected disc space. Contrast myelography (*Fig.* L.4a) may outline the herniation unless the lesion involves the lateral recess when appearances may be normal. Localization of such herniation by CT or MRI scanning (*Fig.* L.4b) offers an improved diagnostic method.

variable disc space narrowing with osteophytic lipping and irregularity of the facet joints. It is important, however, to remember that such changes will be found in the majority of aged spines so that the appearance seen may not account for the symptoms.

Spinal abscesses due to tuberculosis, brucellosis

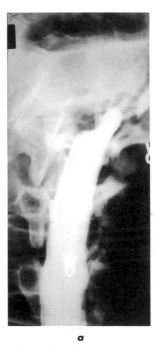

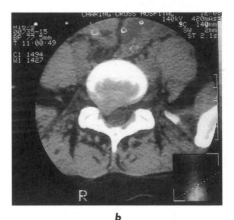

a   *b*

Fig. L.4a. Lumbosacral disc herniation: *a.* X-ray myelogram showing disc bulge and swelling of the S1 nerve root. *b*, CT scan showing posterolateral L5/S1 disc prutrusion.

Spondylosis commonly leads to pain in the neck and back and to root pains in the arm and leg, especially in the elderly. Symptoms may mimic those of an acute disc herniation but there is often a history of chronic or intermittent spinal pain, recurrent sciatica with evidence of osteoarthritis elsewhere in the spine. More than one root may be involved, either simultaneously or at different times, but objective neurological signs are usually less prominent than in younger individuals with acute disc prolapse. Spinal radiographs show

or other pyogenic infections may mimic spondylotic symptoms with local pain, stiffness and sciatic radiation. Sudden onset, or exacerbation, of pain may accompany fracture of the affected vertebra(e). X-rays may initially be normal but a chest X-ray and a CT or MRI scan at the suspect level may be helpful in any suspicious case of sciatica.

Osteomyelitis of the lumbar vertebrae is a rare cause of sciatica. *Fracture-dislocations* also are clinically obvious but *spondylolisthesis* (forward or backward displacement of one vertebra upon its neighbour) can only be diagnosed with certainty by radiography (*Fig.* L.5). The presence of this deformity does not prove that it is the cause of sciatic pain since it may be present without discomfort. When sciatica is caused by spondylolisthesis it is usually bilateral, severe and with marked neurological signs including motor, sensory and reflex changes. Pelvic disease rarely produces sciatica and when it does so the pelvic pathology is usually gross. However, exceptional cases will be overlooked if rectal or vaginal examination is not performed in every case of sciatica in which no cause is apparent. Acute sciatic pain occurring during parturition is usually transient and due to the pressure of the fetal head on the lumbosacral trunk as it crosses the pelvic brim. Permanent paralysis of the muscles distal to the nerve has been reported after prolonged dystocia. Persistent sciatica following parturition is usually due to herniation of a lumbar disc.

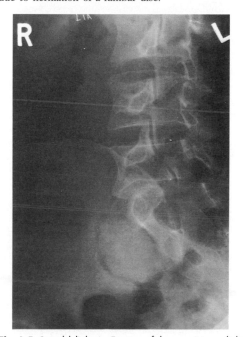

Fig. L.5. Spondylolisthesis: Fracture of the pars intermedialis shown in oblique X-ray of the lumbosacral spine.

Tumours of the sciatic nerve are exceedingly rare; the presence of other evidence of von Recklinghausen's disease—café-au-lait spots and subcutaneous tumours—may suggest this diagnosis, symptoms being due either to increasing size of a neurofibroma or to malignant change.

Extraneural disease may give rise to referred sciatic pain without paraesthesiae or objective neurological signs. Sacroiliac joint disease is a major cause of such pain (*see below*). Tumours of the iliac bones and sacrum may rarely lead to sciatic pain. These can

be demonstrated by X-rays, bone scintigraphy scanning, CT or MRI scanning. Benign osteoid osteomas may respond well symptomatically to aspirin.

Intermittent claudication

CAUSES
Spinal stenosis
Leriche syndrome
Iliac, femoral or popliteal stenosis
Anaemia

The term intermittent claudication is used to describe the development of pains in the leg, usually the calf, brought on during walking, which necessitates limping or rest. It is relieved after 5–15 minutes by rest but recurs after walking a similar distance. With the passage of time the distance walked before pain becomes intolerable usually decreases, progressively restricting exercise tolerance. The condition is due to inadequate arterial blood supply to the leg muscles due to narrowing of iliac, femoral or popliteal arteries. Atheroma with or without thrombosis is the usual culprit but embolism, Buerger's disease and, rarely, syphilitic endarteritis may also give rise to intermittent claudication. Anaemia may also lead to this symptom or may aggravate it.

Physical examination of the affected limbs is usually grossly normal. However, careful examination will reveal absence of pulsation at the dorsalis pedis and posterior tibial arteries. Similarly the popliteal pulse may also be lost though femoral artery pulsation may be reduced or normal. There may however be an audible femoral bruit. After exercise the foot may appear unduly pale; with rest the returning flush of normal colour spreads gradually over its surface.

Similar symptoms, though usually bilateral, may also result from intermittent ischaemia of the cauda equina (spinal claudication). Walking produces characteristic aching in the legs sometimes with paraesthesiae in the feet. Ankle jerks may be lost during exercise. This condition is usually distinguishable from arterial disease by a history of chronic back pain usually with marked radiographic changes of spondylosis and by the presence of peripheral leg pulses with good skin perfusion. This condition is quite common, especially among the elderly. It is important since appropriate spinal surgery may provide effective cure. Myelography, CT or MRI scanning of the lumbosacral spine shows a narrow anteroposterior diameter of the spinal canal (*Fig.* L.6), usually with marked osteoarthritic changes at the intervertebral joints. Often large osteophytes at the apophyseal joints link to form bony bars compressing the cauda equina with further pressure exerted by bulging of the intervertebral disc. Symptoms arise when sufficient stenosis of the spinal canal develops to prevent dilatation of the vasa nervorum during exercise.

attention whenever possible. In the adult, degenerative and inflammatory arthritis, including infection, can usually be diagnosed on the basis of other clinical

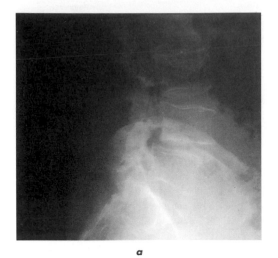
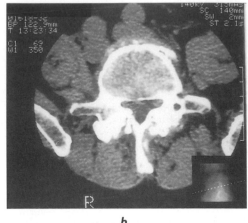

Fig. L.6. Lumbar spinal stenosis: *a*, Lateral X-ray showing spondylosis with grade 1 spondylolisthesis at L5/S1 level. *b*, CT scan showing markedly diminished anteroposterior spinal diameter and apophyseal osteophytes.

Pain in the Hip

CAUSES

Adult
Osteoarthritis
Inflammatory joint disease
Joint infection—tuberculous or pyogenic
Aseptic necrosis
Polymyalgia rheumatica
Bursitis—trochanteric
　—iliopectineal
Enthesopathy—adductor tendinitis
　—pubic tubercle

Child
Perthés's disease
Slipped femoral epiphysis
Joint infection—tuberculous or pyogenic
Juvenile chronic arthritis
Congenital hip dysplasia
Transient osteoporosis
Haemoglobinopathies—aseptic necrosis, synovitis
Familial Mediteranean fever
Henoch-Schönlein purpura
Myeloproliferative disorders

Typically, pain from the hip joint is felt in the groin or perineum, although it may be referred to the greater trochanter. It is aggravated by weight-bearing or exercise and examination reveals restricted movements with pain, especially on rotation. In children hip disease may present with thigh or knee pain.

In children, especially, the diagnosis of hip joint disease is of great importance and requires specialist

features and X-ray changes. A history of acute onset of unilateral hip pain may suggest aseptic necrosis, though X-rays may remain normal for up to 6 months. CT or MRI scanning may reveal a hypodense segment in the femoral head at an earlier stage (*Fig.* L.7).

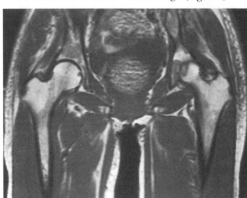

Fig. L.7. MRI showing avascular necrosis of the femoral head as marked.

Polymyalgia rheumatica may present with hip pain and, especially, inactivity stiffness. Usually there are also spinal or shoulder-girdle symptoms and the erythrocyte sedimentation rate will be raised. *Pelvic bursitis* is common and may coexist with X-ray changes of osteoarthritis of the hip. Careful clinical assessment is therefore essential. *Trochanteric bursitis* produces pain aggravated by walking and climbing stairs and there is local tenderness just behind the greater trochanter. This may produce pain when the patient lies on that side. A virtually full, painless range of hip movements is possible but pain may be aggravated by full abduction and adduction of the hip. *Iliopectineal bursitis* occasionally accompanies inflammatory hip disease, producing tenderness over the front of the hip joint, in the groin and pain on forced flexion and extension.

Pain in the Buttock

CAUSES

Sacroiliitis—spondyloarthropathies
Infection—tuberculous or pyogenic
Primary and secondary tumours of pelvic bones
Pelvic fracture (especially due to osteoporosis in the elderly)
Osteomalacia
Paget's disease of bone
Polymyalgia rheumatica
Gluteal or trochanteric bursitis

Sacroiliac joint pain is felt in the buttock, sometimes with radiation down the back of the thigh to the knee but no further. Pain may be aggravated by standing, walking and by twisting the trunk. Inflammatory aseptic sacroiliitis may occur as part of ankylosing spondylitis, when it may be the presenting symptom, or in association with psoriasis, inflammatory bowel disease, acute anterior uveitis or Reiter's syndrome. It may occur alone especially in females. Sepsis of the sacroiliac joint may arise as a result of tuberculous or pyogenic infection. Pregnancy and trauma may lead to subluxation of one or both sacroiliac joints leading to a sensation of uncertainty in the legs or to a feeling of uselessness of the leg(s) immediately after an injury. Clinical signs of sacroiliac joint disease are notoriously unreliable. Induction of local pain by forced abduction of the flexed hips or direct pressure over the sacrum may be helpful in acute cases. Other clinical tests are of little value. X-ray changes generally appear late although in patients with sepsis other abnormalities such as pulmonary tuberculosis, a pointing cold abscess over the joint or in a gluteal fold or abscess formation elsewhere may be found. In the acute phase the investigations of choice are radioisotope bone scanning and CT or MRI scanning.

Osteomalacia should be suspected in malnourished individuals and may give rise to a characteristic stiff gait. In the elderly, *Paget's disease of bone* may produce a local ache, although symptoms are usually due to secondary osteoarthritis and fractures through osteoporotic bone may occur with minimal trauma. Deformity at the hip secondary to softening of the bone due to Paget's disease is known as protrusio acetabuli (*Fig.* L.8). Ischial bursitis is usually associated with prolonged sitting on hard seats, producing tenderness over the ischial tuberosity.

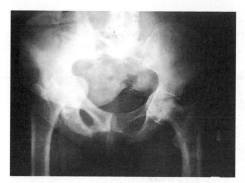

Fig. L.8. Protrusio acetabuli in Paget's disease.

Pain in the front of the thigh

CAUSES

Lumbar root irritation
Hip joint disease
Obturator pain
Meralgia paraesthetica
Tabes dorsalis

In most instances pain is referred from either the lumbar spine or the hip joint. Root lesions at either L2 or L3 may lead to some quadriceps wasting but without detectable sensory loss, weakness or loss of the ankle jerk. Similar features are associated with femoral nerve lesions. A root lesion at L4 produces anterior thigh pain which extends down the front of the shin and in addition the knee jerk may be reduced or lost.

Hip pain of any cause may be referred to the thigh or the knee. *Obturator pain* down the inner aspect of the thigh may arise from the hip joint, the pelvic bones or from within the pelvis. Osteoarthritis of the hip is the most common cause, though tumours of the pelvic bones or fractures in an osteoporotic skeleton must be considered. Occasionally in females ovulation may produce brief but recurrent episodes of obturator pain; rarely obturator hernia or gross neoplastic or inflammatory disease within the pelvis gives rise to persistent pain.

Meralgia paraesthetica arises as a result of compression of the lateral cutaneous nerve of the thigh as it passes under the lateral part of the inguinal ligament. At that point it may become involved in the origin of the sartorius muscle. This compression gives rise both to numbness over the lateral aspect of the thigh and to pain. Pain develops typically on exertion and may be severe enough to produce limping (intermittent claudication) or to halt the exercise. Pain is relieved by rest. Physical examination may or may not demonstrate sensory loss corresponding to the distribution of the lateral cutaneous nerve of the thigh. Symptoms may begin in middle-age especially in association with marked weight gain. Thus dieting may be sufficient to relieve symptoms though in more severe cases surgical decompression of the nerve is necessary.

The 'lightning' pains of *tabes dorsalis* most commonly affect the legs. In contrast to root pain they are usually bilateral and do not conform to any root or peripheral nerve distribution. Although the intensity may vary from trivial to excruciating the episodes are highly characteristic, being of lightning-like short duration and usually affecting an area no larger than the palm of one hand. The affected area may remain hypersensitive for hours after the paroxysm has passed. In addition to lightning pains individuals with tabes may also experience dull aching or boring pains which are persistent rather than episodic. Tabetic pains may precede all other signs and symptoms of the disease. In the presence of such symptoms special attention should be paid to the following: a history of syphilis; absent pupil reactions to light and intact convergence reactions (Argyll–Robertson pupil); loss of knee and ankle jerks; sensory impairment—loss of pain below the knees, over the trunk and inner arms and reduced postural sense peripherally; lymphocytosis in the cerebrospinal fluid; positive serological tests for syphilis in blood and CSF—these may be negative.

Pain in the knee

Pain in the knee may arise because of referral from the spine or hip, ligamentous injury, internal structural derangement, inflammatory or degenerative arthritis, bursitis or underlying bone disease. The presence of soft tissue swelling or effusion indicates the presence of synovitis which may be primary or secondary to these intra-articular lesions. Bony swelling indicates either osteoarthritis or metabolic or malignant lesions.

In many instances isolated knee pain, in both children and adults, not associated with swelling or restriction, is transient and not explained.

Examination of the knee must establish whether symptoms arise from the tibiofemoral, patellofemoral or superior tibiofibula joint and whether or not there is synovitis or hip disease. The anatomy of the knee is illustrated in *Fig.* L.9.

Additional causes of generalized joint disease are considered elsewhere.

Causes

IN CHILDREN (UP TO 15 YEARS OF AGE)
Referred from the hip
Trauma
Chondromalacia patellae
Juvenile chronic arthritis
Infection
  —pyogenic
  —viral

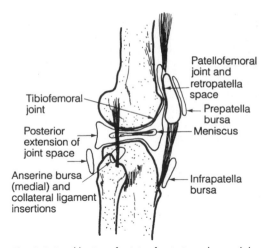

Fig. L.9. Possible sites of origin of pain in and around the knee joint. (Reproduced with permission from Dieppe, Doherty, MacFarlane and Maddison (1985) *Rheumatological Medicine.* Churchill Livingstone, Edinburgh, p. 387, figure 21.29.)

Haemoglobinopathies
Osgood–Schlatter disease
Leukaemia
Rickets
Scurvy
Clutton's joints

IN ADULTS
Chondromalacia patellae
Osteoarthritis
Inflammatory arthritis (*see* p. 346)
Trauma
Internal derangement
Infection
  —pyogenic
  —viral
Intermittent hydrarthrosis
Gout
Pyrophosphate arthropathy (pseudogout)
Synovioma
Malignant tumour of bone
  —primary
  —secondary
Scurvy
Sarcoidosis
Osteochondritis dissecans
Neuropathic (Charcot) joint
Pigmented villonodular synovitis
Synovial chondromatosis
Bursitis
Lipoma arborescens
Lipoarthritis (Hoffa's disease)
Bleeding disorders

IN CHILDHOOD

For the most part chronic arthritis in childhood is analogous to adult disease. In children under 2 years of age sepsis must be excluded with particular care. In some children mono-, pauci- (or oligo-: involvement of fewer than 5 joints) or polyarthritis (involvement of 6 or more joints) occurs, with or without systemic upset; if the condition persists for 3 months or more the term juvenile chronic arthritis (JCA) is used, arthritis being described as 'pauciarticular', 'polyarticular' or 'systemic'. A minority of children progress to develop adult seropositive rheumatoid arthritis and approximately 10 per cent of those with pauciarticular disease, mainly boys, progress to develop ankylosing spondylitis. Rheumatoid factor is almost invariably absent but antinuclear antibodies may be detected. Chronic iridocyclitis must be sought in children with JCA as this may cause painless visual loss.

Plant thorn synovitis follows the introduction of a small sharp object—often the tip of a plant thorn or a needle which penetrates the skin when the child is crawling but breaks off leaving no discernible mark. Persistent low-grade synovitis results, usually necessitating synovectomy in order to remove the foreign body. Pyarthrosis may result from penetrating injury or bacteraemia, especially in the very young child.

Clutton's joints are extremely rare today. Occurring at the age of 8–16 years, these manifestations of congenital syphilis may be misdiagnosed as cases of JCA, hydrarthrosis being present in one or both knees. Serological tests are positive. *Scurvy* is very rare but in infancy may cause intense pain on moving or touching hips or knees. Subcutaneous haemorrhages may be present elsewhere. *Leukaemia* in childhood may cause swelling of the knees and an arthropathy, usually misdiagnosed as JCA.

IN ADULT LIFE

The commonest knee disorder anywhere in the world is *osteoarthritis* which, although essentially a degenerative process, does undergo traumatic or inflammatory episodes with greater pain in the joint and sometimes effusions. Synovial fluid is clear, of high viscosity and low protein content (2 g/dl) and has a low cell count (under 2000/mm³). It may be bloodstained or contain red cells from recent injuries, detached osteophytes or from vascular synovial fringes being torn or stretched. The knees tend to be thickened in osteoarthritis. Bow-legs may predispose to degenerative changes but osteoarthritis may affect the medial compartment of the joint and cause genu varum (knock-knee). Osteoarthritis may be apparently a primary disorder or be secondary to and accompanied by other conditions, such as haemochromatosis, ochronosis, hypermobility syndromes or an inflammatory arthritis, such as rheumatoid arthritis.

Chondromalacia patellae is a premature degeneration of the patellar cartilage often occurring before the age of 30. It may be associated with a mechanical abnormality such as an unduly mobile patella. It has been considered a separate entity from osteoarthritis but tends to progress to osteoarthritis of the anterior compartment of the joint.

Rheumatoid arthritis of the knee is usually easy to diagnose as typical rheumatoid changes are present elsewhere in other joints in most cases, the changes in the hands usually being diagnostic (see *Fig* J.38). When other joints are less obviously affected diagnosis may be more difficult. The joint or joints are painful to move, often swollen, free fluid being palpable in the joint in many cases and bursae around the knee may be affected, particularly the semimembranosus bursa (Baker's cyst) at the back of the knee, which usually communicates with the joint and acts as an over-flow tank. The joint may be tender, particularly on pressure over the medial side. In long-standing cases valgus deformity (knock-knee) is present and the muscles of calf and thigh weak and wasted. The knee may be slightly warmer than normal to the touch but not invariably (*Figs*. L.10, L.11).

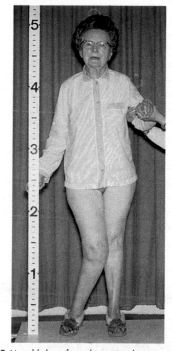

Fig. L.10. Unstable knee from destructive rheumatoid changes.

A similar but usually less active picture is seen in the *spondyloarthropathies*. Knees may be involved in ankylosing spondylitis, usually early in the course of the disease when spinal signs and symptoms are slight or absent, but they may also occur later when spondylitic signs are obvious, effusions sometimes becoming chronic.

In *Reiter's disease* knees are commonly affected early: a history of dysentery or exposure to venereal infection 7–18 days previously is common; in acute arthritis affecting the knees the possibility of psoriatic

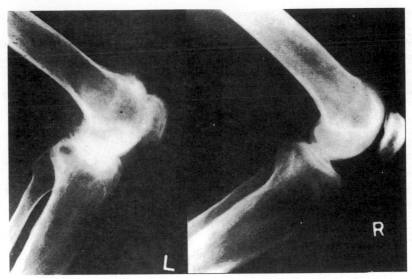

Fig. L.11. Rheumatoid arthritis. Marked active disease on the left side, right side only minimally affected.

arthritis, ulcerative colitis, Crohn's disease and Reiter's disease should be kept in mind.

Trauma may be obvious from the history and from examination, but minor injuries causing damage to collateral ligaments, semilunar cartilage (usually the medial meniscus) and cruciate ligaments, usually the anterior, may cause pain, local tenderness and swelling with limitation of movements and possibly transient effusions.

A *pyarthrosis* or septic joint is usually hot and painful, the patient ill and febrile. The diagnosis may be missed if infection is superimposed on a rheumatoid joint, a not unusual occurrence. Aspiration and culture of joint fluid is obligatory. A gonococcal pyarthrosis is often accompanied by evidence of gonococcal infection elsewhere: urethra, abscesses in the skin and, in women, Bartholin's gland; endocervical and urethral swabs should be taken. Infections elsewhere in the body, usually staphylococcal, may suggest the source of the infection.

In *intermittent hydrarthrosis* effusions occur at fairly regular intervals every 1–3 weeks, lasting only a few days at a time. Effusions may be quite large, are uncomfortable but not agonizing. The fluid, if aspirated, contains less than 6000 cells per mm³, mostly mononuclears. Biopsies reveal only a non-specific synovitis. Some of these cases eventually prove to be part of a polyarthritis, usually rheumatoid arthritis, but others subside spontaneously. It differs from palindromic rheumatism in being confined usually to the knees and in its fairly regular recurrence. Onset is often in adolescence.

Acute gout is uncommon in the knee but when it occurs the joint is agonizing, hot and swollen. The inflammatory fluid contains crystals of monosodium urate. The serum uric acid is almost always raised.

Acute pyrophosphate arthropathy (pseudogout) is, unlike true uratic gout, most common in the knee, crystalline deposits of calcium pyrophosphate dihydrate (CPPD) setting up intense irritation in the joint. Aspirated fluid will usually reveal the typical crystals.

A *synovioma or synovial sarcoma* is a rare but highly malignant tumour arising most commonly in the knee in the synovium or soft tissue around the joint. Pain is not always present, the condition starting as a painless, slowly growing mass which may have been present for several months before being reported. Vague mild pain in the knee may precede any obvious swelling by several months. It may become painful and tender and after a slow start increase more rapidly, and metastases are common. The prognosis is bad. Other varieties of sarcoma may occur in the knee, sarcomatous change in Paget's disease of the lower end of the femur, for instance (*Fig* L.12), but metastatic malignant disease from elsewhere is rare in the knee.

Scurvy is rare today in adults but is seen occasionally in the elderly, alcoholics, food faddists or patients on over-restricted reduction diets. Haemorrhages, subcutaneous and gingival, suggest the diagnosis.

Sarcoidosis may present as a flitting polyarthritis affecting the knees and other joints, lasting several weeks. Joints are affected in 10–30% of patients with sarcoidosis, more often in women. Erythema nodosum and bilateral hilar lymphadenopathy suggest the diagnosis. Effusions are minimal or non-existent and no deformity is left after resolution.

Osteochondritis dissecans is due to separation of avascular fragments of bone and cartilage from the

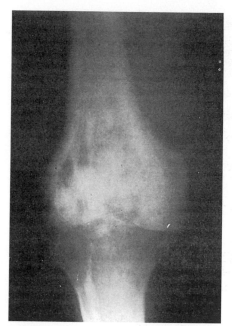
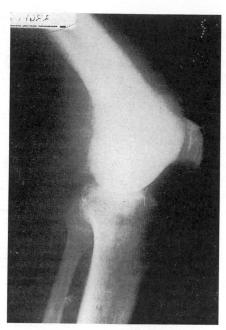

Fig. L.12. Paget sarcoma, lower end of femur.

joint surface. Usually only one knee is involved, pain being slight, but aggravated by exercise. Swelling may be intermittent but the knee may become unstable. It may occur at any age but is most common in the teens. Radiographs show separation of fragments of bone from the joint surface, most commonly over the medial condyle of the femur. The condition often leads to osteoarthritis of the knee later in life.

Neuropathic (Charcot's) knee joints are today a rarity in Europe; in the past they were seen in tabes dorsalis—painless, grossly distorted unstable joints causing extraordinary types of gait. Similar neuropathic knee joints may occur in leprosy and yaws, but syringomyelia affects joints of the upper extremity and diabetes mellitus those of the feet.

Pigmented villonodular synovitis is an uncommon non-malignant condition characterized by marked synovial proliferation and the formation of grape-like masses pigmented with haemosiderin. It usually affects only one knee and though it may sometimes involve bursae, tendon sheath and less often capsule and even bone it is not neoplastic but essentially a chronic synovitis, the aetiology of which is unknown. Repeated bouts of swelling without great pain with heavily blood-stained aspirate in young adults suggests the diagnosis.

Synovial chondromatosis is a benign self-limiting uncommon disorder affecting the young and middle-aged, usually males. Many nodules of metaplastic cartilage form within the synovium and are released into the joint space as loose bodies. The knee is the joint

most commonly involved, usually unilaterally, the patient experiencing discomfort, stiffness, crepitus, swelling and limitation of movement associated with a grating feeling. Some of these loose bodies ossify or calcify and show up typically in radiographs.

Bursitis: There are up to seven bursae around the knee, (see *Fig.* L.9) but not all are present in every individual: (1) the prepatellar bursa; (2) the suprapatellar bursa proximal to the patella behind the quadriceps tendon in front of the distal part of the anterior surface of the femur, communicating with the joint; (3) the subcutaneous infrapatellar bursa anterior to the proximal part of the ligamentum patellae; (4) the deep infrapatellar bursa between the ligamentum patellae and anterior surface of the proximal part of the tibia; (5) the semimembranosus bursa which lies between the semimembranosus and the medial head of the gastrocnemius as they cross one another, usually communicating with (6) a bursa between the medial head of the gastrocnemius and the back of the knee joint which in turn communicates with the knee joint; and (7) the semitendinosus bursa which lies between sartorius, gracilis, semitendinosus and the tibia. Much of the swelling of a knee may be due to inflammation or injury of these bursae rather than the joint itself. In 'housemaid's knee' the prepatellar bursa is swollen and painful, in 'nun's or priest's knee' the infrapatellar bursa, and often the prepatellar also. Inflammation or injury to the semitendinosus bursa may cause pain on the medial side of the knee, not uncommon after athletic activities in persons out of training.

Lipoma arborescens is a benign lipomatous mass which occurs most often in the knee joint and is usually associated with degenerative changes; it causes pain, swelling, restriction of movement and sometimes locking, sometimes with a joint effusion. A visible swelling in the suprapatellar area may become more apparent on flexing the knee.

Hoffa's disease (lipoarthritis traumatica genu), said to be more common in acrobats and ballet dancers, often after trauma or excessive exertion, appears to arise from infrapatellar subsynovial fat becoming swollen and locked in the joint. There is tenderness below the patella but no other physical sign.

Bleeding states may cause a haemorrhagic effusion or frank haemorrhage into a joint: haemophilia, anticoagulant therapy and acute leukaemia are examples. A sudden painful effusion in an arthritic subject on anticoagulants for thromboembolic disease may be due not to the arthritis itself but to a haemarthrosis, the physician having failed to warn the patient that anti-inflammatory drugs and warfarin should not be taken together. Leukaemia itself may also cause pains in the knee from leukaemic involvement of capsule, periosteum and other joint tissues. In hypertrophic pulmonary osteoarthropathy (HPOA) periostitis, sometimes with joint swelling and effusions, accompanies malignant disease or chronic infection at a distant site. Knees and ankles and other joints may become swollen and ache, and effusions may be present in the knees. New periosteal tissue is laid down on bones of forearms, legs below the knees and elsewhere and finger- and possibly toe-clubbing is present. A bronchial carcinoma is often responsible but no malignant changes are present in the joint itself. The changes usually resolve fairly rapidly after removal of the tumour.

Pain in the shin

CAUSES
Referral from the lumbar spine (sciatica)
Referral from the patellofemoral
 joint—usually osteoarthritis
Shin splints
Tabes dorsalis
Periostitis
Hypertrophic pulmonary osteoarthropathy (HPOA)

Most pain is associated with retropatellar osteoarthritis. Discomfort after activity, especially running, is characteristic of shin splints which, if chronic, may lead to radiographically detectable periosteal reaction. HPOA is discussed above.

Pain in the calf

CAUSES
Deep venous thrombosis
Ruptured Baker's cyst
Intermittent claudication

Referral from the lumbar spine (sciatica)
Muscle tension
 —psychological
 —spasticity

If swelling of the calf is also present exclusion of deep venous thrombosis by Doppler technique or venography is the first priority. Even in the presence of known synovitis at the knee demonstration of a Baker's cyst by arthrography or ultrasound does not exclude venous thrombosis.

Pain in the ankle

CAUSES
Arthritis (*see* p. 346)
Ligamentous strain/trauma
Hypermobility syndrome
Achilles tendon bursitis or enthesopathy
Referral from the lumbosacral spine (sciatica)
HPOA

Pain in the foot

CAUSES

Forefoot
Gout
Hallux rigidus
Bunion/hallux valgus
Inflammatory arthritis
Bone or joint infection
Morton's metatarsalgia
Stress fracture
Ingrowing toenail
Ischaemia
Freiberg's disease

Hindfoot
Plantar fasciitis
Achilles' tendonitis/bursitis
Osteochondritis of the navicular (Kohler's disease)
Bone and joint infection

Others
Plantar warts
Stiff flat feet
Oedema
Erythromelalgia
Painful polyneuropathy

Pain in the foot usually arises locally rather than through referral from elsewhere, although root lesions may cause pain along the lateral border of the foot.

Burning pain affecting the 2nd, 3rd or 4th toes which is aggravated by exercise and relieved by rest and removing the shoe is caused by swelling and inflammation of the digital nerve ('digital neuroma'). Usually the cleft between the 3rd and 4th or 2nd and 3rd toes is affected. There may be pain on lateral compression of the metatarsals or tenderness over the adjacent metatarsophalangeal (MTP) joints but there may be no abnormal signs. Surgical excision of the neuroma is curative. Stress fracture of the 2nd, 3rd or

4th metatarsal may also produce forefoot pain which is relieved by rest.

Forefoot pain often arises through deformity (hallux valgus) at the big toe MTP joint with an overlying bunion, stiffness at the same joint (hallux rigidus) with frequent strains due to walking, or inflammatory arthritis at the MTP and toe joints. Rheumatoid disease commonly affects these joints but symmetrical or asymmetrical involvement of toes and MTP joint is also characteristic of seronegative arthritis, the upper limbs being frequently spared. Lesions of the toes including hammer toes and ingrowing toenails are readily apparent. The excruciating podagra of acute gouty arthritis, with surrounding erythema and oedema, is highly characteristic. Bone and joint infections in previously normal feet are rare though opportunistic bone infections may occur in immunocompromised patients including those with human immunodeficiency virus infection.

Pain in the hindfoot is usually attributable to either plantar fasciitis, with pain and tenderness on pressure (especially standing and walking) beneath the calcaneus or Achilles' tendinitis which produces posterior heel pain. Pain at either site impairs or precludes strenuous weight-bearing exercise. Achilles' tendinitis occurs especially in athletes and plantar fasciitis is common in older, overweight, individuals. However, both lesions may occur in young adults in association with seronegative arthritis. In the case of plantar fasciitis X-rays may reveal characteristic plantar spur formation. More rarely osteochondritis of the navicular bone causes transient pain over the inner side of the foot and limb in children between 3 and 6 years. Spontaneous resolution is the rule.

Diffuse pain over the foot may be associated with stiff flat feet (all feet are flat but mobile up to the age of 3 years) and chronic oedema. Burning pain which may be continuous or intermittent may be the presenting feature of erythromelalgia. This uncommon abnormality of superficial blood vessels of the foot may occur in polycythaemia, syringomyelia or in the early stage of chronic arsenical poisoning. It may also occur in normal subjects and may affect the hands. Pain may be severe and is aggravated by heat, dependency and walking. Pain is followed by cutaneous flushing, going on to cyanosis with the pain taking on a pulsatile character. There may be extreme tenderness with oedema and hyperhidrosis. Occasionally Raynaud's phenomenon produces similar episodic pain. Painful polyneuropathy may be attributable to many causes including toxins (especially alcohol) and nutritional deficiencies (especially vitamin B) but is increasingly seen in association with HIV infection. There are usually objective neurological signs.

E. Dudley Hart/Andrew Keat

Leg, ulceration of

Ulceration of the leg may be classified under four headings: (1) *Non-infective ulcers*; these include those that are not due to any specific infection, but which are caused by various factors that interfere with the vitality of the part by injury, poor circulation or deficient innervation of the tissue. (2) *Infective ulcers* resulting from the direct action of a definite specific infection, e.g. tuberculosis or syphilis. (3) *Ulcerating tumours*; these are malignant tumours, which have originated in or invaded the skin. (4) Ulcers associated with leukaemic states and other blood disorders.

Non-infective ulcers

There are usually several aetiological factors at work, of which circulatory disturbance is the most frequent and the most important, and may alone be sufficient cause. With trauma and mild non-specific infection added, the situation is ripe for the development of an indolent ulcer. These conditions obtain in the following varieties:

1. NUTRITIONAL ULCER. Following childbirth or surgical operations, or during the course of recumbency from any disease, especially in patients over the age of 40, there is a liability to thrombosis of the deep veins of the calf. This is manifested by a slight pyrexia, a glossiness, indicative of early oedema, over one ankle joint, an area of tenderness in one calf not present on the opposite side, and pain in one calf on strongly dorsiflexing the foot with the knee straight. The condition may spread into one of the main veins of the leg, and considerable oedema of the limb follows. Such cases, if followed up for a number of years, often develop a chronic oedema, with ulceration subsequently. The ulceration is usually determined by trauma; and some slight knock causing an abrasion which would normally heal is the starting-point of a chronic ulcer.

2. An almost precisely similar condition is caused by *varicose veins* and for the same reason—namely, deficient venous return leading to oedema and circulatory insufficiency (*Fig. L.13*). Not infrequently both factors operate together, and in such cases treatment of the varicose veins is essential and may be sufficient to lead to healing of the ulcer.

These two groups of causes—deep venous thrombosis and varicose veins—account between them for the great majority of leg ulcers seen in practice.

In cases of extreme chronicity the serological tests for syphilis should be made, as this may be a factor, and a biopsy is taken from the edge of the ulcer to preclude carcinoma.

3. ULCERATION DUE TO ARTERIAL DISEASE. Atheroma and thrombo-angiitis obliterans may lead to poor circu-

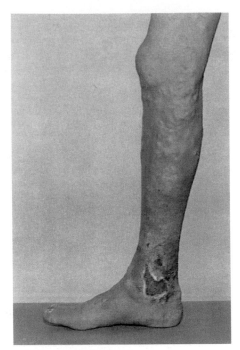

Fig. L.13. Varicose ulcer.

lation and so to loss of nutrition. Ulcerative conditions are common in such cases and even gangrene may result. Such ulceration can start as a result of tissue infarction in large or small blood vessels (arteries or arterioles) due to many causes, thrombotic or embolic. Ulcers over the shin are not uncommon in advanced rheumatoid arthritis, particularly in Felty's syndrome (rheumatoid arthritis with splenomegaly and neutropenia and a tendency to sepsis) (*Fig.* L.14). They also occur in polyarteritis nodosa, scleroderma, systemic lupus erythematosus and allergic vasculitis.

4. LYMPHATIC OBSTRUCTION also leads to loss of nutrition, and ulceration may result. The best instance is seen in elephantiasis due to *Filaria bancrofti*. In Great Britain elephantiasis is rare. Other instances that may be cited are swellings of the leg following a badly united fracture and the cicatricial contractions of extensive burns.

5. DEFICIENT INNERVATION leads to loss of nutrition. Examples are seen in infantile palsy; rubbing of the boot or pressure of an instrument is liable to be followed by an obstinate ulcer. In cases of hemiplegia, even when the patient is lying on a water-bed, ulceration in the form of bed sores will occur much more rapidly on the paralysed side than on the other. Perforating ulcer of the foot is a well-known sequel of *tabes dorsalis* and *diabetes mellitus*.

6. TRAUMA, unless it is continuous, is not alone sufficient to cause an ulcer in healthy people, in whom any abrasion usually heals without trouble. Old ladies,

with thin atrophic skin, may lacerate the tissues over the shin, and the poor blood supply may result in necrosis and subsequent ulceration of the damaged skin. Interference with the normal contraction of scar tissue may also retard healing, as when the lesion is situated over and adherent to a bone.

7. PHYSICAL AGENTS. Burns due to heat or to radium need no elaboration, nor do the ulcers which result from the inadvertent permeation of the subcutaneous tissues by the sclerosing fluids used for the injection of varicose veins. Cold is a factor in the production of ulcerating chilblains, but here once again deficiencies of circulation play a part.

8. DIABETES MELLITUS needs special mention. In this, disease ulceration and gangrene are prone to occur because the resistance of the sugar-laden tissues to infection is lowered, because the arterioles may be occluded by diabetic microangiopathy and because there may be anaesthesia of the foot due to diabetic neuropathy.

9. Varicose or syphilitic ulceration of the leg may be simulated by a *malingerer* who for some reason desires to make out that he is ill; nitric acid or other corrosive may have been rubbed into the leg, or a coin bandaged firmly against the skin, and the diagnosis may be obscure unless the circumstances of the case are well known. Sometimes the diagnosis is suggested by the rectangular or other definite shape of the ulcer itself.

10. BLOOD DYSCRASIAS. Ulcers of the leg may also occur in sickle-cell anaemia, thalassaemia, polycythaemia rubra vera, thrombotic thrombocytopenic purpura and hereditary spherocytosis, all of which should be considered where the aetiology is not evident. Ulceration of the leg, particularly on the lateral aspect, may occur in leukaemia.

Infective ulcers

The legs may be attacked by any form of acute infective ulcer such as *anthrax* or *glanders*, but such an event is rare. *Pyoderma gangrenosa*, frequently affecting the legs but sometimes involving skin elsewhere, may complicate ulcerative colitis or Crohn's disease. The chief ulcers that belong to this group are chronic, and due to syphilis or tuberculosis.

SYPHILITIC ULCERS are the result of gummas which have formed in the subcutaneous tissues. These ulcerated gummas tend to occur in the upper part of the leg and, if in the lower part, on the outer aspect; they are almost always circular, and present a punched-out appearance; they are generally multiple and tend to run into each other, so that the ulcer has a serpiginous outline. They are today rarely seen. Diagnosis can in most cases be made on the distribution and shape of

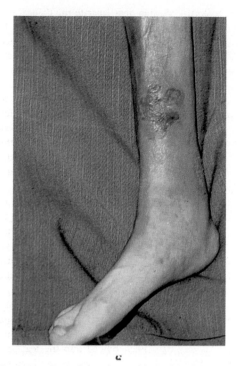
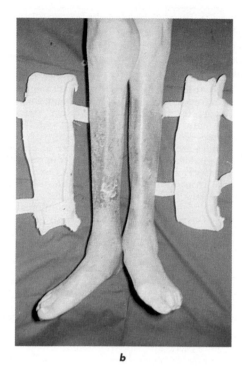

a   *b*

Fig. L.14. *a.* Typical shin ulcer in rheumatoid arthritis. This woman with Felty's syndrome has recurrent shin ulcers due to trivial injuries. She wore these shin pads (*b*) to prevent their recurrence. (*Dr F. Dudley Hart.*)

the ulcer; on the presence of other signs of syphilis; and by finding a positive serological reaction.

There are rare cases of subacute or chronic sores and ulcers of the leg, as of other parts of the body, which have been shown microscopically to arise from various skin fungi. *Blastomycosis, sporotrichosis* and *actinomycosis* of the skin are examples of this group. They are granulomatous eruptions sometimes associated with subcutaneous abscesses and multiple sinuses, sometimes simulating tertiary syphilitic lesions; their exact nature is determined by means of the microscope. Another fungus infection, one occurring in a tropical climate, is *Madura foot*, where the whole foot may become broadened, swollen and distorted by the formation of suppurating granulomatous tissue.

TUBERCULOUS ULCERS usually follow the formation and bursting of tuberculous abscesses, starting either in the subcutaneous tissue or in a bone, and the history may help materially in diagnosis. The ulcer is very chronic, and is characterized by undermining of the skin for a considerable distance from the edge. Lupus vulgaris, a form of primary tuberculosis of the skin, is not often found on the leg, though it may occur there as in any cutaneous area. A useful guiding rule is that lupus never starts later than the age of 20 and lasts for years, whereas a gumma starts at a later period and tends to heal spontaneously. In lupus the chief characteristic is the presence of minute, semi-transpa-

rent nodules at the margin of the ulcer and in the skin around, resembling apple jelly. A particular variety of tuberculous ulcer of the legs is described on page 182 under the heading of erythema induratum scrofulosorum, or Bazin's disease.

Leg ulcers may also be seen in amoebiasis, chancroid, diphtheria, leprosy, yaws, tularaemia, osteomyelitis, kala-azar and granuloma inguinale, all of which should be considered particularly in recent immigrants. The so-called 'phagedenic ulcer' of feet or legs in a chronic lesion caused by mixed bacterial infection that occurs in persons suffering from neglect or starvation.

DYSPROTEINAEMIAS. Leg ulcers may be seen in association with cryoglobulinaemia and macroglobulinaemia.

PYODERMA GANGRENOSUM. In this condition, often associated with ulcerative colitis or Crohn's disease, the ulcers may be multiple and cover large areas of the leg. The ulcers tend to have ragged blue-red overhanging edges and necrotic bases. They often start as pustules or tender red nodules, often from minor trauma.

Ulcerating tumours

EPITHELIOMA may develop in a simple varicose ulcer that has existed for many years (Marjolin's ulcer). The change may be very slow, or rapid. The ulcer spreads, the edges become heaped-up, everted and indurated

(*Fig.* L.15). The groin lymph nodes become enlarged, and if the disease is allowed to progress the bone is attacked. If any doubt arises as to a change in the character of an ulcer, a piece from the edge should be removed for histological examination. The appearance of bare bone at the base of a varicose ulcer should always arouse the gravest suspicion that malignant change has taken place.

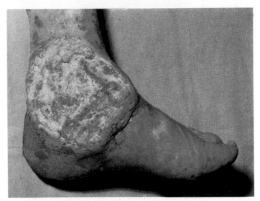

Fig. L.15. Marjolin's ulcer (*Mr Nils Eckhoff.*)

RODENT ULCER (*see also Fig.* F.21) usually attacks the face, though it may be found on any part of the body.

MALIGNANT MELANOMA may ulcerate and bleed (*Fig.* L.16).

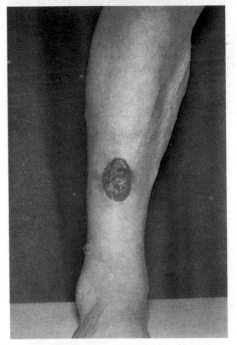

Fig. L.16. Malignant melanoma.

SARCOMA, starting in the deeper tissues, may fungate through the skin and give rise to an irregular breaking-down mass, which is obviously malignant, but may be mistaken for epithelioma unless there is previous knowledge of a malignant bony or soft tissue tumour or unless histological examination is made. Hodgkin's disease and mycosis fungoides may also be associated with ulcers of the leg.

Harold Ellis

Libido, excessive

The desire for sexual intercourse in humans is a biological variable which, like everything else, goes from the diminutive to the excessive. There is no doubt that some people are constitutionally extremely interested in sex and demonstrate excessive libido. Some other individuals use their sexuality in order to increase their own self-esteem and popularity, as in female nymphomania, while the male psychopath may use it to demonstrate his contempt for society. The rapist seems more easily arousable than most, but dispenses with any of the usual forerunning events leading up to sexual intercourse and again may be demonstrating his hatred of women.

The causes of excessive libido are listed in *Table* L.2.

Table L.2.   Causes of excessive libido

Male	Female
Constitutional	Constitutional
Psychological	Psychological
Rapists	Nymphomaniacs
Psychopaths	Manic phase of manic-depressive psychosis
	Menopause
Hormonal	Hormonal
Precocious puberty	Precocious puberty
Adrenogenital syndrome	Adrenogenital syndrome
	Androgen-secreting tumour of adrenal or ovary
	Polycystic ovarian disease
	Androgen therapy
Infections	Infections
Tuberculosis	Tuberculosis
Drugs	Drugs
Alcohol (in small doses)	Alcohol (in small doses)
	Following opioid or benzodiazepine withdrawal

There seems little evidence that exposure of males to erotic stimuli via the cinema, videos, etc. leads to an alteration in sexual behaviour.

Females may show excessive libido during the manic phase of a manic-depressive psychosis or during an evanescent period around about the menopause when they feel that their attractiveness is fading away and 'it is time for one last fling'.

Precocious puberty in a boy (*see* p. 524) or a girl may lead to a libido which is excessive for that individual, in that it is inappropriate for the age. A similar situation may be found in untreated adrenogenital syndrome, commonly due to a 21-hydroxylase defect, when there is a build up of androgens in the adrenal which are the precursors of glucocorticoids. The result is raised testosterone levels in boys and girls, with penile and clitoral enlargement.

Since androgens are important in maintaining libido in women, any situation in which a woman is exposed to excess androgens may promote excessive libido. These include androgen administration, the polycystic ovary syndrome (p. 297) or the very rare case of androgen-secreting tumour of the adrenal or ovary (*Fig.* L.17).

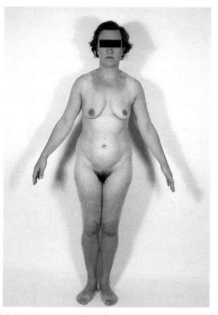

Fig. L.17. Woman with androgen secreting tumour of the ovary. She has a rather masculine habitus, hirsutism and frontal hair recession.

Most infections tend to reduce libido, but curiously it was noticed in both sexes, at a time when chronic tuberculosis was rife, that patients were prone to an increase in their sexuality. Whether this was a true effect of their disease, an attempt to enjoy themselves before a premature death or just secondary to the boredom of being in a sanatorium for months on end it is hard to say.

Alcohol may stimulate libido in both sexes in small doses, but larger amounts, particularly if taken chronically, tend to depress libido. Some cases of increased libido in women have been described following opioid or benzodiazepine withdrawal.

Ian D. Ramsay

Libido, loss of

Libido is the desire to have sexual intercourse. It is promoted by androgens in both male and female, being derived largely from the testes in men and from the adrenal glands in women. Thus hypothalamic or pituitary disease, which reduces gonadotrophin levels in men or adrenocorticotrophic hormone in women, will deprive each sex respectively of their main source of androgen. Similarly testicular disease or damage in a male or Addison's disease in a female will achieve the same effect.

A reduction on gonadotrophins may occur in chronic alcoholics. In addition, cirrhosis of the liver gives rise to an increased oestrogen/testosterone (O/T) ratio in a male which may also lead to a reduction in libido. Similarly an increased O/T ratio is found in thyrotoxicosis. Oestrogen treatment or down-regulation of gonadotrophins by long-acting gonadotrophin releasing hormone analogues in the treatment of carcinoma of the prostate lead to loss of libido.

Hyperprolactinaemia may give rise to a reduction in libido in men by reducing the secretion of gonadotrophins and by blocking the action of gonadotrophins on the testicles. The cause of hyperprolactinaemia may be a pituitary tumour (prolactinoma) or other hypothalamic and pituitary disease leading to lack of prolactin inhibiting factor. Raised prolactin levels may also be found in primary hypothyroidism and renal failure and as a result of drug therapy (*Table* L.3). Anti-androgens used in the treatment of benign prostatic hypertrophy or carcinoma may lead to loss of libido.

Psychological problems are important as causes of loss of libido. Some people just have naturally low levels of libido. Others are anxious or depressed. The menopause in women may be associated with a reduced sex drive which may be partly related to a feeling of unattractiveness and the fact that the reproductive phase of life is over and partly secondary to discomfort on intercourse due to a reduction in vaginal secretion caused by oestrogen deficiency. There is some evidence in the ageing male that libido declines less obviously than do other parameters of sexual function, e.g. morning erections and potency.

Ian D. Ramsay

Table L.3. Causes of loss of libido

Condition	Mechanism
Male	
Endocrine	
Hypothalamic ⎫	Low gonadotrophins and TSH Raised prolactin
Pituitary ⎬ disease	
Thyrotoxicosis	Raised oestrogen/testosterone ratio
Hypothyroidism	Psychomotor retardation, lethargy, raised prolactin
Cushing's disease	Decreased luteinizing hormone
Feminizing tumour of testis or adrenal	Oestrogen secretion
Testicular disease or castration	Reduced testosterone
Ageing	Reduced testosterone
	Increased prolactin
General disease	
General debilitating disease, e.g. chronic infection, cancer	? Psychological
Chronic alcoholism	Reduced gonadotrophins
	Testicular damage
Cirrhosis of the liver	Raised oestrogen/testosterone ratio
Renal failure	General debility
	Raised prolactin
Psychological	
Idiopathic lack of sexual desire	?
Depression	
Anxiety	
Drugs	
Gonadotrophin releasing hormone analogues	Reduced gonadotrophins
Oestrogens	Raised oestrogen/testosterone ratio
	Reduced gonadotrophins
	Increased prolactin
Cytotoxic agents ⎫	
Alcohol ⎬	Testicular damage
Phenothiazines ⎫	
Metoclopramide ⎪	
Haloperidol ⎪	
Pimozide ⎬	Hyperprolactinaemia
Methyldopa ⎪	
Reserpine ⎪	
Cimetidine ⎭	
Spironolactone ⎫	Anti-androgens
Cimetidine ⎪	
Cyproterone acetate ⎬	
Flutamide ⎪	
Finasteride ⎭	
Female	
Endocrine	
Hypothalamic ⎫	Reduced ACTH
Pituitary ⎬ disease	
Hypothyroidism	Psychomotor retardation, lethargy
	Decreased secretion of androgens
Addison's disease	Decreased adrenal androgens
Menopause	Vaginal dryness secondary to oestrogen deficiency
Psychological	
Idiopathic lack of sexual desire	?
Depression	
Anxiety	
Postmastectomy	Worries about loss of feminity, etc.
Drugs	
Cyproterone acetate	Anti-androgen

Lips, affections of

The lips form an important mucocutaneous junction and their proper function is important for feeding and communication. They are subserved by a very large quantity of nerves and hence inflammation can cause disproportionate irritation and pain. The lips are also of considerable cosmetic, psychological and emotional importance. (See *Table* L.4.)

Table L.4. Affections of the lips

Macules
Flat mole (junctional naevus)
Freckle (ephelide)
Peutz–Jegher's syndrome
Telangiectasis
  hereditary haemorrhagic telangiectasia
  liver disease

Papules
Plane warts
Lichen planus
Discoid lupus erythematosus
Pyogenic granuloma
Venous lake
Syphilitic chancre
Actinic cheilitis
  ±solar keratosis
  ±squamous-cell carcinoma

Swollen lips
Trauma, thermal insult
Angio-oedema
Melkersson–Rosenthal syndrome
Crohn's disease

Erosions
Impetigo
Herpes simplex
Hand-foot-and-mouth disease
Secondary syphilis
Erythema multiforme
Fixed drug eruption
Zinc deficiency
Acrodermatitis enteropathica
Pemphigus

Thickening
Atopic dermatitis
Lip-rubbing

Cheilitis
Candidiasis
Contact dermatitis
Lip-licking

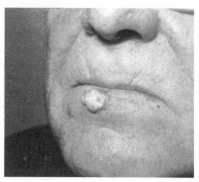

Fig. L.18. Squamous cell carcinoma. (*Dr Richard Staughton.*)

SWOLLEN LIPS

Swollen lips can follow trauma and thermal insult, or be part of an *urticaria*, as *angio-oedema* (*see* p. 26). The *Melkersson–Rosenthal syndrome* comprises permanently oedematous thickened lips (granulomatous cheilitis) with recurrent facial palsy and scrotal tongue. Granulomatous cheilitis is occasionally seen in Crohn's disease (*Fig.* L.19).

MACULES

Macular affections (*see* p. 404) around the lips include flat *moles*, *freckles* and the multiple tiny dark freckles seen in *Peutz–Jegher's syndrome*. Multiple lip telangiectases are seen in *hereditary haemorrhagic telangiectasia* (*see* p. 26) and sometimes with severe liver disease.

PAPULES

The commonest papules on lips are probably plane *warts*, but *lichen planus* papules have a predilection for the lips, as well as plaques of *discoid lupus erythematosus*. *Pyogenic granuloma* can form at this site and in older patients *venous lakes* are commonly seen. The lip can be the site of a primary *syphilitic* chancre. *Actinic cheilitis* is common on the lower lip, especially in seafarers and agricultural workers. The appearance is of atrophy with greyish plaques often surmounted by crusts in cold weather. *Solar keratoses* appear and invasive *squamous-cell carcinoma* (*Fig.* L.18) must be detected early as metastases can quickly occur.

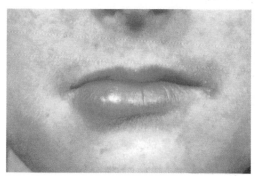

Fig. L.19. Granulomatous cheilitis. Crohn's disease. (*Dr Richard Staughton.*)

EROSIONS

Erosions on lips occur in acute infections such as *impetigo* in children (*see* Fig. C.48), *herpes simplex*, which may be recurrent in adults, *hand-foot-and-mouth disease* and secondary *syphilis*. Erosive dermatoses which affect the lips include *erythema multiforme* (Stevens–Johnson syndrome) (*see* p. 183) and *fixed drug eruption* (codeine and sulphonamides). Chronic erosions around the lips are seen in *zinc deficiency*, *acrodermatitis enteropathica* and *pemphigus* (*see* p. 90).

THICKENED LIPS

Thickening of the skin around the mouth is a characteristic feature of *atopic dermatitis* due to rubbing of the lips with the backs of the hands.

CHEILITIS

When inflammation is confined to the lips, search should be made for occult *candidiasis*, especially in those with dentures and iron deficiency. Chronic *contact dermatitis* can occur at this site, e.g. nickel dermatitis from sucking hairpins, lipstick dermatitis, toothpaste dermatitis and rather surprisingly nail varnish dermatitis. Irritation from excessive *lip-licking* can often be observed in patients with cheilitis and may sometimes be the primary cause.

Richard Staughton

Liver, enlargement of

In adults the liver is about $\frac{1}{36}$; but at birth it is $\frac{1}{24}$; to $\frac{1}{18}$; of the whole body weight, so that in infants and young children it is relatively larger than adults. The normal liver is therefore usually palpable in children. In thin people with lax abdominal muscles the liver is palpable about 1 cm beneath the costal margin and it descends to meet the fingers on deep inspiration. In clinical practice palpation of the liver is an unreliable indicator of actual liver size and the most accurate way of determining this is by percussion. Hepatic dullness extends from the 5th intercostal space in the right nipple line to the 7th intercostal space in the midaxillary line.

In health the edge of the liver is firm and uniform and the surface feels smooth. If the liver is transposed the right lobe is small and the left large. A tongue like projection of the right lobe may protrude from its lower right hand part. This projection, known as *Riedel's lobe* is more common in women than in men. It may cause difficulty of diagnosis, being confused with a mobile kidney, gallbladder or tumour.

Many conditions unconnected with the liver cause an apparent alteration in its size. In emphysema the liver is easily palpable but percussion will reveal that the organ is merely displaced. Deformities of the chest due to rickets or curvature of the spine may depress the liver as may a right subphrenic abscess. It is unusual for enlargement of the liver to lead to upward extension of hepatic dullness because the weight of the liver causes it to descend. Elevation of the upper limit of hepatic dullness occurs when local hepatic disease involves the diaphragm. The best example is an amoebic abscess which may elevate the diaphram. A hydatid cyst may have a similar effect. Loss of hepatic dullness occurs in emphysema principally because of displacement of the liver. Free gas in the peritoneum or distension of the colon may also do this.

Hepatoptosis or *wandering liver* are terms applied to a liver which is found in an abnormal position. This is rare but does occur after therapeutic pneumoperitoneum at laparoscopy. It is usually an

Table L.5. Causes of hepatic enlargement

Hepatitis
Acute
  Viruses
  Drugs
  Alcohol
Chronic
  Lupoid
  HB infection

Venous congestion
Cardiac failure
Constrictive pericarditis
Budd–Chiari syndrome
Veno-occlusive disease
Haemolytic crisis

Fatty liver

Biliary disease
Extrahepatic obstruction
Sclerosing cholangitis
Primary biliary cirrhosis

Infiltration
Malignancy
Granulomatous hepatitis
Amyloidosis

Metabolic
Glycogen storage diseases
Haemochromatosis
Endrocrine diseases

Abscess
Pyogenic
Amoebic

Tropical diseases
Viral hepatitis
Protazoan infections
Helminthic infections

Cryptogenic cirrhosis

asymptomatic condition although the patient may complain of a dragging sensation and heaviness in the right upper quadrant of the abdomen. The liver which is displaced may be thought to be enlarged.

The major categories of disease associated with hepatic enlargement are shown in (*Table* L.5.)

Hepatitis

Acute hepatitis is most commonly due to viral infection (hepatitis A, hepatitis B, hepatitis C, delta virus, hepatitis E), cytomegalovirus, herpes simplex, Epstein–Barr, adverse reaction to a drug, or alcohol. These are fully discussed under JAUNDICE.

Acute hepatitis is invariably associated with hepatic enlargement. The liver is moderately enlarged, usually tender but regular. There are frequently, but not invariably, signs of liver dysfunction including jaundice and in the presence of alcohol abuse there may be stigmata of chronic liver disease. The patient is usually systemically unwell, with anorexia, nausea and weight loss. There may be fever. In alcoholic hepatitis a liver bruit may be audible.

Chronic active hepatitis is also described under JAUNDICE. The usual causes are auto-immune (lupoid hepatitis), chronic hepatitis B and C virus infection and an adverse reaction to drugs. Hepatomegaly is variable in chronic hepatitis. In the early stages the liver is usually enlarged and may be tender. As the disease progresses continuing fibrosis may result in the liver decreasing in size and it becomes impalpable. Liver size can then only be ascertained by percussion. In late stages the stigmata of chronic liver disease develop and splenomegaly and ascites occur as a consequence of portal hypertension. Massive enlargement of the liver associated with hepatitis B and C-related chronic active hepatitis is usually due to a complicating primary hepatocellular carcinoma.

Venous congestion

Venous congestion of the liver results from *obstruction of flow in the hepatic vein*. This may occur at the level of the heart as a consequence either of *right ventricular failure or contrictive pericarditis*. It may occur following *thrombosis of the inferior vena cava* or of the *hepatic vein* (Budd–Chiari syndrome), or there may be an obstruction at the intrahepatic postsinusoidal level.

Venous congestion from *heart disease* causes uniform enlargement of the liver of variable degree. The liver may sometimes be massively enlarged, reaching the umbilicus. In acute heart failure stretching of the hepatic capsule leads to acute pain and tenderness in the right upper quadrant. In chronic heart failure the liver is not usually tender. The presence of a pulsatile liver indicates *tricuspid regurgitation*, as evidenced by a pronounced v wave in the jugular neck veins, cardiac enlargement with a thrill and a pansystolic murmur at the base of the sternum are also evident. Peripheral oedema is usually severe and ascites may occur.

In *constrictive pericarditis* the liver is also considerably enlarged, ascites is often extreme particularly in relation to the degree of peripheral oedema. Jaundice may be prominent and a diagnosis of parenchymal liver disease may be made by the unwary. This should be avoided by the observation that the neck veins are engorged and that the heart is small and 'quiet'.

The *Budd–Chiari syndrome* may present acutely or chronically. Thrombosis of the hepatic vein usually occurs as a consequence of an underlying hypercoagulable state such as polycythaemia rubra vera or thrombotic thrombocytopenic purpura. In some patients the hypercoagulable state is subtle and a bone marrow examination is necessary to make the diagnosis. Antithrombin 3 or protein C deficiency, underlying malignancy (breast, pancreas, lung) or consumption of oestrogens in a relatively high dose are other causes. In the acute disease sudden, painful, massive hepatomegaly develops. Liver decompensation follows and is characterized by jaundice, ascites and splenomegaly due to portal hypertension and (in severe cases) coagulopathy, portasystemic encephalopathy and death. Some surviving patients progress to chronic liver disease associated with marked hepatomegaly, ascites and variceal gastrointestinal bleeding. Rarely the Budd–Chiari syndrome develops insidiously without an initial acute phase. An isotopic liver scan shows diffuse poor uptake, sparing the caudate lobe. The disease is confirmed by hepatic venography and liver biopsy.

Intrahepatic veno-occlusive disease may also occur in hypercoaguable states and presents with painful hepatomegaly. The classical cause is the ingestion of certain plant toxins especially bush tea.

The liver may enlarge suddenly and painfully as a response to venous congestion from *haemolysis*. Haemolytic crises in sickle-cell anaemia and thalassaemia are the best examples.

Fatty Liver

The liver may be enlarged because of excessive deposition of fat droplets. The commonest cause is *alcohol abuse. Protein malnutrition, diabetes mellitus, obesity* and *jejuno-ileal bypass* are others.

The liver is uniformly enlarged, firm but not tender. Signs of hepatic decompensation are absent unless there is pre-existing ethanolic damage.

In acute fatty liver of pregnancy, microvesicular deposition of fat occurs throughout the liver cells. This is a condition which develops in late pregnancy and is associated with liver failure characterized by encephalopathy, coagulopathy and renal failure. The liver is grossly enlarged and tender. The prognosis is poor but Caesarean section and removal of the baby is life-saving.

Biliary disease

Biliary obstruction (cholestasis) can be due to disease affecting the extrahepatic biliary tract, the intrahepatic bile ducts and ductules or the canaliculi.

Extrahepatic biliary obstruction is most commonly due to gallstones within the bile duct or to malignant tumours, either in the pancreas, gallbladder or secondary deposits or within the bile duct itself. Benign structures following operative trauma or sclerosing cholangitis, chronic pancreatitis or infestation by ascaris lumbricoides are less common causes. Patients presenting with extrahepatic obstruction due to impacted gallstones present with right upper quadrant abdominal pain and fluctuating jaundice. The liver is tender and moderately enlarged. A common consequence of choledocholithiasis is infection of bile leading to pain, jaundice and fever with rigors (Charcot's triad).

Biliary infection is unusual in patients with malignant extrahepatic biliary obstruction; such patients present with progressive painful jaundice and the depth of jaundice is usually greater than that associated with gallstones. The liver is uniformly enlarged unless there is metastatic malignant disease. When the obstruction is distal to the cystic duct the gallbladder is also distended and palpable. Courvoisier's law, that 'in a patient with obstructive jaundice a palpable gall bladder is unlikely to be due to stones', is unreliable. Patients with malignant extrahepatic biliary obstruction may have other evidence of neoplastic disease; weight loss is often pronounced. Back pain may occur as a consequence of vertebral or coeliac plexus erosion by tumour. Ascites with a high protein content may be present. The patient with an ampullary tumour may be anaemic because of chronic blood loss from the tumour. Extrahepatic biliary obstruction is considered more fully in under JAUNDICE.

Congenital malformations of the biliary tract are associated with hepatomegaly. In biliary atresia there is failure of development of the extrahepatic biliary tree and the infant develops progressive jaundice and liver failure associated with marked hepatomegaly. The diagnosis is made by radio-isotopic HIDA scan and hepatic transplantation or portoenterostomy (Kasai operation) are life-saving. Other congenital abnormalities of the biliary tree include choledochal cyst, congenital dilatation of the intrahepatic ducts (Caroli's disease), and congenital hepatic fibrosis. *Choledochal cyst* characteristically presents in young women with a triad of jaundice, pain and an abdominal mass. Poor drainage of the biliary apparatus results in recurrent cholangitis and the disease predisposes to the development of cholangiocarcinoma. Primary repair of the cyst is necessary. The cysts may occasionally be intrahepatic when they have to be differentiated from simple cysts or polycystic disease which may be part of a spectrum of polycystic syndromes affecting the liver, pancreas and kidneys. Such cysts do not communicate with the biliary tree. *Caroli's syndrome* is a rare condition associated with intrahepatic cystic dilatation of the bile ductules. Recurrent infection may lead to jaundice and hepatomegaly.

Biliary strictures affecting both the intra- and extrahepatic tree are characteristic of *sclerosing cholangitis* (*Fig*. L.20). This may occur as a consequence of recurrent biliary sepsis, usually associated with bile duct trauma. It may alternatively be a primary condition commonly associated with ulcerative colitis. In primary sclerosing cholangitis males predominate and the disease is extremely variable in its presentation. It is

likely that the majority of patients are asymptomatic for many years. Others present with recurrent jaundice and cholangitis. Examination reveals firm hepatomegaly and in those patients who progress to cirrhosis this may be irregular and associated with other evidence of chronic liver disease. The treatment of sclerosing cholangitis is unsatisfactory. The condition is reviewed more fully under JAUNDICE.

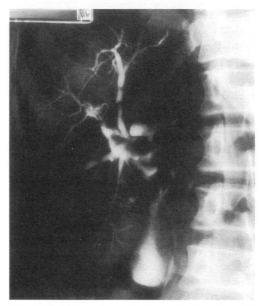

Fig. L.20. Percutaneous cholangiogram showing the typical appearances of intrahepatic primary sclerosing cholangitis in a patient with ulcerative colitis. The biliary tree is beaded with irregularly narrowed ducts.

Chronic intrahepatic cholestasis occurs in *primary biliary cirrhosis*. This is a condition of middle-aged women in which the bile ductules are destroyed by a cell-mediated auto-immune process. The disease is extremely variable in its presentation but it progresses slowly in the majority of patients. Many patients are asymptomatic; the characteristic symptom is that of pruritus. Others present at a late stage with hepatic decompensation or variceal haemorrhage. In the late stages the woman presents with jaundice, xanthelasmata and hepatomegaly which is often marked, irregular and firm (*Fig*. L.21). Splenomegaly and ascites are common and there may be evidence of other auto-immune disease such as thyroiditis, systemic sclerosis or Addison's disease. In common with all chronic cholestatic conditions, pigmentation due to deposition of melanin in the skin develops. Defective copper excretion may occasionally lead to Kayser-Fleischer rings (see *Fig*. J10.). The diagnosis is suggested by cholestatic liver function tests in a woman and is confirmed by the presence of circulating anti-mitochondrial antibodies and a typical liver biopsy appearance

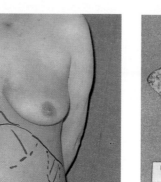

Fig. L.21. Primary biliary cirrhosis. Late disease demonstrating hepatosplenomegaly, ascites and skin pigmentation.

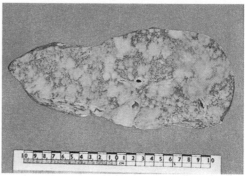

Fig. L.22. Liver almost replaced by secondary deposits. The primary site was a carcinoma of the breast.

characterized by destruction and paucity of bile ductules, granulomata and evidence of fibrosis or cirrhosis.

Other cholestatic conditions are also associated with hepatomegaly, jaundice and pruritus. Rare patients present with *benign recurrent cholestasis* in which severe jaundice and pruritus relapse and remit from birth. Liver biopsy shows only evidence of cholestasis without liver damage. Certain *drugs*, particularly chlorpromazine, tricyclic antidepressants and chloropropamide are associated with cholestasis. Cholestasis may also occur as a non-specific response to severe systemic illness, particularly following operations; the cause is unknown and resolves as the general condition of the patient improves.

Hepatic infiltration

The liver parenchyma may be infiltrated by malignant cells, granulomata or by amyloid.

The commonest of these is *secondary carcinoma*, usually arising from the gastro-intestinal tract, breast, bronchus and kidney (*Fig.* L.22). Symptoms do not develop until very late and comprise right upper quadrant abdominal pain and jaundice. Examination reveals irregular hepatomegaly. The liver is hard and sometimes extremely large, extending into the pelvis. Sudden painful enlargement may be due to bleeding into a secondary deposit. Ascites is common and is associated with a high protein content. There may be evidence of primary disease and it is important in all patients presenting with hepatomegaly to examine the breasts, thyroid and prostate as specific therapy may affect progression both of the primary and of the secondary diseases.

The diagnosis of secondary malignant infiltration is strongly supported by ultrasound or CT scanning of the liver but should always be confirmed by guided needle biopsy or cytology. Once a diagnosis has been achieved it is usually pointless to seek the primary tumour because cure is impossible. The only excep-

tions are those of tumours which might be amenable to hormonal therapy or chemotherapy (prostate, breast, thyroid) and the occasional patient who has a solitary hepatic secondary deposit from a colonic carcinoma. In this situation it may be reasonable to embark upon a colonic resection. Rarely secondary deposits are suitable for hepatic resection.

It is important to differentiate secondary carcinoma of the liver from a *carcinoid tumour* These commonly arise from the small bowel or appendix and may replace large amounts of the liver. A proportion secrete polypeptides and present with the *carcinoid syndrome* which only occurs when the tumour has spread to the liver. Such patients present with flushing and watery diarrhoea and may develop chronic pigmentation of the hands and face. The tumours are often extremely slowly growing and considerable palliation can be achieved either by the use of somatostatin and its analogues, or interferon, by embolization of the tumour via the hepatic artery, or by surgical removal.

Primary hepatocellular carcinoma is comparatively rare in Britain but is the commonest hepatic malignancy worldwide. It is associated with chronic infection with hepatitis B or C and usually develops in cirrhotic patients (*Figs.* L.23, L.24). Other causes of cirrhosis, particularly long-standing alcoholic cirrhosis and, treated haemochromatosis also predispose to the tumour. Patients present with weight loss, abdominal pain and massive hepatomegaly. The liver is greatly enlarged and may or may not be tender. The tumour mass is hard, irregular and sometimes associated with a bruit. There is usually evidence of chronic liver disease. Ascites may either be due to underlying portal hypertension from cirrhosis or as a direct consequence of the primary liver cancer in which event the protein concentration is high (>30 g/l). The diagnosis is made by the finding of increased concentration of circulating alpha-fetoprotein, by liver biopsy or by angiography. The prognosis is very poor.

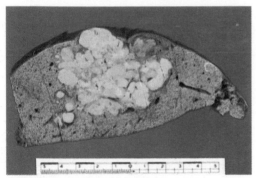

Fig. L.23. An unusual primary hepatoma arising in a previously normal liver.

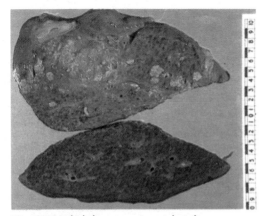

Fig. L.24. Multiple hepatomas in a cirrhotic liver.

Haemangiomas of the liver are relatively common probably occurring in as many as 10 per cent of livers. They are usually asymptomatic. Angiosarcomas occasionally arise from these benign tumours and they are associated with ingestion of plant toxins (aflatoxins), or chronic infestation with liver fluke. Massive enlargement of the liver occurs and health rapidly deteriorates. A liver bruit is often present. The prognosis is very poor.

Benign tumours of the liver are unusual. Adenomas occur in association with the use of oestrogens and in pregnancy. These are usually asymptomatic but may present acutely with massive intraperitoneal bleeding.

Lymphoma may cause hepatomegaly in a variety of ways. The liver may be infiltrated in Hodgkin's disease or non-Hodgkin's lymphoma. The liver is then irregularly enlarged and non-tender. There may be other evidence of lymphoma such as splenomegaly and lymphadenopathy. In other cases infiltration is diffuse and the liver is then smooth, regular, firm and only moderately enlarged. Some patients with lymphoma present as granulomatous liver disease showing little or no hepatomegaly but cholestatic liver function tests. Occasionally patients present as extrahepatic biliary obstruction from lymph node masses particularly arising in the region of the porta hepatis. Lymphoma may present as the Budd–Chiari syndrome as previously described. Occasional patients present with cholestatic jaundice without obvious extrahepatic biliary obstruction and without infiltration. The liver is then enlarged, the patient deeply jaundiced and a biopsy merely shows evidence of intrahepatic cholestasis.

Sarcomas of the liver are extremely rare and cannot be differentiated clinically from carcinoma.

The liver may also be infiltrated in *amyloidosis*. This may either occur as a primary disease or in association with myelomatosis or chronic suppurative disease. The liver is extremely large, smooth, firm and non-tender. In addition the spleen may be enlarged and there may be proteinuria because of renal involvement. The diagnosis may be made by liver biopsy although this can be dangerous because rarely the procedure may cause the rigid liver to split.

The liver may be infiltrated by *granulomata*. There are a wide variety of causes of which the most important are sarcoidosis, tuberculosis, lymphoma, and an adverse reaction to drugs.

The liver is frequently involved in *sarcoidosis* when the alkaline phosphatase concentration is often increased. Symptoms and signs of liver disease are rare and hepatomegaly occurs in only about 20 per cent of patients. Those with enlargement of the liver are often West Indian. The liver may then be considerably enlarged, irregular, and it is usually firm but non-tender. There is often splenomegaly and other features of sarcoidosis including pulmonary infiltration and hypercalcaemia may be evident.

Tuberculosis is also associated with granulomatous liver disease and the liver is commonly somewhat enlarged in this disease. It is usually firm, modestly enlarged but non-tender.

Chronic infection with *schistosomiasis* causes granulomatous infiltration of the liver. The liver is enlarged, firm and non-tender. Pre-sinusoidal portal hypertension causes splenomegaly and oesophageal varices develop. Hepatic synthetic function is maintained until a late stage and jaundice is relatively mild.

Syphilis is now an extremely rare disease in the Western hemisphere. It is associated with hepatomegaly in the secondary stage and in addition tertiary syphilis and the formation of gummas lead to the formation of an irregular rather hard liver similar in appearance and feel to that of cirrhosis.

Metabolic causes

A variety of metabolic, genetic and endocrine disorders are associated with the development of hepatomegaly.

Glycogen storage diseases cause hepatomegaly from birth. Lipid storage disorders such as *Gaucher's disease* are associated with massive hepatosplenomegaly and growth retardation while *Niemann–Pick disease* may have neurological associations including mental retardation.

Haemochromatosis and *haemosiderosis* are disorders associated with accumulation of iron within the liver. Haemosiderosis is commonly associated with multiple blood transfusions often required for haemolytic disorders such as thalassaemia. Iron accumulates within Kupffer's cells. Hepatic function is well maintained and the liver is only moderately enlarged. In contrast, haemochromatosis is a genetic syndrome inherited as an autosomal recessive gene. The condition is associated with alcohol abuse, probably because this also enhances iron absorption. The disease is rare in premenopausal women because of menstrual blood loss. Patients present with hepatomegaly due to cirrhosis. The liver is firm and considerably enlarged. There may be evidence of portal hypertension including splenomegaly, ascites and a proportion of patients present for the first time as a variceal haemorrhage. Iron is also deposited in the skin producing dusky pigmentation. Deposition also occurs in endocrine glands accounting to the common association with diabetes. Marked feminization manifest as gynaecomastia, absent body hair, testicular atrophy and decreased need for shaving are prominent features. Although relatively unusual the diagnosis of haemochromatosis is important because the prognosis is greatly improved by venesection. The diagnosis is made by demonstrating an increased serum ferritin concentration and by liver biopsy. Massive hepatomegaly associated with haemochromatosis may be due to the development of hepatocellular cancer which is a relatively common late complication.

Acromegaly is associated with hepatomegaly without evidence of liver dysfunction. The liver is modestly enlarged but soft. Thyrotoxicosis may also be associated with hepatic enlargement and deranged liver function tests.

Liver abscess

Liver abscesses are either a consequence of bacterial infection or amoebiasis. Pyogenic liver abscess follows portal pyaemia due to diverticulitis, appendicitis, subphrenic abscess, or inflammatory bowel disease. It may complicate biliary disease, usually choledocholithiasis, but sometimes an infected endoprosthesis, sclerosing cholangitis or ampullary tumour. Pyogenic abscesses are commonly multiple and rarely large. They are associated with modest painful hepatomegaly with marked constitutional disturbances including fever with rigors, and jaundice.

An amoebic abscess may be single and large. It commonly follows a history of dysentery and the majority occur in the right lobe. Men are affected more often than women. The patient presents with swinging pyrexia, associated with rigors and tachycardia, a considerably enlarged and very tender liver; there may be a sympathetic pleural effusion.

The diagnosis of liver abscess is made by ultrasound and confirmed by guided aspiration and culture of pus (*Fig.* L.25). Small multiple abscesses may respond to systemic antibiotic therapy and relief of the underlying cause (viz. relief of biliary obstruction, irradication of the primary intra-abdominal sepsis). Larger abscesses are drained either by a percutaneous wide-bore catheter or by formal surgical drainage.

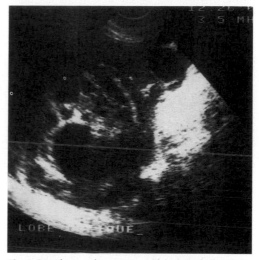

Fig. L.25. Ultrasound examination of the liver demonstrating multiple pyogenic abscesses of the right lobe of the liver.

Tropical diseases

A variety of exotic diseases are associated with hepatomegaly. These include viral hepatitis, protozoan infections including malaria, schistosomiasis, Kala-azar, hydatid and infestations with liver flukes and ascaris lumbricoides.

Acute painful hepatomegaly occurs during the crises of malaria.

Large hydatid cysts can occur within the liver but these are usually asymptomatic and cause no disturbance of liver function. The cysts may achieve considerable size, they are rounded and smooth, and there may be a thrill perceived on percussion (ballottment). The diagnosis is made by plain abdominal X-ray if the cysts are calcified. Ultrasound appearances are extremely characteristic and daughter cysts are often seen (*Fig.* L.26). Needle aspiration is contra-indicated because this may cause infection and spillage of cysts within the peritoneal cavity. The Casoni test is usually positive.

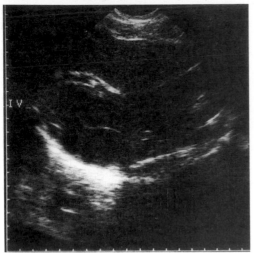

Fig. L.26. Ultrasound examination of the liver revealing classical appearances of hydatid cyst with multiple daughter cysts.

Cryptogenic cirrhosis

A proportion of individuals present with well-established cirrhosis and hepatomegaly without an obvious cause. The majority of these are women and there is no evidence of exposure to alcohol or the hepatitis B or C virus. The smooth muscle antibody and antinuclear factor are negative but there is no evidence of metabolic or congenital liver disease. The clinical findings are variable but include the stigmata of chronic liver disease, evidence of portal hypertension and portosystemic encephalopathy. The size of the liver is variable, ranging from barely palpable to moderately enlarged. The organ is firm, irregular and non-tender (*Fig.* L.27).

K. R. Palmer

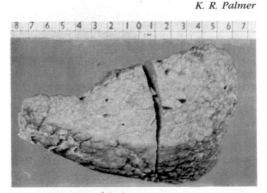

Fig. L.27. Cirrhosis of the liver.

Lymphadenopathy

Although there are a multitude of causes of lymphadenopathy (*Table* L.6) it is usually possible to narrow the differential diagnosis considerably by careful review of the patient's history and clinical examination. The differential diagnosis is very dependent on the patient's age and geographical location. Small soft lymphadenopathy is commonly found in healthy children and young adults particularly in the axillary and inguinal regions. A young adult with significant cervical lymphadenopathy in the UK is likely to have Epstein–Barr (EBV) infection whereas in Africa the commonest cause is often tuberculosis. Local lymphadenopathy may be secondary to local infection or malignancy whereas generalized enlargement is indicative of a systemic disorder. Painful, tender nodes in association with a fever and rash indicate a systemic infection usually of viral aetiology. Firm, painless nodes found in a patient with weight loss or night sweats is likely to be due to malignant disease. Occasionally it is difficult to identify the cause of enlarged lymph nodes and it is then essential to systematically consider all possibilities listed in *Table* L.6.

Infections

Local infections usually result only in regional lymph node enlargement which may be painful. A viral sore throat may cause swelling of the tonsils and tonsillar lymph nodes. Unilateral cervical, axillary or inguinal lymphadenopathy may be due to bacterial or fungal infection in the field of lymphatic drainage.

EBV infection (glandular fever) is a common cause in young adults with generalized lymphadenopathy particularly involving the cervical region. It is clinically very similar to acute cytomegalovirus (CMV) and human immunodeficiency virus (HIV) infection. This latter virus may later cause a persistent painless generalized lymphadenopathy for a period of many months. Acute brucellosis or toxoplasmosis may also produce a similar syndrome although usually without a sore throat.

Tuberculosis usually causes enlargement of a single set of nodes although generalized enlargement is occasionally observed. Primary syphilis may initially result in swelling of the inguinal lymph nodes draining the chancre but generalized lymphadenopathy may be observed in secondary syphilis when the primary lesion has healed. Cat scratch fever often seen in children, presents with an inflamed papule at the site of injury which may be followed by local lymphadenopathy for several months.

Tropical infections such as filiriasis, African trypanosomiasis, and tulareamia may be associated with lymphangitis in association with the primary infection and local lymphadenopathy to which may become generalized later.

Table L.6. Causes of lymphadenopathy

Infections

Viral
Epstein–Barr virus
Human immunodeficiency virus
Cytomegalovirus
Coxsackie
Rubella
Measles

Bacterial
Septicaemia
Local infections
Brucellosis
Tuberculosis
Syphilis
Cat scratch disease
Plague
Scrub typus
Leprosy
Bejel, pinta, yaws
Lymphogranuloma venereum
Granuloma inguinale
Tularaemia
Bartonella
Protozoa
Filaria
Trypanosomiasis
Fungal blastomycosis
Paracoccidiomycosis

Malignant diseases
Secondary deposits from a local malignancy
Hodgkin's disease
Non-Hodgkin's lymphomas
  B-cell
  T-cell
  Mycosis fungoides
  Angioimmunoblastic lymphadenopathy
Chronic lymphatic leukaemia
Acute lymphatic leukaemia
Myeloproliferative disorder
Macroglobulinaemia

Connective tissue disorders
Systemic lupus erythematosis
Rheumatoid arthritis
Drug reactions
Serum sickness

Miscellaneous
Sarcoid

Malignant disease

Malignant disease may spread from a primary site along the draining lymphatics to invade the regional lymph nodes; it is unusual for generalized lymphadenopathy to be secondary to disseminated carcinoma although it is occasionally observed, e.g. melanoma.

Symmetrical generalized painless lymphadenopathy is a common presenting feature of malignancies of the lymphopoietic system, e.g. Hodgkin's disease in a young person or chronic lymphatic leukaemia or non-Hodgkin's lymphoma in an older adult. Macroglobulinaemia, or occasionally myeloma, is characterized by painless generalized lymphadenopathy. Such syndromes may be associated with systemic or 'B' symptoms, i.e. greater than 10 per cent weight loss, fever greater than 38°C or night sweats. These indicate generalized disease and in an individual presenting with only a single group of enlarged nodes is suggestive of more extensive disease. Other malignant disorders of the lymphoreticular system, particularly of T cell origin, have characteristic features. Adult T-cell leukaemia/lymphoma may present with fever, rash and hypercalcaemia as well as extensive hilar lymphadenopathy. Mycosis fungoides is recognizable by the cutaneous deposits which although are initially localized lymphomatous lesions, as the disease progresses it spreads to involve nodes resulting in their generalized enlargement. Acute lymphatic leukaemia, especially in children may present with diffuse lymphadenopathy. Myeloproliferative disorders, e.g. chronic myeloid leukaemia, polycythaemia rubra vera and myelofibrosis are occasionally associated with lymphadenopathy.

Other conditions

Lymphadenopathy can occur in collagenoses, e.g. SLE and rheumatoid arthritis. Sarcoid as well as causing bilateral hilar lymphadenopathy may result in generalized superficial lymphadenopathy. Drugs, e.g. phenytoin may rarely cause lymph node hypertrophy. The unusual condition of angio-immunoblastic lymphadenopathy is often a highly malignant lymphoma but occasionally may be secondary to drugs, e.g. penicillins and sulphonamides.

Splenomegaly may be a feature of any cause of lymphadenopathy. In acute infections it is usually small and soft whereas in long-standing infections or malignancies it is often firm on palpation.

Investigations

These should be directed initially at the diagnosis of the most likely conditions as judged by the history and examination. A full blood count will indicate the presence of a leukaemic process or atypical lymphocytes will reflect an acute viral infection, e.g. EBV or HIV. A chest X-ray may reveal hilar lymphadenopathy or pulmonary pathology, e.g. tuberculosis. A serological search for infections, e.g. EBV and CMV, may indicate active infection if a high titre of a specific IgM is present. Although a bone-marrow aspirate will reveal the presence of leukaemia, a trephine biopsy is much more reliable for diagnosing an infiltrate, e.g. carcinoma or lymphoma.

An abdominal and chest CT scan is a sensitive investigation for identifying pelvic, para-aortic, coelic, mesenteric, hilar or paratracheal node enlargement. If the initial blood tests do not give an early diagnosis it is essential to perform a lymph node biopsy. If the initial histology reveals reactive change only or the presence of granulomas it is often prudent to perform further biopsies if there is a strong indication clinically that the patient may have a malignant condition.

C. A. Ludlam

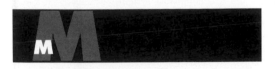

Macules

A macule is a flat circumscribed patch of altered skin colour of *any* size. (In the past the term was often restricted to small lesions less than 2 cm across.) Macules may be red (e.g. rubella), dark red (e.g. purpura), brown (e.g. freckle) or white (e.g. vitiligo). (*See Table* M.1.)

(*See also under* ERYTHEMA.)

Table M.1. Macules

Red macules	Brown macules

1. Exanthems
    Measles
    Rubella
2. Typhoid
3. Drug reaction
4. Macular syphilide (*Fig.* M.1)
5. Tuberculoid leprosy (*Fig.* M.2)
	1. Freckles
	    Sun-induced
	    Xeroderma pigmentosum (*Fig.* S.30)
	    Peutz–Jegher's syndrome
	    Hutchinson's freckle
	2. Flat mole (junctional naevus)
	3. *Café-au-lait* spots
	    Neurofibromatosis (*Fig.* M.4)
	    Albright's syndrome
	4. Mongolian spot
	5. Chloasma
	6. Berloque dermatitis
	7. Postinflammatory hyperpigmentation

Purpuric macules
Inflammatory skin diseases
  Contact dermatitis
  Drug reactions
  Erythema multiforme (*Fig.* E.11)
  Vasculitis
Pigmented purpuric eruptions
  Schamberg's purpura
  Majocchi's purpura
Septicaemia (*Fig.* M.3)
	White macules
	1. Postinflammatory depigmentation
	    Pityriasis alba
	2. Vitiligo (*Fig.* M.5)
	3. Pityriasis versicolor (*see* p. 406)
	4. Naevus anaemicus

Red macules

Redness that is due to hyperaemia and blanches with pressure is known as 'erythema'. A widespread red macular rash occurs at some stage in many infections.

1. *Exanthems—in measles* the rash begins behind the ears and on the forehead in an ill, coughing, febrile child, with conjunctivitis and lymphadenopathy. The rash spreads over the face, neck and extremities and comprises small pink macules which become confluent, turn brown and desquamate. Vesicles on the buccal mucosae (Koplik's spots) are seen just before the rash appears. The pink macules of *rubella (German measles)* also begin behind the ears and spread onto the face, head, neck, and trunk. Occipital lymphadenopathy is common but fever and malaise are mild.

2. In *typhoid*—'rose spots' (0.5 cm red maculopa-

pules) appear in crops on the abdomen, chest and back. Successive crops may come and go for 2–3 weeks.

3. In *drug reactions*—itching and burning are pronounced and lesions may later become elevated (e.g. maculopapular ampicillin rash), purpuric or even bullous.

4. The *macular syphilide* is one of the most characteristic lesions of secondary syphilis. The eruption, named, 'syphilitic roseola', begins as a macular mottling resembling measles, but rather more dusky and distributed over the chest, abdomen and, of great diagnostic importance, on the palms and soles (*Fig.* M.1). Eroded red patches are commonly present on the buccal mucosa. Malaise and lymphadenopathy are common and serology will be positive. A primary chancre will often still be present. Generally about a fortnight after its appearance the rash begins to fade giving place to a papular or follicular eruption on the trunk, limbs, face and neck. Vesicles are never seen, and characteristically the rash does not itch.

It should be distinguished from pityriasis versicolor (*see* p. 406), in which the scaly patches can be demonstrated by scratching and the fungus can be demonstrated microscopically; from drug reactions by their more vivid redness and the presence of itching and burning; from seborrhoeic dermatitis by its scaliness and pinkish-yellow colour; from measles by the coryza, cough and the different distribution; and from pityriasis rosea (*see* p. 585) by the history of the herald patch, the distribution sparing the face and extremities and the characteristic oval lesions, each with their collarette of scaling.

5. In the earlier stages of *tuberculoid leprosy*, red macular areas may appear. These are often isolated and have hyperpigmented borders, and as they expand to their maximum size of 2–10 cm in diameter, the

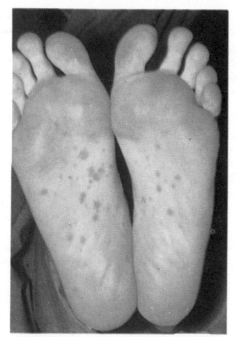

Fig. M.1. Macules on soles—secondary syphilis. (*Westminster Hospital.*)

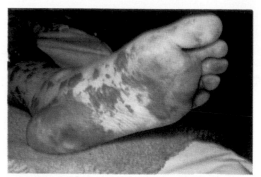

Fig M.3. Meningococcal septicaemia—extensive macular ecchymoses. (*Dr Richard Staughton.*)

centre of lesions becomes depigmented and anaesthetic (*Fig* M.2). In dark skins the red macules are difficult to discern until the central depigmentation makes them obvious.

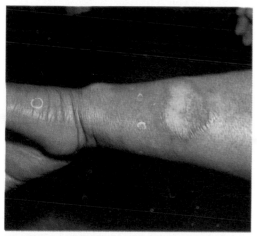

Fig. M.2. Tuberculoid leprosy. (*St John's Hospital.*)

Purpuric macules

Purpuric macules are due to the escape of red blood cells into the skin, and characteristically fail to blanch on pressure. Tiny lesions 1–5 mm are true purpura, larger extravasations are *ecchymoses* (*Fig.* M.3) and associated subcutaneous collections are *haematomas*. Purpura appear suddenly, are painless and change hue from red, to brown, to green and yellow before fading.

Most purpura seen in skin disease is due to damage to vessel walls occurring in a whole variety of inflammatory disorders, e.g. contact dermatitis, drug reactions, erythema multiforme or vasculitis.

The list of possible causes of purpura is extensive (*see* p. 540). There are a few uncommon but characteristic purpuric dermatoses, e.g. the *pigmented purpuric eruptions* occurring much more commonly on the lower than upper extremities, and in males more often than in females. Various patterns are given eponymous titles such as Schamberg's purpura and Majocchi's purpura.

Brown macules

Examples are freckles, flat moles, *café-au-lait* spots, mongolian spots and chloasma.

1. Freckles (ephelides) are small (less than 0.5 cm), brown, roundish macules in areas of sun exposure. They appear in childhood especially in red-haired, fair-skinned individuals and are associated with vulnerability to sunburn. They are particularly florid in the rare *xeroderma pigmentosum*, a condition associated with deficient repair of sun-damaged nuclear protein (*see Fig.* S.30). By their early teens affected children are disfigured by atrophy, telangiectasia and later multiple cutaneous malignancies.

In the *Peutz–Jegher's syndrome* freckles in great profusion on and around the lips are associated with polyposis of the small bowel which may be complicated by recurrent intussusception and melaena. The freckles are smaller than usual and may extend inside the mouth and onto the sides and backs of fingers. *Hutchinson's freckle* is a giant freckle usually on an elderly sun-exposed skin. Pigmentation is variegate and malignant pigment cell tumours often eventually arise within their boundaries.

2. *Flat moles* (junctional naevi) are either present at birth or develop in the first two decades. They have distinct borders and are not uniformly pigmented. They undergo gradual spontaneous involution. Rarely a more rapid involution of moles, both flat or papular, may

be accompanied by a stark chalk-white halo of depigmentation—a halo naevus (Sutton's naevus). This is a dramatic but benign condition.

3. *Café-au-lait spots* are well named and are creamy brown in colour with smooth borders ranging from 1 to 15 cm in diameter. More than six lesions on a child's skin are said to be highly suggestive of the autosomal dominant *von Recklinghausen's neurofibromatosis*. The later appearance of axillary freckling is an even stronger diagnostic pointer (*Fig.* M.4) to the later appearance of multiple pendulous cutaneous nerve sheath tumours. Large brown macules with irregular borders on a child's trunk can also be associated with bone cysts and precocious puberty in girls with *Albright's syndrome*.

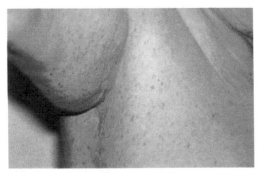

Fig. M.4. Axillary freckling in van Recklinghausen's disease. (*Addenbrookes Hospital.*)

4. *The mongolian spot* is well known to midwives as a marker of Asiatic or Negroid parentage: large brown or slate-grey macules are seen over the sacrum at birth and gradually fade over the first year of life, the colour is due to melanocytes in the dermis.

5. *Chloasma*, a mask-like hyperpigmentation, is common in pregnant women or in those taking oral contraceptives, but occasionally occurs in non-pregnant women, and rarely in malnutrition. The pigment can be quite dark, especially after summer, and is due to excessive retention of pigment by normal numbers of melanocytes. Areas affected are forehead, upper cheeks and moustache area, and are only rarely asymmetrical.

6. *Berloque dermatitis* is an indolent phototoxic dermatitis characterized by browning of the skin of the neck of women at the site of application of perfumes which contain photosensitizing agents, such as bergamot oils.

7. *Postinflammatory hyperpigmentation*—macular hyperpigmentation can follow preceding inflammatory dermatoses and is characteristic of damage to the dermo-epidermal junction, as in lichen planus or fixed drug eruptions. Such 'tattoos' of melanin in the dermal macrophages may take many months to resolve.

White macules

1. Postinflammatory depigmentation may occur following inflammatory dermatoses, such as psoriasis or pityriasis rosea. Perhaps more commonly, many skin diseases fail to tan on a sunny holiday. This is particularly seen over the cheeks and outer arms of children with the eczematous condition *pityriasis alba*.

2. *Vitiligo* usually begins in the second decade as symmetrical chalk-white patches of complete depigmentation around eyes, mouth, genitals and axillae (*Fig.* M.5). White locks of hair may occur but ocular pigmentation is never affected. In dark races lesions are only too obvious but in untanned, pale individuals the use of an ultraviolet light may be necessary to demonstrate the full extent of the disease.

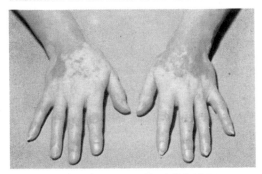

Fig. M.5. Vitiligo. (*Westminster Hospital.*)

3. *Pityriasis versicolor* is becoming a more common cause for medical consultation—the original fawny-pink slightly scaling, round patches on chest and back may not be noticed until, following sun exposure, partial depigmentation of affected areas occurs. The diagnosis can nearly always be made clinically by noting the slight superficial scale and looking at the margin for typical tiny annular lesions. Microscopic examination of scrapings reveals the possible yeast. The most difficult differential diagnosis is postinflammatory depigmentation following guttate psoriasis, but here the small round white macules are scattered uniformly over the body and limbs rather than concentrated in the mantle area.

4. *Naevus anaemicus* is present from birth and may be found at any site as a group of islands of blanched skin. The pigment mechanisms are intact but there is permanent vasoconstriction due to a congenital neurovascular abnormality.

Richard Staughton

Marasmus

Translated literally marasmus is a 'withering' or 'growing lean', so that no more specific application is justifiable beyond that which is WEIGHT, LOSS OF (q.v.). But in common usage the term is applied to progressive emaciation in infants and young children. The alternative description is *infantile atrophy*. Marasmus, then, is the name applied to extreme chronic malnutrition for which numerous causes may be responsible. Actual loss of weight is usually the outstanding criterion; the point at which an infant becomes marasmic is indeterminate, but as a reasonable if arbitrary estimate it may be so described when one-fifth to one-third of his body-weight has been lost. The condition presents an unmistakable appearance. The face, which is pinched and grey, has a curiously senile expression. The eyes and the fontanelles are sunken, the skin is tightly stretched over the bones of the skull, whereas on the limbs and body generally the skin is thin and inelastic through dehydration and loss of subcutaneous fat so that it hangs in festoons on the stick-like arms and legs. The thorax is particularly wasted and the ribs are unduly prominent. The bony fingers are often stuffed into the mouth as if to obtain nourishment. Marasmus has been described as compensated starvation where the child's physiology adapts by limiting body growth and using the less vital body resources to sustain health. The frail balance is disturbed by intercurrent illness such as gastroenteritis, measles or tuberculosis or by incorrect feeding of carbohydrate rather than protein. This decompensation leads to hypoalbuminaemia and the characteristic findings of kwashiorkor. Vitamin and mineral deficiencies also complicate the condition making treatment far more difficult than in uncomplicated marasmus. In the absence of any acute infection the temperature is subnormal and the child is usually apathetic.

Among the very many conditions which may produce this condition are included the following: starvation (either from neglect, extreme poverty or the breakdown of normal civilized behaviour as usually occurs in modern warfare); persistent vomiting (for example, hiatus hernia) or diarrhoea; chronic infections (the urinary tract, tuberculosis, congenital syphilis, AIDS and parasitic infestations); malabsorption—of fat in coeliac disease and cystic fibrosis, of sugar in carbohydrate intolerance, or of protein in protein-losing enteropathy; Hirschsprung's disease; a group of conditions associated with polyuria, that is to say diabetes mellitus, diabetes insipidus, hypercalcaemia, renal acidosis and renal failure; and, rarely in children, thyrotoxicosis, Addison's disease and malignant disease. Severe cyanotic congenital heart disease which is not corrected may be associated with marked failure to thrive.

Starvation comprehends a variety of causes. Because of social and political circumstances the child may simply not receive enough calories. Because of ignorance, feeding may be imperfect both as regards quantity and quality. (*See* Kwashiorkor *below*.) Because of structural imperfections, such as cleft lip, cleft palate, or feebleness from prematurity the infant may be unable to suck. Because of an oesophageal stricture dysphagia may prevent adequate intake of food and persistent vomiting will have a similar disastrous effect.

Chronic infections include serious involvement of the upper renal tract, in which circumstances associated renal failure, for example in advanced bilateral congenital hydronephrosis, may be an aggravating factor. Congenital syphilis was once a potent cause of marasmus although its classic features of snuffles, skin lesions, Parrot's nodes, condylomas and enlargement of the liver and spleen are now rarely seen. Chronic infections associated with the acquired immune deficiency syndrome (AIDS) are the contemporary equivalent. Advanced miliary tuberculosis is now fortunately rare in Great Britain, as is neglected tuberculous disease of bone with its associated discharging sinuses leading to secondarily infected abscess cavities.

Malabsorption is a potent cause of weight loss in children. Cystic fibrosis and coeliac disease are associated with gross steatorrhoea. Disaccharidase deficiency may result in the infant being unable to split disaccharides into absorbable monosaccharides. Lactase deficiency is the commonest example but the enzymes responsible for splitting sucrose and maltose may be affected. Not only is the child prevented from absorbing sugar, but this remains in the small intestine to aggravate the condition by causing diarrhoea by osmosis. Protein-losing enteropathy due to a variety of small intestinal diseases, including Crohn's disease, may result in protein loss into the bowel lumen.

Diabetes mellitus may have a relatively acute onset in children, with thirst, polyuria and severe loss of weight.

Kwashiorkor is a condition seen chiefly in Central Africa but it has been widely described in other tropical and subtropical parts of the world and even in Europe. It is a state produced by gross protein deficiency and is usually due to incorrect feeding. The majority of sufferers are infants under the age of 2 years who, when breast-feeding is discontinued, are placed on a diet mainly of cereals with little if any animal protein; this may be because of shortage of suitable foods or deeply ingrained superstitions. In addition to the failure of growth, there is oedema of the legs, a distended abdomen, and very typical depigmentation of the skin and hair which produces a reddish hue in African babies.

G. S. Clayden

Melaena

Melaena is the term applied to the black bowel motion resulting from haemorrhage which has occurred in the gastrointestinal tract at a high enough level for chemical alteration to take place. It may also occur after swallowing blood derived from haemoptysis or epistaxis. Melaena stools are black, tarry, with a treacly or sticky consistency, rendering it difficult to flush down the toilet. It has been shown by feeding healthy volunteer medical students with increasing aliquots of their own blood, that between 50 and 80 ml are sufficient to cause a melaena stool.

Black or dark stools, simulating melaena, may occur after taking iron preparations by mouth (the iron being converted to the sulphide form), bismuth preparations, licquorice or following the ingestion of charcoal biscuits, black cherries, bilberries or red wine in large quantities, or by the excretion of large amounts of bile pigments. The characteristic thick sticky nature of melaena stools is generally easily differentiated from other causes of black stools, but the diagnosis can be confirmed by laboratory investigation of the stool for the presence of blood.

Melaena is most commonly due to bleeding from the stomach or duodenum, or more rarely from the oesophagus. In such situations it is generally associated with haematemesis, (see p. 253) before the melaena is apparent. If melaena occurs alone from these sources, it generally indicates that the rate of bleeding is relatively slow. Melaena is as serious as haematemesis as an indication of upper gastric haemorrhage; patients with melaena should be investigated and managed as urgently as those with haematemesis. It is possible to judge the severity of a gastrointestinal bleed from the patient's description of the stools.

A detailed account of symptoms such as faintness, sweating and collapse, together with the general assessment of the patient's haemodynamic state allows the clinician to assess the severity of the gastrointestinal bleed leading to the development of melaena. Upper gastrointestinal endoscopy may be required and blood transfusion may be necessary.

The great majority of patients with melaena will have bled from lesions situated in, or proximal to, the duodenum. The commonest cause (perhaps more than 85% of patients) is from duodenal or gastric ulceration, acute gastric erosions and peptic oesophagitis. Bleeding from haemorrhagic erosions associated with the use of non-steroidal anti-inflammatory drugs (NSAIDs) is an increasingly common cause of melaena, especially in elderly patients.

Lesions distal to the duodenum generally give rise to dark or bright red blood in the stools rather than melaena. However, melaena may occur in the relatively uncommon group of causes of the small intestinal bleeding, which include mesenteric thrombosis or embolism, leiomyoma, leiomyosarcoma, or haemangioma of the upper small intestine, the Ehlers–Danlos syndrome, peptic ulcer in a Meckel's diverticulum, Crohn's disease of the small intestine, haemorrhage in typhoid fever from an ulcerated Peyer's patch in the ileum, angiodysplasia of the small intestine, blood dyscrasias resulting in oozing from the intestinal mucosa, or the use of anticoagulant therapy.

Rarely melaena may be associated with small intestinal ulceration in coeliac disease or secondary to drug-induced damage to the small intestine, a rare but increasing occurrence.

R. I. Russell

Memory, disorders of

Disorders of memory (see also CONFUSION) are extremely important in clinical practice because they can be readily tested for and they may be the first indicator of the presence of cerebral disease. It is convenient in everyday clinical practice to divide memory into 'immediate', 'short-term' or 'recent', and long-term' or 'remote'. Immediate memory is assessed by the digit repetition test. Most normal people can immediately recall 6–8 digits presented to them and this reflects the function of a storage mechanism which does not necessarily lead on to a more enduring memory. Short-term or recent memory is clinically assessed by asking the person to memorize the names of several objects, a brief sentence or a name and an address and to repeat these after a few minutes of distraction. Long-term memory is the ability to recall information from the past and includes the process of retrieval of information held in long-term storage. A person with long-term memory loss forgets the names of close relatives, his occupation and schooling and other major events occurring in his earlier life. A related function is that of recognition which is the feeling of familiarity with remembered objects and events. Abnormalities of memory may occur in any or all of these functions and may be psychogenic occurring in healthy people or organic when they are associated with brain disease. The causes of memory loss are given in (Table M.2).

Non-organic memory disturbance

The efficiency of memory is strongly influenced by mood state and a depressed person may perform as poorly as a demented person on tests of memory simply because he or she is retarded and lacks the motivation to take an interest in their surroundings. Similarly a patient who is psychotic may interpret their recall of events by delusional beliefs. In normal people fearful and uncomfortable memories can be coped with by the defence mechanism of denial and repression. This may occur after bereavement or any serious stress. Memory lapses are also common in states of

Table M.2.   Causes of memory loss

Common	Less common
Head injury	Herpes simplex encephalitis
Cerebrovascular disease	Vertebrobasilar disease (transient global amnesia)
Multi-infarct dementia	Tumours of IIIrd ventricle or hypothalamus
Single infarct in region of posterior cerebral artery	Depression (pseudodementia)
Subarachnoid haemorrhage	Fugue states and psychogenic amnesias
Alzheimer's type dementia (and other causes of organic	Malingering
confusion states, see p. 115)	
Thiamine deficiency (Wernicke–Korsakoff Syndrome)	**Rare**
due to alcoholism, malabsorption, carcinoma of the	Bilateral temporal lobectomy for intractible epilepsy
stomach, Hyperemesis gravidarum	Intractible epilepsy
Electroconvulsive therapy	Carbon monoxide poisoning
	Personality disorder
	Pseudologia fantastica
	Ganser state

fatigue. In *Hysterical fugue states* there is a narrowing of consciousness, a move away from normal surroundings and subsequently complete amnesia for these events. The behaviour of the person may appear quite appropriate during the episode which can last from hours to weeks. Such dissociative states may be attempts by people of certain personalities to cope with real or imagined stress. *Pseudologia fantastica* or fluent lying overlaps with the Munchausen syndrome and other factitious disorders. Such patients may claim various degrees of amnesia. The *Ganser state* first described in prisoners awaiting sentence should also be considered an hysterical dissociative state. Two of the main features of the condition are clouding of consciousness and approximate answers (two plus two equals five). Subjects are subsequently amnesic for their abnormal behaviour.

Organic memory impairment

It has long been known that damage to the temporal lobes and to structures in the limbic system, in particular, the hippocampus, amygdala, fornix, mammillary bodies and the dorsal medial nucleus of the thalamus may result in profound amnesia. Bilateral focal lesions affecting these structures, for example, temporal lobe damage following herpes simplex encephalitis or lesions in the mammillary body caused by a thiamine deficiency may cause severe and specific types of memory impairment. Organic memory disturbance may also be a feature of diffuse cerebral disorder perhaps involving quite different brain mechanisms. In some situations frontal lobe dysfunction may contribute to memory impairment. Organic causes of memory impairment include any pathological process that causes bilateral damage to these diencephalic and limbic structures such as head trauma, hypoxia, infarction in the territory of the posterior cerebral arteries and herpes simplex encephalitis. Probably the most commonly encountered form of memory loss, Wernicke–Korsakoff syndrome, is caused by thiamine

deficiency in chronic alcoholism, and less frequently due to carcinoma of the stomach, hyperemesis during pregnancy, malabsorption or dietary deficiency. A similar clinical picture can present with tumours of the third ventricle and hypothalamus, carbon monoxide poisoning, tuberculous meningitis or subarachnoid haemorrhage. The acute effects of thiamine depletion include clouding of consciousness, ataxia and nystagmus (Wernicke's encephalopathy), loss of short-term memory is the principal lasting feature. Patients characteristically retain their long-term memory and can accurately recall events before the onset of the illness. They also have intact immediate memory (digit span) but will be completely unable to store this information for more 1 or 2 seconds. With profound loss of recent memory, patients *confabulate* which is a way of covering up an exposed memory gap. Sometimes confabulation will become fantastic in nature as the patient invents situations in their life. Memory loss in Wernick–Korsakoff syndrome is generally permanent when the cause is alcohol abuse. Transient memory disturbance may occur following *subarachnoid haemorrhage* or *carbon monoxide poisoning*. *Transient global amnesia* describes a memory impairment which starts abruptly and improves over several hours. It generally occurs in middle-aged patients and is thought to be due to bilateral temporal lobe ischaemia caused by vertebrobasilar disease. During on attack the patient is unable to form new memories and their behaviour may be outwardly normal. After recovery the subject is left with a permanent amnesia for the period of the attack. *Closed-brain injury*, chiefly a result of road traffic accidents, but also due to falls, assault and sports injuries are a major cause of organic memory impairment. This may be due to focal or diffuse cerebral damage caused by intracranial haematoma, brain swelling, infection, subarachnoid haemorrhage, hydrocephalus, or to extracranial factors such as hypoxia and hypotension. *Post-traumatic amnesia* refers to the period that elapses between injury and the restoration of normal memory. The duration of post-traumatic amnesia is one indicator of the severity of head injury. Typically patients have impairment in immediate and recent memory following head injury with difficulty in performing digit span as well as tests for words and sentences. Most recovery takes place within 1 year of injury.

D. Blackwood

Menorrhagia

Menorrhagia signifies excessive menstrual flow, or undue prolongation of the time during which it takes place. The patient is free from bleeding during the intermenstrual periods, the term METRORRHAGIA or IRREGULAR UTERINE BLEEDING (q.v.) being reserved for bleeding which occurs between the periods. Careful distinction between these symptoms often serves to distinguish very important conditions, and they should not be confounded with one another. Pure menorrhagia is an important symptom of many well-defined conditions which do not, as a rule, give rise to irregular bleeding. Both these terms must be limited carefully to patients who menstruate, and must not be used for bleeding after the menopause.

The diagnosis of menorrhagia may be difficult because of the absence of anaemia or other signs of severe menstrual blood loss. The diagnosis has to be accepted when the patient complains of having to use more than a dozen and a half pads per menstrual period or when she loses clots or has flooding. Experiments using radioactive chromium to label red cells show that some women may suffer excessive menstrual loss without becoming anaemic, while others who do not bleed so heavily may show all the signs of a severe iron-deficiency anaemia due to chronic blood loss.

Excess of menstrual loss in women without abnormal physical signs is believed to be endocrine in origin and is called *dysfunctional menorrhagia*. Acute endometritis of gonococcal or pyogenic origin tends to cure itself owing to the shedding of the endometrium during menstruation. *Tuberculous endometritis* a rare cause of infertility in the UK. It is due to spread from the Fallopian tubes and is therefore associated with menorrhagia due to the tuberculous salpingo-oophoritis. If a tuberculous infection is suspected the uterine curettings should be examined for the typical tubercles and the organism isolated by culture. Causes of menorrhagia are given in *Table* M.3.

1. Dysfunctional menorrhagia

Menorrhagia of puberty is mainly due to hypofunction of the anterior pituitary body, with consequent failure of ovulation and therefore no corpus luteum. The ovaries contain unruptured Graafian follicles, there is increased oestrogen production, and a lack of the luteal hormone progesterone. These cases often right themselves in time as the pituitary gradually assumes its normal cyclic activities.

Menorrhagia of mature women without obvious lesions of the generative or other systems is thought to be due to an imbalance between the secretion by the ovary of oestrogen and progesterone, with an increase in oestrogen and a complete lack of or a deficiency of progesterone. When there is a complete absence of progesterone in the second half of the menstrual cycle the cycle is referred to as *anovular*, drawing attention to failure of ovulation and formation of a corpus luteum. The condition may be diagnosed by a study of basal temperature charts, there being no postovulatory rise in basal temperature, or by examination of endometrial curettings, which show evidence only of oestrogenic hypertrophy. Sometimes the ovaries become cystic and the endometrium undergoes polypoidal thickening with a characteristic microscopic appearance known as 'Swiss cheese' endometrium or 'cystic glandular hyperplasia'. This condition is known as *metropathia haemorrhagica*. Bouts of amenorrhoea of some weeks are followed by prolonged irregular bleeding, a symptom-complex which does not properly come under the heading 'menorrhagia'.

Menorrhagia in relation to the menopause and in the years preceding is the result of increasing failure of the ovarian functions and consequent upset in balance between the secretion of oestrogen and progesterone.

Polymenorrhoea is the name given to a form of irregular and excessive menstruation in which the cycle is shortened from the usual 28 days to 21 days or even less; this is due to disturbed balance of internal secretions, causing ovulation to occur too early in the cycle; in some cases two corpora lutea have been found at the same stage of development; in many cases fibroids are present.

The function of the thyroid gland can influence the menstrual loss. Menstruation is less or non-existent in cases of hyperthyroidism but menorrhagia occurs as the result of hypothyroidism.

2. Generative system

In considering this, some diseases will be easy to discover, others will require some special method of examination. For instance, of all the causes of pure menorrhagia, *fibromyoma* (fibroids) of the uterus stands out as the only important growth associated with this symptom, and a simple bimanual examination, as a rule, suffices to show that such a tumour exists. The chief characteristics of a fibromyoma of the uterus are these: the uterus itself is enlarged and in almost every

Table M.3. Causes of menorrhagia

1. Dysfunctional menorrhagia	2. In the generative system	3. Circulatory and other systems	4. In the nervous system
At puberty	Fibromyomas	Uncompensated valvular	Excessive coitus
At maturity without	Salpingo-oophoritis	disease of the heart	Prevention of conception
obvious lesions	(chronic)	Cirrhosis of the liver	
In relation to the	Endometriosis	Emphysema of the lungs	*A single excessive period*
menopause, and in the	Adenomyoma	Chronic alcoholism	Fright
years preceding	Tuberculous		Violent emotion
Hyperthyroidism	endometritis	*The blood itself*	Sudden changes of
Hypothyroidism	Intrauterine	Deficient coagulability	temperature
	contraceptive device	Scurvy	Cold bath
		Purpura	Dancing
	Acute infectious diseases	Haemophilia	Hunting
	Influenza	Leukaemia	Gymnastics
	Typhoid		Bicycling, etc.
	Cholera	*High blood pressure*	
	Scarlatina	Arteriosclerosis	
	Variola		
	Malaria		
	Diphtheria		
	Measles		

instance the enlargement is asymmetrical, the typical shape of the organ being altered according to the number and size of the fibroids it contains; as there may be more than one tumour in the uterus, its shape may be exceedingly irregular; the consistence of the tumour is hard and unyielding as a rule, but pathological changes in these tumours are common, some of them leading to softening, others to cystic changes. The tumour and cervix always move together if the organ can be moved at all. The only difficulty in diagnosis, as a rule, lies in distinguishing a fibromyoma of the uterus from an ovarian cyst, and sometimes this is difficult, for it is not always possible to say that a given tumour is actually the enlarged uterus. It must be remembered, however, that the symptom under discussion is menorrhagia, and ovarian tumours almost never give rise to it. Ultrasound scanning is helpful in the diagnosis of fibroids because it is possible by the method to determine if a pelvic swelling is both uterine and solid. If, however, it appears that a swelling is extra-uterine and cystic a diagnosis of ovarian cyst will be made, but it still may be a fibroid which has undergone cystic degeneration and is attached to the uterus by a pedicle (subperitoneal fibroid). If doubt still exists a uterine sound passed into the uterus can be used to determine if the cavity is longer than the normal of 6 cm. Pregnancy must be excluded, of course, before a sound is passed into the uterus. Fibroids that are submucous or intramural enlarge the uterine cavity; ovarian cysts and subperitoneal fibroids do not. Adenomyoma of the uterus produces enlargement as a rule, but cannot be distinguished from fibromyoma until after removal.

Chronic salpingo-oophoritis (in the form of a pyosalpinx, a hydrosalpinx, a tubo-ovarian abscess or a chronic interstitial salpingitis) and *ovarian endometriosis* both give rise to menorrhagia due to pelvic congestion, but dysmenorrhoea, pelvic pain, dyspareunia and backache are usually more prominent symptoms. In either case a firm tender swelling in the pouch of Douglas is felt on bimanual palpation. It is often not possible to differentiate between these two conditions until a laparotomy is performed. Examination of the uterine curettings will reveal a tuberculous origin of the pelvic inflammation.

Retroversion and retroflexion of the uterus may be associated with menorrhagia but, in the absence of other causes, an endocrine imbalance is the reason for the excess menstrual loss, the abnormal position of the uterus merely being coincidental.

Intrauterine contraceptive device. There is almost always some increase of the menstrual blood loss with the use of these devices, and in some cases the loss amounts to menorrhagia.

Exanthemas. The various exanthems are likely to cause menorrhagia but the symptom only occurs during the acute phase of the disease, the periods becoming normal again with improvement in the general condition.

3. Circulatory and other systems

Any lesion of the heart, liver or lungs which leads to back pressure in the venous system may in theory cause hyperaemia of the pelvic organs and consequent excessive menstrual losses. However, it happens very occasionally that menorrhagia is caused by uncompensated valvular lesions of the heart, cirrhosis of the liver or emphysema of the lungs.

Anaemia. The quality of the blood itself may be a cause of menorrhagia if it is deficient in calcium salts or other factors, leading to retardation of the coagulation-time. Modern methods of estimating coagulation-time enable us to distinguish these cases with some certainty, and thus point out a line of treatment. Often, however, there is an underlying cause, such as an endocrine imbalance, which is responsible for both the menorrhagia and the anaemia. Removal of the cause then cures the anaemia.

Thrombocytopenia. Severe menorrhagia may complicate this condition. As soon as it is cured the period loss becomes normal.

4. The nervous system

The nervous system alone is never a cause of menorrhagia. Emotional upsets such as are liable to occur at the time of the menopause may be connected with an endocrine cause of menorrhagia but usually are coincidental.

N. Patel

Metrorrhagia (irregular uterine bleeding)

Metrorrhagia means loss of blood from the uterus between the menstrual periods, and the term should be applied strictly only to irregular haemorrhages during menstrual life. It may be used for losses of actual blood or for blood-stained discharges in which mucus is mixed with blood. There has been a tendency of late to refer only to MENORRHAGIA (q.v.) and to *metrorrhagia*, including all types of irregular vaginal bleeding, whether they occur during menstrual life, before puberty, after the menopause, or during pregnancy. For the purposes of discussion irregular vaginal bleeding will be considered here under three headings: (*A*) Irregular bleeding during menstrual life; (*B*) Irregular bleeding before puberty and after the menopause; (*C*) Irregular bleeding during pregnancy.

A. Irregular bleeding during menstrual life

Causes of irregular bleeding are given in *Table* M.4.

1. Lesions of the uterus and cervix

Those lesions that give rise to metrorrhagia are well defined as a rule, as in the case of carcinoma of the cervix uteri, when the cervix is replaced by a mass of friable growth which bleeds readily on being probed or touched with the finger. A growth of the body of the uterus is more difficult to diagnose and in all instances microscopical examination of material removed by curettage is required; in fact, with the exception of obvious mucous polyps, fibroid polyps and advanced growths of the cervix, all the growths of the uterus require a preliminary histological examination for their exact diagnosis.

The curetted material must be obtained after cervical dilatation, with a sharp curette, and the larger the fragments removed the more easy will be the histologist's work. Anaesthesia is frequently given except in the case of cervical growths. A Danish suction machine (the Vabra) or similar device can be used safely on patients in the outpatient department for diagnostic purposes. The curettings obtained are quite satisfactory for histology. In doubtful cervical growths following colposcopic examination, a rectangular shaped biopsy should be cut out, including some normal tissue if possible. If malignant cells have been seen in a vaginal or cervical smear and the cervix looks grossly normal, intraepithelial diseases of the cervix will be suspected. Several small biopsies of the cervix may be taken from areas which appear abnormal under the colposcope.

Carcinoma of the body of the uterus, carcinoma of the cervical canal, early carcinoma of the cervix, sarcoma of the uterus, chorionic carcinoma, some sloughing fibroids and tuberculous endometritis can be distinguished from one another only by investigations carried out on these lines. The fact that all these lesions produce metrorrhagia and may give rise to haemorrhage on coitus, walking, straining at stool, or bimanual manipulation of the uterus, makes it imperative that there should be histological confirmation of the nature of the lesion before making an exact diagnosis.

Fibromyoma usually causes menorrhagia. Fibroids only produce irregular bleeding when they are submucous and in process of extrusion, when they are infected and sloughing, or when they are actually polypoid. The reason for this is that in these conditions the tumours are always partly strangulated by uterine contractions, and therefore in a state of gross venous congestion; hence they bleed more or less constantly, without provocation. The occurrence of irregular bleeding in a person who is known to have fibroids almost always means one of these conditions, and, commonly, extrusion of the tumour from the uterus. On the other hand, it must not be overlooked that carcinoma may develop in the endometrium with a fibroid also present, or that a fibroid may become sarcomatous, or that a sarcoma may arise *de novo* in the uterus and invade a pre-existing fibroid. Rapid enlargement of a uterus, with irregular haemorrhage, is also very suspicious of a sarcoma, but as it is not uncommon for several fibroids to be present in the same uterus, it is also common for rapid enlargement to occur as a result of cystic changes in one of them, whilst haemorrhage may take place due to extrusion of another.

Table M.4. Causes of irregular bleeding during menstrual life

1. Generative system	2. Endocrine
Malignant growths: Carcinoma of cervix Carcinoma of body of uterus Sarcoma Chorionic carcinoma Carcinoma of Fallopian tube Carcinoma of the ovary	Dysfunctional uterine bleeding Metropathia haemorrhagica Irregular shedding of the endometrium Oestrogen withdrawal bleeding Break-through bleeding from contraceptive pill Granulosa-cell tumour
Benign growths: Submucous fibroid Fibroid polyp Mucous polyp Endometrial polyp	
Inflammatory lesions: Erosion of cervix Endometriosis Tuberculosis of uterus	

Pure *carcinoma of the body of the uterus* rarely produces much enlargement of the organ, and any increase in size is not very rapid. Normally the post-menopausal uterus shrinks considerably in size; thus a uterus of a size which would be regarded as normal in a younger woman indicates abnormal enlargement in a women past the menopause.

Chorionic carcinoma, fortunately a very rare condition, follows hydatidiform mole in about 5 per cent of the recorded cases, and it always follows pregnancy, never having been seen in the uterus where pregnancy could be excluded, although the pregnancy may have occurred some years before. It is associated with profuse bleeding and the rapid development of a foetid discharge due to decomposition of blood and necrosing tissues *in utero*. Carcinoma of the body of the uterus rarely produces foul discharges until the condition is advanced. Secondary deposits of chorionic carcinoma appear as small plum-coloured ulcerating nodules in the vagina and secondaries in the lungs cause haemoptysis. The patient rapidly becomes ill with pyrexia and profound anaemia. A raised level of chorionic gonadotrophin is found in the urine. The diagnosis depends upon the finding of masses of trophoblastic cells in uterine curettings without any evidence of villous formation.

Clear-celled adenocarcinoma of the vagina occurs in teenage girls following high doses of stilboestrol taken by their mothers during pregnancy. The practice, though rare in Great Britain, was common in Boston, USA, several years ago, and the vaginal growths are appearing there now. They tend to occur in areas of vaginal adenosis.

The differential diagnosis of bleeding due to *carcinoma, erosion* and *tuberculosis of the cervix* is often difficult in the early stages. Erosions of the cervix do not as a rule cause bleeding; if there has been irregular bleeding or the cervix bleeds during examination malignancy should be suspected. In advanced cancer the friable hardness of the growth distinguishes it at once from the tough leathery hardness present in erosions. In the former, the growth can be broken down with the finger; in the latter, the soft velvety erosion can be scraped off the tough leathery and fibrous cervix beneath. Whenever there is doubt, colposcopy should be carried out. Tuberculosis of the cervix is usually mistaken for carcinoma, but the difference is clear enough in microscope sections. On occasions sectional biopsy of the cervix reveals a 'carcinoma in situ' or pre-invasive carcinoma. In this condition the epithelial cells throughout the whole depth of the cervical mucosa have the typical appearance of cancer cells but no invasion of the deeper tissues of the cervix has taken place. This condition has been known to become a true cancer, although many years may elapse before this takes place. Only a small proportion of the cases of carcinoma in situ of the cervix becomes invasive cancer even if left untreated. The small possibility of true cancer supervening, however, makes treatment desirable in most cases. They are usually found in the first place by routine cervical smears (*Fig* M.6).

Mucous polyps and *fibroid polyps* are common causes of intermenstrual bleeding, and are usually quite definitive growths. The mucous polyp is soft, strawberry-red in colour, pedunculated, and contains cystic spaces filled with glairy mucus. It rarely gives rise to a malignant growth. The fibroid polyp is hard, and shows the glistening whorled appearance so well known in fibromyomas on section. These growths are liable to infection and sloughing, and are then apt to be mistaken for carcinoma or sarcoma. The microscope alone will enable the difference to be made out.

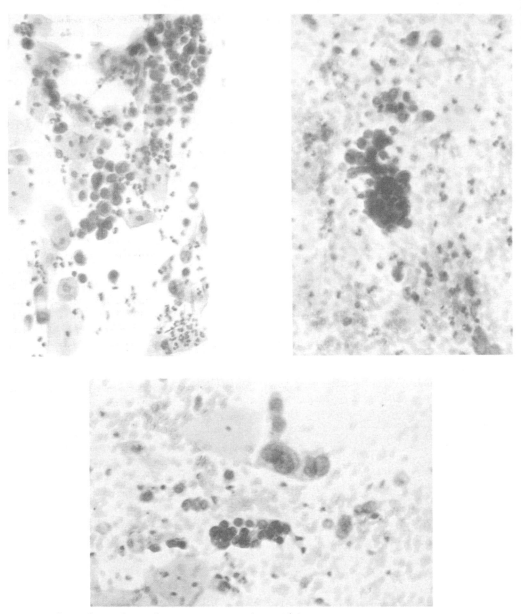

Fig. M.6. Abnormal cervical smear from carcinoma in situ. (*Dr J. Vale.*)

2. DYSFUNCTIONAL UTERINE BLEEDING

Although modern techniques of ovarian steroid estimation in serum allow serial measurements to be made of hormone levels throughout the menstrual cycle, no clear pattern has emerged to explain the mechanism underlying dysfunctional uterine bleeding, except, perhaps, in the case of metropathia haemorrhagica (*see below*).

Dysfunctional bleeding may occur at any age between puberty and the menopause, but 50 per cent occur between the ages of 40 and 50, about 10 per cent at puberty, and the remainder between these ages. Then bleeding is more commonly menorrhagia, although the interval between the bleedings may be shortened. Particularly is this the case in this type of bleeding occurring at the time of puberty and the menopause. The bleeding may be profuse or only slightly in excess of normal. In other cases intermenstrual bleeding occurs, continuing for days or weeks. It is usually preceded by amenorrhoea for some weeks. In a large proportion of these cases ovulation fails to occur. Schröder was able to demonstrate the absence of corpora lutea and the persistence of unruptured follicles in the ovary. This state of excess oestrogen secretion affecting the endometrium leads to marked endometrial hyperplasia (Schröder's disease or metropathia haemorrhagica, (see p. 410). In other cases, however, there is no endometrial hyperplasia present; indeed, the endometrium may be atrophic; again in others the endometrium may be in the secretory phase so that we know ovulation has taken place. In such cases a quantitative imbalance of the sex hormones is assumed, although the cause may lie in the uterine musculature or its autonomic nerve supply. It may be that the close relationship between the pituitary and ovarian functions is disturbed, leading to a temporarily excessive drop in the oestrogen level in the blood because of the inhibition of excessive action of the pituitary gonadotrophins. In other cases it is thought that the endometrium is unable to respond to the stimulation of the ovarian or pituitary hormone in a normal manner (those cases with atrophic endometrium). In other cases irregular shedding of the endometrium takes place leading to prolongation of the desquamative phase of the menstrual cycle. In these cases menstruation is very prolonged, and a late curetting in the bleeding phase reveals islands of secretory endometrium, when normal regenerated endometrium should be found.

There are no gross abnormal physical signs to be found on pelvic examination in cases of dysfunctional bleeding. The diagnosis largely depends on the history and when in doubt curettage. Amenorrhoea followed by prolonged irregular bleeding may be caused by pregnancy and abortion (threatened or incomplete), or by the menopause followed by carcinoma of the body of the uterus. When pregnancy is unlikely, curettage may be indicated to make the diagnosis.

Oestrogen withdrawal bleeding. Women commonly take oestrogen preparations to control menopausal symptoms or to prevent conception. Irregular uterine bleeding may occur while the drugs are being taken or following their withdrawal. In cases where there is doubt curettage should be carried out.

Bleeding associated with ovulation. It is not uncommon for women to bleed very slightly about midway between the periods at the time of ovulation. When this is accompanied by lower abdominal pain (*Mittelschmerz*) the diagnosis is easy.

Bleeding due to granulosa-cell tumour. When irregular bleeding occurs in the presence of an ovarian swelling the possibility of a granulosa-cell tumour arises. Removal of the tumour and histology reveal its nature. The presence of an intrauterine lesion and a non-secreting ovarian tumour must not be overlooked.

B. Irregular bleeding before puberty and after the menopause

The causes of irregular bleeding before puberty and after the menopause are given in *Table M.5*. The bleeding which occurs from the vagina occasionally in newborn infants is usually due to a high concentration of oestrogen in the fetal circulation. It is usually trivial, but a fatal case has been reported. Bleeding later in childhood may be due to sexual precocity when secondary sexual characteristics will be in evidence; or due to a new growth such as an embryonal rhabdomyosarcoma (sarcoma botryoides). Vaginoscopy under anaesthesia (and biopsy if a lesion is found) is essential.

After the menopause the differentiation of *malignant growths, polyps* and *senile endometritis* can only be established by uterine curettage. Carcinoma of the body of the uterus (endometrial adenocarcinoma) is the commonest malignant growth after the menopause. In any doubtful case routine dilatation and curettage of the uterus must never be omitted. Senile (atrophic) vaginitis must not be overlooked as a possible cause; the vaginal walls at the fornices become inflamed and form granulation tissue which may bleed if the surfaces rub together; the surfaces may be partly adherent, and the separation brought about by the examining finger may cause bleeding. Pyometra, or distension of the uterus with pus, may cause haemorrhage, with a foul discharge; although it is almost always due to malignant growth, it may be only the result of infection. The only growth of the ovary which produces uterine haemorrhage is the granulosa-cell tumour. This may occur at almost any age. (*See* PELVIS, SWELLING IN.)

C. Irregular bleeding during pregnancy

In relation to a recent pregnancy, haemorrhage may result from simple subinvolution, from retained products of conception, or from chorionic carcinoma. The differentiation of these conditions can be established only by exploration of the uterine cavity, with, if necessary, the assistance of the microscope. Such conditions may be termed 'secondary postpartum haemorrhage' in cases occurring within a few days of delivery.

Haemorrhage from the pregnant uterus almost always means separation of the placenta or of the embryo from its attachments, but malignant growth of the cervix, erosions and polyps may have to be considered. Haemorrhage from a pregnant uterus is never due to malignant growth of the body of the organ, because pregnancy is impossible with this lesion. There are, however, two great difficulties in connection with pregnancy haemorrhages; these are to differentiate:

Table M.5. Causes of irregular bleeding

Before puberty and after menopause	During pregnancy
Uterine bleeding in the newborn	Threatened, inevitable or incomplete abortion
Malignant growth of the uterus	Carneous mole
Polyps	Hydatidiform mole
Senile endometritis	Antepartum haemorrhage
Senile atrophic vaginitis	Secondary postpartum haemorrhage
Pyometra	Subinvolution
Granulosa-cell tumour of ovary	Chorionic carcinoma
Oestrogen withdrawal bleeding	Extrauterine gestation
	Malignant growth of cervix or vagina
	Erosion
	Polyps

(1) the uterine haemorrhage which occurs along with *extrauterine gestation* from that due to *threatened abortion*; and (2) the bleeding of *placenta praevia* from that due to the *separation of a normally situated placenta*.

In the first case, arising very early in pregnancy, generally when only one menstrual period has been missed, or is overdue, the external haemorrhage occurs when the extra-uterine gestation is separated from its tubal or other attachments and is converted into a tubal mole, when it becomes extruded from the fimbriated extremity of the tube, or when the tube ruptures, events which cause acute pain in the lower part of the abdomen, faintness, and possibly collapse from internal haemorrhage. Along with these the uterus will be found not obviously enlarged, whilst there is some sort of swelling in one or the other posterior quarter of the pelvis. Even if no actual swelling can be defined, bimanual palpation will elicit very marked tenderness, which may be excruciating, due to the presence of blood clot in the peritoneal cavity. In the case of ectopic gestation the abdominal pain is severe. It is often referred to the shoulder. It is much more severe than that experienced in an intrauterine abortion and it almost always precedes the onset of vaginal bleeding; on the other hand the vaginal blood loss in an inevitable abortion is much more than that in ectopic gestation, which is usually scanty. Haemorrhage due to threatened abortion cannot be diagnosed unless the presence of an intrauterine pregnancy can be established; therefore we must look for the definite signs of a normal pregnancy, which in the early months will be: amenorrhoea, morning sickness, breast swelling, darkening of the nipple, dark secondary areola around the nipple, enlargement of the uterus, Hegar's sign, and blue discoloration of the cervix and vaginal walls. Hegar's sign consists in extreme softening of the upper part of the cervix and lower part of the uterine body associated with the as yet unsoftened vaginal portion and globular tense fundus; it is found from the 6th to the 8th week. Ultrasound scanning is very useful because the pregnancy sac can be visualized in the uterus and the size of the embryo measured to make sure of the duration of the pregnancy. The presence of a live fetus can be demonstrated by the beating of the heart with the aid of real-time ultrasound and means that the outlook for continuation of the pregnancy is good. Absence of a pregnancy sac in the uterus with a mass outside of the uterus (sometimes seen to contain a pregnancy sac) make the diagnosis of ectopic pregnancy a certainty. In the case of a positive pregnancy test using methods employing detection of low level of BHCG and a negative ultrasound scan for intrauterine pregnancy, laparoscopy would be advisable to exclude the diagnosis. The diagnosis of inevitable abortion depends upon finding some part of the uterine contents presenting through the dilating cervix. Incomplete abortion is diagnosed by the continuation of bleeding or seeing that not all the products of conception have been passed. Retained products are then confirmed on ultrasound scanning.

If repeated small haemorrhages occur into the chorio-decidual space in early pregnancy a carneous mole results. Unless it is removed by suction or by curettage it may be retained in the uterus for weeks or even months before it is expelled spontaneously (missed abortion). While it remains in the uterus there is a brown or blood-stained vaginal discharge with bleeding intermittently and the uterus ceases to enlarge. On examination the uterus is found to be smaller than it should be for the estimated duration of pregnancy. A pregnancy test may be negative but it is not always so.

A hydatidiform mole should be suspected when rapid increase in size of the uterus occurs during the early months of pregnancy, associated with uterine bleeding. Most cases have a uterus which is larger than would be expected for the dates, but in one-third it is smaller. Sometimes vesicles are passed and the diagnosis is clear. If not, the finding of a high level of chorionic gonadotrophin in the blood or urine and the characteristic 'snow-storm' appearance on ultrasound scanning makes the diagnosis certain. In a normal pregnancy up to 100 000 IU of chorionic gonadotrophin (HCG) are passed in the urine daily. Five times this amount is passed in the presence of a hydatidiform mole. If bleeding continues after evacuation of a hydatidiform mole chorionic carcinoma should be suspected. Chorionic gonadotrophin continues to be produced by the remaining chorionic tissue and high titres are found in blood and urine. Uterine curettage may reveal the malignant tissue unless it is buried deep in the myometrium, in the pelvis or at a remote site such as the lungs. In fact all patients who have a hydatidiform mole removed should be followed up for 2 years with regular urine tests for the beta subunit of HCG, in case of post-molar trophoblastic disease (chorionic carcinoma) develops.

Bleeding due to *placenta praevia* generally does not occur until 30 weeks of pregnancy. Antepartum haemorrhage is likely to be due to placenta praevia if the fetal presenting part is high above the pelvic brim or there is a malpresentation such as a breech or a transverse lie. If the fetal head is engaged in the pelvis antepartum haemorrhage cannot be due to placenta praevia and must therefore be due to accidental haemorrhage, provided that incidental causes such as carcinoma or polyp on the cervix can be excluded. The diagnosis of antepartum haemorrhage has been made much easier with the aid of ultrasound scanning because the placental echo can be seen clearly and the relation of the edge of the placenta to the internal os can be accurately determined. It is not uncommon for a low-lying placenta found in the mid-trimester to be seen on serial scanning to move wholly into the upper uterine segment as term approaches.

N. Patel

Micturition, frequency of

Many urological diseases may present as frequency of micturition. The symptom does not necessarily imply an organic abnormality, but how frequent is 'frequent'? If the normal bladder contains some 300–500 ml, and the amount of urine produced during the day is of the order of 1500 ml, the 'normal' person should pass urine between three and five times daily. As the patient will pass urine less frequently if fluid intake is reduced and insensible loss increased, so will the patient pass urine more frequently if the fluid intake is increased and insensible loss reduced. Frequency is a symptom which we have all experienced during periods of stress, classically before examinations or interviews, but this reflex nervous polyuria may be exaggerated in hysterics. Frequency is also modified by the rate at which the bladder fills, which relates not only to the quantity of fluid drunk but its quality; while water itself is diuretic, the addition of caffeine or theophylline in tea or coffee, or alcohol, will stimulate the urine output.

The consequent rapid filling of the bladder will provoke the stretch reflex to a degree that is far less easily controllable than during slow filling and stretching.

Increased frequency may also relate to general medical conditions described elsewhere, such as diabetes mellitus, diabetes insipidus and chronic nephritis.

Assuming that there is no systemic disorder, continuing frequency relates to: (1) a small bladder capacity; (2) inflammation of the bladder; (3) reduced bladder emptying.

Reduced bladder capacity

Bladder capacity can be reduced by a large intraluminal object such as a large stone or large tumour. These conditions lead simply to a small amount of available effective capacity, the same mechanism that exists in outflow tract obstruction when bladder emptying is incomplete. True reduction in bladder capacity occurs when there is fibrosis of the bladder wall, which may be secondary to the chronic sepsis associated with long-term catheter drainage, tuberculous cystitis or infiltration of the bladder wall with an advanced tumour.

Small bladders may be acquired by habit, where 'habit frequency' is more common in women, especially the older age group, who make use of every opportunity to empty their bladders lest they should run into difficulty with incontinence. After some years of practising this habit the bladder is no longer capable of distention and frequency becomes the rule by day and night.

Bladder contraction also occurs after radiotherapy and as this treatment modality has become more effective in achieving cure in many conditions, such as testicular tumours, some ovarian carcinomas and localized prostatic carcinoma, postradiation fibrosis in the increasing number of survivors becomes a reality, although perhaps a small price to pay for cure of the primary condition.

Inflammation of the bladder

Primary inflammatory conditions of the bladder will give rise to frequency by day and night as will inflammatory processes involving the bladder secondarily, as in pelvic inflammatory disease. Acute appendicitis may also influence bladder behaviour in the short term while carcinoma in adjacent structures, such as the uterus, rectum and colon, may occasionally present as frequency. Diverticulitis coli can of course increase frequency from the secondary inflammatory changes but it is surprising how infrequently this symptom arises, considering how frequently colovesical fistulae develop in apparently unheralded fashion.

Reduced bladder emptying

Outflow tract obstruction in males and females also gives rise to increased frequency by day and night. Nocturia may be the presenting feature of outflow tract obstruction in the male related to prostatic hypertrophy, bladder neck stenosis and detrusor sphincter dyssenergia. It should be borne in mind that this symptom is least affected and corrected by surgical removal of the obstruction.

The presence of a stone in the lower third of the ureter may precipitate reflex frequency of micturition while impaction of the calculus at the uretero-vesical junction may precipitate the most intense frequency, associated with pain in the glans penis or labia and the passage of but a few drops of urine at a time. When a stone is lodged within the bladder, frequency may be a feature by day as the patient moves around and the stone irritates the trigone. This symptom is often relieved at night as the stone rolls back into the bladder proper, an area far less sensitive to stimulation from the sharp points of the calculus.

Lynn Edwards

Micturition, hesitancy

The classical presenting features of outflow tract obstruction are frequency, nocturia, reduction in the flow rate and hesitancy. In hesitancy, the patient feels the desire to pass urine, presents himself in an appropriate place and yet finds that seconds, or even minutes, elapse before the flow starts. Sometimes it is necessary for the male patient to sit down before the stream is initiated.

A distinction must be made between hesitancy and difficulty of micturition. Hesitancy implies a definite time lag between the intended start of micturition and the appearance of the urine at the urethral meatus. In difficulty, the flow is reduced and can often be augmented by abdominal straining. Abdominal straining during the waiting period of hesitancy can often prolong the waiting time.

Difficulty of micturition is caused by: (1) poor bladder contractility and (2) obstruction to outflow.

Poor bladder contractility

Reduced contractility is relatively common in diseases of the nervous system, particularly spinal cord lesions producing a lower motor neurone lesion, such as transverse myelitis, tabes, multiple sclerosis, tumour of the spinal meninges or cord, syringomyelia and secondary deposits in the vertebrae. The level of the lesion is critical and it must involve the cord at the level of the sacral reflex arc. If the lesion is higher than this, the characteristics are of an upper motor neurone lesion, which are frequency, urgency and incontinence secondary to reflex micturition.

Systemic disturbances are also responsible for difficult emptying, for example when there is a peripheral autonomic neuropathy as in diabetes mellitus. Such a neuropathy can often exist in the absence of physical signs of a peripheral diabetic neuropathy. Small vessel disease within the pelvis may reduce the vascular supply to the sacral reflex arc. A lower motor neurone type of lesion is found following prolonged periods of chronic retention when proper detrusor tone is never regained following the surgical relief of the outflow obstruction. A prolonged period of catheter drainage under these circumstances can sometimes cause sufficient restoration of muscle tone to allow normal emptying to occur.

Difficulty of micturition is often seen in herpes zoster lesions affecting the sacral reflex. The same applies to herpes genitalis, a condition which is transmitted by intercourse and which is becoming relatively common in younger women.

Outflow obstruction

Hesitancy and difficulty in women may be secondary to pelvic tumours which push the bladder out of the pelvis and therefore stretch the urethra. It occurs with uterine fibroids or with a retroverted pregnancy. Direct involvement of the urethra by vaginal carcinoma or by a primary urethral carcinoma is rare. Stricture of the urethra in women is far more common than might be suspected and is dealt with fully under (URINE, RETENTION OF). Urethral strictures rarely give rise to true hesitancy in that urine can be felt entering the posterior urethra early enough but the urine then trickles though the stricture zone. A feeling of presence in the urethra proximal to the stricture is often felt. The same symptom is experienced when a stone is impacted along the urethra, or when a well organized blood clot has entered the urethra from a bladder lesion. When there is a urethral obstruction, straining often increases the strength of the stream.

Prostatic enlargement secondary to inflammatory changes can also give rise to hesitancy but pain will also be a feature in these conditions.

Hesitancy and difficulty are rarely observed in children as primary complaints but both may be observed when there is a meatal stenosis or a tight phimosis. In the latter ballooning of the foreskin occurs during micturition.

Lynn Edwards

MICTURITION, PAINFUL
See DYSURIA.

Monoplegia, upper limb

Monoplegia or monoparesis is defined as loss of motor power involving a single limb. In theory a monoplegia or monoparesis can result from damage anywhere in the motor pathway between the motor cortex and the muscles of the affected limb. When the degree of weakness is only slight and associated signs such as increased reflexes are absent, accurate diagnosis may be difficult. For example, localized damage to the hand area of the cortex resulting from a stroke can produce weakness of the hand without any obvious reflex change, mimicking a localized nerve or root lesion. To reach a diagnosis in such a case requires a careful history and a detailed examination of motor function with special efforts being made to delineate the extent and pattern of motor weakness.

A patient may complain of weakness in a limb when in reality the problem is the result of pain, incoordination, loss of sensation, or akinesia and rigidity as in Parkinson's disease. The patient with apraxia of a limb often regards it as weak.

Upper motor neurone

A spastic upper limb monoplegia most commonly results from a lesion affecting the motor cortex or the descending corticospinal fibres in the internal capsule. Cerebral infarction, cerebral haemorrhage or tumour are most likely causes. Muscle atrophy is not a feature and the appearance of the arm is usually normal. In an acute lesion muscle tone may be reduced, but, given time, spasticity develops and the arm adopts a fixed posture, adducted at the shoulder and flexed at the elbow and wrist. Hand movements are usually more severely affected than shoulder movements. Tendon reflexes are brisk and contractures may develop. Even when symptoms are apparently confined to the arm, there may be some degree of facial weakness and the plantar response in the ipsilateral foot may be extensor.

In the patient with a progressive upper motor neurone pattern of weakness, the likeliest cause is an intracerebral tumour and a CT scan is indicated. A similar pattern of weakness may occasionally be seen in multiple sclerosis or rarely in spinal cord tumours.

A spastic upper limb monoplegia may be mistaken for the rigid akinetic arm of a patient with Parkinson's disease. In such cases the arm moves slowly and is thought by the patient to be weak, yet testing usually reveals no significant loss of power. Similarly the tendon reflexes in Parkinson's disease are usually unaffected. Finally, it should be possible to differentiate the rigidity of Parkinson's disease from the spasticity of an upper motor neurone lesion.

Hysterical upper limb monoplegia is rare. In such cases the arm appears normal and muscle tone is not increased. The tendon reflexes remain normal and the plantar responses are flexor. There is often apparent dense sensory loss in the affected arm, usually with a sharp line of demarcation at the level of the shoulder. The most difficult cases are those in which there is some genuine weakness with superadded functional overlay.

Lower motor neurone

A flaccid upper limb monoplegia may result from damage to any part of the lower motor neurone between the anterior horn cell and the muscle. Damage to the lower motor neurone typically is associated with muscle weakness, muscle wasting, decrease in the tendon reflexes and fasciculations. Characteristic changes may be found on electromyographic examination.

Anterior horn cell disorders

Localized loss of anterior horn cells may produce a flaccid weakness of one or other arm. This may be seen as a common after-effect of poliomyelitis and the affected limb is often markedly underdeveloped. In motor neurone disease, localized loss of anterior horn cells may produce progressive lower motor neurone weakness in the arm and this may begin in any of the upper limb muscles. A common pattern is for the weakness to begin in the intrinsic hand muscles with associated muscle wasting. Prominent fasciculations are common in this disorder. Where there is associated damage to the corticospinal tracts, as in amyotrophic lateral sclerosis, the tendon reflexes are brisk despite obvious muscle wasting and fasciculation. This combination of signs is diagnostic.

Localized lesions in the cervical cord may damage the anterior horn cells and produce a lower motor neurone pattern of weakness. This may be seen in syringomyelia and in spinal cord tumours. These may be diagnosed by the associated signs of sensory loss and corticospinal tract signs in the legs. Ischaemic lesions of the cervical cord may produce discrete loss of anterior horn cells, with localized areas of muscle wasting and weakness. This may be one of the mechanisms whereby the lower motor neurone pattern of weakness develops in cervical spondylosis.

Spinal motor root disorders

Localized damage to the spinal roots in the cervical region is common as a result of degenerative cervical spine changes (cervical spondylosis). The C5 and C6 segments are most commonly affected, with muscle wasting and weakness being most prominent in the biceps and shoulder girdle muscles. The biceps and brachioradialis reflexes are depressed and there is often inversion of these reflexes; that is to say, when the biceps tendon is stretched there is no contraction of the biceps muscle but there is a contraction of the finger flexors resulting in finger flexion. Extensive cervical spondylosis sometimes produces quite marked wasting and weakness of many of the upper limb muscles. The cause may be recognized by the associated sensory changes and by the presence of pain. Such cases are usually seen in those who have undertaken heavy manual work, and gross changes are usually confined to those over the age of 50 or 60. Other causes of damage to spinal motor roots are cervical disc prolapse, trauma to the cervical spine, extramedullary spinal tumours and spinal arachnoiditis.

Herpes zoster is occasionally accompanied by paralysis of one or more muscles within the affected segments. In neuralgic amyotrophy there is localized muscle weakness and wasting occurring a few weeks after the development of severe pain in the affected limb. There is some debate as to the localization of damage to the lower motor neurone in neuralgic amyotrophy: in some cases the damage may be in the ventral roots, in some in the brachial plexus and in some in peripheral nerves.

The brachial plexus

Brachial plexus damage on one side may usually be recognized by the distribution of muscle weakness and by the associated reflex and sensory changes.

Damage may occur as a result of an injury at birth. Downward traction on the arm in a breech presentation may rupture the upper end of the plexus (C5–6), with consequent paralysis and atrophy of the spinati, deltoid, brachialis, biceps and brachioradialis. The arm hangs by the side, internally rotated at the shoulder, with the elbow straight and the fingers flexed, the palm of the hand pointed backwards. This is known as Duchenne–Erb paralysis. A similar condition resulting from a fall on the tip of the shoulder is referred to as Erb's paralysis. In both cases the motor disturbances are similar to those produced by a lesion of the 5th and 6th segments of the cervical cord, but there are none of the sensory and pyramidal signs which necessarily occur below the level of the lesion in the latter. A second form of obstetrical palsy, described as Klumpke's paralysis, results from injury to the lower cord of the plexus (C8–T1), by traction on the arm in a vertex or shoulder presentation. Atrophic palsy occurs in the intrinsic muscles of the hand and in the flexors of the wrist and fingers. Horner's syndrome may be present if the roots themselves have been torn. Rarer causes of trauma to the brachial plexus are gunshot wounds or stab wounds. In modern times perhaps the most common traumatic lesion to the brachial plexus is that occurring as a result of a motorcycle accident. In such cases the damage may not only be to the nerves in the brachial plexus but also to the ventral roots themselves which may become completely avulsed from the spinal cord.

Upward spread of an apical bronchial carcinoma may result in erosion into the brachial plexus, most commonly affecting the lower part (Pancoast's syndrome). Metastatic carcinoma of the breast may produce a similar clinical picture and this is often difficult to differentiate from postradiation scarring occurring in a female who has been treated by radiotherapy to the axilla.

The cervical rib

The brachial plexus and subclavian vessels cross the uppermost rib as they pass into the axilla. This may be a normal first rib, an ill-formed rudimentary first rib, or a cervical rib. The last may be a well-developed ossified structure or a fibrous band, but in either case it joins the first thoracic rib lateral to the insertion of the scalenus anterior, at the point where the brachial plexus and vessels pass into the axilla. Such a rib or band tends to angulate the nerves and vessels and to produce friction during respiration and in movements of the shoulder and upper limb, and this in its turn may give rise to pain and paraesthesiae in the ring and little fingers, and atrophic palsy of the small muscles of the hand (see below). But cervical ribs often give rise to no symptoms at all, and though they are present from birth, symptoms, if they do arise, are uncommon before middle life. They tend to be aggravated by carrying heavy weights and by wearing a heavy overcoat. Friction on the plexus causes atrophy and weakness of the interossei, the thenar and hypothenar muscles, and the long flexors of the fingers and wrist. Fasciculation may be seen in the affected muscles, and slight sensory loss is sometimes found in the medial two fingers and the ulnar border of the hand and forearm. To this essentially neurological picture may be added symptoms and signs of vascular origin: Raynaud's phenomenon, persistent cyanosis of the hand, diminution or even loss of the radial pulse. The subclavian artery is subjected to friction and to costoclavicular compression, and this may lead to thrombosis or even to the formation of an aneurysm at the site of compression. If thrombosis occurs, ischaemia gives rise to pallor of the hand, paraesthesiae in all the fingers, claudication of the forearm and hand, and in elderly subjects, to necrosis of the fingertips.

Costoclavicular compression can occur even in absence of cervical rib. The motor features are similar to those of cervical rib, but of milder degree, and vascular symptoms tend to predominate. There is aching pain in the shoulder, paraesthesiae in all the fingers and a feeling of weakness in the limb. These symptoms are intensified by abduction of the arm, by using the hand above the level of the shoulder, as in doing the hair or painting a ceiling, and by recumbency, so that paraesthesiae are worse at night. These symptoms may come on for the first time in middle age after a period of prolonged and unwanted physical work, and more commonly in females than males. A troublesome form occurs in the late stages of pregnancy, usually disappearing after parturition and recurring in subsequent pregnancies; it is related to the postural readjustments which take place in pregnancy. Care must be taken not to confuse these symptoms with those due to compression of the median nerve in the carpal tunnel, for in the latter there are also complaints of paraesthesiae in the hand on waking in the morning, with or without wasting of the thenar eminence. In the carpal tunnel syndrome, however, the paraesthesiae rarely involve the ulnar part of the hand alone.

Peripheral nerve damage

Peripheral nerve damage in the upper limb usually produces localized muscle weakness in the territory supplied by the relevant nerve. Extensive damage most commonly results from lesions in the nerves of the brachial plexus (see above). The term 'mononeuritis multiplex' implies multiple peripheral nerve lesions. It may occur in diabetes but is more commonly seen in connective-tissue disorders such as polyarteritis nodosa.

LOCALIZED WEAKNESS IN PERIPHERAL NERVE LESIONS

The circumflex (axillary) nerve is liable to injury by fractures of the neck of the humerus, by dislocation of the shoulder, by the use of an unpadded crutch, and by penetrating injuries of the axilla and shoulder. The deltoid is paralysed and there is an area of sensory loss over the proximal half of the lateral aspect of the arm. Paralysis of the radial nerve occurs in fractures of the shaft of the humerus, pressure from callus, gunshot wounds of the axilla and arm, and not infrequently from sitting with an arm suspended over the back of a chair. With lesions in the neighbourhood of the shaft of the humerus, the triceps escapes, but there is paralysis of the brachioradialis and of the extensors of the wrist and fingers, with consequent wrist-drop and paralysis of finger extension. There is a somewhat variable loss of cutaneous sensibility over the radial border of the forearm and the radial half of the dorsum of the hand which may be confined to a small patch over the first dorsal interosseous space.

Inability to extend the wrist impairs the mechanical efficiency of the flexors of the fingers, so that the grasp is weakened, a circumstance which may lead to an erroneous diagnosis of a coincident lesion of the median nerve. Wrist-drop is a familiar feature of certain general affections—lead poisoning, leprosy, alcoholic neuritis—but in these conditions the weakness is not wholly confined to the radial distribution.

The posterior interosseous nerve is a branch of the radial nerve in the upper forearm and may suffer entrapment or may become the site of a neurofibroma. There is eventually paralysis of the finger extensors, the thumb extensor and abductor of the wrist. The radial extensor is spared so that there is only partial weakness of wrist extension and no wrist-drop. There is no sensory loss. Spontaneous recovery is unlikely and early exploration is indicated.

Paralysis of the median nerve is usually due to penetrating injuries of the arm or forearm. If the lesion is above the elbow, atrophic palsy involves the pronator teres, flexor carpi radialis, palmaris longus, flexor digitorum sublimis, flexor pollicis longus, pronator quadratus, the inner half of flexor digitorum profundus, the muscles of the thenar eminence and the lateral two lumbricals. Sensory loss and absence of sweating are limited to the median distribution in the hand.

The anterior interosseous nerve is a branch of the median nerve and supplies, essentially, the flexor profundus of the thumb and index finger so that the patient is unable to make a pincer movement (*Fig. M.7*). There is no sensory loss. Lesions usually result from entrapment. Spontaneous recovery may occur, but if there has been none after 2 or 3 months exploration is indicated.

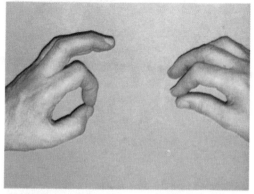

Fig. M.7. Lesion of the anterior interosseous nerve on the right demonstrating the inability to make a pincer movement with the thumb and index finger.

Compression of the median nerve in the carpal tunnel may cause wasting of the muscles of the thenar eminence, with paralysis of abduction and opposition of the thumb, and cutaneous sensory loss over the thumb, index, middle and radial half of the ring finger.

The full-blown picture is rare but milder degrees of compression occur and can be responsible for acroparaesthesiae in the hand even when signs are slight or absent.

The carpal tunnel syndrome occurs mostly in women and usually for no apparent reason. In men there is likely to be a discoverable cause such as arthritis of the wrist, ganglion at the wrist joint, acromegaly or myxoedema. These causes are not, of course, confined to men, and in women pregnancy is another possible precipitating factor.

The earliest symptom is usually intermittent tingling of the fingers of one hand, often waking the patient from sleep. This tingling may spare the little finger and is often most prominent in the ring and middle fingers. If the tingling is severe it is likely to be accompanied by pain in the palm of the hand, sometimes at the elbow or even in the shoulder.

As the condition progresses the patient may find that in the morning the fingers feel swollen and numb. Later, symptoms may occur during the day and may be brought on by use of the hands. Finally, abnormal signs may appear. These consist of weakness and wasting of the abductor pollicis brevis (*Fig.* M.8) and sensory impairment within the distribution of the median nerve in the hand, both of which may be quite mild in degree.

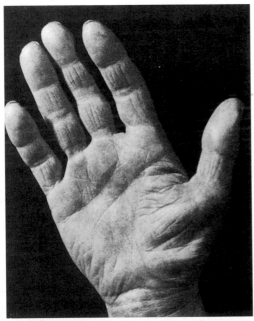

Fig. M.8. Carpal tunnel compression showing wasting of abductor pollicis brevis.

The condition is relieved by division of the flexor retinaculum at the wrist.

The ulnar nerve is frequently injured by penetrating wounds of the forearm, and it is particularly liable to compression where it lies behind the medial epicondyle of the humerus. This occurs particularly if the groove in which it lies is shallow, in which case it is subject to recurrent injury, as in clerks, telegraphists, and others whose occupation entails resting the elbows on a hard table. Cubitus valgus, whether congenital or as a result of a fracture in the region of the elbow, predisposes to this traumatic neuritis. Pain is rare, but paraesthesiae and wasting of the interossei, the hypothenar muscles, and the medial two lumbricals cause discomfort and disability. Sensory loss of ulnar distribution and palpable thickening of the nerve at the elbow afford confirmatory evidence as to the nature of the condition. An occupational palsy of the muscles supplied by the deep branch of the ulnar nerve is seen in long-distance cyclists, who lean heavily on the handle-bars, and also in individuals using files, with the instrument held in one hand, and downward pressure exerted by the hypothenar eminence of the other on the end of the file. Weakness and wasting are confined to the interossei and there is no sensory loss.

Ulnar paralysis can occur in leprosy and may be the sole manifestation.

N. E. F. Cartlidge

Mouth, pigmentation of

The oral mucous membrane contains melanocytes in the basal layer, as a result of neuroectodermal migration in the fetus, which are similar to those present in the skin. Therefore, any condition which causes abnormal pigmentation in the skin can produce similar changes in the oral cavity, although the effects are usually not as marked. The following are important causes of oral pigmentation.

Melanotic naevae

These occur less often than in the skin, with the hard palate and the buccal mucosa being the most commonly involved site. As in the skin, they represent a collection of the normal melanocytes but instead of being evenly distributed in the basal layer, the cells are aggregated together. Depending on their position in relation to the basement membrane, they give rise to junctional naevae, compound naevae, intramucosal naevae and blue naevae. The lesions are generally small, well circumscribed, macular or slightly raised. The majority are pigmented with varying shades of brown, blue or black. The lesions are twice as common in females as in males and tend to occur in middle age.

Malignant melanoma

This is a rare tumour of the oral mucous membrane with a slight male predominance, again occurring in middle age (*Fig* M.9). They are mostly found in the upper jaw, especially the palate, followed by the gingival mucosa. It is more common in the Japanese, Indian and African races and one-third are preceded by a history of oral pigmentation. As in the skin, any oral pigmented lesion which increases in size or changes its surface characteristics or colour and starts to bleed, should be suspected as being a malignant melanoma. Growth of the lesion is followed by destruction of the underlying bone and loosening of the teeth, with rapid spread to the regional lymph nodes. If malignant change is suspected then a wide excision of the lesion should be carried out. Rarely the mouth may be involved with secondary deposits from a cutaneous melanoma.

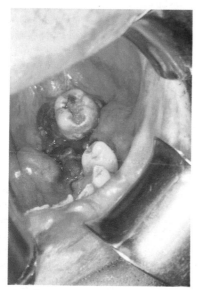

Fig. M.9. Malignant melanoma of the floor of the mouth.

Melanotic neuroectodermal tumour of infancy

This pigmented lesion is invariably noted within the first 6 months of life, the majority of which occur in the anterior maxilla. The tumour grows rapidly in size with underlying bone destruction, and displacement of the developing teeth. The correct diagnosis is essential as the tumour is benign and responds well to simple enucleation.

Peutz–Jegher's syndrome

This inherited condition is characterized by intestinal polyposis and melanotic spots of the face and mouth, with occasionally the hands and feet also being affected. Although it is an inherited condition, a family history will not always be found. There are multiple freckles on the face, especially around the mouth (circum-oral pigmentation), the eyes and the nose. The

polyps in the intestine rarely become malignant as they are hamartomas in origin.

Addison's disease

This condition is caused by bilateral destruction of the supraadrenal glands, the most common cause previously being infection with tuberculosis. Today it is usually caused by auto-immune destruction or an opportunist infection in immuno-deficient patients and more recently, this has been demonstrated in patients suffering from AIDS. The skin becomes pigmented early on in the disease, especially the exposed areas, while the oral cavity shows patchy melanotic pigmentation, which varies in colour from light brown to black. If this disease is suspected then the diagnosis will be verified by measuring the blood pressure which is low, blood urea which is raised and serum sorium, which is lowered, and performing the Synacthen test (measurement of plasma cortisol in response to injection of synthetic ACTH).

Racial

This is the most common cause of oral pigmentation which is most prevalent in the black and Indian races (*Fig.* M.10). However, 5% of caucasian people also show pigmentation of the oral mucosa. The pigment is evenly distributed in the palate, buccal and gingival mucosa. The colour of the pigment is not necessarily related to the colour of the skin.

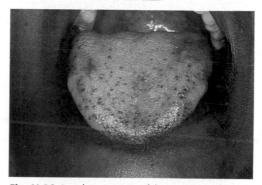

Fig. M.10. Racial pigmentation of the tongue.

Amalgam tattoo

This is a common cause of oral pigmentation and arises by small amounts of amalgam filling material gaining access to the mucosa via a small abrasion during restorative dental procedures or tooth extraction. This produces small regular or irregular areas of pigmentation in the mucosa which rarely require treatment.

Lichen planus

The inflammatory process in this condition may cause some degeneration of the basal layer of the mucous membrane and the pigment released is ingested by macrophages, causing diffuse pigmentation.

Chemicals/Drugs

The metals lead, bismuth and mercury following industrial exposure or their previous use as therapeutic agents can cause blue, brown or black lines characteristically adjacent to the gingival margin. It is felt that these metals formed sulphides following reactions with the dental plaque and were deposited in the gingival mucosa. The drugs in current use which have been reported as causing oral pigmentation are the phenothiazines, antimalarials and the oral contraceptive.

Black hairy tongue

This curious phenomena of unknown origin is characterized by overgrowth of the filiform papillae of the tongue which become stained due to proliferation of chromogenic microorganisms. Heavy smoking and the persistent use of antiseptic mouthwashes have been implicated, but in the majority of cases the cause is unknown (*Fig.* M.11).

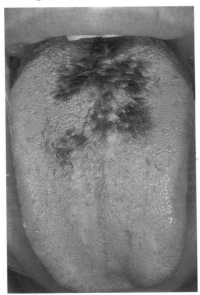

Fig. M.11. Black hairy tongue.

Oral pigmentation has also been found in thyrotoxicosis, malabsorbtion, cachectic states, disorders of iron metabolism and neurofibromatosis.

P. T. Blenkinsopp

Mouth, ulcers in

Mouth ulcers may be classified as follows:

1 TRAUMATIC
2 APHTHOUS
3 ULCERATION ASSOCIATED WITH OTHER MUCOUS MEMBRANES
   (Behçet's syndrome, Reiter's disease)
4 ULCERATION ASSOCIATED WITH SKIN DISEASE
   Lichen planus
   Mucous membrane pemphygoid
   Pemphigus
   Bullous erythema multiforme
5 BLOOD DYSCRASIAS
   Agranulocytosis
   Leukaemia
6 ULCERATION ASSOCIATED WITH GASTROINTESTINAL DISEASES
   Coeliac disease
   Ulcerative colitis
   Crohn's disease
7 ULCERATION ASSOCIATED WITH CONNECTIVE TISSUE DISORDERS
   Lupus erythematosis
8 INFECTION
   a. (Bacterial)
   Acute ulcerative gingivitis
   Syphilis
   Tuberculosis
   b. (Fungal)
   Candida
   c. (Viral)
   Herpes simplex
   Herpes zoster
   Epstein–Barr herpes (infectious mononucleosis)
   Coxsackie (herpangia, hand, foot and mouth disease)
9 TUMOURS
   Squamous-cell carcinoma

1. Traumatic

The diagnosis is usually easy to make because there is a definite history of trauma associated with mastication, ill-fitting dentures or other minor injury to the oral cavity. The ulcers are usually shallow and painful and heal quickly once the noxious stimulant is removed. (*Fig.* M.12). Secondary bacterial infection can occasionally occur, causing an abscess or cellulitis.

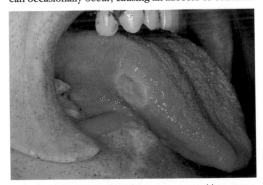

Fig. M.12. Traumatic ulcer of the tongue caused by irritation from a carious tooth.

2. Aphthous ulceration

This is the commonest form of oral ulceration and three types are recognized, depending on the size and number of ulcers. The term ***minor aphthous ulcer*** is given to ulcers less than 5 mm in diameter which occur intermittently as single ulcers or in crops (*Fig.*

M.13). The ulcers take from 1 week to 10 days to heal, and in some patients new ulcers may develop before the original ones have healed so that they are never without ulceration. This type of ulceration tends to commence in childhood and early life and the attacks diminish as the patient becomes older. They are characteristically found on the buccal mucosa, in the sulcus between the jaws and the cheeks, the ventral aspect of the tongue and the floor of the mouth. This condition is often described as recurrent aphthous stomatitis (RAS). The ulcers are round and have an erythematous periphery with a pale central crater.

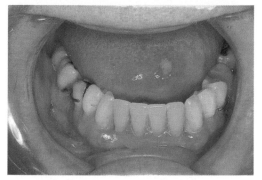

Fig. M.13. Minor aphthous ulcer of the tongue.

Major aphthous ulcers are larger and more persistent and, in addition to the previous sites, may affect the tongue and the palate. They may be up to a centimetre in size and, because of their duration, give concern that the ulcer could be neoplastic.

Herpetiform ulcers are the third variant and here the patient suffers from crops of very numerous small ulcers, which are painful and tend to coalesce into one large irregular area on an erythematous background. Anything from 10 to 100 ulcers may be present at one time.

The cause of aphthous ulceration is unknown, although an auto-immune theory has been advanced. Ten per cent of patients will have an underlying haematological deficiency, especially of vitamin B_{12}, folate or iron; 3 per cent will be suffering from coeliac disease and a few may have Crohn's disease. In some female patients the ulcers are related to the menstrual cycle and will respond to hormone therapy. There is also an association with stress and the cessation of smoking. Aphthous ulceration is thought to be a feature of AIDS, but in the majority cases the cause remains unknown.

3. Ulceration associated with other mucous membranes

BEHÇET'S SYNDROME

This syndrome consists of recurrent aphthous ulceration with also genital and ocular involvement in the form of anterior uveitis. The latter may subsequently cause impairment of vision. The disease characteristically affects young men and there may be associated disease of the skin, joints and nervous system. The cause is unknown, but viral or auto-immune theories have been put forward.

REITER'S SYNDROME

The oral manifestations of this complaint are white circinate lines on an area of erythematous mucosa. These lesions are accompanied by urethritis, arthritis and conjunctivitis. The aetiology is again unknown, but may follow infection with mycoplasma or Shigella.

4. Mouth Ulceration Associated with skin disease

LICHEN PLANUS

Lichen planus is a common condition affecting both the skin and the mouth, although it can affect either in isolation (*see* p. 483). There are several types of oral lichen planus, with the erosive type being characterized by large, irregular areas of mucosal ulceration; the base of the ulcer is often slightly raised with a covering of white to yellow slough. (*Fig.* M.14).

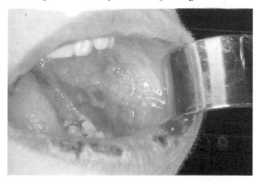

Fig. M.14. Erosive lichen planus affecting the cheek.

Examination of the mouth elsewhere often demonstrates white lacey striations or a desquamative gingivitis. The aetiology of lichen planus is obscure, but it may be mediated by an immunological process, liver disease, drugs (e.g. methyldopa) or in the graft-versus-host reaction (marrow transplantation).

PEMPHIGUS AND PEMPHIGOID

Pemphigus and pemphigoid both may produce oral lesions which commence as bullae when the epithelium separates from the basal layer in pemphigus, and when the epithelium and basal layers separate from the underlying mesoderm in pemphigoid. As a result, the bullae in pemphigus are far more fragile and rupture quickly whereas the bullae in pemphigoid are more resiliant (*Fig.* M.15).

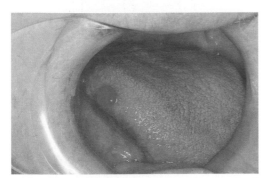

Fig. M.15. Bulla formation on the tongue in a patient with mucous membrane pemphigoid.

In pemphigus there are circulating auto-antibodies against the intercellular attachments of the squamous epithelium but in pemphigoid circulating auto-antibodies are not detectable. They can, however, be found in the basement membrane zone using immunofluorescent techniques.

Pemphigus is a serious mucocutaneous condition, mostly affecting woman in the 40- to 50-year age group, which unless treated may be fatal. The mouth may often be affected first with small bullae or widespread ulceration and loss of the oral epithelium. The diagnosis is made by biopsy of an intact bulla and treatment is by the use of systemic steroids with replacement of fluid and protein in the acute phase.

Benign mucous membrane pemphigoid is a disease of the elderly, which affects the oral mucous membrane and the conjunctiva of the eyes. Anogenital lesions may also occur and minor involvement of the skin may be noted. Because the bullae are more rigid, they tend not to enlarge and rupture late. Once ruptured they leave areas of irregular ulceration, which is accompanied by considerable scarring. The oesophagus and nasopharynx may also be involved, but the most significant aspect of the disease is conjunctival fibrosis leading to visual disturbance.

Examination of the mouth will demonstrate several intact or ruptured bullae during the active phase of the disease and the gingivae may be severely affected with a desquamative gingivitis. Treatment is with topical steroids, although occasionally systematic steroids may be necessary.

BULLOUS ERYTHEMA MULTIFORME

Bullous erythema multiforme or Stevens–Johnson syndrome is the more severe form of erythema multiforme, invariably involving the oral cavity and can be the predominant feature of the attack. The appearance is dramatic because of the severe oral ulceration and the blood-stained and crusted lips. It tends to affect children and young adults and is probably immunologically mediated, via exposure to micoorganisms, e.g.

herpes simplex and mycoplasma, or from drugs, typically the sulphonamides, non-steroidal anti-inflammatory agents, phenytoin and penicillin.

Examination of the skin will demonstrate either extensive erythema, or a macular rash with target lesions exhibiting central bullae formation or ulceration. There is a conjunctivitis, leading to corneal ulceration. In the mouth diffuse inflammation leads to vesicle formation followed by widespread erosions and haemorrhage. Epistaxis commonly occurs. Treatment of the minor case is with topical steroids, but the more severe attack may require systemic therapy. Tetracycline antibiotics should be given if infection with mycoplasma is suspected.

5. Blood dyscrasias

Blood dyscrasias have been discussed under GUMS, BLEEDING, but ulceration of the gingivae is also common, caused by acute local bacterial infection secondary to the abnormal white cell function.

However, it should be remembered that the ulceration may be due to acute ulcerative gingivitis or acute herpetic gingivostomatitis which has arisen *because* of a blood dyscrasia.

6. Ulceration associated with gastrointestinal diseases

Whilst coeliac disease, ulcerative colitis and Crohn's disease can be associated with recurrent aphthous ulceration, these conditions may also show distinctive oral signs. Crohn's disease characteristically produces a 'cobble stone' thickening of the buccal mucosa with hyperplastic folds and fissuring (*Fig.* M.16). Painful ulcers, which are slow to heal, may also be present. Inflammatory bowel disease may also produce the condition of pyostomatitis vegetans, which is characterized by soft hyperplastic mucosal folds between which fissures and ulcers may form.

7. Ulceration associated with connective tissue disorders

Approximately 20 per cent of patients with discoid and systemic lupus erythematosis will show oral ulceration. There may be areas of erythema with erosions and, in some areas, these may resemble lichen planus due to minor striae formation. Frank ulceration may also be present.

The differential diagnosis may be difficult to make but here the lesions often occur on the hard palate, which is rare in lichen planus. The diagnosis is made by biopsy and immunofluorescent studies. Antinuclear antibodies should be looked for in the serum and a history of arthritis and skin rashes should be elicited,

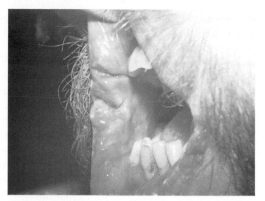

Fig. M.16. Oral mucous membrane showing typical 'cobble-stone' appearance in a patient with Crohn's disease.

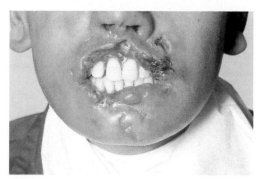

Fig. M.17. Cancrum oris in a patient with acute leukaemia.

particularly an erythematous rash of the face in the butterfly distribution.

8. Infection

A. BACTERIAL

Acute ulcerative gingivitis

Bacterial infection of the oral mucous membrane is rare in normal circumstances, the most important example being acute ulcerative gingivitis, which is associated with large numbers of Vincent's organisms (*Treponema vicentii* and *Fusiformis fusiformis*).

There is haemorrhage, inflammation and the formation of painful, shallow ulcers at the crest of the gingival margin. This eventually leads to destruction and flattening of the interdental papillae. Infection is associated with pre-existing periodontal disease and also any condition reducing host immunity. Patients with leukaemia, AIDS, or those receiving chemotherapy are, therefore, all susceptible and infection may follow an episode of acute herpetic stomatitis.

Acute ulcerative gingivitis in the severely debilitated patient may progress to the destructive condition of **cancrum oris**. This is rare in the developed world, apart from those patients who are immunosuppressed but, still occurs in the Third World as a result of malnutrition and severe viral infections, e.g. herpes and measles. Small areas of gangrene appear in the lips, cheeks or other oral structures, which rapidly progress to larger areas of slough and extensive loss of facial tissue (*Fig* M.17).

Syphilis

The oral cavity may be involved rarely, during the primary stage, to produce a chancre on the lips or the tip of the tongue. Secondary lesions known as the mucous patch are now seldom seen, because of modern effective treatment. Here there is an erosion in the mucous membrane of a few centimetres with a yellowish slough surrounded by erythema. When these areas coalesce they give an irregular shaped ulcer known as the 'snail track' ulcer.

The tertiary stage of syphilis, now rarely seen, produces the gumma, which is a deeply punched-out ulcer caused by central necrosis. These may typically affect the tongue or the palate and in the latter, perforation will produce a central oronasal fistula.

Tuberculosis

With the successful treatment of tuberculosis, oral lesions are rare but, when they do occur, are usually found in the tongue and lips. The ulcer typically shows undermined edges and a granulating floor. The mode of infection is thought to be expectoration of tubercle bacilli from a primary focus in the lungs, which then become implanted in the oral cavity.

B. FUNGAL

Candida (Thrush)

This infection is caused by the yeast-like fungus, *Candida albicans*, which invades the epithelium, causing erythema of the epithelium and a yellow soft plaque, that can be easily removed. This leaves an area of haemorrhagic mucosa or ulceration.

C. VIRAL

The majority of acute infections of the oral mucosa are viral in origin. They tend to effect the younger age groups and are normally associated with constitutional symptoms of fever, malaise and enlarged and tender cervical lymph nodes.

Herpes simplex

The primary infection invariably involves the mouth with many small vesicles, approximately 2 mm in diameter, which are regular in shape and size. The mouth is generally inflamed and in areas the ulcers coalesce to produce irregular raw erosions and a yellow slough (*Fig*. M.18).

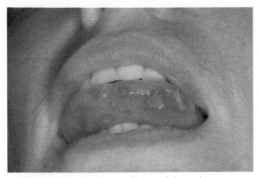

Fig. M.18. Primary herpes infection of the oral cavity.

The gingival mucosa is red and swollen and may bleed even in the absence of ulceration. Herpetic stomatitis may be an opportunist infection and can be severe in immunocompromised patients and patients with AIDS. The lesion of reactivation is known as secondary herpes. The virus which has been quiescent in the trigeminal ganglion becomes active once more, to produce a cold sore or herpes labialis in the distribution of the infected nerve.

Herpes zoster

Herpes zoster causes chicken pox in the patient who has not been exposed to the virus and mouth ulcers are common in this condition. The virus again remains quiescent in the trigeminal ganglion and on reactivation causes painful ulceration within the exact anatomical distribution of the nerve (*Fig.* M.19).

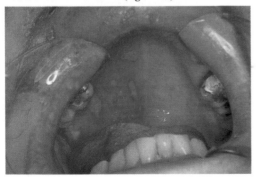

Fig. M.19. Herpes zoster infection in the distribution of the maxillary branch of the trigeminal nerve.

This condition is known as herpes zoster or shingles and on occasions can be an indication of a more serious underlying disease. Again the picture is of erythema, small regular ulcers and pain within the distribution of the nerve affected. If the ophthalmic branch is involved then care needs to be given to the cornea. The infection may be complicated by postherpetic neuralgia.

Epstein–Barr virus

Infectious mononucleosis is caused by the Epstein–Barr virus. There may be characteristic petechiae of the soft palate and pharynx, which are often considered diagnostic.

The patient has a sore throat, the lymph nodes are enlarged and occasionally there is extensive ulceration of the faucies. Ampicillin should not be given for the sore throat as this exacerbates the condition.

Coxsackie

Mouth ulcers arise from infection with the coxsackie virus which causes a febrile illness, lymphadenopathy and ulcers in the region of the soft palate. The ECHO virus causes hand, foot and mouth disease which is a highly infectious condition characterized by small vesicles, leading to ulcers on the hands, the feet and in the mouth. Both these latter infections are trivial conditions and are self-limiting.

9. Tumours

Squamous-cell carcinoma is the most common malignant tumour of the oral cavity and is associated with excessive smoking and alcohol consumption.

The clinical picture of oral carcinoma is very varied but in the advanced case is obvious. There is a friable mass arising in the mucous membrane with a rough, irregular surface, which bleeds easily. There is usually deep, irregular central ulceration with an infected slough at its base. (*Fig.* M.20). Radiographs may show associated bone erosion.

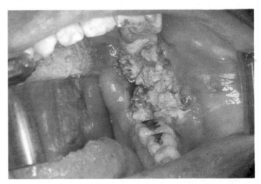

Fig. M.20. Ulcer in the left retro-molar region arising in an extensive squamous-cell carcinoma.

The early lesion may be more difficult to diagnose, showing only an area of erythema or hyperkeratosis, slight roughening of the mucosa and shallow ulceration.

Unfortunately many oral carcinomas are still diagnosed late and therefore, any ulcer which does not heal within 3 weeks, or does not obviously fall into one of the other categories should be submitted to a biopsy.

Other tumours of the oral cavity, both benign and malignant, can undergo ulceration due to trauma or ischaemic necrosis; these are described under JAW, SWELLING OF.

P. T. Blenkinsopp

MOVEMENTS, INVOLUNTARY

See ATHETOSIS; CHOREIFORM MOVEMENTS; TREMOR.

Muscular atrophy

Atrophy of muscles will be considered under the following headings:

1   Atrophy as part of generalized body wasting.
2   Disuse atrophy.
3   Atrophy due to vascular disease in a limb.
4   Atrophy due to damage to the lower motor neurone.
5   Atrophy due to cerebral disorders.
6   Atrophy due to developmental disorders.

1.   General bodily wasting

Muscular atrophy is often seen in general wasting of the tissues due to chronic or subacute disease such as tuberculosis, malignant disease, neglected or undiagnosed diabetes mellitus, hyperthyroidism, malaria, hookworm infestation, conditions associated with chronic diarrhoea and anorexia nervosa. It is also seen in old age.

2.   Disuse

Disuse of a limb gives rise to extreme degrees of wasting. The best example is provided by the results of prolonged immobilization for fractures of the long bones. It also occurs in muscles acting upon a painful or ankylosed joint, and in rheumatoid arthritis. Hysterical paralysis gives rise to wasting only when maintained for a very long time and this is unusual. Voluntary disuse, practised by some eastern cults, can lead to extreme 'withering' of the entire limb, e.g. when penance demands that the arm be held above the head in perpetuity.

3.   Vascular disease

Arterial occlusion is variable in its effects. In tourniquet paralysis, surgical ligation of a major vessel, thrombosis or embolism of the great vessels, the degree of wasting depends on the efficiency of the collateral circulation. In many instances the muscles become fibrosed and hard rather than wasted and flabby. In other cases, there is a true atrophy of muscles due to ischaemia of the motor nerves, as in some cases of Buerger's disease and in polyarteritis nodosa. A special variety of ischaemic palsy, known as Volkmann's contracture, is the result of fractures in the region of the elbow. Oedema and haemorrhage into the soft tissues interfere with the circulation distal to the elbow and cause fibrosis of the flexors of the wrist and fingers, and of the intrinsic muscles of the hand. The affected muscles

are hard in consistency and wasting is comparatively slight owing to replacement with fibrous tissue.

4.   Damage to the lower motor neurone

Lesions of the lower motor neurone are responsible for the majority of cases of muscular atrophy encountered in clinical practice. The muscles are weak, flaccid and wasted. Fasciculation is seen. Electromyography shows fibrillation potentials on mechanical stimulation by the exploring needle and spontaneous fibrillation and fasciculation potentials at rest. The tendon reflexes are depressed or abolished in the affected part unless, as in motor neurone disease, there is a coincident pyramidal lesion, in which case they usually remain brisk as long as there is any power of contraction left in the muscles concerned. It is convenient to classify the causes of this form of atrophy according to whether the lesion is in the anterior horn cells, the motor roots or the peripheral nerves.

Anterior horn cells

Localized damage to anterior horn cells may occur at the site of trauma from fracture-dislocation of the spine or as a result of backward protrusion of an intervertebral disc in the cervical or thoracic regions. Spinal tumours may produce a similar effect. In these instances atrophy is confined to the muscles which are innervated by the affected portion of the cord. Acute poliomyelitis used to be the most common cause of anterior horn cell damage but the incidence of this has been dramatically reduced. The muscular atrophy seen in late cases of polio is often very striking and localized to particular groups of muscles. Other intraspinal lesions that may produce muscular atrophy are

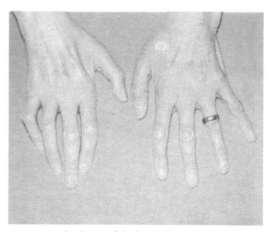

Fig. M.21. The dorsum of the hands showing atrophy of all the dorsal interosseous muscles in a case of progressive muscular atrophy. The wasting of the first dorsal interosseous on the right is particularly marked. The ring and little finger are beginning to adopt the *main-en-griffe* attitude.

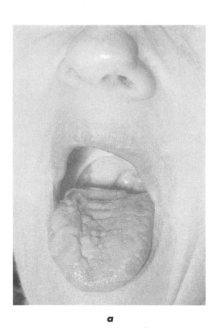

a

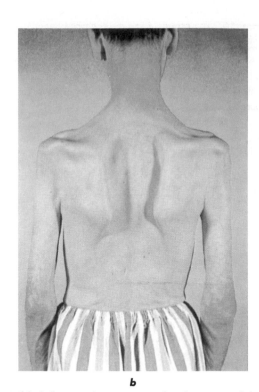

b

Fig. M.22. Progressive muscular atrophy (motor neurone disease) of the bulbar type showing wasting of (*a*) the tongue and (*b*) the shoulder girdle muscles.

syringomyelia, haematomyelia and intramedullary tumours such as ependymomas and astrocytomas; such cases usually have associated sensory loss and other signs of spinal cord damage. Motor neurone disease is a common cause of muscle atrophy in adults. It is prominent in the progressive muscular atrophy form of the disease (*Fig.* M.21) and is also seen in the so-called amyotrophic lateral sclerosis form. Fasciculations are prominent in affected muscles in this condition. In the bulbar form, wasting of the tongue may be obvious. (*Fig.* M.22). The rare syphilitic amyotrophy may mimic motor neurone disease but the tendon reflexes are depressed and serological tests will confirm the diagnosis. Atrophic paralysis of one or more muscles occasionally occurs in herpes zoster; the rash, pain and lymphocytosis in the spinal fluid in the acute phase confirm the diagnosis. Infarction of a localized area of spinal cord consequent upon thromboembolism of a branch of the anterior spinal artery may cause localized damage to anterior horn cells with segmental muscle wasting. This may occur in atheromatous disease, meningovascular syphilis or in association with arteriovenous malformations or tumours of the spinal cord.

Motor roots

Damage to a single motor root seldom causes much atrophy since most muscles are supplied by several

roots. An exception is the first thoracic root which supplies the intrinsic muscles of the hand. Damage to multiple spinal roots may be seen in spinal lesions below the level of the first lumbar vertebra producing damage to the cauda equina. Apart from muscle weakness and wasting there will often be associated sensory loss and sphincteric disturbance; pain is often a prominent symptom. Common causes of cauda equina damage include lumbar spondylosis, lumbar canal stenosis, primary and secondary spinal tumours, and prolapsed lumbar intervertebral discs. More localized damage to spinal roots may be seen in spondylosis and muscle atrophy in the upper limbs may be a feature of cervical spondylosis.

The peripheral nerves

Proximal damage to peripheral nerves may occur at their origin in the brachial or lumbosacral plexus. Malignant infiltration of the brachial plexus typically affects the lower part of the plexus affecting the nerve supply to the intrinsic hand muscles. Malignant infiltration of the lumbosacral plexus may occur but is less common. Pain is a prominent feature. Traumatic avulsion of the plexus in the upper limb is all too common as a consequence of motor-cycle injuries and in some instances the avulsion occurs not at the level of the plexus but at the level of the motor roots.

Table M.6. The causes of peripheral neuropathy

Inherited neuropathies	Chronic acquired neuropathies	Mononeuropathies
Mixed sensorimotor neuropathies:	Carcinoma	Pressure
1. Idiopathic	Paraproteinaemia	Trauma
2. Metabolic	Uraemic	Idiopathic
Sensory neuropathies	Beri-beri	Serum/postvaccinal
	Diabetic	Herpes zoster
Acute acquired neuropathies	Hypothyroid	Neoplastic
Guillain–Barré syndrome	Connective tissue	Leprosy
Porphryia	Amyloid	Radiation
Toxic	Leprosy	Diphtheritic
Diphtheritic		
	Relapsing neuropathies	**Mononeuritis multiplex**
Subacute acquired neuropathies	Idiopathic	Arteritis
Deficiency states	Porphyria	Diabetes
Heavy metals		
Drug intoxication		
Uraemic		
Diabetic		
Arteritic		

Traumatic damage to the lumbosacral plexus is less common. Localized injuries to the plexus or peripheral nerves may occur as a result of stab wounds, gunshot wounds, and fractures and dislocations in the vicinity of motor nerves.

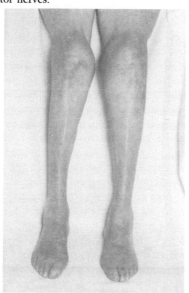

Fig. M.23. Distal muscle atrophy due to peripheral neuropathy.

Compression on motor nerves may produce local damage (so-called 'entrapment neuropathies'). Common sites of damage are the radial nerve in the upper arm, the lower cord of the brachial plexus between the first rib and a cervical rib, the ulnar nerve at the level of the elbow, the median nerve at the level of the carpal tunnel and the lateral popliteal nerve at the level of the neck of the fibula. The causes of peripheral neuropathies, are given in *Table* M.6. Rates of progression vary considerably but the common features are those of diffuse involvement of multiple peripheral nerves. In general the distal parts of the limbs are affected first with muscle weakness and wasting being most obvious in the lower part of the legs and hands (*Fig.* M.23). Signs are usually symmetrical although some types of peripheral neuropathy tend to involve motor fibres more than sensory fibres. But there is usually an associated distal sensory loss which is typically in 'glove and stocking' distribution. Tendon reflexes are almost invariably depressed or absent.

Muscle disorders

Muscular atrophy, although not usually a prominent feature in muscle disease, may be seen in any form of myopathy. (For classification of myopathics *see Table* M.7.) Congenital absence of a muscle may occur and the most common deficiency is the sternocostal portion of pectoralis major. Rupture of a muscle or its tendon may lead to localized atrophy.

5. Cerebral disorders

Although muscle wasting is not a feature of upper motor neurone disturbances, some degree of atrophy may be seen in a hemiplegic patient as a result of disuse. Less common is so called 'parietal wasting' seen in acquired disorders of the parietal lobe, where wasting of a contralateral limb appears out of proportion to the degree of disuse. The mechanism of such atrophy is uncertain.

6. Developmental disorders

Unilateral cerebral disorders which affect the brain before bone growth has ceased may be associated with quite significant atrophy affecting not only muscles but bones and other subcutaneous tissues. The affected limb may be shorter and the hand or foot significantly smaller than its twin. More striking localized atrophy may be seen in patients who have suffered lower

Table M.7.   A classification of myopathies

1. *Inflammatory disease of muscle*
  Polymyositis
  Dermatomyositis
	4. *Metabolic myopathies*
	  Glycogen storage myopathies
	  Carnitine deficiency (and other defects of fatty acid metabolism)

2. *Infective myopathies*
  Trichinosis
  Toxoplasmosis
  Virus infections (e.g. Coxsackie B virus)
	5. *Endocrine myopathies*
	  Thyroid dysfunction
	  Adrenal dysfunction

3. *Muscular dystrophies*
  Duchenne
  Becker
  Fascioscapulohumeral
  Limb girdle
  Oculopharyngeal dystrophy
  Myotonic dystrophy
	6. *Spinal muscular atrophies*
	  Although such conditions are not strictly disorders of muscle they are included because of the frequent difficulty in differentiating them from the true myopathies

motor neurone disturbances affecting a limb before bone growth has ceased.

N. E. F. Cartlidge

Muscular hypertrophy

There is considerable variation in the size of individual skeletal muscles and the assessment of hypertrophy or enlargement may in some instances be very difficult. For example, the normal calf muscles in a leg that has gross wasting of the quadriceps may appear hypertrophied simply because of the relative disproportion.

Exercising muscles can cause them to hypertrophy: this occurs as a result of increase in muscle fibre size secondary to an increase in the number of myofibrils per fibre. Such physiological hypertrophy may be generalized as in body-builders or it may be localized as in those who repeatedly use a particular limb, for example tennis players.

The syndrome of hemihypertrophy is associated with diffuse enlargement of all the tissues of one half of the body, occasionally affecting only the face or one limb. In this condition, the aetiology of which is unknown, the muscles, subcutaneous tissues and bones all appear to enlarge.

Pathological muscle hypertrophy may be classified as in *Table* M.8.

dystrophy. The most commonly enlarged muscle is the gastrocnemius although hypertrophy of the infraspinatus, deltoid, triceps, quadriceps or gluteus muscles may be encountered. The term pseduohypertrophy has been used in reference to Duchenne dystrophy, since in the later stages of the disease the muscles becomes weak but remain enlarged because of replacement of fibres by fat and connective tissues. Often the pseudohypertrophic muscles will have a rather characteristic firm or doughy feeling.

Rapid enlargement of muscles has been described in spinal muscular atrophy, polymyositis, cysticercosis and in certain families with malignant hyperpyrexia.

Diffuse hypertrophy of muscles may occur in myotonia congenita and probably represents work hypertrophy associated with continuous muscle contraction. This produces the so-called 'infant Hercules' appearance. In hypothyroidism, hypertrophy of muscles is more common in children than in adults. Calves, thighs, hands, neck, tongue and face may all enlarge and feel firm or indurated. Often the patient will complain of pain and stiffness and this may be accompanied by proximal muscle weakness. In the DeLange syndrome, hypertrophy of muscles is associated with congenital athetosis and mental retardation.

The early medical literature contains numerous

Table M.8.   Hypertrophy of muscles

1. *Multiple muscle enlargement*
  Duchenne dystrophy
  Becker dystrophy
  Limb-girdle dystrophy
  Spinal muscular atrophy
  Hypothyroidism
  Myotonia congenita
  DeLange syndrome
  Cysticercosis
  Malignant hyperpyrexia
  Hypertrophia musculorum vera
	2. *Localized muscle enlargement*
	  Muscle/tendon rupture
	  Muscle haemorrhage
	  Muscle tumour
	  Myositis ossificans
	  Granuloma
	  Pyogenic abscess
	  Fibrositis

1.   Multiple muscle enlargement

Enlargement of muscles is commonly seen in Duchenne and Becker dystrophy and occasionally in limb-girdle

references to patients whose only abnormality was muscle hypertrophy—so-called 'hypertrophia musculorum vera.' Although many of these cases may have had hypothyroidism or myotonia congenita, there are undoubtedly some families in whom the only abnormal finding is muscle hypertrophy, often particularly marked in the calves and masseters.

2. Localized muscle enlargement

This is most commonly seen in the biceps muscle as a result of rupture of the muscle fibres or tearing of the long head. It may also be seen as a result of a muscle haemorrhage, muscle tumour such as rhabdomyosarcoma, angioma, desmoid or metastatic lesion, or as a result of an infective process such as granulomatous disease or pyogenic abscess. Localized enlargement may occur as a result of trauma leading to myositis ossificans.

D. Shaw

Muscular pain

Pain in muscles is one of the most common of all complaints and may occur either as an ache or as a stiffness or cramp. These two types of muscle pain are usually distinguishable and their causes are different.

Aching Pains

Aches and pains in muscles may be transient, recurrent or persistent. They may be classified as follows:

1 Normal reactions to stress and strain
2 Injuries
3 Pains referred from elsewhere
4 Pains of vascular origin
5 Muscle disorders
6 Neuromuscular disorders
7 Endocrine disorders
8 Drugs
9 Psychogenic or 'functional'

1. NORMAL REACTIONS. Fatigue, unhappiness, anxiety, and particularly depression, may be associated with muscle aches and pains. Few healthy people go through an average day, whatever their occupation or activity, without occasional feelings of muscular discomfort. These are usually suppressed or ignored but in abnormal emotional states they may assume unnatural proportions and become significant and sometimes distressing symptoms. It has been said that 'middle-age is the point in time when emotions become symptoms.' Muscle aches certainly become commoner as individuals become increasingly aware of the ageing process. These aches may be aggravated by postural strain, often resulting from the adoption of fixed positions over prolonged periods.

2. INJURIES. After unduly heavy exertion, muscles may become painful for hours or even days, presumably as a result of small local injuries, tears or haemorrhages, in muscles themselves or at muscle insertions. Injured fibres, particularly at points of attachment to bone, may be acutely painful and tender as in tennis or golfer's elbow, and ligaments may be completely torn across even in the absence of extreme exertion. The largest tendon in the body, the tendo achillis, is particularly liable to rupture in those engaged in sporting activities such as squash or cricket. A patient referred to the author completely severed both his tendons by jumping with excessive exuberance out of bed one sunny morning. The supraspinatas muscle and tendon and the quadriceps are perhaps the most frequently injured; a rupture of the long head of biceps, the rhomboids, major or minor, pectoralis major, rectus abdominus, trapezius, levator scapuli, latissimus dorsi or almost any other muscle or tendon may occur and may mislead the unwary diagnostician. It is important that muscle pain in the chest or abdomen should not be mistaken for pain arising from visceral sources. An unusual cause of muscle pain that may be overlooked is spontaneous haemorrhage of the type that may occur in haemophiliacs or in those on anticoagulant therapy.

3. REFERRED PAIN. Pains apparently arising in muscles are often referred from inflammatory or degenerative disease in nearby joints. Pains in thigh muscles, for instance, may result from hip joint disease and muscle pains in the shoulder girdle, chest or abdomen, from degenerative changes in the cervical, dorsal or lumbar spine. Disease or injury of ligaments may be referred to muscles; injections of hypertonic saline into interspinous ligaments, for instance, may cause pains in muscles several inches away. The cause of the extremely common so-called 'fibrositis' in muscles in the scapular and shoulder regions is still inadequately explained, but undoubtedly the pain is often referred from adjacent spinal joints and ligaments, allegedly triggered in many cases by cold or damp. These 'fibrositic' pains may sometimes be the first signs of an arthropathy such as rheumatoid arthritis, rarely a disseminated connective-tissue disorder such as systemic lupus erythematosus or polyarteritis nodosa, or more commonly in elderly subjects, polymyalgia rheumatica (*see* pp. 354, 382).

4. PAINS OF VASCULAR ORIGIN. The classical example of ischaemic muscle pain is the intermittent claudication experienced on exertion by victims of occlusive arterial disease in the lower limbs. Inflammatory arterial diseases, for example, polymyalgia rheumatica, giant-cell arteritis and polyarteritis nodosa, may also produce pain and tenderness in muscle. In rare instances the increased metabolic demands of exercising muscles may divert blood from others in which perfusion is at a critical level because of arterial disease and ischaemic pain therefore results.

5. MUSCLE DISORDERS. Several inflammatory disorders of muscle are commonly associated with muscle pain and tenderness and should be considered in any

patient who complains of myalgia. In polymyositis and dermatomyositis, over 50 per cent of sufferers will describe pain as well as muscle weakness. The pain is usually a deep aching within the muscles and it is often aggravated by activity. The muscles may be swollen as well as tender. Similar symptoms are seen in a variety of other connective-tissue diseases when there is an associated inflammatory myopathy, for example, rheumatoid arthritis, Sjögrens syndrome, systemic lupus erythematosus, polyarteritis nodosa, scleroderma and mixed connective-tissue disease.

Several epidemics of influenza due to type A or B virus have been described in which there was a rather acute onset of severe myalgia lasting 1 or 2 weeks with creatine kinase often elevated many times above normal. In epidemic pleurodynia, or Bornholm disease, the acute onset of chest and abdominal pain, chiefly at the costal margins and in the subcostal region, is usually the first symptom. Affected muscles are tender to pressure and pain is induced by muscle contraction. The acute pain and fever last several days and after initial recovery one or more relapses are not uncommon. Care must be taken not to confuse one of these relatively benign and reversible syndromes with polymyositis of acute onset.

An unusual type of muscle disease may result from eating undercooked pork infected with the larvae of *Trichinella spiralis*. Muscle pain and stiffness occur particularly in the masseter. There may be associated malaise, fever, periorbital oedema, skin rash and petechial haemorrhages.

Polymyalgia rheumatica should always be considered in older patients in their sixties and seventies complaining of aching pain and stiffness in the shoulder and hip girdle muscles. The pain tends to be worse at night and morning stiffness is a prominent feature.

6. NEUROMUSCULAR DISORDERS. Pains in the muscles may be marked in the early stages of poliomyelitis and are common in the Guillain–Barré syndrome. In acute brachial neuritis or neuralgic amyotrophy severe aching pain in one or both shoulders or arms may precede the development of localized muscle weakness. In diabetic proximal neuropathy pain often accompanies atrophy of the quadriceps or sometimes other muscles. Other neuropathies associated with severe pain include those seen with alcoholism, arsenical poisoning, polyarteritis and porphyria.

7. ENDOCRINE CAUSES. In hypothyroidism muscles may ache and also in acromegaly and hyperparathyroidism. Most endocrine disorders, however, are more commonly associated with weakness than with pain.

8. DRUGS. Severe muscle pains may follow the intramuscular injection of suxamethonium, a muscle relaxant used in anaesthesia; these pains can occur

1–5 days after anaesthesia and are worse if there is earlier resumption of physical activity. A number of drugs may cause an acute or subacute necrotizing myopathy which may be associated with myoglobinuria, sometimes leading to acute renal failure (*Table M.9*).

Table M.9. Drugs capable of causing painful myopathy

Suxamethonium
Clofibrate
Epsilon–aminocaproic acid
Heroin
Amphetamine
Vincristine
Alcohol
Guanoclor
Lithium
Emetine
Cimetidine
Isoetharine
Phencyclidine

9. PSYCHOGENICE. Aching pain in muscles is a common symptom in depression and anxiety and may also be seen in hysteria or in patients who are frankly malingering.

Muscle stiffness or cramps

Ordinary muscle cramps or painful involuntary contractions of muscle are experienced in almost everyone at some time in their lives and in most instances the diagnosis presents no difficulty. Benign muscle cramps most commonly occur after unaccustomed exercise and are usually self-limiting. In some patients, however, these cramps can be persistent and quite incapacitating.

Pathological cramps can be produced by an abnormality anywhere along the final common pathway including the anterior horn cell, peripheral nerve, neuromuscular junction and muscle membrane.

Exertional cramps may be seen in a variety of disorders including cauda equina ischaemia from lumbar canal stenosis, and inborn errors of muscle metabolism such as McArdle's disease or the lipid storage myopathies. In myophosphorylase deficiency and phosphofructokinase deficiency a true contracture occurs with exercise which may be accompanied by myoglobinuria.

Several of the cramping disorders are characterized by myotonia where the patient observes a delayed relaxation after even a single voluntary contraction.

Muscle cramps and spasms may occur either spontaneously or after exercise in a variety of biochemical disturbances. They are most characteristically seen in tetany which may occur with hypocalcaemia, alkalosis or hypomagnesaemia.

Several disorders are characterized by an almost continuous state of muscle activity: these include tetanus, strychnine poisoning and the bite of the American black widow spider. A number of rare neuromuscular disorders are associated with persistent contraction of muscles at rest. These include the symptoms of myokymia, continuous muscle fibre activity and the so-called 'stiff-man' syndrome.

A separate and important group of muscle cramp syndromes are the so-called 'professional' cramps or repetitive strain injury (RSI): the commonest of these is 'writer's cramp'. However, similar localized muscle cramps have been described in typists, telephone operators, painters, tailors, seamstresses, pianists, flautists, violinists, cellists, harpists, drummers, piano players, blacksmiths, filemakers and watchmakers! There is considerable debate as to whether these are occupational neuroses or localized dystonias.

D. Shaw

Muscular tone

The tone of a muscle can be regarded as its resistance to passive stretching. This can only be assessed when the muscle is moved; it cannot be judged on the basis of palpation. Postural tone is that state of partial contraction of certain muscles which is needed to maintain the posture of the body.

The moment a muscle is stretched, receptors in the muscle concerned, particularly in the muscle spindles, transmit afferent stimuli, and reflex partial contraction of the muscle results. The responses to momentary stretching are responsible for the tendon jerks; the responses to more prolonged stretching elicit more complex responses such as tonic contraction.

Forceful continued contraction of a group of muscles, for example, clenching one hand, temporarily causes an increased flow of afferent impulses in the sensory fibres from the spindles. This is associated with exaggeration of the tendon reflexes resulting from increased alpha neuronal discharge This is known as 'reinforcement' which can be helpful in eliciting depressed reflexes.

Muscle tone is normally regulated by reticulo-spinal fibres which accompany the pyramidal tract through the spinal cord and which have an inhibitory effect upon the stretch reflex. This inhibition balances the facilitatory impulses conveyed by the pontine reticulo-spinal and lateral vestibulo-spinal pathways. These in turn are influenced by multisynaptic reflex arcs traversing the cerebellum, basal ganglia and brain stem.

Alterations in muscle tone

RIGIDITY

In this form of increased muscle tone, the muscles are continuously or intermittently tense. The increased resistance to passive movement has an even or uniform quality throughout the range of movement of the limb like that noted when bending a lead pipe. Rigidity is present in all muscle groups, both flexor and extensor, but it tends to be more prominent in those which maintain a flexed posture.

A particular type of rigidity, often encountered in Parkinson's disease, has distinctive characteristics and is described as 'cogwheel'. When the hypertonic muscle is stretched a ratchet-like resistance is felt.

Rigidity is a prominent feature of many extrapyramidal diseases such as Parkinson's disease, Wilson's disease, dystonia musculorum deformans, multiple system atrophy and basal ganglia calcification.

A special type of variable resistance to passive movement is that in which the patient seems unable to relax. This is sometimes called 'gegenhalten' and is seen in diseases of the frontal lobes. A similar difficulty may be observed in children.

The pathophysiology of rigidity is not fully understood though it is generally agreed that it results from lesions of the nigro-striatal system. It can often be relieved by dopamine, dopamine agonists or by stereotactic lesions in the ventrolateral thalamus.

SPASTICITY

This is a form of increased tone resulting from lesions of the pyramidal pathways and the closely associated reticulo-spinal pathways. The stretch reflexes are released from descending inhibitory influences and there is increased excitability of fusimotor neurones and alpha motor neurones. The resistance to passive stretch of muscles affected by spasticity often has a distinctive quality. It may be particularly severe initially and then tend to give way, hence the descriptive term, 'clasp knife rigidity'. The hyperactivity of the tendon reflexes is often accompanied by clonus in which sustained stretch of a muscle evokes repetitive contraction and relaxation.

DECEREBRATE RIGIDITY

A lesion at the mid-brain, at or about the level of the superior colliculus, releases the brain stem, cerebellum and spinal cord from cerebral control. This results in strong continuous contraction in extensor groups of muscles. In such cases all four limbs are rigidly extended, the back is arched and there may be neck retraction.

Although the experimental production of decerebrate rigidity by Sherrington appeared to have a specific anatomical substrate, this does not hold quite true in man; for example, unilateral decerebrate rigidity is not uncommonly seen in the early stages of acute cerebral infarction in the territory of the middle cerebral artery.

Hypotonia

Hypotonia, or flaccidity, implies a reduction in tone. It may be seen in cerebral or spinal shock resulting from acute damage to the brain or spinal cord. It is a common manifestation of cerebellar disease and in this situation is thought to result from diminished gamma efferent activity. It also occurs whenever a lesion interrupts the afferent or efferent pathway of the spinal reflex arc. It is thus seen in damage to the anterior horn cells, spinal roots and peripheral nerves, but it is not a particular feature of muscle disease.

Minor degrees of loss of tone may be difficult to differentiate from normal inherent muscle tone. Gross flaccidity is usually obvious. In the upper limbs lesser degrees of hypotonia can be elicited by asking the patient to hold the arms out horizontally. Tapping the forearms when hypotonia is present will be associated with slow recoil and a wide arm swing.

N. E. F. Cartlidge

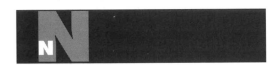

Nails, affections of

The nails become involved in many cutaneous affections, commonly dermatitis, psoriasis, epidermolysis bullosa, pemphigus, exfoliative dermatitis, and rarely in lichen planus (*Fig.* N.1), Darier's disease and alopecia areata. In *dermatitis* (*Fig.* N.2.), when the terminal phalanges of the fingers are affected, there is roughening and ridging of the nail plate, and successive exacerbations of the disease may be recorded by the indentations of the plate so formed. There may also be pitting coarser than that seen in psoriasis (*Figs.* N.3–N.5). In *ringworm of the nails* (*Fig* N.6) caused by *T. mentagrophytes* or *T. rubrum*, one or more of the nails may be involved. The disease affects the plate itself, which first loses its lustre, then becomes discoloured, and finally friable. Often there is heaping up of tissue under the plate. The diagnosis may be confirmed by finding the causal fungus in scrapings of nail material. It is sometimes difficult to differentiate this condition from psoriasis of the nails, especially when, as not infrequently occurs, the nails only are involved. In *psoriasis* one of the most constant features is pitting of the nails (*Fig* N.3), which may take place before any other sign of the disease appears. Other

nail changes in psoriasis are discoloration (*Fig* N.4) and onycholysis (*Fig* N.5) or separation of the nail from its bed; these may be accompanied by or followed by the formation of a granular mass under the nail: in the final stage the nail becomes 'worm-eaten', cracked and split, friable and disintegrated. It is worth bearing in mind that psoriasis of the nails is much more common than ringworm of the nails. In chronic paronychia, which is due to combined candidal and bacterial infection, pockets form under the posterior nailfolds, which will admit the tip of a probe up to an eighth of an inch. (*Fig* N.7). Very occasionally pus may be expressed from these pockets, from which cultures of the yeast may be made. In profile the raised nailfolds over the pockets have a characteristic bolster-like appearance. The changes in the nail plate are secondary. This disease occurs in those who are obliged to keep their hands wet for long periods, notably bar staff, fishmongers and those with 'wet' occupations. It is much commoner in women than in men.

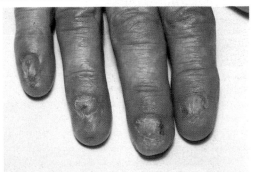

Fig. N.1. Scarring nail dystrophy due to lichen planus. (*Westminster Hospital.*)

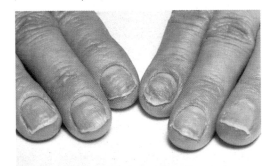

Fig. N.2. Nails in dermatitis showing coarse pitting and cross ridging. (*Westminster Hospital.*)

In *epidermolysis bullosa* the repeated blister formation at the finger ends causes atrophy of the skin and loss of nails. The naked-eye appearances of the nail change may indicate the diagnosis at once, or lesions elsewhere may help one in forming an opinion. In *pachyonychia congenita* the nail plates are thick, hard and firmly attached to the nailbeds. It may be

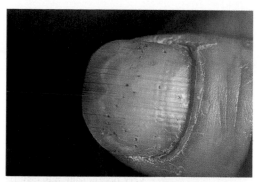

Fig. N.3. Psoriasis, showing pitting of nail.

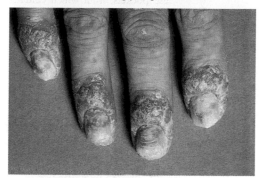

Fig N.4. Psoriasis, showing discoloration, distortion and thickening of nail plate. (*Westminster Hospital.*)

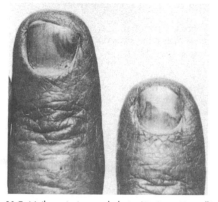

Fig. N.5. Nail psoriasis: onycholysis. (*Dr Peter Hansell.*)

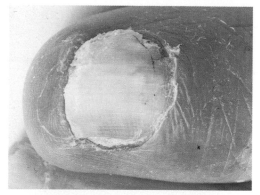

Fig. N.6. Ringworm of nail. (*Westminster Hospital.*)

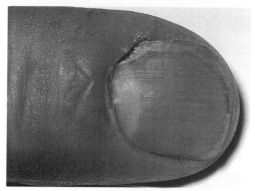

Fig. N.7. Paronychia—chronic stage. (*Westminster Hospital.*)

associated with follicular, keratotic grey-coloured papules on the extensor surfaces. Blistering and maceration with secondary infection may take place around and between the toes and leucokeratosis of the tongue may be present. In congenital ectodermal defect the nails may be absent; more often they are short and fail to reach the free edge of the digit.

Trophic changes in the nails are not at all uncommon, and while they sometimes occur in general illness more often they are of unknown aetiology. Transverse furrows (*Beau's lines*) usually follow acute illnesses. They are formed at the time of the illness but will not appear on the nail plate for about 6–8 weeks and then move steadily forward with the growth of the nail, finally being lost at 5-6 months (*Figs* N.8, N.9).

Longitudinal ridging more often has no apparent cause (*Fig.* N.10). Brittleness (*onychorrhexis*) or softness of the nails with splitting or terracing of the free edge is more common in women than in men. The cause is unknown but repeated wetting and drying may be a factor of importance. It has been thought to be aggravated by the use of nail varnish and varnish removers, but many cases occur in women who do

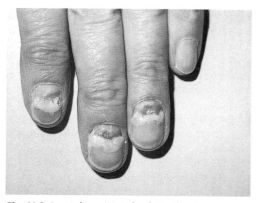

Fig. N.8. Beau's lines. (*Dr Richard Staughton.*)

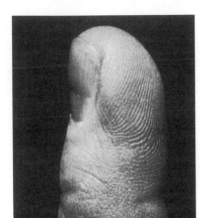

Fig N.9. Beau's lines: side view. (*Dr Peter Hansell.*)

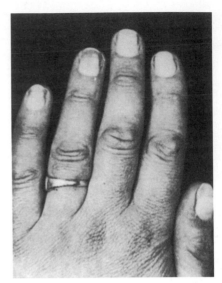

Fig. N.11. Leuconychia totalis. (*St John's Hospital.*)

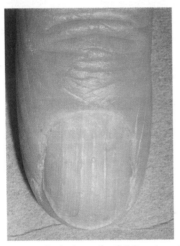

Fig. N.10. Longitudinal ridging of nail. (*Westminster Hospital.*)

not use nail polish. Spoon nails (*koilonychia*) occur in anaemia due to iron deficiency and are part of the Plummer–Vinson syndrome. In hypo-albuminaemia the appearance of paired narrow white bands running transversely across the nail plate has been described. The nails may appear white in some cases of hepatic cirrhosis; all degrees of whiteness may be found in chronic congestive heart failure, pulmonary tuberculosis, diabetes, rheumatoid arthritis and some forms of carcinoma. Red half-moons are seen in some cases of cardiac failure. Hypertrophy of the nails (*onychauxis*) occurs more often on the toes and may lead to onychogryphosis.

Leuconychia totalis (*Fig.* N.11) is a rare congenital anomaly in which the whole nail plate is white. Leuconychia striata and punctate (white lines or dots) are much more common but are of no significance.

In leuconychia the changes are in the nail plate itself. Whitening from other causes is due to changes in the nailbed.

The nails may be shed in many acute skin diseases that involve the fingers, notably in exfoliative dermatitis, and this also occurs occasionally in severe secondary syphilis. In X-ray burns affecting the fingers the nails may be destroyed.

Onychia, or inflammation of the nail, is usually septic in origin, but may be the result of trauma or contact with irritants at work. It usually terminates in shedding of the affected nail. *Paronychia*, or whitlow, is usually obvious, but a primary chancre of the finger may sometimes imitate it.

Trauma is responsible for many nail deformities. Single injuries produce haematomas which may lead to temporary nail loss or to permanent splits if the nail matrix is injured. Repeated minor traumas may be inflicted in several ways. Probably the commonest is nail biting where the usual deformity produced is a short ragged nail and is often complicated by the appearance of periungual warts (*Fig.* N.12). Hang nails are spicules of hard material from the edges of the nailfolds and are often due to nail biting and may give rise to minor local sepsis. Excess manicuring, especially pushing back the cuticle, may lead to cross ridging of some nails and a similar appearance is produced by a habit tic of playing with the nails (*Fig.* N.13). Ill-fitting footwear is responsible for ingrowing toenails and probably for most cases of onychogryphosis; it may also lead to repeated shedding of selected nails, usually the great toenails (e.g. in roller-skating shoes) (*Fig.* N.14).

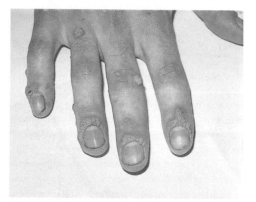

Fig. N.12. Periungual warts. (*Dr Richard Staughton.*)

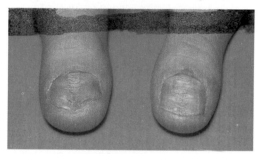

Fig. N.13. Traumatic nail dystrophy due to habit tic. (*Westminster Hospital.*)

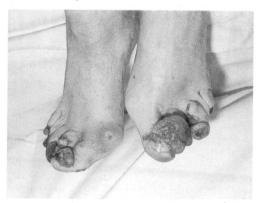

Fig. N.14. Onychogryphosis. (*Dr Alistair Carruthers.*)

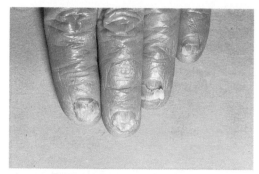

Fig. N.15. Nail dystrophy due to impaired peripheral circulation. (*Westminster Hospital.*)

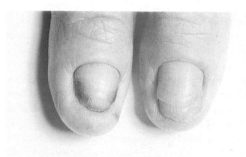

Fig. N.16. Yellow nail syndrome. (*Westminster Hospital.*)

Impaired peripheral circulation is also responsible for numerous cases of nail dystrophy. The most characteristic follows Raynaud's phenomenon of many years' duration and consists of thin nails, ridged longitudinally and in places showing partial onycholysis. There are variations in colour on the nail surfaces, some areas being redder than normal and others paler. The thin ridged nail is brittle and is therefore usually kept cut short by the patient (*Fig.* N.15).

In the *yellow nail syndrome* all nails take on a pale yellow or greenish-yellow colour (*Fig.* N.16). The nails grow very slowly. The cuticles are deficient and the nail plate is overcurved in its long axis. The nails may come loose from their beds and be shed but are slowly replaced. The condition is often accompanied by lymphoedema and various pulmonary abnormalities may be present including chronic bronchitis, bronchiectasis or pleural effusion.

Haemorrhages below the nail are common. They may be the result of trauma or disease and may be petechial (splinter) or more extensive. Haemorrhages are common in fungus infections of the nail plate, psoriasis and dermatitis. Splinter haemorrhages are terminal arterial emboli in the nailbed and consist of a homogeneous mass of blood embedded in a layer of squamous cells adherent to the undersurface of the nailbed. They occur in infective endocarditis, a few cases of uninfected mitral stenosis, septicaemia, and rarely in peptic ulcer, hypertension and malignant neoplasm. They may, however, occur with jarring trauma as in hockey players, and at times for no apparent cause in healthy persons.

Peter D. Samman

Napkin (perineal) eruptions

Napkin dermatitis, at least in transient form, occurs in all babies at some stage. It is usually responsive to emollients and home remedies. Most examples are caused by irritation of the skin due to prolonged contact with urine or faeces and are favoured by infrequent nappy changes, particularly when occlusive plastic pants are worn. The convexities are affected by shiny red plaques, sometimes eroded, which spare the flexural creases. If the flexures are the main site of inflammation secondary *candidiasis* should be suspected and a search made at the edge for typical 'satellite pustulation'. *Infantile seborrhoeic dermatitis* is an acute self-limiting red scaly eruption in which the napkin area is usually severely affected. The condition begins with cradle cap and spreads to the face, chest, back and limb flexures as well as the napkin area. Despite the widespread eruption, infants show little sign of discomfort. This is in marked contrast to those infants with *atopic dermatitis*, who may also have a napkin eruption, but who are distressed by itch and sleep poorly.

Irritable children with erosions and papules around their napkin areas should be carefully examined for *scabies* (*Fig.* N.17)—other common sites for burrows are anterior axillary folds, wrists, finger webs, ankles, palms and soles. Nursing mothers may have burrows around their nipples as well as the usual sites. *Molluscum contagiosum* causes persistent irritating papules around the ano-genital area in both children and adults. Patients are frequently atopic and individual lesions may heal spontaneously, sometimes with considerable purulent reaction or a stark halo of eczema.

Earlier editions of this book dwelt on the details of the nappy rash seen as a manifestation of *congenital syphilis*. The new epidemic raging in American cities, especially New York, may herald outbreaks elsewhere. Affected infants are irritable, feed poorly and have a purulent nasal discharge. Peri-anal and peri-oral erosions and rhagades are prominent and highly infectious. At 2 months of age the napkin area as well as palms and soles may be affected by a new pinkish rash resembling the rash of secondary syphilis in adults.

In the extremely rare *acro-dermatitis enteropathica* zinc absorption is deficient. Affected infants have diarrhoea and characteristic peri-orificial erosions, which may spread on to the limbs, sometimes in a livedoid pattern. Similar lesions can occur in zinc-deficient premature babies. If a napkin eruption becomes purpuric, *Letterer–Siwe disease* (histiocytosis) should be suspected. Other flexures, the gums and external auditory meatuses should be inspected for lesions.

White patches in the perineum can be due to *vitiligo* which may begin in childhood and has a predilection for genital skin.

Lichen sclerosus of the vulva (white spot disease) is rare in infancy, but young children are affected. The physical signs of a porcelain-white, scarred, purpuric vulva may lead to suspicions of molestation.

Hyperpigmentation is most commonly due to the *Mongolian spot*, a reliable marker of Negroid or Asiatic parentage, which causes considerable and

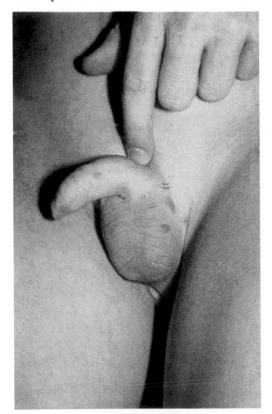

Fig. N.17. Scabies. (Dr A. Carruthers.)

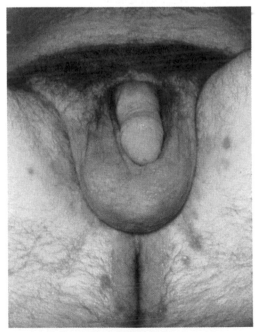

Fig. N.18. Flexural psoriasis. (Dr Richard Staughton.)

extensive bluish pigmentation of the sacral napkin area and is due to dermal dendritic pigment cells.

In *adults* the perineum may be involved in numerous dermatoses with scaly eruptions, e.g. tinea (*see Fig.* S.9), erythrasma, candidiasis or psoriasis (*Fig.* N.18). The area can be infested in *pediculosis pubis*, as well as scabies. *Molluscum contagiosum* can cause irritating papular lesions. Venereal warts are increasing in frequency and can be a marker of other sexually transmitted infections or cervical intraepithelial neoplasia in women. *Syphilitic chancre* occurs more commonly within the anal canal or vagina, but rarely syphilitic *condyloma acuminata* may be seen on the perineum. In *pruritus ani* lichenification from scratching and rubbing will be seen. There may be a complicating contact dermatitis due to one of the topical remedies employed (e.g local anaesthetics, local antibiotics or lanolin).

R. Staughton
G. S. Clayden

Nasal deformity

Nasal deformity can be congenital, acquired or developmental. The skeleton of the nose consists of bone in the upper third and cartilage in the lower two thirds. The septal cartilage should articulate with the columellar cartilages which form the division between the nostrils.

Congenital abnormalities of the nose are rare. Arhinia (absence of the nose) is almost unknown and a bifid nose is rarely seen (*Fig.* N.19). The more usual type of congenital nasal abnormality is the bony cartilaginous hump. Many regard this as a sign of distinction but others dislike it and want it corrected by cosmetic rhinoplasty (*Fig.* N.20). The commonest acquired nasal deformity is the fractured nose. Severe trauma fractures the nasal bones and this presents as an obvious deformity, accompanied by epistaxis and bruising of the eyes (*Fig.* N.21). It is easily seen on X-ray, although X-rays are unreliable in the primary diagnosis of a fractured nasal bone because of the multiple vascular markings in normal nasal bones.

The nose is the most prominent part of the face in the Caucasian and is frequently struck during falls in childhood. While the septal cartilage can be fractured by a severe blow, a commoner clinical situation is for a green-stick fracture to occur in childhood. During growth spurts, the nose then apparently grows squint. The patient may either present with a squint nose or nasal obstruction due to internal derangement of the septal cartilage.

Severe trauma to the nose, or a septal excision operation carried out with excessive zeal, can cause a saddle nose (*Fig.* N.22). This does not usually cause nasal obstruction and is corrected by inserting a bone

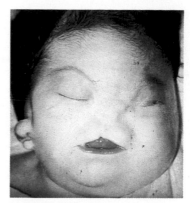

Fig. N.19. Arhinia—This child had multiple craniofacial and other abnormalities and has since died.

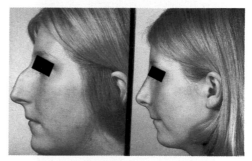

Fig. N.20. Bony cartilaginous hump. Congenital bony cartilaginous hump (a). Corrected by rhinoplasty (b).

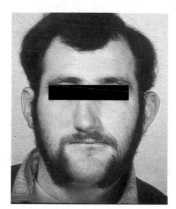

Fig. N.21. Fractured nasal bones.

graft into the nasal dorsum. A saddle nose can also be caused by congenital syphilis, but this is almost unknown now. The most usual cause of a saddle nose in conjunction with a systemic illness is polychrondritis or a nasal granuloma such as Wegener's granulomatosis.

The skin of the nasal tip is normally thicker than the skin of the nasal dorsum due to an increased volume of sebaceous tissue. A relatively common development abnormality of this part of the nose is for the sebaceous tissue to hypertrophy with age, producing an ugly

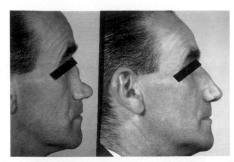

Fig. N.22. Saddle nose—The cause of this was an SMR operation for a septal haematoma (*a*). Corrected by the insertion of a bone graft (*b*).

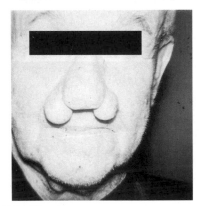

Fig. N.23. Rhinophyma.

deformity of the tip of the nose known as rhinophyma (*Fig*. N.23).

A. G. D. Maran

Nasal discharge

The causes of nasal discharge are listed in (*Table* N.1.)

Congenital. Choanal atresia by blocking the posterior choana prevents the normal nasal mucus stream from reaching the pharynx, so that anterior nasal discharge is the result. Infections ensure that the discharge is mucopurulent at times.

Infective. The common cold and the prodromal stages of the infectious fevers give rise to clear mucoid discharge. When and if secondary bacterial infection follows the discharge becomes increasingly purulent. Purulent discharge, either unilateral or bilateral, occurs in sinusitis, the origin of the discharge indicating the sinus or sinuses involved. The maxillary sinuses open into the middle meatus, so pus is seen there and on the floor of the nose. Pus from the anterior ethmoids is also found in the middle meatus but that from the posterior ethmoids or sphenoid comes down the postnasal space. If the pus is especially foul smelling it has probably arisen in the maxillary antrum as a result of dental infection. Caseous sinusitis or rhinitis

Table N.1. Conditions causing nasal discharge

Congenital
Choanal atresia

Infective
Acute rhinitis
Sinusitis
Enlarged adenoids
Caseous rhinitis
Atrophic rhinitis
Fungus infections
Chronic infective granulomas
  Syphilis
  Tuberculosis
  Leprosy
Rhinoscleroma

Trauma
Foreign body
Rhinolith
Inhaled irritant gases or vapours
Fractured anterior fossa
Excessive cold

Hypersensitivity
Vasomotor rhinitis
Perennial nasal allergy
Seasonal nasal allergy (pollinosis)
Nasal polyps

Neoplastic
Carcinoma
  Nasal fossa
  Nasopharynx
  Sinus
Malignant granuloma
Wegener's granuloma

Old age
Senile rhinorrhoea

follows inspissation of pus and possibly fungus infection. The material is whitish, cheesy and foul smelling. Even more foul smelling are the crusts and dry discharge of atrophic rhinitis. In these patients the nasal fossae are unduly wide and the mucosa thin and devoid of mucus cells. The especially disgusting odour is called 'ozaena'.

Pathogenic fungi and yeasts cause nasal infection and discharge, mainly in tropical countries but, of course, nowadays occasionally in this country in immigrants and returning travellers.

To summarize the nasal symptoms of the main fungal diseases: *Rhinosporidiosis* predominantly affects the nasal mucosa where the characteristic lesion is a bleeding polyp containing the sporangium from which spores spread via the lymphatics. It chiefly affects the peoples of Sri Lanka or India. Phycomycoses cause serious disease often starting with granulomatous lesions in the nose and considerable mucoid discharge. This fungus occurs in tropical areas.

Aspergillus infection, sometimes contracted from captive birds, is characterized by a watery mouldy smelling discharge and a greyish membrane on the mucosa.

Actinomycosis, showing the typical 'sulphur granules', rarely but sometimes affects the sinuses and nose. There is a woody mass and multiple sinuses from which the pus exudes.

Candida albicans occurs commonly in the mouth and occasionally in the nose in the young and those in a poor state of general health. The white patches can be removed without bleeding.

The pathology of fungus diseases is complex. Many start with nasal discharge and bleeding. Diagnosis is by identifying the fungus in scrapings or by biopsy.

Secondary syphilis affects the nose, causing a simple catarrhal rhinitis; the diagnosis is usually suggested by other lesions. *Tertiary syphilitic gummas* affect the nose very commonly with destruction of bone and cartilage; secondary infection causes offensive discharge and there is bleeding and often the later development of atrophic rhinitis.

Lupus vulgaris is probably the commonest tuberculous infection of the nose. There is nasal discharge and the typical lesion, a reddish firm nodule, is found at the anterior end of the nasal septum which may later perforate.

Leprosy occurs in the nose as almost the earliest sign of the disease. Nodular thickening of the mucosa with inflammation and obstruction are associated with discharge. Later perforation of the septum and destruction of tissue allows for secondary infection and very offensive discharge.

Rhinoscleroma is a progressive granuloma beginning in the nose in an atrophic form with ozaena. Nodules later form and there is considerable scarring. Diagnosis is by biopsy and by the identification of the Frisch bacillus and Russell bodies.

AIDS is associated with a watery nasal discharge which is frequently found concomitantly in the disease.

Trauma. A unilateral nasal discharge in an infant or child is pathognomonic of a foreign body, often a piece of foam rubber or paper inserted into the nasal fossa. Small hard objects may remain in the nose for some time before symptoms occur. A rhinolith may develop in these circumstances if calcium salts are deposited around the foreign body.

A clear watery discharge following a head injury must lead to thoughts of a fracture of the anterior fossa or cribriform plate. Such a discharge will increase on leaning the head forward or on compression of the jugular veins. The presence of sugar in this fluid confirms that it is cerebrospinal fluid. This can be confirmed by isotope tests.

Hypersensitivity. Copious clear mucoid nasal discharge almost as freely flowing as water is present in nasal allergy and may be associated with violent attacks of sneezing, lacrimation and conjunctival injection. The diagnosis is confirmed by the history and by RAST and PRIST tests. Nasal allergy is liable to be confused with less non-specific vasomotor rhinitis, which is also very common. Numerous factors are present in the aetiology of this troublesome condition and these include changes of environmental temperature and humidity, mechanical irritation from dusts and vapours, psychological factors, pregnancy and drug reactions. The patient with vasomotor instability not infrequently carries a box of paper tissues. The diagnosis is made after excluding nasal allergy.

Neoplastic. Malignant nasal disease may cause nasal discharge, sometimes relatively clear to start with but later almost always offensive and thick. The presence of blood must always raise the question of malignancy. The growth may be in the nasal fossa, sinus or in the nasopharynx. Nasal discharge stained with blood occurs and when one of the sinus ostia becomes blocked infection follows. If an undue amount of blood is found in a sinus undergoing lavage when there has been no undue trauma the sinus must be carefully investigated for a growth. Diagnosis is by a CT scan and biopsy.

Malignant or non-healing granuloma, sometimes called 'midline granuloma', is a slowly progressing ulceration of the face starting in the region of the nose. The chronic inflammatory reaction naturally produces discharge. They may represent a special form of malignant lymphoma and must be differentiated from Wegener's granuloma by their clinical and histological characteristics.

Wegener's granuloma affects kidneys, lungs and respiratory tract including the nose. The lesions are giant-celled granulomas and there is never the gross destruction seen in malignant granuloma.

Old Age. Senile rhinorrhoea, due probably to the failure of the vasomotor control of the mucosa, is common and sometimes distressing in the elderly. There are no physical signs apart from the nasal drip.

Although nasal discharge may be of various different characters, the cause can usually be arrived at by the history and simple clinical examination. Three clinical situations, however, require special management.

A unilateral, blood-stained discharge might be the prodromal bleed of an epistaxis but the possibility of a tumour or granuloma of the nose or sinuses must be ruled out by nasal endoscopy and flexible endoscopy of the nasopharynx.

A clear nasal discharge after trauma is cerebrospinal fluid rhinorrhoea until proved otherwise. Although assessment of sugar content of the discharge with a clinistix is a useful indicator, a definitive diagnosis cannot be made without assessment by CT scan and injection of fluorescein or radioactive albumin to the CSF with subsequent measurement in the nose.

A. G. D. Maran

Nasal obstruction

All the conditions mentioned in the section on nasal discharge are likely to cause nasal obstruction owing to the associated inflammation and oedema of the mucous membrane. There are, however, some disorders which simply cause a blockage of one or both nasal passages and are less commonly associated with discharge.

These can be listed (*see below*) and should be read in conjunction with the list of the causes of nasal discharge.

CONGENITAL
Choanal atresia
  Bilateral
  Unilateral
Deviated nasal septum
INFLAMMATORY
Adenoids
Trauma
Haematoma of septum
Deviated nasal septum
HYPERSENSITIVITY
Vasomotor rhinitis
Atopic rhinitis
Rhinitis medicamentosa
NEOPLASTIC
Benign tumours
  Papilloma
  Fibroma
  Osteoma
  Fibroangioma of puberty
  Teratoma
  Nasal polyps
Malignant tumours
  Nasopharyngeal carcinoma
  Squamous carcinoma of the nose and sinuses
  Adenocarcinoma of the nose and sinuses
  Malignant melanoma of the nose and sinuses
  Transitional cell carcinoma of the nose and sinuses

Choanal atresia (*Fig.* N.24), when bilateral, causes complete nasal obstruction at birth and must be relieved at once if the infant is to live. Unilateral choanal atresia is sometimes not discovered until later. Soft rubber or plastic catheters are often employed to assess the patency of the nasal fossae. Malleable silver probes bent into a smooth curve with a radius of about 5 cm are preferable and can be passed painlessly along the floor of the nose. They do not kink and curl up like the thin soft catheters and by palpation it is possible to say if the blockage is fibrous or bony in nature.

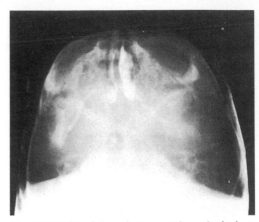

Fig. N.24. Bilateral choanal atresia. Radiograph of infant's skull with radio-opaque dye outlining the nasal fossae. The dye is held up by the membranous obstruction to the posterior choanae.

Many deviated nasal septa originate at the time of birth when the infant's skull is compressed as it passes through the birth canal. The components of the bony septum are forced out of alignment and, during the development of the nose and upper jaw until about 18 years of age, the septum gradually deviates. The angles of maximum deviation are along the cartilage/vomer and ethmoid/vomer junctions and at the lower border of the vomer where it meets the maxillary and palatine crests.

This deviation can be seen with a nasal endoscope. It will often be found that the inferior turbinate in the concavity of the deviation will have hypertrophied thus increasing the obstruction. It is important to remember that the spur of the deflected septum may obscure other pathology behind.

Adenoid enlargement is probably the commonest cause of nasal obstruction in childhood. These lymphoid masses usually regress at about 8–10 years of age but may cause nearly complete obstruction in the young. It is sometimes possible to see them with a postnasal mirror in co-operative children. If there is doubt as to the size of adenoids a soft-tissue lateral radiograph is helpful (*Fig.* N.25).

Trauma frequently causes nasal obstruction without discharge. Immediate mucosal swelling and depressed nasal bones after a blow may cause very considerable blockage. A haematoma of the septum is characteristic as there is a swelling, soft to gentle palpation, on each side. This may resolve spontaneously but the pressure may cause cartilage necrosis and later a collapsed septum or infection may supervene with a septal abscess and an increased likelihood of cartilage necrosis. Though not dissimilar in appearance the abscess is more tense and the nose is very tender. Both must be evacuated. The deviated nasal septum following trauma is more likely to show a corrugated

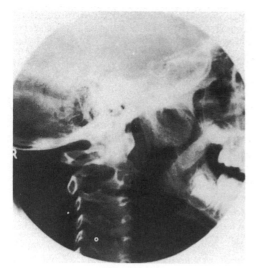

Fig. N.25. Enlarged adenoids. (*Dr Lorna Davison.*)

appearance as the component parts of the septal skeleton may overlap and the fibrosis after fracture may lead to considerable anatomical abnormality and difficulty in corrective surgery.

Vasomotor rhinitis has been mentioned in the section dealing with nasal discharge, but it commonly occurs without discharge, causing nasal obstruction. Not infrequently patients notice that at one time one nasal passage is more obstructed and within hours the problem is worse on the other side. This alternating obstruction is merely an exaggeration of the normal nasal cycle which passes unnoticed in those with clear noses but becomes obvious in the partially obstructed. On examination, the inferior turbinates may be enormous and in chronic cases show a 'mulberry' appearance.

Rhinitis medicamentosa may be the cause of very acute nasal obstruction. The nasal mucosa is very red, swollen and the turbinates rather firm to palpation. The condition is caused by rebound vasodilatation following the too-frequent use of constrictor drops which have to be used more and more often to obtain relief. There is often some psychological instability in these patients.

Atopic rhinitis is seasonal if associated with a grass allergy (hay fever) or episodic if associated with other contact allergens (cats, dogs, etc.). The release of histamine and other related substances from the degranulated mast cells cause mucosal oedema, vasodilatation and hypersecretion. The patient will always be aware of the cause and conversely, if he is not, the diagnosis is probably not atopic rhinitis; it is more likely to be vasomotor rhinitis.

Benign nasal tumours are not common but cause nasal obstruction and can nearly always be seen on nasal examination in the outpatients. Papillomas may arise on Little's area at the anterior end of the nasal septum. They are typically wart-like in appearance and bleed easily. Fibromas and osteomas are rare. The bleeding nasal fibroma, almost confined to adolescent boys, is a fibroangioma and usually arises from the roof of the nasopharynx. Torrential haemorrhage may occur if the surface is breached. Benign teratomas of the nasopharynx occur. The simplest is the 'hairy nasal polyp' which is usually a pedunculated dermoid. It can be seen hanging below the level of the soft palate or in the postnasal space. Other dermoids and teratomas are more complex and usually associated with extensive deformities of the head.

Nasal polyps are very common and are of unknown aetiology. They are not due to atopy as was formerly thought. They are known to be associated with aspirin sensitivity and over 50 per cent of patients have associated asthma. They are probably the result of an abnormality of arachidonic acid metabolism with either an excess of leukotrienes or a deficiency of prostaglandins. They must be removed surgically and their recurrence rate is significantly lowered by the continual use of steroid nose drops.

Malignant tumours of the nose, as opposed to the sinuses, are rare. Tumours nearly always begin in the ethmoid or maxillary sinuses and it is only when the tumour exists from the sinus 'box' that the patient gets symptoms which may be related to the eye, the cheek, the palate and alveoli or the nasal cavity, depending on where the tumour comes out of the box.

A. G. D. Maran

Nasal regurgitation

Regurgitation of food through the nose may be only a temporary accident, the result of an unsuccessful attempt to stave off a sneeze, a cough or a burst of laughter when the mouth is full of food or fluid; or it may result from an explosive return of gas from the stomach or oesophagus, particularly after drinking gassy fluids. Pathological regurgitation of food through the nose results from three main groups of causes:

PERFORATIONS OF THE PALATE
Congenital
   Cleft palate
   Congenital short soft palate
Trauma
   Oro-antral fistula after dental extraction
   Palatal fenestration following surgery for
   malignancy of maxillary antrum
   Gunshot wounds
Inflammatory
   Destruction or perforation of palate due to
   syphilis, tuberculosis or leprosy
Malignant disease

FIXATION OF THE PALATE

PARALYSIS OF THE PALATE

Postdiphtheritic paralysis
Damage to the nucleus of the 10th nerve
  Postero-inferior cerebellar artery thrombosis
  Tumours of the medulla
  Bulbar palsy
  Poliomyelitis
  Landry's ascending paralysis
Posterior fossa lesions
  Tumours
  Syphilitic meningitis
  Glomus jugulare tumour
  Hydrocephalus
Extracranial lesions
  Malignant disease
  Posttonsillectomy weakness

Examination of the roof of the mouth and the soft palate should be sufficient to determine the causes of regurgitation in the first group. Congenital short soft palate may be suspected but is less easy to assess without cine-radiography to demonstrate palatal competence. An oral-antral fistula (usually postsurgical) is revealed by direct inspection. In these cases usually only a small amount of food or, more usually, liquid comes through the nose.

Fixation of the palate may occur from the scarring of syphilis, lupus or leprosy (now all uncommon in the Western world), scarring after extensive palate surgery in severe cleft-palate cases and, rarely, palatal scarring after badly performed tonsillectomy. These fix the palate so that it cannot be drawn up to close the nasopharynx.

In the majority of the third group other symptoms and signs will be present with 10th nerve paralyses of the larynx and paralysis of the 5th nerve and other nerves depending on the extent of the lesion. Diphtheritic paralysis may involve the soft palate alone and usually recovers in time.

Malignant disease of the nasopharynx is characteristically silent and insidious—palatal palsy (sometimes part of 'Trotter's triad' of deafness, trigeminal pain and palatal palsy) may be an early sign and is due to local infiltration rather than to involvement of the nerve-trunks.

Paralysis of the palate, when bilateral, may be difficult to notice at rest but it remains immobile on phonation and is even more obvious if the patient is made to gag. In addition the patient is unable to blow up a balloon. When the paralysis is unilateral the normal side is drawn up like a curtain and the uvula is displaced to the normal side.

Harold Ellis

Nausea

Nausea is the unpleasant sensation experienced by patients who are usually about to vomit. The causes of nausea are therefore very similar to that of vomiting and are listed on p. 711. Nausea is characterized by an unpleasant, 'sick' feeling with a revulsion for food and abdominal fullness. The patient feels that he is about to vomit but does not actually do so. Other sensations or phenomena which accompany nausea are a desire to swallow, a certain amount of sweating, hypersalivation and lightheadedness.

When the patient is nauseated there is an associated decrease in gastric tone and an inhibition of gastric peristalsis with increased duodenal tone. Nausea may result from unpleasant or frightening emotional experiences, from a variety of psychological causes, from stimuli arising from intra-abdominal viscera or a variety of visual, oral, olfactory or tactile sensations which are unpleasant, and from stimulation of the labyrinths.

Although nausea is intimately bound with the act of vomiting, there are certain circumstances when nausea is more prominent than the vomiting. This occurs, for example, with certain *drugs* such as salicylates, digoxin, non-steroidal anti-inflammatory agents, opiates, oral contraceptive pill, some antibiotics and many of the cancer chemotherapeutic agents. Nausea may be a prominent feature of *motion sickness*. Early morning nausea is a feature of *pregnancy*, *anxiety states* and *alcoholism*. Nausea may have *psychogenic* origins and this is seen, for example, in people who are averse to certain foods and feel nauseated on sitting at table, the nausea which occurs in certain stressful situations many of them of a domestic or social reason. Patients with *migraine* may suffer intense nausea and not necessarily vomit. Intense nausea is one of the earliest features of *viral hepatitis* and precedes other features of the disease such as abdominal pain and the development of icterus. Patients in severe *right-sided heart failure* with hepatic congestion will also complain of nausea.

Ian A. D. Bouchier

Neck, engorged veins in

For practical purposes, the jugular venous pressure may be regarded as raised if jugular pulsation is visible, or the internal jugular vein is seen to be distended, with the patient sitting erect. This is more reproducible than the older criterion of 4 cm above the sternal angle with the patient lying at 45 degrees, and a grossly elevated venous pressure is less likely to be missed. The first major distinction is between *non-pulsatile* and *pulsatile* elevation of the venous pressure.

Non-pulsatile elevation of the jugular venous pressure

This is due to obstruction of the jugular or brachio-cephalic vein, or, most commonly, of the superior vena cava. Causes of this are listed below:

Common

Thrombosis following pacemaker implantation
Bronchial neoplasm
Mediastinal tumour, e.g. lymphoma, thymoma

Less common

Fibrosing mediastinitis
Right atrial or pericardial tumours
Late complication of Mustard's operation for transposition of the great arteries

The diagnosis of venous obstruction can be confirmed by venography; the cause of the obstruction may be more difficult to diagnose, and needs careful study of the chest radiograph supplemented by tomography and, perhaps, CT scanning.

Pulsatile elevation of the jugular venous pressure

This is much more common. Causes include:

Common

Congestive cardiac failure
Over-transfusion
Cor pulmonale/right heart failure
Tricuspid regurgitation

Less common

Pericardial effusion
Massive pulmonary embolism
Constrictive pericarditis
Tricuspid stenosis

Rare

Restrictive cardiomyopathy
Carcinoid syndrome
Right atrial tumours

Analysis of the venous waveform helps to identify the cause of the elevation (*Table* N.2.). A 'normal' jugular pulse has three 'humps' (the a,c and v waves) and two 'dips' (x and y descents). The a wave is transmitted atrial systole, the c wave occurs early in systole as the tricuspid valve closes and braces back towards the atrium, and the v wave is produced by the filling of the atrium from the venae cavae followed by the emptying of the atrium after tricuspid valve opening (*Fig.* N.26). The relation of this pattern to those found in disease is not always straightforward. Where an increased load on the right heart develops gradually, as in pulmonary stenosis or some forms of pulmonary hypertension, the right atrium has time to hypertrophy and there may be a *prominent a wave*. If the tricuspid valve becomes incompetent, the jugular

pulse shows a systolic pulsation in time with the arterial pulse. This is traditionally called a v wave, though its timing and cause are both different from the 'normal' v wave. The v waves of tricuspid regurgitation are often striking in appearance and readily palpable.

Cannon waves are also prominent systolic waves appearing in the venous pulse, but these are due to

Table N.2.   Abnormalities of the jugular venous pulse

Cause	Most prominent feature
Congestive failure	Raised mean pressure with early diastolic descent
Tricuspid regurgitation	Systolic v waves
Right atrial hypertrophy	Presystolic a waves
Complete heart block, ventricular tachycardia, pacemaker, etc.	Cannon waves (sporadic or regular sharp v waves)
Constrictive pericarditis	Very high pressure, sharp early diastolic descent
Tricuspid stenosis	High pressure, slow diastolic descent

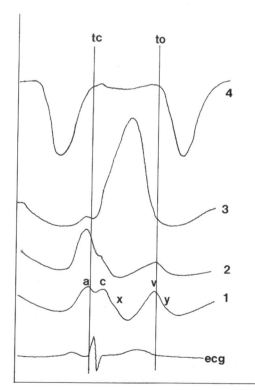

Fig. N.26. Diagram to show the relationship of different jugular waveforms to the cardiac cycle. ecg = electrocardiogram; tc = tricuspid valve closes; to = tricuspid valve opens. 1, Normal trace to show a,c,v waves and x and y descents. 2, Exaggerated a wave due to right atrial hypertrophy. 3, Tricuspid regurgitation wave (note different timing from normal v wave). 4, Prominent y descent in severe cardiac failure, pericardial effusion or constrictive pericarditis.

contraction of the atrium against a closed tricuspid valve. Classical cannon waves are seen in patients with complete heart block and atrioventricular dissociation when the atria and ventricles contract at their own independent frequencies; when atrial and ventricular contraction coincide, cannon waves are seen as striking, sharp pulsations in the jugular pulse. Cannon waves may also occur in patients in junctional rhythm and in those with a permanent ventricular pacemaker who have preserved retrograde atrioventricular conduction; in such cases retrograde atrial activation and cannon waves may occur in a series of consecutive beats. The murmur of tricuspid regurgitation is, of course, absent.

When the mean jugular venous pressure is considerably raised, the sudden fall in pressure (and consequent collapse of the vein) as the tricuspid valve opens at the beginning of ventricular diastole (y descent) is usually the most prominent feature of the venous pulse. In patients with *tricuspid stenosis* this fall in pressure occurs more slowly as the right ventricle fills via the stenotic valve. In patients with *constrictive pericarditis* the y descent is usually prominent, but a proportion of patients show a more pronounced dip in early systole (x descent), possibly because ventricular contraction causes a transiently negative intrapericardial pressure. This may also be seen in *pericardial tamponade*, although many cases simply show a prominent y descent. Patients with constrictive pericarditis or pericardial tamponade may also show a paradoxical elevation of venous pressure on inspiration (Kussmaul's sign). The probable mechanism is compression of an engorged liver in a patient unable to increase the right ventricular stroke volume.

D. De Bono

Neck, stiff

The important causes of stiff neck may be classified as follows:

Congenital

Congenital torticollis or wryneck
Congenital deformities, e.g. Klippel–Feil

Acquired

ACUTE

Exposure to cold
Positional
Intracerebral and subarachnoid haemorrhage
Cerebral tumour

Infective

Reflex spasm due to adenitis from otitis media, tonsillitis, etc.
Abscess in the neck

Traumatic

Fractures of cervical spine
Dislocations of cervical spine
Subluxations of cervical spine
Strains of cervical spine
Injuries to muscles and soft tissue

Degenerative

Acute painful episode in cervical spondylosis

Malignant

Multiple myeloma
Primary or metastatic neoplasm

Acute systemic infections

Meningitis
Typhus
Brain abscess
Poliomyelitis
Psittacosis
Arbovirus infections (e.g. sandfly fever)
Leptospirosis
Tetanus, etc.

Hysteria

CHRONIC

Degenerative

Cervical spondylosis

Arthritic

Chronic juvenile arthritis (Still's disease)
Rheumatoid arthritis
Ankylosing spondylitis
Other spondylarthropathies

Infective

Tuberculous disease of the spine

Post-traumatic

Untreated acute traumatic lesions
Contractures following burns, nerve injuries, etc.

Congenital

With the exception of congenital lesions, contractures and possibly some late cases of untreated injury and a few cases of arthritis, all these conditions are usually painful at some stage.

Congenital torticollis or wryneck is due to a contraction of the sternomastoid muscle on one side, generally considered to be the result of an injury during labour, possibly ischaemic in nature. The muscle stands out as a tight band in the neck, and its contraction leads to a characteristic deformity. The head is pulled down towards the affected side, and the face and chin are tilted towards the opposite shoulder. (*see Fig. S.39*). The movements of the head are necessarily restricted owing to the shortening of the muscle, and in long-standing cases this leads to a marked asymmetry of the face. The consequences are not limited to the head and neck, for the spine shares in the general obliquity, and shows marked lateral curvature in old cases.

In the klippel–feil syndrome there is a congenital fusion of one or more cervical vertebrae resulting in a short, thick stiff neck, the head set low on the shoulders. Other coexisting abnormalities are common: undescended scapulae (Sprengel's deformity), platybasia, etc.

Acquired

Exposure to cold or sleeping in a cramped position may give rise to a transient stiff neck associated with no other symptoms. There is generally a distinct history of the patient waking up in the morning with a stiff neck, and the diagnosis is made by exclusion.

A cold draught on the neck when driving in a car or from air-conditioning may result in an acutely painful stiff neck for a short time.

Cerebral or subarachnoid haemorrhage. Conscious patients who have had intracranial bleeding usually complain of headache and stiffness of the neck, and after subarachnoid haemorrhage the main physical sign is marked neck rigidity and pain on trying to move the head. A brain tumour may cause a stiff neck by causing meningeal irritation from bleeding into the subarachnoid space, by direct meningeal involvement or by causing cerebellar herniation through the foramen magnum.

Inflammation of the lymph nodes and the cellular tissues of the neck may cause local stiffness, whether the infecting focus be a boil or carbuncle, or a carious tooth, an inflamed tonsil, pediculosis capitis, or other similar cause. In a mild case the neck can be moved, but movement is painful and therefore it is held stiffly. With a more severe reaction reflex muscle spasm is present.

Injuries to the neck. These vary from soft-tissue injuries and strains to fractures and dislocations. Although some are rapidly fatal, subluxation may occur without cord involvement, the only symptoms being stiffness and pain. Readily missed cases and permanent disability may result if the condition is not diagnosed and treated. The deformity is rendered more obvious when the spine is X-rayed in the flexed position, and may be missed in extension.

New growth in one of the cervical vertebrae may cause progressive stiff neck, and generally much local pain on movement; the diagnosis may suggest itself when the patient is known to have had a primary neoplasm elsewhere, especially a carcinoma of the breast, lung, prostate, kidney or the thyroid gland; cases of primary new growth of the vertebra (apart from multiple myeloma deposits), are fortunately rare.

Acute systemic infections. Many acute infections are accompanied by a stiff neck (meningism), particularly in children; pneumonia, once a common cause in childhood, is now much less so. Fever is almost always present. Meningitis from any cause, bacterial or viral, almost always causes some neck rigidity. Neck stiffness may be an early prodromal sign in paralytic or non paralytic poliomyelitis and changes in the cerebrospinal fluid are found. Phlebotomus (sandfly) fever, an arbovirus infection, presents as fever, malaise, myalgia and sometimes headache, in some cases with findings of an aseptic meningitis. Stiffness of the neck may be an early sign of tetanus, but other signs, such as trismus (inability to open the mouth due to tonic contraction of the jaw muscles) rapidly appear (*see* p. 679).

In hysteria. A theatrical and over-dramatic symptom of neck stiffness is accompanied by other features of hysteria but not by any objective physical signs of organic disease.

Chronic

Degenerative. The commonest cause of stiffness of the neck is degenerative disease of bone, joint and cartilage, i.e. cervical spondylosis. This is a common disorder of the group of patients over 60 years of age. Pains are commonly referred from the painful stiff neck into the occiput and out towards the shoulders.

As few radiographs of the neck are normal in this age-group care should be taken in relating radiological findings to symptoms.

Arthritis. Stiffness of the neck is less common in rheumatoid arthritis of adult life than in chronic juvenile arthritis (Still's disease). It is more common, however, in cases of ankylosing spondylitis, where the neck and head may be held in a completely fixed position (*Figs.* N.27, N.28). A similar picture may more rarely be seen in the spondylarthritic varieties of psoriatic arthropathy, Reiter's disease and the arthropathy associated with ulcerative colitis and Crohn's disease.

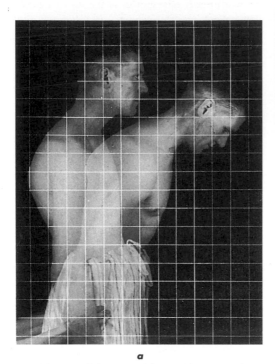

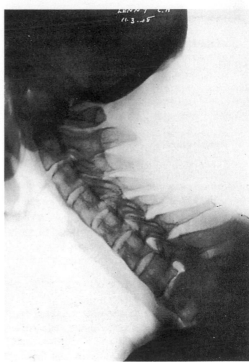

a

b

Fig. N.27. a. Ankylosing spondylitis. Double-exposure showing neck in full flexion and extension. b. Radiograph of same patient showing typical anterior ligamentous calcification.

Atlanto-axial subluxation in rheumatoid arthritis is not uncommon in advanced cases and leads to stiffness of the neck and a characteristic posture (*Fig.* N.29).

Such subluxation occurs, but less often, in ankylosing spondylitis.

Cervical caries (*Fig.* N.30). The greatest care must be taken not to overlook tuberculous disease of the cervical vertebrae as a cause of reflex muscular rigidity of the neck. Pain and rigidity are among the earliest signs; the pain is increased by the least movement, and the child—for it is generally a child that is affected—takes the greatest precaution to avoid any movement, even holding the head between the two hands. The position of the head varies; it is most often held very stiff and straight, the natural backward curve of the neck being lost. In the late stages there may be an angular or lateral curve.

Post-traumatic. A neck may remain stiff from previous injuries. The diagnosis will be given by the history, but nervous overtones may cause persistence of symptoms, particularly in medico-legal cases where compensation is involved.

Harold Ellis

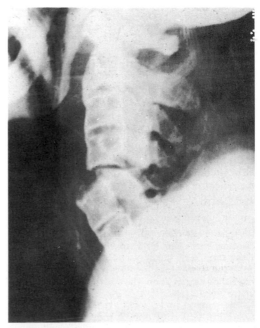

Fig. N.28. A broken neck in ankylosing spondylitis. Such rigid necks are more prone to such traumatic lesions than are normal supple ones. (*Courtesy of the Gordon Photographic Museum, Guy's Hospital.*)

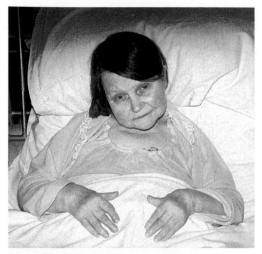

Fig. N.29. Advanced rheumatoid arthritis with atlanto-axial subluxation.

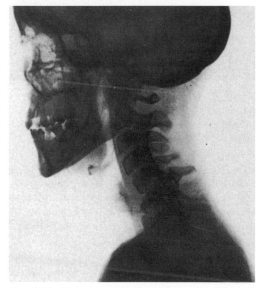

Fig. N.30. Cervical caries showing collapse of bodies of 6th and 7th cervical vertebrae. (Dr T. H. Hills.)

Neck, swelling of

See also THYROID ENLARGEMENT

Anatomy

The neck on either side is divided into anterior and posterior triangles by the sternomastoid muscle arising from the sternum, sternoclavicular junction and medial third of the clavicle below and being inserted into the mastoid process of the temporal bone above. At the upper end of the anterior triangle the digastric muscle defines the lower borders of a subsidiary space known as the 'digastric triangle', and at the lower end of the posterior triangle the posterior belly of the omohyoid

muscle defines the upper border of a subsidiary space known as the 'supraclavicular fossa'.

The sternomastoid muscles are enclosed within the deep cervical fascia which splits to embrace them. If even a part of a mass in the neck overlaps either border of the sternomastoid muscle then, by putting one or other of these muscles into contraction, the relation of the mass to the sternomastoid muscle and so to the deep fascia can readily be determined. This method is applicable to practically all masses in the neck except the majority of those situated in the midline. The right sternomastoid muscle is put into contraction by rotating the head to the left while resistance is applied to the chin and vice versa; both sternomastoids are made to contract when the forehead is pressed forwards against resistance.

Lumps in the neck arising from structures superficial to the deep cervical fascia are not specific to the neck. Thus, sebaceous cysts, lipomas, carbuncles and so on are common, particularly in or deep to the skin at the back of the neck. It is the masses deep to the deep cervical fascia which have particular relevance in regard to the neck and it is the differential diagnosis of these that must be considered.

It is conventional to divide swellings in the neck into midline swellings and lateral swellings, but this is a little misleading as nearly all so-called 'midline swellings' deviate slightly to one side or the other. They can, however, be divided appropriately into masses arising from unpaired midline structures and masses arising from paired lateral structures.

1. Masses arising from unpaired midline structures

A. THYROGLOSSAL CYST

The thyroid gland is developed from an epithelial-lined duct which grows downwards from the region of the foramen caecum of the tongue, passing close in front of and then behind the hyoid bone, and so towards the site of the adult isthmus from which the lateral lobes expand. A cyst may form in any part of this track by failure of obliteration of the duct, but the most common site is at the lower border of the hyoid bone, anterior to the thyrohyoid membrane. These cysts usually appear at about puberty and enlarge to a variable size slightly to one or other side of the midline. They are fluctuant, globular masses which, if superficial, may transilluminate. If the jaw is held open and the tongue steadily protruded, the swelling will rise in the neck demonstrating its attachment to the hyoid bone (*Fig.* N.31). These cysts occasionally become infected and may rupture, leading to a fistula.

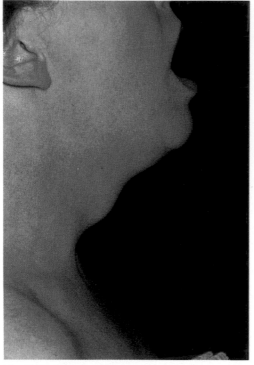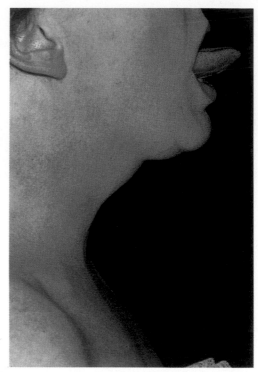

Fig. N.31. Thyroglossal cyst showing elevation on protruding the tongue.

B. SWELLINGS ARISING FROM THE ISTHMUS OF THE THYROID GLAND

All those pathological conditions described on page 662 and giving rise to swellings of the thyroid gland can arise in the isthmus. It should be repeated once more that practically all thyroid swellings move up and down on deglutition owing to their intimate relation to the larynx and upper part of the trachea, the movements of which they following during this act.

C. PHARYNGEAL POUCH (*Fig.* N.32).

At the back of the inferior constrictor muscle of the pharynx there is a triangular area (Killian's dehiscence), between the upper border of the transversely running fibres of the cricopharyngeus below and the lower border of the obliquely running fibres of the thyropharyngeus above, where the wall is deficient in muscle. Through this defect, a pouch of mucosa, covered only by the fascia propria of the pharynx, may protrude. This pouch gradually enlarges, usually towards the left side of the neck, and tends to fill up when food or fluid is swallowed. At first this is just a nuisance and gives rise to an uncomfortable feeling on swallowing together with a rapidly developing swelling which may be emptied by pressing on the mass. Later, the mass becomes sufficiently large to press upon the

oesophagus, against which it lies, to produce severe dysphagia with inanition.

Food is apt to stagnate within the pouch and this leads to diverticulitis which may spread giving rise to pharyngitis or oesophagitis, and so adding to the burden of dysphagia. This condition may appear at any age, but usually arises during the 3rd and 4th decades. Treatment, after attention to the nutritional needs of the patient, is by surgical excision.

D. RARE CASES OF SWELLING ARISING IN MIDLINE STRUCTURES

i. Subhyoid bursa, a cystic swelling arising behind the hyoid bone and indistinguishable clinically from a thyroglossal cyst.

ii. Perichondritis of the thyroid cartilage.

iii. A carcinoma of the larynx, trachea or oesophagus penetrating the walls of these viscera and protruding to one or other side.

iv. The so-called 'Delphic lymph node', which lies in the midline on the thyrohyoid membrane, may enlarge in carcinoma of the thyroid gland and may be the first evidence of this disease.

v. Laryngocele (*Fig.* N.33).

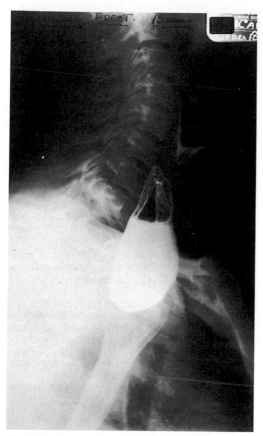

Fig. N.32. Pharyngeal pouch filled with barium. Lateral view.

2. Masses arising from paired lateral structures

A. LYMPH NODES

The commonest swellings in the neck are undoubtedly due to pathological processes arising in the lymphatic nodes, usually secondary to some inflammatory or neoplastic process in one of the organs which they drain, but sometimes, as in the lymphomas, appearing to arise primarily within these nodes.

The distribution of the lymphatic nodes in the neck is variable, but the general disposition is as follows. In the upper part of the neck there is a horizontally disposed system consisting of the submental, suprahyoid, submaxillary and upper deep cervical groups. The names of these groups indicate sufficiently their situation except for the upper deep cervical group which is situated in relation to the internal jugular vein where it is crossed by the posterior belly of the digastric muscle. One important node of this group—the jugulo-digastric node—is particularly significant in relation to pathological conditions of the tongue and tonsil. These nodes all drain from before backwards.

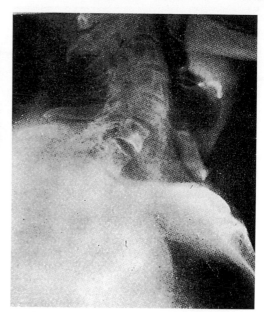

Fig. N.33. Lateral view of left-sided laryngocele.

In addition to the horizontal system, there is a vertical system ranged along the internal jugular vein. At the upper end there is the upper deep cervical group, common to both systems, and at the lower end the lower deep cervical group with subsidiary groups in between. The lower deep cervical group of lymph nodes is in relation to the internal jugular vein where it is crossed by the posterior belly of the omohyoid, and one large node of this group—the jugulo-omohyoid node—is again of significance in relation to pathological processes in the tongue receiving lymphatics from this organ without the interposition of any intervening lymphatic nodes; so that, for instance, a carcinoma of the side of the tongue can give rise to secondary deposits in the supraclavicular fossa, where this node is situated, without the enlargement of any of the systems in the upper part of the neck. It remains to mention the Delphic node on the thyrohyoid membrane already referred to. The differential diagnosis of the various types of enlarged lymph nodes is described on page 402.

B. THYROID SWELLINGS

These, which are the second commonest cause of swellings situated laterally in the neck, are fully described on page 662. Nearly all these swellings move up and down with deglutition, by which property they may be recognized. There are, however, some exceptions to this rule. If the mass is very large and fills one or both anterior triangles and perhaps the midline as well, there may not be room for the thyroid to move on deglutition. Again, in certain types of carcinoma with infiltration of the pretracheal muscles the growth may not move on deglutition. This is because the larynx, which causes the thyroid to move, cannot itself do so as there is no elasticity left in the infiltrated pretracheal muscles. Indeed it is this tethering of the larynx by infiltration of the surrounding structures which leads to dysphagia in carcinoma of the thyroid, as can readily be appreciated by anyone who attempts to swallow while holding down his thyroid cartilage by placing a finger on its upper border. Sometimes in a nodular goitre the excursion of the mass on swallowing or on coughing may be so considerable that it rises up from 'plunging down' into the superior mediastinum or retroclavicular spaces during these movement. This so-called 'plunging goitre' is only a type of retrosternal or retroclavicular goitre with an abnormally free range of movement. Its very mobility argues that it will probably be a simple matter to deal with surgically.

C. MORE RARE CASES OF SWELLING LATERALLY PLACED IN THE NECK

i. *Branchial cyst*. This is a congenital condition believed to arise in the remains of the second branchial cleft and giving rise to a cystic swelling in the lateral part of the neck. Another theory is that it represents cystic degeneration within a lymph node. The condition may arise at any age, but usually occurs in young people and is rare after the age of 40 (*Fig*. N.34). The swelling, which varies in size, usually protrudes into the anterior triangle from the deep surface of the upper part of the sternomastoid muscle. It is usually rather soft and fluctuates readily, but it is generally too deeply situated to demonstrate translucency. Occasionally these cysts become infected, when the differential diagnosis from breaking-down tuberculous nodes may be difficult.

Ordinarily the sternomastoid muscle tends to spread over and be attached to a mass of breaking-down tuberculous nodes, whereas it is inclined to go into spasm and retreat from an inflamed branchial cyst. However, the diagnosis can usually be determined by aspiration, which will yield either tuberculous pus or, on the other hand, purulent fluid containing numerous cholesterol crystals which is typical of an inflamed branchial cyst.

Although not strictly a swelling in the neck, it should be mentioned here that the unobliterated second branchial cleft, instead of forming a cyst, may communicate with the exterior, usually just medial to the sternal head of the sternomastoid muscle below and into the pharynx in the supratonsillar fossa above, forming a *branchial fistula*.

ii. '*Sternomastoid tumour.*' As a result of birth or intra-uterine injury, some fibres of the sternomastoid muscle may be torn and a haematoma appears in this muscle. This gives rise to a lump which may persist and prevent the proper development of the muscle, leading to torticollis (wryneck).

iii. *Cervical rib*. Another congenital abnormality which may give rise to a swelling in the supraclavicular fossa is cervical rib. The swelling may be due to the rib itself or there may be a pulsatile swelling due to a 'post-stenotic' dilatation of the subclavian artery.

iv. A rare congenital abnormality is *cystic hygroma*, a lymphangiomatous condition arising usually in the supraclavicular fossa of infants. It forms a soft, fluctuating, translucent and painless swelling which may grow rapidly. These masses are liable to attacks of infection.

v. *Aneurysm and arteriovenous fistula*. The large vessels of the neck are liable to the same pathological changes as vessels elsewhere. Aneurysms may occur in the cervical part of the subclavian artery, or the carotid arteries. A penetrating injury of the neck, as by a metallic fragment, may damage both the carotid artery and the internal jugular vein, leading to an arteriovenous fistula.

vi. *Carotid body tumour*. This is a rare lesion arising in the chromaffin tissue situated at the bifurcation of the common carotid artery. It appears at any time after infancy as a very firm 'potato-like' tumour in close association with the carotid sheath so that pulsation is usually, but not invariably, transmitted to it (*Fig*. N.35). Its steady growth over a period of years serves to distinguish it from tuberculous cervical adenitis with which it may readily be confused. Carotid angiography demonstrates the diagnostic splaying apart of the internal and external carotid arteries at their origins by the tumour mass at the bifurcation.

vii. *Swellings of the submandibular salivary gland* arise in the digastric triangle and are described on page 580. Ludwig's angina is an acute inflammatory process of the cellular tissue around the submaxillary gland, usually arising from the floor of the mouth or the teeth. The physical signs extend into the floor of the mouth and give rise to considerable oedema which, without treatment, may spread to the glottis and demand tracheotomy.

viii. *Actinomycosis* is a chronic inflammatory swelling of the cellular tissue about the angle of the mandible. The diffuse induration with the eventual development of multiple sinuses and the accompanying trismus should make the diagnosis obvious.

Late in the disease, 'sulphur granules' containing the streptothrix may be discharged, but the diagnosis should not await bacteriological confirmation which may be equivocal in the early stages.

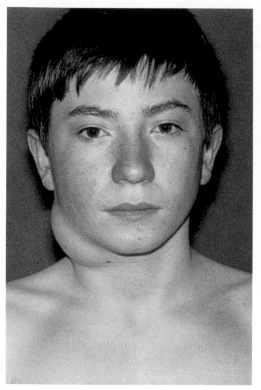

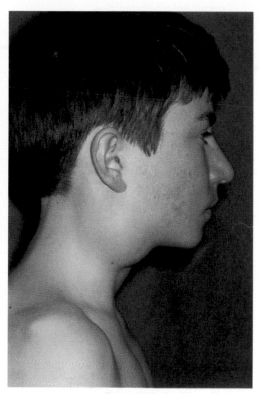

Fig. N.34. Branchial cyst.

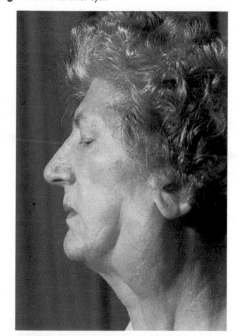

Fig. N.35. Carotid body tumour. (*Professor G. Westbury.*)

ix. *Spinal abscess*. In certain cases of tuberculosis of the cervical spine, the abscess may track from the retropharyngeal region laterally, and present as a fluctuant mass in the upper part of the posterior triangle and deep to the insertion of the sternomastoid muscle. The accompanying stiffness of the neck, together with the general evidence of a chronic infection, should alert the examiner to this possibility. If untreated, the abscess breaks down, discharges and forms multiple sinuses in the apex of the posterior triangle.

Harold Ellis

Nipple, abnormalities of

Deformities of the nipple may be classified as follows:

Congenital

Congenital absence
Supernumery
Congenital inversion
Bifid nipple

Acquired

Acquired inversion
Plasma cell mastitis
Mammillary duct fistula
Duct ectasia
Tumour
   Retro-areolar carcinoma
   Paget's disease

Congenital abnormalities

Rarely there can be complete absence of the development of the breast and the nipple. This may be associated with failure of development of the pectoral muscles when the condition is known as Holland's syndrome. Supernumery nipple areolar complexes are quite common, running down the milk line from the subclavicular area across the lateral part of the abdomen, ending in the region of the anterior superior iliac spine (*Fig*. N.36). Congenital inversions of the nipples are common and must be distinguished from the acquired inversion of the nipple associated with either carcinoma of the breast or duct ectasia. A bifid nipple is a rare but well-recognized entity.

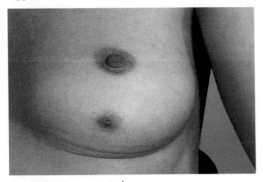

Fig. N.36. Accessory nipple.

Acquired abnormalities

Acquired inversion of the nipple may be a consequence of duct ectasia/plasma cell mastitis syndrome (*see section on* BREAST LUMP). In this condition the inversion of the nipple is usually bilateral, central and slit-like. Apart from this, acquired inversion of the nipple is usually of sinister significance and may represent a retro-areolar carcinoma, or even the first sign of a cancer in one of the outer quadrants of the breast (*Fig*. N.37).

Paget's disease of the nipple (*Fig*. N.38) is a relatively rare presenting sign of carcinoma of the breast and may be an eczematous condition affecting the nipple and areola. This is usually associated with an intraduct element of carcinoma invading along the terminal portions of the lactiferous ducts to infiltrate the dermis of the nipple and areola. If this eczematous condition is unilateral and not associated with patches of eczema elsewhere on the body, then it should be treated seriously by an immediate biopsy. The histological appearance is characteristic with foamy cells with large atypical nuclei seen scattered throughout the dermis and subdermal layers (*Fig*. N.39).

Mammillary duct fistula is a sequel of periductal mastitis and presents as a discharging sinus at the

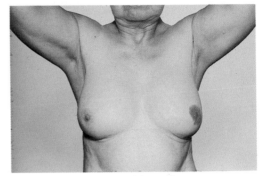

Fig. N.38. Paget's disease of the nipple.

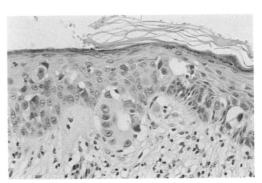

Fig. N.39. Histological appearance of Paget's disease of the nipple.

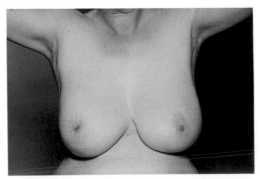

Fig. N.37. Nipple inversion and skin dimpling associated with a carcinoma of the breast.

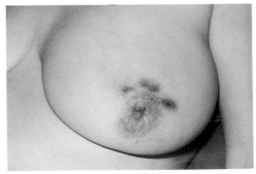

Fig. N.40. Multiple mammillary fistulae.

areolar margin (*Fig*. N.40). This complex of diseases is described under BREAST LUMP.

Michael Baum

Nipple, discharge from

Discharge from the nipple may be divided into three classes:

1. Normal discharges

A discharge of milk from the breast during pregnancy is not uncommon especially in multiparae; both then and during lactation it is usually of small amount except when the child is put to the breast, but occasionally the flow at other times may be sufficient to be distressing.

2. Normal discharges at abnormal times

A secretion similar to colostrum sometimes occurs from the breasts of both sexes in the newly born and again at puberty; it is due to endocrine stimulation but it may predispose to a true infective mastitis, when the breast, already tender and swollen, becomes hot and red, and the discharge may change from being clear to purulent.

Occasionally the normal secretion of milk during lactation is prolonged for many months or years after the stimulus of suckling has been removed. This is probably due to some endocrine abnormality and, apart from being a serious nuisance and sometimes a source of anxiety to the patient, has no sinister significance. It usually resolves spontaneously and unpredictably after a varying period with or without the aid of endocrine therapy. Women with prolactin-secreting tumours of the anterior pituitary may present with galactorrhoea and amenorrhoea.

3. Abnormal discharges

A. SEROUS FLUID

A discharge of serous fluid from the nipple is a common accompaniment of duct ectasia or epithelial hyperplasia.

B. Pigmented fluids

i. *Green fluid*. When the colour is due to melanin or pigments other than derivatives of haemoglobin, its admixture with yellow serum gives to the resultant discharges a green colour of varying shades. If the discharge is very dark, dilution with water will disclose the green colour. In cases of real difficulty the discharge may be submitted to spectroscopic or chemical assay for haemoglobin. Such discharges have precisely the same significance as the non-pigmented serous discharges discussed above.

ii. *Haemorrhagic*. Blood-stained discharges can usually be recognized on sight; the colour is red to black, and again if there is real doubt the final arbiters are the microscope and the chemical test. Blood-stained discharges are indicative of duct papilloma, epithelial proliferation, and intraduct carcinoma, in that order of frequency.

The nipple should be examined through a magnifying glass and a bead of blood or a speck of clot may reveal from which of the twenty or so ducts the bleeding is arising. Such evidence is important in determining from which section of the breast the bleeding is originating. Having examined the nipple thus, it should be wiped clean and (with the breast rendered moderately tense by an assistant if available) the tip of the finger is pressed on to the breast at successive sites, working spirally from the nipple, and paying particular attention to the subareolar region, where the source of the bleeding lies in the majority of cases. By this means it will be found possible to cause blood to issue from the nipple on pressure over quite a restricted area, whereas pressure elsewhere has no effect. If the affected duct has been previously identified the significant area will be found to lie in the segment of the breast drained by that duct, and the pathological region is confirmed. The segment of the breast affected should be removed by local operation, and the pathological condition causing the bleeding determined by naked-eye inspection and histological study. Further treatment depends upon the nature of the lesion so determined. Solitary papillomas adjacent to the nipple are the commonest cause of this symptom, and if removed in this way bleeding seldom recurs.

Should it be impossible to localize the origin of the bleeding, and with care and practice this is most unusual, the diagnosis depends on an assessment of probabilities. The younger the patient the more likely is the cause to be benign; the older the patient the more likely to be malignant. Mammography is valuable in demonstrating or excluding an occult neoplasm as the source of the haemorrhage. Where the discharge of pigmented fluids from multiple ducts associated with duct ectasia is profuse and embarrassing, total excision of the subareolar duct system (Hadfield's operation) will affect a cure.

4. Grumous material

The discharge of 'cheese-like' material or material having the consistency of toothpaste or putty, grey or green in colour, indicates the condition known as 'comedo mastitis'. This is another variant of the duct ectasia/periductal mastitis complex (*see p. 83*).

5. Pus

Pus, or pus mixed with milk, generally indicates acute suppurative mastitis; the other signs of inflammation or abscess are well marked as a rule, so that there is no difficulty in arriving at a diagnosis. A *tuberculous lesion* also causes a discharge of pus, and it may simulate carcinoma; the discharge may contain demonstrable tubercle bacilli, but specific bacteriological culture, together with a radiograph of the chest, will very likely be required before a positive answer on the nature of the infection can be given.

Michael Baum

Nodules

Nodules are larger than papules (more than 5 mm in diameter) but are distinguished by depth rather than by diameter. They may be free in the dermis or fixed to overlying skin or underlying subcutaneous tissue. Possible causes are legion (*see Table* N.3) but persistent non-tender nodules should always be biopsied.

1. Neoplasms

Nodules are a stage in the development of tumours, both benign and malignant (p. 601). Many nodular skin neoplasms are aetiologically related to sun exposure. Modern man has a startling appetite for recreational ultraviolet light exposure hence the prevalence of sun-induced skin tumours is increasing and the age of incidence is falling. A high index of suspicion should be maintained when examining nodules on sun-exposed skin—especially in the presence of obvious solar skin damage—accelerated 'ageing', deep furrows on the back of the neck, pale 'younger' looking skin in the shaded eye sockets and under the point of the chin, solar elastosis (*Fig*. N.41) and solar keratoses on forehead, backs of hands and pate. The commonest tumour is a basal-cell *carcinoma*, beginning as a small, rounded, pearly, translucent papule, showing telangiectasia (*Fig*. N.42). These may not ulcerate for a long time and nodulo-cystic lesions grow as solid tumours composed of lobulated masses of cells in which cystic degeneration may occur. Enlarging lesions eventually ulcerate centrally, where a haemorrhagic crust forms. A *squamous-cell carcinoma* is a harder, fleshy nodule, often with overlying scale, occurring in the same sites and, in addition, the lower lip. Draining lymphadenopathy may indicate metastases or secondary infection. A *kerato-acanthoma* is a neat, dome-shaped nodule which grows alarmingly in weeks on exposed skin of face and limbs. A juicy hyperkeratotic central plug forms which may discharge later, giving the lesion the appearance of a giant molluscum contagiosum. Kerato-acanthoma is a benign tumour which eventually involutes spontaneously after some 3 months. Nodular

Table N.3.   Causes of nodules

1. **Neoplasms**
   Basal-cell carcinoma (*Figs* F.209 in 12e, F.210 in 12e, F.25, N.43)
   Squamous-cell carcinoma (*Fig*. L.18)
   Kerato-acanthoma (*Fig*. S.31)
   Malignant melanoma (*Fig*. S.27)
   Lymphoma
   Kaposi's sarcoma (*Fig*. A.19)
   Dermatofibroma
   Pyogenic granuloma (*Fig*. N.44)
   Keloid (*Fig*. K.1)

2. **Vasculitis**
   Erythema nodosum
   Nodular vasculitis
   Wegener's granulomatosis
   Polyarteritis nodosa (*Fig*. N.44)
   Temporal arteritis

3. **Chronic inflammation**
   Sarcoid
   Rheumatoid nodules
   Bromoderma
   Acne (*Fig*. N.45)

4. **Metabolic**
   Xanthoma (*Fig*. C.13)
   Gouty tophus
   Lipoid proteinosis
   Pretibial myxoedema

5. **Infections**
   Mycobacteria (*Figs* N.48, N.49)
   Fungi (*Fig*. S.7)
   Leprosy
   Treponema
   Infestation (*Figs*. N.17, P.43, V.5)

6. **Miscellaneous**
   Heberden's nodes
   Chondrodermatitis nodularis chronica helicis (*Fig*. N.50)

malignant melanomas are usually ominously obvious though the amelanotic variant is often first diagnosed by the histopathologist. Early changes in moles which can point to malignant change include haemorrhage, loss of hairs growing from the mole, pigment spilling into surrounding skin, ulceration and inflammation. *Lymphomatous* infiltrates in the skin are often nodular and the later stages of *cutaneous T-cell lymphoma* (mycosis fungoides) are nodular and tumorous. *Kaposi's sarcoma* comprises slow-growing port-wine-coloured plaques and nodules, particularly on the lower limbs (*see Fig*. A.19). A more aggressive form occurs widely on the body in HIV-positive individuals (and is now an accepted AIDS-defining diagnosis).

The commonest benign nodular neoplasm is a *dermatofibroma* (histiocytoma) developing as a firm red/brown nodule in the upper dermis fixed to overlying skin usually on the legs. Histology shows a dense proliferation of fibrocytes, which may represent a tissue reaction to a preceding insect bite.

A *pyogenic granuloma* (*Fig*. N.43) is a firm, small, cherry-red pedunculated nodule of hypertrophic

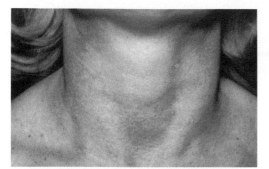

Fig. N.41. Solar elastosis. (*Westminster Hospital.*)

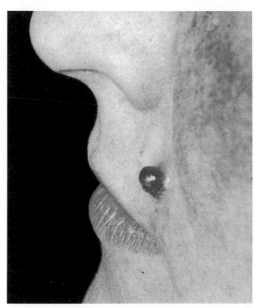

Fig. N.43. Pyogenic granuloma. (*Dr Peter Hansell.*)

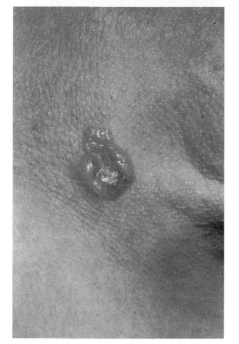

Fig. N.42. Basal cell carcinoma. (*Dr Richard Staughton.*)

granulation tissue, which bleeds easily on slight trauma and occurs most frequently on the lips and extremities. Its rapid growth and characteristic collarette are helpful diagnostic pointers.

2. Vasculitis

Skin nodules can be caused by swollen, inflamed, dermal blood vessels and are particularly seen on the legs. Small vessels are involved in *erythema nodosum*, larger in *nodular vasculitis* and *Wegener's granulomatosis*, and arteries in *polyarteritis nodosa* and *temporal arteritis*.

Erythema nodosum occurs most often in females in their second and third decades as crops of painful, tender, red nodules, on the shins, 1–8 cm in diameter, which heal over several weeks without breaking the surface, and going through the colour changes of a bruise. A cause for this reaction can be found in half the affected individuals. Examples include sarcoidosis, inflammatory bowel disease, infections (streptococcus, tuberculosis, leprosy and deep fungus) and drugs (sulphonamides and thiazides).

Nodular vasculitis is also more common in women but later in life in their third and fourth decades. The calves are the usual site of well-demarcated, bluish, fixed, subcutaneous nodules. Underlying tuberculosis must be excluded, but often a cause is not determined. *Polyarteritis nodosa* (*Fig.* N.44) affects adult men and nodules usually occur along the course of arteries. There is severe illness with fever, arthralgia, hypertension, peripheral neuropathy and eosinophilia. Nodular lesions may be seen along retinal arteries. The prognosis is related to the degree of renal vascular involvement. In *giant-cell arteries* exquisitely tender, nodular swellings occur most commonly along the course of the temporal artery. Sometimes extensive ischaemic scalp ulceration is seen. Early recognition and treatment is important as irreversible retinal artery thrombosis, and consequent blindness, can occur.

3. Chronic inflammation

Non-infectious granulomatous nodules are seen in sarcoidosis, rheumatoid arthritis, bromoderma and around ruptured pilo-sebaceous glands in acne. *Sarcoidosis* usually begins in early adult life, most commonly in women, especially negroes and Irish, with groups of purplish papules and nodules on the face or extensor aspects of the extremities. Erythema nodosum is common. The nodules of *rheumatoid arthritis* occur over the bony prominences at points of pressure,

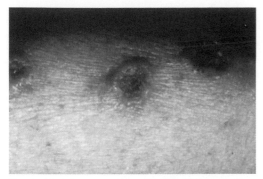

Fig. N.44. Polyarteritis nodosa. (*Dr Richard Staughton.*)

especially just below the elbow. They are painful, very rarely ulcerate and vary in size from a pin-head to 2 cm in diameter. When present they indicate seropositivity (Rose-Waaler or latex). Reaction to ingested bromides and iodides (bromoderma, iododerma) can rarely produce dramatic purplish, nodular and vegetative lesions on the face of infants or extremities of adults. They may persist for long periods until recognized. Firm, suppurating nodules are seen in *nodulo-cystic acne vulgaris* (*Fig.* N.45), due to granulomatous reactions around ruptured, swollen sebaceous glands. Similar lesions in the axillae, groins and peri-anal skin are seen in *hidradenitis suppurativa* (*Fig.* N.46), but these abscesses are based on apocrine glands. Young adults are chiefly affected and the nodules are accompanied by draining sinuses.

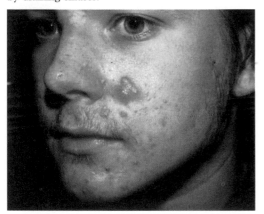

Fig. N.45. Nodulo-cystic acne vulgaris. (*Dr Richard Staughton.*)

4. Metabolic

Deposition of *metabolic products* in the dermis may cause nodular swelling. These begin as papules and include xanthoma, pretibial myxoedema, gouty tophi and lipoid proteinosis. Xanthomas are reddish-brown nodules of varying size usually found on the elbows and knees and dorsa of hands and feet. They betoken underlying disturbance of carbohydrate/lipid meta-

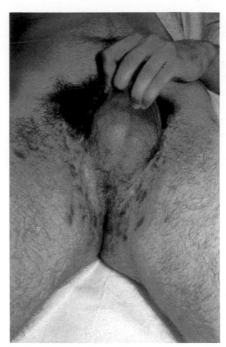

Fig. N.46. Hidradenitis suppurativa. (*Dr Richard Staughton.*)

bolism usually primary but sometimes secondary, e.g. uncontrolled diabetes.

Gouty tophi are hard yellow-white waxy nodules, on the helix or antihelix of ear, palms or soles, tarsal plates of eyelids and tendons of hands or feet. Sometimes tophi ulcerate and discharge cheesy material containing crystals of sodium biurate.

Lipoid proteinosis is a very rare inherited tendency to infiltrate the skin and mucosa with a hyaline material (muco-polysaccharide). Affected patients have a hoarse voice and characteristic beading along eyelid margins.

In *pretibial myxoedema* firm red nodules or plaques arise on lower legs, over the front of the shin and on the dorsa of the feet; hair and follicle orifices are grossly hypertrophied giving a *peau d'orange* appearance.

5. Infections

Nodules due to infection are less common in western countries, except for the ubiquitous furuncle or boil. Boils appear chiefly on the face, neck and buttocks and are painful red nodules, often with a yellow pustule at the apex. The cause is a follicular infection with *Staphylococcus aureus*, and lesions may be recurrent for many weeks or months. They are more frequent in diabetic and debilitated people.

Any organism which induces a chronic granulomatous tissue reaction seems particularly prone to produce skin nodules (*see Table* N.3).

A. MYCOBACTERIA

Lupus vulgaris (*Fig. N.47*) is now extremely uncommon. Small, softish, reddish-brown or yellowish nodules appear on the face or mucous membrane in childhood. When examined compressed under a glass slide (diascopy), the nodules have a typical 'apple jelly' appearance. The nodules progress and slowly coalesce over very many years to form annular scaling plaques with central atrophy and fibrosis. More common now are nodules caused by infections with atypical mycobacteria, for example *fish-tank granuloma* (*Fig. N.48*). Usually a finger is abraded against an infected fish-tank and soft subcutaneous nodulo-cystic lesions develop. These are followed by a succession of nodules appearing along a lymphatic chain (sporotricoid spread). In *swimming pool granuloma* lesions are smaller papulo-nodules on elbows, knees or any skin area traumatized against an infected pool wall – sporotricoid spread does not occur.

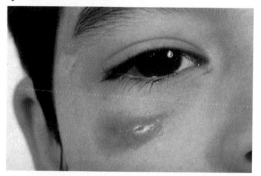

Fig. N.47. Lupus vulgaris in a young Asian immigrant. (*St Stephens Hospital.*)

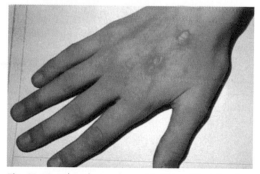

Fig. N.48. Fish-tank granuloma. (*Dr Richard Staughton.*)

B. FUNGI

In the UK, fungi and other infections in the immunosuppressed particularly those with HIV disease, should be thought of as the cause of nodules. *Actinomycosis* causes abscesses around carious teeth, tonsils or gastrointestinal tract. The pus contains 'sulphur' granules of the penicillin-sensitive 'ray fungus', *Actinomyces israeli*. *Cryptococcosis* (torulosis) occurs in all parts of the world, usually involving the central nervous system, where meningitis, abscess or brain tumour may be suggested. Sometimes transient skin nodules occur. *Sporotrichosis* begins with a skin nodule at the site of injury of hand or forearm, in contact with infected wood, soil or plant. There may be a considerable local inflammation before the characteristic succession of nodules appears up the draining lymphatic chain. Occasionally a superficial dermatophyte infection elicits so violent a reaction that a boggy nodulopustule, rather like a carbuncle, develops. This is called a *kerion* and usually occurs in a hairy area, e.g. scalp or beard (*Fig. N.S.7*).

C. LEPROSY

At the later stages of *lepromatous leprosy* dull, red-brown nodules or plaques may be seen in symmetrical distribution on limbs, face and ears. There may be hypopigmented anaesthetic macules elsewhere on the body, impaired eyebrow growth and the diagnosis is made by finding acid-fast organisms in tissue smears.

D. TREPONEMA

Late *syphilis* can produce nodular skin lesions. For example, nodulo-ulcerative tertiary syphilis is characterized by groups of crusted copper-coloured nodules which spread peripherally and heal centrally in bizarrely shaped patterns. Sometimes these ulcerate and are seen on the face, trunk or limbs. The solitary syphilitic gumma begins as a dermal or subcutaneous bluish-red nodule. Later this sloughs to produce a punched-out ulcer with a rubbery necrotic base and may cause gross tissue destruction. In secondary *yaws* exuberant moist red nodules, rich in *Treponema pertenue*, may occur widely particularly in the groins and at the angles of the mouth (their resemblance to raspberries gives rise to the alternative name 'framboesia'). Juxta-articular nodules can occur in the tertiary stage of yaws.

E. OTHER INFECTIONS

Leishmaniasis (Baghdad boil) is common in young adults and children in the Middle East but can be seen in European holidaymakers on their return from the south shore of the Mediterranean and the Middle East. Pruritic papules slowly develop into ulcerating nodules on exposed sites following the bite of an infected phlebotomus fly. Giemsa staining of material readily reveals the intracellular parasite. *Onchocerciasis* (see p. 519) gives rise to pruritus and indolent non-tender nodules varying in size from 0.5 to 5 cm on head, shoulders and trunk. These nodules contain the adult worm. In *loaiasis*, or Calabar swelling, transient hot skin-coloured nodules occur on the face and extremities. *Tick bites* can be the cause of remarkably persistent dermal nodules.

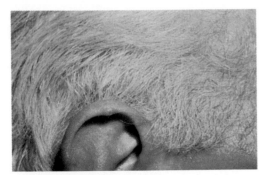

Fig N.49. Chondrodermatitis nodularis chronica helicis. (*Dr Richard Staughton.*)

6. Miscellaneous

Heberden's nodes, small bony swellings on the terminal interphalangeal joints, are more common in women. They are a sign of osteoarthritis. *Chondrodermatitis nodularis chronica helicis* is the descriptive title given to a not uncommon exquisitely painful nodule, which occurs in the upper third of the helix of the ear (*Fig. N.49*). The lesions are probably due to pressure, like a corn, causing underlying perichondritis with fibrinoid degeneration of the cartilage.

Richard Staughton

Nystagmus

Nystagmus refers to an oscillatory movement of the eyes which is often rhythmic and repetitive. A classification is presented in *Table* N.4. It is sometimes present with the eyes at rest, but it may only appear when the eyes are moved conjugately. Nystagmus of pathological significance must be differentiated from end-point nystagmoid jerks at extremes of gaze deviation and from the few unsustained nystagmoid jerks that may be observed at the completion of a lateral or vertical eye movement. Searching eye movements are seen in those who are born blind or who have lost the power of fixation as a result of a lesion at the macula. These eye movements are wide ranging and slow as if the eyes are seeking something they can never find. Voluntary nystagmus is rare but some individuals can produce rapid oscillations of the eyes at will and this may be mistaken for true nystagmus. These movements tend to be of high frequency and cannot be maintained for long periods.

Physiological nystagmus occurs in normal subjects as a result of either a visual (optokinetic) or vestibular (caloric/rotational) stimulus.

Pendular nystagmus, which is pathological, is characterized by oscillations of equal velocity and results from long-standing ocular disorders with impaired macular fixation from early in life. It may indeed be congenital. A similar syndrome has been described

Table N.4. Classification of nystagmus

Physiological
Optokinetic
Vestibular (caloric/rotational)

Pathological
Pendular
Phasic (jerk)
  Horizontal
  Rotatory (rotational)
  Vertical
Dysconjugate

in miners (miner's nystagmus) though this is rare. Congenital nystagmus is not always of the pendular variety and in the condition called 'spasmus nutans' the nystagmus is associated with nodding movements of the head.

Phasic (jerk) nystagmus has fast and slow components alternating in opposite directions and by convention the direction of nystagmus is taken to be that of the fast component. The plane of the nystagmus may be horizontal, vertical or compound, the latter giving rise to rotatory nystagmus. Vestibular nystagmus occurs when there is damage to the labyrinth, vestibular nerve or vestibular nuclei. The nystagmus is most prominent on looking away from the side of the lesion with the fast phase directed away from the side of the lesion. The nystagmus remains unidirectional no matter what the direction of gaze. Vestibular neuronitis or ischaemic lesions of the vestibular nerve or labyrinth are the common causes. Toxic damage to the vestibular nuclei, as seen in aminoglycoside ototoxicity, may be associated with nystagmus. Oscillopsia, that is an illusion of movement of the visual field, is often a prominent concomitant of this type of nystagmus. Positional nystagmus is induced by abrupt alteration in the position of the head (the so-called 'Hallpike' or 'Nylen' manoeuvre). It is seen in benign positional vertigo, after damage to the vestibular apparatus subsequent to head injury, and in central disorders affecting the brainstem vestibular/cerebellar connections.

Gaze peretic nystagmus is associated with variation in the direction of nystagmus in relation to direction of gaze. The fast phase is always in the direction of gaze. It results from disturbance of the brainstem centres controlling conjugate gaze. It is seen in drug intoxication from anticonvulsants or sedatives and also after alcohol. It is most commonly horizontal. Vertical gaze paretic nystagmus is most commonly seen in patients who also have horizontal nystagmus. When occurring in isolation vertical nystagmus is a useful localizing sign. Upbeat nystagmus most commonly occurs with lesions of the mid-brain at or about the superior colliculus, whereas downbeat nystagmus is most frequently associated with disorders at or around the foramen magnum such as the Arnold–Chiari malformation. Multiple sclerosis and brainstem vascular events are other causes.

Convergence or retractory nystagmus is characterized by rhythmical convergence or retraction movements of the eyes when the subject attempts to look upwards. It is usually associated with impairment of upward conjugate gaze and results from a lesion such as a pinealoma at the level of the superior colliculous. See-saw nystagmus is characterized by rhythmical movements of the eyes in opposite directions. Whilst one eye elevates the other drops and the movements are often associated with inward or outward rotational elements as well.

There is no convincing evidence that lesions at any level lower than the medulla or cerebellar tonsils ever produce nystagmus. Other eye movement disorders that need to be differentiated from nystagmus include ocular dysmetria, opsoclonus and ocular bobbing.

S. T. D. Roxburgh

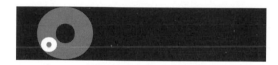

Obsessions

Minor degrees of obsessional symptoms are extremely common in the general population and only a very small proportion of these seek medical advice. Obsessions may refer to thoughts, images, impulses or acts. This last category, obsessional acts or rituals, are usually described as compulsions. What distinguishes obsessions from other sorts of preoccupation are the following characteristics: they intrude repeatedly into a patient's mind against his will; the patient, however, recognizes that these thoughts are his own even though he finds the thoughts unpleasant or silly; finally, the patient is unable to quietly tolerate the intrusive thoughts but is compelled because of them to perform rituals and to resist the thoughts themselves. Obsessions are thus quite different from delusions because the obsessional person has good insight. In everyday language many activities when engaged in excessively, are referred to as 'compulsive'; these include eating, gambling, drinking, drug abuse and some forms of sexual behaviour. However, these are best not considered as true compulsions because they lack the essential quality of being the result of intrusive thoughts resisted by the patient. Obsessional individuals do not derive pleasure from their symptoms.

In contrast to obsessional traits which are common, obsessive compulsive disorder is uncommon. The most common obsessions are repetitive thoughts of dirt contamination which may lead to excessive washing rituals, repetitive thoughts of violence and an unreasonable fear of harming somebody else (for example making it impossible for the obsessional person to drive a car for fear they may knock somebody down). Obsessional ideas may take the form of doubts and the subject will develop rituals of checking door locks, switches and taps many times before bringing themselves to leave the house or retire to bed. Rituals may take the form of mental activity such as repeatedly counting to a certain number thus causing a slowing down of all normal activities. Such a person may take hours to dress in the morning.

There is no clear dividing line between an obsessional trait and obsessional neurosis. The former is a normal personality variant which may be advantageous in many walks of life where meticulousness is essential. Obsessions become disabling when they are associated with marked anxiety, when rituals are very time consuming or bizarre and normal routine at home and at work is interfered with. A subject with obsessional fear of contamination may have to avoid meeting people and shaking hands, eating food prepared by anyone but themselves and may spend many hours repeatedly washing themselves and their clothes, to the extent that their hands become excoriated.

An obsessional disorder may develop for the first time during a depressive illness (*see* DEPRESSION) or depression may exacerbate an underlying obsessional trait. Obsessional thoughts in depression may be hypochondriacal with thoughts of having cancer, obsessional brooding about financial ruin or impending doom. Obsessional thinking and associated rituals improve as the depression is treated. Stereotypal and sometimes bizarre ritualistic behaviour is common in schizophrenia but is usually related to delusional beliefs. However, schizophrenia and obsessive compulsive disorders are sometimes diagnosed in the same person.

D. Blackwood

Oedema, dependent

The fact that oedema typically 'pits' on pressure is because the fluid can be easily displaced from one part of the subcutaneous tissue to another. It is this free mobility of the fluid within the tissues that is responsible for the fact that, whenever there is a significant expansion of the extracellular fluid volume, the excess fluid accumulates under the influence of gravity in the dependent parts of the body. The term 'dependent oedema' has, therefore, no specific diagnostic significance and its only value is as a reminder to beginners to look for oedema in those parts of the body which are dependent at that time. Thus, a decrease in ankle oedema after a night's rest is not necessarily a sign of improvement; in such circumstances, the oedema may well have moved and be found in the back and sides of the calves and thighs. This behaviour of the oedema fluid accounts for an occasional curious finding such as rings of oedema around the olecranon processes; this can be due to the patient spending much of his time in bed leaning forward with his elbows on a bed table in front of him.

The causes of oedema, nearly always dependent, are discussed under OEDEMA, GENERALIZED.

Peter R. Fleming

Oedema, generalized

Generalized oedema is due to an increase in the volume of extracellular fluid. This is brought about by excessive renal tubular reabsorption of sodium and water; the mechanism of this reabsorption is complex and the renin–angiotensin–aldosterone system is only one of the factors involved. The accumulation of fluid in the extravascular space which causes oedema is determined by the relationship between the hydrostatic and oncotic pressures in the capillaries and the interstitial tissue. Thus, a rise in capillary hydrostatic pressure due, for example, to venous obstruction and a fall in capillary oncotic pressure, as a result of hypoalbuminaemia, increases the net movement of fluid from the capillaries to the tissues. When sufficient fluid has been transferred in this way—at least 5 litres in adults—clinically detectable oedema results. Another factor concerned in the transfer of fluid across capillary walls is their permeability; in practice, an increase in this is more important in the production of localized rather than generalized oedema. Impairment of the lymphatic drainage of tissues is also a cause of localized oedema (*see* ARM; LEG, OEDEMA OF). In any patient with generalized oedema, fluid may also accumulate in serous cavities in the form of ascites and pleural or pericardial effusion.

Gravity determines the fact that, in any situation in which sodium and water retention occurs, the oedema fluid tends to accumulate in the dependent parts of the body (*see* OEDEMA, DEPENDENT). This tendency is so marked that, even in normal subjects, a little ankle oedema is common following prolonged periods of immobility in the seated position. It is particularly common during long journeys by air and, sometimes, by train or coach; it is probable that this is mainly due to a reduction in lymphatic drainage which is critically dependent on muscular activity. Also, in about 90 per cent of pregnant women, slight oedema is present at term and is, in fact, associated with a more favourable outcome to the pregnancy than when no oedema is present. The pathological situations in which generalized oedema most commonly occurs are heart failure and renal, hepatic and, less often, gastrointestinal disease. These, and other less common causes of oedema, are discussed below.

Heart failure

The oedema of *heart failure* is typically dependent, affecting particularly the ankles and, in recumbent patients, the sacral region. Despite this clear evidence of a hydrostatic component in determining the site of the oedema, the rise in central venous pressure in heart failure is a minor factor in the production of the oedema, compared with the reduction in renal blood flow and glomerular filtration rate and the increase in tubular reabsorption of sodium and water. These mechanisms operate whatever the cause of the heart failure but, in cor pulmonale, an additional factor may be a movement of fluid from the cells to the interstitial tissue; this is believed to occur in order to provide more buffers for the associated respiratory acidosis. The oedema is usually symmetrical but, sometimes, it is more marked in the left leg than the right; this is thought to be due to pressure on the left common iliac vein by the right common iliac artery as it crosses it. It is heart failure which is the mechanism of the oedema of so-called 'wet beri-beri, due to a dietary deficiency of thiamine, and also of the oedema seen commonly in severe anaemia from any cause.

Renal disease

Slight transient generalized oedema is a characteristic feature of *acute poststreptococcal glomerulonephritis* but this is not due to the proteinuria, which is of no more than moderate severity. It is in the *nephrotic syndrome* that hypoalbuminaemia, due to heavy proteinuria, is severe enough to lower the intracapillary oncotic pressure to a level at which oedema occurs. In this condition the urinary protein loss is usually more than 3 g per 24 hours and the serum albumin below 30 g per litre. It is probable that the hypovolaemia resulting from massive loss of fluid from the capillaries stimulates the renin–angiotensin–aldosterone system and this leads to renal retention of sodium and water. The oedema is usually dependent but, in children, it may be as prominent in the trunk and face as in the legs (*Fig.* O.1); the external genitalia are commonly very swollen. Spontaneous disappearance of the oedema is not necessarily a good sign as, with advancing renal failure, the fall in glomerular filtration rate may markedly reduce the amount of protein lost.

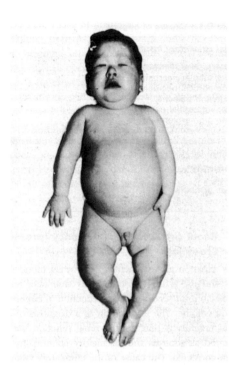

Fig. O.1. Massive oedema and ascites in the nephrotic syndrome. (*Dr. P.R. Evans.*)

There are numerous conditions which can cause the nephrotic syndrome. In children, by far the commonest cause is *minimal change nephropathy*, in which, as the name implies, the glomeruli are nearly normal on light microscopy but show characteristic changes on electron microscopy; clinically the most typical feature is the complete remission produced by steroid therapy. In adults, *membranous* and *proliferative nephropathy* are at least as common as the minimal change lesion and these three conditions together represent about three-quarters of all cases of the nephrotic syndrome. Less common causes include *focal glomerulosclerosis*, a condition of unknown aetiology with patchy glomerular scarring without previous inflammatory changes, *systemic lupus erythematosus*, *amyloidosis* and *diabetic nephropathy*; oedema is quite common in diabetics even in the absence of heavy proteinuria, perhaps due to microvascular disease. There is also a recognized association of the nephrotic syndrome with *malaria* due to *Plasmodium malariae* and with *malignant disease*, especially adenocarcinoma and lymphoma. The high venous pressure of *constrictive pericarditis* is also known occasionally to cause the nephrotic syndrome which has also been seen in *cyanotic congenital heart disease*. Renal vein thrombosis *per se*, however, is no longer thought to be a cause but rather a complication of the nephrotic syndrome. A number of *drugs and*

other substances are known to cause a membranous glomerular lesion and proteinuria heavy enough to cause oedema; these include mercurials, gold, penicillamine and captopril. A specific allergy is probably responsible for the nephrotic syndrome associated with certain foods, pollens, penicillin, bee stings and poison ivy.

Liver disease

Fluid retention is common in hepatic failure in which it is due to impaired protein synthesis and consequent hypoalbuminaemia. The changes in renal function are similar to those in the nephrotic syndrome. Both oedema and ascites can occur, often together, but one can be present without the other. Any form of cirrhosis may be the underlying disorder but *cryptogenic* and *alcoholic cirrhosis* and *chronic active hepatitis* are those most likely to be associated with oedema.

Protein-losing enteropathy

Protein may be lost from the body not only in the urine but also via the gastrointestinal tract. Marked hypoalbuminaemia can develop, causing oedema and, sometimes, ascites and pleural effusion. This situation arises particularly with *intestinal lymphoma* and *giant hypertrophic gastritis* (*Menetrier's disease*) but has been seen in many other disorders such as *coeliac disease, ulcerative colitis, Crohn's disease, tumours of the stomach and colon* and *intestinal allergies*.

Other causes of oedema

Oedema, more or less generalized, is a recognized feature of a number of other conditions, all rather rare in Britain. *Malnutrition*, of course, is far from rare in developing countries where it is an all too common cause of oedema. It is usually due to dietary deficiency of protein, causing hypoalbuminaemia, and is a constant feature of kwashiorkor. A condition affecting emotionally labile women of reproductive age is known, non-committally, as *idiopathic oedema*. The distribution of the oedema is curious, affecting particularly the face, hands, breasts, thighs, buttocks and abdominal wall and, hardly ever, the ankles. The aetiology is unknown but in some cases it may follow the use of diuretics in an attempt to lose weight; in that case it would be described as 'rebound' oedema. Oedema of the face, hands and ankles sometimes occurs at *high altitudes*. It may or may not be accompanied by the more severe manifestations of acute mountain sickness, such as pulmonary oedema, and is relieved by a spontaneous diuresis on return to a lower altitude. Very rarely oedema may occur in diabetics on first being given *insulin*; this resolves completely in a week or so.

Peter R. Fleming

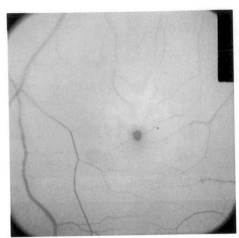

Fig. O.15. Occlusion of the central retinal artery.

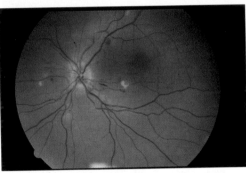

Fig. O.16. Hypertensive retinopathy. (*See also* p. 473)

deflections at these points. In ischaemia haemorrhagic exudates and cotton wool spots may occur. There is pupilloedema in accelerated hypertension.

Optic disc cupping

Excavation of the optic disc, optic disc cupping, occurs in chronic glaucoma (*Fig.* O.5). There is enlargement of the cup associated with thinning of the normally pink neuroretinal rim with associated peripheral visual field loss. The cupping is particularly evident in the vertical meridian. The excavation of the optic disc in cases of glaucoma may be distinguished from the physiological cup by the fact that it extends to the beyond the physiological norm, ie >60% of the size of the disc in the vertical meridian. The retinal vessels bend sharply over the edge, and may disappear from view behind the overhanging margin of the disc reappearing on the base of the cup. The lamina cribrosa is clearly seen and the disc becomes white and atrophic.

Optic atrophy (*Fig.* O.17)

Pallor of the disc signifies atrophy of the disc. The causes are listed in *Table* O.3.

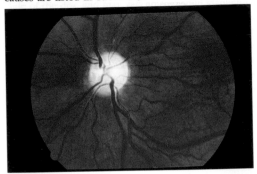

Fig. O.17. Optic atrophy.

Table O.3. Causes of optic atrophy

Congenital
Secondary to raised intracranial pressure
Secondary to retinal disease, e.g. central retinal
  artery occlusion
Choroiditis
Retinitis pigmentosa
Secondary to optic neuritis or neuropathy, e.g.
  ischaemic optic neuropathy,
Neuritis
Secondary to optic nerve compression, e.g. (tumours—
  meningioma, pituitary tumours),
  (dysthyroid disease),
  (secondary to trauma).
Toxic neuropathy (drugs, heavy metals),
Vitamin B1 deficiency.

Peripapillary atrophy

Atrophy of the tissues around the disc occurs with age. In younger patients it is most frequently seen with myopia (i.e. myopic crescent) (*Fig.* O.6). This is usually found on the temporal side of the disc and may vary in size and extent from a thin crescent to a large atrophic area around the whole disc.

Retinal abnormalities

1. VASCULAR DISEASES

Central and branch retinal vein occlusion (Fig. O.14).
Both central and retinal vein occlusion are associated with degenerative arterial disease, systemic hypertension and conditions associated with increased whole blood viscosity, e.g. polycythaemia. Distal to the occlusion there are numerous scattered haemorrhages, dilated tortuous veins and retinal oedema. In central retinal vein occlusion the disc is oedematous. Central retinal vein occlusion is associated with severe visual loss with little prospect of visual recovery. Branch retinal vein occlusion has a much more favourable prognosis.

Central and branch retinal artery occlusion (Fig. O.15)

Arterial occlusion of the retina is most commonly embolic from carotid artery disease. The infarcted retina appears pale and the choroid appears through the thinnest area of the retina as a cherry-red spot. No visual recovery is likely. The pallor of the inner retina slowly clears and secondary atrophy of the optic disc develops.

Diabetic retinopathy (Fig. O.18)

This is a common cause of blindness and is very common in long-standing diabetes mellitus. The capilla-

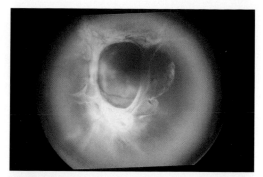

Fig. O.20. Traction retinal detachment in a diabetic.

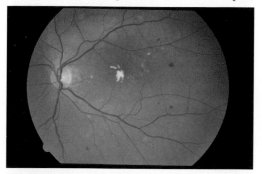

Fig. O.18. Diabetic retinopathy.

ries of the retina are involved and microaneurysms develop. Visual loss may occur due to leakage of fluid from the abnormal capillaries with the development of retinal oedema or the complications of retinal neovascularization which arise in response to widespread capillary occlusion. Such new vessels bleed easily causing vitreous haemorrhage (*Fig.* O.19) and may give rise to fibrous proliferation which may cause traction retinal detachment (*Fig.* O.20).

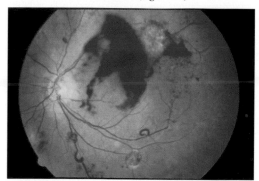

Fig. O.19. Vitreous haemorrhage in diabetes.

Hypertensive retinopathy (Fig. O.21)

Hypertension leads to secondary arterial changes with fibrous replacement of the media of small arterioles. This is readily demonstrated in the retina. The arteries become narrow and the normally transparent arterial wall becomes more visible. This appears as silver- and

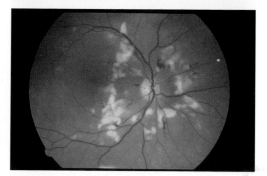

Fig. O.21. Hypertensive retinopathy.

copper-wiring and arteriovenous nipping where veins are compressed by crossing arteries. In more severe hypertension there is retinal ischaemia and loss of the integrity of the small vessels resulting in the appearance of retinal oedema exudates and cottonwool spots which can be confused with diabetic retinopathy. In malignant hypertension papilloedema is also evident.

Retinal vasculitis

There are many systemic associations with retinal vasculitis which is manifest by perivascular sheathing by inflammatory cells. Common associations are sarcoidosis and syphilis.

2.   MACULAR DISEASES

Age-related macular degeneration

This is the commonest cause of blindness in Western countries. It is due to age-related changes in the most metabolically active part of the eye, the retinal pigment epithelium. Changes occur within the retinal pigment epithelium and smaller vessels of the choroid, and the fundus changes include atrophy and clumping of the pigment and atrophy and sclerosis of the choroidal blood vessels. Drusen (hyaline deposits) between the retinal pigment epithelium and choroid also appear (*Fig.* O.22). In some patients, sudden visual loss results in haemorrhage in subretinal neovascularization. Occasionally laser treatment may halt the progress of subretinal neovascularization, otherwise no treatment is available for this condition. Patients often benefit however from low visual aids.

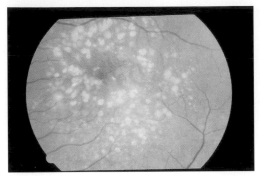

Fig. O.22. Age-related macular degeneration.

Macular oedema

Macular oedema may be caused by many disease processes all of which have in common a breakdown of the blood retinal barrier with an increase in extracellular fluid within the retina. The retinal capillary endothelium and the retinal pigment epithelium form this barrier and diseases affecting either may cause oedema with accompanying visual loss. The main causes are due to retinal vascular disease such as retinal vein occlusion and diabetic retinopathy.

3. PERIPHERAL RETINAL ABNORMALITIES

Retinal detachment

The retina may become detached from the underlying retinal pigment epithelium by various mechanisms:

1. Most commonly, fluid vitreous tracks through a break or tear in the retina progressively lifting the retina around the break. The area of detachment slowly spreads until the whole retina is detached (*Fig.* O.23). Unless the retinal break is sealed surgically the eye will be blind. Retinal breaks are most common in myopic patients and may follow trauma.

2. Traction forces from the vitreous may pull the retina off. This may occur in conditions where there is fibrous proliferation within the eye which may occur in advanced diabetic retinopathy or following penetrating injuries of the eye.

3. The retina may detach because it is pushed off either by a tumour of the underlying choroid (*Fig.* O.24) or by subretinal exudate which may complicate inflammatory choroidal disease or vascular anomalies.

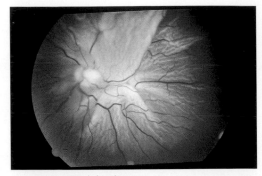

Fig. O.23. Retinal detachment.

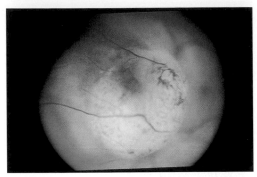

Fig. O.24. Retinal detachment due to underlying tumour.

The detached retina has a grey appearance and the retinal vessels are tortuous and thin and appear dark in colour.

Retinitis pigmentosa

This is a group of hereditary diseases affecting the photoreceptors and retinal pigment epithelium. Night blindness and constriction of the visual fields is variably progressive (tunnel vision) leading eventually to blindness. The earliest fundus changes occur in the equatorial zone with areas of hyperpigmentation (typically in a bone corpuscular pattern) which spread to involve the whole fundus. Waxy pallor of the disc and gross attenuation of the retinal arterioles are also features (*Fig.* O.25).

Choroiditis

Active choroiditis manifests itself as a greyish-white, ill-defined, slightly raised area. Overlying vitreous opacities are commonly associated with such areas of active choroiditis. When healed, the patch appears white because there is atrophy of the choroid and overlying retinal pigment epithelium. Such scars are generally surrounded by clumps of dense pigment (*Fig.* O.26).

Eales's disease

This rare disorder manifests itself as recurrent intraocular haemorrhages in young adults and is generally attributed to retinal phlebitis. Sudden obscuration of

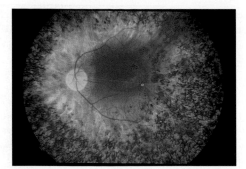

Fig. O.25. Retinitis pigmentosa.

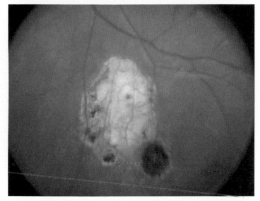

Fig. O.26. Scars from old choroiditis. (*Institute of Ophthalmology.*)

vision results from haemorrhage into the vitreous. Recurrence is the rule, and proliferative retinopathy may ensue with fibrovascular membrane formation and traction retinal detachment.

S. T. D. Roxburgh

Orthopnoea

(*See also* DYSPNOEA)

A patient is said to have orthopnoea if he experiences breathlessness especially when lying down. Most patients suffering breathlessness at rest are more comfortable in the sitting position, but a clear history of intense breathlessness in the recumbent position is particularly characteristic of left ventricular failure, mitral stenosis and other conditions which cause pulmonary venous hypertension. The paroxysmal nocturnal dyspnoea of patients with left ventricular failure is at least partly related to posture in bed. Orthopnoea, and episodic breathlessness at night, is also a common feature of asthma.

Anne Cockcroft

Otorrhoea

Otorrhoea (aural discharge) may arise from the external meatus or the middle ear itself. In rare cases discharge

of fluid may originate in nearby structures. It is important to note the duration of the discharge, whether it is continuous or intermittent, its character, colour, amount and whether it is inoffensive or offensive.

Careful aural toilet with a sucker and examination with a good light are necessary for a diagnosis.

The various causes of discharge may be listed (*Table* O.4).

Table O.4. The causes of otorrhoea

External meatus
Wax
Localized boils or furuncles
Otitis externa
   Reactive—eczematous or atopic
   Infective
     Bacterial
     Fungal
     Viral
   Malignant
Trauma—blood
Salivary fistula (rare)
Branchial fistula (very rare)

Middle ear
Acute otitis media
Chronic otitis media
   Tubotympanic otitis media
   Attic disease
Mastoiditis
Mastoid cavity infection
Tuberculosis
Malignant disease
Eosinophilic granuloma
Wegener's granuloma (very rare)
Fracture of temporal bone
   Cerebrospinal fluid
   Blood
Radionecrosis

External meatus

Wax (cerumen) is so variable in colour and consistency that it may be mistaken for other substances. It may be present in small flakes only which, by epithelial movement, are carried out of the meatus. It may collect in hard masses or may be semi-liquid and yellow in colour when it can truly be called a discharge. In children, perhaps as a result of fungal infection, the wax may form as a yellowish-grey material with the consistency of toothpaste, completely blocking the meatus and causing deafness. Keratosis obturans is a condition where wax and desquamated squamous epithelium forms an adherent mass in the bony meatus, sometimes even causing bony erosion. This condition may be associated with bronchiectasis and sinusitis. In most cases, however, wax causes no symptoms at all until water from swimming or bathing makes it swell to occlude the meatus and cause sudden deafness.

Otitis externa is a common disease and is sometimes a straightforward allergic reaction. The sorts of things that incite an allergic eczematous reaction are hairsprays, perfumes and ear drops, especially those containing neomycin. Some wax solvents can also cause enough irritation to create an eczema.

The most common cause of otitis externa, however, is a breakdown in the migratory mechanism of the skin of the deep meatus. Elsewhere in the body where skin divides, movement, clothes, friction and washing get rid of the dead skin. The external meatus is one-and-a-half inches long, therefore is not exposed to any of these factors and so a different mechanism must exist to get rid of the dead epithelium. The epithelium in the area has the property of migrating dead epithelium from the deep meatus to the wax glands in the outer half-inch of the ear canal. If, for any reason, this migratory process breaks down, then dead epithelium collects in the deep meatus. This acts as an excellent culture medium for bacteria if it is moistened with water from bathing or from a swimming pool. Secondary bacterial infection occurs and creates the symptoms of pain and discharge. Treatment consists of removing the dead epithelium and keeping the ear in a sterile condition until the migratory process recovers in a number of months.

The overuse of ear drops can lead to the fungal otitis externa. This usually presents as moist, whitish debris like damp blotting paper. *Aspergillus niger* infection will show black spots; the other common fungus is *Candida albicans*.

Two types of viral infections can cause an otitis externa. The commonest is a herpetic infection which causes severe pain and may sometimes be accompanied by facial paralysis (Ramsay–Hunt syndrome). The other type is myringitis bullosa haemorrhagica, which is often seen in conjunction with the flu virus. Blood blisters form on the drum and lead to a serosanguinous discharge and bouts of severe pain.

In many cases it is not possible, because of the oedema, to see the tympanic membrane. It is most important, however, to differentiate between otitis externa and otitis media as soon as possible and it must be remembered that as the discharge of the latter may set up a secondary otitis externa both conditions may coexist. The pain of external otitis is chiefly felt on moving the pinna, while in otitis media it is pressure above and behind the ear that is painful. If in addition to the characteristic pain the patient has good hearing and a positive Rinné test, even though the meatus may be almost completely occluded, the condition is not otitis media. If the meatus is completely blocked efforts must be made to clear a very small air passage to the drum, so that this most important differentiation can be made.

Malignant otitis externa is caused by *Ps. pyocyaneus* and is a very severe, sometimes fatal infection which occurs in elderly, immunocompromised and nearly always diabetic patients. Green purulent discharge and much oedema precede osteomyelitis of the temporal bone and base of skull.

Salivary fistula leading into the cartilaginous meatus may follow injury that involves the ear, the temporo-mandibular joint and the parotid gland. Discharge may be caused by a first branchial arch sinus, which classically communicates with the bony cartilaginous junction and may travel into the parotid and underneath the facial nerve.

Middle ear

Acute otitis media rarely gives rise to discharge until the tympanic membrane ruptures with sudden relief from pain. There may be a little blood followed by mucopurulent discharge which may be profuse and may continue for some days before (in most cases), stopping spontaneously. If the meatus is carefully cleaned the discharge will be seen to be pulsating as it comes out of the perforation. The pus is usually inoffensive and mucopurulent and the organism is a streptococcus, pneumococcus or haemophilus.

In chronic suppurative otitis media (CSOM) it is of great importance to differentiate between the safe tubotympanic otitis media and the potentially serious attic disease. Tubotympanic otitis media is often accompanied by an anterior or a central perforation of the pars tensa of the drum. There is a constant moist discharge, usually related to a blocked Eustachian tube. There is a mucositis of the mucosa of the middle ear and often an accompanying otitis externa. It is a very difficult condition to eradicate and should be kept under control with ear drops and occasional antibiotic therapy. If the perforation in the drum can be closed the ear dries up.

Attic disease is due to cholesteatoma. The origin of cholesteatoma is not known but it may be related to childhood serous otitis media that remains untreated. It is also a disease related to poor socioeconomic circumstances. It is a collection of keratin which has enzymes in its matrix that can dissolve bone. The cholesteatoma, therefore, destroys the attic region of the middle ear and can extend into the mastoid, may paralyse the facial nerve and make form a fistula into the lateral semicircular canal. It can also erode the floor of the middle fossa, causing an extradural abscess or even a brain abscess and meningitis. It is essential to make the diagnosis of cholesteatoma and have it eradicated by mastoid surgery.

Aural polyps develop from granulation tissue which, in turn, signifies an underlying osteitis of the tympanomastoid bone. Polyps may bleed easily to the touch and must be distinguished from glomus tumours.

Glomus tumours usually present, however, with no previous history of chronic otitis media where its polyps are nearly always associated with long-standing ear problems. The presence of a polyp usually indicates that the patient will have to undergo some form of mastoid surgery at some time.

Acute mastoiditis may complicate a case of acute otitis media. The mastoid air cells are filled with pus as well as the middle ear, so that if after cleaning the meatus it immediately refills with pus. Mastoid infection is now much rarer than previously because of better social environments and more aggressive treatment of ear disease in children.

Malignant disease presents with granulations in the middle ear and deep meatus and a blood-stained mucopurulent discharge. Diagnosis is by biopsy as in the case with Wegener's granuloma. Eosinophilic granuloma (or histiocytosis X) affecting the ear presents with granulomatous polyps and discharge. Osteolytic skeletal lesions in skull and elsewhere give an indication of the diagnosis but biopsy is also required.

Osteoradionecrosis occurring months or years after radiotherapy in the area of the ear may present with suppuration following sequestration of dead bone. There is also atrophy of the organ of Corti and deafness.

Blood and cerebrospinal fluid, both originating from outside the middle ear but presenting as a middle-ear discharge, may result from trauma. Simple trauma to the meatus or a ruptured drum usually bleeds slightly. The drum may be damaged by direct trauma from a penetrating injury. Otitic barotrauma, air pressure changes in diving, aircraft or bomb blast injuries, may rupture the membrane, the tear being usually in the posterior half of the drum. It may also be ruptured by syringing. More serious trauma with fractures of the temporal bone, often so fine that they do not show on X-ray, lead to bleeding and, if the meninges are torn, a cerebrospinal fluid leak.

A. G. D. Maran

Overactivity

The causes of overactivity may be classified as follows:

Common causes

Mania
Organic brain disease (*see* CONFUSION)
Delirium
Agitated depression
Anxiety neurosis
Schizophrenia
Hyperthyroidism
Hyperparathyroidism
Drugs
  Caffeine intoxication
  Withdrawal from: sedatives, hypnotics, anxiolytics, alcohol

Abuse of: hallucinogens (LSD), amphetamine, cocaine, phencyclidine
Akathisia and restless leg syndrome
Attention-deficit hyperactivity disorder in children

Less common causes

Post head injury (in children)
Anorexia nervosa
Temporal lobe epilepsy (postictal confusional state)
Neurosyphilis

Disorders of movement may frequently provide valuable clues about a diagnosis especially when a patient is confused, mute or otherwise unable to give a clear account of symptoms. Disorders of movement include *overactivity, underactivity* (*see* p. 680) and abnormal *involuntary movements*. Overactivity describes behaviour where there is an increase in physical activity, overtalkativeness and sometimes aggressiveness. The subject may make exaggerated gestures and facial expressions and at interview have difficulty in sitting still feeling impelled to move about the room, their attention easily distracted by external stimuli. This type of overactivity typically occurs in *mania* when it is associated with elevated or irritable mood, pressure of speech and flight of ideas, grandiose plans and, in severe forms, grandiose or paranoid delusions. Sleep is disturbed and patients may remain awake and active all night with apparently undiminished energy levels next morning. Libido and appetite may both be increased. Such a typical presentation of a manic illness presents few diagnostic problems especially if there is a history of previous mood swings or a family history of affective disorder. Restless overactivity may also be drug-induced or a feature of organic brain disease. Both *acute* and *chronic organic confusional states* (*see* CONFUSION) may present with irritability, restlessness and excitement and this can be particularly marked in states of *drug intoxication* and withdrawal from *alcohol and sedatives*. In the early stages of *Alzheimer's type dementia* a state may develop resembling mania and the diagnosis should be made from the history of increasing memory impairment. *Neurosyphilis* could also present in this way and associated signs such as Argyll Robertson pupils, peripheral neuropathy, and evidence of dementia combined with serological tests will confirm the diagnosis. Patients with *temporal lobe epilepsy* may rarely develop *postictal confusional states* with overactivity, irritability or senseless aggression. These episodes are usually brief and in the context of a known history of epilepsy. *Akathisia* is a particular form of restlessness found frequently in Parkinson's disease and as a side-effect of antipsychotic medication. Subjects are unable to remain still through a subjective sense of unease and restlessness. They have an urge to get up to move their feet and legs or rock the body. Restless legs may keep them awake at night and be troublesome to a partner. If caused by drugs a dose reduction may alleviate the symptom and anticholinergics should also be tried.

Overactivity may be a main presenting feature of *agitated depression* when the subject's complaint of worry is reflected in their appearance, thought content and behaviour. The person will appear restless, tense and fidgety, constantly seeking reassurance, because of feelings of guilt about the past and uncertainty about the future. Agitation may also be a principal feature of an *anxiety neurosis*, and in patients with *schizophrenia*. In all these psychiatric conditions and in physical illnesses including *hyperthyroidism* and *hypoparathyroidism*, agitation may be associated with signs of increased autonomic activity including sweating, tachycardia, palpitations, shallow breathing and gastro-intestinal disturbance.

Overactivity without significant mood disturbance can be a feature of *anorexia nervosa*. These patients will exercise relentlessly and methodically in order to keep their weight low. The exercise may take the form of housework or regular training in a gym, or various sports.

Hyperkinesis is the commonest and most disruptive sequela of *head injury* in children. Features include restlessness and impulsive disobedience at home and at school, sometimes with explosive outbursts of anger. A similar pattern of hyperactivity and resistance to discipline has been observed in children with epilepsy and after *encephalitis lethargica* although fortunately epidemic encephalitis has now largely disappeared. Both organic and psychogenic factors are involved and the pre-traumatic personality of the child and the family setting may be as important as the severity or nature of head injury. The *attention-deficit hyperactivity disorder* in children is viewed as a developmental abnormality presenting around the time the child enters school or earlier, with inappropriate degrees of inattention, impulsiveness and hyperactivity. The disorder is manifest in all situations including home, school and in play activity. There may be inappropriate running about in the classroom, fidgetyness, and over talkativeness. These children tend to be academic underachievers with low self-esteem, low mood and temper outbursts. There is an increased likelihood of 'soft' neurological signs including poor coordination. Enuresis and encopresis are more common. Children may show features of conduct disorder and impairment of social and school functioning persisting throughout childhood.

D. Blackwood

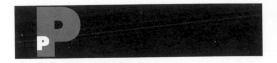

Pain, psychogenic

Pain is the commonest complaint brought to a doctor, and is probably the most complex of subjective experiences. Its primary role as an indicator of physical damage is obvious, but emotional elements heavily influence the presentation and behaviour in almost all acute and chronic pain conditions. The *pain threshold* varies little among individuals but can be readily changed by factors like drugs, emotions, activity, distraction and suggestion. The *complaint of pain and its presentation* is affected by such diverse antecedents as age, sex, social class, culture, personal and family experiences of illness, personality traits, life events and circumstances. Thus the presentation of pain as a symptom for which relief is sought frequently depends less upon severity than background factors, while the timing of presentation may be determined by prevailing circumstances. The differential diagnoses of psychogenic pain are listed in *Table* P.1.

Table P.1. Differential diagnosis of psychogenic pain

Commonest
Psychological aspects of 'organic' pain
   Alteration of the pain threshold
   Personality traits
   Life events and stresses
   Interpersonal mechanisms
   Intrapsychic mechanisms

Common
Anxiety state
Neurotic depression
Alcoholism
Drug dependence
Drug withdrawal syndrome
"Masked depression" pain syndromes, especially
   atypical facial pain
Hypochondriasis

Rare
Hysteria
Briquet's syndrome (somatization disorder)
Malingering
Cryptic organic pain
   Thalamic pain
   Migrainous neuralgia
   Basilar migraine
   Myofascial pain
   Chronic paroxysmal hemicrania
   Reflex sympathetic dystrophy
   Ectopia cerebelli
   Syndrome of painful legs and moving toes
   Causalgia
   Soft-tissue injury
Unexplained pain

Before describing the presentation of psychogenic pain it is necessary to review the *roles of pain* beyond its strictly sensory response. Pain is a very powerful method of expression which is utilized in various ways. *Interpersonal mechanisms* include securing gains, control or help: pain features prominently in sick role (illness) behaviour attracting attention and care from others, avoiding responsibilities within the family or at work, earning a living through allowances, benefits and compensation. In the psychosexually immature, pain may prove an effective means of engaging/disengaging the opposite sex, while in some marriages stability may only be maintained if the couple relate to each other through adopting carer–invalid roles, the 'pain full' marriage. Pain also mediates *intrapsychic mechanisms*, as a method of coping with other powerful unpleasant feelings. Chronic pain may be suffering self-imposed by an individual seeking to atone for a mistake: identification in mourning or following serious illness in a loved one may lead to a sharing of the pain and protection from the full impact of loss or anticipated loss; finally pain is closely tied psychoanalytically to anger and hostility, and for some individuals unable to ventilate those feelings, pain may be the product of suppression.

The other psychological component common to all pains is *personality*, with traits exerting various influences upon presentation. Anxiousness exacerbates pain through heightened awareness and direct tensing actions, and this in turn increases anxiety. Depressiveness also increases the awareness of pain and reduces the ability to cope, although sometimes the opposite occurs. The pain-prone personality encapsulates a group of individuals who can only relate and cope through suffering; depressiveness accompanied by pessimism, stoicism and masochism are the cardinal traits identified in this minority of cases. Much more frequently encountered are obsessional and hypochondriacal traits where the experience of pain is dwelt upon and emphasized, and hysterical and somatizing traits where pain experience and behaviour is exaggerated; such individuals are typically more aware, more demonstrative, more persistent and/or more communicative about their pain than is normal.

That all pains are influenced, or have the potential to be influenced by personality, and can be employed for functions other than their obvious role makes a nonsense of the traditional dichotomy that has been imposed between organic and psychogenic pain. However, notwithstanding the artificiality of this division the evaluation of how much of the presentation is psychogenically determined can be assisted by considering the features of the symptom that characterize a psychological element (*see Table* P.2).

A practical problem arising from the organic–psychogenic pain dichotomy is that some cases do not fit either category. The assumption that because a pain does not have an established physical

Table P.2. Characteristics of psychogenic pain

Precipitant
Absent; trivial; life event

Onset
Often vague

Site
Indefinite, poorly localized or fluctuating
Does not adhere to recognized clinical distribution
May be the site of previous damage
May lie on rather than in the body

Description
Can be bizarre but more often unclear, atypical and changing
Several sorts of pain plus other changes of sensation not uncommon
Behaviour and disability incongruous with description

Sleep
Usually unaffected by pain

Exacerbating factors
May be aggravated by a wide range of differing stimuli—or may be completely uninfluenced

Relieving factors
Rarely responds to standard treatments (such as rest, heat or analgesics)—indeed these may exacerbate the pain
Often completely unresponsive to interventions, sometimes helped by unusual therapies

Associated psychological factors
Emotional reactions often denied or minimized.
Emotional response may be excessive for circumstances

Clinical findings
Over-reaction to examination or the prospect of examination
Increased sensitivity to light touch or gentle pressure
Fluctuating, inconsistent findings
Inappropriate reports of pain on pseudo testing
Limitations evident on direct examination disappear when patient undertakes normal activity: may require distraction techniques to elicit

basis it is necessarily psychogenic—or even worse 'imaginary'—reflects misplaced confidence in our technical capabilities and more importantly, risks doing the patient a gross disservice. The 'not proven' verdict should be invoked more than it is with *unexplained pain* differentiated from psychogenic pain which is a diagnosis based upon positive findings and not solely by exclusion of organic possibilities.

Psychological aspects of pain should be considered routinely in three clinical situations.

1. When there is an *established physical cause for the pain but an exaggerated, prolonged or abnormal response*, the personality and background of the patient and any functions the pain may mediate require evaluation. Sometimes the explanation may be determined by cultural factors such as mourning or childbirth practices, while in other cases a superimposed emotional disorder may be diagnosed, but most frequently the answer lies in function and/or personality. Once identified, management should take such factors into

account, and not pursue uncritically the path of escalating analgesia.

2. Pain frequently presents in the setting of a *primary psychiatric disorder* being associated most notably with states of excessive anxiety. Anxiety generates muscle tension and may thus directly cause tension headaches, neck stiffness, chest pain, back pain and limb muscle pains. Anxiety probably also contributes to the aetiology of some common pain-associated syndromes like temporomandibular joint syndrome, irritable bowel syndrome and premenstrual tension, as well exacerbating or precipitating organic pains such as migraine, angina pectoris, ulcerative colitis and peptic ulcer. Hysteria, malingering and hypochondriasis can all present with pain, most frequently sited on the head or lower back, then the abdomen and next the pelvis in women and chest in men. Feigned pain to obtain opiates is a ploy adopted by drug addicts, while musculoskeletal and abdominal pain commonly occur in drug-withdrawal states, real or simulated. In alcohol dependence calf pain and burning soles of the feet typically indicate a peripheral neuropathy. Pain is very rarely reported as a psychotic phenomenon in either schizophrenia or major depression, indeed there is evidence that pain is reported less frequently in these disorders.

3. Finally there are *the presentations of pain which are unexplained by physical and psychological evaluation*. Such cases may require further specialist assessment to consider causes that are difficult to establish, for example thalamic pain, basilar migraine, migrainous neuralgia, myofascial pain, chronic paroxysmal hemicrania, reflex sympathetic dystrophy and ectopia cerebelli—and sometimes impossible to confirm, for example causalgia, and various soft-tissue injuries. In these circumstances trials of treatment may be worth implementing when suspicions are raised but convincing evidence is not forthcoming.

Treatment response has also proved the basis by which an interesting group of pain conditions has been identified. The fact that it is antidepressant treatment has led to these disorders being regarded as psychogenic—masked depressions or depressive equivalents, in spite of major depressive disorder being diagnosed in only 13 per cent of cases in one large study and the analgesic action of these drugs being unrelated to the presence of depressive features and also evident in true neuropathies such as in diabetes. The commonest presentation is *atypical facial pain*, a usually unilateral, deep, boring, continuous pain located in the cheek and around the orbit; other characteristic presentations are in the mouth and on the tongue or lips (oral dysaesthesia) where the pain is usually burning in character and associated with altered sensation, a bad taste and reduced production of saliva; atypical toothache (odontalgia) and on the perineum or scrotum, where adjectives like tugging, drawing, burning, stretching, and boring are frequently applied. Even when depressive mood, ideation and outlook are inapparent these patients frequently give an account of social withdrawal, loss of interests and pleasures in life, their pain occasionally exhibits diurnal variation and sometimes early morning wakening is present. A family or personal history of depression is elicited more often than would be expected by chance and, untreated, there is a significant risk of suicide. Compared with other psychogenic and unexplained pain syndromes these patients are more frequently women who are peri- or postmenopausal, they have fewer life stresses and a good premorbid personality, and their pain serves no obvious function. While these conditions remain poorly understood and potentially dangerous if unidentified, their response to antidepressant medication is gratifyingly frequent and complete, so paradoxically the outlook is generally better than in many other presentations.

George Masterton

Pallor

Pallor is a very subjective sign indicating a reduction in skin or mucous membrane colouring. It usually refers to a generalized reduction rather than localized depigmentation as in vitaligo.

Pallor may be a congenital characteristic resulting in an individual always looking pale even when healthy.

Anaemia, for any reason, is the commonest cause of pallor. Pallor of the conjunctivae or mucous membranes is a very unreliable indication of a reduced haemoglobin except when there is severe anaemia. Pallor may be accentuated in hypopituitarism when in addition to the anaemia there is a reduction in skin pigmentation.

A reduction in blood flow to the skin will result in acute pallor. This can arise either due to hypotension as in shock or due to hypothermia.

Any increase in the thickness of the skin, particularly the epidermis will tend to obscure the haemoglobin in the capillaries resulting in pallor. Skin thickness is increased in acromegaly and myxoedema.

C. A. Ludlam

Panic

Panic is an extreme form of anxiety characterized by (1) severe, acute, brief attacks and (2) the feeling of loss of personal control. The symptoms are predominantly the somatic (especially cardiovascular) features of anxiety and hyperventilation so that a primarily physical presentation is common. The emotions experienced are stark and distressing: terror, fear of dying, going mad or losing control. Attacks may be triggered by specific stimuli or be unpredictable and life frequently becomes dominated by the apprehension of the acute distress and helplessness engendered. Panic attacks are common, occurring at some time in 10 per cent of the adult population and to a persistently disabling degree in one in five of those affected. The causes of panic are listed in *Table* P.3.

Table P.3. Causes of panic

Commonest
Normal
Stress related
Anxiety
? Primary panic disorder

Less common
Drugs
   Stimulants
   Hallucinogens
Drug withdrawal
Physical disorders
   Hyperthyroidism
   Hypoglycaemia
   Phaeochromocytoma
   Carcinoid syndrome
   Asthma
   Menière's disease
   Temporal lobe epilepsy
   Migraine
Psychiatric disorders
   Phobia
   Depression
   Chronic hyperventilation syndrome
   Post-traumatic stress disorder

Rare
(as for ANXIETY *see* p. 29)

There are a number of *physical conditions* which enter the differential diagnosis. Hyperthyroidism and phaeochromocytoma can mimic closely while, particularly in a diabetic or partial gastrectomy patient, the possibility of hypoglycaemia should be excluded. Other episodic medical conditions that can be confused with somatic presentations of panic attacks are migraine, Menière's disease, temporal lobe epilepsy and carcinoid syndrome. Not uncommonly patients with these conditions develop genuine panic attacks as an emotional reaction to the uncertainty they experience: they may begin to report symptom differences between attacks which can confound the physician unless he is aware of the possibility of a superimposed panic disorder. In addition to the symptom content, the brief duration of panic attacks (usually lasting a few minutes) is a pointer in distinguishing panic from most physical disorders.

Panic attacks are frequently predominant features in the setting of other *psychological conditions*. In phobias panic is often experienced when exposed to the phobic stimulus, but anticipating or even thinking about exposure may trigger panic. Panic attacks occur, and may occasionally be the presenting complaint in depressive illness, or develop subsequently during recovery; episodes occurring regularly early in the day are a clue, but usually there are readily identifiable features of depressive change evident in the history and mental state. Hyperventilation may be involved in the development of panic attacks, and may also be exacerbated by them.

Panic attacks are induced by stimulants, both illicit drugs like amphetamine and cocaine and the socially acceptable caffeine—a note of coffee consumption is worth taking. Drug withdrawal also precipitates episodes, perhaps most commonly implicated are the benzodiazepines.

Finally the relationship between *anxiety* and panic is disputed. It is evident that patients who suffer from generalized 'free floating' anxiety are likely to experience panic attacks of varying degree and frequency, while patients having panic attacks get appreciably anxious about these alarming experiences, and commonly develop a secondary chronic anxiety state or agoraphobia. The controversy stems from the American view that panic disorder is a separate diagnostic entity, based essentially on the discovery that tricyclic antidepressant drugs have a specific anti-panic action in patients without clinically apparent depression. While British psychiatry has not yet cleaved panic from anxiety, panic attacks have now become regarded as a distinct focus for research and if putative differences in inheritance, pathophysiology, natural history and treatment responses are confirmed, the status of panic is likely to change from a subcategory of anxiety to independence as an emotional disorder.

George Masterton

Papules

Papules are solid, circumscribed elevations of the skin up to the size of a split pea (5 mm). Similar lesions, if larger, are nodules (*see* pp. 458, 601) or tumours. Papules are usually round or oval in shape but they may be irregular and in lichen planus are polygonal. Their colour can vary and may be white, red, brown, yellow or violaceous. Their profile may be domed, pointed or flat-topped, and their surface smooth, warty or scaly. Papules may be transitional lesions, becoming vesicles or growing into nodules and tumours, or breaking down into ulcers (*Table* P.4).

White or pearly papules

Milia are tiny firm papules filled with white solid material, most often found on the face and, once

Table P.4. Papules

White	Yellow
Milia	Xanthelasmas (Fig. C.13)
Keratosis pilaris	Naevoxanthoendothelioma
Phrynoderma	Pseudoxanthoma elasticum
Molluscum	Sebaceous adenoma
contagiosum.	Fordyce's disease
Syringomas	
Lipoid proteinosis	

Brown	Red
Acrochrodia (skin tags)	Guttate psoriasis (Fig. P.6)
(Fig. P.1)	Pityriasis lichenoides
Viral warts	chronica
Seborrhoeic warts	Pityriasis lichenoides acuta
Plane warts	Pityriasis rosea
Venereal viral warts	Acne vulgaris
Lichen amyloidosis	Dermatitis (Fig. P.21)
Darier's disease (Fig. P.2)	Eczema
Acanthosis nigricans	Lichen simplex chronicus
Dermatosis papulosa	Papular syphilide
nigra (Fig. P.3)	Campbell de Morgan spots
Tuberous sclerosis (Figs.	Angiokeratoma of Fordyce
P.4, P.5)	

Violaceous
Lichen planus (Fig. P.7)
Kaposi's sarcoma (Fig. A.19)
Malignant melanoma (Fig. S.27)
Blue naevus

present, persist until incised. They may also follow blister formation (e.g. porphyria cutanea tarda and epidermolysis bullosa). They consist of keratin.

Keratosis pilaris is a common condition of children and young adults and consists of rough firm white papules, approximately one mm in diameter, found over the lateral upper arm and the anterior thighs above the knees. The buttocks are occasionally involved. They give the skin a nutmeg grater-like feeling, and are occasionally surrounded by an inflammatory halo. They are caused by keratin plugs in the ostia of hair follicles. The development of keratosis pilaris is determined by a dominant gene and the condition is closely related to ichthyosis and atopic dermatitis. It can also occur in vitamin A deficiency (*phrynoderma*).

Molluscum contagiosum occurs as pearly white or skin-coloured papules, 2–10 mm in diameter. They have a smooth shiny surface with central umbilication. In children, especially atopics, lesions may be widespread on the face and limbs; in adults they are more common around the genitals and should be suspected when chronic inflammatory lesions appear at this site. They are caused by a DNA virus of the pox group and are spread by auto-inoculation, hence their frequently clustered grouping.

Syringomas usually occur on the upper cheeks just below the eyes as smooth white oval papules 2–4 mm in length. Lesions accumulate over the years, and must be differentiated from *xanthelasmas* which are yellower and larger. In *lipoid proteinosis* pearly translu-

cent white papules occur widely on mucous membranes and skin, particularly the eyelid margins.

Brown papules

Viral warts are a common cause of brown skin-coloured papules, and occur particularly over the dorsa of fingers and on the soles. Flat *plane warts* can also occur on the backs of hands and may form subtle tan papules over the chin and cheeks, especially in young women. They must be differentiated from *basal-cell papillomas* (seborrhoeic warts) which occur at an older age, and are more profuse on the trunk than on the limbs or face. These warty lesions grow to form large brown plaques but they begin as light brown tiny verrucous papules scattered widely on the chest and back.

Venereal viral warts are usually small, brown, flat-topped and smooth with an angular outline, in contrast to *condylomata acuminata* seen in secondary syphilis, where extensive crops of soft, skin-coloured or pink pedunculated papules or nodules, covered with tiny moist papillary projections, occur on the genitalia, scrotum and peri-anal region (and also between the toes and at the angles of the mouth). The serology will be positive.

An *acrochrodion* (skin tag) (*Fig.* P.1) is a tiny brown pedunculated soft papule with a narrow neck found in the flexures of patients from middle age onwards. Lesions may be numerous around the neck, axillae and groins. They are more profuse in the obese and are particularly marked in *acanthosis nigricans* (*See* p. 600). In *Darier's disease* papules are brownish, perifollicular, and covered by a brown-grey crust (*Fig.* P.2). Papules may be grouped or accumulate into sheets, and the sites of predilection are the seborrhoeic areas of scalp, behind the ears, naso-labial folds, mid-back and interscapular regions. They may be crusty on the scalp, and vegetating in the intertrigenous areas. Palmar pits and notching of the nails are common. The disease often flares during the summer months and is dominantly inherited.

Dermatosis papulosa nigra is the rather grand and cumbersome title of tiny common jet black papules over the cheeks of Negroes (*Fig.* P.3). In *lichen amyloidosis* multiple, closely spaced, uniform, rounded, hard papules, that may be red, brown or skin-coloured, occur over the anterior shins or rarely more widely. The lesions are intensely pruritic, resistant to treatment and not associated with systemic amyloidosis. Even more rare are the brown skin-coloured papules crowded around the nose seen in *tuberous sclerosis* (*Fig.* P.4) the so-called *adenoma sebaceum of Pringle*. These usually begin in childhood and may be associated

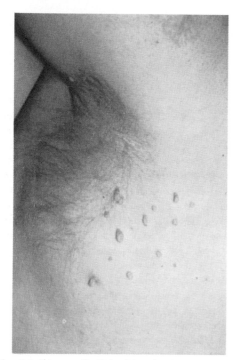

Fig. P.1. Skin tags. (*Dr Richard Staughton.*)

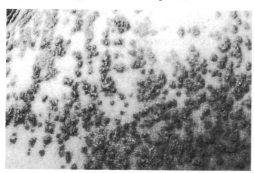

Fig. P.2. Darier's disease.

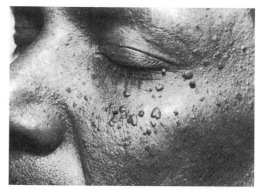

Fig. P.3. Dermatosis papulosa nigra.

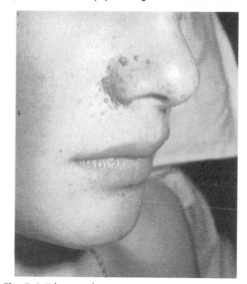

Fig. P.4. Tuberous sclerosis.

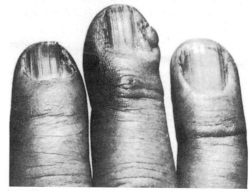

Fig. P.5. Periungual fibromas associated with tuberous sclerosis.

with mental deficiency, epilepsy, tumours and cysts of kidneys and cardiac and periungal fibromas (*Fig*. P.5).

Violaceous papules

Flat-topped shiny polygonal papules are the hallmark of *lichen planus* (*Fig*. P.7). The colour is characteristically lilac-pink. The papules are smooth and not crusted and may be crossed by tiny white lines known as 'Wickham's striae'. Papules are intensively irritating and may appear in areas of skin damage, the Köbner phenomenon. The eruption is usually symmetrical, particularly on the flexural aspects of wrists and fore-arms, anterior and inner aspects of calves and ankles, and over the upper abdomen and lumbar region. In Caucasians a delicate white lace-like pattern is common on the buccal mucosa and this is an important diagn-ostic sign. Similar lesions may be present on other mucous membranes (medial aspect of labia majora, glans penis). Lesions may be simulated by a lichenoid drug eruption. This was particularly common during the Second World War; when all troops were given mepacrine as an antimalarial, a proportion developed an eruption identical to idiopathic lichen planus. Antidiabetic drugs, beta blockers and gold have also been implicated in lichenoid eruptions. A unique contact-allergic reaction to chemicals used in the colour developing process can produce a lichen planus-like eruption on the hands and wrists of those working in the industry.

Dark blue or blue-black papules or nodules can be due to *blue naevus, melanoma* or *Kaposi's sarcoma*. A blue naevus most commonly occurs on the hands, forearms or face and the lesion is sharply outlined and usually less than 1 cm in diameter. It has an oval contour and is firm on palpation. The lesions remain unchanged over many years. A *malignant melanoma*, rare before puberty, by contrast grows either horizontally (superficial spreading melanoma) or vertically (nodular melanoma). Pigmentation is often variegate and may diffuse into the surrounding skin (pigment spillage). Lesions may ulcerate and very occasionally may be fleshy and amelanotic. Regional lymphadenopathy, diffuse melanosis and melanuria are late findings. In *multiple idiopathic haemorrhagic sarcoma of Kaposi (See Fig. A.19)* purplish macules appear usually over the feet and ankles of elderly patients of Jewish or Italian lineage. Gradually lesions become elevated to form multiple papules and later soft nodules, plaques and angiomatous tumours. They may ulcerate, bleed and crust. A more generalized, aggressive and metastasizing form of the disease is endemic in East Africa and has been seen increasingly in AIDS sufferers in the last decade.

Yellow papules

Xanthelasmas are found on the upper cheeks and eyelids in middle-aged men and women. Investigation should exclude hyperlipidaemia, coronary artery disease, diabetes, myxoedema or primary biliary cirrhosis. *Naevoxanthoendothelioma* (juvenile xanthogranuloma) occur as rounded yellow firm papules or nodules over extensor surfaces within a few weeks of birth. They involute spontaneously in 1–3 years and are not associated with underlying lipid abnormalities. The skin of the neck and axillae may be covered in sheets of yellowish papules in *pseudoxanthoma elasticum*. This is inherited as an autosomal recessive condition and is a generalized defect of support tissue. There may be associated tears in Bruch's membrane in the eye and aneurysms of small and large arteries.

Tiny yellow papules on the face and forehead of older people can be caused by *sebaceous adenoma*. They are usually flat-topped with an erythematous halo and a tiny central depression. They must be differentiated from molluscum contagiosum, which are more rapidly growing and numerous, and early basal-cell carcinoma, which is more translucent in colour and is associated with telangiectasia and slow growth with ulceration. Discrete tiny yellow papules 1–2 mm in diameter can be due to ectopic sebaceous glands visible on lips or mucous membranes, penis and vulva—*Fordyce's disease*.

Red papules

Several of the commoner skin diseases have papular elements or a papular stage in their evolution, e.g. psoriasis, acne, dermatitis and chickenpox, *Psoriasis* (*see* SCALY ERUPTIONS p. 583) may present as myriads of tiny flat, pink papules scattered widely over the body and limbs; this cutaneous reaction pattern is known as *guttate psoriasis* (Fig. P.6) and may follow a streptococcal infection. This eruption occurs in adolescence and may clear over a few weeks, but papules can amalgamate into the more characteristic plaques. *Pityriasis lichenoides chronica* produces lesions somewhat like guttate psoriasis but with more confluent papules. Each is surmounted by a mica-like scale which can be detached en masse. This occurs in young individuals and may persist for months or even years; an acute form (pityriasis lichenoides acuta) exists where chickenpox-like inflammatory lesions predominate, though mixed forms exist. The eruption of *pityriasis rosea* occurs over the T-shirt area (trunk, upper arms and tops of thighs) and the elements run in Lange's lines of cleavage resulting in the typical 'Christmas tree' arrangement of dozens of oval, salmon-coloured macules. These scale from within outwards, leaving a characteristic collarette of scale near their margins. The eruption is often preceded by a 'herald patch', which is a larger, but otherwise typical lesion, often situated on the trunk. Sometimes, especially in coloured children, the lesions may be more papular, not unlike lichen planus or papular syphilide.

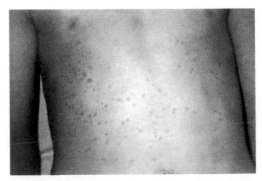

Fig. P.6. Guttate psoriasis. (*Dr Richard Staughton.*)

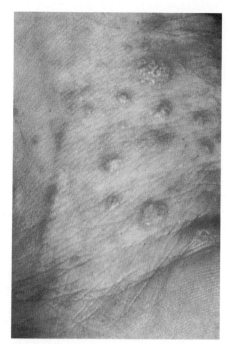

Fig. P.7. lichen planus. (*Westminster Hospital.*)

Comedones are the cardinal signs of *acne vulgaris* and these may progress to papules, pustules, cysts and scars. Consequently the lesions of acne vulgaris are follicular and this differentiates them from the papules of rosacea which are not.

Dermatitis and *eczema* often have a papular phase before the lesions progress to vesicles and weeping. When eczema becomes chronic, the skin becomes thickened and leathery with exaggerated skin markings (lichenification). In *lichen simplex chronicus* which has some eczematous features, large oval patches of skin-coloured lichenified papules are seen on the typical areas (nape of neck, ankles and perineum) (*Fig.* P.7.) The condition is most common in women between the ages of 30 and 50 and is severely pruritic.

In a *papular syphilide* papules are shiny or scaly but the colour is of a copper-red hue. The palms, soles and forehead are particularly affected and there is no pruritus. Other features of secondary syphilis may be present, e.g. fever, lymphadenopathy, patchy alopecia (*see* p. 17) and 'snail-track' erosions in the mouth and genital areas.

Campbell de Morgan spots are cherry-red and smooth-surfaced. They can be seen in most elderly people on the trunk and proximal parts of the limbs. Similar but slightly smaller and scaly lesions are *angiokeratoma*; these are common on the scrotum of old patients (angiokeratoma of Fordyce) and rare in the bathing trunk distribution in Anderson–Fabry disease.

Richard Staughton

Paranoid disorders

The causes of paranoid disorders are listed below:

Sleep deprivation
Severe stress (hospital/prison)
Immigrant status
Paranoid personality
Organic mental disorder
    Alzheimer's type dementia
    Multi-infarct dementia
    Huntington's chorea
    Brain tumour
    Temporal lobe epilepsy
    Drug abuse (amphetamines, cocaine, phencyclidine, cannabis)
Deafness (especially in the elderly)
Alcohol-induced psychosis
Hypothyroidism
Cushing's syndrome
Mania
Depressive illness
Schizophrenia
Monosymptomatic delusions

In everyday language paranoid ideas are considered synonymous with unpleasant persecutory ideas. However, in a stricter sense the word paranoid denotes *self reference* so that paranoid delusions may be persecutory, grandiose or hypochondriacal. The majority of paranoid beliefs do involve ideas of persecution taking the form of delusions or over-valued ideas and these have little diagnostic significance. Ideas of persecution develop in normal individuals deprived of sleep or at times of great stress. Quite commonly they may be a transient phenomena in immigrants living in a new and strange environment without home supports, suffering from 'culture shock'. Other predisposing factors include deafness especially when accompanied by failing physical powers and loneliness in the elderly although curiously blindness does not appear to be such a strong predisposing factor as deafness. Paranoid ideas may become more evident as age advances in individuals who have long-standing personality traits of undue sensitivity and wariness in relationships. Such people may have few friends and social supports. There is a tendency for those with paranoid illnesses to be single, divorced or widowed, perhaps because they tend to be 'loners'. Simple persecutory delusions may occur in the early stages of a dementia or due to a brain tumour or drug abuse particularly with stimulants such as amphetamines.

In paranoid disorders the following delusional themes are frequently encountered: erotic, grandiose, jealous, persecutory and somatic. When organic brain disease, drugs, social isolation, severe sensory deprivation in old age have been excluded as causes, the clinician should look for mood change to suggest depressive or manic aetiology, and assess the presence of features such as hallucinations and thought disorder which might indicate a schizophrenic illness.

There will remain a perplexing group of patients expressing strange paranoid beliefs who defy a classical diagnosis. These patients may present in middle age with clear-cut delusions of persecution and reference but no other symptoms to give a clue as to the underlying diagnosis. Treatment should be with antipsychotic medication and in some cases the diagnosis will be clarified by follow-up when affective or schizophrenic symptoms may then be manifest. However, a group of patients will continue over the years to consistently report *monosymptomatic delusions of a paranoid nature* without showing deterioration in other aspects of their mental life. The term 'paraphrenia' is sometimes used for paranoid illness presenting for the first time in middle or old age. *Erotomania (de Clerambault syndrome)* describes a paranoid illness usually in women who develop an unshakeable conviction that a man, usually an authority figure, is in love with her, and may develop elaborate erotic delusions and cause considerable social disruption in attempting to come to the attention of the object of her feelings. It is commonly associated with schizophrenic or affective psychosis. In *delusional jealousy* a spouse will become unreasonably suspicious concerning their partner's fidelity. It takes the form of an overvalued idea when the subject can be temporarily reasoned out of their conviction or it may be held with delusional intensity when, despite evidence to the contrary, the spouse remains intensely jealous and preoccupied. Morbid jealousy sometimes is associated with alcoholism, schizophrenia and affective illness, it may occur in psychopathic persons and sometimes the absence of any other psychiatric pathology. The symptom is a cause of domestic violence and not infrequently homicide.

Hypochondriacal delusions similarly are a common presenting symptom in schizophrenia and in depressive illness but they may be the only feature of a chronic paranoid illness in which the subject will be convinced of infestation of the skin by insects, or their bowel by worms, that their body gives off a bad smell, or that part of their body is not working (intestines, the stomach or brain) or is not there at all (nihilistic delusions). The patient's preoccupation may centre around the teeth, gums, mouth and face and until the delusional quality of the belief is recognized it may lead to excessive medical and surgical referrals and requests for investigations. These delusions may be accompanied by social phobias if the abnormal belief includes a conviction that part of the body is deformed or to sexual difficulties if the delusions relate to the sexual organs.

In *Capgras syndrome* the patient becomes convinced that someone close to them, often a spouse, has been replaced by a double who resembles the spouse in appearance but is really an imposter. This is most commonly a symptom in a schizophrenic illness.

An unusual feature of paranoid psychosis is that in rare instances paranoid beliefs are contagious and are taken up by the healthy partner of the psychotic patient. This particularly occurs if the partner is relatively isolated and dependent on the sick person who often has paranoid schizophrenia. A *folie à deux* situation may persist for years maintaining stability in the partnership each reinforcing the other's beliefs. Separation leads to complete loss by the normal partner of the paranoid ideas.

D. Blackwood

Paraplegia

Paralysis of both legs may occur with damage to any part of the neural pathways between the motor cortex supplying the legs and the muscles of the legs themselves. In practice paraplegia most commonly results from disorders of the spinal cord, spinal roots or peripheral nerves. If the onset is acute it can be difficult to distinguish spinal from neuropathic paralysis because the initial spinal shock results in the abolition of reflexes and is associated with flaccidity. In acute spinal cord disorders with damage to the corticospinal tracts the paralysis affects all muscles below a given level and it is often associated with sensory loss below the same level. Frequently there is accompanying bladder and bowel paresis.

In peripheral nerve disorders motor weakness tends to involve the distal muscles of the legs rather than the proximal ones and sphincter function is usually spared. Sensory loss, if present, is also more prominent in the distal parts of the limbs.

For clinical purposes it is helpful to separate the acute paraplegias from the chronic. The former should always receive urgent attention, otherwise neurological damage, in particular loss of sphincter control, may become permanent even in surgically remediable conditions. It should be noted that in several disorders, for example multiple sclerosis and spinal cord compression, the onset of paraplegia may be either sudden or gradual.

The most common cause of acute paraplegia is spinal cord trauma usually combined with fracture-dislocation of the spine. Spontaneous haematomyelia or spinal cord infarction resulting from thrombosis of one of the arteries supplying the spinal cord are less common causes. Postinfectious myelitis, acute demyelination and epidural abscess or tumour with spinal cord compression, tend to develop rather more slowly, usually over hours, days or even longer. Epidural or subdural haemorrhage from bleeding disorders or anticoagulant therapy may cause acute paraplegia, often associated with severe pain. Loss of power in the legs due to acute poliomyelitis or acute idiopathic postinfectious polyneuritis may at times be very difficult to distinguish from that resulting from spinal cord pathology.

In adults, multiple sclerosis, subacute combined degeneration, spinal cord compression from tumours, cervical discs and cervical spondylosis, epidural abscess, motor neurone disease, syringomyelia and degenerative disease of the lateral columns represent the most frequently encountered forms of spinal paraplegia of gradual onset. Several varieties of polyneuropathy and polymyositis must also be considered in the differential diagnosis of such paraplegias. Parasagittal tumours compressing bilaterally the motor cortex representing both legs are another rare and readily overlooked cause of paraplegia. Finally, the possibility that paraplegia is a manifestation of hysterical illness should be borne in mind.

D. A. Shaw

Pelvis, pain in

In practice, pelvic pain can usually be classified under six headings, namely:

(1) *Deep-seated pain*;
(2) *Referred pain*;
(3) *Spasmodic pain*;
(4) *Backache or sacralgia*;
(5) *Mid-cycle ovulation pain (Mittelschmerz)*;
(6) *Pain related to varicosity*.

All women at some time experience pelvic pain associated with events such as menstruation, ovulation or sexual intercourse. Although only a few women seek medical advice for such pain, it is the commonest reason for laparoscopy examination in the UK. In many of these cases a cause is not found. It is recognized that the incidence of anxiety and depression is high in women with unexplained pelvic and abdominal pain but it is necessary to carry out a detailed examination to exclude the other causes of pain.

1. DEEP-SEATED PAIN is aching in character, continuous, and may be acute in onset or chronic in duration. It is the result of congested blood vessels and oedema of the pelvic organs, most commonly the result of inflammation. In acute inflammation the pain is severe, elicited by lower abdominal pressure and thereby made worse. Infection of the pelvic organs gives rise to *local peritonitis*, and hence the severe pain. Chronic dull aching pain is caused by chronic salpingo-oophoritis (pyosalpinx, hydrosalpinx, ovarian abscess or chronic

interstitial salpingitis), whether gonococcal, tuberculous or pyogenic in origin or following labour or abortion, by endometriosis of the ovaries and by chronic pelvic appendicitis or diverticulitis. It may also occur as the result of infection of the pelvic cellular tissue, parametritis, following labour or abortion. More severe pain may be due to a twisted or infected or ruptured ovarian cyst or to a ruptured ectopic pregnancy.

Sometimes there is no evidence of infection or other disease to account for chronic pelvic pain. Although congestion due to unrelieved sexual stimulation is suggested as the reason there are not always good grounds for saying this. It is unlikely that retroversion or retroflexion of the uterus causes pelvic pain; they may occasionally give rise to backache. Culdocentesis (puncture and aspiration of the pouch of Douglas), ultrasound scanning and laparoscopy are used to diagnose pelvic lesions, but generally a careful history and examination make such procedures unnecessary. When no lesion is found but the patient still complains these procedures may be used to exclude pathology.

2. REFERRED PAIN may appear to arise in the pelvis when the true cause lies elsewhere, pain being referred through spinal segments T10–L3, as, for instance, from a spinal tumour, or in tabes dorsalis.

3. SPASMODIC PAIN in the pelvis is nearly always due to painful uterine contractions when it is of genital origin. The exception to this is the spasmodic pain which occurs in connection with *tubal gestation*, as a rule in the few days which precede tubal abortion or rupture of the tube. The only way to diagnose between this tubal pain and that due to uterine contractions is by a careful consideration of the history of the case, and the finding of a definite tubal swelling by bimanual palpation. Even then the diagnosis may be difficult. Laparoscopy is indicated when doubt persists. Spasmodic pain due to *uterine contractions* is caused by: the onset of abortion or labour; spasmodic dysmenorrhoea (p. 157); attempted expulsion from the uterus of a growth such as a fibromyoma; 'after-pains' following labour; the presence of a contraceptive device in the uterus.

The differential diagnosis of these conditions is easy, but it may be difficult to be sure that the pelvic pain has a uterine origin, for sometimes spasmodic pain may be referred to the pelvis from such relatively distant causes as appendicitis, intestinal, renal or bilary colic, leaking gastric ulcer, ruptured tubal gestation, twisted ovarian pedicle, haemorrhage into a Graafian follicle, leakage or rupture of an ovarian cyst or pyosalpinx, dyspepsia or flatulent distension of the bowels.

4. BACKACHE or SACRALGIA is a common complaint in many cases of pelvic disease, but as a sole symptom

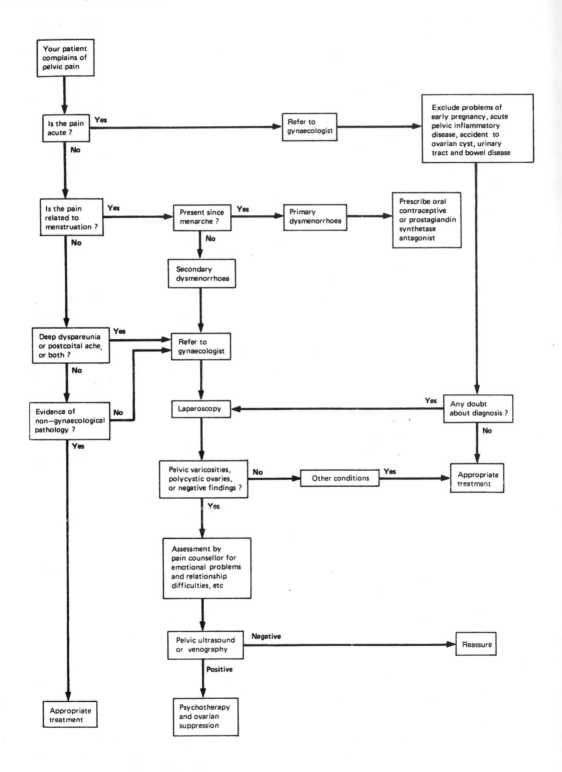

Fig. P.8. Algorithm for diagnosis of pelvic pain. (Reproduced with permission from Beard R. W. *et al.* (1986)) Pelvic pain in women. (*British Medical Journal* **293**, 1161)

is most unlikely to be due to a pelvic lesion. It is true that in such cases the pain may be worse at the time of menstruation but the same applies to those cases which have an orthopaedic origin. Before the pelvic contents can be suspected there should be present other symptoms of pelvic disease, and it will be found, almost invariably, that the backache is only a secondary or minor complaint. The presence of such conditions as (1) a heavy congested retroverted uterus with prolapse; (2) large, or impacted ovarian or fibroid tumours; (3) a retroverted gravid uterus impacted in the pelvis; (4) a pelvic haematocele; (5) pelvic endometriosis or chronic salpingo-oophoritis make the association more likely, particularly if the backache is low down. Most backaches in women are at a high level in the small of the back or lumbar region and are of orthopaedic origin; pain arising in the pelvic organs is at a lower level in the back, over the sacrum. Sometimes a large cervical erosion with surrounding parametritis is the only finding, and in many of these cases adequate treatment of the erosion cures the backache. Pelvic congestion, the result of coitus interruptus or other unsatisfactory sexual relationship, particularly if a retroversion is present, may be responsible. A backwardly displaced uterus, however, without some other complicating factor is hardly ever the cause of backache. In some cases where slight prolapse is present in addition, if the uterus is replaced and a ring inserted, the backache will be cured. Dyspareunia is often present in such cases owing to the prolapse of one or both ovaries. The back should be examined and any abnormal posture, limitation of movement, tenseness of the back muscles or tender areas should be noted. In such cases an orthopaedic cause is more likely, although a pelvic cause may be responsible for the assumption of abnormal postures to secure comfort. In cases of impacted tumours the pain may be due to actual pressure on the sacral nerves at their exits, in which case pain will be felt down the inner sides of the thighs and back of the legs. In advanced cases of carcinoma of the cervix, backache is a complaint, but it is always associated with pain in the buttock, due to involvement of the sacral plexus, and the pain radiates down the legs. Secondary deposits in the lumbar spine may be the cause.

Probably not more than a very small minority of backaches are of genital origin. It may result from some urinary irritation due to oxalates or coli bacilluria; it may accompany a calculus in the ureter or some lesion of the renal pelvis, though as a rule, in renal cases, the pain is situated rather higher up. Caries of the spine low down, growth in the spine or in the spinal cord membranes, might also cause it, or it may result from inflammation or strain of the sacro-iliac joint, displaced disc, rectal growth, haemorrhoids, proctitis or scybala. Injuries to the lumbar spine, including strain and subluxation as well as damage of a minor character to the erector spinae and other muscles causing muscle fatigue, have to be remembered in this connection. A correct diagnosis cannot be made without a complete examination of all adjacent structures, combined with careful urinary analysis.

5. MID-CYCLE OVULATION PAIN (MITTELSCHMERZ). Some women habitually experience some dull pain in the midline or in one or other iliac fossa at about the time of ovulation about 14 days before the next period. In others the pain may be experienced for a few cycles only. Occasionally slight vaginal bleeding accompanies the pain. The timing of the pain and the absence of any abnormal pelvic findings usually make the diagnosis clear.

6. PAIN RELATED TO VARICOSITY. Recent work suggests that in some women with pelvic pain it is possible to demonstrate congestion of the pelvic veins using examinations such as pelvic venography. These women tend to be in their early thirties and the pain is often described as dull and aching with sharp exacerbation. The diagnosis is made based on history, and on clinical examination, tenderness could be elicited at a point located two-thirds from the junction of anterior-superior spine to the umbilicus. Initial results suggest that progesterone therapy in this group of patients helps to alleviate the problem (*Fig.* P.8) indicates the algorithm for diagnosis of pelvic pain.

N. Patel

Pelvis, swelling in

The following list tabulates the many swellings which may rise up out of the pelvis into the abdomen or which may appear to be pelvic when they are really primarily abdominal:

BLADDER
Simple distension. New growth

VAGINA
Haematocolpos
Hydrocolpos

UTERUS
Pregnancy: normal or abnormal, or associated with
   tumours of the uterus or ovary
New growths: fibromyoma, adenomyoma
   sarcoma; carcinoma; chorionic carcinoma;
   haematometra; pyometra

OVARY
Cyst. Solid new growths

FALLOPIAN TUBES
Salpingo-oophoritis
Hydrosalpinx
Pyosalpinx
Tubal gestation

Progressive extrauterine gestation
Carcinoma

PELVIC PERITONEUM
Encysted peritoneal fluid
Haematocele due to extrauterine gestation
Haematocele due to haemorrhage from a corpus
  luteum
Pelvic abscess
Ascites
Hydatid cyst
Retroperitoneal lipoma or sarcoma

PELVIC CELLULAR TISSUE
Cellulitis; pelvic haematoma

APPENDIX VERMIFORMIS
Abscess, appendicitis with pregnancy

PELVIC BONES
New growths

OMENTUM
New growths; cysts

PHANTOM TUMOUR

PANCREATIC CYST

MESENTERIC CYST

KIDNEY
Tumour; hydronephrosis; pyonephrosis
  Pelvic kidney

SPLEEN
Enlargement; displacement

URACHUS
Cyst

SIGMOID COLON
Diverticulitis; carcinoma

The use of ultrasound in the diagnosis of pelvic swellings

Ultrasonography can be extremely useful in the diagnosis of swellings in the pelvis. The examination is always made with a full bladder which can be easily identified. The uterus can be seen and the cavity measured. A pregnancy may be seen within the uterine cavity, the fetus measured and the beating of the fetal heart established, denoting viability. Uterine and extra-uterine swellings can be seen and their size, shape and consistency (solid or cystic) determined—in the case of a cystic swelling, whether it is uni- or multi-locular. With the help of this information and the clinical findings an accurate diagnosis should be possible.

The commonest difficulty which arises in the diagnosis of pelvic swellings is to differentiate between the *distended bladder*, *pregnant uterus*, *ovarian cyst* and *uterine fibromyoma*, and the commonest mistakes are made between these swellings. The *distended bladder* is the easiest to dispose of, the passage of a catheter settling the question; yet neglect of this simple procedure has led to the abdomen being opened.

The history is of value in differentiating pelvic swellings, for amenorrhoea is the rule in pregnancy,

menorrhagia in fibromyoma, and no change in menstruation with ovarian tumours. These assumptions are correct in almost 99 out of every 100 cases, but exceptions do exist. The cardinal point in diagnosis is not to think of the possible fallacies until the common rule has been considered thoroughly. Normal menstruation during pregnancy is virtually unknown. That haemorrhages occur during the early months of pregnancy is true, but in most cases these haemorrhages represent threatened abortion, and not menstruation. Fibroids are associated with haemorrhages in the case of interstitial or submucous growths; but there may be no disturbance of menstruation with subperitoneal fibroids. Ovarian tumours only cause amenorrhoea when they are bilateral and destroy all ovarian tissue; as long as a small piece of ovarian tissue remains menstruation should occur normally. In the case of granulosa-cell tumours of the ovary irregular haemorrhage may occur from the uterus even after the menopause, or before puberty; these tumours secrete the follicular hormone, oestrogen, which causes the uterus to hypertrophy and the endometrium to undergo changes like those of the proliferative phase of the menstrual cycle; hence irregular haemorrhage after the menopause may be a symptom of this type of ovarian tumour.

Palpation of these tumours may be fallacious; in the early months of pregnancy the uterus may fluctuate like a cyst; a softened fibroid may do the same; or a tense ovarian cyst may feel so hard as to be mistaken for a fibroid. While the presence of the sound of the fetal heart is characteristic of pregnancy, its absence cannot be taken as evidence of a fibroid or of an ovarian tumour. It is not always possible to hear the fetal heart even in advanced pregnancy without the aid of an ultrasonic device such as the 'Doptone'. If the pedicle of a tumour can be felt definitely attached to one uterine cornu it is strong presumptive evidence of an ovarian tumour. When small tumours are in question the first point which arises is: Can the tumour be separated from the uterus bimanually? If so, it can be neither a fibromyoma of the uterus nor a normal uterine pregnancy. This point can only be made out by careful bimanual examination, and requires considerable skill in some cases. A pedunculated fibroid is, of course, extra-uterine and may have the same anatomical arrangement to the uterus as an ovarian tumour. If it is a fibroid that has undergone cystic change the physical signs are identical to those of an ovarian cyst and only a laparotomy will reveal the true state of affairs.

Early pregnancy in a retroverted uterus should not give rise to diagnostic difficulties if it is remembered that the soft, cystic fundus is felt through the posterior fornix, that the cervix looks down the vagina or forwards to the symphysis, and that the posterior mass is continuous with the cervix. If the retroverted uterus is associated with bladder distension the picture is usually clear enough. The history of urinary retention followed by constant dribbling of urine (distension with overflow), amenorrhoea, other signs of pregnancy, the presence of two tumours—one in front, tense, tender and elastic, the other behind, soft and cystic—and finally the passage of a catheter will settle the question. The diagnosis of solid ovarian tumours is not always possible, for the pedicle is often short, and the tumour is then so close to the uterus that the two cannot be separated. They are therefore likely to be mistaken for fibroids of the uterus. They do not often cause menorrhagia, however, and this should be remembered as a cardinal point.

Large tumours arising in the pelvis are not often difficult to differentiate from one another, bearing in mind that ovarian tumours, uterine fibroids and pregnancy are the common conditions occurring. It cannot be repeated too often that amenorrhoea stands for pregnancy, and occasionally for ovarian tumours when bilateral; menorrhagia goes with uterine fibroids except in the case of subperitoneal tumours. Exceptions to these general statements are uncommon, and mistakes in diagnosis will occur but seldom if they are borne in mind. Ascites has to be differentiated from ovarian cysts. In general, ascites give dullness in the flanks on percussion, with resonance over an area somewhere about the umbilicus, while ovarian cysts give dullness over the front of the abdomen, with resonance in the flanks. When ascites exist along with ovarian tumours the free fluid may be so large in amount that the tumour cannot be felt; as a rule, however, it can be touched on dipping through the fluid. Ascites with an ovarian tumour does not necessarily mean malignancy. Fibroma of the ovary, or a simple ovarian cyst with a twisted pedicle, may also be accompanied by some fluid. Ovarian fibromas may be accompanied by a large amount of ascites and bilateral pleural effusions (Meigs' syndrome).

When *pregnancy is associated with a tumour*, the diagnosis may be difficult. This does not lie in the recognition of the pregnancy; amenorrhoea, breast changes, fetal movements and the fetal heart will usually make that clear enough; it lies in deciding the nature, or even the presence of a tumour along with the pregnant uterus. In the early months, when the presence of two tumours can be demonstrated, the diagnosis is easier, but in the later months the great size of the abdomen, and the way in which the swellings merge into one another may obscure the picture. The relation to the uterus, whether a part of it, or attached to it by a pedicle; the feel of the tumour,

whether solid or cystic, soft or hard; and the previous history, will assist in making out the nature of the growth. Fibroids are likely to soften and degenerate during pregnancy, so that they are liable to be mistaken for ovarian cysts.

In the case of ovarian *tumours*, it is often impossible to be sure of the exact nature of the growth until this has been decided microscopically after removal. Because of this doubt there should be no undue delay in the removal of an ovarian tumour larger than the size of an orange or one that is growing. Small follicular cysts may be left as they are harmless and eventually disappear. Fixation of the growth in the pelvis, obvious ascites, unilateral oedema of the leg, emaciation of the patient, abdominal pain and rapid growth in size of the abdomen point to malignancy.

In the case of definite *uterine tumours*, the diagnosis of malignant growths is not often difficult because they cause irregular bleeding in addition to uterine enlargement, but the diagnosis should always be confirmed by microscopic examination of curetted fragments. Fibroids are only likely to be mistaken for malignant growths when they produce constant bleeding as a result of extrusion, infection and sloughing. Rapid growth of a fibroid is more likely to be the result of degenerative changes, such as formation of cysts or necrobiosis, than to the developing of a sarcoma or other malignant growth along with it. Growth of a fibroid after the menopause, however, should make one consider sarcomatous change in it.

With small tumours confined to the pelvis, or rising only a little above the brim, diagnosis is often difficult. In practice, however, *extra-uterine gestation* and its resulting blood-tumour stand out pre-eminently as a swelling which must be recognized at once if treatment is to be successful. Before rupture or abortion has occurred a tubal gestation is essentially a small tumour in one posterolateral corner of the pelvis, attached to the uterus, indefinite in consistence, remarkably tender, and perhaps—though not always—associated with amenorrhoea of short duration and acute attacks of pain in the pelvis. Definite signs of pregnancy may be entirely wanting but a pregnancy test will be positive. It may be mistaken for a chronic salpingo-oophoritis, a small cystic ovary, a small pedunculated fibroid or a small ovarian dermoid. The differential diagnosis may be difficult, but attacks of pain unassociated with menstruation are not likely to occur in any of the above conditions; the pains are usually the result of over-distension and stretching of the tube from haemorrhage into its wall or lumen around the fertilized ovum. Unless the swelling is tender (often very tender) it is not likely to be due to a tubal pregnancy. When tubal abortion has occurred, or tubal rupture, the signs of internal bleeding accompanied by sudden pain and collapse, with haemorrhage from the uterus or the passage of a decidual cast, usually make an unmistakable picture. Intraperitoneal haemorrhage is more commonly severe and copious with tubal rupture than with tubal abortion. If the patient recovers from the initial bleeding the clinical picture may be that of a retro-uterine or peritubal *haematocele*. The uterus is pushed forwards and upwards against the symphysis pubis, and the mass of blood clot can be felt posteriorly bulging the posterior fornix and also the anterior wall of the rectum. It is very tender. Tubal abortion is most likely to be mistaken for an ordinary uterine abortion; but the presence of a tender mass on one side of the uterus, with a closed cervix and a negative ultrasound scan, and the absence of uterine contractions or extrusion of any products of conception, should make the case clear. Pain is much more severe but external bleeding is much less in extra-uterine pregnancy. The essential point in diagnosing an ectopic pregnancy is to approach every woman of child-bearing age who complains of irregular bleeding and abdominal pain with the possibility in mind. No two cases are alike and there are more exceptions to the rule in the symptomatology of this condition than in any other.

Progressive extra-uterine gestation is a rare occurrence, and is the result of continued growth of an embryo after a partial separation from the tube as a result of rupture, or extrusion from the fimbriated end (abortion). The continued enlargement of a mass beside the uterus, with amenorrhoea and progressive signs of pregnancy, are the most characteristic points. Abdominal pain in late pregnancy is a characteristic feature. The uterus may be felt in the pelvis separate from the fetal sac. The diagnosis, however, is difficult, because there is always some effused blood which obscures the outlines of the uterus, and makes it appear to be a part of the pelvic mass. The fetus is often situated high above the pelvis and it tends to lie transversely facing downward. A radiograph reveals the fetus adopting a position that is characteristically odd, the spine hyperextended or acutely flexed and the head and limbs at unusual angles to the trunk. If, on a lateral view, radiography shows fetal parts overlapping the maternal spine the pregnancy must be extra-uterine. Ultrasonography will establish the absence of an intra-uterine gestation and also the size of the uterus, which never exceeds that of a 5 months' gestation even in the presence of a full-term extra-uterine pregnancy, and the cervix does not soften to the same degree. In those cases where the fetus lies in the front of the false sac it will feel very superficial owing the absence of uterine wall in front of it, and between it and the examining hand. The fetus is, however, often difficult to palpate, due, perhaps, to the placenta in front, which may give rise to a loud vascular souffle just medial to the anterior superior iliac spine on the side from which it derives its main blood supply (via the ovarian vessels).

The swellings due to *salpingo-oophoritis* are usually easy to distinguish. They form fixed tender masses in the pelvis, seldom of any definite shape, but occasionally presenting the characteristic retort shape, with its narrow end near the uterus, which the tube assumes when distended with fluid. The history is usually that of an acute illness at some period, with pain in the pelvis, rise of temperature and peritoneal irritation. It is preceded, as a rule, by uterine discharge and menorrhagia. This inflammatory disturbance in married women is associated with long periods of infertility, owing to the sealing up of the tubes. In the chronic state pelvic pain, congestive dysmenorrhoea, dyspareunia, vaginal discharge, menorrhagia and infertility are complained of. The signs of suppuration, pyrexia, leucocytosis, wasting and daily sweating are usually absent and the pus in the tubes is sterile.

A large *pelvic abscess* may accompany salpingo-oophoritis, or may occur alone without infection of the tubes, as we see occasionally in puerperal septic infections. When it does occur, it is of course peritoneal; it fixes the uterus in a central position, bulges into the posterior fornix and rectum, tends to rupture into the rectum, before which occurrence there is a copious discharge of mucus per anum, is acute in onset, and accompanied by signs of local peritonitis. A swinging temperature, leucocytosis, sweats and the symptoms of fever are present, all suddenly improving when the abscess discharges itself. It is likely to be confounded with *pelvic cellulitis*, in which the uterus is fixed in a laterally displaced position. This swelling bulges one lateral fornix and extends right out to the lateral pelvic wall, tends to burrow along the round ligament to the groin, and may point there like a psoas abscess, is slow in onset, chronic and not accompanied by signs of local peritonitis. It always follows labour, or abortion, whereas pelvic abscess of peritoneal origin may occur with salpingo-oophoritis or appendicitis, quite apart from pregnancy. Pelvic cellulitis never bears any relation to salpingo-oophoritis. It may take many weeks to resolve, which it usually does without pointing.

Encysted peritoneal fluid, hydatid cysts and *retroperitoneal lipomas* are generally diagnosed as ovarian cysts, and their true nature is only discovered at operation. There are no definite signs by which these conditions may be diagnosed, and as they all require operative treatment, postoperative diagnosis meets their requirements. Encysted peritoneal fluid due to tuberculosis may be suspected if tuberculous lesions are present elsewhere in the body. They lack the definite outline of an ovarian cyst and are often semiresonant on percussion.

Distension of the vagina by menstrual fluid is not likely to be mistaken for anything else, if only on account of the absolute closure of the atretic membrane which gives rise to it. This condition is often referred to as 'imperforate hymen'. This is not correct because the atresia is at a higher level in the vagina than the hymen which is always perforate. Haematocolpos is practically the only central tumour occurring between the rectum and the bladder reaching from the hymen to the pelvic brim. It presents in girls about the age of 16 or 17 years who complain of acute retention of urine due to the fact that the swelling fills the pelvis and the distended bladder in front is forced upward into the abdomen. Primary amenorrhoea is present although monthly symptoms without loss of blood may have taken place. Two swellings are present; the tender distended bladder in the lower abdomen reaching as high as the umbilicus and the distended vagina filled with menstrual fluid in the pelvis. The uterus can usually be felt like a cork movable upon its upper extremity. The lower pole of the haematocolpos presents a blue-coloured swelling at the vulva. A similar swelling may be found on rare occasions in newborn girl babies: the vagina is filled with a milky fluid (hydrocolpos).

Urachal cysts occur in front of the uterus and in close relation to the bladder; but in spite of this they are usually mistaken for ovarian cysts. It is to be remembered, however, that ovarian cysts are only likely to get in front of the uterus when they are large, but dermoid cysts of the ovary of small size occasionally do so. Urachal cysts rarely attain a large size.

Appendicitis with pregnancy occurs occasionally, and may be mistaken for such a condition as torsion of an ovarian pedicle. The swelling due to appendix inflammation is, however, in close relation to the anterior superior spine of the ilium, and apparently adherent to the iliac fossa. The lump is ill-defined, and rarely fluctuates unless there is a large abscess. The acute onset may be similar to that of torsion of an ovarian pedicle. There is usually a definite fluctuating tumour when an ovarian cyst is present, and some interval between it and the iliac crest can usually be felt.

Phantom tumours are due to diaphragmatic contraction, causing the abdominal wall to bulge. They are usually mistaken by patients for pregnancy, but are not accompanied by any of the signs of pregnancy. Amenorrhoea must be excepted from this, however, because these cases usually occur about the menopause. Their true nature can usually be discovered by making the patient breathe normally, relaxing the diaphragm; but if any doubt exists, the protrusion will disappear under an anaesthetic. Ultrasonography will also be quite normal.

Growth of the pelvic bones are very rare tumours, usually cartilaginous or sarcomatous. They are only likely to be mistaken for adherent inflammatory masses due to salpingo-oophoritis. They will be found to be continuous with the bones forming the pelvis, and when growing from the sacrum may have the rectum in front of them; all other pelvic tumours have the rectum behind them. In most cases of this nature the uterus and adnexa can be palpated bimanually, and shown to be free from disease and unconnected with the mass. When complicated by the presence of a pregnant uterus their true nature may be difficult to determine unless examination reveals that they are absolutely fixed and the continuous with the bones of the pelvis.

Many of these lesions are not primarily pelvic, but they are included in the list because they are liable to be mistaken for pelvic tumours. Thus, renal, splenic, or pancreatic tumours may reach the pelvic brim, but the history ought to show that they have grown down from above, not up from below. Renal swellings may be associated with urinary changes, or absence of urinary secretion on the affected side as detected by the cystoscope or an intravenous pyelogram. Malformations of the genital tract are associated with developmental abnormalities of the renal tract. It is not uncommon to find a solitary pelvic kidney in patients with congenital absence of the vagina and uterus. Splenic enlargements may be associated with bloodchanges. Pancreatic cysts are the least likely to be mistaken for pelvic swellings, but they have been difficult to distinguish from ovarian tumours with long pedicles.

N. Patel

Penile sores

Sores on the penis may be present on the thin mucous covering of the glans or prepuce, or on the cutaneous surface of the body of the penis; they are more common in the former situation.

Ulceration in the neighbourhood of the glans penis may be due to:

Balanitis
Herpes genitalis
Soft sore
Granuloma venereum (inguinale)
Lymphogranuloma inguinale (venereum)
Chancre
Epithelioma
Papilloma

Gummatous ulceration
Tuberculous ulceration
Injury, for example from a bite

Balanitis

If inflammatory processes have been allowed to continue beneath the prepuce, ulceration and excoriation of the mucous membrane covering the glans penis or lining the prepuce will occur, accompanied by a stinking, purulent discharge. Multiple shallow ulcers are formed, rapidly coalescing and causing considerable discomfort. The prepuce often becomes swollen and oedematous, preventing retraction, so that a condition of phimosis occurs, or, if retraction has taken place, the analogous state of paraphimosis, almost strangulating the end of the penis and even causing it to become gangrenous. Care must be exercised in diagnosing a simple balanitis from one accompanying acute gonorrhoeal urethritis or an underlying syphilitic or soft chancre. The so-called balanitis circinata is part of Reiter's syndrome, occurring in association with urethritis, arthritis, conjunctivitis (often slight and transient) and buccal ulceration. In Behçet's syndrome also ulcerative penile and scrotal lesions may occur in association with buccal ulcers. With an acute urethritis there will be a history of infection and pain along the course of the urethra during micturition; the intracellular gonococcus may be identified in a Gram-stained smear of the discharge.

If a chancre exists under the swollen phimosed prepuce there is often a tender spot about the corona or at the fraenum. With a soft sore consecutive sores may appear about the orifice of the prepuce, while the inguinal nodes are much more likely to be inflamed or to suppurate than with simple balanitis. A syphilitic chancre obscured by a phimosis can usually be felt distinctly under the skin, and causes a comparatively small amount of discharge, while the inguinal nodes become enlarged but do not suppurate. The interval of about 4 weeks from the time of the possible source of infection until the appearance of the sore will suggest, and the finding of spirochaetes (*Treponema pallidum*) in the fluid expressed from the ulcer will prove, the diagnosis. In later cases, enlargement of the inguinal nodes, secondary cutaneous rash, sore throat and positive serological reactions will be present.

A form of balanitis which is frequently very obstinate to treatment may occur in patients with diabetes mellitus. The main causative organism is *Candida albicans*. Phimosis appearing in an adult male is often due to unsuspected diabetes; the urine should always be tested for sugar.

Herpes genitalis

Herpes may attack the genital organs as part of a herpes zoster which is unilateral. This is a rarity compared with herpes simplex, which is now regarded as an important sexually transmitted disease. Recent work has implicated *Herpes simplex virus* Type 2 in the aetiology of uterine cervical cancer. The disease begins as a patch of erythema on the inner surface of the prepuce or on the glans penis, followed by vesicles and pustules; the latter become rubbed by the clothes, and form small ulcers. Herpes of the genital organs tends to recur, so that a previous history of a similar attack is often forthcoming. If seen during the vesicular stage no difficulty will be met with in the diagnosis; but if suppuration has followed, it must be diagnosed from a venereal sore. Soft chancres are usually deeper, with marked edges; their bases are sloughing, and they are usually accompanied by a bubo, which is exceptional with herpes. A syphilitic chancre is usually single, indurated and raised, and is accompanied by the typical multiple, discrete nodes in the inguinal region. It should be remembered that syphilis may become inoculated upon a herpetic patch or that herpes may appear in an area already infected with syphilis.

Soft sores or chancroids

Soft sores or chancroids of the penis occur almost invariably from infection during sexual connection. The incubation period is short, a vesicle occurs in 2 days, and this breaks down rapidly to form a rounded or oval ulcer with undermined edges and a yellowish sloughing base. The ulcers appear usually on the mucous surface of the glans, fraenum or corona, and are multiple, direct inoculation occurring from each ulcer to the contiguous part. They may cause rapid destruction of tissue, perforating the fraenum or spreading over the surface of the glans. The soft sore must be differentiated from others occurring on the glans, and above all from a syphilitic chancre, and serum from the edge of the lesion should be examined for *Haemophilus ducreyi* (Ducrey's bacillus) as well as by dark-ground illumination for *Treponema pallidum*. At the same time it must be remembered that besides the infection with chancroid, a simultaneous infection with syphilis may have taken place, so that a soft sore may ultimately become indurated and assume the character of a primary syphilitic lesion. The chancroids are multiple, are accompanied by a good deal of thin, purulent discharge, and by a painful swelling of the inguinal nodes, usually of one side, which have a marked tendency to suppurate. On the other hand, a syphilitic chancre is single, is raised and indurated, has little discharge, and is accompanied by enlarged but firm and indolent nodes in both inguinal regions; the incubation period of a syphilitic chancre is from 21 to 28 days. The multiple ulcerations caused by herpes are more superficial, and rarely cause a bubo.

Granuloma inguinale

Granuloma inguinale (granuloma venereum) is a chronic granulomatous ulceration which may affect the perineum and the inguinal regions as well as the penis. It occurs in tropical countries and is mildly contagious. The lesion on the penis starts as a papule which appears after a few days' or weeks' incubation period and breaks down to form a superficial ulcer. Examination of the discharge shows intracellular capsulated bacteria known as Donovan bodies (*Donvania granulomatis*). Lymph nodes are not involved.

Lymphogranuloma venereum

Lymphogranuloma venereum (lymphogranuloma inguinale) is also commoner in the tropics, and is a chronic condition characterized by a small initial lesion on the penis with marked glandular enlargement in the groins and severe constitutional disturbances. The nodes tend to break down and form sinuses. The lesion on the penis appears, after an incubation period of about a week, as a vesicle, papule or ulcer, and it tends to disappear by the time the lymphatic nodes are enlarged. It is due to a filter-passing organism which is a member of the *Chlamydia* group and can be diagnosed by complement fixation reactions, demonstration of specific skin reactivity (Frei's test), and a biopsy of the primary lesion or lymph node. It must be distinguished from chancroid and from granuloma venereum. Rectal stricture and effusions into joints are other lesions caused by this disease.

Chancre

Chancre—the initial lesion of syphilis—generally appears on the penis, and is most common in the neighbourhood of the fraenum or coronary sulcus. A chancre appears about 25 days after infection as a reddened patch, which becomes raised above the surface of the mucous membrane, with distinctly indurated margins. The central part breaks down into an ulcer (*Fig.* P.9), discharging a thin, purulent fluid, and at the same time the inguinal nodes of both sides become palpable, slightly enlarged, but discrete, and with no tendency to suppurate. The chancre increases but slowly in size, or may occasionally become smaller without any treatment, and after a further lapse of from 4 to 6 weeks the typical secondary symptoms make their appearance: namely, a roseolar rash on the chest, abdomen, face and thighs, general adenitis, and mucous patches about the faucial pillars and tonsils,

accompanied by low pyrexia. The diagnosis of the primary lesion of syphilis frequently presents no difficulties, the indurated character of the sore, the date of its appearance after infection, and the presence of firm, indurated nodes in the inguinal region being distinctive. If the character of the sore is not distinctive it is necessary to differentiate it from other lesions of the penis. Careful search must be made by dark-ground illumination for the *Treponema pallidum* in the serum expressed from the sore; negative serological reactions in the early stage of the disease are not reliable. If the sore is syphilitic, the secondary manifestations of the disease will follow, provided that the doubtful ulcer is not treated as a chancre.

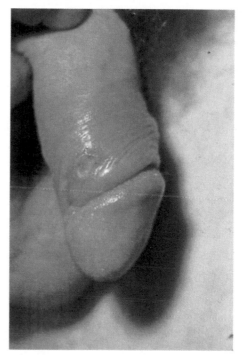

Fig. P.9. Primary chancre of the penis.

A chancre may be simulated by an inflamed soft sore; soft sores are, however, frequently multiple, appear within a few days of infection, and are accompanied by painful enlargement of the inguinal lymphatic nodes, which are particularly prone to suppurate. It must not be forgotten that a double infection may have occurred, so that a soft sore may show little inclination to heal or, becoming indurated, may present the features of a chancre after about 3 weeks, followed later by the symptoms of constitutional syphilis.

Epithelioma of the penis in the early stage may be confused with syphilitic chancre. In epithelioma there is no history of infection; it occurs usually in elderly uncircumcised patients, and there is frequently a greater destruction of tissue than in syphilis. The inguinal nodes are not enlarged until the sore has been present for some weeks, and there are no secondary lesions such as the faucial ulceration and cutaneous rash. Diagnosis is confirmed by histological examination of a biopsy specimen.

Perhaps the greatest difficulty in the diagnosis of a chancre is experienced when it is hidden beneath an inflamed and phimosed prepuce. There is a purulent and foul discharge from beneath the oedematous and swollen prepuce; the inguinal nodes are enlarged from the associated sepsis. If a chancre is present it can frequently be felt as an indurated area under the prepuce, while if it has been present for some time the secondary lesions of syphilis may be present. If any doubt exists as to whether an indurated subpreputial area is an early epithelioma or a syphilitic sore, the prepuce should be split up along the dorsal aspect under anaesthesia, the ulceration inspected, a small piece submitted to microscopical examination if necessary or some serum expressed from the ulcer examined on a dark stage for *Treponema pallidum*.

Epithelioma

Epithelioma (squamous-celled carcinoma) is the commonest form of malignant growth of the penis (*Fig. P.10*). It arises most frequently from the inner aspect of the prepuce, or from the mucous membrane of the glans, as a small, raised ulcer with friable, irregular edges. It is rarely present before the age of 40, and frequently occurs on the site of previous ulceration or long-standing irritation; it is unknown where circumcision has been performed in infancy, although later circumcision does not confer this near-total immunity. An *epitheliomatous ulcer* increases in size gradually in spite of various forms of treatment, and with it is frequently associated enlargement of the inguinal lymph nodes. At first the nodes may be enlarged from septic infection, but later from malignant infiltration. An epitheliomatous ulcer may in some cases be confused with a chancre; but the friable, irregular edges of the former, the liability to bleed, and the gradual progressive increase in size in spite of treatment, in an elderly patient, together with the extensive induration of the base, should give rise to grave suspicion of malignant disease. Microscopical examination of a small piece removed from the edge of the ulcer will give direct evidence of epithelioma.

Carcinoma of the penis may also occur in a *papillary form* which grows to produce a large cauliflower excrescence. In this type any enlargement of the inguinal nodes is more likely to be due to infection than to metastasis.

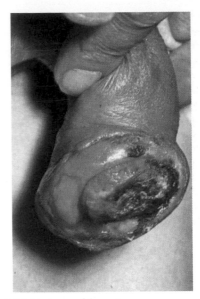

Fig. P.10. Carcinoma of the penis.

Papillomas

Papillomas (venereal warts or condylomata acuminata) occur on the glans and contiguous surface of the prepuce and are most frequently found on the corona. They are simple papillomas, usually multiple, and are distinguished from epithelioma by the absence of induration in the base.

Gummatous ulceration

Gummatous ulceration of the penis occurs today with great rarity, resulting from the disintegration of a small gumma of the glans or prepuce, frequently in the position of an old scar. A gumma begins as a small, elevated nodule, which, if left untreated, softens and discharges its contents, leaving an ulcer bounded by thin edges and with a yellowish, sloughy base.

Tuberculous ulceration

Tuberculous ulceration of the penis is rare, and is generally associated with advanced tuberculous infiltration elsewhere. Tuberculous ulcers are usually shallow, with thin overhanging edges, painful and multiple. The diagnosis is clinched by discovering tubercle bacilli in films made from the discharge.

Injury

Injury is an uncommon cause of a penile sore but in one case under the care of Sir Eric Riches an epithelioma of the penis followed a bite from a pig!

Harold Ellis

Penis, pain in

Pain in the penis is a symptom which occurs not only in association with lesions of the penis or urethra, but also as a referred pain from disease of the prostate, bladder or kidney. Penile pain may be present either during or immediately after micturition, or may be entirely independent of the act. If pain is felt only during micturition there is probably some inflammatory lesion of the urethra or prostate; if it occurs immediately after the flow of the urine it suggests some lesion in the urinary bladder; pain present quite apart from micturition may be due to various diseases of the penis, bladder, ureter or kidney.

The term 'pain', too, is a relative quantity, varying with the nervous susceptibility of the patient, for what is pain in one may be merely discomfort in another, so that the patient's description may have to be discounted to a certain extent by the clinician.

A. Causes of pain in the penis experienced during micturition

1. DISEASES OF THE URETHRA

Acute inflammation, gonorrhoeal or other
The passage or impaction of a calculus
Stricture of the urethra
Injury of the urethra
Foreign body in the urethra

2. DISEASES OF THE PROSTATE

Acute prostatitis
Prostatic carcinoma
Prostatic abscess

3. DISEASES OF THE BLADDER

Acute cystitis
Vesical calculus
Papilloma
Pedunculated carcinoma

1. Diseases of the urethra

The commonest cause of pain in the penis *during* micturition is acute inflammation of the urethra, usually gonorrhoeal, but may result from other organisms, and this is particularly common following catheterization (*see* URETHRAL DISCHARGE). In the earliest stages of an acute urethritis, before any marked urethral discharge is apparent, there is usually a sense of smarting or tingling in the terminal urethra, more marked as the discharge increases, when it is of a burning or scalding character. The pain during micturition within a few days of sexual connection is frequently the earliest symptom of urethral infection; a purulent discharge from the urethra is usually present when the patient comes under observation.

The *passage of a calculus* through the urethra cases a sharp, cutting pain along the urethra, the cause of which is apparent when the calculus is voided. Occasionally it may happen that micturition occurs in these cases in the dark, or that urine is not passed into a vessel, so that the calculus is not actually seen by the patient; but if there is a history of previous renal descent of a stone or symptoms pointing to vesical calculus, the sharp urethral pain during micturition occurring upon one single occasion is significant of the passage of a calculus. A stone may, however, pass into the urethra during micturition and become *arrested* at some narrowed portion of the canal, usually at the membranous portion or at the distal end, when a sudden, sharp pain is felt in the urethra, and at the same time the flow of urine is partially or completely stopped before the bladder has been emptied, further efforts to expel urine resulting only in a forceless stream; the whole length of the urethra should be examined by passing the finger along its course, when a stone may be actually felt; or the calculus may be seen through an endoscope or identified on a plain radiograph.

Occasionally a calculus may remain in the urethra, becoming gradually enlarged in size and causing pain on micturition. These calculi usually lie in the dilated posterior urethra behind a stricture in the bulb.

Urethral stricture occasionally causes pain in the urethra during micturition, especially if the calibre is small, and if there is septic infection or ulceration of the urethral mucosa behind the stricture, but as a rule stricture causes but little pain; gradually increasing difficulty in micturition, feeble stream and dribbling of urine from the meatus after the stream has terminated are common symptoms; the diagnosis will be confirmed by the obstruction offered to the passage of a full-sized bougie or, better, by direct observation of the urethra through a urethroscope under water distension.

Injury of the urethra may cause pain during micturition. The urethra may be injured by a fall on the perineum, by a kick or blow, or by the faulty or careless passage of instruments; it may also be injured or lacerated in association with a fracture of the pelvis. The urethra may be merely bruised, lacerated on one aspect or completely ruptured. If it is lacerated by direct injury blood usually appears at the external urinary meatus, together with a contusion in the perineum or along the course of the urethra; any attempt at micturition causes pain in the penis, while urine may or may not be expelled from the meatus, depending upon the extent of the injury, or may be extravasated into the perineal or scrotal tissues (*Fig. P.11*). As a rule there will be no difficulty in the diagnosis, but in any suspected case the greatest care should be exercised in passing an instrument into the urethra.

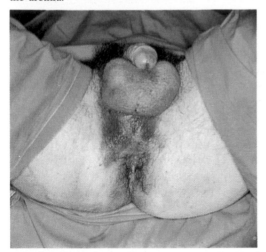

Fig. P.11. Traumatic rupture of the urethra showing blood from meatus and perineal haematema limited posteriorly by the attachment of Colles' fascia.

A *foreign body* in the urethra may cause considerable pain. In some cases the history will be clear; for instance the end of a catheter or bougie may have broken off within the urethra; but in others, especially in weak-minded individuals, no history of the insertion of a foreign body in the urethra will be forthcoming. Urethroscopy will show the foreign body; various articles have been found in the urethra, such as a wax taper, a seed of barley with its barb, a hairpin, a small shell, a nail and a glass tube used to contain hypodermic tablets.

2. Diseases of the prostate

Acute prostatitis and *prostatic abscess* both give rise to pain during micturition in addition to increased frequency and difficulty during the act. Both are usually sequelae of an acute urethritis, and whereas an acute prostatitis is accompanied by a temperature raised to 100–101°F (38°C), a prostatic abscess causes the usual rise and fall common to septic processes. The diagnosis of the two conditions is made by careful rectal examination, the acutely inflamed gland presenting a much enlarged, smooth-surfaced prominence in the rectum, while if an abscess is present a softer acutely tender area in the inflamed gland can usually be detected. An acute prostatitis may accompany a haematogenous bacterial urinary infection as distinct from a venereal urethritis.

Adenomatous enlargement of the prostate gives rise to no penile pain during micturition; but pain in the penis is present during micturition occasionally in cases of *prostatic carcinoma*, owing to the direct infiltration of the urethral mucous membrane. Prostatic carcinoma is by no means uncommon (indeed, it is the sixth commonest cause of death from cancer in the United Kingdom), and while in its general symptoms it resembles those of prostatic adenoma, there is a marked difference found on digital examination of the gland per rectum. The carcinomatous gland presents rounded areas of densely infiltrated tissue, in contradistinction to the elastic, uniform feel of the adenomatous variety; the whole gland becomes fixed and immovable, and in advanced stages distinct infiltration of the lateral pelvic lymphatics and soft tissues may be felt extending laterally from the affected organ. It is often tender on palpitation.

Care must be taken not to mistake the hard nodules felt in a prostate containing *calculi* for carcinoma; with calculous disease the gland is not fixed and is only slightly enlarged. During the passage of a catheter through the prostatic urethra distinct grating may be felt if any calculus has ulcerated the urethral wall. Radiography will distinguish the two conditions (*See Fig.* K. 15) but they may coexist.

3. Diseases of the bladder

Diseases of the bladder may cause penile pain during micturition under certain circumstances, although it is much more common to find that pain in vesical disease follows the completion of micturition. In *acute cystitis*, penile pain is present throughout micturition, due to the intense congestion of the vesical mucous membrane of the trigone and around the internal urethral orifice. The other symptoms of acute cystitis, namely suprapubic pain, pyrexia, increased frequency of micturition and the presence of pus and blood in the urine, suggest the diagnosis.

Pain during micturition in other vesical lesions is caused whenever there is sudden obstruction to the normal flow or urine by the impaction of something against the internal urethral orifice. This may occur with a small *calculus* or with a *pedunculated tumour*, whether simple or malignant, when during micturition the flow is arrested suddenly, accompanied by a shooting pain in the urethra, while after an interval of a few seconds the stream may be established. With vesical calculus the urine may be normal or may contain pus and blood if the bladder has become infected; there is penile pain after micturition, and the stone will be seen both on plain X-ray of the pelvis and with a cystoscope. With a simple villous papilloma there is no pain unless part of the fimbriated portion of the tumour engages in the urethral orifice during micturition, but there are usually recurrent attacks of profuse haematuria, while with a carcinoma there is increased frequency of micturition, with pain following the act and more frequent haematuria. Upon rectal examination the base of the bladder may be felt to be infiltrated, but by far the most valuable means of diagnosis between the three conditions is by cystoscopy, when a calculus or villous tumour is seen readily, whilst a pedunculated carcinoma appears as a dark red tumour covered with stunted processes.

B. Penile pain following micturition

This symptom is common to many lesions of the urinary bladder, more especially those in which there is ulceration or infiltration of the basal areas. The particular pain felt by the patient is described as a sharp pricking or tingling at the terminal part of the penis on the cessation of micturition, lasting some minutes and causing a desire to squeeze the glans. It was thought to be diagnostic of vesical calculus, but this is far from being the case, for it may be due to almost any affection of the trigone.

The common causes of pain in the penis following upon micturition are:

1. VESICAL
Calculus
Tuberculosis
Tumour (carcinoma, papilloma)
Acute cystitis
Bilharzia

2. URETERIC
Calculus in lower end
Tuberculous ureteritis

3. PROSTATIC
Acute inflammation
Abscess
Calculus
Carcinoma

4. VESICULAR
Acute seminal vesiculitis

5. RECTAL
Carcinoma

6. ANAL
Fissure or ulcer
Inflamed haemorrhoids

1. Diseases of the bladder

A *calculus* in the bladder, unless it is trapped in the pouch behind an enlarged prostate or in a diverticulum, causes pain in the glans penis after micturition. It may exist without causing cystitis, although commonly there is some degree of pyuria when the case is first seen. There is increased frequency of micturition during active exercise or during the jolting of travelling, but not during complete rest unless cystitis is marked.

The terminal drops of urine during micturition are often tinged with blood, and on some occasions there may have been a sudden stoppage of the stream during micturition. In some cases there is a history of acutely painful colic due to the descent of a stone from the kidney without the subsequent passage of a calculus in the urine. Patients subjected to vesical stone have usually reached the later part of life in this country, although bladder stones in children are still common in tropical parts, and although the symptoms are as a rule sufficiently marked to render the diagnosis easy, sometimes they may be so few that vesical calculus is unexpected, or the symptoms are so like those caused by other lesions of the bladder that error is easy. The great majority of vesical calculi are radio-opaque and can be seen on a plain X-ray of the pelvis. In such a case it is advisable to examine the interior of the bladder with a cystoscope, by which means stones can be seen, their approximate size determined, and any other conditions of the bladder accompanying or simulating calculus may be diagnosed with certainty.

Vesical tuberculosis is usually secondary to tuberculous disease in some other part of the genito-urinary tract, particularly the kidney. It causes marked penile pain after micturition, together with pyuria and a tinge of blood in the terminal drops of urine; the frequency of micturition is increased during both day and night, and is uninfluenced by rest, thus differing from the increased frequency of calculous disease. Vesical tuberculosis occurs in young adults and is usually associated with renal tuberculosis in which symptoms referable to the bladder are commonly present before the bladder is attacked by disease. In a young patient in whom increased frequency of micturition, pyuria and penile pain are present, a search should be made for any tuberculous focus, especially in the kidneys by excretion urography, and in the epididymes, prostate or seminal vesicles, or for marked thickening of the terminal ureter as felt per rectum, and a careful search should be made for tubercle bacilli in the urine. The deposit from three early morning specimens should be examined, and if this is negative, search should be continued by culture. A cystoscopic examination may be necessary to determine the extent of the disease.

Vesical tumours. Carcinoma of the bladder occurs in a papillary or a solid form. Papillary carcinoma is at first non-infiltrating, while the solid nodular and ulcerative types and adenocarcinoma are infiltrating. They begin most commonly in the base of the bladder, except the urachal adenocarcinoma, which arises in the dome; the submucous coat and the muscular wall become infiltrated by malignant cells so that contraction of the bladder during micturition causes pain referred to the terminal portion of the urethra. All forms occur in elderly patients, mostly men, and give rise to increased frequency of micturition during both day and night, and to haematuria. They also often give rise to renal pain when the infiltration has extended to the ureteric orifice in the bladder.

The incidental cystogram of intravenous urography (*Figs*. P.12, P.13). may sometimes afford visual proof of the deformity the new growth is producing or of a filling defect in the otherwise regular contour of the bladder.

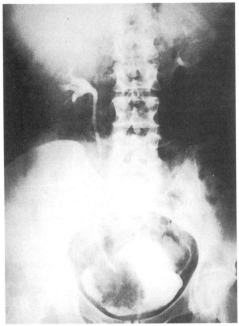

Fig. P.12. An intravenous pyelogram and cystogram taken 20 minutes after injection. There is a filling defect on the right sides of the bladder due to a large benign papilliferous tumour. Both kidneys are normal.

Under anaesthesia the base of the bladder may be felt per rectum to be thickened, or lymphatic infiltration may be felt in the lateral pelvic space, and a cystoscopic examination, together with biopsy, will usually clear up the diagnosis.

Whereas solid infiltrating growths of the bladder give rise to penile pain after micturition from the direct infiltration of the vesical walls, the pedunculated papillary carcinoma and the simple villous papilloma may occasionally give rise to sharp penile pain during micturition from blocking of the internal urethral orifice by a process of growth. The occurrence of this, together with attacks of profuse haematuria, is suggestive of a pedunculated growth. On cystoscopic examination the carcinomatous pedunculated tumour is seen to be covered by blunt, stunted processes, whereas the innocent villous papilloma presents much more delicate fimbriae.

Acute cystitis causes tingling pain in the penis

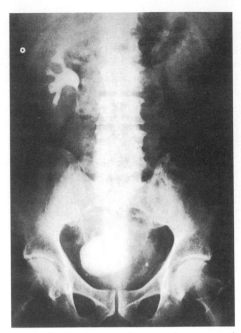

Fig. P.13. An intravenous pyelogram and cystogram taken 20 minutes after injection. There is a solid defect in the left side of the bladder caused by an infiltrating carcinoma. The left ureter is obstructed and there is no function in the obstructed left kidney.

after micturition from the inflammatory infiltration of the trigonal area. The mode of onset, the character of the pain and other symptoms of cystitis will point to the cause of the pain.

Bilharzia haematobia gives rise to clinical symptoms very similar to those of vesical tuberculosis. The history of residence in an infected district (e.g. Egypt or East Africa), microscopical examination of the urine for ova, and the typical cystoscopic appearance of the bladder establish the diagnosis.

Radiographs may show calcification of the bladder or ureters and pyelography often demonstrates stricture formation and gross dilatation of the ureters (*Fig*. P.14).

2. Ureteric lesions

Ureteric lesions not infrequently produce pain in the glans penis after micturition, and may cause considerable difficulty in the diagnosis from vesical disease.

When a *calculus* becomes impacted in the narrowed terminal or intramural portion of the ureter, symptoms are produced almost exactly similar to those of vesical calculus or tuberculosis, namely increased frequency of micturition, pain in the glans penis after micturition, and a small amount of pus and blood in the urine. Intimate knowledge of the history of the illness will often be of value in these cases; the first attack of pain is usually described as being sudden,

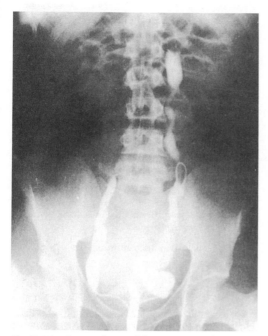

Fig. P.14. Dilatation of ureters following stricture of their lower ends in a case of vesical schistosomiasis. From a man of 20 who lived in East Africa.

and felt in the renal angle posteriorly, passing forwards above the iliac crest and spine and finally becoming localized at the situation of the external abdominal ring. The calculus may become impacted in the terminal inch of the ureter, when, in addition to this pain, there will be increased frequency of micturition and penile pain, and possibly haematuria. With ureteric calculus there is usually aching pain in the kidney of the affected side from the dilatation of its pelvis. The diagnosis of these cases is not difficult if a careful inquiry is made into the history and symptoms, and so long as it is remembered that increased frequency of micturition and penile pain may be caused by ureteric impaction of a calculus; a good radiographic examination of the pelvic areas may show the shadow of a stone. Indeed, some 90 per cent of these calculi are radio-opaque but, when small, may mimic phleboliths or be obscured by gas shadows or underlying bony structures (*Fig.* P.15). The stone itself may be felt occasionally as a small, painful nodule on pelvic examination, especially in women. A cystoscopic examination also affords valuable information, not only in excluding vesical lesions, but by giving a distinct indication of ureteric calculus by the marked congestion and dilatation of the blood vessels in the immediate vicinity of the ureteric orifice. An intravenous pyelogram may demonstrate obstruction of the ureter and confirm that the calculus lies in its lumen. A small bougie passed into the ureter may meet with obstruction in its passage; a

stereoscopic radiograph of the pelvis with an opaque bougie passed into the ureter will show the shadow to be in the immediate line of the ureter (*Fig.* P.16).

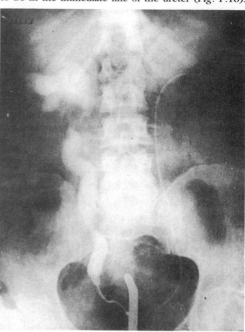

Fig. P.15. Dilatation of the right ureter due to a calculus impacted at its lower end.

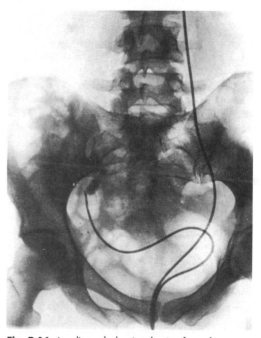

Fig. P.16. A radiograph showing the tip of a radio-opaque catheter obstructed by a calculus in the right ureter.

Ureteritis descending from infection of the renal pelvis may give rise to slight penile pain and to increased frequency of micturition, and thus simulate vesical disease before the bladder is actually infected. This is seen most commonly in the *tuberculous* form, but is present in a less marked degree with infection by other organisms, of which the most common are *Escherichia coli communis* and *Streptococcus faecalis*. In the non-tuberculous form the ureter may be felt per rectum to be slightly thickened, but the cystoscopic appearance of the inflamed ureteric orifice is distinctive. In *descending tuberculosis* from the kidney, the ureter may be felt as a firm, infiltrated cord on the bladder base, the penile pain and increased frequency of micturition are more marked, the kidney may be felt enlarged and tender, and tubercle bacilli will be found in the urine. Apart from this, typical changes in the ureteric orifice are seen on cystoscopic examination, the orifice being pulled up or retracted or horseshoe-shaped, and usually occupying a position slightly above and outside the situation of the normal orifice, due to the actual shortening of the ureter by infiltration of the submucous coats. The rigid 'golf-hole' ureteric orifice is a late manifestation caused by contraction of scar tissue around it and in the ureter above it.

3. Diseases of the prostate

These often cause pain in the penis immediately following micturition. This is seen most commonly with acute inflammation or abscess in the gland as a sequela of acute gonorrhoea or septic urethritis. In either case there is penile pain, sometimes associated with erection, but little difficulty will be experienced in the diagnosis on due consideration of the symptoms and upon rectal examination.

Prostatic calculi are not uncommon there may be a single calculus or a nest of them in the prostate. They may ulcerate into the urethra so that small calculi may be passed in the urinary stream, or some may pass back along the dilated prostatic urethra into the bladder. If a calculus projects from the prostate into the urethra it causes pain in the penis after micturition. A diagnosis of prostatic calculus is often made by the grating sensation imparted to a catheter in traversing the prostatic urethra, whilst on rectal examination the calculus may be felt as an isolated hard nodule in the gland (where it may mimic prostatic carcinoma), or, if more than one is present, by the crepitation of one upon another on digital pressure in the rectum. A radiograph of the pelvis will show the shadows of prostatic calculi at the level of the upper part of the pubic symphysis (see *Fig. K.* 14).

4. Diseases of the seminal vesicles

These are seldom present without accompanying disease of the prostate of bladder. Acute vesiculitis may follow urethritis and give rise to pain after micturition, but in most cases it will be associated with prostatitis. Similarly, tuberculous nodules in the vesicle will be associated with foci in the epididymis, prostate or bladder.

5, 6. Diseases of the rectum and anus

These may occasionally give rise to penile pain following micturition, apart from any infection of the bladder or prostate. Thus an infiltrating carcinoma in the anal canal, a rectal fissure or an inflamed haemorrhoid may occasionally cause pain in the penis, but in each the local symptoms of the trouble will be the more marked, and little difficulty will be found in the diagnosis if a local examination is made with care.

C. Pain in the penis apart from micturition

Under the above divisions the symptom of penile pain has been considered in relation to the act of micturition, and it remains to consider some conditions giving rise to pain in the penis *apart from urination*. These include certain local lesions of the penis and urethra, and also the pains referred from disease elsewhere. Although a local lesion may cause little more than discomfort in many patients, in some it is described as pain, the degree of which depends upon the nervous susceptibility of the individual. Thus penile pain may be present with *acute urethritis*, with *balanitis* in association with *phimosis*, with *paraphimosis*, or with the *lymphangitis* of the organ due to a septic sore or abrasion of the skin or mucous membrane. In some instances *herpes* of the prepuce or penile skin causes distinct pain. Any infiltration of the cavernous tissue of the penis causes pain during erection of the organ; thus during an attack of acute urethritis the symptom known as *chordee* arises from this cause. It may occur in a chronic form in Peyronie's disease (chronic indurative cavernositis), a condition of unknown aetiology but similar to, and sometimes associated with, Dupuytren's contracture and retroperitoneal fibrosis. In this condition erection is not only painful but may be accompanied by lateral deviation of the organ. Another condition causing the same trouble arises from the organization of a haematoma in the cavernous tissues of the penis following upon a local injury, due either to external violence or arising during forcible attempts at coitus. A similar condition may arise spontaneously in blood diseases, especially *lymphatic* or *myelocytic leukaemia*.

Epithelioma of the penis on rare occasions gives rise to pain the organ.

Pain may be felt in the penis in some cases of *renal colic*, in which case it is classed as a referred pain. Thus in the acute colic accompanying the passage of a calculus, blood clot or debris of caseous material, aching pain may be felt in the penis quite apart from the increased desire to pass urine. Penile pain is, however, only a minor detail in the presence of the severe pain in the loin, and along the course of the ureter, and is often only lightly alluded to or revealed on direct questioning of the patient.

Finally, pain in the penis may be based on an anxiety state or some other mental cause rather than organic disease.

Harold Ellis

Perineal pain

Pain in the perineum is a symptom often mentioned by patients in giving their history of some affection of the genito-urinary apparatus or of other organs, but usually only as a dull aching, of which little notice is taken, as it is generally of minor degree in comparison with other more striking symptoms. The complaint of perineal pain *per se* does not convey much information to the clinician, and it is practically never present as the only symptom in a case. It may be a manifestation of an anxiety state.

Aching in the perineum is frequently present in diseases of the following organs:

PROSTATE
Acute or subacute inflammation
Abscess
Chronic prostatitis
Tuberculosis
Calculus
Adenomatous enlargement
Carcinoma

SEMINAL VESICLES
Acute inflammation
Tuberculosis

TESTICLE
Congenital misplacement in perineum

URINARY BLADDER
Cystitis
Tuberculosis
Calculus
Carcinoma

URETHRA
Gonorrhoea
Injury and rupture
Stricture with extravasation or urethral abscess
Fistula
Calculus impacted in bulbo-prostatic portion

ANAL AREA
Haemorrhoids
Fissure
Follicular abscess
Carbuncle
Ulcer
Carcinoma

VAGINA
Acute inflammation
Inflammation or abscess of Bartholin's glands
Cystocele
Epithelioma

CUTANEOUS DISEASES
Intertrigo
Diabetic inflammation
Condylomas

From the foregoing list it will be seen that aching in the perineum occurs with numerous different lesions, but other symptoms discussed elsewhere are in almost every case more marked. In prostatic disease it is an indication of inflammation rather than of enlargement. In clinical practice it is most commonly found to be due to chronic inflammation of the prostate gland. Examination of the secretion expressed after prostatic massage will show the presence of many pus cells.

Harold Ellis

Perineal sores

Ulceration may be present in the perineum as the result of:

1   Cutaneous inflammation or injury
2   Urethral suppurations or fistulas
3   Prostatic suppuration
4   Anal fistula
5   Syphilis
6   Granuloma venereum (inguinale)
7   Lymphogranuloma inguinale (venereum)
8   Epithelioma and other cutaneous cancers
9   Carcinoma of the urethra

1.   Cutaneous inflammation or injury

An ulcer in the perineum may result from *direct injury* to the area, or from inflammatory *infection of the sebaceous* or *hair follicles*. An ulcer from these causes may be placed at the centre or to one side of the perineum, is movable on the deeper parts, and shows no track into which a probe can be passed. In women, ulceration of the perineal area may be associated with *gonorrhoeal* or *septic vaginal discharge*. It may also arise from severe scratching caused by the irritation of such skin infections as *tinea cruris* or *pruritus ani*.

2.   Urethral suppurations or fistulas

During the progress of an acute urethritis a glandular follicle may become infected. The suppurative process leading from this in the bulbous urethra may extend towards the perineum and open externally, leaving a small fistula which may or may not discharge urine during the act of micturition. In a similar manner urinary fistulas may result from inflammatory processes behind a urethral stricture, and in an old-standing case it is not uncommon to find a urinary calculus in the dilated portion of the urethra behind the stricture. When the urethral suppuration is acute and an abscess bursts in the perineum, the diagnosis will be obvious, and the ordinary treatment for an abscess, in addition to that of the acute urethritis, will usually suffice to cure the condition. If the perineal wound discharges urine this occurs as a rule only during the act of micturition, as there is no interference with the vesical sphincter; a stricture of the urethra, not necessarily of sufficient degree to cause severe interference with micturition, will generally be seen on endoscopic examination, the sloughy granulations behind it denoting the position of the urethral opening of the fistula.

3. Diseases of the prostate

An abscess or tuberculous focus in the prostate may occasionally discharge in the perineum, and remain as a sinus. An abscess in the prostate arises practically always from some infection in the posterior urethra, from venereal causes, or after septic instrumentation. It is accompanied by urethral discharge, or there is a history of a recent infection, whilst per rectum the prostate may be felt to be inflamed, or scarred from the shrinkage of the abscess cavity.

When a tuberculous cavity in the prostate opens in the perineum there is advanced tuberculous disease, so that little difficulty will be found in arriving at a diagnosis. A tuberculous prostate is very rarely a primary condition, but in most cases is secondary to disease in the kidney, epididymis or bladder, so that examination of these organs will in nearly all cases give evidence of tuberculous disease and indicate the nature of the perineal fistula. Palpation of the prostate per rectum may reveal the rounded nodular deposits of tubercle in the gland.

4. Anal fistula

An ulcer on the perineum may be present as the result of an anal fistula—commonly from perianal suppuration and occasionally as a tuberculous infection. The history of pain on defecation followed by the rupture of a suppurating focus and the history of passage of flatus or faecal matter from the fistula are usually present, or a probe may be passed into the fistula and felt by a finger passed into the rectum.

Perianal and perirectal abscesses, fissures and fistulas may occur in Crohn's disease, especially when the colon is involved, and less commonly in ulcerative colitis.

5. Syphilis

Syphilis may cause ulceration on the perineum either as a chancre or as mucous tubercles. A *chancre* at this site is rare. It forms a small ulcer with slightly indurated borders, indolent in character, and accompanied by slight enlargement of the inguinal lymph nodes. A chancre of the skin may not possess the usual features of a genital chancre, and is not usually diagnosed with certainty until the secondary lesions of syphilis become apparent; but an ulcer with raised, infiltrated edges, which shows no tendency to heal under aseptic precautions, should always give rise to a suspicion of syphilis. The *Treponema pallidum* should be looked for, under darkground illumination, and serological tests for syphilis performed.

Condylomas may be present about the perineum in association with active syphilis. They may extend from the anal or vulval orifice, and form oval or rounded, flat-topped, sessile masses, covered by macerated greyish epithelium, or they may be ulcerated on the surface. The accompanying signs of syphilis will indicate the diagnosis.

Soft sores may occur in the perineum as well as on the scrotum or the vulva; they are generally venereal, but are not in themselves syphilitic; they are generally multiple, are apt to be foul, and cultures from them yield Ducrey's bacillus (*Haemophilus ducreyi*).

6, 7. Ulceration of granuloma inguinale

Ulceration of granuloma inguinale sometimes attacks the perineum, and fistulas there can be caused by lymphogranuloma venereum (*see* PENILE SORES).

8, 9. Epitheliomatous ulceration

Epitheliomatous ulceration of the perineum is seen as a direct spread of a growth of the anus or vulval area, when the diagnosis presents no difficulty. An epithelioma may develop in the scar of some former cutaneous affection, particularly in long-standing fistula in ano, in which case an ulceration may exist showing the usual characteristics of a cutaneous epithelioma. The inguinal nodes may be enlarged early from the inflammatory absorption, or later by invasion with malignant disease. Other cutaneous cancers, malignant melanoma and basal-cell carcinoma, may also occur in this situation. In case of doubt a fragment may be removed for microscopical examination. In late cases of carcinoma of the urethra following urethral stricture malignant ulceration spreads to the perineum by direct extension.

Harold Ellis

Peristalsis, visible

(*See also* BORBORYGMI.)

Usually visible peristalsis is pathological. However, in a number of conditions the normal movements of the bowel may be visible; these circumstances are divarication of the abdominal recti muscles, an incisional or massive umbilical hernia containing bowel, and extreme thinness of the abdominal parietes—the result of emaciation or, rarely, congenital absence of the recti. It is not uncommon to see visible peristalsis within the sac of a very large ventral or inguinoscrotal hernia (*Fig.* P.17). In all these circumstances the diagnosis can be made at inspection and the patient is otherwise symptomless. In all other situations, visible peristalsis is pathological and may be of two types, gastric and intestinal.

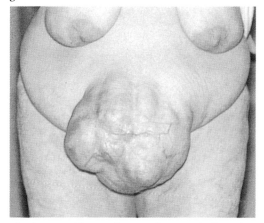

Fig. P.17. Visible peristalsis was obvious in this large thin-walled umbilical hernia.

Gastric peristalsis

Gastric peristalsis takes the form of a comparatively large swelling in the upper abdomen showing slow waves of peristalsis which progress from under the region of the left ribs, slowly downwards and to the right. This swelling indicates obstruction to the gastric outlet. There may be other signs of gastric dilatation and distension, particularly a loud succussion splash (*Fig.* P.18). Typically there is a history of the vomiting of large amounts of liquid in a projectile manner which may contain fragments of food ingested 24 hours or more previously. The diagnosis can be confirmed by the passage of a nasogastric tube, which will yield a pint or more of fluid several hours after the last food or drink has been taken; the aspirate has a typical stale, unpleasant smell and may contain recognizable particles of food eaten even several days before. A barium X-ray examination will clinch the diagnosis by demonstrating the gastric retention and dilatation. An X-ray taken 6 or 8 hours after the ingestion of the barium is particularly valuable since this will confirm the extent of gastric holdup (*Fig.* P.19). In doubtful cases of visible gastric peristalsis, the sign may be accentuated by asking the patient to swallow several glasses of soda-water. In the normal subject no peris-

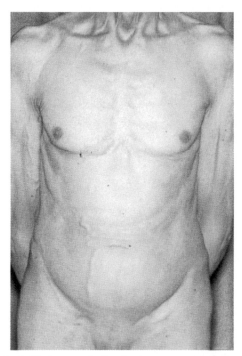

Fig. P.18. Gross gastric dilatation due to a stenosing duodenal ulcer. The stomach was visible, gave a loud splash, and showed typical gastric peristalsis.

talsis is seen, but in cases of pyloric obstruction, previously invisible peristalsis may now become obvious.

In congenital hypertrophic pyloric stenosis of

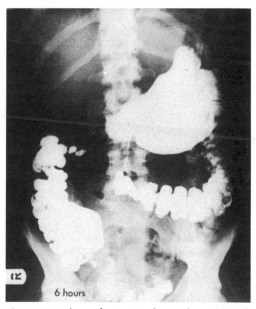

Fig. P.19. Six hours after ingesting barium this patient, with gross pyloric stenosis due to duodenal ulceration and with obvious visible gastric peristalsis, still has considerable residue in the stomach. Note that the barium which has escaped through the stenosis has already reached the splenic flexure.

infancy not only can gastric peristalsis be seen after a drink from a bottle but the hypertrophied pylorus can often be felt. This interesting and eminently treatable condition becomes apparent not immediately, but some 4 weeks after birth.

Visible intestinal peristalsis

Visible intestinal peristalsis is a feature of advanced intestinal obstruction with the limitations discussed above. As a pathological entity it will not occur alone but is accompanied by colicky abdominal pain, abdominal distension, vomiting and absolute constipation. The discussion of the differential diagnosis of the different causes of the symptoms will be found elsewhere. If the small intestine alone is involved, the waves are multiple and run more or less transversely across the abdomen—the ladder pattern; when the colon is obstructed, peristalsis takes the form of vertical waves, especially in one or both flanks, but this is much more rarely seen. Plain radiographs of the abdomen taken in the erect and supine positions are invaluable; the first demonstrate multiple fluid levels, the second the distribution of gas shadows within the dilated loops of bowel which will often enable the clinician to determine whether small or large bowel is obstructed. (*See also* p. 117 and *Figs.* C.26, C.27).

Harold Ellis

Phobias

A phobia is a persistent, irrational, morbid fear of a specific object, situation or activity that induces a compelling desire to avoid that stimulus. This reaction is acknowledged as inappropriate or disproportionate, but nevertheless the individual is unable to desist from avoidance behaviour because of the anxiety that develops when exposure occurs or is anticipated. In effect phobias are negative obsessions. The causes of phobias are listed in *Table* P.5.

Most people probably harbour mild phobic responses to such common stimuli as harmless insects and snakes, spiders, dogs, small furry animals, lifts, heights, air travel, darkness, tunnels, blood, vomiting, dentists—and even doctors! All are catalogued by classically derived prefixes which can be employed to impress. Typically these exaggerated fears can be overcome if necessary, place no limitations upon lifestyle and are often regarded as socially acceptable reactions, so treatment is rarely sought or required. Clinically appreciable phobias are reported in about 8 per cent of the adult population, about 1 in 40 cases being severely disabling.

1. SIMPLE PHOBIAS (monophobias) become a medical problem when either they are intense and distressing or impair social functioning—common

Table P.5. Causes of phobias

Commonest
Primary phobia
Anxiety

Less common
Drugs
  Alcohol abuse
  Hallucinogens
  Sympathomimetics
  Stimulants
Drug withdrawal
Psychiatric disorders
  Depression
  Panic
  Schizophrenia
  Paranoid disorder
  Obsessive compulsive disorder
  Post-traumatic stress disorder
  Personality disorder
    Avoidant
    Schizoid

Rare
Neurological disorders
  Brain tumour
  Cerebrovascular disease
  Multiple sclerosis
  Epilepsy
  Head injury

examples include the pregnant women who cannot permit venepuncture, the businessman who cannot fly when his job demands it, the child who will not leave home because of the neighbour's dog. In children this type of development is usually brief and overcome with reassurance, but in adults specialist assistance and behaviour therapy are more likely to be required. Secondary simple phobias are uncommon: in schizophrenia a phobia can represent the response to an unrevealed delusion and remits when the delusion subsides, while in obsessional neurosis phobias frequently develop in the context of cleaning rituals with the patient avoiding objects or situations through which contamination is feared.

2. ILLNESS PHOBIAS differ in that the phobia consists of endless ruminations about the possibility of suffering from a disease rather than primary avoidance. The patient will seek reassurance from the doctor that they do not have the disease, which contrasts importantly with hypochondriacal delusions where the patient is already convinced the disease is present. Common illness phobias concern cancer, heart disease and venereal disease but any disorder can become implicated—and particularly when attracting media attention, hence topical illness phobias include AIDS, radiation and food additives. Illness phobias are more common in patients with appreciable obsessional or hypochondriacal traits in their personality and often signify an underlying stress. The presentation is distinguishable from obsessional ruminations in that the patient feels no tension to resist their thoughts, and from

hypochrondriasis in that there is a single concern with reassurance often effective. Illness phobias can be the presenting feature of a primary depressive illness when they respond to antidepressant treatment; but if unrecognized, phobias may progress to frank hypochondriacal delusions in depressed patients.

3. While simple phobias are the most common form of the disorder, AGORAPHOBIA tends to be the most incapacitating and accounts for over half the phobic presentations to specialists. The essential features of agoraphobia are a marked fear of being alone accompanied by apprehension of becoming helpless in, or unable to escape from, a public place. Life becomes increasingly constricted as fears about streets, travelling, shopping, crowds and enclosed or open spaces take root: typically the patient will battle unsuccessfully and present when virtually restricted to their home or dependent upon others for accomplishing routine daily activities. This condition is twice as common in women than men, usually develops in early adult life and is associated with personality traits of passivity, dependence and anxiousness. A precipitant which may threaten the individual's security is often evident—commonly a social change such as marriage, divorce, bereavement, childbirth; less commonly an incapacitating, unpredictably episodic illness such as asthma, epilepsy or Menière's disease, and sometimes a more persistent physical change, for example, following a head injury or other brain disease, amputation, transplantation or other forms of major surgery. Once established for about a year, agoraphobia usually persists with remissions and relapses linked to life stresses.

Agoraphobia is almost always accompanied by other neurotic features—panic attacks, free-floating anxiety, neurotic depression, hyperventilation, obsessions and depersonalization are all frequently reported. As with simple phobias, schizophrenia or obsessional neurosis may occasionally be underlying, but the commonest cause of secondary agoraphobia is depressive illness.

Sometimes it can be impossible to decide clinically whether the patient has depression with secondary agoraphobia or agoraphobia with secondary depression, although evidence of agoraphobic changes over months or years would point to the latter. In circumstances of uncertainty it is worthwhile prescribing an antidepressant drug as secondary agoraphobia will remit.

Finally it is advisable to inquire about health and education problems in the children of agoraphobic women. Children may not be going to school either because their mother would be stranded at school or, more seriously requires them as a crutch at home:

sometimes school phobia or other neurotic problems emerge, and occasionally the child can form the initial presentation.

4. SOCIAL PHOBIAS are especially common in adolescents. The patient avoids social situations because of the intense fear of behaving in an embarrassing or humiliating manner, and the feeling of being under scrutiny by an audience who are able to detect minor signs of their anxiety. Common social phobias are speaking, eating, drinking, writing or blushing in public, and using public lavatories. Usually the patient has a single phobia linked to a specific situation but occasionally all forms of social contact are avoided and the patient leads the life of a recluse.

Many social phobics treat their fear and anxiety by using alcohol or tranquillisers and consequently some present with alcohol or drug dependence. Other phobias can coexist, although agoraphobia tends to develop later in life: incidentally agoraphobics also fear groups of people but their phobia centres upon the mass of people while social phobics are apprehensive of the individuals within the crowd. Again schizophrenia and obsessional neurosis may underlie a social phobia, although in depressive illness unresisted social withdrawal is commoner and motivated by anhedonia rather than fear. In more profound social phobia the possibility of a developing schizophrenic illness should be kept in mind, particularly if the patient is less concerned about their impoverished lifestyle than would be anticipated, and for some patients with avoidant personality disorder social phobias establish a persistent, unwelcome impairment of life, with work and relationships grossly affected. However such patients are rare, and the majority of social phobics have an excellent outlook often with a minimum of advice and assistance.

George Masterton

Photophobia

Photophobia, or intolerance of light, needs to be carefully distinguished from blepharospasm (a reflex spasm of the orbicularis, usually due to some conjunctival or corneal irritant, which can be annulled by a drop of amethocaine).

Photophobia is found in albinos (who are dazzled by the excess of light reaching their retinas), in cases of acute iritis, keratitis and congestive glaucoma, and it can be allayed by dark glasses or an eye-pad. It should be emphasized that dark glasses are generally worn for cosmetic or psychopathic reasons.

Photophobia is also a feature of subarachnoid haemorrhage and meningitis, although headache and other cerebral symptoms will predominate.

S. T. D. Roxburgh

Pica

Dirt eating is seen in children with emotional deprivation especially between the ages of 2 and 5 years; it is interpreted as the child's symbolic response to a lack of maternal affection and care. It may lead to poisoning if noxious substances are eaten accidentally or to obstruction of the stomach if multiple foreign bodies are eaten, such as pebbles. If the swallowed material is fibrous it may bind together to form a bezoar which forms a cast of the stomach with consequent obstruction. A variant of pica is trichophytomania where hair is pulled out and eaten with the formation of a trichobezoar.

Severe learning difficulties at all ages may be associated with pica. Iron deficiency, especially when the haemoglobin falls below 7 g/l, is associated with pica and is thought to represent a primitive craving for iron-containing soil. Although this may have been an important survival feature of the species, it is impossible to prove. Lead poisoning is associated with pica and may greatly add to the intake of lead if it is available in the child's environment in the form of paint on toys or cots, or pieces of crumbling paintwork in old houses. The relationship between pica and learning difficulties, iron deficiency and lead poisoning is complex but investigation should always be performed to take account of this interrelationship.

G. S. Clayden

Pilimiction

Pilimiction, that is the passage of hairs in the urine, a rare condition which almost invariably signifies that the patient has a pelvic dermoid cyst that has become inflamed, thereafter opening into the bladder and discharging its contents via the urinary passages, has been observed in men, but it is less uncommon in women. Subacute or acute cystitis accompanies the event with vesical pain, frequency of micturition and pyuria. The obvious fallacy in diagnosis arises from the possibility of contamination in the urine of hairs which were not, as supposed, passed per urethram.

Harold Ellis

PLASMA
  ALBUMIN
  BILIRUBIN
  CALCIUM
  CREATININE
  ENZYMES
  GLUCOSE
  MAGNESIUM
  PHOSPHATE
  POTASSIUM
  SODIUM
  TOTAL PROTEIN
  UREA
  URIC ACID
See APPENDIX.

Pleural effusion

Pleural effusion, the presence of fluid lying between the visceral and parietal pleura, is common and may be associated with a large number of conditions. Pulmonary embolic disease, cardiac failure, malignant pleural infiltration and pneumonia are the four most important conditions which are responsible for more than 90 per cent of pleural effusions seen in clinical practice.

Physiology of the pleura

In health the two pleural surfaces are in close contact but separated by a thin layer of fluid. Estimates of the volume vary but quoted figures range from 1 to 20 ml with an electrolyte content similar to serum and a low protein concentration. The fluid is formed by transudation from the parietal pleura and is absorbed by the visceral pleura. It is in a dynamic state with some two-thirds of the fluid being absorbed and replaced every hour.

The pleura transmits the forces generated by the respiratory muscles to the lungs and there is a negative pressure within the pleural space of about −5 mmHg. Capillary fluid and gas would enter the pleural space were it not for a number of balancing factors including a hydrostatic pressure difference between the parietal capillaries and the capillaries of the visceral pleura which are supplied by the low pressure pulmonary arterial system. Plasma oncotic pressure is the same in both sets of capillaries (about 35 mmHg) while pleural osmotic pressure is only about 6 mmHg due to its low protein content.

Thus fluid is driven in sequence from the parietal pleural capillaries to the pleural space and then on to the visceral pleural capillaries and lymphatics resulting in a continuous transfer of low protein fluid.

In the case of gas entering the pleural space there is a driving force of about 40 mmHg (atmospheric pressure−pleural pressure + pleural capillary blood gas tension) which assists gas absorption, as occurs in closed pneumothoraces.

Clinical features

The symptoms associated with the accumulation of fluid in the pleural space depend upon the cause, volume and rate of formation of fluid. Small effusions are often symptomless and even quite large effusions can cause little disability provided the fluid has accumulated slowly. Effusions caused by inflammatory disease often present with pleuritic pain which may be relieved as the fluid accumulates. Large effusions eventually cause symptoms including dry cough, shortness of breath, initially on exercise and later at rest, together with dull, aching discomfort over the affected side of the chest.

The clinical findings are influenced by the size and site of the effusion. Most effusions occupy the dependent part of the pleural space and so when the patient is sitting, the characteristic findings of stony dullness to percussion and distant or absent breath sounds are most prominent at the lung bases. Bronchial breath sounds or aegophony may be heard directly above an effusion. Large effusions displace the mediastinum towards the unaffected side unless the underlying lung is fibrosed from previous inflammation (tuberculosis) or collapsed due to a proximal bronchial lesion. Very large effusions may displace the mediastinal contents to produce an area of dullness at the opposite base close to the midline (Grocco's sign).

Radiological features

Effusions may be small, moderate, large, encysted, mediastinal or subpleural. Small effusions may be difficult to detect clinically but can be seen radiographically as non-specific blunting of the costophrenic angles. Moderate sized free effusions cast a characteristic homogeneous shadow over the lower lung fields obscuring the diaphragm and cardiac silhouette. At the upper border of the effusion there is decreased density of the radiographic opacification with a superior concave curvature which appears to reach its highest level in the axilla when seen on PA films or posteriorly on lateral films. In fact the level of the effusion is horizontal and the radiographic appearances are artefactual due to the increased distance traversed by the radiation. Massive effusions cause complete opacification of the hemithorax often with very marked displacement of the mediastinal structures to the opposite side. Sometimes the fluid collects in the pleural cavity under the lung adjacent to the diaphragm, the so-called diaphragmatic or subpulmonary pleural effusion. The upper margin of the fluid shadow runs parallel to and may be mistaken for an elevated diaphragm. On the left side the apparent separation of the transradiant gastric 'air bubble' from the transradiant lung tissue may draw attention to the effusion. If the presence of fluid is in doubt, a lateral decubitus film may help to differentiate between effusion or pleural thickening when, in the former, the fluid is seen to shift to the lateral chest wall or mediastinum. Interlobar pleural effusions are quite commonly seen as an extension of an effusion and result in a characteristic ovoid

homogeneous shadowing with well-demarcated margins lying in one of the interlobar fissures. Interlobar effusions may mimic tumours and occur particularly in cardiac failure when clearance following diuretic treatment gives rise to the term 'vanishing pulmonary tumour'.

Encysted effusions can give rise to diagnostic difficulties especially if they lie posteriorly and cause homogeneous shadowing suggesting consolidation when seen on posteroanterior films. The nature of the abnormality becomes apparent in a lateral view when opacification is seen to lie posteriorly.

Etiology

The majority of pleural effusions are related to increased pleural capillary permeability and occur in response to inflammation (both infective and other), ischaemia (pulmonary infarction) and pleural neoplasia. The clinical findings may provide some diagnostic clues as may radiology which will also localize the position of the fluid and reveal its extent. In most cases the fluid must be examined cytologically, biochemically and be cultured for organisms.

Table P.6. Causes of pleural transudates

Increased hydrostatic pressure
Congestive cardiac failure
Constrictive pericarditis
Pericardial effusion
Restrictive cardiomyopathy
Massive pulmonary embolism

Decreased capillary oncotic pressure
Nephrotic syndrome
Malnutrition
Protein-losing enteritis
Cirrhosis
Hepatic cirrhosis

Other causes
Myxoedema
Ascites due to ovarian tumour (Meig's syndrome)

The appearance of the freshly aspirated fluid can be informative. It is usually straw-coloured or cloudy but can be frankly purulent (empyema), blood-stained (haemothorax) or opalescent (chylothorax). Blood-stained effusions are relatively common and, setting aside trauma to the chest or accidental haemorrhage resulting from a traumatic pleural tap, is most commonly seen in malignancy or pulmonary infarction. A pleural fluid red cell count of less than 10 000 RBC per ml is not diagnostic but more that 100 000 RBC per ml is significant.

The pleural fluid formed through normal capillary membranes is a transudate with a low protein content whereas fluid formed through abnormally permeable capillary walls contains a higher concentration of protein. The distinction between a transudate and exudate

Table P.7. Causes of pleural exudates

1. Pulmonary embolism/infarction

2. Neoplasia
Mesothelioma/adenocarcinoma of pleura
Lymphoma
Bronchial neoplasm with local spread
Metastases
   Thoracic primary
   Secondary—breast, gastrointestinal or ovary

3. Infections
Pneumonia—sympathetic effusion or empyema
Tuberculosis
Atypical mycobacterial infection
Subphrenic abscess
Hepatic
Hydatid disease (lung or liver)
Actinomycosis
Aspergillosis in immunosuppressed patients
Coccidioidomycosis
Blastomycosis

4. Connective tissue diseases
Rheumatoid arthritis
Systemic lupus erythematosus
Sjögren's syndrome
Wegener's granulomatosis
Rheumatic fever
Postmyocardial infarction syndrome (Dressler's)

5. Other causes
Recurrent polyserositis
Yellow nail syndrome
Drugs—eosinophilic reactions induced by a range of
   drugs (sulphonamides, salicylates, beta blockers) or
   the lupus syndrome (isoniazid, phenytoin,
   hydralazine)
Chylothorax
Industrial exposure to asbestos
Radiation
Sarcoidosis
Oesophageal perforation

may be obvious on clinical grounds, for instance when there is cardiac, renal or hepatic failure. By convention a transudate has a specific gravity of less than 1·016 or a protein content less than 30 g/l. However, up to 30 per cent of transudates are shown to have a specific gravity in excess of 1·016 and 10 per cent have a protein content greater than 30 g/l. An improved discrimination between transudate and exudate can be achieved by considering the pleural fluid lactic dehydrogenase (LDH) level, where activity in excess of 200 iu or pleural fluid/serum LDH ratio greater than 0·6 is characteristic of an exudate.

The pleural fluid cytological findings in benign effusions are variable. Mesothelial cells and macrophages are found in most transudates. Mesothelial cells predominate in exudates especially when due to pulmonary infarction. Neutrophil polymorphonuclear leucocytes are frequently present in sterile and infected effusions associated with pulmonary inflammation. The exception to this pattern is tuberculosis where an initial neutrophil excess is quickly replaced by lymphocytes which may account for between 80–100 per cent of all

the cells present in the effusion. Lymphocytic pleural effusions are not specific to tuberculosis and occur in sarcoidosis or some forms of malignancy (e.g. lymphoma).

A high pleural fluid eosinophil count is seldom associated with allergy but is seen in occasional pulmonary infarcts, malignancy or simply when there has been bleeding into the pleural space.

Malignant cells are present in about two-thirds of cases where there is malignant invasion of the pleura. The appearances are often diagnostic of the cell type and when due to metastases often can reveal the site from where the primary tumour has arisen.

Other useful characteristics of the fluid include measurements of pH and blood glucose. A low pH (pH less than 7·30) is occasionally seen in tuberculosis or in parapneumonic effusions prior to the onset of frank empyema. A pH greater than 7·40 is most frequently found in malignancy. The presence of a low pleural fluid glucose (less than 1·7 mmol/l or 13 mg/100 ml) and normal serum glucose suggests rheumatoid pleural disease; although rarer cases of tuberculosis, malignancy and empyema may also be found to have a low pleural fluid glucose.

Tables P.6 and P.7 summarize the causes of pleural effusions.

P. R. Studdy

Pleural rub

The diagnostic sign of pleurisy is a rub of a creaking superficial nature usually located close to the site of pain.

The pleura is a double serous membrane separating the lung from the chest wall and mediastinum. The pleural surface consists of a uniform layer of mesothelial cells supported on a connective tissue framework well supplied with capillary and lymph vessels. The parietal pleura is innervated with pain-sensitive nerve fibres supplied by the intercostal and phrenic nerves, and is exquisitely sensitive to painful stimuli.

In health the visceral and parietal pleural surfaces are smooth, glistening and separated by a small amount of fluid, allowing low friction movement of the lungs with respiration.

In contrast, if the pleural surfaces become thickened or roughened by inflammation or neoplastic infiltration, movement with breathing will cause increased friction, which may be heard with a stethoscope. Patients commonly complain of thoracic pain on breathing or coughing. On auscultation sounds of varying intensity may be heard during inspiration and expiration, often described as having a leathery or creaking quality that may be exaggerated when the stethoscope is applied firmly to the chest wall. Pain associated with a pleural rub may vary in degree from lancinating discomfort during slight inspiratory effort to a less sharp 'catch' of pain at the end of maximum inspiration. Pleural pain is often reduced by breath holding or exerting firm pressure over the affected thoracic segment. Except when it involves the diaphragm, the affected pleura typically underlies the area in which pain is perceived. The central portion of the diaphragm is innervated from the third and fourth cervical posterior nerve roots running via the phrenic nerve. Pain caused by diaphragmatic pleural irritation is often referred to the neck and shoulders.

A pleural rub may last for as little as a few hours in short-lived inflammatory conditions such as pneumonia, to months or even years in patients with more chronic causes of pleurisy. Typically, as the pleurisy settles, the pain and physical signs including the rub become less obvious, although in some patients the rub may persist after the pain has gone and occasionally a loud rub may persist indefinitely.

Most pleuritic conditions giving rise to pain and auscultatory rub are inflammatory in origin. Infection associated with community acquired pneumonias, especially pneumococcal, mycoplasma and other 'atypical' infections, may present with severe pleurisy and a pleural rub accompanied by signs of pneumonic consolidation. Pulmonary infarction secondary to pulmonary embolism is another frequent cause, and is especially common following major surgery, in patients with underlying abdominal malignancy when thromboembolism may be the first sign of gastric or pancreatic carcinoma, or in females taking oestrogen preparations. Tumours invading the chest wall typically cause a continuous persistent pain, but may occasionally present with pleurisy and a pleural rub. Rather less frequently, a pleural rub may occur in association with asbestos-induced pleural disease, or connective-tissue diseases such as systemic lupus erythematosus, or rheumatoid arthritis. Recurrent pleurisy at the same site should suggest bronchiectasis, and at different sites, broncho-pulmonary aspergillosis. If pleurisy progresses to a pleural effusion the sharp pain and pleural rub largely disappear to be replaced by a dull and more constant ache and heaviness.

The pain of pleurisy may be mimicked by a number of chest wall conditions, such as rib fractures, intercostal muscle pain due to tearing or strain, Tietze's syndrome, and neurogenic causes such as intercostal nerve root compression and herpes zoster. Pain due to intercostal muscle strain and tears can be quite sharp, may be caused by coughing and can result in shallow breathing. However, local tenderness over the affected site is common and typically no pleural rub is heard.

Epidemic myalgia (pleurodynia, Bornholm disease, devil's grip, epidemic dry pleurisy), is an acute febrile viral illness affecting skeletal muscle characterized by an abrupt onset of intense pain in the lower chest or upper abdomen. In about 25 per cent of patients headache, malaise, anorexia, sore throat and deep myalgia precede the onset by 1 or 2 days. The afflicted patient complains of a fever of 38°C–40°C and multiple paroxysms of excruciating pain lasting from a few minutes to several hours. The illness is often biphasic with an initial bout of pain and fever settling, only to recur after a day or two. The acute illness usually settles within a week, but rarely patients have several recurrences over a period of several weeks. The illness may be accompanied by myocarditis or pericarditis.

Epidemic myalgia is caused by enteroviruses usually Coxsackie B3 or B5 but also Coxsackie A or echoviruses. The incubation period is short, about 3–5 days, and as with other enteroviral infections the majority of illnesses occur in the summer and autumn. A specific diagnosis can be made by isolating virus from the throat and faeces during the acute illness, or demonstrating a rising titre of serotype-specific neutralizing antibodies in acute and convalescent sera. The level of creatine phosphokinase in the serum may also be elevated, reflecting injury to striated muscle. Confusion with acute myocardial infarction is inevitable in those patients presenting with abnormal electrocardiograms and raised creatine phosphokinase. The condition may also be confused with pre-eruptive herpes zoster, although in the latter condition pain is more constant and no pleural rub detected.

Recurrent polyserositis (familial Mediterranean fever), is an autosomal, recessive, recurrent inflammatory disease of unknown cause, characterized by recurrent inflammation of serous membranes. Attacks occur at irregular intervals from several days to several years with pleurisy, abdominal and joint pain, and other systemic symptoms which typically settle spontaneously within 12–48 hours. This condition usually manifests in children, is recognized in many parts of the world, but is largely restricted to ethnic groups originating in the eastern Mediterranean area.

Investigation of patients presenting with pleurisy and a pleural rub will almost inevitably include a chest radiograph which is frequently useful in showing a primary lung condition. If the chest X-ray is normal, or if it only shows a small pleural reaction, it may be important to consider the possibility of a pulmonary embolism, and further examination of the legs, together with scanning may help in coming to a therapeutic decision. If pulmonary embolism is considered unlikely, and in the absence of any other features, it is reasonable to make a provisional diagnosis of viral pleurisy, and to treat with patient with adequate analgesia.

P. R. Studdy

Pneumaturia

The passage of gas per urethram, either with or independently of urine, is a rare but striking peculiarity, particularly when it occurs in males. It may be due to one or other of two distinct groups of causes, namely:

1 Communications between the rectum, caecum, vermiform appendix or other part of the alimentary canal and the bladder, ureter or renal pelvis, either directly or via an intermediate gas-containing abscess cavity.
2 Infection of the bladder or other part of the urinary tract by gas-producing microorganisms.

When the cause lies in the first group, the patient is apt to pass faecal material as well as gas. It should be added, however, that the passage of gas without faeces per urethram by no means excludes a fistulous communication between some part of the alimentary canal and the urinary tract: the fistula may be of such a character that while gas can traverse it faeces cannot. It may also happen that a lesion such as appendicitis or, most commonly, acute sigmoid diverticulitis has led to the formation of a local abscess which, owing to infection by the *Escherichia coli*, contains gas; this abscess may open into the bladder and cause the discharge of pus and gas, but no faeces, per urethram. The same applies to similar abscesses which though not arising primarily in connection with the bowel nevertheless contain gas from infection by the *E. coli*— for instance, a suppurating hydatid or ovarian dermoid cyst, or a pyosalpinx. Rectal, vaginal, abdominal, barium-enema X-ray, intravenous pyelographic and cystoscopic examinations may yield the diagnosis, but on occasion doubt will persist as to whether the gas is finding its way into the urinary passages from some external source, or whether it is being produced in situ, for certain organisms, notably *E. coli* and *Aspergillus aerogenes*, produce gas when they grow in urine, as may various *yeasts* in patients with glycosuria.

If no sign of a fistulous communication between any part of the bowel or a gas-containing abscess cavity with the urinary tract can be distinguished on cystoscopic examination, it may be with confidence presumed that the pneumaturia is due to infection. Such patients are usually elderly female diabetics with considerable glycosuria. The infecting organisms are usually *E. coli.*, *A. aerogenes*, *yeasts* or combinations of these.

The urine in such a case contains pus, sugar, and albumin. It may be acid, and not foul-smelling or ammoniacal; on the other hand, it may sometimes be so foul and faeculent as to arouse unwarranted suspicion of a communication between the colon and the bladder. A cystoscopic examination will serve to exclude a fistulous opening into the bladder, but it may be much more difficult to exclude a similar communication with the higher parts of the urinary tract, especially the renal pelvis. Such a condition is very rare, so that urinary infection is the more probable unless there is a known or recognizable cause for communication between the bowel and the renal pelvis, such as a carcinoma.

Harold Ellis

Polydipsia

The primary stimulus to the sensation of thirst is dehydration, which gives rise to an increase in the plasma osmolality of the blood passing through the thirst centre in the hypothalamus. An increase in plasma osmolality can also be achieved by increasing the solute load, for example by drinking salt water. The sensation of thirst must be distinguished from a dry mouth caused by Sjögren's syndrome, or mouth breathing or by drugs (monoamine oxidase inhibitors, the belladonna group, e.g. atropine, or astringents such as alum, gallic acid, tannic acid or perchloride of iron). Apparent thirst may also be due to a psychiatric disorder, when it is called psychogenic polydipsia.

True polydipsia due to dehydration may be associated with disorders which cause polyuria (*see below*), such as diabetes mellitus, cranial diabetes insipidus, nephrogenic diabetes insipidus and diuretic therapy. Other causes of dehydration not associated with polyuria include inadequate fluid intake, excessive loss of fluid from the skin (fever, thyrotoxicosis), from the stomach (repeated vomiting), from the bowel (diarrhoea) and into serous-lined cavities, as in acute peritonitis.

Ian D. Ramsay

Polyuria

The term 'polyuria' signifies a larger than normal daily volume of urine. There is considerable variation from subject to subject in the amount of urine passed, but a urinary output of more than 2·5 litres per 24 hours is nearly always abnormal. Polyuria must not be confused with frequency of micturition due, for example, to prostatic hypertrophy or cystitis. Also, although polyuria will almost always lead to a complaint of nocturia, many individuals complaining of the latter have no increase in the total output of urine but show a reversal of the normal diurnal variation in urine flow; this is the case in most cases of sodium and water retention as in cardiac failure or the nephrotic syndrome, in suprarenal disorders, and in chronic renal failure. Polyuria may be due either to an increased solute load with obligatory water loss or to a primary water diuresis and will be discussed under these headings. The main causes are summarised in *Table P.8*.

Polyuria due to increased solute load

Any osmotically active solute will produce a diuresis if present in excess in the distal tubular fluid. For example, the massive protein breakdown occurring in a large *haematoma* may be associated with a diuresis, urea itself being the active solute. It is also the mechanism of *diuretic therapy* in which the solute concerned is sodium. *Diabetes mellitus* is much the commonest pathological condition in which this type of polyuria occurs. The daily urine volume is often 4 litres or more and polyuria and excessive thirst are the most common symptoms; in children, previously dry at night, enuresis may be an early symptom of diabetes. The diagnosis is usually straight forward. In *chronic renal failure* the total solute load may be normal but the reduction in the number of nephrons results in a greater than normal load per nephron and consequent polyuria which is usually only of moderate severity. The polyuria which may follow the relief of chronic *urinary tract obstruction* is also partly due to this mechanism but some defect of concentrating power may also be present. Diuresis is also common during recovery from *acute tubular necrosis*; this is partly due to the elimination of water and electrolytes retained during the phase of oliguria and partly to incomplete recovery of tubular function.

Table P.8. Causes of polyuria

Due to increased solute load
Diabetes mellitus
Diuretic therapy
Chronic renal failure
Following relief of obstruction
During recovery from acute tubular necrosis
Resolving haematoma

Due to water diuresis
Psychogenic polydipsia
Cranial diabetes insipidus
Nephrogenic diabetes insipidus
  X-linked
  Potassium depletion
  Hypercalcaemia
  Drugs
  Sickle-cell anaemia
  Early chronic pyelonephritis

Other causes
Following fevers
After attacks of migraine, etc.
Paroxysmal tachycardia

Polyuria due to water diuresis

The simplest cause of this is an increased water intake which may reach pathological dimensions is the condition known as *psychogenic polydipsia* or *compulsive water-drinking*. This is a hysterical manifestation and simulates diabetes insipidus. The differentiation is discussed below but, clinically, marked fluctuations in urine output would strongly suggest psychogenic polydipsia. Patients with Sjögren's syndrome may try to relieve the dryness of their mouths by drinking large volumes of water, with a consequent modest polyuria.

The urine is normally concentrated in the distal tubules and collecting ducts. Antidiuretic hormone (ADH) is secreted by the posterior pituitary in response to a rise in plasma osmolality; its action is to increase the permeability of the tubular epithelium to water. The effect of this is to increase the transport of water from the tubular lumen into the hypertonic renal medulla through which these tubules pass. Thus a pathological water diuresis may be due either to failure of secretion of ADH or to failure of the renal tubules to respond to its action.

Cranial (neurogenic) diabetes insipidus is often caused by an identifiable lesion of the hypothalamus or pituitary or both, but in about one-third of cases no such cause can be found. Tumours in that region are a common cause and include craniopharyngioma, pinealoma, glioma and metastases from distant primary growths. Diabetes insipidus may also follow trauma to the skull (including operative), infections such as exanthemas in childhood, or be due to infiltration with granulomatous lesions such as sarcoidosis or histiocytosis X. In such cases other evidence of hypothalamic-pituitary disease may well be present. Occasionally diabetes insipidus is complicated by a destructive lesion of the 'thirst' centre in the hypothalamus so that polydipsia does not accompany the polyuria; water loss is severe and hypernatraemia with brain damage may result. There is a very rare familial form of cranial diabetes insipidus, inherited as an autosomal dominant trait; even rarer is the DIDMOAD syndrome (Diabetes Insipidus, Diabetes Mellitus, Optic Atrophy, Deafness), with autosomal recessive inheritance.

Failure of the renal tubules to respond to the action of ADH is termed *nephrogenic diabetes insipidus*. A familial form is seen in males only, inherited as a sex-linked recessive (X-linked). It may also be a part of other renal tubular defects such as the Fanconi syndrome with cystinosis and proximal renal tubular acidosis (Type 2); it can also occur in renal amyloidosis, myelomatosis and hyperglobulinaemia.

The differentiation of the two types of diabetes insipidus from each other and from psychogenic polydipsia may be difficult. This is because a prolonged water diuresis from any cause may lead to partial resistance to the action of ADH. Thus deprivation of water in psychogenic polydipsia may not cause immediate cessation of the polyuria although there will usually be a considerable reduction. In diabetes insipidus, nephrogenic or of cranial origin, the polyuria will continue despite water deprivation and the patient becomes very thirsty and ill; the test is not without its dangers in this situation. Further information may be obtained from the administration of desmopressin, an ADH analogue. This will clearly have no effect in nephrogenic diabetes insipidus but will reduce the urine output in cranial diabetes inspidus and in psychogenic polydipsia; once again the result may not be clear-cut and the effect of desmopressin may not be apparent for several days. There is a danger that, in psychogenic polydipsia, the continued ingestion of large amounts of water after the administration of ADH may cause water intoxication.

Several other conditions cause nephrogenic diabetes insipidus. Polyuria is a common feature of the renal lesion of *potassium depletion*, this condition might be suspected if muscular weakness is a prominent complaint or the deep reflexes are absent. Potassium depletion may be due to chronic diarrhoea, diuretic therapy, primary aldosteronism, excessive doses of corticosteroids and alkalosis from any cause; it is particularly seen in the type of Cushing's syndrome produced by an ACTH-secreting bronchial carcinoma. The polyuria fails to respond to desmopressin but is reversible if the potassium balance can be restored to normal.

Hypercalcaemia also can cause a water diuresis and might be suggested by associated abdominal pain and vomiting. Thus polyuria may be a feature of primary hyperparathyroidism, vitamin-D intoxication, sarcoidosis, multiple bony metastases or primary tumours secreting a parathormone-like substance. The renal lesion is reversible unless severe nephrocalcinosis has developed or renal calculi have produced irreversible damage. As in hypokalaemia there is no response to ADH. A reversible nephrogenic diabetes insipidus can also be produced by a number of drugs including lithium carbonate, demeclocycline, amphotericin B, glibenclamide and gentamicin.

Other conditions in which failure of urinary concentration occurs are *sickle-cell anaemia* and chronic *pyelonephritis* at an early stage. The polyuria due to the latter must not be confused with the osmotic diuresis of chronic renal failure discussed above.

Transient polyuria

Polyuria lasting for a few hours only can occur in various circumstances. It is rarely of any great significance and indeed is often physiological. The diuresis which follows excessive water drinking needs no comment. The same applies to polyuria in the course of

diuretic therapy, although the diuretic effect of such substances as tea or coffee may occasionally provoke a complaint from a patient who has not realized the association. *Cold* weather may also induce polyuria as a result of reduced fluid loss from the skin; travellers returning from a long stay in the tropics and accustomed to a large fluid intake may occasionally complain of polyuria on return to a colder country. It is this contrast with previous oliguria that partly explains the polyuria following *fevers*; there may also be a temporary impairment of ADH secretion.

Polyuria can also occur following various stressful situations and has been described after attacks of *migraine*, *asthma* and *angina*. A more striking polyuria may occur during and after attacks of *paroxysmal tachycardia*. Any dysrhythmia, supraventricular or ventricular, which lasts for more than half an hour may produce this effect. This is probably due to the release of atrial natriuretic peptide; this is probably due to the release of atrial natriuretic peptide.

Peter R. Fleming

Popliteal swelling

Popliteal swellings may be divided into:

1. FLUID SWELLINGS

Bursa
Morrant Baker's cyst
Varicose veins
Abscess
Aneurysm

2. SOLID SWELLINGS NOT CONNECTED WITH BONE

Enlarged lymph nodes
Malignant tumours
Innocent tumours

3. SOLID SWELLINGS CONNECTED WITH BONE

Exostosis
Sarcoma
Periostitis
Separation of the epiphysis

1. Fluid swellings

BURSAE

There are six primary bursae associated with muscles and tendons around the knee. Communications between two bursae and between a bursa and the knee joint are common.

The semimembranous bursa on the posterior aspect of the knee is often enlarged. When the leg is extended it stands out as a tense fluctuating swelling on the inner side of the popliteal space: on flexion it disappears completely. It may be found enlarged in young athletes and cause no symptoms whatever. On account of its fairly frequent communication with the knee joint it may be distended when that joint is the seat of an effusion, acting, as it were, as an overflow tank. Where the joint condition is an acute one the bursa may be very tender. In rheumatoid arthritis it is common for fluid to pass from joint into bursa but not in the reverse direction, a ball-valve mechanism apparently operating.

The bursae under either of the two heads of the gastrocnemius muscle or those connected with the insertion of the semitendinosus may be enlarged similarly, but these are rare.

MORRANT BAKER'S CYST

This is a herniation of the synovial membrane and only occurs in connection with chronic inflammatory changes in the joint, most commonly in rheumatoid arthritis, but the semimembranous bursa is usually also affected and is also distended. The extension from the joint tends to spread along fascial planes and may point at varying distances from its origin. The 'cysts' may be multiple. Such extensions of the knee joint may sometimes rupture and cause an inflammatory reaction in the calf muscles which may be mistaken for a deep venous thrombosis. Arthrography may be of help in diagnosis.

VARICOSE VEINS

Varicose veins are often present in the popliteal space; the diagnosis presents no difficulties, as the veins in the lower part of the leg will also be varicose. They become much more obvious when the patient stands.

These are the most common causes, the conditions which follow being much more rarely encountered.

ACUTE ABSCESS

This is recognized by the signs of acute inflammation; the skin is red and oedematous, the pulse and temperature are raised, and the swelling is very painful. The knee is kept flexed in order to minimize the tension of the part. The abscess may be caused by suppurating lymphatic nodes or by suppurative periostitis or necrosis of the lower end of the femur. In the former case the abscess will be superficial, and in the latter deep to the popliteal vessels.

ANEURYSM OF THE POPLITEAL ARTERY

This gives rise to an expansile pulsating tumour, the pulsation being synchronous with the heart's beat. Pressure on the femoral artery above will cause a diminution in size of the swelling and cessation of pulsation. The pulse at the ankle on the affected side

may be smaller than that on the opposite, and delayed. If a stethoscope be placed over the swelling a distinct bruit can be heard.

The complaint of the patient will probably be of pain, which may be referred down the leg if either popliteal nerve is pressed on, or in the site of the swelling if the bone is eroded. Varicose veins are almost always present on account of pressure on the popliteal vein. Owing to its pulsatile character an aneurysm is not often mistaken for anything else, but every swelling that pulsates is not an aneurysm. A soft vascular sarcoma growing from the end of the femur may be pulsatile, and over it a bruit may be heard, but the tumour is not as compressible as an aneurysm is and the effects on the distal pulse are not so marked. A radiograph will usually settle the question at once. Distinction must also be drawn between a tumour that pulsates and a tumour to which pulsation is communication. For instance, an abscess or a solid swelling lying over the popliteal artery may appear to pulsate, but the movement is heaving in character and not expansile. In the rare event of an aneurysm having become filled with clot it might be taken for a solid tumour growing either from the soft parts or from the bone. Finally the aneurysm may present on the medial side of the lower end of the thigh, anterior to the tendon of the sartorius.

2. Solid swellings not connected with bone

ENLARGED NODES

It is not common to find the popliteal nodes enlarged from any cause. It is possible that they may become infected with pyogenic organisms from a sore on the back of the leg.

TUMOURS

Tumours are rare. They may be innocent, e.g. *lipoma* and *neurofibroma*; or *sarcomatous*, starting in the connective tissue of the popliteal space, or attached to one of the muscles. The innocent tumours are of long history and well defined; the malignant, rapidly growing and infiltrating.

A lipomatous mass, either in the popliteal fossa or on the medial aspect of the knee, is not infrequently present in osteoarthritis of this joint, and is part of the general fatty infiltration which gives rise inside the joint to the *lipoma arborescens* of the synovial membrane.

3. Solid swellings connected with bone

In all cases of bony tumour a radiograph should always be obtained.

INNOCENT TUMOURS

Cancellous exostoses may be found, generally in children and young adults, growing from the region of the epiphysial cartilage of the femur. There may be others in other parts of the skeleton, and sometimes several members of the family are similarly affected. The swelling is of slow growth, well defined and rarely gives any trouble. It is most often found at the inner side of the popliteal space. There is one thing that may be confounded with it, namely, *ossification of the insertion of a tendon* or muscle. The adductor longus muscle is the one most commonly affected (rider's bone).

Osteoclastoma is prone to occur in the bones around the knee joint and may cause an asymmetrical expansion of the cortex presenting in the popliteal fossa. Usually expansion of the bone can be detected on other aspects and the shell may be so thin in some places if the condition is advanced that 'eggshell crackling' can be elicited. The radiographic appearances are typical—the expansion and thinning of the cortex, the absence of new bone formation and the trabeculation.

MALIGNANT TUMOURS

These include osteosarcoma, fibrosarcoma arising from the fibrous periosteum and metastases from neoplasm elsewhere. Here, as in giant-cell tumour, enlargement of the bone is not usually confined to the popliteal space. The diagnosis from inflammatory lesions can be very difficult even with a radiograph, and is often impossible without. The type of osteosarcoma which shows a palisade of bony spicules perpendicular to the line of the cortex is easily diagnosed by radiography, but it must be remembered that a sarcoma may present itself with an obvious clinical swelling and yet with little or no radiographic changes. This usually but not always denotes a *fibrosarcoma of the periosteum*, particularly if a thin line of periosteal new bone is laid down. Occasionally a small central area of erosion with a clinical swelling may indicate the presence of a bone sarcoma of the osteolytic type. Although there may be marked swelling, there is usually less effusion into the joint than is the case if the lesion is inflammatory. Computerized tomography is useful in providing accurate anatomical delineation of the tumour mass. Serological tests and a biopsy of the diseased part should be done in all doubtful bone lesions. A *gumma* is indicated by dense sclerosis around the lesion, clear-cut central softening without erosion, and regular bone formation. For further details and illustrations *see* the article on BONE, SWELLING OF.

PERIOSTITIS

Popliteal necrosis with abscess formation may give rise to a large swelling. The signs of inflammation will usually be well marked and accompanied by constitutional symptoms and leucocytosis. Chronic periostitis, or chronic abscess of the bone, or central necrosis, may be extremely difficult to distinguish from a malignant growth. A radiograph should be taken, and if necessary an incision made down to the tumour for a piece to be removed for histological examination.

SEPARATION OF THE EPIPHYSIS

In the somewhat rare accident of separation of the lower epiphysis of the femur the lower fragment becomes displaced backwards, forms a prominence in the popliteal space, and presses on the vessels sometimes to a dangerous extent. It is unlikely that such a condition would present itself as a doubtful popliteal swelling for diagnosis.

Harold Ellis

Porphyrias
See Appendix.

Posture, abnormal

The term 'posture' refers to the position either of one particular part of the body such as an arm or leg or to the position of the body as a whole. Abnormalities of posture may thus be limited to either individual parts of the body or to the appearance of the whole body.

A variety of factors may produce abnormalities of posture:

Pain

The position of a limb or the neck or back may be influenced by pain. The posture of the neck and back in particular may be affected when there is pain and paraspinal muscle spasm secondary to disc disease. The most obvious abnormalities are seen in patients with cervical spine disorders.

Skeletal abnormalities

Abnormalities of either bones or joints may produce postural changes; most obvious are those in the hands resulting from the deformity of rheumatoid arthritis.

Hysteria

Some of the most bizarre postural abnormalities may be seen in patients with hysteria. These abnormalities may affect head position, spine, gait or limbs. It is common for organic disorders such as dystonia in the early stages to be mistaken for hysteria.

Neurological disorders

Postural abnormalities are typical of a variety of neurological disorders.

In the unconscious patient, abnormalities such as decorticate or decerebrate posturing of the limbs may have diagnostic value.

In the conscious patient, disorders of the basal ganglia produce some of the most characteristic abnormalities of posture. Dystonia may affect the body as a whole in the generalized dystonic disorders such as dystonia musculorum deformans. Focal dystonias may produce a local abnormality such as spasmodic torticollis or writer's cramp. Parkinson's disease is associated with a very characteristic flexed posture in the late stages. In athetosis and chorea, postural abnormalities may be seen in addition to the involuntary movements.

In spasticity of severe degree the limbs adopt the characteristic hemiplegic posture with a flexed upper and an extended lower limb. In lower motor neurone motor disorders, with decrease in muscle tone, limb posture may be abnormal, most evidently during movement. Postural changes in walking are also evident in cerebellar disturbances.

In neonates, abnormalities of posture, particularly in the assessment of so-called 'floppy' infants, may give valuable information particularly when looking for evidence of developmental delay.

In neurological disorders, abnormalities of posture are often overlooked as they are masked by other more obvious signs of the underlying disorder, such as disturbances of power, coordination and muscle tone. The above examples should serve to emphasize the importance of assessment of posture.

N. E. F. Cartlidge

Premenstrual syndrome

During the premenstrual week most women experience symptoms which indicate that a period is imminent, but the majority are perfectly able to tolerate them, accepting them as one of the features of being a woman. The symptoms include bloating, cramping, pain and tenderness in the breasts, temporary gain in weight and some swelling of the hands and feet. When they are associated with emotional tension, bad-temper, nervousness, irritability, headache, lack of concentration, depression and insomnia, sufficient to interfere with the normal enjoyment of life, the condition is referred to as 'premenstrual tension'. Although it is recognized that crimes and suicide are committed by women more frequently in the week before a period, premenstrual tension cannot reasonably be submitted as being an excuse for criminal behaviour. The cause of premenstrual tension is thought to be an obscure disturbance of endocrine balance, acting through a redistribution of water from the blood vessels into the tissues of the body. Progesterone by injection (100 mg daily) or by suppository (400 mg), norethisterone (5 mg twice daily), diuretics, oral contraceptives, bromocriptine, pyridoxine and monoamineoxidase inhibitors have all been tried in attempts to relieve the condition, with varying success. Recent reports suggest that oestrogen implants inverted subcutaneously are helpful in the management of this condition.

N. Patel

Priapism

'Priapism' (*see also* PENILE PAIN) signifies erection of the penis, persistent, of troublesome degree and not necessarily accompanied by sexual desire. Though generally spoken of in connection with the male sex, a precisely similar affection may occur in the female clitoris. The symptom is not often by itself of diagnostic importance. Though it may be due to a considerable number of different conditions, the ultimate cause is usually thrombosis in the vascular spaces in the cavernous tissue which are found to contain thick black grumous blood.

The important causes are:

1   After injury to the upper dorsal region of the spinal cord. The damage may have produced fracture-dislocation of the spine with paraplegia, in which case the diagnosis will be obvious; short of this, however, a minor degree of injury, with contusion and small haemorrhages into the substance of the cord, may be followed by painful priapism, persisting sometimes for weeks before recovery occurs. Cerebrospinal syphilis or tumour may also rarely be responsible.

2   In leukaemia; apart from obvious change in the penis—cavernous haemorrhage or the like—priapism has been noted in both myelocytic and lymphatic leukaemia even before the other symptoms and signs have led to a haematological diagnosis. The cause of the priapism in leukaemia is obscure, but the diagnosis is suggested by the concomitant splenomegaly and/or lymphadenopathy adenopathy and is confirmed by the haematological findings.

3   Sickle-cell anaemia.

4   New growths of the urethra, either primary or secondary to carcinoma of the bladder or testis.

5   Trauma with haematoma formation.

Chronic intermittent priapism is the term used to describe frequently repeated erections which are of long duration but lack the persistence of true priapism. The attacks occur in the night and may or may not be associated with sexual desire. They are due to nerve irritation arising from lesions of the central nervous system or from local lesions in the posterior urethra, prostate or seminal vesicles. In elderly men they are frequently associated with enlargement of the prostate.

Seldom will priapism be the only symptom in the case; the diagnosis will be made from the history and from the other symptoms.

Harold Ellis

Pruritus ani

Pruritus ani, the sensation of itching around the anal verge, is a common symptom. In more than half the patients, no obvious cause can be found (idiopathic pruritis) but in every case the following checklist should be considered:

1   The pruritus may be the result of a general disease associated with itching (*see* PRURITUS, GENERALIZED). Examples are lymphoma, advanced renal failure, severe jaundice and diabetes mellitus. The latter is often associated with *Candida albicans* infection (thrush) and this may occur, of course, in the nondiabetic patient. Moreover, *Candida* is often a secondary invader on any moist and excoriated skin and so may well not be the primary cause of the condition.

2   The localized itching may be due to a skin disease which happens particularly to affect the perianal region. Examples are scabies, where characteristic lesions may be seen elsewhere in the body, notably between the fingers and on the anterior aspects of the wrists, pediculosis pubis, where the parasites may be noted in the anal region, as well as in their usual site in the pubic hairs, and fungal infection. The latter is particularly to be thought of where the skin lesion has a well-defined border at its lateral extent. Other lesions may be found between the toes and in the groin and proof may be obtained by examination of scrapings from the affected skin.

3   Any cause within the anus or rectum which produces moisture and sogginess of the anal skin is liable to cause pruritus ani. These lesions include prolapsing piles, prolapse of the rectum, anal fissure, anal fistula, anal papillomata or condylomata, carcinoma or benign tumours of the rectum, colitis or colonic Crohn's disease (*Fig*. P.20). Anal incontinence due to sphincteric injury may result in constant soiling of the perianal skin. Careful inspection of the anal verge, digital examination of the anal canal, proctoscopy and sigmoidoscopy, where necessary, will rapidly expose the underlying cause of this condition.

Excessive sweating, especially in hot weather and in hairy men, may be associated with pruritus ani, especially in subjects who wear thick and rough undergarments.

Pruritus ani is unusual in children and, when it occurs, a well-recognized cause is infestation with threadworms (*Enterobius vermicularis* or *Oxyuris vermicularis*). Characteristically the worms migrate to the anal verge especially at night and scratching results in auto-infection. The parasite is white and about 6 mm long with the thickness of cotton thread. The parasites may be noted at the anal verge or seen at proctoscopy. If the diagnosis is suspected but no parasites immediately seen, a wash-out of the rectum with normal saline should be inspected against a black

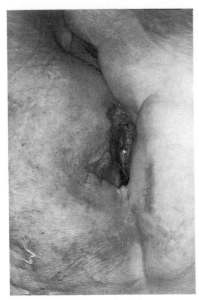

Fig. P.20. Severe pruritus ani extending forward to the vulva in a young girl with extensive Crohn's disease of the distal colon and rectum.

background when the white parasites can be detected. It should be noted that threadworm infection may also occur in adults.

Idiopathic pruritus is diagnosed when no obvious cause can be found. A number of theories have been suggested, which include allergy, that the original cause has now disappeared but the pruritus has persisted because of continued scratching of the anal region by the patient, irritation of the perianal skin by faecal contamination even when no gross soiling is evident, or some psychogenic cause.

Harold Ellis

Pruritus, generalized

Pruritus, or itching, is that sensation of the skin which excites the urge to rub or scratch. It is sensed by undifferentiated endings of unmyelinated C-fibres at the dermo-epidermal junction; the fibres pass centrally with pain fibres and itching appears to be caused by stimuli too weak to cause pain. Itching is most pronounced in those areas served by the greatest number of pain-conducting fibres, e.g. around the lips and nose, and in the anogenital area. For the same reason, itching is more easily provoked in the flexures than on extensor surfaces and this may be a factor in the localization of atopic lichenification. Response to itch stimuli, like pain, is immensely variable between individuals. The threshold for pruritus can be lowered by warming the skin, by stimulants such as dexedrine and caffeine, and by emotional tension. It is probable that rubbing a particular area may 'facilitate' the itch pathway which would explain why itching may be worsened by scratching: the so-called 'itch-scratch cycle' as seen in pruritus ani and lichen simplex chronicus. The causes of pruritus are listed in *Table* P.9.

Table P.9. Causes of pruritus

Itchy dermatoses
Infestations (scabies, lice, insect bites) (Figs. N.17, P.43, V.5)
Dermatitis—all causes (Fig. E.5)
Lichen planus (Fig. P.7)
Prickly heat
Urticaria (Fig. W.2)
Dermatitis herpetiformis
Pemphigoid gestationis
Cutaneous T-cell lymphoma (Fig. P.22)
Onchocerciasis

Generalized pruritus
Senile asteatosis
Liver: obstructive hepatopathy
Kidney: renal failure, hyperparathyroidism
Blood: polycythaemia, anaemia, iron deficiency
Endocrine: hyperthyroidism, myxoedema
Lymphoma; liver secondaries; T-cell leukaemia
Pregnancy: last trimester (especially in atopics)
Psychological: delusional state of parasitosis
Drugs, gold salts, detergents, de-greasing agents

Some dermatoses are tremendously pruritic and the debilitating nature of a chronic, nagging pruritus, depriving the patient of sleep, may easily be underestimated by physicians. The degree of pruritus is seldom of great diagnostic help, largely because of variability of individual response, the possible exception being *cutaneous syphilis* which never itches. In general the most itchy dermatoses, apart from the infestations, are *dermatitis* of all causes particularly atopic dermatitis (*Fig.* P.21), *lichen planus, prickly heat, urticaria, dermatitis herpetiformis, pemphigoid gestationis* and *cutaneous T-cell lymphoma*. Faced with a scratching patient the most important condition to rule out is an *infestation* e.g. scabies on the patients, lice on his clothes, fleas, insects and bed bugs in his environment.

One condition often forgotten by Western physic-

ians is *onchocerciasis* (estimated by WHO recently to affect 20 000 000 people in the world), where pruritus may be intense, and localized to the legs and buttocks or involve the whole body. Onchocerciasis occurs in a broad belt world-wide from 19 degrees north to 15 degrees south, and scattered foci in Mexico, Central and South America, the Yemen and parts of Saudi Arabia. Onchocercoma nodules containing the adult worm (*see* p. 461) may be found around the pelvic girdle or on the head and neck, and the diagnosis will be confirmed by finding microfilariae from skin snips.

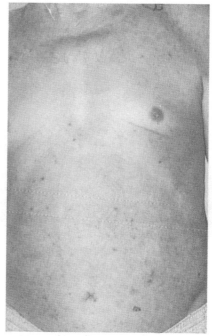

Fig. P.22. Generalized pruritus due to follicular lymphoma. (*Dr. Richard Staughton.*)

The term *generalized pruritus* is usually reserved for those patients in whom no cutaneous lesions are present except those due to scratching. In the elderly the most common cause is a subclinical dryness of skin, *senile asteatosis* due to inadequate secretion of sebum and sweat. A subtle scaling may be seen, and perhaps an eczema craquelé on the anterior shins or forearms. Nevertheless in any patient with generalized pruritus without cutaneous cause, the following possibilities should be considered:

Liver disease. Pruritus is severe in obstructive jaundice, but in hepatitis and primary biliary cirrhosis can begin before icterus is obvious.

Renal disease. The skin in advanced uraemia may be intensely pruritic and in patients on dialysis sudden shifts in electrolytes may cause pruritus, as may secondary hyperparathyroidism.

Blood disease. Pruritus is common in polycy-

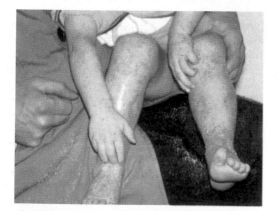

Fig. P.21. Atopic dermatitis. (*Addenbrooke's Hospital.*)

thaemia rubra vera and also in iron deficiency, even without anaemia.

Endocrine disease. Generalized itching is occasionally a presenting feature of hyperthyroidism, and can accompany the dry skin of myxoedema. Diabetes mellitus is said to cause generalized pruritus, but this is more often found to relate to localized infection with candida, e.g. candidal vulvo-vaginitis.

Malignancy. Generalized pruritus, sometimes with prurigo nodules, can be the presenting feature of underlying cancers especially lymphomas (*Fig.* P.22). T-cell leukaemia, particularly the Sezary syndrome, produces a notoriously itchy erythroderma.

Pregnancy. Itching is common during the last trimester of pregnancy and a proportion of patients, probably atopics, will produce prurigo nodules on arms and legs. The itch disappears after parturition.

Psychological. Scratching may be associated with delusions, particularly that parasites are crawling over the skin, a symptom which may indicate serious underlying mental disturbance.

Richard Staughton

Pruritus vulvae

Pruritus vulvae may be defined as a sensation of itching of the vulva which necessitates scratching or rubbing for its relief.

In younger women, before the menopause, infection of the vagina and vulva with *Candida albicans* (thrush) is common and often associated with taking the combined contraceptive pill. The pruritus is intense and the condition may be recognized by the typical curdy, white discharge which adheres to the vaginal wall. There may also be a watery discharge. Even when the typical discharge is not present, it is worth taking a swab for culture and microscopic examination and, because the infection is commonly found in early diabetes, the urine should always be tested for sugar. Vaginal discharge from any cause may be responsible for pruritus, as may infection from the urinary tract. The mucoid discharge from an erosion, however, does not usually cause pruritus, and infection with *Trichomonas vaginalis* is more inclined to give rise to vulval soreness.

In older women, after the menopause, the vulva shows either lichenification from rubbing and scratching, or the thickened white skin of vulval dystrophy. In some cases, in the absence of abnormal physical signs, apart from scratch marks, the onset of pruritus may have followed an emotional shock. In other cases the pruritis may be due to simple uncleanliness from the accumulation of sweat, sebaceous material or smegma, particularly in the obese. General diseases such as diabetes, anxiety states, jaundice, leukaemia, chronic nephritis and Hodgkin's disease must be excluded.

Sometimes the vulva is red, inflamed and excoriated with a weeping discharge due to contact with clothing, lotions or ointment to which the skin is allergic. Such contact dermatitis can be due to nylon, detergents used for washing clothes or lotions with scent in them. Withdrawal of the precipitating cause lends to instant relief providing scratching can be avoided. Sometimes scratching alone will remove the protective cover of the skin from superficial nerve endings so as to stimulate further scratching. Unless the vicious circle is broken, pruritis continues.

Chronic vulval dystrophies are a common cause of pruritus vulvae, which may be intense, in later life. In a typical case, the skin of the whole vulva excluding the vestibule, is thickened and white, or thin and red, with cracks and fissures. The condition may involve the clitoris, the perineum and the perianal skin, in addition to the labia majora and minora. Names such as atrophic vulvitis, kraurosis, lichen sclerosus and leucoplakia have been given up for hypoplastic and hyperplastic dystrophy, according to the microscopical appearances on biopsy. It is common to find both kinds of dystrophy on the same vulva and it is then called 'mixed'. Hyperplastic dystrophy is liable to have atypical cells in the epidermis and such a finding is regarded as being premalignant. Carcinoma in situ and Paget's disease are also found on the vulva. They both cause pruritus and need biopsy for diagnosis. Because the histology varies in different parts of the vulva and at different times, several biopsies need to be taken from each side and repeated from time to time. Conservative measures, including the use of 1 per cent hydrocortisone cream, are adopted for dystrophies without cell atypia, but excision of the affected area has to be undertaken when atypia denotes premalignancy.

N. Patel

Ptosis

Ptosis is the term applied to drooping of the upper eyelid with inability to elevate it to the full extent. (*Fig.* P.23). The commonest form is a congenital defect and if the pupil is in consequence covered urgent surgical correction is indicated to prevent amblyopia. The acquired kind is usually caused by *paralysis of the III nerve*, when it may also be associated with paralysis of other ocular muscles, either external or internal.

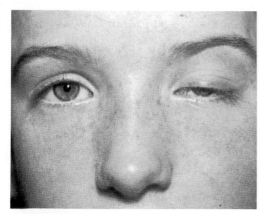

Fig. P.23. Ptosis.

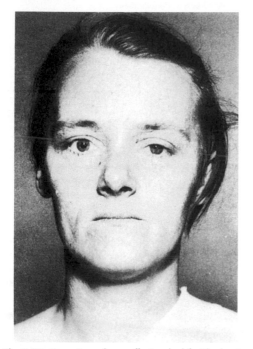

Fig P.24. Horner's syndrome affecting the left side showing ptosis, enophthalmos and small pupil. (Dr. R. G. Ollerenshaw, Manchester.)

In *paralysis of the cervical sympathetic*, slight ptosis may be associated with diminution in the size of the pupil on the affected side, retraction of the eyeball or 'enophthalmos' and absence of sweating—Horner's syndrome. (*Fig*. P.24). Ptosis occurs in *myasthenia gravis* and is diagnosed using the Tensilon test.

Ptosis, associated with oedema and infiltration of the lids, is also found in *inflammatory disorders* of the conjunctiva and upper lids. Gross oedema may occur in angioneurotic oedema. It also follows direct injury of the elevating muscle or its nerve supply following lid laceration or blunt trauma.

Congenital ptosis is often bilateral, and associated with smoothness of the upper lids and absence of all the usual cutaneous folds. The levator palpebrae may be absent or ill-developed, and efforts to open the eye are made by the occipito-frontalis muscle.

In the condition called 'jaw winking', movements of the jaw, especially lateral movements, cause the lid to rise.

S. T. D. Roxburgh

Ptyalism

Ptyalism means excessive secretion of saliva. It is not always easy to determine if there really is excess, or if the patient is merely allowing the normal volume of saliva to dribble from the mouth. Thus the difficulty may be solely that of swallowing the normal secretion, as in bulbar paralysis. There may be both excess of secretion and difficulty in swallowing, as in mercurial stomatitis. In other instances there is too much secretion but no difficulty in swallowing, as in functional or hysterical ptyalorrhoea. The first step towards ascertaining the cause is to inquire as to any *medicine* or *drug* the patient may be taking orally or applying externally.

Mercury was the most important of these when the drug was used in the treatment of syphilis; its effects were worst when the mouth was not kept clean. Iodides, bromide and arsenic were in the past often responsible.

If the salivation is not attributable to any drug it may be the result of one of the many forms of *general stomatitis*.

The nature of a severe stomatitis will be ascertained by local examination; by bacteriological examination of swabbings from the mouth; by serological tests for syphilis; or by microscopical examination of a fragment of the affected tissues. Tuberculous stomatitis is one of the rarer but severe forms; it may be primary but is more often associated with pulmonary tuberculosis.

If drugs and general stomatitis can be excluded, local examination may still serve to detect a cause acting by reflex irritation of the 5th nerve, especially:

A jagged carious tooth
A stump left beneath a dental plate
A broken or ill-fitting dental plate
A foreign body impacted in the gum
An ulcerating tumour of the oral cavity

If appropriate examination serves to exclude these, the salivation, apparently rather than actually increased, may be found to result from *mechanical difficulties in swallowing* (*see* DYSPHAGIA). The excessive salivation seen in many cases of advanced carcinoma of the oesophagus results from the oesophago-salivary reflex; a constant excess flow of saliva is secreted in an attempt to 'swallow' the obstructing bolus of tumour in the gullet.

In the absence of an obvious local structural lesion, apparent salivation may be due to inability to swallow, as in cases of:

Parkinsonism
Bulbar paralysis
Pseudo-bulbar paralysis
Bilateral facial paralysis
Myasthenia gravis
Hypoglossal nerve paralysis

The differential diagnosis of these conditions is discussed elsewhere. It is only in bulbar and pseudo-bulbar paralysis that the dribbling of much saliva is a prominent symptom. Pseudo-bulbar paralysis, being of cortical and not of medullary nuclear origin, does not exhibit wasting of the tongue.

Slovenliness and lack of cerebral control are responsible for the slobbering and salivation of some elderly or mentally handicapped patients.

Harold Ellis

Puberty, delayed

Delayed puberty is rather more common in boys than in girls and may be defined as the total absence of sexual development in a boy over the age of 15 years or in a girl who is more than 14. Constitutional delayed puberty accounts for half of the male cases, but is much less likely to be the cause in a girl, in whom well over 80 per cent will have some pathological condition. For practical purposes the first sign of puberty in a girl is the appearance of pubic hair or a breast bud, whereas in a boy enlargement of the testicles is the earliest sign, before rugosity of the scrotum or pubic hair growth. Pre-pubertal testes are less than 2 cm in length. A length of more than 2·5 cm indicates that pubertal testicular stimulation is taking place. Alternatively the size of the testes may be compared with a Prader orchidometer. A volume of more than 4 ml indicates pubertal change. The causes of delayed puberty are listed in *Table* P.10.

Constitutional delayed puberty

Constitutional delayed puberty accounts for half of the cases in boys and only 16 per cent in girls. There is often a family history and there may be an indication of a recent slowing of growth. This may, in fact, be the normal pre-pubertal deceleration of growth. Bone age is delayed and is usually appropriate for testicular size, which is usually reasonable. So long as the penis is not very small and there is no anosmia it is reasonable to review these patients every 6 months, especially if the testosterone response to human chorionic gonadotrophin is appropriate for the bone age. If the boy is

Table P.10. Causes of delayed puberty

Constitutional

Hypothalamic syndromes
Lack of gonadotrophin-releasing hormone
Laurence–Moon–Biedl syndrome
Prader–Willi syndrome
Lyndi's syndrome

Destructive lesions of hypothalamus and/or pituitary
Craniopharyngioma
Chromophobe adenoma
Prolactinoma
Optic chiasma glioma
Meningioma
Trauma
Vascular lesions
Granulomas
Infections

Isolated pituitary deficiencies
Growth hormone
Luteinizing hormone (fertile eunuch syndrome)

Gonadal abnormalities
Anorchism
Ovarian dysgenesis
  Turner's syndrome
  Pure dysgenesis
Noonan's syndrome (boys and girls)
Klinefelter's syndrome (rarely causes delayed puberty)
Auto-immune ovarian failure
Resistant ovary syndrome
Hormonal
  Masculinizing tumour of ovary
Destructive lesions
  Castration
  Mumps (damage occurs very rarely in children)
  Tuberculosis
  X-irradiation
  Cytotoxic therapy

Adrenal disease
Congenital adrenal hyperplasia
Cushing's syndrome

Thyroid disease
Hypothyroidism
Hyperthyroidism

Chronic disease
Anorexia nervosa
Malnutrition
Tuberculosis
Severe uncontrolled diabetes
Chronic renal failure
Cyanotic congenital heart disease
Cystic fibrosis
Gluten enteropathy and other malabsorption
  syndromes
Connective-tissue diseases

Drugs
Girls
  Androgens
  Anabolic steroids
Both sexes
  Excess thyroid hormones

becoming embarrassed by his lack of sexual development and if his height is adequate, one may consider low doses of anabolic agents. Similarly oestrogens may be used in girls. Generally speaking, however, these individuals usually develop perfectly normally, albeit in their late teens or even in their early twenties.

Hypothalmic and pituitary causes

Altogether abnormalities of the hypothalamus and pituitary account for approximately one-third of cases of delayed puberty in both girls and boys. The cause may be a space-occupying lesion, trauma or the result of infection or granulomatous infiltration involving the hypothalamus or the pituitary or both. The hormone defects in these cases tend to be multiple, so that in addition to delayed puberty due to lack of gonadotrophins there may be short stature due to growth hormone deficiency, lethargy and weakness due to lack of ACTH and cold insensitivity due to low TSH levels. However, patients with solitary growth hormone deficiency (see p. 619) may present not only with short stature (and often obesity) but also with delayed puberty, though sexual development usually occurs normally later on. Chromophobe adenomas and prolactinomas may cause hypogonadism due to the secretion of high levels of prolactin. High prolactin levels may also be produced by lesions which interfere with the production of prolactin inhibiting factor (dopamine) or its delivery to the pituitary.

Hypothalamic lack of the releasing hormone for gonadotrophins (GnRH) accounts for about 7 per cent of all cases of delayed puberty. This may be due to a midline developmental defect, since in some of them anosmia due to hypoplasia of the olfactory bulbs is present (Kallmann's syndrome) and there may be cleft palate and hare lip. These patients tend to be tall because of their hypogonadism.

Male patients have been reported with isolated luteinizing hormone deficiency. They are tall with eunuchoidal skeletal proportions and are sexually immature. Full maturation can be achieved by injections of human chorionic gonadotrophin (HCG).

In some cases of the Laurence–Moon–Biedl syndrome (see p. 722) a hypothalamic deficiency of GnRH has been shown. This also occurs in the Prader–Willi syndrome (see p. 629), and in the Lyndi's syndrome of male hypogonadism and congenital ichthyosis.

Gonadal abnormalities

A primary gonadal abnormality is responsible for over a third of cases of delayed puberty in girls, but in little over 5 per cent of boys. The commonest cause in girls is *Turner's syndrome* (see p. 622) in which ovarian dysgenesis is classically associated with the karyotype 45/XO. Unlike most other patients with hypogonadism the girl is short and there are usually several physical abnormalities, such as a webbed neck, a low hair line postero-laterally, an increased carrying angle of the elbows, short 4th and/or 5th metatarsals and metacarpals, a shield-shaped chest with widely spaced nipples, pigmented naevi, renal anomalies, coarctation of the aorta, atrial and ventricular defects and aortic stenosis. In about a quarter of patients not all the cell lines carry the karyotype 45/XO. They are mosaics and cells may be XO/XX, XO/XXX or XO/XX/XXX. Patients with mosaicism tend to be taller than those with XO Turner's syndrome and the physical features outlined above may be less apparent. The serum gonadotrophins, LH and FSH, will be elevated. Buccal smear examinations will usually show absent Barr bodies, indicating the presence of one X chromosome, but if there is any doubt full karyotyping should be done, as there could be mosaicism.

In a small number of cases of ovarian dysgenesis there are none of the features of Turner's syndrome, the stature is normal and the appearance female, though hypogonadism is present ('pure dysgenesis'). Half of the patients have a normal female karyotype, 46/XX; in the other half the karyotype is male, 46/XY. Serum gonadotrophins are high. It is advisable in these patients to do a laparoscopy in order to confirm dysgenesis of the ovaries

Noonan's syndrome (see p. 622), which looks superficially like Turner's syndrome, may occur in both sexes and may present with delayed puberty.

In the *resistant ovary syndrome* the ovaries fail to respond to gonadotrophins, probably owing to lack of receptors, and an adolescent girl may present with lack of pubertal development.

In a small proportion of girls suffering from autoimmune disease (of the adrenals, thyroid and parathyroid especially) delayed puberty may be due to autoimmune ovarian failure; antibodies against the ovaries can be demonstrated in the serum.

In boys *anorchism* will cause delayed puberty, but will usually have been investigated long before the expected age of puberty because of the absence of testes in the scrotum. High levels of LH and FSH in the blood will confirm the diagnosis.

In both sexes surgical removal of the gonads (castration), for whatever reason, will lead to delayed puberty. *Mumps* usually only damages the post-pubertal gonad and *tuberculosis* has become rare in the developed world. *Irradiation* for the treatment of lymphomas is becoming a more common cause of hypogonadism, particularly in girls. The Leydig cells of the testis seem to be more resistant. *Cytotoxic chemotherapy* may cause gonadal damage.

A *masculinizing tumour of the ovary* will cause delayed puberty in a girl because of the suppression of gonadotrophins by the excess androgens. Secondary sexual hair and even hirsutism will be present and there may be clitoromegaly.

Adrenal disease

In girls *congenital adrenal hyperplasia* (*see* p. 298) or *Cushing's syndrome* (*see* p. 721) may lead to failure of breast development and to primary amenorrhoea because of the production of excess amounts of androgen. Pubic and axillary hair will almost always be present, for the same reason. A boy with either of the above two conditions may be thought to be well developed, but examination of his testes will show them to be small because of suppression of pituitary gonadotrophins by the excess androgens. In *Cushing's syndrome* in both sexes the hyperproduction of cortisol also may have an effect in reducing gonadotrophin secretion.

Thyroid disease

Where *hypothyroidism* is associated with delayed puberty in a girl it is usually due to auto-immune ovarian failure. Hypothyroidism is, in fact, more often associated with precocious puberty (*see below*). *Hyperthyroidism* in a child of either sex may lead to delayed puberty due to suppression of gonadotrophin release.

Chronic disease

Chronic debilitating diseases of any type, particularly those causing poor nutrition, may cause delayed puberty by interfering with the hypothalamic control of pituitary gonadotrophins. *Anorexia nervosa*, occurring in about 1 per cent of all teenage girls in Western society, may be missed as a diagnosis, but a careful history may reveal abnormal eating habits and fads and evidence of vomiting or purgation. Fine 'lanugo' hair may be seen over the body (*see* p. 177).

Malnutrition such as marasmus and kwashiorkor, will be obvious causes of delayed puberty in underdeveloped countries. *Tuberculosis, chronic renal failure, cyanotic congenital heart disease, connective-tissue disease* and severe *uncontrolled diabetes* should present no problem in diagnosis. Patients with *cystic fibrosis*, in addition to having chronic respiratory infections, may also have evidence of gastrointestinal malabsorption due to pancreatic enzyme deficiencies. *Gluten enteropathy*, occurring in approximately 1 in 2000 children, may be more difficult to recognize as a cause of delayed puberty. Bowel symptoms may be very subtle, but the diagnosis should be suspected in a short child who has a protubertant abdomen and scanty subcutaneous fat elsewhere. Low red cell folate and poor xylose absorption are useful screening tests, but the definitive investigation is a small bowel biopsy by Crosby capsule. In gluten enteropathy the villi are flattened.

Drugs

In girls the administration of either *androgens* or *anabolic steroids* will lead to suppression of sexual development due to inhibition of gonadotrophin release. Pubic and axillary hair will, however, usually be present. In both boys and girls, the ingestion of excess *thyroid hormones* in the treatment of hypothyroidism or thyroid cancer may lead to delayed puberty owing to the inhibition of gonadotrophin release.

Ian D. Ramsay

Puberty, precocious

Before puberty, blood levels of luteinizing hormone (LH) and follicle stimulating hormone (FSH) are low and are poorly responsive to administered gonadotrophin-releasing hormone. At the time of puberty, by a mechanism which is ill-understood, gonadotrophin secretion begins to increase and gonadal stimulation occurs, with a consequent rise of testosterone in boys and of oestradiol in girls. In both sexes puberty is preceded by an increase in the production of the adrenal androgens dehydroepiandrosterone and androstenedione. The causes of precocious puberty are listed in *Table* P.11.

In 95 per cent of girls the first sign of puberty, which is either breast bud or pubic hair development, appears between the ages of 8·5 and 13 years. Puberty is precocious if either of these two events occurs before the age of 8 in a girl. Menarche occurs in 95 per cent of girls between the ages of 11 and 13 years.

In 95 per cent of boys the testes begin to enlarge between the ages of 9·5 and 13·5 years (mean 11·6 years) and reach adult size between the ages of 13 and 17 (mean 14·9 years). Pubic hair growth develops after testicular enlargement has begun, so it is rare before the age of 9·5 years. Testicular growth is stimulated by the action of FSH on germinal epithelium and of LH on Leydig cells. The testosterone produced by the Leydig cells is responsible for the growth of the penis. Puberty is precocious in a boy if any of the above-mentioned changes takes place before the 9th birthday.

Precocious puberty can be either a true puberty or a false pseudo-puberty. In true puberty the changes proceed in the normal physiological manner, albeit at an early age. In false puberty, on the other hand, changes such as secondary sexual hair growth and enlargement of the phallus occur because of abnormal androgen production and gonadal function is, in fact, inhibited. A rare intermediate variety may be produced by non-pituitary gonadotrophin-secreting tumours.

Constitutional precocious puberty

This is much the commonest cause of precocious puberty, especially in girls, where it accounts for 80

Table P.11. Causes of precocious puberty

True
Constitutional
Cerebral
  Hypothyroidism
  Hydrocephalus
  Encephalitis
  Meningitis
  Tuberose sclerosis
  Neurofibromatosis
  Cerebral tumour
  Pineal tumour
  Craniopharyngioma
  Hamartoma
  McCune—Albright syndrome (polyostotic fibrous
    dysplasia with cutaneous pigmentation)
  Russell–Silver syndrome
Gonadotrophin-producing tumours
  Hepatoma
  Hepatoblastoma
  Teratoma
  Chorionepithelioma

False
Adrenal
  Congenital adrenal hyperplasia
  Tumours
  Cushing's syndrome
Testicular
  Leydig cell tumour
  Leydig cell hyperplasia
Ovarian
  Granulosa cell tumour
  Androblastoma
  Lipoid cell tumour
  Chorionepithelioma
  Benign ovarian cyst
Drugs
  Androgens
  Anabolic steroids
  Oestrogens

Cerebral

Hypothyroidism is included under cerebral causes of precocious puberty because it seems likely that the mechanism is via the stimulation by thyrotrophin releasing hormone (TRH) of gonadotrophins in addition to TSH and prolactin.

A wide variety of other cerebral conditions can give rise to precocious puberty if the area posterior to the median eminence, including the mamillary bodies and the posterior part of the floor of the 3rd ventricle are involved.

The *McCune–Albright syndrome* is only tentatively included under cerebral causes of precocious puberty because it has been postulated that there may be inappropriate secretion of hypothalamic releasing hormones in this condition. The syndrome is rare and is much more common in girls than in boys. Precocious puberty is usual, but other endocrine abnormalities such as thyrotoxicosis, hyperparathyroidism and Cushing's syndrome may occur. One of the characteristic features is polyostotic fibrous dysplasia which may be unilateral. There are pigmented areas on the skin roughly corresponding to the underlying bony lesions.

Patients with the Russell–Silver syndrome (*see* p. 619) may develop early puberty. The cause is unknown.

Gonadotrophin-producing tumours

These are exceedingly rare and produce testicular enlargement in boys and vaginal bleeding in girls as the first sign. They are usually malignant.

Adrenal causes of false puberty

The secretion of excess androgens by the adrenal causes false puberty. The growth of secondary sexual hair is stimulated and the phallus enlarges. Gonadotrophins, however, are suppressed so the testes remain small in a boy and periods do not develop in a girl. Adrenal tumours and Cushing's syndrome can be distinguished from congenital adrenal hyperplasia by the presence of raised plasma 17-hydroxyprogesterone and urinary excretion of pregnanetriol in the latter when it is due to a 21-hydroxylase defect and by normal suppressibility of urinary 17-oxosteroids.

Testicular causes of false puberty

Testicular Leydig cell tumours causing false puberty are exceedingly rare. Occasional cases of Leydig cell hyperplasia have been described. Tumours are usually palpable but occasionally may be small. However, a useful clue to the presence of a testicular tumour is that the contralateral testis is even smaller because gonadotrophins are suppressed. In most cases the condition is fully established by the age of 6 years.

per cent of cases. Early puberty in boys is five times less common than in girls and in boys a pathological cause is found in 50 per cent. A family history of precocious puberty may be found, though the majority of cases are sporadic. Ovarian cysts may be detected in girls by rectal examination or on ultrasound. They should not be confused with granulosa cell tumours.

Other variants of premature puberty may be present. *Premature adrenarche* is characterized by the early growth of pubic hair and a slightly advanced bone age. There are no other signs of premature sexual development and full puberty develops at the normal age. *Premature thelarche* refers to the early development of breast tissue often in the second year of life. It usually regresses spontaneously within 2 years but may lead on to a full early puberty.

The important implication for a child who enters early puberty is that, because bone maturation is advanced, final adult stature may be below that predicted for an offspring of that family.

Precocity is marked: the physique is muscular, body-hair growth is considerable, the voice is strikingly gruff and manly and the penis and prostate are enlarged. In half the cases there may be grossly overt psycho-sexual behaviour. Because the tumour is secreting testosterone, high levels of 17-oxosteroids are not always found in the urine, but raised plasma testosterone is diagnostic.

Ovarian causes of false puberty

Ovarian tumours account for only a few per cent of cases of precocious puberty in girls. They usually present at about the age of 4 with irregular vaginal bleeding, breast development and pubic and axillary hair growth. There may be abdominal pain and the tumour may be palpable. The usual type of tumour producing endocrine effects is a granulosa cell tumour. This is usually benign, but about a fifth are malignant.

Androgen-producing tumours of the ovary (andro-blastomas) cause heterosexual precocious puberty with the development of secondary sexual hair, hirsutism and virilization.

Drugs

The accidental or deliberate ingestion of oestrogens (commonly mother's contraceptive pills) by girls may lead to vaginal withdrawal bleeding and to some breast development. Androgens and anabolic steroids may cause secondary sexual hair growth and phallic enlargement.

Ian D. Ramsay

Pubic hair, loss of

The amount of pubic hair varies from individual to individual and is less in some races than others, for example in orientals compared with caucasians. In the female the secretion of the adrenal androgens, androstenedione and dehydroepiandrosterone, is responsible for the development of pubic hair, via their peripheral conversion into testosterone. In the male the secretion of testosterone by the testis and its conversion to dihydrotestosterone brings about pubic hair growth. Bearing these facts in mind, it can be seen that any disease process which affects the adrenal gland in a female or testicular function in a male may lead to loss of pubic hair. The causes of loss of pubic hair are listed in *Table* P.12. Thus hypothalamic or pituitary disease may cause loss of adrenocortico-trophic hormone (ACTH) or of the gonadotrophins, luteinizing hormone being the one responsible for testosterone production by the testis. Primary disease of the adrenals such as Addison's disease will cause loss of pubic hair in females, whereas in males destruction by disease or removal of the testes will lead to

pubic hair loss. The testes can be damaged by mumps or orchitis in adult life, by trauma or by cytotoxic drugs. The testes may be removed surgically or their function inhibited medically in the treatment of prostatic carcinoma. In this condition the loss of pubic hair may also be caused by the administration of oestrogens. Oestrogens may sometimes be secreted in a male by a Leydig secreting tumour of the testis. Other conditions which can lead to a rise in the ratio of oestrogen to androgen in the male include cirrhosis of the liver and haemochromatosis.

Table P.12. Causes of loss of pubic hair

Males	Females
Hypothalamic disease	Hypothalamic disease
Pituitary disease	Pituitary disease
Testicular disease, damage or removal	Addison's disease
	Hypothyroidism
Oestrogen therapy	Hypoparathyroidism
Cirrhosis of the liver	Alopecia universalis
Haemochromatosis	
Hypothyroidism	
Thyrotoxicosis	
Hypoparathyroidism	
Alopecia universalis	

In addition to adrenal and testicular androgens, other hormones affect the growth of pubic hair. The low calcium levels of hypoparathyroidism may lead to coarse and scanty pubic hair, while there is loss of genital hair in hypothyroidism and, in some cases of thyrotoxicosis, loss of pubic hair has been described. Finally, pubic hair may disappear completely in the condition of alopecia universalis.

Ian D. Ramsay

Pulse, character of

One of the observations which should always be made when feeling the arterial pulse is its character. By this is to be understood the shape which would be inscribed by an instrument recording the movement of the artery. The most important deviation from the normal character is in the rate of rise of the pulse. This, together with variations in the amplitude, often referred to as the volume, of the pulse, produces patterns which are characteristic of various cardiac lesions—usually of the valves. These observations are best described in simple, unambiguous terms; thus the pulse volume should be referred to as 'small', 'normal' or 'large' and not as 'good' or 'poor'; the latter term, in particular, should be avoided if only because, if the patient should hear it used, he or she is likely to be unfavourably impressed. Another term to be avoided is 'thready' pulse, which is meaningless.

The most common abnormality in the character of the pulse is a rapid rate of rise. The most typical form of this is the pulse of aortic regurgitation. This pulse is of large volume and is described as *collapsing*; this term is hallowed by tradition but it is actually the rapid rate of rise rather than a 'collapse' which is detected by the fingers. In doubtful cases the character of this pulse can be accentuated by feeling with the palmar surfaces rather than the tips of the fingers and then elevating the patients arm rather sharply. Another term used to describe this pulse is *water-hammer*. It was Sir Thomas Watson who, in 1844, first used this term, explaining that a water-hammer was a 'toy formed by including a small quantity of fluid in a glass tube exhausted of air and hermetically sealed'; inversion of the tube produced a sudden impact very like this pulse. Occasionally the term *Corrigan's pulse* is used but, in fact, the palpable pulse received very little attention in Corrigan's description. The feature which he emphasized was the easily visible pulsation in the carotid arteries characteristic of gross aortic regurgitation. In such cases the pulse can sometimes be seen in the nail-beds as capillary pulsation; this is due to vasodilatation which is common in this condition. If this vasodilatation is replaced by vasoconstriction, which occurs if heart failure develops, much of the collapsing quality of the pulse is lost and the diastolic blood pressure, typically very low in aortic regurgitation, rises considerably. Other causes of a collapsing pulse are a large persistent ductus arteriosus and arteriovenous fistula and some other rarer congenital lesions such as pulmonary atresia with a large ventricular septal defect and persistent truncus arteriosus. The collapsing pulse must be distinguished from a large volume pulse with a normal rate of rise as with bradycardia from any cause or ageing inelastic arteries. As has been said, the typical collapsing pulse is of large volume. A pulse of similar quality with normal or small volume is felt in such conditions as gross mitral regurgitation, hypertrophic obstructive cardiomyopathy and fixed subvalvar aortic stenosis. This type of pulse is sometimes described as *jerky*.

Unlike subvalvar aortic stenosis, aortic valve stenosis causes a *slow-rising* pulse. The volume of the pulse is usually small and this type of pulse is more easily missed than is the collapsing pulse. Sometimes a notch is felt low down on the upstroke of the pulse so that there appears to be a very small impulse followed by a much larger one. If this is the case, the pulse is described as *anacrotic* (an abbreviation of anadicrotic meaning 'twice-beating on the upstroke'). This pulse can often be felt in the radial and brachial arteries but it is much more easily detected in the carotids where it is often accompanied by a systolic thrill—the palpable counterpart of the murmur transmitted to the neck. A variation of this pulse is

when the notch is very much higher on the upstroke, producing the impression of two more nearly equal impulses. This is the *bisferiens* pulse and is felt when aortic stenosis is accompanied by aortic regurgitation of at least moderate severity. This type of pulse is rather uncommon and must not be confused with one in which a small notch is felt at the very apex of the pulse; this is sometimes felt in aortic regurgitation, especially if the palpating finger is applied more firmly than usual. A very well-marked bisferiens pulse is very occasionally visible in the carotid arteries.

The terms 'bisferiens' and 'dicrotic' have exactly the same meaning—twice-beating—the former being Latin and the latter Greek. However, the *dicrotic* pulse, in the sense in which the term is used today, is unlike the bisferiens pulse in that the second impulse is very much later, being a diastolic event, and is due to the dicrotic wave and notch sometimes recorded graphically in the arterial pulse. If is of no particular diagnostic significance but it tends to be found in young people with a rather low cardiac output and higher than normal peripheral vascular resistance.

Peter R. Fleming

Pulse rate, abnormal

In normal adults the resting pulse rate varies from about 60 to 100 per minute. This does not imply that rates outside this range are necessarily abnormal; for example, a rate of 40 or so is quite common in athletes in training and, at a first consultation with its associated anxiety, a rate of over 100 would not necessarily be remarkable.

Bradycardia

Bradycardia may be due either to a slow rate of discharge of the sino-atrial node or to various disorders of impulse formation or conduction. It should not be diagnosed solely from the rate as felt at the radial pulse as, in various conditions such as atrial fibrillation or extrasystoles, only a proportion of the beats may reach the wrist; the true heart rate can then be determined only by auscultation. The causes are summarised in *Table* P.13.

Sinus bradycardia is not uncommon in otherwise normal individuals especially during sleep when rates as low as 30 to 40 have been recorded during continuous monitoring. The pulse rate may also be slow during convalescence after influenza and other fevers. In acute nephritis bradycardia is probably a reflex result of the acute hypertension. A similar mechanism operates in cases of phaeochromocytoma releasing predominantly noradrenaline; the paroxysms of hypertension are associated with striking bradycardia unlike the type of attack due to release of adrenaline. Brady-

Table P.13. Causes of bradycardia

Sinus bradycardia
Athletics
Reflex
Obstructive jaundice
Myxoedema
Anorexia nervosa
Hypothermia
Aortic stenosis
Drugs, e.g. beta-blocking agents

Sick sinus syndrome

Junctional rhythm

Conduction defects
2 : 1 atrioventricular block (or higher degrees of partial a-v block)
Complete heart block

cardia is also a well-recognized, but far from constant, finding in obstructive jaundice and when the intracranial pressure is raised for any reason; in the latter case the slow rate may be due to direct stimulation of the vagal centre. Myxoedema is another cause of bradycardia which may be profound in myxoedema coma. The pulse is also often very slow in anorexia nervosa. The only valve lesion to be associated with a slow pulse is aortic stenosis; in some severe cases a rate as low as 50 may be found even in the presence of left ventricular failure. As in myxoedema, the reduced metabolic rate of hypothermia, either accidental or induced, is associated with bradycardia; even in atrial fibrillation, a common complication of hypothermia, the ventricular rate is quite slow. As a transient phenomenon, bradycardia occurs in carotid sinus syncope and in vasovagal attacks in general. Few drugs cause bradycardia. It is, however, a constant finding in patients on beta-blocking agents. Bradycardia may also be found after large doses of cholinergic drugs, such as carbachol, and anticholinesterases, such as neostigmine. In digoxin intoxication, also, sinus bradycardia may be seen.

The *sick sinus syndrome* is caused by impairment of sino-atrial node function. It is thus characterized by sinus bradycardia (*Fig.* P.25), sinus arrest, which may cause Stokes–Adams attacks, and sino-atrial block (*Fig.* P.39). The latter, like sinus bradycardia, may occur normally during sleep and is a result of failure of transmission of a sinus impulse to the atria; a whole electrocardiographic complex is thus deleted. With 2:1 sino-atrial block the electrocardiogram resembles sinus bradycardia but exercise or atropine will cause the rate suddenly to double. A well-known association of the sick sinus syndrome is the occurrence of paroxysms of atrial fibrillation, often with a slow ventricular rate, and atrial flutter, the so-called bradycardia-tachycardia syndrome.

Junctional rhythm, originating in the atrioventricular node or the main bundle of His, is a common dysrhythmia. It is most often due to digoxin but may occur after myocardial infarction or in healthy individuals; the rate is usually around 60. The atria and ventricles contrast simultaneously so that, clinically, the diagnostic feature is a cannon wave in the jugular venous pulse with each beat. In the electrocardiogram the P wave is inverted in Leads II, III and aVF and may be just before, incorporated in or just after the QRS complex (*Fig.* P.26). Junctional rhythm is rarely of any serious significance.

Disorders of the atrioventricular conducting system are an important cause of bradycardia. In first-degree heart block, with prolongation of the P–R interval as the only abnormality, the heart rate is normal. The pulse is slow and regular, however, if second-degree heart block has progressed to 2 : 1 block. This is the case whether the conduction defect has progressed via Wenckebach periods (Mobitz Type I) or is the more serious Mobitz Type II block. Clinically these two types can be differentiated by the response to exercise or atropine. In Type I block, conduction improves and a normal heart rate results (*Fig.* P.40); an increase in the severity of the block is the rule following these manoeuvres in Type II block. A 2 : 1 block is most often diagnosed from the electrocardiogram (*Fig.* P.27).

In *complete heart block* atrioventricular dissociation is present and the ventricular rate is that of a pacemaker somewhere in the conducting system distal to the block. The site of this pacemaker can be determined approximately from the surface electrocardiogram. If the QRS complexes are of normal configuration, the pacemaker must be above the bifurcation of the main bundle; a pacemaker in one or other bundle branch produces complexes with the pattern of bundle-branch block. Precise localization of the site of the block is possible by intracardiac electrocardiography. The commonest cause of heart block is fibrosis of the atrioventricular bundle and its branches; the cause of this fibrosis is not known and the remaining myocardium is usually healthy. Ischaemia, particularly myocardial infarction, is a less common cause as are digoxin intoxication and cardiomyopathy of almost any type; cardiac amyloidosis is particularly likely to be associated with conduction defects. Even less common causes include myocarditis, particularly diphtheritic and, in South America, trypanosomiasis (Chagas' disease); calcification of the atrioventricular rings in and around the aortic valve may encroach on the bundle and cause heart block. Congenital heart block is a rare condition; the ventricular rate is usually rather faster than in the acquired variety.

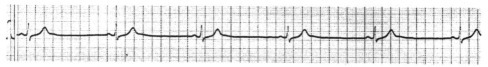

Fig. P.25. Electrocardiogram (head II), showing profound sinus bradycardia at a rate of 31 per minute, in a man, aged 61, complaining of recurrent syncope. A 2:1 sino-atrial block was suspected but the rate increased gradually during exercise and after atropine.

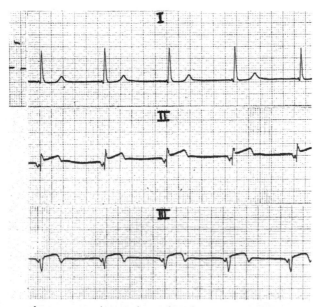

Fig. P.26. Electrocardiogram of a woman, aged 66, 24 hours after inferior myocardial infarction. Apart from the changes of recent infarction, the P wave is inverted in Leads II and III and closely precedes the QRS complex. Junctional rhythm at a rate of 60 per minute.

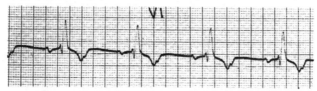

Fig. P.27. Electrocardiogram of a woman, aged 58, admitted following a Stokes–Adams attack. The record shows a 2:1 atrioventricular block with right bundle-branch block; the unconducted P waves deform the upstroke of the T waves of the preceding QRS complex.

The commonest symptom of heart block is the Stokes–Adams attack, particularly if the degree of block is changing. Established complete heart block may also cause some reduction in exercise tolerance with fatigue, dyspnoea and even heart failure. The diagnosis of Stokes–Adams attacks is discussed under FAINTS. Clinical diagnosis of complete heart block is almost always possible. Apart from marked bradycardia with a ventricular rate around 30 or 40 or less, the diagnostic signs include 'a' waves in the jugular venous pulse at a faster rate than the arterial pulse with, in addition, cannon waves occurring whenever atrial and ventricular systole happen to coincide. On auscultation the first heart sound varies markedly in intensity, the louder sounds occurring when ventricular systole follows closely upon atrial systole, so that the atrioventricular valve cusps are wide apart when the ventricles contract (*Fig.* P.28) (*see also* HEART SOUNDS). Occasionally it may be possible to hear separate atrial sounds. It is obvious that, when complete heart block is complicated by atrial fibrillation, none of these signs, which result from a coordinated atrial contraction, is present. An ejection systolic murmur is commonly present due to the large stroke volume which is also the reason for the wide pulse pressure; these two signs are present in bradycardia from any cause. In the electrocardiogram P waves and QRS complexes can be identified with no mathematical relationship between the atrial and ventricular rates.

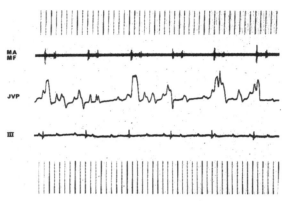

Fig. P.28. Phonocardiogram, jugular venous pulse and Lead III of the electrocardiogram of a man, aged 47, with long-standing complete heart block. In the first and last beats the P waves closely precede the QRS complexes and the first heart sound is loud. In the third beat the P wave coincides with the QRS complex and a tall cannon wave is present in the venous pulse. Smaller cannon waves are seen from time to time and a waves can also be identified occurring 0.14 second after each P wave. Time-marker 0·2 and 0·04 second.

Tachycardia

Tachycardia may be due to an increased frequency of discharge of the sino-atrial node—sinus tachycardia—or to a dysrhythmia. Dysrhythmias causing an irregular pulse are discussed under PULSE, RHYTHM OF. In this section only those dysrhythmias producing a rapid regular pulse will be discussed in any detail. The common causes of tachycardia are summarized in *Table* P.14.

Table P.14. Causes of tachycardia

Sinus tachycardia
Anxiety
Febrile conditions
Hyperthyroidism
Drugs, e.g. sympathomimetic agents
Reflex, e.g. heart failure, hypertension

Supraventricular tachycardia
a-v re-entrant tachycardia
Atrial and junctional tachycardia
Atrial flutter
Atrial fibrillation

Ventricular tachycardia

Sinus tachycardia is present in most febrile conditions due to a direct effect of the pyrexia on the sino-atrial node. In tetanus the rapid pulse is probably due to involvement of the autonomic nervous system by the toxin. In a few infections, such as typhoid, the rise in pulse rate may be rather less than expected from the degree of fever; this relative bradycardia may be of some slight diagnostic significance. The sino-atrial node is affected directly in a number of other situations in which tachycardia is prominent. These include hyperthyroidism in which there is also the reflex effect of the high cardiac output discussed below, phaeochromocytoma secreting predominantly adrenaline, anxiety states and other conditions, such as severe pain, in which there is a raised level of circulating catecholamines. Da Costa's syndrome, known also as cardiac neurosis and effort syndrome, is an important cause of moderate tachycardia persisting sometimes for many years. Various drugs including atropine and sympathomimetic agents such as ephedrine and isoprenaline also produce tachycardia which is also a characteristic feature of poisoning by tricyclic antidepressant drugs.

Sinus tachycardia can also be caused by reflex mechanisms. In conditions causing a rise in right atrial pressure the sinus rate is increased via the Bainbridge reflex. Hypotension from any cause or, more precisely, a fall in pulse pressure, also causes tachycardia via baroceptors in the aortic arch and carotid sinus; this is the mechanism, for example, of the tachycardia during the straining period of a Valsalva manoeuvre. In high-output states the tachycardia is probably secondary to the tendency of the right atrial pressure to rise as a result of the increased venous return; therefore, the pulse rate is rapid in hyperthyroidism, severe anaemia, pregnancy, beri-beri, widespread Paget's disease and arteriovenous fistula. If such a fistula is accessible, the effect of the high cardiac output can be convincingly demonstrated by the abrupt fall in pulse rate which results from digital occlusion of the fistula. In cardiac failure the tendency to a reduction in pulse pressure, acting on the aortic and carotid baroceptors, combines with the rise in right atrial pressure to produce considerable tachycardia in most, although not all, cases. Tachycardia is also a feature of severe myocardial disease even in the absence of frank failure; thus it is found in most cases of myocarditis and in some cases of ischaemic heart disease. Hypotension due to extracardiac factors is also a cause of tachycardia which is seen in shock and as a result of the administration of vasodilating agents.

Disproportionate tachycardia on exertion, with

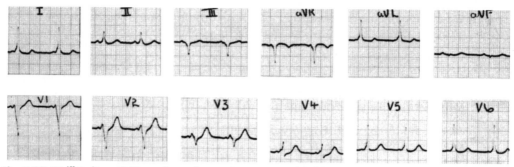

Fig. P.29. Wolff–Parkinson–White syndrome showing short P–R interval and broad QRS complexes. The slowly rising initial part of the QRS complex (the delta wave) is well shown in Leads aVL and V6.

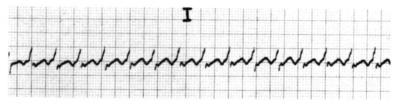

Fig. P.30. Atrial flutter with 2:1 atrioventricular block; the atrial rate is 340 per minute and the ventricular 170 per minute. The baseline is nowhere iso-electric.

a normal resting pulse rate, is seen in patients less severely affected by the conditions discussed above and is also a measure of an individual's lack of training. Physical fitness can be roughly quantified by the amount of work which can be done at any given heart rate.

The sleeping pulse rate is sometimes recorded as an aid to the diagnosis of hyperthyroidism. Tachycardia persisting during sleep certainly favours the latter as against nervous tachycardia, but it must be remembered that, in most organic diseases causing tachycardia, it is likely to persist during sleep.

Lesions of the vagus nerve may occasionally cause tachycardia which has been described with subtentorial tumours and in various types of peripheral neuropathy including alcoholic and diphtheritic. There is also a rare primary disorder of the sino-atrial node (sinus node re-entry) in which tachycardia is a feature.

There are several varieties of *supraventricular tachycardia*. The most common is *a-v re-entrant tachycardia* which occurs when there is a conducting pathway between the atria and ventricles in addition to the atrioventricular node. This is either in, but functionally separate from, the node or is anatomically separate as in the pre-excitation syndromes. Differences in the conductivity and refractoriness of these two pathways can result in a circus movement with an impulse re-entering the atria from the ventricles via one pathway and then being transmitted again to the ventricles via the other. There is usually no other evidence of heart disease and paroxysms of tachycardia occur throughout life. The attacks begin abruptly, sometimes as a result of sudden alarm but often without

apparent cause, and the patient complains, with more or less emphasis depending on his or her temperament, of palpitation and lightheadedness. The associated anxiety may cause hyperventilation and paraesthesiae in the fingers or even frank tetany may occur; in such cases it is clearly important to distinguish cause from effect in the manifestations. The attack may last for minutes, hours or, rarely, for days and ends as abruptly as it began. Prolonged attacks, lasting for a week or more at a very fast rate, can cause cardiac failure even in otherwise normal individuals but this resolves rapidly and completely once the attack is over. In older patients more serious symptoms may occur; in particular, ischaemic pain is common even though the associated coronary artery disease may be quite mild. Paroxysms of a-v re-entrant tachycardia are common in the pre-excitation syndromes of which the Wolff–Parkinson–White syndrome is the most common. In this the P-R interval is pathologically short and the initial part of the QRS rises or falls slowly to form the so-called 'delta' wave (*Fig. P.29*). In paroxysms of tachycardia in such cases the QRS assumes a normal configuration. This condition is often benign but paroxysms of atrial fibrillation with a very rapid ventricular rate can occur and sudden death, due probably to ventricular fibrillation, has been reported.

Atrial and *junctional tachycardia* due to enhanced automaticity of a focus in the atria or atrioventricular junction are much less common than a-v re-entrant tachycardia. They may occur in paroxysms but are more often sustained for long periods. There is often some degree of atrioventricular block which never occurs in a-v re-entrant tachycardia and there is usually associated heart disease such as ischaemia or cardiomyopathy; digoxin toxicity may also cause such dysrhythmias.

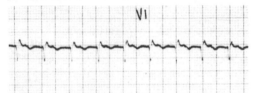

Fig. P.31. Supraventricular tachycardia at 160 per minute, probably junctional as P waves cannot be certainly identified, in a patient 1 week after inferior myocardial infarction.

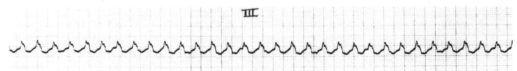

Fig. P.32. Ventricular tachycardia at 190 per minute in a patient a few hours after a myocardial infarction. Low-amplitude deflections which are probably P waves at a slower rate can be seen between some of the ventricular complexes; this confirms the ventricular origin of the dysrhythmia.

Faster atrial rates than those found in the tachycardias already considered produce *atrial flutter*. The atrial rate is often around 300 per minute; this is faster than the bundle can conduct and some degree of atrioventricular block is almost invariable. A 2:1 ratio is most common, producing a regular ventricular rhythm at about 150 per minute. This particular rate is rather characteristic of atrial flutter as it is faster than most sinus tachycardias and slower than many other supraventricular tachycardias. It may be possible to see atrial waves at twice the rate of the arterial pulse in the jugular venous pulse but this requires a good deal of experience—or imagination! The diagnosis can be made with near-certainty by studying the effect of pressure on the carotid sinus. In atrial flutter the degree of atrioventricular block is increased with, characteristically, an abrupt halving of the pulse rate. In sinus tachycardia carotid sinus pressure produces a more gradual slowing and in other supraventricular tachycardias the attack is either terminated or continues unabated. In atrial flutter the electrocardiogram shows rapid regular flutter waves with QRS complexes at half or a quarter of the atrial rate. The atrial rate is so rapid that, in most leads, the flutter waves produce a continuous 'saw-tooth' appearance of the baseline (*Fig* P.30). The absence of any iso-electric segments in the baseline has been suggested as a diagnostic criterion of flutter. There is, however, no real justification for this view and many authorities prefer to use the term 'flutter' for all supraventricular dysrhythmias with an atrial rate of 250–350 per minute. The causes of atrial flutter are similar to those of atrial fibrillation (*see* p. 535) except that it is not so common in mitral valve disease or hyperthyroidism.

Atrial fibrillation presents with an irregular tachycardia and is discussed at length in the section on PULSE, RHYTHM OF.

The electrocardiographic diagnosis of a supraventricular tachycardia depends on finding a regular tachycardia with P waves which are abnormal both in their timing in relationship to the QRS and in their shape (*Fig*. P.31). The QRS complexes are usually normal, although they may be widened and deformed as a result of aberrant ventricular conduction and resemble bundle-branch block.

Ventricular tachycardia is a much more serious affair than its supraventricular counterparts. Although it can occur in patients with otherwise normal hearts there is usually serious underlying heart disease. Much the commonest cause is ischaemic heart disease and it is particularly common after myocardial infarction when it can cause serious deterioration in the patient's condition and may be a forerunner of ventricular fibrillation. Ventricular tachycardia also occurs in a group of syndromes characterized by a prolonged Q-T interval in the electrocardiogram and, sometimes, congenital deafness. In ventricular tachycardia the rate is very variable; most commonly around 180 per minute, it may be as low as 100 or less, in which case some prefer to use the term 'idioventricular rhythm' rather than 'tachycardia'. The electrocardiogram shows broad, often notched, QRS complexes with no preceding P waves; a variation in which the QRS axis changes gradually and repeatedly so that the complexes appear to twist around the baseline is known as 'torsades de pointes'. In the usual type it may sometimes be possible to identify P waves separately at a slower rate; in this case the diagnosis of ventricular tachycardia is certain (*Fig*. P.32). Otherwise there can be confusion with supraventricular tachycardia with aberrant ventricular conduction. This is a difficult diagnostic problem as the certain identification of P waves in such a record may be impossible.

See also PULSE, RHYTHM OF.

Peter R. Fleming

Pulse, rhythm of

An absolutely regular pulse is rare. Even in normal sinus rhythm slight fluctuations in rate can be detected by measuring successive R–R intervals in the electrocardiogram. This can hardly be detected by palpation of the pulse, however, and this section will deal with irregularities which are apparent clinically. When examining the pulse, it is necessary first to determine whether it is regular or irregular and, if the latter, whether any pattern can be detected within the irregularity. Complete clinical analysis of an irregular pulse includes inspection of the jugular venous pulse and auscultation at the apex beat in addition to feeling the arterial pulse. The venous pulse provides evidence of the presence and frequency of atrial contractions; auscultation allows the detection of ventricular contractions too feeble to produce a pulse at the wrist. Many dysrhythmias can be diagnosed clinically but electrocardiographic confirmation is always desirable if possible. In some cases the diagnosis can only be made from the electrocardiogram and, in a few, only with considerable difficulty.

There are two main mechanisms which can produce an irregular pulse. The first is a disorder of impulse formation in which, most commonly, an abnormal (ectopic) pacemaker drives the ventricles either directly or via the atrioventricular bundle. The other mechanism is a disorder of conduction in which a block develops somewhere along the long pathway from the sinoatrial node to the ventricular myocardium; if this block is intermittent, an irregular pulse is likely to result. The common causes of an irregular pulse are summarized in *Table* P.15. For a more detailed discussion of the genesis of dysrhythmias *see* PULSE RATE, ABNORMAL (p. 527).

Table P.15. Causes of an irregular pulse

Disorders of impulse formation
Sinus arrhythmia
Ectopic beats (supraventricular or ventricular)
  Escape beats
  Extrasystoles
  Parasystole
Atrial fibrillation
Atrial flutter with varying atrioventricular block

Disorders of conduction
Sino-atrial block
Partial atrioventricular block
  Mobitz Type I (Wenckebach)
  Mobitz Type II

Apparent irregularity in normal rhythm
Pulsus alternans
Pulsus paradoxus

Disorders of impulse formation

The rate of discharge of the sino-atrial node can vary, more or less rhythmically, in many normal subjects; this condition, termed *sinus arrhythmia*, is quite benign and hardly justifies classification as a 'disorder'. The fluctuations in rate are most commonly in phase with respiration, the rate increasing during inspiration and slowing during expiration. This is very common in children and is due to reflex variations in vagal tone (*Fig.* P.33). The *absence* of respiratory sinus arrhythmia is sometimes of some slight diagnostic significance in a child as this is a feature of a large atrial septal defect. There are also two, much rarer, types of non-respiratory sinus arrhythmia. In one the cycles of tachycardia and bradycardia are much longer and are quite unrelated to respiration; the P waves of the electrocardiogram are normal and constant in configuration. In the other type the P waves vary slightly in shape and the irregularity is believed to be due to changes in the site of the pacemaker within the sino-atrial node itself. The irregularity in respiratory sinus arrhythmia is exaggerated by deep breathing and, in all types, is abolished or markedly reduced by exercise or other causes of tachycardia.

Ectopic beats are a very common cause of an irregular pulse. They are due to the discharge of an abnormal pacemaker in the atria, atrioventricular junction (AV node and main bundle of His) or ventricles. Apart from their site of origin, they can be classified as escape beats, extrasystoles and parasystoles. *Escape beats* should be regarded as a protective mechanism against asystole. They arise either from the atrioventricular junction or from the ventricles and occur whenever, for any reason, there is a prolonged pause in the activity of the sino-atrial node. Thus they may be seen in sinus bradycardia and during the slow phase of sinus arrhythmia. They are difficult to recognize clinically but can be identified in the electrocardiogram by the abnormally long pause preceding an ectopic beat identified, as described below, as junctional or ventricular in origin.

Extrasystoles most frequently arise from the ventricles but atrial and junctional extrasystoles are also common. If a ventricular extrasystole occurs early in diastole, ventricular filling will be incomplete and the contraction may fail to open the aortic valve; even if it does so, the pulse may be so feeble that it does not reach the wrist. Thus, in the radial pulse a 'dropped beat' will be noticed; on auscultation the extrasystole will be heard either as the first sound only or as both sounds. Ventricular extrasystoles occurring later in diastole are more likely to produce a palpable impulse at the radial pulse. Often an extrasystole follows each sinus beat to produce pulsus bigeminus or coupled beats; this is often a result of digoxin overdosage. The patient with extrasystoles may have noticed no abnormality or he may complain of palpitation described in terms such as to indicate a momentary disturbance in the action of the heart; expressions such as 'my heart missed a beat' or 'my heart seemed to

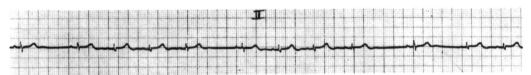

Fig. P.33. Electrocardiogram showing gross respiratory sinus arrhythmia. The cycle lengths vary from 0·7 to 1·24 seconds.

turn over' are not uncommon. In the electrocardiogram ventricular extrasystoles are identified by the bizarre configuration of the QRS complex and by the absence of a P wave (*Fig* P.34). The pause following the extrasystole is usually fully compensatory, that is the sum of the R–R intervals preceding and following the ectopic beat equals two complete cycles. Rarely, if the sinus rate is slow, interpolated ventricular extrasystoles occur—the only true 'extra' systole. Occasional ventricular extrasystoles are usually benign and do not necessarily indicate organic heart disease; they are more common following over-indulgence in tea, coffee, alcohol or tobacco. Frequent ventricular extrasystoles occurring at rest are of more importance and probably indicate heart disease of some kind; however, their exact significance is uncertain and, provided that the standard investigations, including an exercise electrocardiogram, are normal, a good prognosis can be given. They are certainly of more serious significance following myocardial infarction, when, if they are multifocal, or appear in salvoes, or are so premature as to deform the T wave of the preceding complex (R-on-T), they may presage ventricular tachycardia or fibrillation.

from a ventricular extrasystole by the finding of an ectopic P wave preceding the QRS (*Fig*. P.35). The pause following a supraventricular extrasystole is usually less than fully compensatory. Supraventricular extrasystoles are nearly always benign but if they are frequent, for example in a patient with mitral stenosis, they may indicate that atrial fibrillation is impending.

With extrasystoles in general, the interval between a sinus beat and an extrasystole—the coupling interval—is remarkably constant, implying that the discharge of the ectopic focus is in some way dependent on the preceding sinus beat. This is not the case in the phenomenon known as *parasystole*. In this situation an ectopic focus, most often in the ventricles but occasionally in the atria or atrioventricular junction, discharges at its own intrinsic rate regardless of the rate of the sino-atrial node or other dominant pacemaker. The ectopic focus is 'protected' from discharge by the normal sinus beats so that, whenever the ectopic discharge finds the ventricles in an non-refractory state, an ectopic beat appears. The diagnosis is made from the electrocardiogram by finding ectopic beats with varying coupling intervals and a succession of interectopic intervals all of which are multiples of

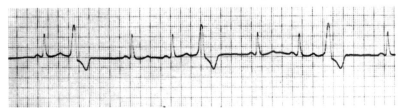

Fig. P.34. Electrocardiogram showing ventricular extrasystoles producing pulsus bigeminus.

Atrial and junctional (supraventricular) extrasystoles produce very much the same symptoms and signs as ventricular. The electrocardiogram shows abnormal P waves indicating the site of the ectopic focus; with junctional extrasystoles the P wave is typically inverted in Leads II, III and aVF. The form of the QRS complex is usually normal as the impulse reaches the ventricles via the normal conducting pathways. Occasionally, however, if the supraventricular extrasystole is very premature, one or other branch of the bundle may still be partially refractory so that intraventricular conduction proceeds abnormally and the configuration of the QRS is bizarre, simulating bundle-branch block. This phenomenon is known as 'aberrant ventricular conduction' and can only be decisively distinguished

a single shorter interval—the intrinsic cycle length of the ectopic focus (*Fig*. P.36).

The clinical diagnosis of extrasystoles is usually easy but, if they occur frequently, they may be difficult to distinguish from atrial fibrillation. Exercise will usually abolish extrasystoles and, if anything, cause greater irregularity in atrial fibrillation. The jugular venous pulse may also be helpful as cannon waves are a constant finding in junctional extrasystoles and may occur in other varieties also, if atrial and ventricular systole happen to coincide. A cannon wave implies an effective atrial contraction and therefore rules out atrial fibrillation.

Progressively more rapid rates of discharge of an ectopic atrial focus lead to atrial tachycardia and atrial

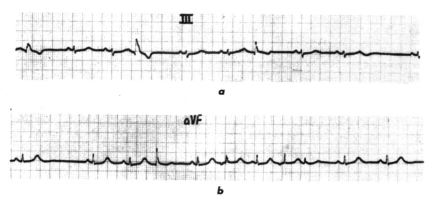

Fig. P.35. Electrocardiogram showing frequent supraventricular extrasystoles conducted normally or with ventricular aberration. *a*, The first, fourth and seventh complexes are supraventricular in origin, despite their abnormal configuration, as shown by the preceding P waves which deform the T waves of the previous complexes. The long pause at the end of the strip is preceded by an ectopic P wave which is completely blocked. *b*, The sixth and eighth complexes are supraventricular extrasystoles conducted normally, the fourth and ninth show ventricular aberration.

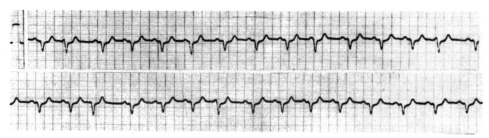

Fig. P.36. Two strips of continuous record showing junctional parasystole with retrograde block. The sinus P waves continue uninterruptedly with a cycle length of 0·7 second. The second, tenth and fourteenth complexes in the upper strip and the third and seventh in the lower are junctional in origin. The interectopic intervals are 5·76 seconds (=2×2·88) and 2·88 seconds. Later in the same record an interectopic interval of 31·5 seconds (=11×2·86) was found.

flutter which can be regarded as a series of atrial ectopic beats. In these conditions the ventricular rhythm is usually regular but when the rate of discharge of the ectopic focus exceeds about 400 per minute, coordinated atrial depolarization and contraction are impossible and *atrial fibrillation* results. The supraventricular impulses impinge, more or less at random, on the atrioventricular node, finding it and the remainder of the conducting tissue more or less refractory at any given time so that the ventricular response is totally irregular.

Atrial fibrillation is an extremely common finding in almost any type of heart disease. Probably the commonest cause is rheumatic heart disease, especially mitral valve disease; it is much less common, except as a terminal event, in isolated aortic valve disease. In hyperthyroidism, also, it is a well-known complication, especially in the toxic nodular goitre of older subjects. It is not very common in uncomplicated angina, but it occurs quite frequently after myocardial infarction and when failure develops. In hypertensive heart disease, as well, it is rather unusual except late in the course of the disease. Other conditions characterized by chronic atrial fibrillation, as distinct from the transient type to be discussed below, are constrictive

pericarditis, invasion of the pericardium by bronchial carcinoma or other mediastinal tumours, tumours of the heart itself, many varieties of cardiomyopathy and atrial septal defect, but not other types of congenital heart disease. Idiopathic or 'lone' atrial fibrillation, with no other evidence of heart disease, is well recognized but rather rare. Infections, particularly respiratory, can precipitate atrial fibrillation, especially in patients predisposed by rheumatic heart disease. Once the infection is over, sinus rhythm may be restored, either spontaneously or by direct-current shock. Return to sinus rhythm is also possible if atrial fibrillation has been caused by myocardial infarction and is almost the rule in thyrotoxic atrial fibrillation once the patient is euthyroid. Other causes of transient atrial fibrillation include pulmonary embolism (although it is rather unusual in chronic cor pulmonale), sick sinus syndrome, alcohol abuse, thoracotomy for any purpose, electric shock and hypothermia, either accidental or induced. It can rarely be caused by drugs such as digoxin and anaesthetic agents.

The development of atrial fibrillation will usually cause the patient to complain of palpitation, and failure may be precipitated in patients with severe heart disease. This is particularly the case in mitral stenosis in which the rapid ventricular rate, by restricting the time available for ventricular filling, causes a steep rise in left atrial pressure and may precipitate pulmonary oedema (*Fig*. P.37). Once the ventricular rate has been brought under control by digoxin, most patients with atrial fibrillation have few, if any, symptoms attributable to the dysrhythmia. The pulse is totally irregular and rapid in uncontrolled atrial fibrillation. The true ventricular rate can be determined only by auscultation as many of the impulses fail to reach the radial pulse; it is usually around 160 per minute. The difference between the rates as determined at the radial pulse and by auscultation—the pulse deficit—is some measure of the lack of control. Once the ventricular rate is under control there is no pulse deficit and the irregularity of the pulse, although still present, may be less easy to detect. The other diagnostic feature is the absence of evidence of atrial systole; no 'a' waves are seen in the jugular venous pulse and the presystolic murmur of mitral stenosis disappears as does an atrial gallop rhythm if one has been heard previously. The electrocardiogram shows three diagnostic features; a totally irregular ventricular rhythm, absence of P waves and their replacement by 'f' waves, fairly large in amplitude if the atrial fibrillation is of recent onset and becoming smaller as the months and years go by (*Fig*. P.38).

The ventricular rhythm will be regular only if every other beat is dropped as in 2:1 atrioventricular block or if the block is complete and a lower pacemaker is driving the ventricles. Any other pattern of failure of conduction will cause an irregular pulse.

Sino-atrial block is a rather rare conduction defect in which the impulse fails to pass from the sino-atrial node to the atrial myocardium. Clinically occasional dropped beats are noted or, if 2:1 sino-atrial block is present, a regular slow pulse (*Fig*. P.39). The patients may be symptom-free but Stokes-Adams attacks can occur. The condition can occur in the absence of other evidence of heart disease especially during sleep but is quite often associated with ischaemic heart disease or, as a transient phenomenon, with acute rheumatic carditis. It is one of the typical features of the sick sinus syndrome and can also occasionally be produced by digoxin.

Partial atrioventricular block can also produce an irregular pulse. In Mobitz Type I (Wenckebach) second-degree block conduction in the atrioventricular bundle becomes progressively more impaired from beat to beat, as shown by an increasing P–R interval in the electrocardiogram, until conduction fails completely and a ventricular beat is missed (*Fig*. P.40). Thus, in the radial pulse, every third, fourth or fifth beat

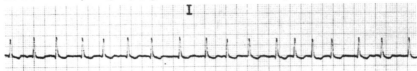

Fig. P.37. Atrial fibrillation with a ventricular rate of 140 per minute. Recorded from a man, aged 51, with mitral stenosis who was in pulmonary oedema at the time. He became virtually symptom-free when the ventricular rate was controlled with digoxin.

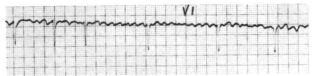

Fig. P.38. Electrocardiogram showing atrial fibrillation with a ventricular rate of 60 per minute. The f waves are well shown as is usually the case in Lead VI.

Atrial flutter, although usually associated with a regular ventricular rhythm, may produce an irregular pulse if the degree of atrioventricular block is variable. Clinically this is very difficult to distinguish from atrial fibrillation and, indeed, at fast atrial rates the two conditions merge in so-called 'flutter-fibrillation'. This unsatisfactory term should be avoided if possible; if each of the varying R-R intervals is a multiple of the interval between two 'f' waves, flutter should be diagnosed. Atrial flutter is considered at greater length in the section on PULSE RATE, ABNORMAL.

Disorders of conduction

Failure of transmission of the impulse from the sino-atrial node to the ventricles causes 'dropped beats'.

may be dropped; there is also a slight progressive increase in ventricular rate during the runs of conducted beats but this cannot be detected by palpation alone. This type of atrioventricular block is relatively benign and may be a transient occurrence in myocardial infarction or digoxin intoxication. Normal conduction is almost always restored by exercise, atropine or any other measure which increases the atrial rate (*Fig*. P.40). Mobitz Type 2 second-degree block is a much more serious condition. In its mildest form beats may be dropped intermittently, as in Type 1, but without any previous lengthening of the P-R interval; later 2:1 or 3:1 block with a slow regular ventricular rhythm is common. Increasing the atrial rate, by any means,

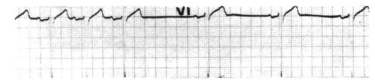

Fig. P.39. Electrocardiogram showing the sudden development of 2:1 sino-atrial block. From a woman, aged 59, with severe hypertensive and ischaemic heart disease.

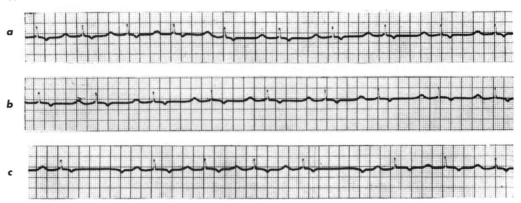

Fig. P.40. Electrocardiogram showing Type I (Wenckebach) partial atrioventricular block. In *a*, the P–R intervals progressively lengthen until conduction fails and a QRS complex is deleted. In *b*, recorded 1 min after 1 mg of atropine intravenously, the Wenckebach periods have ceased but the P–R interval is prolonged to 0·25 seconds. In *c*, another minute later, atrioventricular conduction is normal.

increases the severity of the block. (*See also* PULSE RATE ABNORMAL).

Two mechanical causes of a palpably irregular pulse should be mentioned. *Pulsus alternans* is characterized by a regular rhythm with alternation in amplitude of the equally spaced beats. It may be easily palpable but, more often, is detected by sphygmomanometry. As the cuff pressure is lowered, half of the beats are heard at the higher systolic pressure and, as the pressure of the smaller amplitude beats is reached, the rate seems suddenly to double. A run of pulsus alternans is often initiated by an extrasystole but it must not be confused with pulsus bigeminus. Nor should it be confused with electrical alternans in which the QRS complexes alternate in amplitude; the two conditions may coexist, however. Though rather rare, pulsus alternans is an important sign of left ventricular failure.

Pulsus paradoxus is a feature of constrictive pericarditis, high-pressure pericardial effusion and other, less common, conditions in which the primary abnormality is failure of the ventricles to fill adequately (restrictive cardiomyopathy). It is also important evidence of the severity of an attack of asthma. The normal tendency of the pulse-pressure to fall slightly during inspiration is much exaggerated so that, in a gross example, the arterial pulse may become impalpable during inspiration. At first the impression is of a grossly irregular pulse but there is little difficulty in relating the changes to the phases of respiration; the diagnosis

is confirmed by finding other evidence of pericardial constriction. This includes a rise in the, already elevated, venous pressure on inspiration instead of the usual fall. This behaviour of the venous pressure, known also as Kussmaul's sign, is much commoner than a paradoxical arterial pulse and is truly paradoxical, or the opposite of the normal. The arterial changes are an exaggeration of, not opposite to, the normal; the term 'paradoxical' was applied because the heart's action appeared to have ceased during inspiration and yet, *paradoxically*, heart sounds could still be heard normally at this time.

Peter R. Fleming

Pulses, unequal

A thorough physical examination should include palpation of all the easily accessible arterial pulses. The pulses on the two sides should be compared and, in the arms at any rate, inequalities should be confirmed by sphygmomanometry. It must be remembered that, in normal subjects, the blood pressure in the right arm may be slightly higher than that in the left; this difference is, however, rarely palpable. It is always worth recording the arteries in which the pulse has been felt, if only for future reference; the significance of an absent pulse is much greater if it is known to have been present on a previous occasion.

The pulse in one or other radial artery may be reduced or absent as a result of a minor *congenital abnormality* in the course or calibre of the vessel. Other congenital conditions in which the radial pulses may be unequal include a few cases of *coarctation of the aorta*. In 2 per cent of cases the lesion is proximal to the left subclavian artery so that the pulses in the left arm are weaker than those in the right; in addition stenosis of the origin of a subclavian artery is a rare complication of coarctation. *Supravalvar aortic stenosis* is another, very rare, cause of unequal pulses; in this condition the blood pressure in the right arm is often a good deal higher than that in the left and the difference may be palpable. There is no convincing explanation for this finding.

Inequality of pulses previously known to be equal is a most important sign. In the legs *atherosclerosis* of the larger arteries is the commonest cause and the level of occlusion should be sought by comparing the pulses in the femoral, popliteal, posterior tibial and dorsalis pedis arteries. Another cause of unequal pulses, usually in the legs, is *Buerger's disease* although some authorities doubt the existence of this condition as a separate entity. Atherosclerosis is less common in the vessels of the upper limbs but can certainly involve the branches of the aortic arch and cause inequality of the brachial and radial pulses. Giant-cell *arteritis* and other inflammatory diseases of arteries occasionally cause occlusion of major limb vessels.

Arterial embolism is an important cause of unequal pulses in the upper or lower limbs. The three commonest sources of such an embolism are the left atrium in atrial fibrillation, particularly in association with mitral valve disease; vegetations in infective endocarditis of the mitral or aortic valve; and mural thrombus laid down on the endocardial surface of a myocardial infarct. Less common causes of systemic embolism are left atrial myxoma, left ventricular endocardial thrombus in a ventricular aneurysm or in dilated cardiomyopathy, thrombus detached from an atherosclerotic plaque in the aorta, and a so-called 'paradoxical embolus' passing from veins in the legs via a patent to the systemic circulation. This last occurs only if the pressures on the right side of the heart have been raised, often by a previous pulmonary embolism.

Frequent palpation of the arterial pulses is most important when *dissecting aneurysm* of the aorta is suspected. As the dissection proceeds along the length of the aorta the branches may be occluded one by one over a period of a few hours; the process may be capricious, branches past which the dissection has spread unexpectedly remaining patent. If re-entry occurs, the pulse may return in arteries previously occluded.

Takayasu's disease, or the 'pulseless disease', is a rare form of arteritis involving the branches of the aortic arch. Apart from inequality in the pulses in the arms or, perhaps more commonly, obliteration of the pulses in both arms, signs and symptoms of cerebral ischaemia are common. Takayasu's disease is one of the causes of so-called 'reversed coarctation', a not very satisfactory term implying diminished or absent pulses in the arms with normal femoral pulses. This situation can also occur as a result of *aortic aneurysm*, particularly of the arch, in which unequal pulses in the arms may be of diagnostic importance.

Occlusion of a subclavian artery by external pressure, as by a *cervical rib* or a *tumour* in that region, must be remembered. In cervical rib particularly, pain, paraesthesiae and weakness and wasting of the small muscles of the hand, due to compression of the 1st thoracic root, are common associated features.

Finally, such obvious causes of unequal pulses as previous *subclavian-pulmonary anastomosis* for cyanotic congenital heart disease or brachial *arteriotomy* must be mentioned.

Peter R. Fleming

Pupils, abnormalities of

Abnormalities of the pupil may be classified as irregularities in shape or irregularities in size and movement.

1. Irregularities in shape

The normal pupil is circular or slightly oval with its longer axis horizontal. Its outline may become irregular due to an adhesion between the iris and the lens, most commonly the result of previous iritis. Such adhesions are most evident when the pupil is dilated. A similar irregularity sometimes occurs in association with the persistence of a pupillary membrane, a congenital defect in which the adhesions are distinguished from inflammatory adhesions by the fact that they arise from the anterior surface of the iris at a slight distance from the pupil and not from the posterior surface or the extreme edge.

Irregularities in the shape of the pupil may result from injury, such as rupture of the sphincter and tearing of the root of the iris from its ciliary attachment, referred to as iridodialysis, dislocation of the lens, or partial adherence to an old perforated corneal ulcer. A concussion injury may cause a dilatation of the pupil, regular or irregular, and with or without associated loss of reflex movement. Rarely a traumatic meiosis may be seen. Irregularity of shape after injury may give an important clue as to whether perforation of the globe has occurred, since incarceration of the iris in a corneal wound will necessarily cause distortion of the pupil.

The circular shape of the pupil is lost in coloboma or as a result of surgery in the form of iridectomy.

2. Irregularities in size and movement

Pupillary size and equality are dependent on a balance between the action of parasympathetic nerve fibres which innervate the constrictor of the pupil (carried by the third cranial nerve) and of the sympathetic fibres responsible for pupillary dilatation (the cranial sympathetic supply). Slight inequality in the size of the pupils (anisocoria) is observed frequently and may be of no pathological significance. Pronounced difference in the size of the pupils is likely to be symptomatic of an organic lesion. In cases where the abnormal pupil is the smaller, the condition is usually due to hyperaemia of the iris resulting from iritis, paralysis of the cervical sympathetic or the use of a miotic drug such as pilocarpine. In cases where the abnormal pupil is the larger, the dilatation is usually due to stimulation of the sympathetic (the so-called 'reverse Horner syndrome'), the use of a mydriatic such as atropine, paralysis of the fibres of the third cranial nerve, or increased ocular tension, as in glaucoma.

The pupil varies in size depending on age. In infancy it is small and it becomes larger during young adult and middle life. It becomes small again in old age. As a general rule the pupil is smaller in hypermetropic and larger in myopic eyes. In pontine haemorrhage there is bilateral pupillary constriction.

Variations in pupillary movement may occur spontaneously as in hippus, when the pupils are seen to constrict and dilate together without any obvious stimulus being applied. This is simply an exaggeration of physiological movements of the pupil. Otherwise movements of the pupil occur as a result of one of the pupillary reflexes of which there are four:

i   The light reflex.
ii The near reflex (accommodation).
iii The reflex to sensory stimulation.
iv Psychic reflexes.

The reflex to light and the near, or accommodation, reflex both cause pupillary constriction on each side; the sensory and psychic reflexes cause pupillary dilatation. The former reflexes are mediated by the third cranial nerves and the latter two by the sympathetic supply to the iris. Some abnormalities of the pupil and their reflexes are illustrated in *Table* P.16.

A third nerve palsy results in dilatation of the pupil with absence of response to both direct and consensual light stimuli and to accommodation. Damage to the sympathetic supply to the head results in a Horner's syndrome with a small pupil in association with ptosis. The pupillary light reflex and the accommodation reflex are preserved. However, the pupil will have some impairment of dilatation in response to shading the eye. The Adie pupil seen as part of the Holmes–Adie syndrome is characterized by a large pupil which reacts slowly on accommodation and shows incomplete response to a bright light. The pupil will usually constrict to dilute (2·5 per cent) methacholine indicating supersensitivity. The Adie pupil is thought to result from degeneration of postganglionic neurones in the ciliary ganglion. It is most commonly seen in young women in the second and third decades of life and is usually asymptomatic though occasionally photophobia may be a symptom. The pupil gradually becomes smaller with the passage of time. Argyll-Robertson pupils are typically small and irregular and may be bilateral or unilateral. There is loss of the pupillary light reflex but often preservation of the accommodation reflex. They occur most often in neurosyphilis but sometimes also in diabetes. Damage to the afferent limb of the pupillary light reflex, as in an optic nerve lesion, results in an afferent pupillary defect. Complete transection of the optic nerve results in ipsilateral loss of the direct light reflex, with loss of the consensual light reflex in the opposite eye. In these circumstances the pupils are often equal. Less severe damage to the optic nerve may result in minor impairment of the pupillary light reflex which

Table P.16. Pupillary disorders

Unilateral	Light reaction	Associated signs
IIIrd nerve palsy	Negative	Ptosis (may be complete)
		External ophthalmoplegia
Horner's syndrome	Poor dilatation to shade	Ptosis (always partial)
		Anhidrosis
		Enophthalmos
Holmes–Adie syndrome	Slow reaction	Constriction to methacholine
Bilateral		
Argyll Robertson	Negative	Depigmented iris
Metabolic coma	Positive	Coma
Midbrain compression	Negative	Coma plus or minus lateralizing signs
Pontine stroke	Negative	Coma
		Hyperventilation
		Hyperpyrexia

may be detected only by the so-called 'swinging flashlight' test. A bright light is shone into the affected eye and maintained until the pupillary constriction is static, then into the unaffected eye with a similar reaction. But, when the light is once more shone into the affected eye, the pupil may initially dilate before constricting. This lag in response is diagnostic of a partial optic nerve lesion.

N. E. F. Cartlidge

Purpura

(*See also* BLEEDING; BRUISES)

The presence of purpura usually indicates thrombocytopenia (*Table* P.17) although there are additionally, non-thrombocytopenic causes (*Table* P.18). In any patient with purpura due to a reduced platelet count it is important to ascertain the cause and severity because purpura usually indicates a severe haemorrhagic potential. Whereas purpura on the skin is not life-threatening, thrombocytopenia can result in rapidly fatal intracranial or massive gastrointestinal haemorrhage. Purpura usually indicates a platelet count less than 30×10^9/l. Platelet functional disorders, e.g. thrombasthenia or platelet storage pool disorder, do not usually result in purpura unless there is a secondary provocative stimulus, e.g. protracted coughing. The presence of purpura in an individual with a normal platelet count is indicative of a vasculitis. Whereas thrombocytopenia results in flat purpura lesions, those due to a vasculitis are often slightly raised and on some occasions may be up to 1 cm in diameter.

Table P.17. Causes of thrombocytopenia

Impaired production of platelets
Congenital megakaryocytic abnormalities
  Wiscott–Aldrich
  May–Hegglin anomaly
  TAR (thrombocytopenia with absent radii)
Marrow hypoplasia
Aplastic anaemia
Megaloblastosis
  B_{12}/folate deficiency
  Folate antagonists
Toxins
  Chemotherapy
  Drugs
    Phenylbutazone
    Sulphonamides
    Choramphenicol
    Procainamide
    Thiazides
    Oestrogens
  Ethanol
  Ionizing radiation
Infiltration by
  Leukaemia
  Lymphoma
  Myeloma
  Carcinoma
Paroxysmal nocturnal haemoglobinuria
Myelodysplasia

Increased utilization/destruction of platelets

Immune-mediated
  Acute ITP
  Chronic ITP
Secondary to immune abnormalities
  SLE
  Chronic lymphatic leukaemia
  Hodgkin's disease
  Non-Hodgkin's lymphoma
  Hyperthyroidism
Drugs causing immune destruction
  Quinine
  Gold
  Penicillins
  Para-amino salicylatic acid
  Rifampicin
  Methyldopa
  Heparin
Neonatal thrombocytopenia
  Maternal auto-antibody
  Maternal iso-antibody
Post-transfusional purpura
Disseminated intravascular coagulation
  Pregnancy-associated conditions
    Eclampsia
    Abruptio placentae
    Retained dead foetus
  Septicaemia
  Hypothermia
  Asphyxia
  Cardiopulmonary arrest
Local thrombosis
  Massive thromboembolism
  Giant haemangiomas
Thrombotic thrombocytopenic purpura (Moschcowitz syndrome)
Haemolytic uraemic syndrome
Virus
  Rubella
  CMV
  EBV
  HIV
  Herpes
Other infections
  Toxoplasmosis
  Syphilis

Abnormality of distribution of platelets
Splenomegaly
Massive transfusion

Table P.18. Non-thrombocytopenic causes of purpura

Vasculitis
  Henoch–Schönlein purpura
  Systemic lupus erythematosus
  Drugs

Mechanical
  Coughing
  Orthostatic
  Senile

Steroid-induced

Scurvy

Factitious purpura

C. A. Ludlam

Pustules

A pustule is an elevation of the skin containing pus, differing from a vesicle or bulla only in its contents.

Pustules may develop from vesicles that have become purulent or from papules. They may develop so rapidly that their origin cannot be observed. They vary in colour from bright yellow to cream, orange, grey or green. Examination with a hand lens may show them to arise in hair follicles, but they may occur on normal skin or around sweat pores (*Table* P.19).

Table P.19. Pustules

1. Pustules of infectious origin
Staphylococcal
  folliculitis, boils, carbuncle, ecthyma (Fig. P.42),
  hordeolum, sycosis barbae
Candidiasis
Dermatophyte
Gonococcal septicaemia (Fig. P.44)
Gram-negative folliculitis (Fig. P.41)
Anthrax
Glanders
Smallpox
Chickenpox (Fig. V.4)
Pustular syphilide
Jacuzzi folliculitis

2. Sterile pustules
Pustular psoriasis
  localized, generalized (Figs. P.45, P.46)
Facial
  acne, rosacea, peri-oral dermatitis (Fig. P.47)
Itchy
  dermatitis herpetiformis, swimmers' itch
Widespread
  miliaria, drug-induced, Behçet's disease, subcorneal
  pustular dermatitis

1. Pustules of infectious origin

Pustules are usually the result of staphylococcal infection, especially *staphylococcal folliculitis*. Organisms may be introduced usually from outside by friction or occlusion but may also be blood borne from a distant focus. Lowered local resistance to the ubiquitous staphylococcus is probably the commonest cause, but colonization of the carrier sites of anterior nares and inner thighs with virulent organisms can be the source of recurrent cutaneous staphylococcal infections. Folliculitis is particularly common in the hospital setting where the occlusive effect of plastic-covered mattresses is combined with the prevalence of virulent, and sometimes resistant, staphylococci.

A boil (furuncle) is a deeper staphylococcal follicular pustule or abscess. The neck, buttocks and face are the commonest sites for boil formation. There is often considerable acute inflammation surrounding boils and lesions can be hot and very tender. The central painful papule undergoes rapid necrosis, a yellow pustule is formed, which becomes boggy, fluctuates and ultimately ruptures and discharges pus. In many cases a hard 'core' of necrotic material is extruded before healing takes place. Occasionally the contents of the boil are absorbed before rupture occurs

and the lesion regresses, a 'blind-boil'. After poulticing a boil a ring of small satellite boils may form around the original lesion. Boils beginning in the hair follicles of the eyelid are known as *styes* (hordeolum).

A *carbuncle* resembles a boil but the infection spreads to the deeper tissues and when rupture occurs there may be several openings onto the skin. Boils may follow one another in series for many months, when the condition is known as *chronic furunculosis*.

Sycosis barbae is staphylococcal folliculitis of the hairy areas of the face, including the eyebrows. It differs in no way from the other forms of staphylococcal folliculitis; it may be localized to small areas or it may affect the whole of the face and neck. The pustules are grouped on a bright erythematous base and in the centre of each pustule there is a hair which pulls out easily. It must be distinguished from the more common seborrhoeic sycosis in which the predominating lesions are red papules with little or no pustule formation. In all forms of staphylococcal folliculitis the diagnosis is fairly simple. Only rarely do other organisms, e.g. streptococcus or Gram-negative organisms (*Fig.* P.41), produce similar lesions.

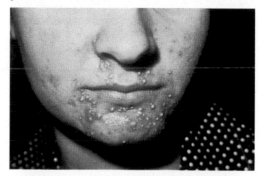

Fig. P.41. Gram-negative folliculitis in acne patient on long-term tetracycline. (*Dr Richard Staughton*)

An *ecthyma* begins as a burning painful vesico-pustule on an erythematous base, either singly or as sparse lesions scattered over buttocks and lower legs (*Fig.* P.42). Later deep-crusted ulcers form which heal slowly with considerable scarring. Patients are usually young women, debilitated by anaemia or systemic illness or are suffering from HIV disease. Streptococci or staphylococci may be cultured.

Boils in the axillae and groins can be the presentation of *hidradenitis suppurativa*, an intractable purulent condition affecting the apocrine sweat glands.

Recurrent purulent skin infections in a child, especially with crops of pustules in the webs of fingers and on wrists, is sometimes a feature of neglected *scabies* (*Figs* N.18, P.43, V.5). Pustules are also a feature of secondarily infected dermatitis, and can be particularly widespread in *atopic dermatitis* (Fig. P.21).

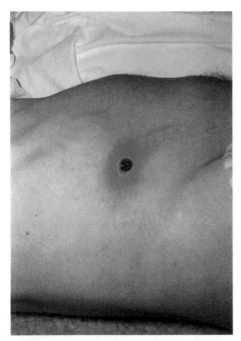

Fig. P.42. Ecthyma. (Dr Richard Staughton.)

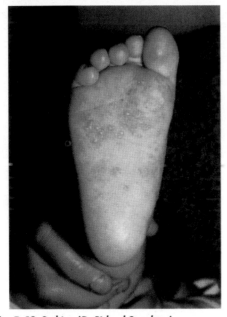

Fig. P.43. Scabies. (Dr Richard Staughton.)

Satellite vesico-pustules at the edge of a moist eroded patch are highly suggestive of *candidiasis* (thrush). This particularly favours damp, intertriginous areas, such as the submammary, perineal and perioral folds of skin. Scrapings from lesions warmed with 10 per cent potassium hydroxide show small oval budding thin-walled spores on microscopy; culture shows *Candida albicans*.

Some *dermatophyte* species appear to proliferate deep in hair follicles, especially *Trichophyton mentagrophytes*. Inappropriate treatment of superficial fungal infections with topical corticosteroids often leads to an apparent initial improvement of the condition but fungal growth persists deep in hair follicles and a curious resistant pustular eruption may result—so-called *tinea incognito*.

Characteristic discrete inflammatory pustules which may become haemorrhagic, accompany the fever, arthritis and tenosynovitis of *gonococcal septicaemia*. The representative photograph (*Fig.* P.44) should be studied carefully, as recognition of this skin lesion can lead to making this important diagnosis at an earlier stage, particularly in women who may have little in the way of genital symptoms.

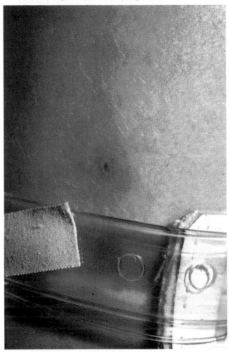

Fig. P.44. Gonococcal septicaemia with haemorrhagic pustule near wrist. (Dr Richard Staughton.)

Anthrax infection of the skin in its localized variety takes the form of a carbuncle-like inflammatory lesion caused by *Bacillus anthracis*. It is contracted from cattle, from their hides or hairs or rarely from shaving brushes. It attacks an exposed area of skin and the incubation period is from 1 to 3 days. The first sign is a small, itching red macule, not unlike a flea bite. In 2 days a papule forms which rapidly becomes a pustule; this soon ruptures and sometimes blood as well as pus is extruded. There results a gangrenous ulcer which in a simple case heals in a few weeks. In severe cases there may be grave constitutional symptoms with septicaemia and rapid death, and sometimes there are multiple skin lesions. It must be distinguished from a carbuncle and extragenital syphilitic chancre. Scrapings from the lesion contain the causal organism in large numbers. Anthrax is mostly an occupational disease in handlers of hides or wool ('wool sorter's disease').

Glanders is a disease of horses, mules and donkeys which very rarely affects humans, and then only those in contact with these animals. The main lesion is an ulcerating pustule. It is not unlike a carbuncle in its early stages and occurs on exposed areas of skin. The general symptoms are those of septicaemia and there is always a purulent nasal discharge. The presence of *Pseudomonas mallei* in this or material from the ulcers or pustules is diagnostic. The disease is almost invariably fatal.

The pustule was an important manifestation of *smallpox*. After an incubation period of 8–12 days the disease began with fever, headache, backache and vomiting. On the third and fourth days there was macular erythema and after a few hours shotty papules developed. These became vesicles and by the fifth day pustulated. The rash was most profuse on the head and limbs and there was only one crop of lesions which matured in 'majestic' concert. The vesicles were tough, firm and often multilocular and showed definite umbilication. By the time the pustules formed the umbilication was less well marked. In severe cases there was confluence of the pustules, particularly on the face. The mucous membranes were often involved as well. As a rule the temperature fell slightly with the eruption but rose again on the eighth or the ninth day when the pustules ruptured. In the final stage the pustules dried up to form brown crusts. Pitting or scarring was the rule. Previous vaccination modified the course of the disease considerably and there was a type of the disease known as *alastrim* (variola minor).

Chickenpox can be distinguished by the usually milder nature of disease, which is vesicular rather than pustular, and its profusion on the trunk rather than the extremities. In chickenpox the eruption comes out in successive crops and the vesicles are unilocular, fragile and do not exhibit umbilication. In spite of these differences, mild smallpox and severe chickenpox were difficult to differentiate.

Other viral diseases causing pustules are *vaccinia, cowpox and orf.* In the so-called *pustular syphilides* there are no true pustules, their resemblance to pustules being only superficial; on incision they will be found to be solid and contain no pus. The histology is diagnostic, and the serology will be positive.

Perhaps the most modern form of folliculitis is a new epidemic of *Pseudomonas folliculitis* that has been described in those indulging in jacuzzi bathing

and is inoculated on to the skin by the high-pressure water jets.

2. Sterile pustules

Pustules do not always indicate cutaneous infection and can arise during inflammatory dermatoses. These are often referred to as 'sterile' pustules as routine bacteriological examination of the pus always yields negative results. The classical example is *pustular psoriasis of palms and soles* (acrodermatitis perstans) where bright yellow sterile pustules arise within well-demarcated areas on palms and soles (*Fig.* P.45). As they age the pustules change to dark-brown macules and eventually peel off. The condition is commonest in middle-aged women and is notoriously resistant to conventional treatment. Only 25 per cent of such patients have evidence of psoriasis elsewhere on the body. On very rare occasions psoriasis may produce widespread sheets of sterile yellow pustules, associated with considerable toxicity and fever. This can occur spontaneously, with hypocalcaemia, or as a rebound phenomenon in patients whose severe psoriasis was hitherto suppressed by oral steroids or cytotoxic drugs. The condition is referred to as *generalized pustular psoriasis* (of von Zambusch), and until the advent of cytotoxic drugs the toxicity and mortality were high (*Fig.* P.46).

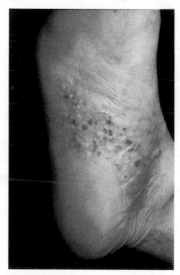

Fig. P.45. Pustular psoriasis of palms and soles. (Dr Richard Staughton.)

Sterile pustules on the *face* are seen in *acne, rosacea* and *perioral dermatitis.* In *acne* these are associated with evidence of comedones (open, closed or 'ice-pick', scarring), acne papules and perhaps acne cysts (*Fig.* P.41). The distribution is more peripheral on the face than *rosacea,* where pustules surround the 'muzzle' area, and are associated with vascular

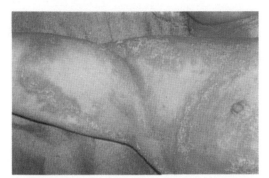

Fig. P.46. Generalized pustular psoriasis (of von Zambusch).

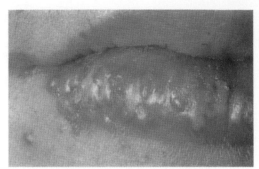

Fig. P.48. Herpes labialis. (*Westminster Hospital.*)

changes (erythema, flushing, telangiectasia) as well as papules and sometimes hypertrophied and patulous pilosebaceous pores on the nose (rhinophyma). *Perioral dermatitis* is a modern condition unknown before the introduction of fluorinated topical corticosteroids—the pustules are tiny and surmount painful small red papules, which abound around the mouth. A further diagnostic feature is a background of perioral erythema with a halo of pallor around the lip margins (*Fig.* P.47).

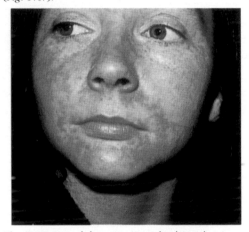

Fig. P.47. Perioral dermatitis. (*Dr Richard Staughton.*)

Unilateral pustules near the lips may have developed from *herpes simplex* vesicles, and tend to be greyish in colour. The grouped distribution and a history of recurrent lesions or recent respiratory tract infection are suggestive (*Fig* P.48).

If pustules are extremely pruritic consideration must be given to infestation or *dermatitis herpetiformis*. Scabies has already been mentioned; the burrows can become pustular, but in *swimmer's itch*, 12 hours after freshwater bathing, itchy weals may appear on the legs and later vesico-pustules appear. Scrapes from these may reveal the causative bird or mammal schistosomes which have been inoculated. In *dermatitis herpetiformis*, the greyish vesico-pustules are transient because of rapid deep excoriation. They occur

on forehead and scalp, shoulders, buttocks, natal cleft and knees. Diagnosis is often delayed.

Widespread pustulosis over the chest and back may follow a febrile illness or travel to a tropical environment with *miliaria* (*see* p. 642). A similar mono-morphic pustulation of face and upper trunk is prone to develop 4–8 weeks after administration of systemic steroids or ACTH, or more rapidly after iodides or bromides. A widespread sterile pustulosis of the skin is a recurrent feature of *Behçet's disease*, where deep painful ulcers develop on the orogenital mucosae. A dermatologist's finest hour comes with the diagnosis of the extremely rare *subcorneal pustular dermatitis* of Sneddon and Wilkinson. Here the pustules are very superficial and often form rings or gyrate patterns in flexures or flexor aspects of extremities. The condition affects middle-aged women and the cause is unknown. Again the pustules are sterile.

Richard Staughton

Pyrexia, prolonged

Fever is a controlled elevation of body temperature brought about by thermoregulatory reflexes. This distinguishes fever from hyperthermia, which is an uncontrolled rise in temperature as a consequence of thermal overload as in heat stroke or the loss of thermoregulatory function; malignant hyperthermia is a rare genetically determined disorder of muscle metabolism causing a very high temperature after general anaesthesia. Certain cytokines (e.g. interleukins 1 and 6, tumour necrosis factor) produced by inflammatory cells act as endogenous pyrogenic mediators. There is evidence that the fever response may be beneficial in cases of infection and fever is a cardinal sign of inflammation, whatever the cause may be.

A fever may be described as prolonged if it persists beyond 3 weeks. It may be persistent, remittent, swinging up and down but remaining above normal, or intermittent, with periods of normal temperature between febrile episodes. In many cases the cause may be obvious, but in others further investigation is required, for instance:

Blood counts; a high polymorphonuclear leucocytosis is not invariably present with local abscess formation but a full blood count may help to explain many fevers.

Serum agglutination tests, for instance, for typhoid fever, paratyphoid fever, abortus fever, listeriosis, etc.

Blood cultures.

Urine cultures.

Bacterial examination of exudates.

Lumbar puncture, revealing, for example, unexpected meningeal infection.

X-ray examination of the thorax, kidney, colon, and elsewhere, to identify or exclude infection or neoplasm.

Computed tomography, bronchoscopy, sigmoidoscopy, endoscopy.

Blood and tissue cultures, from bone, spleen, liver or other tissues, for infective organisms and biopsy for evidence of malignancy or specific inflammatory tissue changes.

Causes of prolonged pyrexia

The list of conditions that may cause prolonged pyrexia is lengthy. The relative frequency of the different causes varies greatly from country to country and, to a less extent, from time to time. The more common conditions to consider are:

1. Specific fevers

Viral:
  Infectious mononucleosis
Salmonella:
  Typhoid
  Paratyphoid
Rickettsia:
  Epidemic and scrub typhus
  Rocky Mountain spotted fever
  Q fever
  Trench fever
Legionella:
  Legionnaire's disease
Chlamydia:
  Psittacosis
Fungus:
  Coccidioidomycosis
  Histoplasmosis
Spirochaete:
  Syphilis
  Leptospirosis
  Lyme disease
Brucella:
  Abortus and melitensis fever
Tuberculosis
Listeriosis
Streptobacillary rate-bite fever
Tularaemia

2. Bacteraemia

Staphylococcal
Streptococcal
Meningococcal
Gonococcal
Coliforms
Infective endocarditis

3. Localized infection

Prostatic abscess
Ischiorectal abscess
Pyosalpinx
Suppurating ovarian cyst
Parametritic abscess
Empyema of the maxillary antrum,
  frontal sinus or ethmoidal air cells
Osteomyelitis
Infected lymph nodes in neck, axilla, groin
Mammary or submammary abscess
Empyema thoracis
Lung abscess
Hepatic abscess
Renal abscess
Splenic abscess
Empyema of gallbladder
Suppurative cholangitis
Suppurative pyelephlebitis
Subdiaphragmatic abscess
Bronchiectasis
Appendix abscess
Perinephric abscess
Diverticulitis
Lumbar and iliac retroperitoneal abscess
Psoas abscess
Actinomycosis of jaw, cheek, neck, lung, liver, spine or caecum

4. Infective and inflammatory conditions

Pyelonephritis and other urinary infections
Papillary necrosis
Chronic cystitis
Chronic cholecystitis
Phlebitis
Thyroiditis
Pneumonia and pneumonitis
Bronchopneumonia
Parametritis
Vesiculitis
Dysenteric colitis, bacillary or amoebic
Ulcerative colitis
Crohn's disease (regional enteritis)
Pancreatitis
Familial Mediterranean fever
Sarcoidosis

5. Non-purulent hepatic affections

Cirrhosis
Secondary carcinoma
Hepatitis, subacute and chronic

6. The connective tissue disorders

Rheumatoid arthritis
Rheumatic fever
Systemic lupus erythematosus
Polyarteritis nodosa and other arteritides
Polymyositis and dermatomyositis
Giant-cell arteritis
Still's disease (childhood and adult)

7. Blood diseases

Aplastic anaemia
Agranulocytosis
Lymphatic, myeloid or monocytic leukaemia,
    acute or chronic
Haemolytic anaemias

8. Diseases of tropics and subtropics

Trypanosomiasis
Malaria
Kala-azar
Plague
Relapsing fever
Filariasis
Leprosy
Schistosomiasis

9. Meningeal and cerebral haemorrhage

10. Skin conditions

Pemphigus
Severe or exfoliative dermatitis
Bullous pemphigoid

11. Malignancy

Lymphoma (e.g. Hodgkin's disease, lymphosarcoma)
Sarcoma
Carcinoma

12. Allergic (antigen-antibody reactive) conditions

Henoch-Schönlein syndrome
Allergic skin rashes
Post-cardiac injury syndrome

13. Factitious pyrexia produced by malingerers

14. Drug reactions

Sulphonamides
Antibiotics
Arsenicals
Iodides
Barbiturates, etc.

Such a list is bound to be incomplete and cannot be comprehensive. Space does not permit a full descrip-

tion of each of the diseases mentioned, but the following are some of the salient points:

1. Specific fevers

Infectious mononucleosis is today one of the commonest causes of prolonged fever in children and young adults, and diagnosis is often difficult. Paul–Bunnell or 'Monospot' tests are useful after the first 2 weeks or so in diagnosis. These are tests for heterophile antibodies; several specific antibodies against components of the Epstein–Barr virus have also been identified.

Infectious mononucleosis should be seriously considered in any prolonged low-grade fever with malaise and loss of weight in children and young adults for lymphadenopathy, splenomegaly and typical blood counts are not invariably present in all cases or may have been present earlier and have disappeared. Some authors consider infectious mononucleosis a clinical syndrome rather than a single entity, as the same picture can be due to the Epstein–Barr virus (EBV), the cytomegalovirus (CMV) or toxoplasma, but only the EBV variety gives a positive Paul–Bunnell test; full serological tests should therefore be done in all cases.

Typhoid fever suggests itself when a patient, previously in good health, suffers from a progressive fever of considerable and increasing degree with a pulse-rate that is relatively slow in relation to the temperature, the illness starting with headache and malaise but without any conspicuously abnormal signs. During the first week, the temperature rises each night to a slightly higher level than that of the previous night until a maximum is attained and maintained during the second week, after which there is a progressive diminution during the third week until normal temperature is reached again. Diarrhoea may occur with foul-smelling stools of pea-soup consistency, but constipation is more usual. Abdominal pain is usually confined to the right lower quadrant. The headache, which is in most cases a conspicuous feature, persists for about a week when it almost invariably ceases, thus contrasting with the headache of tuberculous meningitis. Blood cultures are positive in the first 10 days and in acute relapse, similar cultures later on proving negative although urine and faecal cultures may by then be positive. The spleen becomes palpable early in the disease and remains so until defervescence; it enlarges again in a relapse. Typical typhoid rose spots appear—chiefly on the abdomen, less often on the chest or back, and seldom on the limbs—from the seventh day onwards and in successive crops. They are about 2 or 3 mm in diameter, rose red, fading on pressure and without a central punctum. The majority of patients, but not all, develop a rise in agglutinins against the O antigens of the typhoid bacillus during the course of the disease. Another help in diagnosis is the absence of leucocytosis, and in the differential leucocyte count the lymphocytes are relatively increased, the polymorphonuclear cells being absolutely reduced. The leucocyte count may, however, be influenced by complications. Rigors are exceptional, a fact which sometimes helps in diagnosis from conditions such as septicaemia and malaria.

Some difficulty arises in the diagnosis of those cases in which there has been previous immunization of the patient by antityphoid inoculations; the fever is then of shorter duration and the illness relatively mild.

The Rickettsial disorders are numerous, ranging from epidemic typhus to trench fever. Different Rickettsiae are transmitted by lice, fleas, ticks and mites via man, wild rodents, domestic animals and cattle. In the history of mankind they rank high as a cause of epidemic disease causing great suffering and death, but they do not usually persist beyond 20 days and rarely cause prolonged fever.

Legionnaire's disease usually resolves or proves fatal within 3 weeks but the pneumonia caused many extend to lobes of both lungs and prolong the febrile disorder. The causative organism resembles a Rickettsia in some cultural characteristics, but it is larger in size and does not react with the standard Rickettsial antigens in complement fixation tests.

Psittacosis or *ornithosis* is transmitted to man from parrots and the parrot family, pigeons and a number of other birds, including ducks, turkeys and chickens. It is due to a Gram-negative obligate intracellular parasite, *Chlamydia psittaci*, formerly classified as a virus. The illness may be transmitted from the patient to others by contact. Clinically the illness is similar to typhoid fever, with liability to serious pulmonary complications. The fever lasts about 3 weeks, tending to end abruptly followed by slow convalescence, but may last for as long as 3 months. When the disease is contracted from parrots or parakeets it tends to be more severe and prolonged. The diagnosis is suggested in a patient with an illness that bears a general resemblance to typhoid fever but whose blood does not give the agglutination test and especially if there has been contact with a recently imported parrot, budgerigar or pigeon. The organism may be isolated from the blood or sputum. A rising titre of complement-fixing antibody in the patient's blood is useful in diagnosis.

Secondary syphilis may be a febrile illness. The diagnosis becomes obvious when the rash is associated with a fading primary sore, typical snail-track ulcers of tonsils, fauces and pharynx, and generalized enlargement of most of the palpable lymph nodes. Spirochaetes may be isolated from the skin lesions.

Lyme disease is caused by a tick-borne spirochaete, *Borrelia burgdorferi*. Cases have been reported from most parts of the USA, Scandinavia and Europe. Early disease is characterized by the annular skin lesion, erythema chronicum migrans (ECM). At this stage there may be fever, lymphadenopathy, myalgia and arthralgia. A history of tick-bite is often obtained. After several weeks of this flu-like illness neurological, cardiac and joint changes can develop— the latter often becoming permanent. The diagnosis can be confirmed serologically and by culture of the organisms or their demonstration in skin biopsies of ECM.

Abortus fever is a not uncommon cause of prolonged unexplained pyrexia, lasting usually for several months and occasionally for a year. It is due to infection by *Brucella abortus*. This organism causes fatal abortion in cows, and apart from the geographical circumstances the fever is identical to Mediterranean fever in which the disease is communicated by goat's milk. Infection may arise from ingestion of milk or the handling of infected animals or excreta. This infection may underlie obscure, long-continued febrile illness either in children or in adults. There are no characteristic symptoms, although arthritis is a frequent accompaniment. Diagnosis is usually by agglutination tests, rarely by blood cultures. Rarely it causes endocarditis, sometimes fatal. Cultures taken from bone marrow or liver may be positive when blood cultures are negative. Brucellar infections are particularly persistent, probably due to the intracellular location of the organism in the reticulo-endothelial tissues.

Melitensis, Mediterranean or *Malta fever* is one of the most prolonged of the fevers due to a known specific organism, in this case *Brucella melitensis*. In the undulant form of the disease successive exacerbations of pyrexia may prolong the illness into the sixteenth, eighteenth or twentieth week or longer (*Fig. P.49*). It may simulate typhoid fever, including the enlargement of the spleen and the paucity of abnormal physical signs, but there are no rose spots or other eruption. The diagnosis may be suggested by geographical factors—recent residence, for instance, in some part of the Mediterranean coast or islands, or Spain, Portugal, the Canary Islands or parts of South America, especially if the patient has been taking goat's milk, by which the infection is transmitted. The diagnosis is established by serum-agglutination tests, which may be positive from the fifth day onwards, the patient's diluted blood serum agglutinating cultures of *Br. melitensis*. Blood cultures should be done. *Brucella suis* infections, contracted from pigs, are also diagnosed by agglutination tests and blood cultures.

Tuberculosis. Tuberculous lesions often occur

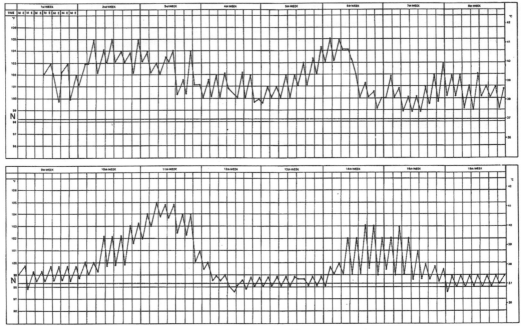

Fig. P.49. Temperature chart of a case of Mediterranean fever of undulant type (*Br. melitensis*).

without pyrexia. On the other hand, the occurrence of some degree of fever without any apparent cause may be the sole evidence of such disease, especially the miliary form. Pulmonary tuberculosis is almost invariably pyrexial but in an earlier stage there are often long periods of apyrexia even when the tuberculous process is active, with brief febrile spells. Tuberculous disease of the joints may be apyrexial unless secondarily infected. Glandular tuberculosis is less likely to be pyrexial when the nodes involved are cervical or bronchial than when the mesenteric and other abdominal nodes are caseous and softening ('tabes mesenterica'), when there may be, and usually is, prolonged pyrexia. The diagnosis may be easy if there is ascites in a child or if there are palpable abdominal masses, but it may be difficult in the absence of lumps and ascites in a condition of ill health with pyrexia and with vague abdominal pains which may be mistaken for some other non-tuberculous abdominal disease. The patient is usually young, and in European countries, may be an immigrant. The presence of enlarged cervical lymph nodes supports this diagnosis.

Listeriosis is an infectious disease of animals and man of world-wide distribution due to a Gram-positive bacillus, *Listeria monocytogenes*. Clinically it may present as a meningitis or resemble infectious mononucleosis with pharyngitis and diffuse lymphadenopathy, influenza or miliary tuberculosis. Untreated severe cases with meningitis often prove fatal. It may occur in infancy or in pregnancy. Diagnosis rests on isolating the micro-organisms, which resemble diphtheroid bac-

illi in culture, and on rising agglutination titres in the serum.

Streptobacillary rat-bite fever is due to bites from rats and, sometimes, mice, cats, dogs and weasels. It is caused by *Streptobacillus moniliformis* or *Spirillum minus* and is characterised by acute febrile attacks at fairly regular intervals of a few days. These persist for from two to ten months.

Tularaemia is uncommon in England, but cases have occurred amongst those handling live rabbits—for instance in bacteriological laboratories. It is a specific infectious disease due to *Pasteurella (Francisella) tularensis*, transmitted from rodents by ticks, or deer flies, by the handling or ingestion of infected animal tissues or by inhalation of infected aerosols. It is not transmitted directly from human to human. A sore on a finger is commonly the start, the sore becoming a small ulcer in a day or two, with associated enlargement of the epitrochlear and axillary lymph nodes; a chill or rigor is usual, and pyrexia continues for 2 or 3 weeks with marked prostration followed by slow convalescence. There may be erythematous blotches on the skin, or even purpura. Swallowing a very large number of bacilli may cause a typhoid-like disorder with high fever, abdominal pain and toxicity. Lung involvement may occur and enlargement of cervical glands. Rigors initially in severely ill patients may be followed by pyrexia persisting for several weeks. The diagnosis can be confirmed by a skin test which becomes positive in the first week, or the organism can be recovered from a mucocutaneous ulcer or regional lymph node, and occasionally from sputum on appropriate culture. Specific agglutinins appear in the serum within 8–10 weeks of onset of the illness, which is severe and prolonged, but the prognosis is good.

2. Bacteraemia

Disseminated infection may occur in association with a local lesion and metastasize to new areas. This may occur with many organisms. As an example, in *meningococcal infection* meningitis is not always present. In the early stages patients are acutely ill, with fever, chills, arthralgia and myalgia, particularly severe in the legs and back. They are very prostrated, hypotensive and 70 per cent develop a characteristic petechial rash (*Fig*. P.50). Meningococci are cultured from the blood and sometimes from scrapings from the skin lesions, and from the cerebrospinal fluid in cases with meningitis. A rare form of chronic meningococcaemia occurs which lasts for weeks or months and is characterized by fever, rash and arthritis or arthralgia.

Infective endocarditis. The comparatively rare acute or malignant endocarditis is due to infection by one of the pyogenic bacteria, such as haemolytic *Streptococcus*, *Pneumococcus*, *Gonococcus* and *Staphylococcus*. Many other organisms may cause endocarditis: *Corynebacterium diphtheriae*, Brucella and numerous others have been reported. Pseudomonal endocarditis may follow open-heart surgery. The type formerly termed the 'subacute' variety occurs in a subject with chronic valvular disease of congenital or rheumatic origin when the organism is usually *Streptococcus viridans*. Patients present with cardiac symptoms, anaemia, cerebral vascular lesions, or most commonly with pyrexia of unknown origin, a feature which arouses suspicion when progressive anaemia of normocytic and orthochromic type develops. The white cell-count is variable, a polymorphonuclear leucocytosis up to about 9–12 000 per mm^3 is common. Other diagnostic features are an enlarged spleen, clubbing of the fingers in half the subacute cases, rarely in the malignant type, petechial haemorrhages under the nails (*Fig*. P.51). and in the retina and conjunctiva and Osler's nodes (*Fig*. P.52). Emboli may occur in any organ or tissue. Red blood cells in the urine are invariable in greater or lesser degree.

Blood cultures should be done immediately as treatment must not be delayed. The patient, if over middle age, if not immediately treated, may be cured of the infection but die of cardiac failure due to the damage to the heart.

3. Localized infection

Many cases of continued fever are due to localized infection, i.e. abscess formation. Elicitation of local

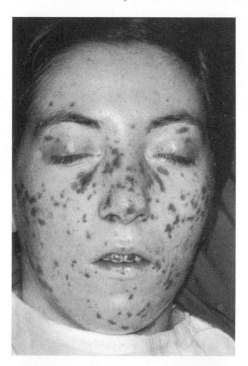

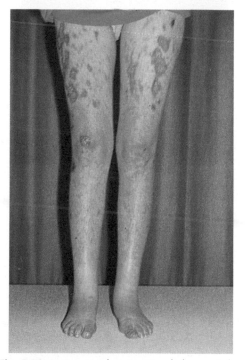

Fig. P.50. Meningococcal septicaemia which presented as subarachnoid haemorrhage and purpuric rash.

signs, in addition to pyrexia and other evidence of generalized systemic illness, will give the diagnosis, but it may be long delayed.

Rectal or vaginal examination should serve to

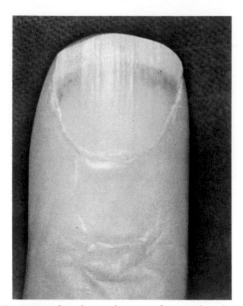

Fig. P.51. Splinter haemorrhages in infective endocarditis. (*Dr R. G. Ollerenshaw, Manchester Royal Infirmary.*)

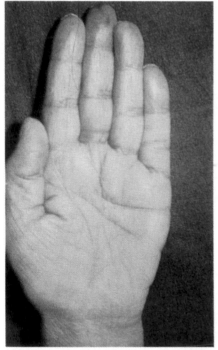

Fig. P.52. Large Osler's node on the tip of middle finger in a case of infective endocarditis. (*Dr R. G. Ollerenshaw, Manchester Royal Infirmary.*)

detect *prostatic abscess, periproctal abscess, ischiorectal abscess, pyosalpinx, suppurating ovarian cyst* or *parametritic abscess*, all of which are likely to cause local pain in the perineum, anal region, sacral region, back or lower abdomen.

Empyema of the maxillary antrum, when acute,

causes pain and tenderness over the affected maxilla with oedematous swelling of that side of the face, but in chronic cases the symptoms may be much less definite. The diagnosis may be suggested by facial pain, local swelling and perhaps an intermittent purulent discharge from one nostril. Radiographs and antral aspiration will confirm the diagnosis.

Empyema of a frontal sinus may be acute or chronic, causing pyrexia in either case. The diagnosis may be suggested by complaint of local headache above the eyes, generally on one or other side of the midline rather than central, especially if the headache is associated with local tenderness to percussion. Identification becomes easy if the abscess points above the inner canthus of the orbit near the root of the nose; but doubt may persist for a long time. Difficulty in diagnosis applies still more to *empyema of the ethmoidal* or *sphenoidal sinuses* in which few objective signs are to be expected. The patient may complain of severe frontal headaches, often worse in the morning and passing off later in the day; and a purulent nasal discharge may be present; pyrexia may be only slight, but is generally persistent.

Suppurating lymph nodes will be diagnosed from the character of the tender swellings that precede the skin-reddening and the actual formation of an abscess; the site is likely to be neck, axilla or groin, and there will usually be an indication of the source of the trouble in the form of a septic focus in the skin corresponding to the lymph drainage of the node concerned—impetigo, a septic cut or wound or a whitlow. One source of trouble that may be overlooked is *pediculosis* of the scalp; it should be suspected if there is irritation of the back of the neck at the roots of the hair in association with enlargement of the occipital as well as of the cervical lymph nodes.

Mammary and *submammary abscess* may be of chronic type and cause pyrexia without much pain.

Empyema thoracis is generally easy of diagnosis. The abnormal physical signs at the base of one lung suggest the presence of fluid; on needling the chest pus will be found. The condition may be simulated by subdiaphragmatic abscess, but X-ray examination will usually help in distinguishing the two. In some cases both conditions are present. Difficulty in diagnosis may on occasion be considerable when the empyema is interlobar, or between the pericardium and the pleura, or between the diaphragm and the lower lobe.

Lung abscess may be single or multiple, and may be part of a blood-borne or local infection or be associated with a bronchial neoplasm. Much of the fever and acute systemic upset in the last case is due to infection rather than the primary neoplasma. Imaging will help in the differential diagnosis.

Hepatic abscess, especially amoebic, may be a subacute or chronic rather than an acute condition, with fluctuating pyrexia persisting for months. The diagnosis may be suggested by complaint of pain or tenderness over the lower part of the right chest in front or behind, by dullness at the base of the right lung, or by friction sounds over the liver. A history of amoebic dysentery is not always forthcoming. Pain is in some instances referred to the right shoulder. When pyrexia and rigors are the only objective features malaria is simulated, but a high polymorphonuclear leucocytosis is against this diagnosis. The diagnosis of hepatic abscess is clinched by needling the liver and finding pus, often chocolate coloured; on rare occasions this may be coughed up as the result of ulceration through the diaphragm and pleura into a bronchus.

Empyema of the gallbladder. Jaundice is generally absent. Pyrexia may be considerable and prolonged, and rigors are to be expected. The diagnosis depends largely upon the patient's complaint of pain in the right hypochondrium associated either with enlarged gallbladder or with acute pain and tenderness on palpation of the gallbladder region below the tip of the right 9th rib cartilage.

Suppurative cholangitis is the result of extension of pyogenic infection up the hepatic ducts into the biliary canals within the liver. It generally is associated with obstruction in the bile duct by stone or growth. When the infection has extended to become suppurative cholangitis the patient becomes increasingly ill. The supervention of cholangitis may be indicated by progressive, soft, uniform and tender enlargement of the liver, associated as a rule with jaundice. Recurrent rigors are almost invariable.

Suppurative pylephlebitis arises from infection somewhere in the periphery of the portal area—for example, previous appendicitis. It is often fatal. The liver becomes studded with multiple small abscesses around the intrahepatic subdivisions of the portal vein. The liver becomes progressively, smoothly and uniformly enlarged, and generally tender; jaundice is present in less than half the cases. The high degree of pyrexia, the rigors, the asthenia and wasting all indicate that the patient has developed some form of septic extension of the original disease. There is a high degree of leucocytosis.

Subdiaphragmatic abscess is often difficult to diagnose even with full X-ray examination. Since the pus is often spread in a thin layer between the liver and the diaphragm or between the spleen and the diaphragm, attempts to locate it by needling are frequently unsuccessful. There may be no abnormal physical signs, but more usually infection of the pleura through the diaphragm leads to impaired percussion note at the base of one lung accompanied by pleuritic friction and râles.

Bronchiectasis may be responsible for prolonged periods of pyrexia with afebrile intervals of varying length. The pyrexial bouts are due either to invasion of the pus-containing cavities by fresh organisms or to recrudescence of infection already present, possibly brought about by impaired bronchial drainage. The abnormal physical signs in the lungs, the abundant foul sputum and the clubbed fingers indicate the diagnosis. Not infrequently there is considerable inflammation in the lung tissues around the area of bronchiectasis, the so-called 'peribronchiectatic pneumonitis'. In any patient where consolidation, often with pleurisy, recurs repeatedly in one area of the lung, this condition should be suspected.

Appendix abscess may be easy to diagnose on palpating the tender swelling in the right iliac fossa. In other locations the abscess may be difficult to diagnose; rectal examination leads to the detection of the abscess when it descends into the pelvis. Pyrexia ceases as a rule when the pus obtains free drainage, so that it is exceptional for appendix abscess to be the cause of prolonged pyrexia.

Perinephric abscess may cause pyrexia of considerable degree, possibly lasting for several weeks. Pain in the loin is almost always present, eventually with tenderness to palpation in both the loin and the lumbar region, but it is often absent in the early stages, and may not appear until the patient has been febrile for some weeks. There may be no defined swelling but only a sense of resistance evident when, with the patient recumbent, the examiner places one hand behind each loin with the fingertips external to the erector spinae muscles, and then makes as if to raise the patient from the bed though without actually lifting him: the fingers on the affected side will not feel the hollow of the loin as clearly as will those on the sound side. The signs may be yet more striking if the patient lies prone. If the patient is well enough to sit up in bed with the back bared and the observer then looks down his spine from above, it may often be apparent that the loin on the sound side is slightly concave, while that of the perinephric abscess side is either flat or slightly convex; only in pronounced cases does the loin show a distinct convexity. Perinephric abscess is generally the result of pyogenic infection within the kidney; or it may be due to pus tracking up behind the colon from appendicitis or it may be a delayed result of a loin injury, a haematoma due to the injury becoming infected and slowly forming a perinephric abscess weeks or months after the trauma. In many cases the history is obtainable of a suppurative process a short time previously. Pre-existing neutropenia, or corticosteroid therapy, will in these cases, as in all infective processes, predispose to abscess formation.

Diverticular abscess may be subacute and yet cause prolonged pyrexia. It is generally situated in the left lower part of the abdomen producing a tender swelling that may simulate carcinoma. It is preceded by chronic bowel symptoms, constipation and colic. Bleeding may occur, sometimes profusely. It is a disease of the second half of life.

Psoas abscess results from tuberculous spinal disease; the condition may be apyrexial, but, like any other form of tuberculosis, it may cause protracted irregular pyrexia. Pain localized to some part of the back and stiffness of the corresponding part of the spine in a child are suggestive features. Radiographs must be taken (*Fig.* P.53). On the other hand, the diagnosis may remain unsuspected until a tender swelling appears above or below one groin as the abscess tracks down from the spine along the course of the psoas muscle ultimately giving fluctuation from above to below the inguinal ligament.

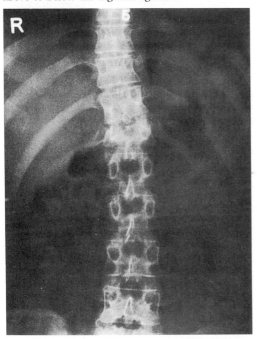

Fig. P.53. A radiograph from a case of spinal caries involving the 11th and 12th dorsal and 1st lumbar vertebrae.

Actinomycosis is diagnosed by the discovery of the organism. It may be in the discharge from a sinus communicating with the focus infected, generally the cheek, jaw, neck, lung, liver, caecum or spine. It may, however, occur anywhere in the skin or viscera, and the disease is likely to be missed if specific bacterial investigation is not undertaken. An actinomycotic ischiorectal abscess, for instance, may be regarded as of merely pyogenic origin. There is diffuse infiltration

of deep as well as superficial parts, liability to discharge through one or more sinuses, and a suggestive purplish red colour of the skin adherent to the lesion. The course is chronic, often apyrexial, but frequently there are periods of pyrexia.

4. Infective and inflammatory conditions

Coliform infection of the urinary tract may be chronic and apyrexial but is liable to exacerbations with prolonged pyrexia, aching or pain in one or both loins, frequency of micturition, and pain during micturition. It may exist, however, especially in children, with so few symptoms of urinary disease that its responsibility for continued pyrexia may be missed.

Chronic or recurring pyelonephritis is more common in women than men but may be associated with an enlarged prostate or urethral stricture. The patient is ill, with rigors and high, long-continued pyrexia; the urine is purulent and yields a positive culture of the causative organism or organisms. In papillary necrosis the renal calices become clubbed and pyuria is common even when urine cultures are sterile. Prolonged fever is not uncommon. It may be due to prolonged taking of compound analgesic tablets or diabetes mellitus.

Gallstones may be silent causing no symptoms or they may be associated with irregular and sometimes prolonged pyrexia and with bouts of pyrexia in attacks of biliary colic.

Phlebitis in a superficial vein is indicated by tenderness, with or without redness and swelling along the course of the vein; pyrexia of variable degree and duration accompanies the disorder in the earlier stages, but usually subsides in a few days. The diagnosis is much more difficult when the inflamed vein is deeply situated. Intra-abdominal phlebitis may be responsible for both continued pyrexia and vague but possibly severe abdominal pain in certain cases for which no explanation is forthcoming. *Thrombophlebitis migrans* occurs uncommonly. Venous thrombosis in the pelvis, not necessarily associated with obvious femoral or popliteal thrombosis, may account for pyrexia after childbirth.

Thyroiditis, an inflammatory but noninfective condition, may cause the complaint of sore throat, the thyroid itself being painful and tender.

Parametritis is diagnosed by pelvic examination. It is likely to be the after-effect of recent labour and is often associated with continued pyrexia, pain in the pelvis and lower part of the back. Abscess formation may occur. Elderly women are apt to develop a purulent form of endometritis, sometimes pyrexial, with pelvic pain, bearing-down pain, pain in the back, a foul vaginal discharge often bloodstained, the condition simulating advanced carcinoma of the body of the uterus.

Vesiculitis, though it may be of local origin, is generally due to gonococcal infection of the seminal vesicles. The complaint is mainly of hot burning pain in the rectum aggravated by defecation; proctitis, or carcinoma of the rectum or acute prostatitis are simulated. Diagnosis is established by rectal examination, the finger locating a tender swelling in the vesicles.

Colitis, whether infective or ulcerative, will be suggested by a history of diarrhoea with the passage of blood and mucus associated with more or less pain along the course of the colon, particularly the descending colon; carcinoma or diverticulitis may be simulated. The diagnosis is confirmed by endoscopy, barium enema and/or bacteriological studies.

Crohn's disease (regional enteritis) should be suspected when there is a history of chronic intermittent diarrhoea, fever, loss of weight and abdominal pains or distension. Barium studies are necessary. Intermittent small-bowel obstruction is common.

Pancreatitis, when subacute or chronic, is very difficult to diagnose. It is sometimes but not always pyrexial. It may simulate other abdominal lesions such as gallstones. Glycosuria in association with pyrexia and a dull aching pain in the abdomen across the site of the pancreas may be suggestive, but the symptoms are generally too vague to be characteristic. There is often a curious dull-brown pigmentation of the skin. Chronic pancreatitis should be suspected in a patient with recurrent abdominal pain, particularly if the pain or tenderness extends to the left of the midline, if gallstones are present, and if there have been bouts of overconsumption of alcohol. Radiographs may show pancreatic calcifications. Repeated serum amylase estimations taken within 12 hours of an acute episode are elevated in most cases, but as more acinar and ductal cells are destroyed these become less evident. After acute pancreatitis suppurative pancreatitis may occur in the second or third week with return of fever.

Familial Mediterranean fever (paroxysmal polyserositis, periodic fever) is an unherited disease of unknown aetiology characterized by acute episodes of self-limited fever with signs of inflammation of peritoneum, pleura and joints, such febrile episodes recurring irregularly and unpredictably. The disease occurs most commonly in patients of Mediterranean or Middle-East origin, particularly in Sephardic (but not Ashkenazic) Jews, Armenians, Turks, Arabs, Greeks and less commonly in Italians and others. In the acute attacks fever may reach 40°C (104°F) but symptoms of peritonitis or 'pleurisy' usually subside within 48 hours. Small pleural effusions may occur. Abdominal symptoms

occur most often, occurring in over 95 per cent of patients, sometimes mild but sometimes with severe localized pain which spreads over the whole abdomen, associated with abdominal distension and muscle rigidity and sometimes ileus, so that an acute surgical emergency may be suspected. Acute arthritis is less common, usually affecting one joint, the knee in most cases. Such arthritic episodes usually last only a few days but may occasionally last for weeks or even months. The onset of this disorder is usually in childhood or adolescence, but it may come on at any age, males more often being affected than females. Amyloidosis is a complication commonly seen in Israel, less commonly in USA. The prognosis depends on the development, or absence, of amyloidosis. In about 25 per cent of cases transient inflammatory skin lesions like erysipelas occur, usually below the knees.

Sarcoidosis, a chronic granulomatous inflammatory condition, may cause prolonged fever, sometimes with relatively little systemic upset. Hilar glandular enlargement on X-ray examination, erythema nodosum, a weakly positive or negative tuberculin test and a positive Kveim test are diagnostic findings.

5. Non-purulent hepatic affections

Quite apart from fever that occurs in obviously infective lesions of the liver, such as hepatic abscess, acute viral hepatitis, cholangitis and pylephlebitis, pyrexia, generally without the ordinary concomitants of fever, often occurs when the liver tissue is affected by lesions which are not obviously pyogenic, particularly *cirrhosis* and *carcinoma*. Laennec's (alcoholic) cirrhosis, post-necrotic and biliary cirrhosis may all be accompanied by prolonged fever as may *chronic active hepatitis*, a disorder induced by the hepatitis B or C virus or by autoimmune aetiology or precipitated by various drugs including methyldopa, isoniazid and nitrofurantoin. Hypergammaglobulinaemia is a striking feature. Liver biopsy is necessary to confirm the diagnosis. Rapidly growing neoplasms are sometimes accompanied by pyrexia. The appetite may be fairly good, and the patient may even be carrying on his ordinary work although his health is failing.

6. The connective-tissue disorders

Rheumatoid arthritis. In some cases prolonged fever is a part of the clinical picture of rheumatoid arthritis.

Systemic lupus erythematosus may for many months present as pyrexia, often accompanied by skin rashes and symptoms relating to locomotor and other tissues. The high ESR and joint pains may lead to confusion with rheumatoid arthritis (*Fig.* P.54).

Polyarteritis nodosa and other arteritides, such as giant-cell arteritis or Wegener's granulomatosis, may cause prolonged fever, though the latter is often rapidly

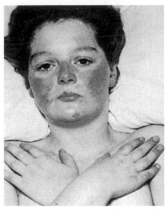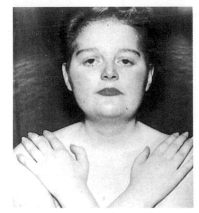

Fig. P.54. Female patient with prolonged fever and flitting joint pains due to systemic lupus erythematosus. The contrast is striking between the red butterfly rash of the disorder and the Custingoid appearance on full steroid therapy 1 month later.

fatal in a few weeks or sometimes less. *Polymyositis* and *dermatomyositis* may also be associated with fever, as may, though rarely, *systemic sclerosis (scleroderma)*.

7. Blood diseases

Any one of the severe blood diseases may be associated with prolonged pyrexia: diagnosis depends upon other factors, particularly the blood count, as in *leukaemia*. In agranulocytosis and aplastic anaemia infection is responsible for the fever, but in any severe prolonged anaemia, particularly in childhood, prolonged pyrexia may be seen. In previous times, for instance, untreated Addisonian anaemia was a febrile disease. Febrile episodes occur also in haemolytic anaemias.

8. Diseases of tropics and subtropics

Trypanosomiasis is a parasitic infection occurring particularly in Africa where *Glossina palpalis*, the tsetse fly, abounds; the bite of this insect spreads the disease, sleeping sickness, by invasion of the central nervous system. It is not always pyrexial and at times malaria may be simulated. The trypanosome may be identified in blood-films, lymph node aspirates, more rarely bone marrow, or, in the final sleeping stage, in the cerebrospinal fluid. There is no distinctive feature on the temperature chart.

Malaria. The main types are the benign tertian (*Plasmodium vivax* or *Plasmodium ovale*), in which rigors occur on alternate days with a maximum temperature of 39·4–40°C (103–104°F) (*Fig*. P.55) and complete freedom on the intermediate days, the quartan (*Plasmodium malariae*) in which there are 2-day intervals so that the paroxysms occur every fourth day (*Fig*. P.56) and the malignant tertian (*Plasmodium falciparum*) in which the fever is often more irregular. The intervals between the attacks of fever vary in accordance with the time that successive generations of the various strains of parasites take to mature. A patient may be infected by one set of bites by a mosquito with a tertian or quartan ague and become subsequently infected by other mosquitoes with either tertian or quartan parasites so that there is a mingling together of the effects of different generations of *Plasmodium* and the patient would have a daily (quotidian) paroxysm (*Fig*. P.57). Similarly, infection by two lots of parasites might result in a complicated clinical picture in which the attacks of pyrexia might be irregular or almost continuous. As a rule, a paroxysm with its various cold, hot and sweating stages lasts about 8 hours. The diagnosis of malaria will be confirmed by the discovery of parasites in the blood (*Figs*. P.58–P.60).

One remarkable feature is that malaria may remain latent for many years, particularly with *P. malariae*. Considering the large number of serving men infected in the last war, however, relapses of malaria 1 year after returning home have been rare. Reappearance is brought about by general deterioration in health or through some intercurrent illness.

Kala-azar (visceral leishmaniasis). There is no characteristic chart, the pyrexia, often extreme, being of a swinging but continued type. Great enlargement of the spleen with continued pyrexia would suggest the diagnosis, which is confirmed by discovering Leishman–Donovan bodies from material obtained by splenic or sternal puncture. It was not uncommon on the Mediterranean coast and may even today, though rarely, be acquired on a short Continental holiday.

Plague is also epidemic; its type are various, the two best known being the bubonic and the pneumonic. The diagnosis depends on discovering plague bacilli (*Pasteurella pestis*) in fluid obtained by aspirating a bubo or from the sputum by special bacteriological methods. The pneumonic form is the more acute and it may simulate lobar pneumonia; the bubonic form is of longer duration with a lower grade of pyrexia.

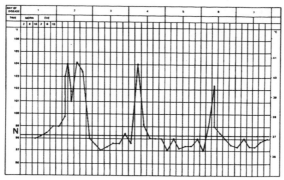

Fig. P.55. Case of simple tertian malaria, showing the attacks occurring every third day. (*London School of Tropical Medicine.*)

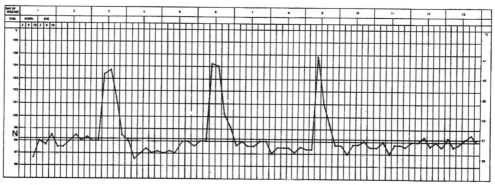

Fig. P.56. Temperature chart from a case of quartan malarial fever, the attacks recurring every fourth day. (*London School of Tropical Medicine.*)

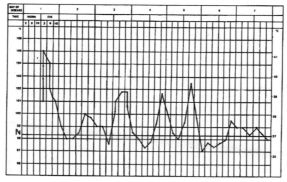

Fig. P.57. Temperature chart from a case of malaria to illustrate quotidian fever due to double tertian infection. (*London School of Tropical Medicine.*)

Both cholera and plague when they occur in England tend to be in persons coming from India or the East, particularly members of ships' crews.

Relapsing fever was at one time prevalent in Great Britain and acquired the name 'famine fever' from the circumstances of its occurrence. It is due to infection with *Borrelia recurrentis* introduced by an infected louse being crushed against an abrasion or wound. Many strains are also conveyed by ticks and the disease transmitted by their bites. The course of the disease is characteristic. There are outbreaks of high pyrexia (*Fig.* P.61) associated with extreme prostr-

ation and severe illness lasting 5 or 6 days, alternating with complete intermission of about the same duration. There may be an indefinite number of relapses before death or recovery. The spirochaete may be identified in a blood-film shortly before the febrile paroxysm, but not in the intervals.

Schistosomiasis is widely spread through Egypt, Zimbabwe and certain other parts of Africa. Involvement of the urinary tract with *S. haematobium* is extremely common in these countries. *S. mansoni* affects the colon more and is associated with splenome-

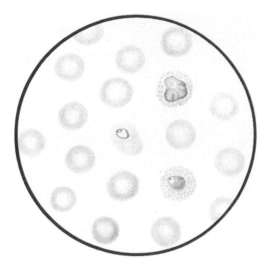

Fig. P.58. *Plasmodium vivax*: causing benign tertian malaria. Three stages of development of the ring-parasite (schizont) are shown: as the ring grows it expands the red corpuscle and produces multiple small dots of dark pigment which distinguish it from the *Plasmodium malariae* of quartan fever, in which case the pigment is in larger spots, few in number. No crescents are formed. (Stained by the Wright–Romanowsky method, and viewed under the $\frac{1}{12}$-in oil-immersion lens.)

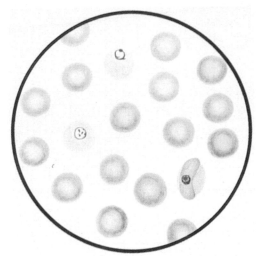

Fig. P.60. *Plasmodium falciparum*: causing malignant malaria. Two stages of the ring-parasite (schizont) and one crescent (gametocyte) are shown. (Stained by the Wright–Romanowsky method, and viewed under the $\frac{1}{12}$-in oil-immersion lens.)

hyperthermia, often without the other symptoms usually associated with fever. As a rule death or recovery renders such types of pyrexia of short duration, for instance in cases of pontine haemorrhage. Sometimes, however, the patient may survive long enough to come into the category of cases of prolonged pyrexia.

10. Skin conditions

These are discussed in the article on BULLAE (p. 88); there is less tendency to pyrexia in dermatitis herpetiformis, herpes gestations and erythema iris than in acute and subacute pemphigus. Pemphigus is always a serious and often a fatal malady, the skin blebs being but a local manifestation of some severe but ill-defined systemic reaction. Eosinophilia is usual. Any diffuse inflammation of the skin, from acute psoriasis to a gold dermatitis, may be accompanied by fever.

11. Malignancy

Lymphomas, of different kinds, including Hodgkin's disease, may be associated with prolonged fever, the Pel–Ebstein type depicted in *Fig.* P.62 being seen typically in this condition though not confined to it. Lymphosarcoma may be associated with prolonged pyrexia, as may carcinoma, particularly if associated with sepsis, as is seen not infrequently in the bronchus and large intestine. Infection is not necessary for pyrexia to be present; high fevers are occasionally seen in primary and secondary carcinoma where no sepsis exists, and a low-grade pyrexia is common. Particularly likely to be accompanied by prolonged pyrexia are hypernephroma, hepatoma, secondary carcinoma in the liver and widespread metastatic disease.

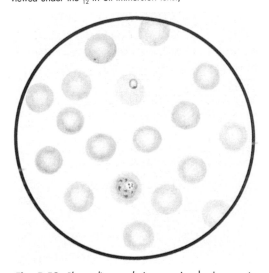

Fig. P.59. *Plasmodium malariae*: causing benign quartan malaria. Two stages of development of the ring-parasite (schizont) are shown: as the ring grows it does not expand the red corpuscle as does that of benign tertian (*Plasmodium vivax*), and the pigment particles are in the form of relatively large dots, few in number, instead of the multiple tiny dots of *Plasmodium vivax*. Crescents are not formed. (Stained by the Wright–Romanowsky method, and viewed under the $\frac{1}{12}$-in oil-immersion lens.)

galy. Pyrexia over long periods is not uncommon with either type of infection.

9. Meningeal and cerebral haemorrhage

Almost any pathology that interferes radically with the heat-regulating centres in the brain may cause

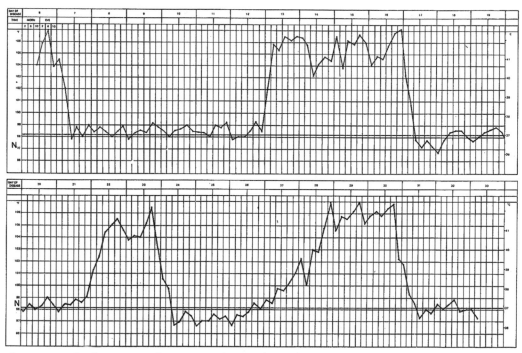

Fig. P.61. Four-hourly temperature chart in a case of severe relapsing fever.

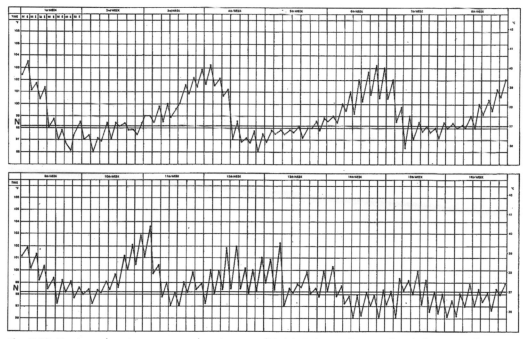

Fig. P.62. Morning and evening temperature charts in a case of Hodgkin's disease, illustrating the Pel–Ebstein type of recurrent or periodic pyrexia that may occur in this disease.

12. Allergic (antigen–antibody reactive) conditions

Being inflammatory disorders, these are often pyrexial. This is seen, for example, in Henoch–Schönlein syndrome (anaphylactoid purpura) and various skin allergies. The postcardiac injury syndrome may occur after any injury to the heart, whether it be an operation, stab-wound or myocardial infarction (Dressler's syndrome).

Fever, pericarditis, pleurisy and pneumonitis may occur 2 or more weeks after the injury and recurrences are common.

13. Factitious pyrexia produced by malingerers

From time to time there arise cases in which illness is simulated by a patient who deliberately deceives by one or other of various devices, such as dipping the thermometer bulb in a cup of tea, holding it against a hot-water bottle or rubbing it violently against the blankets. It is said that some have the art of squeezing the bulb between the fingers or between the teeth with just sufficient force to raise the temperature, but without breaking the glass; on suspicion of such a possibility the temperature is taken preferably per rectum under careful scrutiny. If a factitious pyrexia is suspected the patient may be left unattended on the first occasion and, if the temperature is raised, it is taken again immediately under close observation. A marked difference between the two readings strongly suggests that the first reading has been faked. Cases are also recorded where patients have deliberately infected themselves to produce a fever.

14. Drug reactions

In any persistent unexplained fever where drug treatment is being given the possibility of therapy being the cause should be considered. Fever occurring in the treatment of pulmonary tuberculosis, for instance, may be due to isoniazid, aminosalicylate, streptomycin, or all three drugs. Antibiotics, sulphonamides, arsenicals, iodides, barbiturates and many others may be responsible. When in doubt the motto should be, if possible, 'Stop treatment'.

Gordon Duff

Pyrexia without obvious cause

1. Fever in children

Temperature-regulating reflexes may be underdeveloped or poorly-controlled in children and infants. Body temperature is apt to be disturbed in children by causes that would not produce pyrexia in an adult; hence transient, irregular or recurrent rises of temperature in a child may often be of little significance. Immediately after birth temperatures of around 38°C (100·4°F) are not uncommon and are physiological, but fever may persist with birth injuries associated with intracranial bleeding. In small children *excitement* is apt to produce transient hyperthermia. A bout of bad temper, coughing or crying or moderate or severe exertion may have a similar result and so may any gastrointestinal

upset. In none of these is it necessary to implicate an infective process.

Nevertheless, if such rises of temperature persist it is unwise to regard them as purely trivial; there are three conditions in particular that need to be specially borne in mind: (1) *Urinary infection*; (2) *Upper-respiratory-tract infection*; (3) *Exanthemas and the infectious diseases of childhood* before their specific rashes or other clinical features appear.

URINARY INFECTION

Usually due to *E. coli*, this is only too easily missed in a child, for there may be no symptoms attracting attention to the urinary system. The presence in the urine of leucocytes makes the diagnosis likely, though it needs culture of a clean specimen of urine to establish it.

Upper-respiratory-tract infections

These include tonsillitis, acute pharyngitis and rhinitis, and otitis media. Although symptoms usually point to the cause of the fever, in a small child this is not always so; the child has fever, is distressed and apparently in pain, but cannot indicate to the parents where the trouble lies.

Of the many other causes of fever in childhood, starvation, dehydration and acidosis should be mentioned. Tuberculosis in lung, lymph nodes or elsewhere is much less common now than previously but is still common in many parts of the world. The only sign of tuberculous disease initially in a child may be unexplained fever, but the same is true of a large number of infective processes. Of course, bacterial meningitis should always be borne in mind in a listless child with fever. Evidence of meningism, photophobia and skin lesions should be sought.

2. Pyrexia in adults

The types of obscure pyrexia in adults fall into two main groups: (1) *Transient or short pyrexia*; (2) *Continued pyrexia*.

TRANSIENT OR SHORT PYREXIA

This is usually due to one of a number of mild viral or bacterial infections, the common cold, sinusitis, nasopharyngitis, mild pyelonephritis and a host of others. It is as well to remember that drugs may themselves cause fever, and that the curative drug may sometimes maintain the fever it was used to cure. It is also as well to remember that products of tissue destruction may cause fever, as after myocardial infarction, pulmonary infarction, gangrene and tissue necrosis, and accumulation of blood in body cavities, gut, joints or elsewhere.

CONTINUED PYREXIA

This may occur in any of the large number of conditions listed under PYREXIA, PROLONGED. In Great Britain today one thinks primarily of the more common conditions: coliform and other infections of the urinary tract, infectious mononucleosis, carcinoma (particularly of the bronchus), Hodgkin's disease, non-Hodgkin lymphoma, leukaemia, tuberculous disease, chronic sepsis (as in sinusitis), abortus infections and so on. Fever may also be associated with AIDS with its intercurrent infections. With air travel readily available, malaria, kala-azar, or any other tropical disease may be imported overnight, and with a large immigrant population from overseas conditions such as amoebiasis, schistosomiasis and leprosy may be encountered in the ordinary out-patient clinic.

3. Fever in the aged and debilitated

Febrile disorders are often missed in the elderly, the debilitated and immunosuppressed individuals (such as those receiving steroids), as infections may be accompanied by much less fever than usual. In some cases absence of fever in the presence of acute infection carries a bad prognosis.

Gordon Duff

Pyuria

Pyuria means no more than the presence of pus in the urine. It will be present when there are infective processes affecting the urinary tract, in some chronic non-infective conditions such as bladder carcinoma in situ and interstitial cystitis, and occasionally following the rupture of an abscess outside the urinary tract into the system. The quantity of pus may vary; when present in large quantities it forms a thick, grey or yellow sediment. The sediment of urate crystals is usually pink or red in colour and clears when the sample is warmed to body temperature; the sediment of phosphate is cleared by the addition of acetic acid: pus in the urine will be unchanged by both these tests.

When the urine is alkaline, pus cells tend to aggregate either into a dense viscid deposit or into large clumps, the deposit or clumps separating to leave a slightly turbid supernatant. On microscopy, pus cells are seen as rounded multi-nucleated bodies about twice the size of a red cell. As pus cells are, in fact, protein, dip-stick testing is almost invariably positive for this substance; this test will also be positive if there are abnormally large numbers of epithelial cells in the sample so that microscopy of a urine sample is the only reliable simple test for the presence of pus.

The site of the pus-producing lesion cannot be determined simply by examination of the urine. The general and specific history of the individual case are essential although, in general, vesical lesions are often consequent upon renal lesions, particularly when these are infective. For example, when a pyelitis arises as a result of haematogenous spread, the initial symptom may be frequently due to cystitis. In time, the hyperpyrexia, rigors and sweating attacks of pyelitis become manifest, together with severe loin pain on the affected side. A pyonephrosis need not necessarily present with pyuria if outflow from the kidney is blocked for one reason or another, such as a stone.

Special Investigations

Imaging

If the patient is investigated during an acute illness associated with pyuria, imaging investigations of the urinary tract may give specific answers with regard to the site of the pus. The kidney which is the seat of acute pyelitis will appear larger on *ultrasound examination* and the fluid in the collecting system will appear less transonic than normal urine, implying turbidity.

Urography during an acute episode of pyelitis may show spasm of the collecting systems on the affected side, or dilatation if there is sufficient oedema of the pelvi-ureteric junction to obstruct the outflow of urine; complete cessation of renal function is occasionally observed in acute interstitial bacterial nephritis.

Cystoscopy

Instrumentation of the lower urinary tract has little to commend it during an acute illness as the risk of septicaemia is considerable. However, following appropriate antibiotic therapy and resolution of gross infection, cystoscopy under further intravenous antibiotic cover may give useful information.

It is most likely that the bladder will be the source of pyuria but if the viscus is normal on cystoscopy, inspection of the two ureteric orifices may yield valuable information.

A ureterocele is seen as a bulge above and lateral to the ureteric orifice, disappearing as the pressure inside the bladder increases with filling.

A refluxing ureter is wider than it should be and often placed far lateral. The ureteric efflux may be thick and turbid, and exuding like toothpaste from the orifice if the urine production from that side is diminished.

The ureteric orifice may be oedematous if pyelitis has extended along the whole length of the ureter as secondary ureteritis.

The ureteric orifice in **chronic tuberculosis** is characteristically 'golf-ball' in appearance.

Tiny nodules resembling sand granules are seen around the orifice in **schistosomiasis**.

The areas above and lateral to the orifices are those characteristically affected by early **carcinoma in situ**, looking very much like inflammatory patches.

Interstitial cystitis (Hunner's ulcer), presents as a red vertical line on the posterior wall of the bladder; this line extends into a split as the bladder is distended and rivulets of blood are seen on the back wall of the bladder, falling down as a curtain into the area behind the trigone.

The following is a classified list of the causes of pyuria:

A FROM DISEASES OF THE URINARY ORGANS

1 RENAL
  Pyelitis
  Pyelonephritis
  Renal abscess
  Renal papillary necrosis
  Pyonephrosis
  Tuberculosis
  Calculus
  Medullary sponge kidney

2 URETERIC
  Calculus
  Megaureter
  Ureteric foreign body
  Vesico-ureteric reflux

3 VESICAL
  Cystitis
  Tuberculosis
  Calculus or foreign body
  Ulcer—simple, epitheliomatous
  Tumour—sloughing papillary or solid carcinoma
  Diverticula
  Bilharzia haematobia
  Trichomoniasis
  Carcinoma in situ
  Interstitial cystitis

4 URETHRAL
  Urethritis
   specific
    gonococcal
    chlamydial
    trichomonal
    monilial
    non-specific
  Stricture
  Calculus or foreign body

5 PROSTATIC
  Prostatis, acute or chronic
  Prostatic abscess
  Calculus
  Prostatic epithelial tumour

6 VESICULAR
  Seminal vesiculitis, acute or chronic vesicular abscess

B FROM DISEASES OUTSIDE THE URINARY ORGANS
  Leucorrhoea
  Balanitis with phimosis
  From the extension of inflammatory processes to the bladder, or the rupture into the bladder or urethra of an abscess such as:

  Prostatic abscess
  Appendicular abscess
  Iliac or pelvic abscess
  Abscess due to colonic diverticulitis
  Psoas abscess
  Pyosalpinx
  Carcinoma of the uterus, rectum, caecum, sigmoid or pelvic colon
  Ulceration of the small intestine, tuberculous or dysenteric

A. URINARY TRACT PYURIA

The kidneys

Recurrent attacks of **pyelitis** are commonest in childhood, during pregnancy and after childbirth. In childhood, pyelitis secondary to reflux often remains undetected and therefore untreated; **chronic pyelonephritis** in later life is a serious complication.

The kidneys may be infected: (1) *through the blood stream*—It is surprising that they are not infected more frequently, remembering the enormous renal blood flow and the oft-repeated transient bacteraemia associated with normal eating; (2) *by direct spread from the bladder* which can occur if there is vesico-ureteric reflux; (3) *by infections ascending through peri-ureteric lymphatics* from an infected bladder or from a para-vesical structure; or (4) **by direct spread** from the bladder along submucosal planes.

Outflow tract obstruction will predispose to ascending infection, particularly if the bladder has to contract violently in order to expel urine. This explains the occasional association of pyelitis with **prostatic hypertrophy** and almost certainly accounts for the increase of incidence of **pyelitis in pregnancy**. It is unusual for both kidneys to be affected simultaneously but it is certainly true to say that once a kidney is damaged it is more likely to be a seat of infection on subsequent occasions.

Congenital abnormalities in themselves will not predispose towards sepsis, but if there is interference with free drainage in a **horseshoe kidney** (*Fig.* P.63), an **ectopic kidney** or a kidney with a degree of **pelvi-ureteric junction obstruction**, it may be the seat of infection more frequently than a normal system. A **duplex kidney** may become infected in one or other of its moieties.

Vesico-ureteric reflux arises because the intramural course of the ureter is short and the normally acute 'ureterovesical angle' is lost. The normal 'hydraulic valve' which prevents reflux is not therefore present and there is no obstruction to the retrograde passage of urine. At the same time, acute cystitis may in itself alter the efficiency of this ureterovesical angle

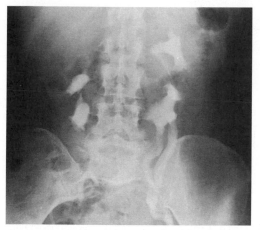

Fig. P.63. Horseshoe kidney. The classical malrotation is shown. The picture is complicated by a duplex left kidney with distal obstruction of both ureters.

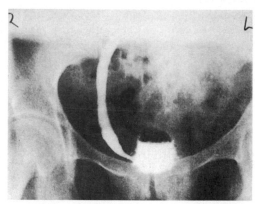

Fig. P.64. Vesico-ureteric reflux shown during a voiding cystogram.

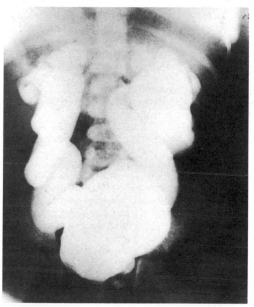

Fig. 65. Bilateral vesico-ureteric reflux with gross hydro-ureter due to congenital valve of the posterior urethra in a boy of 5 years.

so that reflux can occur secondary to the primary cystitis.

Cystoscopy of a patient with reflux often shows a small saccule or shallow diverticulum above and lateral to the ureteric orifice. It seems more likely that this is part of the original maldevelopment than a traction diverticulum.

Megaureter in children is a condition in which the whole of the ureter may be dilated, although the condition more commonly affects the distal ureter only. A megaureter may be obstructed or non-obstructed, and may reflux or may not; paradoxically, an obstructed megaureter may also reflux, with relative obstruction to the passage of urine from upper tract to bladder but a facilitated passage from lower tract to upper.

Megaureter is physiological during pregnancy, either as a result of direct obstruction from the gravid uterus or secondary to the progestogen effect of a maintained pregnancy. Whatever the aetiology of megaureter the resulting stasis predisposes to sepsis, stone formation, squamous metaplasia, and so on. Reflux may occur in severe cases of outflow tract obstruction where the intravesical pressure rises to a level that overcomes the resistance of the most normal ureteric orifice.

Reflux is demonstrated by a micturating cystogram (*Fig.* P.64), by radioisotope investigation during micturition and also by ultrasound assessment. Reflux is sometimes severe enough to cause gross distention of the upper urinary tract especially when there is congenital outflow obstruction as in urethral valves (*Fig.* P.65).

The congenital megaureter megacystis syndrome arises because of improper development of the urinary tract and the ureteric orifices are widely patent (*Fig.*

P.66), a similar picture may be seen in severe chronic retention when dilatation of the bladder and ureters has occurred beyond the point of recovery when the obstruction is relieved.

PYELITIS

Haematogenous pyelitis arising as an entity separate from other urinary tract pathology is not unusual following acute febrile illness or secondary to suppuration elsewhere in the body. The organisms responsible are usually *Escherichia coli*, *Proteus* and *Klebsiella*; *Pseudomonas* is common as a hospital-based infection as is the increasingly common multiple-resistant *Staphylococcus aureus*.

The symptoms of **acute pyelitis** are severe. There

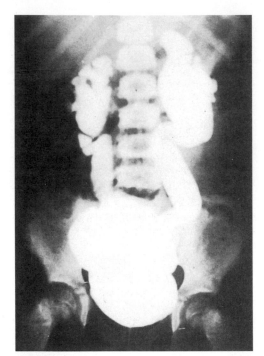

Fig. 66. Bilateral vesico-ureteric reflux in the megaureter mega-cystis syndrome.

is loin pain, symptoms of an associated acute cystitis, hyperpyrexia, tachycardia, rigors and sweating. The urine is turbid, opalescent, may be bright red from haematuria, positive for protein and microscopy reveals large numbers of free bacteria with pus cells and red cells. The patient may be oliguric because of fluid loss.

While examination reveals a high white cell count and ESR, urography may show reduced function on the affected side; calculi will almost always show up as radiopaque bodies overlying the urinary tract.

Chronic pyelitis is dangerous because there may be few symptoms early in the course of the disease. Slight stinging during micturition and vague pain in the renal areas may be ignored and general malaise, lassitude secondary to anaemia, a low-grade persisting pyrexia and hypertension are often presenting features. The urine classically has a specific gravity of 1010, the blood urea and plasma creatinine are raised and creatinine clearance significantly diminished. Excretion urography may be impractical because of poor renal function but delayed films will show irregularity and blunting of the calyces, cortical atrophy and a reduction in renal size. The physical signs of hypertension may be manifest.

RENAL ABSCESS

Renal abscesses follow acute haematogenous infections and are initially situated in the peripheral area of the cortex. There are general symptoms and signs of a systemic abscess, with acute tenderness in the loin, developing into a mass with an overlying hyperaemic skin. It is rare for renal abscesses to discharge spontaneously through the skin as they are usually seen and treated well before this happens. Occasionally they may discharge into nearby viscera, the ascending or descending colon and the second and third parts of the duodenum, depending on the side affected. It is uncommon for a left-sided abscess to involve the tail of the pancreas. An abscess may occasionally follow a renal infarct.

RENAL PAPILLARY NECROSIS

Renal papillary necrosis is common in **diabetics**. It is now rarely seen following **phenacetin abuse** as the substance was withdrawn following the discovery of the association between its abuse and renal failure. The renal papillae undergo avascular necrosis and separate from the kidney. They may be passed as sloughs, in which case the patient may present with ureteric colic, or retained within the pelvicalyceal system, where they calcify. An acute bacterial infection often supervenes and presentation with an acute pyelitis or cystitis is not unusual.

Urography shows several changes depending on the severity of the process; in the early stage, a line of contrast can be seen crossing the base of each papilla; as the papilla sloughs it may be seen as a filling defect within a dilated calyx; later still a triangular zone of calcification lying within the pelvicalyceal system is readily apparent. Bilateral renal papillary necrosis can lead to progressive renal failure and death from uraemia.

PYONEPHROSIS

In pyonephrosis, the urine within an obstructed pelvicalyceal system becomes infected, usually secondary to congenital pelvi-ureteric junction or impaction of a stone at the junction. Obstruction of a ureteric orifice by stone or tumour, or ureteric involvement from a primary bladder or primary uterine carcinoma, are less common causes of pyonephrosis. The symptoms are not as severe as those of an acute pyelitis and more gradual in their onset. Examination almost invariably shows tenderness in the affected loin, together with a palpable renal mass.

Radiological examination often reveals the presence of a stone while renal function is rarely preserved. The quickest way of proving the diagnosis is by establishing a nephrostomy under local anaesthesia and ultrasound control; this will not only allow aspiration of pus for diagnostic and therapeutic purposes but will also provide drainage of the system. Nephrectomy is usually required together with appropriate management of the precipitating cause.

RENAL TUBERCULOSIS

This disease, once commonplace, is now relatively rare and there must always be the danger that the diagnosis will be missed unless it is remembered that all cases of persistent sterile and acid pyuria must be considered as tuberculosis until disproved by the examination of no fewer than three early morning urine samples. Even this number may be insufficient to exclude the diagnosis with certainty and as many as 12 could be reasonably cultured for tubercle bacilli if the clinical suspicion of the disease is relatively high.

The miliary form of tuberculosis, once seen in childhood, is now extremely rare; it is not associated with urinary symptoms. Renal tuberculosis, however, is still very much a reality, the kidney at first being attacked by a tuberculous infection on a microscopic basis, the resulting small tuberculous nodules eventually coalescing to form an area of caseation, which then bursts into the renal pelvis by direct ulceration into a calyx. The transitional cell lining of the pelvis and ureter are subsequently infected with tubercle bacilli, becoming thickened by submucosal infiltration and by oedema.

The symptoms prior to discharge into the urinary tract may be very slight; aching in the loin may be the only symptom and albuminurea the only finding once the septic focus has discharged. The symptoms mimic a low-grade pyelitis and cystitis; aching in the renal area increases, while frequency of micturition, discomfort while passing urine and polyuria occur.

The urine is pale, acid, of low specific gravity and turbid; tubercle bacilli may sometimes be found after appropriate staining of a centrifuged sample.

Cystoscopy may show areas of oedema within the bladder and sometimes small tubercles are visible, while the ureteric orifice is usually oedematous and pouting into the bladder. The 'golf-ball' change is seen in long-standing disease when fibrosis has caused contraction of the orifice. Digital examination per rectum or per vaginam may reveal thickening of the bladder wall and pencil-like thickened ureters are occasionally felt as they hook their way into the bladder base.

Urography may show reduced function on one side, together with cavities, ureteric dilatation, and a thick-walled bladder. The caseating areas occasionally undergo calcification, these areas being poorly defined, contrasted with the clear-cut margins or a renal calculus. Calcific caseous debris is sometimes seen passing along the ureter, with a dilated column of contrast proximal. Renal tuberculosis should be considered strictly in relation to the rest of the genito-urinary system, the male frequently having lesions in the bladder, epididymis, prostate and vesicles while the female may have tuberculosis secondarily in the Fallopian tubes. Evidence of former disease in the spine, joints, chest or mesenteric lymph nodes may also be noted.

RENAL CALCULUS

The symptoms of stones will depend on their site, size and pathological effects (*Fig.* P.67). Renal stones may be asymptomatic. A stone floating free within the renal pelvis may cause intermittent obstruction and loin pain; a stone in the ureter presents as acute ureteric colic. Macroscopic haematuria is rare but microscopic bleeding is almost invariable. Secondary infection is most likely to occur if calculi impact at a narrow area— a calycine neck, the pelvi-ureteric junction, the ureter as it crosses the iliac vessels or at the uretero-vesical junction. Ninety per cent of renal calculi are radio-opaque; all stones are shown on ultrasound of the kidneys or on CT scanning.

MEDULLARY SPONGE KIDNEY

This is a congenital abnormality which probably represents a minor form of polycystic kidneys. The condition is not always bilateral and is often associated with the unusual physical sign of body hemihypertrophy. Unless the family history is known, the condition usually presents as renal angle pain, pyuria, supervening upper tract sepsis and ureteric colic. The stones may erode into the pelvicalycine system and from there make their way along the ureter. The radiological changes are pathognomonic of the condition, showing the typical 'bouquet of flowers' sign (*Figs* P.68–P.70).

Ureteric disease

URETERIC CALCULUS

Most ureteric calculi will pass of their own accord once they have passed the pelvi-ureteric junction. This is the rule in 95 per cent of cases if the stone is less than 1 cm in diameter. It is probable that acute ureteric colic is the most severe pain known to man (or woman), the severe pain starting on the affected side radiating upwards to the renal area and downwards towards the bladder and into the testicles or labia. It is surprising how many ureteric stones are, in fact, asymptomatic and present as an incidental finding. Complete blockage of a ureter by a calculus is unusual but, if it happens, it can result in a nonfunctioning and atrophic kidney. The lower down the ureter the stone impacts, the more lower urinary tract symptoms will be manifest; a stone impacting very near to the

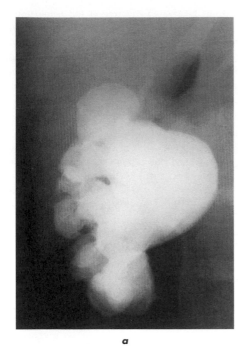
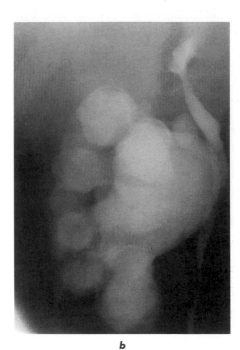

a   b

Fig. P.67. Staghorn calculus. *a*, plain X-ray. *b*, after contrast—the calculus fills the whole of the lower moiety of a duplex kidney. The small upper moiety is remarkably normal.

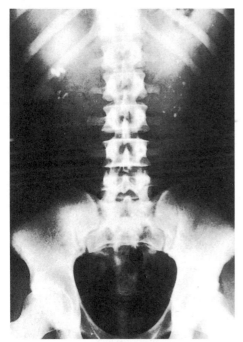

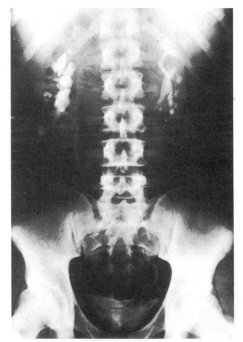

Fig. P.68. Multiple small bilateral renal calculi in a case of medullary sponge kidney.

Fig. P.69. Excretion pyelogram in the same case as *Fig.* P.68, showing caliceal saccules which contain the stones. From a boy of 16.

bladder can exactly mimic an acute cystitis, with supervening pyelitis, except that there is no pyrexia unless the obstructed and retained urine becomes infected.

Calculi are well demonstrated by urinary tract ultrasound; most stones show on plain X-rays; ultrasound will also give an accurate picture of the degree of upper tract dilatation.

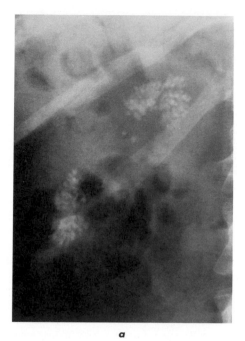 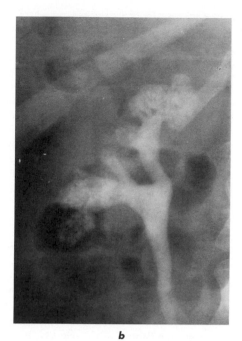

a   *b*

Fig. P.70. Medullary sponge kidney. *a*, Plain X-ray showing nephorocalcinosis. *b*, after contrast—'bouquet of flowers' appearances of upper and lower groups of calices.

URETERIC FOREIGN BODIES

It might seem inappropriate to discuss foreign bodies within the ureter but with the increasing frequency of endoscopic stone surgery, iatrogenic foreign bodies are now introduced with increasing regularity. One of the disadvantages of overvigorous ultrasound stone destruction is fragmentation of the metal probe-tip; these metal fragments may embed in the mucosa of the ureter and predispose to pyuria.

It should be noted that non-absorbable suture materials should never be used to close surgical incisions in the ureter; they form an excellent nidus for calculus formation.

Vesical diseases

Pyuria will be present in any lesion of the bladder which is associated with inflammation. This applies to acute and chronic bacterial infections, parasitic infections, the presence of stone, primary and secondary malignant disease, squamous metaplasia, leucoplakia and interstitial cystitis.

CYSTITIS

Cystitis may be acute or chronic and, while both forms are usually associated with infection by a microorganism, a true infective cause is not essential as any process which produces congestion of the bladder will give rise to cystitis.

In **acute cystitis** the mucosa of the bladder is oedematous and congested, leading to epithelial desquamation, pyuria, haemorrhage, the development of small abscesses within the mucosa and occasionally to areas of ulceration. The changes are sometimes sufficiently severe to cause sloughing of the whole of the mucosa of the bladder, with profuse haemorrhage.

The symptoms of acute cystitis are well known: there is frequency, urgency, dysuria, perineal pain and pain in the suprapubic area, haematuria and pyuria. The diagnosis of an acute bacterial cystitis depends on the positive culture of an infective organism.

While the precipitating cause may be evident in some cases, such as lower tract instrumentation, overvigorous intercourse, or acquired urethritis, many cases cannot be attributed to a specific event. An attack of **acute abacterial cystitis** may exactly mimic a true cystitis; the inflammatory agent in these cases must be a chemical irritant which is irrigated into the bladder by the turbulent urine flow associated with distal urethral stenosis in women. A causative organism can never be found, but red cells and pus cells are frequently present on urine testing. The condition is most frequently seen in young women after they become sexually active, but is also common in perimenopausal women. The name 'honeymoon cystitis' is often given to the condition but it seems rather inappropriate nowadays. Because of the common incidence of the condition at the extremes of reproductive life it seems reasonable to postulate distal urethral stenosis as a very real aetiological factor, the stenosis arising because of the hormone imbalances which occur at these two stages of a woman's development.

Chronic cystitis may follow an improperly or inadequately treated acute episode. While the symptoms are less severe, increased frequency or micturition, pyuria, and a persisting alkaline urine are noted. It is often seen with some form of urinary obstruction or retention and is sometimes found in cases of urinary incontinence, of whatever cause. The main differential diagnosis is from pyelitis, which can also cause increased frequency of micturition with pyuria, but the urine is usually acid, pale, generally turbid and has little inclination to form a deposit; an important second diagnosis is tuberculous cystitis.

The differential quantities of pus and protein present in the urine can act as a useful diagnostic test—in upper tract infections there is more albumin than the pus will account for, and on microscopy casts of varying kinds of forms are found in addition to pus cells; in cystitis, the amount of albumin is far less and the cellular elements do not form casts in themselves. At cystoscopy, the bladder wall is red, smooth and oedematous; in pyelitis, the cystoscopic appearance of the bladder is normal apart from possible modifications in the appearances of the ureteric orifices, the efflux of which is often cloudy as it contains more particulate matter.

TUBERCULOSIS

This is part of a tuberculous infective process affecting the whole of the urinary system, together with the reproductive system of both sexes. Frequency is the predominant presenting symptom, by day and by night, associated with a minor discomfort usually felt at the end of the urethra. A few drops of terminal haematuria are often observed. Pyuria is constant. **Vesical calculus** and **vesical carcinoma**, particularly carcinoma insitu present in a similar fashion. **Bladder calculi** are usually found in older patients with symptoms of outflow tract obstruction or a history of previous lower urinary tract instrumentation and catheterization. Calculi in the bladder often give pain only on movement; haematuria in calculous disease is observed throughout the stream and is often a more regular occurrence than with carcinoma.

The symptoms of bacterial cystitis may supervene in both calculus and carcinoma, accompanied by frequency, urgency and painful micturition by day and night. Vesical carcinoma may be felt per rectum, especially when the patient is thin and the tumour is extensive. The early stages of tuberculous cystitis are characterized cystoscopically by the appearance of greyish tubercles in the submucosal coat of the bladder, particularly around the ureteric orifice; at this stage frequency of micturition may be the only symptom but as the disease progresses, the tubercles enlarge, coalesce and eventually ulcerate, by which time pus and blood will both be present in the urine; tubercle bacilli should show up on special staining. The bladder becomes extremely small, with micturition occurring every 15 minutes or so throughout the 24 hours.

As a general diagnostic rule, any patient with increased frequency of micturition and a sterile acid urine should be considered as suffering from tuberculosis until disproved; as noted previously, as many as 12 negative early morning sample cultures may be required before the clinical suspicion of tuberculosis can be dismissed. Tuberculosis within the bladder is often associated with tuberculosis in the Fallopian tubes, vas, epididymis, prostate and seminal vesicles.

Tuberculosis in the bladder usually arises secondarily from an infection in the upper tract. A caseous lesion, however small, in the kidney ruptures and discharges its contents into the renal pelvis so that the urothelium of the pelvis, the ureter and the bladder become affected in turn. The primary site may similarly be within the epididymis, infection ascending through the vas deferens to affect the bladder, seminal vesicles and prostate. Prostatic tuberculosis is rare but may involve the bladder by direct ulceration. As with simple infective pyelitis, renal tuberculosis may present with lower urinary tract symptoms; the amount of blood present in the urine is usually less than if the bladder is chiefly involved and blood will, of course, be noted and found throughout the urinary stream. In renal tuberculosis there may be tenderness in the loin, while the kidney may be more readily palpable than usual and the distal end of the lower ureter can sometimes be felt on rectal or vaginal examination.

It is not, however, critical to establish whether the kidneys or the bladder are the primary sites of the disease and in many cases it is impossible to do this. Intravenous urography or ascending ureterography may give useful information with regard to the state of the upper tract; cystoscopy in renal tuberculosis may show pathological changes surrounding one ureter but not the other. The affected ureter is primarily oedematous, the wall is thickened and patulous; later on, the orifice becomes rigid and patent, representing the 'golf-hole', and drawn up towards the affected kidney by fibrotic shortening of the ureter. The final stage of vesical tuberculosis is a small thick-walled bladder (the 'golf ball').

VESICAL CALCULUS

Calculus in the bladder often presents as simple bacterial cystitis and under these circumstances there is little that will distinguish cystitis from many other form except, perhaps, the urine may be loaded with crystals. An increase in the amount of blood after exercise is noted frequently, while pyuria is usually constant. Haematuria may occur after exercise, as it does in joggers.

The constant symptoms of vesical calculus are frequency and discomfort during the daytime, especially when erect and moving, penile pain after micturition and haematuria. Except for those patients who have had indwelling catheters or complex lower urinary tract surgery, vesical calculus is almost always secondary to sepsis and stasis from outflow obstruction. Management must not only aim to remove the calculus but also to eliminate the source of obstruction. A suspected calculus will almost always show on plain pelvic X-ray or ultrasound. It may not always be possible to determine whether a stone lies within a diverticulum except by cystoscopy.

Stones which form in the upper tract and pass into the bladder without producing the symptoms of ureteric colic are almost always small enough to pass per urethram, unless the bladder outlet is obstructed. Radiolucent stones within the bladder, such as uric acid stones, are unusual as they accumulate calcium once within the viscus and take on a laminated appearance; if a pure uric acid stone is present within the bladder, it will not show on plain X-ray but will probably be detected as a filling defect at urography.

ULCERATION OF THE BLADDER

This occurs secondary to chronic cystitis, following traumatic cystoscopy, secondary to a long-standing stone and as a consequence of radiotherapy for pelvic malignancy. **Hunner's ulcer (interstitial cystis)** is a disease peculiar to women, causing severe frequency, pain on micturition, urgency with incontinence, and occasional haematuria. The diagnosis is established cystoscopically when a vertical ulcer is usually observed on the posterior bladder wall; the ulcer splits as the bladder is distended, resulting in a curtain of blood rivulets falling down the posterior wall. Biopsy of the area, usually taken to exclude malignancy, shows chronic inflammatory changes with a heavy mast-cell infiltrate. Calcium encrustation occurs, so that pyuria and calcific debris are often seen. The bladder capacity in this condition is relatively small and therapy often consists of forcible distention.

Tuberculous ulceration, **malignant** ulceration and ulceration secondary to **radiotherapy**, have similar presenting symptoms of frequency, haematuria, urgency and additional pain at the termination of micturition. The cystoscopic appearances of these different ulcers are not always easy to distinguish and multiple biopsies are often necessary in order to establish the diagnosis with certainty.

MALIGNANT ULCERATION OF THE BLADDER

Malignant ulceration of the bladder and papillary transitional cell carcinoma of the bladder are common conditions, giving rise to irregular haemorrhage, which is often profuse and almost always painless. Well-differentiated tumours tend to protrude into the bladder lumen, supported by a pedicle of rather narrow size, which accounts for the fact that the surface is often necrotic and ulcerated, giving rise to pyuria in conjunction with haematuria. The pathognomonic symptom is painless haematuria but increased frequency can occur if the tumour, or tumours, are sufficiently large to disturb bladder capacity. Pain is unusual unless infection is secondary. Tumours are often multiple because of the 'field change' that occurs within the whole of the transitional cell lining of the urinary tract—the urothelium.

When tumours are less well-differentiated and situated near the ureteric orifices, there may be ureteric obstruction and loin pain secondary to distention of the affected upper tract. Diagnosis can almost always be established preoperatively by a combination of urography and ultrasound examination of the urinary tract.

Endoscopic examination of the bladder is conclusive, and with the advent of continuous-irrigation instruments the presence of a bleeding lesion offers no handicap to the endoscopist.

When the tumours are large, clumps of the frondlike tumours may separate and be present in the urine; cytological examination of voided samples is relatively unsatisfactory if the tumour is well-differentiated as the cells are barely different from normal bladder epithelial cells. As soon as relative de-differentiation occurs, cytological examination of the urine is a useful diagnostic and monitoring tool.

It is probably true to say that the more poorly differentiated a transitional cell carcinoma, the more solid-looking it becomes. The solid carcinomas are nodular, sessile, often solitary and involve the trigone rather than affecting the lateral walls. Ureteric obstruction is a frequent complication and early invasion of the muscle wall occurs. The presence of a mass on bimanual palpation reveals that the tumour is probably beyond the scope of endoscopic resection, while fixity to the pelvis implies inoperability.

DIVERTICULUM OF THE BLADDER

A bladder diverticulum may give rise to intermittent or persistent and excessive pyuria together with increased frequency, pain and difficulty with micturition. The last symptom relates to the outflow tract obstruction. A common symptom is that bladder emptying is often followed quickly by the need to empty the bladder again; as the bladder 'empties' it expels as much urine into the diverticulum as it does through the urethra, so that when the sphincter apparatus has closed, urine flows back into the bladder cavity from the distended diverticulum.

The diagnosis is established by urography or ultrasound, but the size of the orifice into the bladder is rarely established without endoscopic examination. A cystogram gives a reasonable idea of the size of the diverticulum but an exaggerated impression may be obtained because of the magnification seen on this kind of X-ray, and the relatively forceful distention which occurs during the examination.

SCHISTOSOMIASIS

This causes pus in the urine when the small submucosal nodules, the 'sandy' patches, ulcerate into the bladder. Ova are often observed in the urine, together with pus and blood, but microscopic examination of a 'squashed rectal-snip' is pathognomonic. Complement fixation testing is specific. In advanced cases, calcification, appearing as a ring in the bladder wall, may show on plain X-ray while urography shows upper tract dilatation, due to the presence of uretero-vesical stricture. Complication of the disease process by carcinoma is all too common and is to some extent related to the duration of the disease; the consequent bladder carcinoma frequently affects young people.

TRICHOMONIASIS

This condition is relatively rare in males but may be acquired from an infected partner. The pyuria is relatively symptom free but trichomonads are found on staining the urine, or motile organisms are seen in centrifuged urine deposits. They can also be found in urethral discharge, semen, or fluid massaged from the prostrate.

Urethral causes

Urethral pyuria will be caused by any condition which causes a purulent urethritis. A profuse discharge, together with a history of recent unprotected sexual contact, are enough to provide the diagnosis but urethritis may be secondary to cystitis as well as the converse. The symptoms of urethritis are discharge, urethral pain and occasional initial haematuria; if there is also increased frequency, suprapubic pain and bleeding throughout the stream, cystitis is probably present as well. The pyuria of urethritis is usually confined to the initial sample of urine; in cystitis,

the mid-stream sample will be contaminated as well. Urethral calculi, foreign bodies, and self-inflicted urethral trauma will also cause purulent urethritis.

Prostatic causes

Acute prostatitis presents with increased frequency, perineal and suprapubic pain, discomfort on micturition, pyuria and even acute retention. Prostatitis may arise by haematogenous spread or may complicate cystitis or urethritis. Rectal examination reveals a large prostate which is exquisitely tender, to the degree that touching the oedematous gland causes acute reflex contraction of the external sphincter and straightening of the hips.

Prostatic abscess usually follows an acute urethritis which has affected the posterior urethra and caused an acute prostatitis. It may be secondary to a sexually transmitted infection, such as gonorrhoea or chlamydia, and may also follow instrumentation of the urethra. The prostate is intrinsically infected subclinically and endoscopy can trigger this infection, however carefully performed. Acute prostatitis may result in the formation of an abscess, almost always unilateral, which may discharge spontaneously into the urethra, bladder or rectum unless de-roofed by transurethal resection. Acute prostatitis presents with increased frequency of micturition, perineal and hypogastric pain, fever, rigors and difficulty with micturition. The abscess can be felt as a soft area within the tender and oedematous prostate.

Prostatic calculi are frequent but prostatic abscesses complicating calculi are relatively unusual, as are abscesses related to genito-urinary tuberculosis. Involvement of the prostate is a very late manifestation of this disease, presenting as increased frequency, perineal pain, difficulty with micturition and a sudden episode of initial haematuria.

Pyuria is invariable following prostatic surgery whether covered by prophylactic antibiotics or not; the healing cavity of a prostatectomy, carried out transurethrally or retropubically, can take as long as 8 weeks to epithelialize and pyuria during the whole of this period is common.

Vesicular causes

Seminal vesiculitis often accompanies acute prostatitis and often causes persistent symptoms following gonococcal or non-specific urethritis. It is a very rare complication of prostatectomy but an abscess may develop if the openings of the vesicles are involved in the cicatrization process postoperatively. Tuberculous vesiculitis also occurs.

The symptoms of vesiculitis are pain in the bladder area, in the perineum, and in the low back.

Pyuria may be scant but if the channels between the vesicle and urethra are free it may be profuse; haematospermia is not infrequent while ascending inflammation of the vas and acute epididymitis are often associated. The inflamed vesicle can be felt above the prostate on rectal examination. While massage can produce a bead of pus at the urethral meatus, it is difficult to distinguish this sign from the similar phenomenon encountered in acute prostatitis.

B. PYURIA CAUSED BY DISEASES OUTSIDE THE URINARY SYSTEM

The commonest cause of pyuria is the improper collection of a sample, in that the urinary meatus, in the male or female, is improperly cleaned prior to collection. If the sample has been connected appropriately, pyuria can occur by secondary inflammatory changes within the bladder, prostate or urethra, from septic foci or malignant processes outside. In the male, retained secretions behind a phimosis can result in pyuria; and an excess of physiological discharge in the female may do the same. If there is persistent doubt with regard to the presence of pyuria in a woman, suprapubic fine-needle aspiration of a bladder, well distended with urine, is a relatively safe method of establishing the diagnosis with certainty.

The presence and spread of inflammatory processes outside the urinary tract into the urinary passages will cause pyuria, as will the **rupture of an extra-vesical abscess**. When the symptoms suggest urinary trouble, such as increased frequency, urgency, pain on micturition and haematuria, and are followed by the sudden appearance of a quantity of pus in the urine, there is a strong possibility of the rupture of an extra-urinary abscess into the bladder or urethra or very rarely into the ureter, provided that the sudden emptying of a renal abscess or pyonephrosis can be eliminated. This spontaneous discharge is often associated with a relief of the primary symptom. The history will often give some indication of the primary diagnosis, of which the most frequent are prostatic abscess, appendix abscess, pyosalpinx, psoas, iliac and pelvic abscess and an abscess around a carcinoma or diverticulitis of the colon, the last of these being the commonest of all.

Pyuria in acute appendicitis. If the appendix is in its usual position the bladder is rarely affected, but if the appendix passes downwards across the pelvic brim it is not unusual to find that the patient complains of frequency and pain on micturition when appendicitis occurs. If the appendix is severely inflamed it may adhere to the bladder and both pus and blood may be present in the urine; if cytoscopy is carried out, a localized area of congestion will be seen on the right lateral wall. Very occasionally, a small abscess may develop in the adhesions between the appendix and the bladder, and if this abscess discharges into the bladder pyuria results and an entero-vesical fistula is established. Diagnosis in the case of a dependent appendix is difficult; the pain is much lower in the pelvis than is usual with appendicitis while the lower urinary tract symptoms point to a bladder disorder; the onset of the condition is, however, gradual and there is an elevation of temperature and pulse rate with right-sided abdominal rigidity; none of these is present in acute cystitis and the possibility of an alternative acute intra-abdominal lesion has to be considered. A right-sided pelvic abscess arising from a burst appendix may rupture into the bladder. The usual history of acute appendicitis is accompanied by the presence of a mass in the right iliac fossa or the pelvic space, bimanually palpable if in the later. Pyrexia continues and is associated with rigors. If the abscess discharges into the bladder, the fever resolves and a large quantity of pus appears in the urine. Rectal examination reveals not only the tenderness of acute appendicitis but considerable thickening relating to the thick wall of the abscess cavity.

Pyosalpinx may cause cystitis by direct spread of the inflammatory process to the bladder and may eventually rupture. There has usually been a history of profuse vaginal discharge associated with constant aching in the pelvic region and in the lower back; there are often frequent attacks of severe pain and malaise at variable intervals, together with an intermittent pyrexia. Periods may be profuse, frequent, and more painful than usual, while vaginal examination reveals fullness or a mass in one or both vaginal fornices.

Psoas and iliac abscesses may rupture into the bladder, and the former has been known to discharge into a ureter. There is a swelling in the iliac fossa and sometimes in the inguinal region, and clinical and radiological evidence of spinal osteomyelitis, together with lateral displacement of the psoas shadow.

Diverticulitis of the pelvic colon often becomes adherent to the bladder and if peridiverticular abscesses form these may rupture into the bladder, causing pyuria and formation of an entero-vesical fistula. Pneumaturia, the passage of flatus per urethram, is pathognomonic but it is surprising how rarely it occurs; the appearance of solid faecal particles in the urine is more common; when air is passed in the urine the stream hisses or whistles. The main differential diagnosis of pneumaturia is an acute cystitis with a gas-forming organism, particularly in diabetic patients. A colo-vesical fistula occurs far more frequently following rupture of a peridiverticular abscess than by direct extension of a colonic carcinoma.

Carcinoma of the pelvic structures often involves the bladder by direct extension. This is particularly true of carcinoma of the cervix and of the rectum but may also happen from carcinoma of the pelvic colon, sigmoid and caecum. Spread of disease to the bladder occurs relatively late and the symptoms of the primary condition have usually given a clear indication of the diagnosis before pyuria results. Involvement of the bladder is first shown by frequency, dysuria, and urgency, while the presence of blood and pus in the urine are late features, representing ulceration through the whole thickness of the bladder wall. Utero-vesical and vesico-vaginal fistulae may result from extension of primary tumours from either of these two structures into the bladder; the pathognomonic symptom is continuous incontinence by day and night. It is hardly likely that this incontinence will need to be distinguished from that secondary to an ectopic ureter as this will be evident from birth. Penetration of the bladder by a carcinoma of the rectum or colon will give rise to pneumaturia and the passage of pus, blood and faecal debris in the urinary stream. Occasionally the urine flow passes in the other direction and the urine output falls while the passage of watery stools, alternating with reasonably well-formed motions may occur.

Tuberculosis, or **dysenteric ulcers** of the intestines and **caecal actinomycosis** are rare causes of pyuria. In the last of these, the fungus, instead of infiltrating the skin and pointing in the groin externally as it usually does, extends downwards into the pelvis and opens into the bladder or rectum; the diagnosis depends on the discovery of ray fungi in the urine and it is unlikely that they would be found unless specifically sought. Actinomycosis of the kidney is usually mistaken for tuberculosis until the fungi are discovered by microscopy.

The commonest causes of the intermittent appearance of large amounts of pus in the urine are pyonephrosis, diverticulum of the bladder and vesico-colic fistula. The presence of a persistent low-grade pyuria which cannot be explained otherwise may indicate carcinoma *in situ* of the bladder or urinary tract tuberculosis.

Lynn Edwards

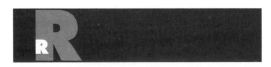

Rectal bleeding

Bleeding from the rectum is one of the commonest symptoms and also the most commonly mismanaged. The majority of patients with rectal bleeding are found to have haemorrhoids as the underlying cause. Hae-

morrhoids are cushions of erectile tissue containing extensive arteriovenous anastomoses and when traumatized arterial bleeding results. Usually the bleeding is of a minor nature; there is light staining of the lavatory paper following defaecation. Rarely profuse bleeding leading to hypovolaemic shock can occur. The possibility of a neoplasm must always be a consideration irrespective of the age of the patient. Although the incidence of rectal carcinoma is highest in the sixth and seventh decades it is not uncommon in younger age groups. The presence of malignancy must be considered particularly when there are constitutional symptoms or there is a history of recent irregularity of bowel function. Profuse mucous discharge in association with bleeding is consistent with a villous adenoma or carcinoma and a history of bloody diarrhoea is most consistent with a diagnosis of inflammatory bowel disease.

Approximately 80 per cent of rectal neoplasms are within range of digital examination and a per rectal examination should be conducted in all patients with rectal bleeding. If a lesion is palpated an assessment should be made of its mobility and fixity to surrounding tissues. A highly mobile lesion is indicative of a benign adenoma whereas any degree of fixity is strongly suggestive of invasion and hence of malignancy. Haemorrhoids, in contrast, are not usually palpable and not tender on palpation in the absence of strangulation. Undue local tenderness suggests the presence of underlying fissure, infection (intersphincteric abscess) or haematoma.

Sigmoidoscopy is an essential step in the exclusion of (*a*) carcinoma and (*b*) inflammatory bowel disease and where there is dispute over the macroscopic appearances biopsy is mandatory. The presence of oedema, erythema or a shallow discrete ulcer, usually confined to the anterior rectal wall, are features which may be indicative of the solitary rectal ulcer syndrome. This is a benign condition associated with excessive defaecation straining and can readily be confused with carcinoma on its sigmoidoscopic appearances.

The diagnosis of haemorrhoids largely rests on the appearances at proctoscopy. Most commonly the right anterior haemorrhoid is noted to be enlarged and congested and is the putative cause of bleeding since it is rare to see the active bleeding source at the time of the examination.

Patients with a history of blood mixed in with the stool or where there is a major loss of altered or of venous blood may require more detailed investigation which will include barium enema and colonoscopy. If angiodysplasia is to be excluded arteriography may be necessary. Finally rectal bleeding may be readily confused with bleeding from the upper gastrointestinal tract and small intestine; this is dealt with under MELAENA.

Classification of major causes of rectal bleeding

ANAL CAUSES

Haemorrhoids
Anal fissure
Anal fistula
Perianal haematoma
Condylomata
Trauma
Malignancy
  Squamous carcinoma
  Adenocarcinoma
  Paget's disease
  Malignant melanoma
  Bowen's disease
  Basal cell carcinoma

RECTAL CAUSES

Angiodysplasmia
Ischaemia
Infective (e.g. tuberculosis)
Inflammatory (e.g. ulcerative colitis)
Solitary rectal ulcer syndrome
Trauma
Neoplasia
  Adenoma
  Carcinoma
  Malignant melanoma

COLONIC CAUSES

Diverticular disease
Infective (e.g. dysentery)
Inflammatory
Angiodysplasia
Intussusception
Ischaemia
Neoplasia
  Adenoma
  Carcinoma

GENERAL CAUSES

Clotting deficiencies
Anticoagulants
Uraemia

(See under MELAENA for other causes particularly related to disorders in the upper gastrointestinal tract and small intestine).

M. M. Henry

Rectal discharge

Secretion from sweat glands in the perianal area and from the anal glands is a common and normal phenomenon which rarely gives rise to significant problems. Profuse mucous secretion, however, often causes considerable discomfort and pruritis ani as a consequence of inflammation of the perianal skin. Such secretion is commonly observed with *haemorrhoids* particularly where there is a combination of *prolapse* with a weak internal anal sphincter. More serious *pelvic floor disorders* (e.g. complete prolapse, solitary rectal ulcer syndrome) may be responsible for profuse and sometimes blood-stained mucous secretion which can be incapacitating. *Inflammation* of the rectal mucosa from ulcerative colitis or Crohn's disease of the rectum may similarly produce a mucous discharge which is usually blood-stained and accompanied by diarrhoea. The existence of *neoplasia* should always be suspected since copious secretion is a particular feature of villous adenomas of the rectum in which the potassium loss may be sufficient to induce hypokalaemia. Carcinoma may also be a cause of mucous secretion although bleeding is usually a more prominent feature and there may be constitutional symptoms.

A purulent discharge is usually caused by *anal* and *perianal sepsis*. On inspection of the perineum, a small opening discharging pus to the side of the anus is highly suggestive of fistula. The diagnosis can be confirmed by palpation and observation at proctoscopy of the internal opening. Ulcerating and purulent perianal lesions should raise the possibility of Crohn's disease, anal tuberculosis or of sexually transmitted disease (e.g. AIDS, syphilis, gonorrhoea). Where there is doubt, bacteriological examination of the pus and histological examination of the biopsy from the perianal skin should be performed. Anal neoplasms and condylomata can be responsible for an offensive purulent discharge; the diagnosis is apparent on inspection but biopsy is always mandatory even if simple condyloma is diagnosed since malignant development can occur with this lesion.

Classification of major causes of rectal discharge

DISCHARGE OF MUCUS

Haemorrhoids
Rectal prolapse
Solitary rectal ulcer syndrome
Villous adenoma
Carcinoma rectum
Proctitis

DISCHARGE OF PUS

Anal fistula
Perianal Crohn's
Anal tuberculosis
Anal neoplasms
Anal fissure
Syphilis
Gonorrhoea
Condyloma accuminata
AIDS

M. M. Henry

Rectal mass

Every medical practitioner should be aware of the importance of conducting a digital examination of the anal canal and rectum in all patients with anorectal symptoms since the majority of rectal neoplasms are well within reach of the examining finger. The relevance of performing a rectal examination as part of a general examination in a patient without rectal symptoms is less clear. Since rectal cancer is a common malignancy in patients aged over 60 years, a strong argument can be made that all patients in this age group should undergo rectal examination as part of any general physical examination. Clearly, if there are urinary symptoms, a digital assessment of the prostate is highly relevant and similarly digital examination of the rectum (and, where relevant, vaginal examination) may be valuable in patients with pelvic or perineal symptoms.

Digital examination of the rectum should be conducted, where possible, with the patient lying in the left lateral position and should not be attempted until a full inspection of the perineum has been conducted to exclude fissure or other pathology which might give rise to severe pain on palpation. Initially, a digital assessment is made of anal sphincter tone which may be increased in the presence of fissure and decreased in functional disorders such as anorectal incontinence. Each quadrant of the anus and rectum should be examined sequentially. Within the anus, lesions may extend caudally from the rectum and vice versa. In the normal state, haemorrhoids are not palpable and no specific structure is palpated until the examining finger reaches the rectum. In women, the cervix frequently projects into the anterior rectal wall and is readily palpable; this is frequently mistaken by some clinicians for a rectal neoplasm. In men, the prostate is easily palpable anteriorly. Laterally, the ischial spines may be palpated and this may be of value in the location of the pudendal nerves (to provide a pudendal nerve blockade). Posteriorly, the 'shelf' created by the levator ani, and in thin subjects, the bony coccyx may be palpable.

Intrinsic lesions

If a mass is perceived on digital examination, it is not always possible to decide on palpation alone if the lesion is intrinsic or extrinsic. The differentiation may only be possible after sigmoidoscopy and histological examination. The consistency and mobility may closely relate to the diagnosis. Hence, a *benign villous adenoma* will feel soft, fleshy and highly mobile. In contrast, a *carcinoma* may feel hard with obvious fixation of the mucosal lesion to the underlying muscle or perirectal fat. Sometimes nearby *extrarectal lymph nodes* containing secondary tumour deposits may be palpable.

A circumferential stenosis of the rectum may be seen following *trauma* (e.g. previous surgery) or be a complication of: (*a*) *infection* (e.g. lymphogranuloma); (*b*) *inflammation* (e.g. ulcerative colitis) or (*c*) *ischaemia*. Digital examination under these circumstances is usually accompanied by marked tenderness and pain. *Anal neoplasms* may extend into the lumen of the anus and upwards into the rectum, in which case there may be a marked stenosis and the examination will cause pain.

Extrinsic lesions

Rectal examination is a simple clinical means of diagnosing the presence of *pelvic pus* or *pelvic tumour*. A tender mass in the presence of oedematous rectal mucosa suggests a collection of pus whereas a hard, fixed extrinsic mass in which there is no mobility of the rectal wall or uterus would be strong evidence in favour of pelvic malignancy. Infection may arise secondary to gynaecological or intestinal sepsis but may be secondary to an anal fistula where pus has tracked superiorly to create a collection above the levator musculature. Such fistulas are important to recognize since their treatment is complex. *Benign enlargement of the prostate* may give rise to symmetrical hypertrophy of the gland in which the midline sulcus is preserved. *Malignant enlargement* gives rise to a mass which is denser, asymmetrical and the midline sulcus is invaded.

A mass which is clearly situated posterior to the rectum arises in the potential space ventral to the sacrum and coccyx bounded distally by the levator ani and proximally by the pelvic peritoneal reflection. The important primary distinction is whether the lesion is solid or cystic; this may require ultrasound examination for confirmation. The majority of solid lesions are *chordomas* and a cystic lesion is usually one of the following: (*a*) *epidermoid cyst*; (*b*) *mucus secreting cyst*; (*c*) *teratoma*; (*d*) *teratocarcinoma* or (*e*) *meningocele*. Neurogenic and osseous tumours are rare in this region. Clinically, presacral masses usually present with a history of low back pain radiating to the rectum and buttocks. Pressure on the bladder may lead to urinary retention and constipation is a frequent symptom. On sacral radiographs, presacral lesions may show up as an area of calcification with rarefaction of the sacrum; if there is bony destruction malignancy should always be suspected. A barium enema should always be performed to exclude colonic communication with the mass and similarly, communication with the subarachnoid space should be excluded by CT, MRI or lumbar myelography.

Classification of major causes of rectal masses

INTRINSIC CAUSES
Rectal neoplasia
  Benign
   Polyps
   Leiomyoma
  Malignant
   Carcinoma
   Carcinoid
   Leiomyosarcoma
   Lymphoma
   Melanoma
Anal neoplasia
  Benign
   Condylomata
   Polyps
  Malignant
   Adenocarcinoma
   Squamous carcinoma
   Melanoma
   Bowen's disease
   Paget's disease
   Basal cell carcinoma
  Infection
   Lymphogranuloma
   Tuberculosis

EXTRINSIC CAUSES
Infection
  Pelvic abscess
  Anal fistula with supralevator extension
Tumour
  Secondary spread to pelvis/pouch of Douglas
  Carcinoma prostate
Gynaecological causes
  Carcinoma body uterus
  Carcinoma cervix
  Carcinoma ovary
  Fibroid uterus
  Ovarian cyst
  Pyosalpinx
  Ectopic gestation
  Endometriosis
Presacral lesions

PRESACRAL (RETRORECTAL) CAUSES
Congenital
  Epidermoid cyst
  Teratoma/carcinoma
  Meningocoele
  Chordoma
Causes arising from bone/cartilage
  Osteogenic sarcoma
  Ewing's sarcoma
  Osteochondroma
  Myeloma
  Giant cell tumour
Neurological causes
  Neurofibroma/sarcoma
  Neurilemmoma
  Ependymoma
  Neuroblastoma
Miscellaneous

Lymphoma
Lipoma
Fibroma/sarcoma
Haemangioma

M. M. Henry

Rectal tenesmus

Rectal tenesmus is a non-specific term employed to describe a state in which there is either difficulty with, or repeated, painful and sometimes *futile* defaecation. A similar condition has been described affecting micturition and is referred to as urinary tenesmus (or strangury). The repeated defaecation is often accompanied by the passage of mucus and/or blood and this collection of symptoms should be distinguished from the symptom of diarrhoea. In the latter, there is either a complaint of stool of loose consistency or there is increase in frequency, but, in contrast to patients with tenesmus, defaecation is usually productive of stool.

As with all rectal symptoms, there may be a sinister underlying cause and a full clinical assessment, which includes digital examination of the anus/rectum and sigmoidoscopy, is essential.

Inflammatory and infective causes (proctitis)

Proctitis (*see* RECTAL ULCERATION) may be inflammatory (e.g. ulcerative colitis. Crohn's disease) or infective in origin. The tenesmus may be associated with constitutional symptoms (e.g. malaise, weight loss, anorexia) and with severe diarrhoea. In patients with ulcerative colitis, the bleeding may be substantial, so leading to severe anaemia. The diagnosis is readily made by sigmoidoscopy, biopsy and, where relevant, by stool culture. Less commonly perianal sepsis (e.g. fistula) can cause tenesmus. The diagnosis is suggested either by the presence of extreme tenderness on digital examination of the anus or by the presence of a sinus/ fistula opening in the perianal region.

Neoplastic causes

Benign (e.g. villous adenoma) or malignant lesions of the rectum or anus frequently cause tenesmus. An extensive villous adenoma of the rectum is notorious as a cause of excessive secretion of rectal mucus, which is sufficiently rich in potassium to lead to hypokalaemia. Adenocarcinoma of the rectum may similarly be responsible for the secretion of mucus but to a lesser degree. Rectal bleeding is a more pronounced feature in the history; the bleeding may be bright or dark red, may be mixed in with the stool, and accompanies defaecation. In the case of advanced malignancy the rectal symptoms may be accompanied by constitutional symptoms, such as weight loss. Squamous carcinoma of the anal margin should be recognizable on simple inspection of the anal verge and examination of the inguinal region may reveal lymphadenopathy in the presence of metastatic spread to the regional nodes.

Mechanical causes

Tenesmus occasionally results from a poorly understood condition in which the pelvic floor and external anal sphincter musculature fail to relax or may actively contract during attempted defaecation. Under normal circumstances these muscles relax reflexly to enable easy passage of the faecal bolus through the anal canal. This condition is usually diagnosable only either by conventional electromyography or by defaecography and may be associated with a solitary rectal ulcer as seen on sigmoidoscopy (*see* RECTAL ULCERATION). The cause is usually not known, but occasionally pelvic floor 'spasticity' is identified in patients with multiple sclerosis and the symptom of tenesmus may be the first symptom noted by patients with demyelinating diseases.

Minor anorectal disorders, particularly in an acute presentation (e.g. perianal thrombosis), may cause tenesmus since the lesion within the anus may cause stimulation of anal sensory receptors at and below the dentate line which gives rise to a false impression that there is faecal matter present within the anus and lower rectum.

M. M. Henry

Rectal ulceration

Normally a diagnosis of rectal ulceration will be made from the macroscopic appearances of the rectum at either sigmoidoscopy or radiologically at barium enema. Only under certain circumstances (*see below*) will an ulcer be palpable.

The clinical distinction between inflammatory bowel disease and infection can rarely be made on macroscopic appearances alone. Hence ulcerative colitis or shigella infection may both give rise to: (*a*) shallow ulceration; (*b*) granular appearances; (*c*) haemorrhagic friable mucosa and (*d*) oedematous mucosa in the rectum. The presence of pseudopolyps is more closely allied to ulcerative colitis but these rarely occur in the rectum and are more a feature of colonic disease. Bacterial infections tend to be of more sudden onset and are often associated with severe abdominal pain. Patients with ulcerative colitis develop symptoms usually over a prolonged period and rarely complain of significant abdominal pain. The presence of multiple yellowish-white plaques varying in size from a few millimetres to 15–20 mm in diameter may be suggestive of pseudomembranous or antibiotic-associated colitis. The latter condition is now recognized to be a toxin-

mediated disease induced by *C. difficile* following exposure to antibiotics. The organism is a component of the normal flora of approximately 30 per cent of healthy adults but exogenous infection can probably occur as well.

Where ulceration is observed sigmoidoscopically, a portion of mucosa should be biopsied in most instances. Unfortunately, the discrimination between infection and inflammation is not always possible on the microscopic appearances alone; particularly in the early stage of inflammatory disease. The diagnosis in these patients will depend on bacteriology of the stool. If the stool culture is negative, the microscopic appearances will be important in the distinction between Crohn's proctitis and ulcerative colitis. The presence of granulomas, fissures, transmural inflammation and an anal lesion would provide strong evidence in favour of Crohn's disease. A non-specific microscopic inflammation may also be a feature of postirradiation proctitis and can often only be distinguished by the history alone. The list of infective agents which can give rise to a proctitis is legion; only the more important are listed below. If rare organisms are cultured such as the protozoan cryptosporidia or viruses (e.g. cytomegalovirus, herpes simplex), the possibility of immune deficiency (e.g. AIDS, leukaemia) should always be considered.

Ischaemia rarely affects the rectum but when present is usually prevalent in older age groups, is of sudden onset and is associated with profuse bleeding and abdominal pain. The diagnosis is confirmed by barium enema in which the characteristic appearances of 'thumb-printing' are observed principally in the descending and sigmoid colon.

The ulcer of the solitary rectal ulcer syndrome and the ulcerating lesion associated with some rectal carcinomas are often both readily palpable on rectal examination. Both may feel indurated with fixity to extrarectal tissues and the sigmoidoscopic appearances can be identical. Adequate biopsy is essential to enable the diagnosis to be made since the presence of carcinoma will require radical surgical measures. Ulceration may rarely be traumatic in origin either as a result of self-mutilation or because digitally assisted evacuation is the only means by which the voiding of rectal contents can be achieved.

Classification of major causes of rectal ulceration

Inflammatory
   Ulcerative colitis
   Crohn's disease
   Radiation

Infective
  Shigella
  Salmonella
  Campylobacter
  Tuberculosis
  Gonococcal
  Amoebiasis
  Pseudomembranous colitis (*Cl. difficile*)
  Lymphogranuloma
  Schistosoma
  Syphilis
  Herpes simplex
  Enterovirus
  Cytomegalovirus
Solitary rectal ulcer syndrome
Trauma
Malignant ulcer
  Carcinoma
  Leukaemia
Ischaemia

M. M. Henry

Reflexes, abnormalities of

Reflex activity, loosely defined as an involuntary response to the passage of nervous impulses through a reflex arc, enters into a wide range of somatic and visceral functions both in health and disease. A comparatively small number of these reflexes are used in the practice of clinical neurology (*Table R.1*). Only tendon stretch reflexes and the superficial reflexes will be discussed here.

Table R.1. Reflexes that may be used in neurological practice

1. *Autonomic and related sensory reflexes*
   The axon reflex
   Blood pressure responses to postural change
   Valsalva's manoeuvre

2. *Primitive reflexes*
   For example, pout reflex, grasp reflex

3. *Pupillary reflexes* (see page 539)

4. *Tendon or stretch reflexes*

5. *Superficial reflexes*

The tendon reflexes

In normal man muscles contract when stretched by a sharp tap on the tendon of insertion. Anatomical factors limit the application of this test to only a number of muscles (*Table R.2*). These tendon stretch reflexes are monosynaptic. The reflex pathway ascends from the muscle through the posterior roots, passes forward to the anterior horn cells of the same segment and descends to the muscle or muscles concerned via the motor nerve.

Table R.2. Clinically useful tendon reflexes

Reflex	Roots
Biceps	C5 and 6
Triceps	C7
'Supinator'	C6
Knee	L3 and 4
Ankle	S1

Exaggeration of tendon reflexes

There is considerable normal variation in the briskness of tendon reflexes and the judgement as to whether a tendon reflex is pathologically brisk can be exceedingly difficult. Generalized increase in the tendon reflexes occurs in excitement, anxiety, thyrotoxicosis and in certain intoxications, such as amphetamine poisoning. Diffuse increase in the reflexes may also be seen in generalized damage to the upper motor neurone, as in hydrocephalus. Localized exaggeration of tendon reflexes is a valuable sign of damage to the pyramidal pathways in which case it may be associated with loss of the abdominal and cremasteric reflexes and an extensor plantar response.

Depression or loss of tendon reflexes

This may occur as a transient event in shock, haemorrhage, cerebral and spinal concussion, deep anaesthesia, severe general infections, diabetic coma, potassium intoxication (in uraemia) and overdosage with drugs which depress the central nervous system. Localized loss of reflexes due to local disease affecting the reflex arc is of considerable localizing value in neurology. Any part of the reflex arc may be interrupted leading to loss of the appropriate tendon reflex.

1. DISEASE OF MUSCLE

Depression or loss of reflexes occurs as a late event in any form of myopathy.

2. DISEASE OF PERIPHERAL NERVES

Damage to either the motor or sensory peripheral nerves may lead to loss of tendon reflexes. This may occur where the damage is localized to an isolated peripheral nerve or where the damage occurs as part of a generalized peripheral neuropathy.

3. DAMAGE TO THE MOTOR OR SENSORY SPINAL ROOTS

Damage to either the afferent or efferent part of the spinal reflex as a result of root damage is a common cause of loss of a localized tendon reflex. Common causes are cervical and lumbar spondylosis, cervical and lumbar disc disease and intraspinal tumours. Tabes dorsalis produces areflexia due to damage to the posterior nerve roots

4. DISEASE OF THE SPINAL CORD

Damage within the spinal cord, either within the dorsal root entry zone or between the dorsal root entry zone and the anterior horn cell, or in the anterior horn cell itself, may produce loss of the tendon reflex. This may occur in intraspinal lesions, such as syringomyelia or intramedullary tumours, and it is also seen in diffuse damage to the anterior horn cells as occurs in motor neurone disease or poliomyelitis.

The tendon reflexes are lost in the Holmes–Adie syndrome. Typically the patients are young women who are found, incidentally, to have an Adie pupil and loss of tendon reflexes in the legs. The cause of the loss of tendon reflexes is uncertain.

In some instances, even in an apparently relaxed patient, it may be impossible to elicit tendon reflexes without there being any obvious pathological abnormality.

N. E. F. Cartlidge

Regurgitation

In regurgitation the patient is aware of food that is passed from the oesophagus into the mouth. There is therefore relaxation of the upper oesophageal sphincter to allow the contents of the oesophagus to enter the mouth. It is important to distinguish between regurgitation, reflux and vomiting. In vomiting the food passes through open lower and upper oesophageal sphincters and is the consequence of forceful contractions of the abdominal wall and the stomach muscles. Reflux is the passage of food from either the duodenum or the stomach into the oesophagus. If the food fails to pass the upper oesophageal sphincter, then the patient is said to be suffering from gastro-oesophageal reflux. If, however, the food passes into the mouth then the term regurgitation can be used. Thus reflux and regurgitation are often used synonomously. While regurgitation can be regarded as a classical symptom of oesphageal disorder, it is not necessarily so and this is seen to best effect in infants where regurgitation can be a common and normal phenomenon and is related to the passage of gastric contents into the child's mouth.

Patients who complain of regurgitation will often indicate that there is a postural element with the symptom being most marked by change of position, particularly when bending forward and often on physical exercise. The symptom occurs classically in *achalasia* (or achalasia of the cardia, or cardiospasm). In this motor disorder of the oesophagus there is a reduction in the number of ganglion cells which innervate oesophageal musculature. This is particularly so in the region of the lower oesophageal sphincter. The patient is usually between 20 and 40 years of age and classically describes dysphagia, painful swallowing and regurgitation. The regurgitation of food into the mouth at nighttime can be associated with inhalation pneumonia and bronchopneumonia. Halitosis may be a symptom. The diagnosis is made manometrically when reduced contractions in the body of the oesophagus will be noted. The resting pressure in the lower oesophageal sphincter is usually elevated and fails to fall, as is normal with swallowing. A poorly contracting, dilated oesophagus will be seen on barium swallow with the non-relaxing lower oesophageal sphincter giving the appearance of a 'beak' on the X-ray. Oesophagoscopy is usually unnecessary but is useful to exclude the association of a squamous carcinoma of the oesophagus which is a recognized complication of achalasia.

Gastro-oesophageal reflux is often known as reflux oesophagitis. The two terms are not necessarily synonymous because reflux into the oesophagus from the stomach is not necessarily associated with inflammation. By definition in reflux oesophagitis there is the regurgitation of fluid from the stomach into the oesophagus. The cause for the reflux is not always clear.

Reflux is associated with a reduced tone in the lower oesophageal sphincter which has inappropriate relaxation. In addition to this it has been claimed that the secondary peristaltic clearing mechanisms in the oesophagus are inadequate. In other words instead of refluxed material being promptly cleared back into the stomach it remains for a longer period than normal in the oesophagus thereby causing symptoms and possibly inflammation. It is controversial whether in patients with severe reflux there is an element of ineffective clearing of the oesophagus. Reduced lower oesophageal sphincter pressure has been seen following ingestion of fat and alcohol. Smoking also tends to cause relaxation of the oesophageal sphincter as do drugs such as morphine, pethidine and diazepam. Carminatives such as coffee will cause a temporary relaxation of the sphincter.

Whether or not a *sliding hiatus hernia* is associated with regurgitation is a much more controversial issue. It is true that regurgitation, gastro-oesophageal reflux and a hiatus hernia may coexist, but the two conditions can exist independently and many authorities believe that the position of the lower oesophageal sphincter in relation to the diaphragm is irrelevant in the genesis of the symptoms from hiatus hernia. Patients with a sliding hiatus hernia in which the gastro-oesophageal junction lies in the thorax above the diaphragm complain of heartburn, dysphagia and reflux. A small percentage of the patients may actually have a haematemesis. The hiatus hernia may be diagnosed on endoscopy or on a barium swallow and meal.

Evidence of reflux may be obtained by various tests in which the oesophageal pH is measured. There are tests available to measure oesophageal pressures, sphincter function, and the ability of the oesophagus to clear material in its lumen. It must be emphasized, however, that the demonstration of a hiatus hernia is no guarantee that it is the cause of oesophageal reflux or of the symptoms.

A picture very similar to achalasia is produced by *Chagas' disease* due to *Trypanosoma cruzi* which is encountered in South and Central America. The disease is characterized by a megaoesophagus, megacolon and severe cardiac dilatation and dysfunction. It is the cardiac complications of the disease which usually brings the patient to medical attention but occasionally the oesophageal symptoms may be dominant and they are then identical to that of classic achalasia.

Other motor disorders which may occasionally cause dysphagia include the *collagen vascular disorders* such as *scleroderma*, *diabetes mellitus*, and *alcoholic neuropathy*. In these conditions reflux or regurgitation is not a prominent feature, dysphagia or heartburn being more frequently the predominant symptoms.

It is well worth stressing that in many patients who have a complaint of reflux as manifested by heartburn or occasionally regurgitation of food into the mouth, no clear aetiological factor can be determined. Tests of oesophageal motor function and 24-hour monitoring of oesophageal pH will very often not demonstrate any evidence of abnormality despite the patient complaining of quite severe symptoms. These are important considerations in deciding whether or not a patient with the symptoms of regurgitation and who has a hiatus hernia demonstrated should be subjected to surgery.

Ian A. D. Bouchier

Rub, pericardial

A pericardial rub, once identified as such, is pathognomonic of acute pericarditis. A rub has a characteristic 'creaking' or 'leathery' character but this quality does not certainly differentiate it from a cardiac murmur. A typical rub is virtually continuous throughout the cardiac cycle but three components have been identified; systolic, early diastolic and, if the patient is in sinus rhythm, late diastolic. If all three components are heard there is little doubt about the diagnosis but the to-and-fro cadence of the systolic and early diastolic components can sometimes be confused with the murmurs of aortic stenosis and regurgitation. If the rub is heard in systole only, as is often the case when the

pericarditis is resolving, it may often be confused with a murmur.

A rub may be heard anywhere over the precordium. It may be markedly influenced by respiration and posture although the changes are not predictable and, to be sure of not missing a rub, it is necessary to auscultate in all phases of deep respiration and with the patient in several postures. Sometimes it may be possible to increase the intensity of a rub by increasing the pressure with which the stethoscope is applied to the chest. In practice, there is rarely much difficulty in identifying a pericardial rub but there may occasionally be confusion with the 'scratchy' murmur of Ebstein's anomaly or the late systolic murmur of mitral valve prolapse. When doubt remains, the passage of time will usually resolve the issue as pericardial rubs are evanescent and usually disappear within a few days.

The causes of pericarditis are discussed under CHEST PAIN (p. 98).

Peter R. Fleming

RUB, PLEURAL
See PLEURAL RUB.

Salivary glands, pain in

Pain in one or other of the major salivary glands is associated with enlargement of the affected organ itself (*see* SALIVARY GLANDS, SWELLING OF). For practical purposes, this symptom is confined to the parotid and submandibular salivary glands. Painful enlargement of the sublingual gland is rare; it is occasionally seen as a manifestation of mumps, together with painful enlargement of the other glands, and in the unusual condition of an advanced carcinoma of the gland itself or invasion from adjacent structures. This gland will not be considered further.

The painful salivary swellings may be classified thus:

PAROTID GLAND

Mumps (epidemic parotitis)
Acute bacterial suppurative parotitis—postoperative, dehydration, following radiotherapy
Parotitis association with duct obstruction (calculus, trauma)
Carcinoma (primary or spread from another focus)

SUBMANDIBULAR GLAND

Mumps (rare)
Inflammation associated with duct obstruction
Carcinoma

MUMPS

Mumps (epidemic parotitis) is a viral disease which is transmitted by droplet infection. It is the commonest cause of a painful parotid swelling.

Children are most often affected. There is usually prodromal fever with malaise. Only one gland may be involved, or both may be affected simultaneously, or one gland may become enlarged after the other. The swelling progresses for several days with marked tenderness of the gland and thickening of the overlying skin. There is characteristic uplifting of the lobe of the ear and stiffness of the jaw. Rarely, the submandibular glands may also become swollen and this may also unusually implicate the sublingual glands.

After 7–10 days, the swelling gradually subsides. There may be an associated acute orchitis, which may be bilateral, and which may proceed to testicular atrophy. A rare complication is pancreatitis.

ACUTE SUPPURATIVE PAROTITIS

Acute parotitis as a complication of major surgery is now quite unusual (*Fig.* S.1): This is because it results from postoperative dehydration in a patient with poor oral hygiene and septic dental stumps. Nowadays this condition is usually obviated by adequate fluid replacement and by both pre- and postoperative oral care. Acute parotitis is also occasionally seen as a complication of the severe dehydration in conditions such as typhoid fever and cholera. Radiotherapy to the parotid region may result in damage to the gland, reduction in its secretion and a propensity, therefore, for ascending infection to occur.

On examination the whole of the gland is enlarged with a tender red swelling of the side of the face. This may progress to overlying cellulitis. Pus can be expressed from the parotid duct on the affected side. Because of the dense overlying fascia, which confines the enlarged gland, pain may be intense. There are the associated features of severe infection with pyrexia and toxaemia.

PAROTITIS ASSOCIATED WITH DUCT OBSTRUCTION

Obstruction of a salivary duct, from any cause, results in a typical syndrome in which the gland becomes painful and swollen at meal times, due to the increased secretion of saliva being unable to discharge through the duct. Between meals, as the saliva gradually escapes, the swelling and pain subside. Frequently, inflammation of the obstructed gland occurs as a result of ascending infection from mouth organisms. Under these circumstances, there may be the associated features of infection (*Fig.* S.2a) and there may be a discharge of pus from the mouth of the duct.

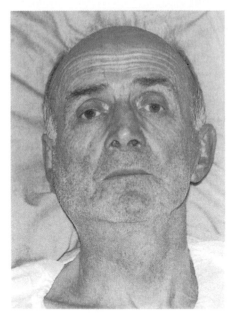

Fig. S.1. Acute postoperative right-sided parotitis following gastrectomy for gastric carcinoma.

Although less common than in the submandibular duct, calculi in the parotid duct are not rare. They tend to be smaller and less radiopaque than in the submandibular duct or gland so that only larger ones are seen on a plain X-ray of the region. A sialogram may be necessary to identify the stone, which will then be seen as a filling defect.

Other causes of parotid duct stenosis are trauma from the irritation of an adjacent tooth stump or, occasionally, from traumatic division of the duct, for example following a knife laceration of the cheek.

SUBMANDIBULAR CALCULUS

Calculi are the commonest cause of a painful swelling of the submandibular gland and account for some 95 per cent of all salivary stones. There are several reasons for the comparative frequency of stones in the submandibular gland and its duct. Its secretion contains more mucus than the parotid duct so that it is more viscid. Its duct is longer and slopes upwards from the gland so that there is more tendency for a small concretion to remain within the duct. Furthermore, its orifice, being on the floor of the mouth, is more exposed to trauma than that of the parotid duct. The aetiology of these stones remains subject of debate. Their size varies from minute to the size and shape of a date stone. Numbers vary; there may be a single stone in the duct or the gland itself may contain numerous stones throughout a dilated duct system (sialectasia).

The classical story of swelling and pain associated with food is elicited in the history. The gland itself

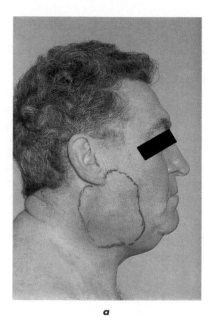

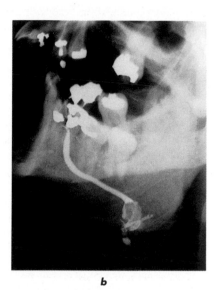

a   b

Fig. S.2. a, Parotitis secondary to calculus obstruction. The outline of the gland has been marked with a skin pen. Note that the whole gland is diffusely enlarged. This is in contrast to a tumour of the gland, which produces a localized swelling. The overlying skin is reddened. b, Sialogram of the submandibular salivary duct. The arrow demonstrates a large filling defect produced by an impacted calculus. (*Westminster Hospital.*)

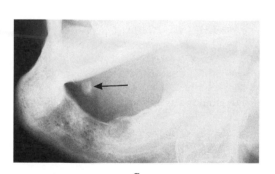

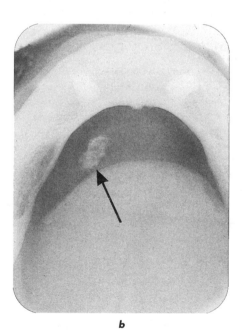

a   b

Fig. S.3. Radiopaque submandibular salivary calculus demonstrated on an oblique lateral view of the mandible (a), and, in another case (b) on a floor of mouth view. In both cases, the stone has been arrowed. (*Addenbrooke's Hospital.*)

can be felt as a tender enlargement on bimanual palpation with one finger below the angle of the jaw and the other in the sulcus between the tongue and the mandible. Occasionally a calculus can be seen to extrude through the duct orifice at the side of the base of the fraenulum linguae. At other times it may be palpated along the course of the duct in the floor of the mouth or stones may be felt in the gland itself. Pus may be expressed from the duct orifice by pressure on the gland.

Submandibular calculi are nearly all radiopaque and can be visualized on a plain X-ray of the floor of the mouth (*Fig.* S.3).

CARCINOMA OF THE SALIVARY GLANDS

In its late stages, a carcinoma of the salivary gland (commonest in the parotid, less often seen in the submandibular gland and rare in the sublingual gland) will invade adjacent tissues and produce severe pain. Invasion of a salivary gland from an adjacent tumour, for example a carcinoma of the floor of the mouth, a squamous carcinoma of the overlying skin or a malignant melanoma, will be associated with intense pain.

Harold Ellis

Salivary glands, swelling of

The salivary glands are subject to swelling due to inflammation and new growth in the same way as any other organ. In common with other externally secreting glands they are also subject to swelling resulting from retention of secretion. This most commonly occurs as a result of blockage of a duct by a stone. Parotid swelling with fever, often with lacrimal adenitis and uveitis (Mikulicz's syndrome) may occur in leukaemia, Hodgkin's disease, tuberculosis, systemic lupus erythematosus and sarcoidosis. Confusion in diagnosis may result from the close proximity of the lymphatic nodes; in the case of the submandibular gland, the lymphatic nodes may be right in the centre of the salivary tissue. The different salivary glands do not exhibit the same liability to each lesion, the submandibular for instance being the most liable to calculus formation, while inflammatory lesions are only common in the parotid. Mumps is the commonest cause of all parotid swellings; it may occasionally involve other glands than the parotid, but this is a rare exception and usually occurs only after the parotid is first attacked. Here, as in all diagnosis, it is important to decide the exact anatomical site of the lesion before considering its pathology. For example, swelling of the loose tissues over the jaw from alveolar inflammation may mimic parotitis. A useful point in this connection is that a generalized parotid swelling tends to lift the auricle away from the head and inspection of the orifice of Stensen's duct within the mouth will usually reveal some abnormality (*see Fig.* S.1) If lymphatic nodes are suspect as a site of swellings, the presence of other enlarged nodes or of a primary lesion should be sought.

Sialography may prove helpful. Radiopaque contrast is injected into the appropriate orifice (Wharton's or Stensen's, the lingual ducts are not suitable for injection). The branching system of ducts is well visualized in the radiograph. Blockage by a stone or by growth, sialectasia (dilatation and beading of the duct system, especially in the parotid gland), or the presence

Table S.1. Lesions of the salivary glands

Salivary gland	Acute unilateral enlargement	Acute bilateral enlargement	Chronic unilateral enlargement	Chronic bilateral enlargement
Parotid	Non-specific infective parotitis (rarely bilateral)	Mumps. (One side usually appears first, second commonly appears 24–36 hours later, but occasionally up to 4–5 days later)	(1) Progressive—growth or inflammation. May involve part of gland only; differentiate from preauricular adenitis by searching area drained, etc. (*see below*)	Sarcoidosis
		Both of these show signs of inflammation with much pain. In both, orifice of Stensen's duct is red and pouting	(2) Intermittent—sialectasia (calculus uncommon)	
Submandibular	As for parotid, but both very rare. *N.B.* Inflammation of submandibular lymphatic nodes common		(1) Progressive—growth (rare) (2) Intermittent—stone. Swelling occurs at mealtimes when the flow of saliva is stimulated, but the gland is permanently swollen when condition is of long standing. Stone may be palpable in duct and will show on X-ray. Orifice of duct inflamed	
Sublingual	Uncommon. Ranula was originally thought to be due to retention of secretion in this gland, but retention in adjacent simple mucous glands is the more probable explanation			
All glands	Mikulicz's syndrome—characterized by chronic painless swelling of all the salivary glands and the lacrimals. This occurs in Hodgkin's disease, tuberculosis, leukaemia, sarcoidosis and systemic lupus erythematosus			

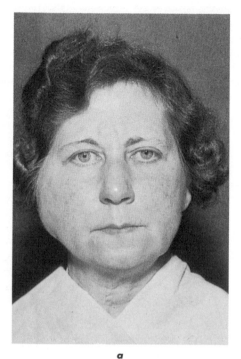 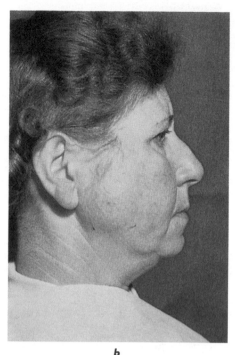

a   b

Fig. S.4. Mixed parotid tumour (pleomorphic adenoma). Courtesy of the Gordon Museum, Guy's Hospital.)

Parotid tumours

The histology of salivary tumours is complicated and will not be discussed. It is sufficient to mention the so-called 'mixed tumour', which is better termed a 'pleomorphic adenoma' (*Fig*. S.4). which is benign as a rule although locally recurrent owing to inadequate removal. Characteristically the tumour arises as a lobulated mass, noticed first when about the size of a cherry, and of variable consistency. If there is much myxomatous degeneration, the lump will appear to be fluctuant; if chiefly composed of fibrous tissue it will be hard yet elastic. The lump is painless and is typically situated between the ascending ramus of the mandible and the mastoid process, although no part of the parotid is exempt from this change and these tumours may be found as low as an inch below the angle of the mandible. Women between the ages of 30 and 50 and men between 45 and 60 are the usual sufferers and a frequent history is that the lump, over a period of years, shows a progressive slow increase in size. Involvement of the facial nerve or fixity to the skin and involvement of the cervical lymph nodes indicates that the growth is a carcinoma.

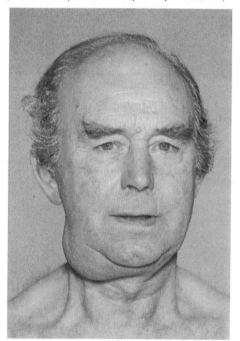

Fig. S.5. Pleomorphic adenoma of the submandibular salivary gland.

of a fistula is the lesion most likely to be demonstrated in this way (*see Fig*. S.2b).

The lesions of the salivary glands are summarized in *Table* S.1.

The submandibular salivary gland (but not the sublingual gland), may also be the site of both the pleomorphic adenoma and carcinoma, but much less commonly than the parotid (*Fig*. S.5).

Sarcoidosis

In sarcoidosis asymptomatic enlargement of the parotid, sublingual and submaxillary glands occurs in about 6 per cent of cases. Spontaneous resolution often occurs. The glands are not tender. Facial palsy may occur with parotid enlargement. The syndrome of fever, uveitis and lacrimal and salivary gland enlargement is known as 'uveoparotid' fever or 'Heerfordt's' syndrome.

Harold Ellis

Scalp and beard, fungous affections of

Tinea capitis

Tinea capitis is mainly a disease of childhood. It is contracted by direct contact. The hair follicles are first

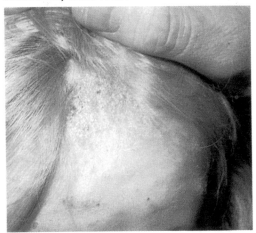

Fig. S.6. Tinea capitis: *Microsporum canis*. (Dr Richard Staughton.)

infected, causing small, red, scaly patches in which hairs break off short, rather like down-trodden stubble (*Fig.* S.6). The patch extends at the periphery and further patches appear on other parts of the scalp. Itching may or may not be present and the degree of scaliness varies from a fine branny desquamation to heaped-up masses of soft scale. Diagnosis is confirmed by microscopic examination of a few stumps that have been soaked in 10 per cent potassium hydroxide and in this way the spores of the fungus are also seen. Scalp examination using an ultraviolet lamp (Wood's light) can be most helpful, as infections with small-spored fungi cause green fluorescence (*Table* S.2).

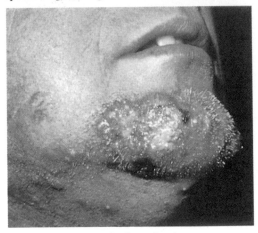

Fig. S.7. Kerion. (*Dr Richard Staughton.*)

Other diagnostic features are the age of the patient and a possible history of contact with a known case; but it must be remembered that the disease is relatively uncommon today. Most species of dermatophyte can cause tinea capitis (except *Trychophyton concentricum* and two common causes of tinea pedis, *Epidermophyton floccosum* and *Trychophyton mentagrophytes* var. *interdigitalis*). Anthropophilic species are the most common, but there is considerable variation from country to country and year to year as to which species predominate. All can produce tinea of glabrous skin and nails as well. Anthropophilic species generally cause a balding but little surrounding redness, whilst animal fungi (zoophilic species) causes moderate to severe inflammation (*Table* S.2).

Tinea capitis must be differentiated from *seborrhoeic dermatitis* where there may be diffuse

Table S.2. Fungous affections of scalp or beard

		Fluorescence with Wood's light	Clinical features	Usual geographical location
Small spored	M. audounini	+	Scaling bald patches	Canada, USA, Nigeria
	M. canis	+	Inflammatory scalp ringworm	Worldwide
Large spored	T. violaceum	−	Black dot fungi	S. America, E. Europe, Far and Middle East
	T. schoenleinii	−	Favus with scutuli	Iran, Iraq, Pakistan, Greenland
	T. tonsurans	−	Scaling bald patches. Occasionally kerion	Mexico and Peru

fine scaling but no broken-off hairs. In scalp *psoriasis* there are well-demarcated areas of scale heaped over red plaques through which the hairs grow undisturbed.

In large-spore ringworm of the scalp the infection may be so severe that multiple abscesses form around the hair follicles, invading underlying tissues. This is known as a *kerion* (*Fig.* S.7) and its appearance is reminiscent of a carbuncle, save that tenderness is less marked.

Tinea barbae

Tinea barbae is perforce a disease of the adult male, and confined almost exclusively to agricultural workers who contract the disease from infected cattle. It may take the form of superficial patches with folliculitis, or more usually a deep suppurative type (*see* kerion *above*). *Trichophyton verrucosum* and *Trichophyton mentagrophytes* are responsible for the majority of cases. Anthropophilic species are occasionally causes, and *Microsporum canis* can affect eyebrows and eyelashes.

Richard Staughton

Scaly eruptions

Scales are dried-up thin plates of keratinized epithelial cells which occur as a result of an alteration of the normal keratinization process. Normally, as the epithelial cells become slowly impregnated with keratin, their nuclei are lost; eventually they desquamate invisibly from the surface and are responsible for the majority of house dust. When the process is abnormally speeded up keratinized cells may reach the surface of the skin before losing their nuclei and adhere together in abnormal clumps which appear white or silvery rather than translucent and are shed as visible scales. This can occur in many chronic inflammatory conditions of the epidermis, particularly psoriasis. When the rate of epithelial turnover is markedly slowed, e.g. in myxoedema, severe malnutrition or ichthyosis, keratinized cells may accumulate abnormally at the skin surface, which again loses its translucency and is shed in large abnormal pieces. Epithelial neoplasms may make large quantities of abnormal scale, e.g. viral warts, cutaneous horns, squamous-cell carcinomata.

Scales vary in size and colour and may be dry, moist or greasy. Scaling may occur in localized patches or be generalized over the whole skin surface. It may occur with or without obvious underlying erythema and inflammation. The major causes of scaly skin conditions are listed in *Table* S.3.

Table S.3. Scaly eruptions

Red scaly plaque
Psoriasis (Fig. S.8)
Eczema
   discoid, lichen simplex chronicus, atopic eczema,
   contact dermatitis
Dermatophyte infection (*Figs* S.9–S.11)
Lichen planus (*see Fig.* P.7)
Seborrhoeic wart
Solar keratosis
Bowen's disease

Red scaly rash
Seborrhoeic dermatitis (Fig. S.12)
Infantile seborrhoeic dermatitis
Psoriasis (Fig. P.6)
Keratoderma blenorrhagica
Parapsoriasis
   chronic superficial scaly dermatitis
   mycosis fungoides
Pityriasis versicolor
Pityriasis rosea
Secondary syphilis

Scaly papules
Guttate psoriasis (*see Fig.* P.6)
Pityriasis lichenoides chronica
Darier's disease (*see Fig.* P.2)

Red Scaly Plaque

The differential diagnosis of a red, scaly plaque is a common clinical problem. If consideration is given to the site, size, shape and quality of the plaque a diagnosis can frequently be reached. *Psoriasis* is one of the commonest of skin diseases and is also the most scaly (*Fig.* S.8). Individual plaques can be any size and can on occasions be isolated, although search in the sites of election of the disease (scalp, elbows, knees, sacrum) often reveals additional affected areas, which may not have been mentioned by the patient. Plaques have distinct, abrupt edges and are of uniform height (usually 1–2 mm), surmounted by a uniform coating of silvery scales. The scales may have been removed by bathing, emollients or treatments and if so can easily be produced by gently scratching with the fingernail; if such scratching is continued small bleeding points will eventually be revealed.

Plaques of 'dry' chronic *eczema* can be seen in

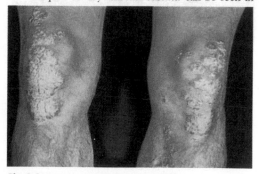

Fig S.8. Psoriasis. (*Westminster Hospital.*)

all varieties of endogenous and exogenous eczema, but most particularly as coin-sized fairly well-demarcated patches on the lower legs in middle-aged adults with *discoid eczema*; as well-demarcated, thick, lichenified plaques, with geographical outlines, on the nape of the neck, dorsa of feet and backs of hands, usually in asymmetrical distribution in *lichen simplex chronicus*; poorly demarcated thick scaly plaques over the knuckles, dorsa of hands and ankles in *atopic eczema*; in poorly demarcated beefy red scaly plaques in *contact dermatitis*, under wrist-watch buckle in *nickel dermatitis*; in poorly demarcated pink plaques with branny scales, mid-chest, mid-back, anterior hairline or nasolabial folds in *seborrhoeic dermatitis*.

Dermatophyte infection can cause isolated red scaly plaques, usually with central clearing, a raised red edge with an advancing scaly border—zoophilic fungi causing considerable inflammation and rapidly expanding rings, anthropophilic species being more indolent (*Fig*. S.9–S.11).

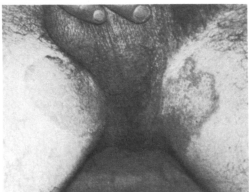

Fig. S.9. Tinea cruris. (*Dr Peter Hansell.*)

The red plaques of *lichen planus* are seldom very scaly unless on the lower legs, where they can be surmounted by considerable dry, hard, adherent verrucous scales. The underlying plaques are bluish and have a distinct polygonal outline. Oral lace-like lesions confirm the diagnosis.

Seborrhoeic warts, virtually universal on the trunks of elderly people, though surmounted by greasy scales, are usually varying shades of brown, but when irritated or secondarily infected can become red and inflamed.

On the sun-exposed skin of dorsa of hands, forehead, cheeks, pinnae and pate small thin red plaques covered with hard, irregular abrasive scale can be due to *solar keratoses*. Larger, eroded beef-red plaques may be variably scaly and due to *Bowen's disease*.

Red Scaly Rash

The diagnosis and treatment of red scaly rashes is probably the commonest cause of dermatological

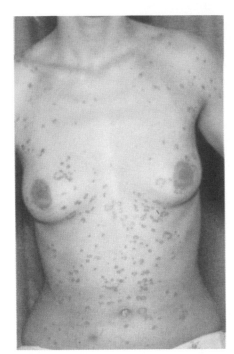

Fig S.10. Animal ringworm of body: *Microsporum canis*. (*Westminster Hospital.*)

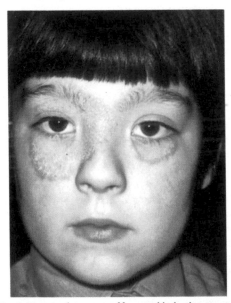

Fig. S.11. Animal ringworm of face. (*Addenbooke's Hospital.*)

referral. In *seborrhoeic dermatitis* (*Fig*. S.12) lesions are distributed in the 'seborrhoeic' areas (scalp, anterior hairline, behind ears, in external auditory meati, in eyebrows, nasolabial folds, mid-chest and mid-back). The patches are fawn-red in colour, variably itchy, poorly demarcated and often accentuated around hair follicles. One variety occurs in neonates, usually beginning with a severe cradle cap before 3 months of age—*infantile seborrhoeic dermatitis* which, though extensive and upsetting for parents, seldom causes much upset or irritation in affected babies. In adults the condition is chronic and relapsing: exacerbations are now thought to be related to the amount of pityrosporum yeast present on the skin. The yeast is lipophilic and nutrients are provided by sebum, cosmetic creams or sun tan oils. There is often an accompanying scaling dandruff (pityriasis capitis) sometimes causing very thick adherent scales and hairfall (pityriasis amientacea). This can occur as a sole manifestation of seborrhoeic dermatitis.

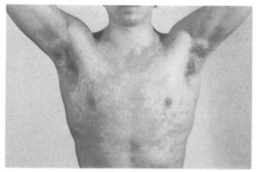

Fig. S.12. Seborrhoeic dermatitis. (*Addenbrooke's Hospital.*)

Psoriasis occurs in some 2 per cent of the population and, though showing some familial tendency, is of unknown aetiology. The usual pattern is a bout of *guttate psoriasis* (see below) in adolescence followed at a variable time by the appearance of chronic plaque disease which may wax and wane throughout most of adult life. Some plaques resolve leaving absolutely no trace; others can persist indefinitely. Itch is fortunately rare and lesions are less common on exposed than covered sites, which may in part be due to the effects of ultraviolet irradiation. Lesions often occur in areas of skin damage (Köbner phenomenon). Manifestations of the condition can clear for many years, only to recur 'out of the blue', or following infections or acute emotional upset. Some 10 per cent of patients will have nail changes—thimble pitting, onycholysis and subungual hyperkeratosis (*see* p. 437). Approximately 2 per cent will have psoriatic arthropathy—classically of sacroiliac and distal interphalangeal joints. Rare complications include exfoliative erythroderma or generalized pustulation (*generalized pustular psoriasis of von Zambusch*).

The diagnosis is usually easy but certain varieties of psoriasis pose difficulties: for example, *flexural psoriasis* where the scaling may be less obvious but plaques have a similar well-demarcated appearance; psoriasis on the glans penis, again where scaling is less obvious, and gyrate psoriasis where lesions adopt bizarre shapes and often spread widely over the body. *Keratoderma blenorrhagica* is a cutaneous reac-

tion pattern comprising thickly scaled, red plaques often in bizarre shapes and occurring chiefly on soles, palms and genitalia. Lesions have a great similarity to psoriasis but follow urethritis and are accompanied by uveitis, fever, arthralgia and sacroiliitis. This symptom complex is called *Reiter's syndrome*, and many authorities believe that it only occurs in those with the psoriatic genotype.

Parapsoriasis is the name given to lesions looking very much like psoriasis but having subtle differences in morphology and sometimes ominous differences in progression. The most benign variety of parapsoriasis is *chronic superficial scaly dermatitis* (digitate dermatitis). Here pink, lightly scaled oval lesions occur on the trunk and are usually arranged along Lange's lines of cleavage. Each lesion is not as thick as a psoriatic plaque and its scale is less profuse. They are likened to finger-daubs, hence digitate dermatitis. Lesions are remarkably constant, remaining in exactly the same site for decades. They are variably pruritic and respond well to ultraviolet light, only to recur in exactly the same site. The prognosis is benign.

Mycosis fungoides (cutaneous T-cell lymphoma) begins with red scaly patches on the body, which at this stage are very difficult to differentiate from eczema, being poorly demarcated, pruritic and variably scaled. They are less well demarcated and thinner than psoriatic plaques, but they may show serpiginous borders reminiscent of tinea corporis, from which they can only be differentiated by negative scrapings and lack of responsiveness to antifungal remedies. They are, however, remarkably persistent and after years may become infiltrated plaques, and later tumours which ulcerate and eventually involve internal lymphoreticular tissue and can be fatal. Helpful diagnostic features in the early red scaly lesions include lesions of very different sizes, bizarre serpiginous outlines and the difference in colour between individual lesions. Multiple biopsies may be necessary to establish the diagnosis.

The rash of *pityriasis versicolor* begins as pink or tan flat, annular lesions with superficial branny scaling. They usually begin on the shoulders, back and mid-chest and can spread to involve large areas; after sun exposure affected areas turn white (*see* p. 406). Scrapings of the scale reveal on microscopy the responsible lipophilic yeast. The scaly patches in *pityriasis rosea* tend to be more oval and arranged in linear distribution along Lange's lines of cleavage on the chest, back and proximal limbs. The face and extremities are spared. The prodromal larger herald patch may be seen and inspection of individual oval lesions reveals the scale to be concentrated in a collarette just inside the edge.

If lesions extend to palms and soles and are accompanied by malaise, lymphadenopathy, fever and a sore throat *secondary syphilis* should be suspected. The plaques are less pink and more of a ham colour. There is often patchy alopecia, 'snail-track' ulceration of the oral mucosa, the serology will be positive and a primary chancre may still be present.

Scaly papules

Guttate psoriasis is most commonly seen in adolescents several weeks after a streptococcal sore throat. Myriads of tiny pink flat-topped papules erupt widely over the trunk and limbs; the face, palms and soles are usually spared. The papules are all of the same age and gradually become scalier and may enlarge or coalesce into plaques. After several weeks or months the eruption subsides but chronic plaque psoriasis may supervene (*see* Figs. P.6, S.8).

The eruption must be differentiated from *pityriasis lichenoides chronica*, which affects an older age-group, does not follow a streptococcal sore throat, and where individual papules are covered by a single translucent 'mica' scale which detaches *en masse*, also where lesions are less numerous and in varying stages of evolution in different sites.

In *Darier's disease* the red papules are acuminate and perifollicular. They are often covered with a greasy brown scale and are concentrated in seborrhoeic areas including the scalp; accompanying notched nails and pitted palms are common (*see* p. 482).

Scaly palms

A unilateral scaly palm is the hallmark of *tinea manum*. The colour is of a dull lustreless greyish red and the scaling fine and concentrated in skin creases. There may be associated fungal onychodystrophy of one or many fingernails and signs of tinea elsewhere on the body. The condition is often of very long standing. Bilateral scaly symmetrical palms can be inherited as a familial trait in the extremely rare *tylosis palmaris*. The hyperkeratosis is tightly packed and yellowish in colour. Even more rare is one lineage from the north-west of England, with association of tylosis with carcinoma of the oesophagus. Similar yellowish, thick hyperkeratosis of palms is seen in *pityriasis rubra pilaris*, an uncommon condition which may be seen at all ages and accompanied by a widespread psoriasiform rash with follicular accentuation.

Scaly scalp

The scalp is one of the sites of election of *psoriasis*, where well-demarcated plaques of thick scale cause surprisingly little disturbance of hair growth. The shedding of large amounts of silvery scales from these lesions is often a source of great embarrassment for patients. *Seborrhoeic dermatitis* causes a more confluent scaly eruption and the scales are greasier and more adherent. Corroborative evidence should be sought of seborrhoeic dermatitis in the classic areas elsewhere on the skin. *Tinea capitis* usually causes asymmetrical scaling eruptions of the scalp. The hairs are usually broken off close to the surface, giving a stubbled appearance (*see* Fig. S.6).

Scaling of whole skin surface

Inflammatory skin conditions can on occasions affect the whole skin surface causing an erythroderma; when large amounts of scale are shed the term *exfoliative erythroderma* is applied. This may develop from extension of a previously diagnosed skin condition, e.g. psoriasis, or present in this manner when the diagnosis may be more difficult to establish. Possible causes include drug allergy (e.g. gold, antimalarials, sulphonamides, fansidar), severe contact dermatitis, atopic dermatitis, seborrhoeic dermatitis, psoriasis, underlying lymphoma and the Sézary syndrome.

If exfoliation is unaccompanied by underlying erythema then the cause may be an *ichthyosis*. In this the keratinization process is slowed down and scale is 'retained'. The commonest variety is a congenital *ichthyosis vulgaris*, but rarer forms exist.

Richard Staughton

Scrotum
See Hemianopia.

Scrotum, surface affections of

The skin of the scrotum may be involved in many generalized or widespread eruptions, such as drug eruptions, exanthemas or exfoliative dermatitis. On the other hand it may be the only area affected. Owing to the heat, moisture and mobility of the part, it is particularly liable to become chafed. In a bedridden patient it may be irritated by urine or faeces, or the drugs they may contain (e.g. danthron breakdown products). Acute dermatitis and intertrigo are common on scrotal skin. (*See Table* S.4.)

Acute dermatitis of the scrotum frequently follows over-treatment; the thin skin is particularly sensitive to medicaments such as those used in the treatment of pediculosis pubis or tinea cruris. *Seborrhoeic dermatitis* may affect the scrotum and be confused with *tinea*. The latter nearly always affects the neighbouring groin skin (*Fig.* S.10), has a well-defined wavy edge, and shows mycelia when the scales are examined under the microscope; moreover, patches of white macerated or scaly skin produced by the same fungus can often be found elsewhere, e.g. between the toes. It is when a seborrhoeic dermatitis of the scrotum

Table S.4. Surface affections of the scrotum

I   Generalized eruptions affecting scrotal skin
e.g. drug eruptions, exanthema, exfoliative
dermatitis

II   Confined to scrotum
a. Rashes
Irritant dermatitis
Seborrhoeic dermatitis
Tinea cruris (Fig. S.9)
Erythrasma
Psoriasis (Fig. N.19)
Syphilis
b. Malignancies
Bowen's disease, basal-cell carcinoma
Extramammary Paget's disease
c. Ulcers
Behçet's syndrome
Herpes simplex
d. Papules
Angiokeratomas of Fordyce
Scabies (Fig. N.18)
Hidradenitis suppurativa (Fig. N.47)
e. Erosions
Herpes simplex
Fixed drug eruption
f. Thickening
Lichen simplex

and groin is mistakenly treated for tinea (e.g. with Whitfield's ointment) that a particularly acute and painful dermatitis can occur.

Erythrasma occurs as a discoid plaque of a beefy, brownish-red colour covered with fine scales; unlike tinea there is no central healing and the plaques are uniform in appearance. They fluoresce pink under Wood's light and culture reveals the causative *Corynebacterium minutissimi*. Plaques of *psoriasis* can affect the scrotum, especially in flexural psoriasis (*see Fig. N. 19*). Scaling is less prominent at this site but plaques will have the typical well-defined edge and salmon pink colour. There should be evidence of psoriasis elsewhere on the body (e.g. elbows, knees, sacrum and scalp) (*Fig. S.8*).

Syphilis gives rise to moist papules or serpiginous, erythematous patches and ulcers; however, in contrast with dermatitis, the whole of the scrotal skin is not affected, itching is absent and the serology will be positive. Hard and soft chancres may affect the scrotum as well as other parts of the genitals; the differential diagnosis is discussed under SCROTUM, ULCERATION OF.

Boils, warts, sebaceous cysts and tumours are referred to under TESTICULAR SWELLING. Some scrotal neoplasms may cause non-healing erosive and ulcerating lesions; for example, *Bowen's disease, basal-cell carcinoma* and rarely *extramammary Paget's disease*. Moles and malignant melanomas can also occur on scrotal skin.

Ulceration of the scrotum may be a feature of

Behçet's syndrome, the features of which are recurrent orogenital ulceration, together with iritis, keratitis, diffuse pustulation, polyarthritis, thrombophlebitis, and sometimes neural infarcts.

Small angiomas are very common on the scrotum in elderly persons: they are called *angiokeratomas of Fordyce*. Small nodules on the scrotum and penis are characteristic of *scabies* (*see Fig. N.18*). Discharging nodular lesions on the scrotum, spreading into the groins and often affecting the axillae, are seen in *hidradenitis suppurativa* (Fig. N.47).

Recurrent erosions in the same site can be caused by both *herpes simplex* and *fixed drug eruptions*. In the former case multiple vesicles and minimal scarring will be seen. In the latter case considerable post-inflammatory hyper-pigmentation is the rule, and a carefully taken drug history will usually reveal the culprit (e.g. codeine, laxatives, and sulphonamides).

In *lichen simplex chronicus* the habit of regular rubbing and scratching leads to considerable thickening and lichenification of the skin; this is common in peri-anal skin but also occurs on the scrotum.

Richard Staughton

Scrotum, ulceration of

Ulceration of the scrotum occurs in association with:

1   New growth:
Carcinoma
Papilloma
2   Fistula
3   Syphilis
4   Testicular disease:
Inflammatory
Tuberculous
Syphilitic
Malignant growths
5   Suppurating cysts
6   Infected haematocele
7   Irritants and corrosives, such as mustard gas
8   Behçet's syndrome, herpes simplex, candidiasis.

1. New growth

Carcinoma of the scrotum, formerly known as 'chimney-sweep's cancer', or 'tar-worker's cancer', is by no means limited to these occupations, but is certainly more common in men engaged in work in which they are exposed to much irritation from solid particles or from noxious fumes. Hence the disease is, or was, most commonly seen amongst chimney-sweeps, employees in gas works, paraffin, tar and chemical works, and coal mines and in mule-spinners in the cotton trade. It often begins as a small subcutaneous nodule, over which the skin is thinned and adherent; the nodule enlarges slowly, and the thinned covering gives way to form an ulcer with thickened irregular edges and a tendency to bleed on slight injury. The ulcerated area extends both radially and into the tissues of the scrotum, later involving the testes. The inguinal nodes become enlarged soon after active ulceration begins, at first from inflammatory causes, later from malignant infiltration and, untreated, themselves ulcerate; this indeed is the common mode of death in this condition, from repeated haemorrhages. In other cases a scrotal epithelioma begins in a *wart* or *papilloma*, which may have been present for years with only slight increase in growth (*Fig.* S.13). These soft papillomas are not unusually the starting-point of malignant change, when they become more vascular, while the surface epithelium becomes thinned and easily excoriated. A small amount of foul discharge is present, often encrusted into a scab, which on removal leaves an ulcer with indurated, everted edges, with the gradual progress of a cutaneous epithelioma. Any ulcer on the scrotum, especially if indurated or readily caused to bleed, must be looked upon with extreme suspicion and immediately subjected to biopsy for microscopic examination. It is not unusual, however, for a large mass of nodes to be found in the groin when the primary lesion is very small and almost imperceptible. The scrotum must be examined very carefully in such cases lest the primary lesion be missed.

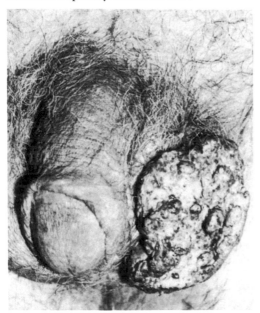

Fig S.13. Epithelioma of scrotum.

2. Fistula

Fistulas may occur in the scrotum and cause ulceration. Sinuses occur in association with tuberculosis or syphilitic disease of the testes, but fistulas may follow urine extravasation, or burrowing from rectal suppuration. An abscess may form and open through the scrotal skin from a peri-urethral abscess accompanying an acute urethritis or formed by septic infection behind a urethral stricture. In either case a small amount of urine may leak through the opening during micturition while the history of urethral discharge, or of difficulty in micturition and other symptoms of stricture, will point to the diagnosis.

3. Syphilis of the scrotum

This may be present either as a primary chancre or as a mucous tubercle. A *primary chancre* in this situation is by no means easy to recognize unless other signs of syphilis are present; but the presence of a cutaneous sore which does not show much inclination to heal under antiseptic dressings should always give a suspicion of syphilis. There is often only slight induration of the ulcer compared with that of a penile chancre, but the edge is raised and of a rolled appearance. The inguinal lymph nodes are enlarged and discrete, and some 5 to 6 weeks after the commencement of the ulcer the usual secondary symptoms of syphilis become manifest.

Mucous tubercles may be present on the scrotum, usually on the femoral aspect. They may extend directly from the anal area. No difficulty will be met with in the diagnosis, as other signs of syphilis are obvious.

4. Testicular disease

In some cases extension of disease in the testicle may involve the coverings of the scrotum, and may even perforate them to form a scrotal sore. This sequence occasionally occurs with: (1) A testicular abscess; (2) Tuberculosis of the epididymis; (3) Gumma of the testis; (4) Malignant disease of the testis.

A *testicular abscess* is somewhat uncommon, but may arise from direct extension from the urethra via the vesiculae seminales and vasa deferentia or by a haematogenous infection during the course of a specific fever, such as scarlet fever, mumps or typhoid fever. With urethral disease, the primary trouble may be due to gonorrhoea, or more frequently to a septic urethritis from the introduction of infected instruments. In cases in which the infective process extends from the urethra the epididymis is affected first, while in the metastatic cases the body of the testis usually shows the first sign of enlargement. If the vas has been divided as part of the operation of prostatectomy, or sometimes following vasectomy for sterilization, the swelling and possible abscess will occur in the upper part of the scrotum at the site of the division. These acute inflammations of the testis occasionally suppurate, when the scrotal tunics become inflamed and adherent, whilst softening occurs later, and unless surgically relieved the abscess opens through the skin, leaving an ulcer, and a sinus discharging pus. An unusual form of abscess of the testicle is caused by a *suppurating dermoid cyst* of the testicle, and may discharge through the scrotal coverings to form an ulcer.

Tuberculosis of the testicle rarely occurs as a primary disease but more often as a secondary deposit in association with tuberculosis elsewhere in the genito-urinary tract. Testicular tubercle almost always begins as a nodule in the epididymis, but in the later progress of the disease may extend into the testis proper. If the tuberculous nodule progresses rather than undergoes cure, the scrotal skin becomes adherent, thinned, and finally perforated, leaving a shallow ulcer with thin, undermined edges and discharging thin pus. The ulcer in this case is most likely to be on the posterior aspect of the scrotum. Occasionally the necrotic epididymis fungates through the opening in the scrotum, appearing as a greyish, sloughy projection from the cutaneous opening—the so-called 'hernia testis'.

A *gumma of the testis* (once common, now very rare), causes a swelling in the body of the testis rather than in the epididymis. A gumma which remains unrecognized or untreated may soften and ulcerate through the scrotal skin in a manner similar to tuberculous disease, leaving a clearly defined ulcerated area with sharply cut margins and a wash-leather-like sloughy base. Such ulcers are usually placed on the front of the scrotum. The gummatous granulation tissue may fungate through the scrotal aperture, forming a yellowish necrotic mass.

The diagnosis of these three conditions may produce some difficulty in the earlier stages (*see* TESTICULAR SWELLING), but in the advanced stage now under consideration, when an open scrotal sore is present, the diagnosis is easier.

The *opening of a testicular abscess* on the scrotum leaves a small sinus discharging pus and accompanied by a general enlargement of the organ. Preceding the rupture of the abscess there is acute pain in the testicle, with rise of temperature, rigors and general signs of suppuration, which are much diminished as soon as the abscess bursts or is incised. There is often a urethral discharge, which, however, is frequently much lessened with the onset of the acute epididymitis, with distinct thickening of the cord and aching pain in the neighbourhood of the external abdominal ring. In metastatic cases the abscess occurs during the progress of an acute fever. The general history is one of acute pain beginning in the testicle, with rapid and extremely tender swelling of the organ, followed by abscess formation.

In *tuberculosis of the testis* the progress is much more gradual. A nodule may have been present in the epididymis for some time, gradually enlarging, but causing very little pain; in some cases a nodule may have been present for months without any apparent change, and then it may enlarge rapidly, involve the scrotal tunics, and discharge its contents. By the time the disease has reached this stage it is probable that evidence of tuberculosis will be found in other organs, particularly the other testis, prostate, seminal vesicles or bladder. The affected testicle usually presents several nodules in the epididymis, tender on pressure, whilst small nodules may also be felt in the vas deferens.

The opening remaining from the discharge of a *gummatous orchitis* is usually a rounded ulcer with sharply cut edges and yellowish base. The whole testis is enlarged and practically painless. The cord is not thickened, and there is no evidence of disease in the other testicle, prostate or seminal vesicles. There is probably a history of syphilis, and other tertiary syphilitic lesions may be present elsewhere, such as gummatous periostitis.

A *hernial protrusion of necrotic testicular tissue* may be present either with tuberculous disease or from a gumma. In tuberculosis the mass is greyish and necrotic, discharging thin pus, and there will be evidence of tuberculous disease in the underlying testis and other genital organs. Tubercle bacilli very rarely may be found in the discharge. A distinctive feature of the gummatous hernia testis is found in the appearance of the cutaneous opening; if the fungating mass is pushed aside the opening in the scrotal skin will be seen to be cleanly cut and to encircle the protruding tissue tightly. The fungating hernia testis of tubercle or syphilis must also be diagnosed from other conditions producing a raised tumour on the scrotum. An epithelioma of the scrotum has raised borders, but the centre is excavated, and there is rarely any enlargement of the testis. A sloughing papilloma of the scrotum may more nearly reproduce the appearance, but the tumour and the skin are freely movable on the underlying testis, while in hernia testis the mass is connected with the testicle, and the tubular structure of the latter is often apparent on picking up a small fragment of the fungating tumour.

New growths of the testis seldom cause ulceration of the scrotum because they have generally been removed by operation before so late a stage is reached; any variety, however, whether seminoma or teratoma, may cause local recurrence in the scar, with ulceration; the diagnosis depends upon histological examination, either of the tumour previously removed or of a biopsy from the edge of the recurrence. Occasionally fungation of the tumour is seen through the scar of the biopsy site in the scrotal skin when there has been delay in carrying out definitive treatment, a state of affairs which should never be allowed to happen.

5. Cysts of the scrotum

A sebaceous cyst in the scrotal skin may suppurate and leave an open sore. The areas remaining present raised borders, and are easily mistaken for an early epithelioma. An accurate history of the previous swelling in the skin is of little assistance in these cases, but microscopical examination of a piece removed from the margin of the ulcer will exclude malignancy. A suppurating cyst in the scrotum is less common than epithelioma.

6. Haematocele

A haematocele which becomes infected may form an abscess which bursts through the scrotal coverings. It may have a superficial resemblance to a gumma.

7. Mustard gas

Mustard gas caused most troublesome ulceration of the scrotum, as of other parts, during the war of 1914–18; but the diagnosis is easy if the correct history of exposure to this or some other irritant is available.

8. Behçet's syndrome

Behçet's syndrome causes painful ulcerative lesions of the scrotum as well as the penis, unlike the lesions in the vulva and vagina, which are often painless and therefore often missed. Behçet's may be accompanied by abscess or herpes-like lesions of the scrotum. Herpes simplex, both types I and II, may cause vesicular lesions less commonly, and very rarely candidiasis.

Harold Ellis

Self-harm, deliberate

Deliberate self-harm, sometimes termed parasuicide, remains the commonest reason for emergency hospital care in young adults, accounting for 10 per cent of all acute admissions or about 100 000 cases each year in England and Wales.

The initial management is of course the medical and/or surgical evaluation and treatment of the physical presentation. Psychosocial assessment of the behaviour takes place subsequently when the patient is fit to be interviewed, which may not coincide with when physical evidence of toxicity has subsided.

The first psychological task is to confirm whether deliberate self-harm actually took place, and to accomplish this the account of an individual close to the patient is always desirable and may prove essential. The types of self-harm are listed in (*Table* S.5.).

Table S.5. Types of self-harm

Commonest
Deliberate
Less common
Experimental
Accidental
Feigned
Self-mutilation in the mentally impaired

Feigned self-poisoning is by no means rare, suspicions being raised by atypical symptoms, responses or behaviour and the absence of confirmatory physical signs or evidence. Such patients may be habitual self-poisoners who eventually only go through the motions, or may be a self-referral from out of town with a dramatic story and no corroboration available when the possibility of Munchausen's syndrome should be considered. Gains from simulating self-harm may sometimes emerge later from another source.

Experimental self-poisoning is usually evident from the drugs taken and the account of somebody present at the time. Commonest are illicit substances such as opiates, barbiturates, amphetamines, magic mushrooms and solvents, but prescribed drugs, particularly minor tranquillizers, hypnotics, analgesics, anticholinergics and inhalers are taken for this purpose and proprietary medicines such as Actifed and Benylin may also be abused. It should not be uncritically assumed that the employment of an illicit substance necessarily implies that the purpose of the act was for recreation— the circumstances must also be taken into account.

Accidental self-poisoning can be harder to establish and if doubt persists the patient should be considered to have acted deliberately. This problem occurs most commonly when the patient's judgement was impaired by alcohol, drugs, or other physical causes of confusion, with an invariably sketchy recall of events. The most difficult situation is the depressed elderly individual recently prescribed antidepressants, when heavy reliance has to be placed on a relative's observations of changes in behaviour and mental functioning in the days leading up to the overdose: such presentations are not uncommonly caused by good compliance with a large dose of medication leading to anticholinergic-induced confusion. The necessity for an independent account is crucial in cases where accident is asserted by the patient, as this may be a ploy for evading recognition in an acutely suicidal person.

Deliberate self-harm or *self-mutilation in people with more profound degrees of mental impairment* is usually regarded as distinct from parasuicide in that these patients have diminished judgement which raises doubts their capability to form intent. However self-injurious behaviour should never be assumed to be acceptable or normal in the mentally handicapped: its origins may lie in factors as diverse as epilepsy, manic depressive psychosis, understimulation and relationship problems within the family.

Table S.6. Profile of suicidal risk factors

1. *Circumstances surrounding the act*
   Evidence of planning and timing
   Evidence of precautions against discovery
   No communication or seeking help afterwards
   Suicide note, will, gifts, insurance changes

2. *Self-report about the act*
   Expectations of fatality
   Concepts of method's lethality and reversibility
      (more important than quantity taken)
   Intention/motive(s)

3. *Sociodemographical variables*
   Male
   Middle-aged or elderly
   Widowed,* divorced,* separated* or single
   Unemployment*
   Social isolation or rejection*
   Financial difficulties*

4. *Physical variables*
   Any disabling, painful, chronic or life-threatening
      illness*
   Epilepsy

5. *Psychological variables*
   Family history of suicide
   Previous deliberate self-harm or psychiatric history
   Alcoholism or drug addiction
   Personality disorder
   Schizophrenia (especially during a quiescent phase)
   Depression especially if
   a. suicidal ideation/impulses
   b. pessimism
   c. self-denigration
   d. hypochondriacal or guilt delusions
   e. self-neglect
   f. sleep disturbance
   g. mood is cycling
   h. early stages of treatment
   Hopelessness—may be the single most important
      predictor, irrespective of mood state

* Especially if this represents recent, abrupt change.

Having ascertained deliberate self-harm has occurred the next step is *to evaluate the act*, and it is important to appreciate that parasuicide is a common endpoint of behaviour, not a medical diagnosis. The circumstances surrounding the act are a pointer to the degree of suicide intent while the events leading up to taking the decision also help to establish motive(s). It is crucial to understand that the majority of patients who deliberately harm themselves have no wish to kill themselves: other common motives include ridding oneself of unpleasant feelings, escaping from a stressful situation, obtaining help (the classic 'cry for help'), and as a form of communication with another person.

Next, precipitating and vulnerability factors should be inquired about in the patient' social and personal history. Symptoms of mental illness, especially depression should be specifically sought. Recent life events, especially losses and interpersonal difficulties,

are particularly important. Other background factors that are associated with increased suicidal risk are presented in *Table* S.6. Finally, mental state assessment should seek objective evidence of mental illness as well as considering continuing suicidal risk. How the patient views their action and their future are essential inquiries; hopelessness is consistently reported to be strongly associated with subsequent self-harm and suicide.

This interview is often more difficult than usual situations because it rarely takes place at the patient's request. Resentment at the suggestion of a psychiatric label, embarrassment about the behaviour with fear of the consequences, and unwillingness to disclose the true motive may all lead to poor compliance while the lingering effects of alcohol or drugs may subtly impair the mental state. Nevertheless, it is important to persevere for three purposes: (1) the identification of treatable mental disorder; (2) the identification of issues where intervention may help the patient and thus (hopefully) reduce the likelihood of recurrence; and (3) the evaluation of suicidal risk.

Much effort has been spent upon refining methods of identifying high-risk groups with the aim of preventing suicide but this has proved of little practical value because suicide is a very uncommon early outcome even among patients who have demonstrated high lethality in their attempt. Default rates in follow-up are around 50 per cent and treatment interventions have generally proved ineffective in preventing recurrent parasuicide, even when social stressors are alleviated and the patient reports improved satisfaction with life. The problem may be that not enough is understood yet about this behaviour when the circumstances do not fit the medical model, i.e. is not a failed attempt at suicide in a person suffering from serious mental illness.

George Masterton

Sensation, abnormalities of

Sensory disturbances are referred to in many sections of this book but it is convenient to consider the subject as a whole under the present heading.

Terminology

The inaccurate application of an exact terminology gives rise to so much confusion in the literature that it is often preferable to describe sensory experiences and sensory findings in plain language. 'Paraesthesia' is used for sensations of tingling, pins-and-needles, subjective numbness and feelings of cold and heat whether they appear spontaneously or as a result of touching or manipulating the part. Since the term covers so many different sensations, it should be avoided when precise descriptive work is required, as for instance in case histories.

Anaesthesia means 'without feeling', but neurologists use it for loss of sensibility to light touch; partial reduction of such sensibility is called 'hypoaesthesia' or 'hypaesthesia'. Analgesia (loss of pain) and hypoalgesia or hypalgesia (reduction of pain sensibility) are useful terms, free from ambiguity. Thermanaesthesia and thermhypaesthesia (loss of, and reduction of, temperature sensibility) are explicit if inelegant. These cutaneous sensibilities together with those derived from the special senses are called 'exteroceptive'. 'Proprioceptive' sensibility is concerned with information received from the labyrinths and from muscle and joint receptors. Vibration sense is difficult to classify and is of no apparent value to the individual, but its loss may help to localize a lesion, especially of the spinal cord.

Hyperaesthesia, hyperalgesia and hyperthermaesthesia refer to increased sensibility to touch, pain and temperature respectively. Increased sensibility to proprioceptive stimulation has not been described.

Anatomy and physiology

The four common cutaneous sensations—touch, pain, heat and cold—together with the deep sensations of pressure and proprioception are referred to as the somatic sensations. These are consciously appreciated in all parts of the body and have a common pathway within the nervous system. An appropriate stimulus generates an impulse at the periphery which passes into the central nervous system, is relayed by the thalamus, and thence, by a final relay, is passed to the appropriate part of the cerebral cortex. In simple terms, the pathway for somatic sensation is subserved by three orders of neurones: the first-order neurone is concerned with transmitting information from the periphery to the spinal cord; the second-order neurone transmits information from the spinal cord to the thalamus, and the third-order neurone transmits information from the thalamus to the cerebral cortex.

Receptors

Information to the first-order neurones comes from a variety of receptors. Every sensation depends on impulses excited by the adequate stimulation of these receptors, which comprise two main groups—those in skin and those in the deeper somatic structures. Many morphological variants have been described, although with a few exceptions it has not been possible to ascribe specific functions to each. Although individual cutaneous sensory receptors are most sensitive to a particular form of natural stimulation, this specificity is not absolute and other forms of stimulation may also excite the receptors.

Transmission of information from receptors

Stimulation of a sensory ending gives rise to a receptor potential which appears at the specialized end of an afferent nerve fibre. This is not an all-or-none phenomenon, but varies in amplitude and time course and may be rapidly dissipated even though the stimulus continues, with resulting falling away of the firing frequency in the nerve fibre. Impulses from the receptors travel centrally through the first-order neurones, the cell bodies of which are in the dorsal root ganglia. The fibres are of varying calibre and are classified into groups A, B and C. Group C comprises unmyelinated axons, with diameters ranging from less than 1 μm up to 2 μm, and with conduction velocities of from 0·7 to 2 m/s. A and B fibres are myelinated, those in the B group being the preganglionic neurones of the autonomic nervous system of mammals. The (myelinated) axons of the A group have been subdivided into groups alpha, beta, gamma and delta, with alpha A fibres having the fastest conduction velocity and delta A fibres the slowest.

Different types of fibres transmit different sensory modalities. Alpha and beta fibres transmit information from tactile receptors, whereas gamma and delta fibres transmit heat, cold and certain information concerned with pain. The ratio between receptors and neurones varies: Pacinian corpuscles, which are sensitive to displacement and vibration, have a one-to-one ratio with primary afferent fibres; that is to say, the peripheral end of a single fibre branches to supply one receptor.

The afferent pathways to the spinal cord

The afferent sensory fibres from the various receptors pass up the differing peripheral nerves and enter the spinal cord via the dorsal roots. To understand the variety of peripheral nerve disturbances that may occur requires knowledge of the anatomy of the distribution of peripheral sensory nerves and sensory roots. It should be emphasized that there is considerable overlap in the peripheral nerve distributions and in the dermatome distributions.

There is some evidence to suggest that a number of afferent fibres enter the cord in the ventral roots. The significance of these is uncertain but their presence may be responsible for the persistence of pain in some patients after dorsal rhizotomy.

Somatic sensory pathways

All the somatic sensory pathways are crossed and terminate in the opposite sensory cortex in the cerebral hemisphere. Three anatomically separate pathways may be recognized.

Dorsal column medial lemniscus pathway

Input to this pathway within the spinal cord is via large thickly myelinated fibres which pass through the medial division of the dorsal spinal nerve root to enter the dorsal white column of their own side, dividing into ascending and descending branches. The descending branches establish reflex connections by sending collateral branches into the dorsal grey column; the ascending branches are the first link in the sensory pathway. At their entrance these ascending fibres are situated immediately medial to the dorsal horn, but during their course up the spinal cord they are steadily pushed to a more medial position because the fibres entering at succeeding rostral levels intrude between the ascending fibres and the dorsal horn. As a consequence of this, the fibres occupying the most medial part of the dorsal column in the upper cervical region will belong to the sacral roots, whilst the fibres from the upper extremity are found most laterally. The fibres terminate at the cervico-medullary junction in the nucleus gracilis and nucleus cuneatus. The fibres terminate synaptically on to the second-order neurones in the gracile and cuneate nuclei and the axons of these neurones curve ventrally and medially, crossing the midline, and the turn upwards to form a prominent bundle of fibres, the medial lemniscus.

The classical view is that the impulses ascending in the fibres of the dorsal columns mediate the sensations of touch, deep pressure, vibratory sense and sense of position of joints and are particularly important for sensory discrimination. During the past few years this view has been challenged and, although the matter is far from certain, it appears that the dorsal columns mediate sensory signals necessary for complex discriminative tasks.

The segmental somatotopic organization present in the dorsal columns and their nuclei is maintained in the medial lemniscus as it ascends to the thalamus where the fibres enter the ventro-posterior lateral nucleus which contains the cell bodies of the third-order sensory neurones.

SPINOTHALAMIC PATHWAY

This transmits impulses which are concerned with the appreciation of heat, cold and pain. It also provides an alternative pathway for touch sensibility—so-called crude or coarse touch. The first-order neurones have their cell bodies in the dorsal root ganglia and their fibres are thinner than those of the dorsal column medial lemniscus pathway; some, indeed (the C fibres),

have no myelin at all. They enter the spinal cord in the lateral part of the dorsal root and divide into short descending and ascending branches. The ascending branches run for one or two segments in the posterolateral column before synapsing with second-order sensory neurones which lie deep in the dorsal column. The axons then cross the midline, the so-called ventral white commissure, and ascend in the ventrolateral white column as the spinothalamic tract. Some authors recommend that the spinothalamic tract can be divided into a lateral and a ventral portion, but this is probably an unnecessary subdivision. Some of the spinothalamic fibres give off collaterals to certain nuclear regions such as the reticular formation.

In the brain stem the spinothalamic tract lies lateral to the medial lemniscus which it accompanies to terminate in the thalamus in the ventroposterior lateral nucleus. Important features of the spinothalamic pathway include the following:

1. The second-order neurone fibres cross the midline only one or two segments above the level of entry of the dorsal root fibres.
2. The site of decussation of the fibres in the cord exposes them to damage by expanding ventral cord lesions.
3. Fibres concerned with pain and temperature sensibility are situated dorsally to those involved with touch and pressure.
4. The spinothalamic tract is less compactly organized than the medial lemniscus, being intermingled with other ascending pathways giving off collaterals to the brain stem reticular formation.

THE TRIGEMINOTHALAMIC PATHWAY

This pathway carries information from the distribution of the trigeminal nerve which serves most of the skin of the face, the forehead as far as the vertex, the mucous membranes of the nasal cavities, paranasal sinuses, mouth, tongue and parts of the pharynx, the teeth and gums, and part of the dura mater.

About half of the fibres entering in the trigeminal nerve divide into a branch which terminates in the chief nucleus of the trigeminal nerve and the other half descends in the spinal tract to end in the spinal nucleus. The chief nucleus, which is in the lateral part of the pons, contains the second-order neurones concerned with tactile and postural sensibility; it gives rise to fibres which cross the midline to ascend near the medial lemniscus. The nucleus of the spinal tract, which extends downwards in the lateral part of the medulla to about the level of C2, contains the second-order neurones concerned with pain and temperature sensibility. The ophthalmic division of the trigeminal nerve terminates in the more caudal part and the mandibular division terminates in the most cephalic part of the nucleus. Second-order neurones cross to the quintothalamic tract which ascends close to the spinothalamic tract. Both sets of second-order neurone fibres terminate in the ventroposterior medial nucleus of the thalamus.

A small group of trigeminal first-order sensory fibres terminate in the mesencephalic nucleus and are thought to be important in proprioceptive reflexes concerned with chewing and regulating the strength of the bite.

The thalamus and thalamocortical projections

The third neuronal link in the ascending somatic sensory fibre system is made up of neurones the nuclei of which are in the thalamus. The axons of these neurones transmit impulses to the cerebral cortex.

As previously mentioned, the ventrolateral posterior nucleus of the thalamus receives fibres from the medial lemniscus; the fibres from the gracile nucleus end most laterally and those from the cuneate nucleus most medially. The exact area of termination of the spinothalamic fibres has been the subject of much controversy, although many believe that they terminate in the ventroposterior lateral nucleus. There is now a considerable amount of information to suggest that the medial part of the posterior complex of the thalamus represents a terminal area of spinothalamic fibres and the available physiological evidence suggests that this nucleus has a role in central pain mechanisms.

The somatosensory cortical areas

From clinical and physiological observations it has been known for many years that the postcentral gyrus in man is the main (primary) somatosensory area. Another area beneath the lower end of the postcentral gyrus is known as the secondary somatosensory area. Since the work of Penfield, it has been known that there is a clear somatotopic representation in the sensory cortex. The first sensory area appears principally to reflect activity in the dorsal column medial lemniscus system and also in the associated trigeminal system. The thalamic relay for these impulses passes through the internal capsule.

There is still debate as to whether thermal and painful stimuli are related to the first cortical somatosensory area. Some evidence suggests that there is such a relay to the second somatosensory cortical area, although our understanding of the sensory cortex is hindered by its complexity. What is known so far of the somatosensory cortical areas is that they are not functionally equivalent and each has specific tasks.

However inadequate our understanding of the sensory cortex, one thing is clear: provided that the subcortical structures—especially the thalamus—are intact, certain sensations such as pain, touch, pressure and extremes of temperature can reach consciousness.

The accurate localization, however, as well as the patient's ability to make sensory discriminations, depend on the integrity of the sensory cortex. This is a fundamental distinction and will be discussed further when considering individual sensory syndromes.

Patterns of sensory disturbance

MONONEUROPATHY

Changes in this instance will vary, depending on whether the nerve involved is predominantly motor, sensory or mixed. In sensory nerves the area of touch loss is usually more extensive than the area of pain loss. Because of overlap from adjacent nerves the area of sensory loss following damage to a cutaneous nerve is always less than its anatomical distribution. Deep pressure and joint position senses remain intact because they are mediated by nerve fibres from the subcutaneous structures and joints. Particular types of pathological lesion may differentially affect the fibres in a sensory nerve. Compression typically disturbs large touch and pressure fibres and leaves intact small pain, thermal and autonomic fibres. Lesions of the brachial or lumbosacral plexus may be differentiated from multiple peripheral nerve involvement by the distribution of the sensory and motor loss.

POLYNEUROPATHY

In most instances of polyneuropathy the longest and largest fibres tend to be involved. The sensory loss is most severe over the feet and legs and less severe over the hands, and the trunk and face are usually spared except in the most severe cases. Typically, the sensory loss involves all the modalities, although this varies depending on the type of neuropathy. The term 'glove and stocking' sensory loss draws attention to the distal pattern of involvement. However, it is an inaccurate term as the border between normal and abnormal sensation is not sharp and the sensory loss shades off gradually. In hysteria the border between normal and abnormal sensation is usually sharp.

RADICULOPATHY

Irritative symptoms may be present when the dorsal roots are the subject of traction or compression. This shows itself as pain which is often limited to the dermatome belonging to the affected root. In some root disorders pain is absent and paraesthesiae in the dermatome distribution are present. Damage to a dorsal root will result in loss of sensory modalities of all types within the distribution of the dermatome. Because of overlap between dermatomes, interruption of one single dorsal root will often give no definite sensory loss. When two or more roots have been completely divided, the zone of sensory loss is usually greater for pain than for touch. Surrounding the area of complete loss will be a zone of partial loss.

Spinal cord syndromes

LESIONS OF THE DORSAL HORN (THE TABETIC SYNDROME)

Lesions of the dorsal horn produce syndromes similar to those seen in lesions of the dorsal roots. Depending on the number of segments involved, there will be a segmental sensory loss affecting vibration and position senses in particular. Accompanying this may be pain which often is called 'lightning pain'. This repeated severe pain is described as occurring at right angles to the skin and penetrating through the affected limb. Most commonly this syndrome results from neurosyphilis, although it may be seen in diabetes mellitus.

TRANSVERSE CORD LESIONS

A complete transverse lesion of the spinal cord will be associated with loss of all forms of sensation below the segmental level which corresponds to the lesion. There may be a narrow band of hyperaesthesia at the upper margin of the level of sensory loss. Loss of pain, temperature and touch sensation is usually evident two or three segments below the level of the lesion, whereas vibratory and position sense is less easy to delimit. A compressive cord lesion is usually associated with ascending loss of sensation as the outermost fibres carrying pain and temperature sensation are from the legs. A lesion expanding from the centre of the cord, such as an intramedullary tumour, will tend to involve the innermost fibres carrying pain and temperature sensation and thus there may be relative sparing of the most superficial fibres from the sacral segments; this may lead to so-called 'sacral sparing'.

HEMISECTION OF THE SPINAL CORD (THE BROWN-SÉQUARD SYNDROME)

Occasionally in spinal cord disorders pathology is limited to one side of the spinal cord. Loss of pain and temperature sensation is found on the opposite side and the upper margin of this is usually two or three segments below the level of the lesion. Proprioceptive sensation is affected on the same side as the lesion and an associated motor paralysis occurs on the same side. Touch sensation is not involved, because the fibres are distributed in both posterior columns and the spinothalamic pathway on both sides of the cord. In clinical practice a complete hemisection of the spinal cord is rarely seen, although a partial syndrome occurs in multiple sclerosis.

CENTRAL SPINAL CORD LESIONS (THE SYRINGOMYELIC SYNDROME)

A central spinal cord lesion characteristically will involve the pain and temperature fibres as they cross in the anterior commissure. Typically, these modalities are affected on one or both sides over a number of dermatomes, with relative preservation of tactile sensation (so-called dissociated sensory loss). Abolition of tendon reflexes in the affected segment is usually seen. The commonest cause of this syndrome is syringomyelia but intramedullary tumours, such as gliomas or ependymomas, may also produce it.

THE POSTERIOR COLUMN SYNDROME

In lesions preferentially affecting the dorsal columns there is loss of vibration and position sense below the level of the lesion, with preservation of pain, temperature and touch. When such sensory loss affects the legs there is typically a sensory ataxia and a positive Romberg's sign. Sensory loss of this type in the hands produces clumsiness when manipulating small objects and inability to recognize shapes such as coins in the pocket. Tingling and pins-and-needles sensations are common and patients often complain that the hands and feet feel swollen or tight.

THE ANTERIOR CORD SYNDROME

In anterior cord disturbances there is typically damage to the spinothalamic tracts producing pain and temperature loss below the level of the lesion.

Brain stem syndromes

Because of the complex structure of the brain stem, with multiple ascending and descending tracts intermingled with a variety of cranial nerve nuclei, lesions result in far more complex clinical pictures than those which may be seen in spinal cord disorders. A characteristic feature of a medullary or lower pontine lesion is that the sensory disorder is crossed, i.e. there is loss of pain and temperature sensation on one side of the face and on the opposite side of the body. This results from involvement of the trigeminal tract or nucleus, resulting in ipsilateral facial sensory loss, and of the lateral spinothalamic tract, resulting in contralateral loss of sensation of the trunk and limbs. Higher in the brain stem, the trigeminothalamic and lateral spinothalamic tracts run together and a lesion will therefore produce contralateral loss of pain and temperature sense on the whole of the opposite side of the body. In the upper brain stem the spinothalamic tract and the medial lemniscus become confluent, so that a lesion at this level may cause contralateral sensory loss of all types.

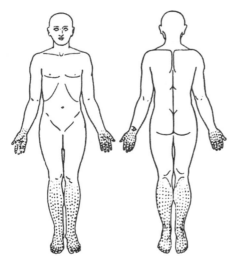

Fig. S.14. Peripheral neuritis. 'Glove and stocking anaesthesia'. Cotton-wool and pin-prick sensibility impaired or lost over the dotted areas. This is associated with hyperalgesia of the underlying muscles.

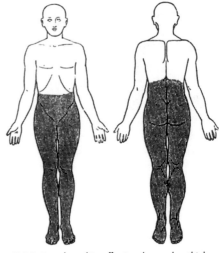

Fig. S.16. Dorsal myelitis affecting the cord as high as the 9th dorsal segment. The shaded parts are insensitive to touch, pain and all degrees of temperature.

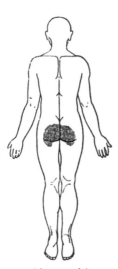

Fig. S.15. Comminuted fracture of the sacrum, with injury to the 3rd, 4th and 5th sacral roots, complete loss of sensibility to touch, pain, heat and cold resulted in the shaded area.

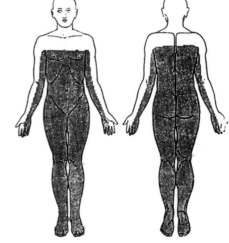

Fig. S.17. Fracture-dislocation of the cervical spine. The shaded area represents the loss of sensibility to touch, pain, heat and cold.

Thalamic disorders

Thalamic sensory disorders usually result from discrete cerebral infarcts. A destruction of the entire thalamic area receiving sensory fibre systems would be expected to result in an impairment or loss of somatic sensation in the whole of the opposite half of the body. In documented cases where such a lesion was identified, the perception of pain has often been found to be only slightly affected. Position sense typically is affected more profoundly than any other sensory function. Pure lesions of the ventroposterior lateral nucleus of the thalamus will be associated with contralateral sensory disorders of the limbs and trunk, whereas involvement

In brain stem lesions there is frequently bilateral involvement and a variety of syndromes have been described involving sensory, motor and cerebellar dysfunction accompanied by cranial nerve palsies. Lesions, particularly vascular lesions, are rarely discrete and it requires a detailed knowledge of the anatomical structure of the brain stem to achieve accurate localization. Another point of practical importance is that partial involvement of the sensory tracts may produce sensory impairment which may mimic lesions in the cord.

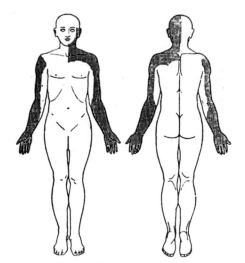

Fig. S.18. Syringomyelia. The shaded parts show the areas of dissociated anaesthesia, i.e. of thermo-anaesthesia and analgesia. This was associated with atrophic palsy of the upper extremities.

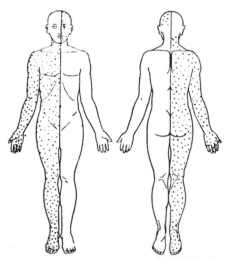

Fig. S.19. Thrombosis of the left posterior inferior cerebellar artery. The dotted areas show the regions of dissociated anaesthesia, i.e. loss of sensibility to pain and temperature of all degrees.

of the ventroposterior medial nucleus will produce sensory impairment of the contralateral face.

In thalamic disorders there is often accompanying spontaneous pain or discomfort. These thalamic pains are often very intense and occur in paroxysms affecting the opposite side of the body. They typically are more pronounced in the face, hand or lower leg and are uncommon on the trunk.

Cortical disorders

Circumscribed lesions of the postcentral gyrus will be followed by localized sensory loss in parts of the opposite half of the body. This is typically a loss of discriminatory sensory function and includes loss of position sense, impaired ability to localize touch and pain stimuli, elevation of the two-point threshold, and astereognosis. In acute lesions of the parietal cortex there may appear to be impairment of pain sensibility, but this is rarely prominent or persistent.

Occasionally sensory seizures are seen in lesions of the sensory cortex although these are rare. Typically, they show themselves as a wave of sensory irritative symptoms spreading over the body in accordance with the somatotopic organization of the sensory cortex.

Simulated sensory loss

A variety of sensory disorders may be simulated. Patients may complain of the sensory loss but more commonly it is found incidentally during examination. The area of sensory loss is usually sharply demarcated and, in other than medical personnel, does not conform to a recognized anatomical distribution. Characteristically pain loss is the most striking feature and loss of position sense is uncommon. Bearing in mind the difficulties of the sensory examination it is probably safer to ignore sensory findings that do not fit with any other neurological abnormalities that are present. Often it is possible to make a positive diagnosis of a simulated sensory loss because the individual's knowledge of anatomy is not sufficient to enable him to get it right. For example, anybody who is found to have unilateral loss of vibration sense on the skull can be confidently diagnosed as simulating. It must be added, however, that the positive finding of non-organic sensory loss does not necessarily indicate that the whole of the neurological problem is simulated. Sensory loss that is simulated is often added on to symptoms and signs as part of a functional overlay.

Figs S.14–S.19.) illustrate some of the sensory syndromes discussed above.

N. E. F. Cartlidge

Sexual dysfunction

Most commonly advice is sought for problems arising in the context of heterosexual relationships. For women the two main categories of complaint are disorders of arousal and disorders of orgasm during sexual intercourse. For men complaints can be grouped as *erectile impotence* (when erection cannot be obtained or maintained), *premature ejaculation* and *retarded ejaculation*. There appear to be quite marked differences between men and women in their expectations from sexual intercourse, the majority of men complaining of problems with erection or ejaculation and only a minority seeking help on account of lack of interest or enjoyment of sex. An approach to understanding sexual dysfunction must take account of the social, psychological, physiological and drug-induced effects which may all influence the sexual response so that when advice is sought for sexual problems from patients with multiple sclerosis, hypertension, epilepsy, colostomy, mastectomy and with many other physical conditions the clinician must consider the effects of the reaction of the patient and their spouse to the disability as well as the direct physiological disturbances and the effects of medication.

Disorders of arousal and orgasm in both men and women are most commonly connected with psychological and emotional factors. Particularly in the young there may be *anxiety* about sexual prowess and performance. Negative feelings about intercourse may arise in people with *obsessional personalities* because of a general fastidiousness and a fear of losing control of feelings and bodily functions. *Fear of pregnancy* is possibly the most widespread and realistic inhibiting factor and unpleasant sexual experience in childhood may lead to difficulties in establishing normal relations in adulthood. It is also normal for many women to achieve orgasm only through sexual activities other than full intercourse. In women, pain during intercourse (dyspareunia) may result from vaginal infection or other pathology in the pelvis, there may also be inadequate lubrication of the vagina particularly in postmenopausal or lactating women. In some women there is a tendency to develop spasm of the pelvic floor muscles during intercourse resulting in *vaginismus* which makes intercourse painful or impossible.

Failure to achieve orgasm (anorgasmia) may be the outcome of dyspareunia or occasionally severe physical malformation of the genital tract but in the majority of cases there appears to be no good physical or psychological reason for their inability to achieve orgasm. Women depend on tactile stimulation for arousal, and anorgasmia may be due simply to poor technique by the partners.

Libido may be severely impaired in *depressive illness*. *Chronic alcoholism* may cause erectile impotence in the man and in the woman, impaired arousal due to revulsion towards her partner. Organic causes of impotence include *autonomic neuropathy* (e.g. diabetes mellitus), *spinal cord damage* and sometimes central nervous system impairment as in *tumours* in the region of the third ventricle and *temporal lobe epilepsy*. Endocrine disorders include primary and secondary *hypogonadism*. The only drugs which clearly and directly interfere with vascular mechanisms leading to erection are the *ganglian blockers*. Adrenergic blockers interfere with ejaculation and drugs may interfere with the male sexual function by effects on the central nervous system, on blood pressure, or endocrine effects. For example, the re-

duced libido in some patients with temporal lobe epilepsy has been attributed to the effect of anticonvulsant drugs in lowering testosterone levels.

Medical advice may be sought by homosexuals because of sexual and relationship difficulties and these may be exacerbated by the attitudes of society. A group of sexual disorders which may lead the person into trouble with their partner or with the law are the disorders of sexual preferences (the *paraphilias*) which include abnormalities of the sexual object (*fetishism, paedophilia*) and abnormalities of the sexual act (*exhibitionism, voyeurism, frotteurism and sadomasochistic sexual practices*). Fetishism and sadomasochism may be quite common and easily concealed in a stable relationship. Help may be sought only when such practices cause strain in a heterosexual or homosexual partnership. Fetishism occurs almost only in men and describes the use of objects such as clothing, parts of the body or specific textures such as rubber, leather or plastic to stimulate erection. Sadomasochism related to sexual arousal occurs in both men and women and has a role more frequently in fantasy than in reality. The sadist inflicts pain and the masochist adopts a passive role as in sexual practices involving bondage. Generally these practices do not lead to conflict with society. A medical opinion is most likely to be sought with sexual offenders, the common deviations being *exhibitionism and paedophilia*. Exhibitionism or *indecent exposure* is the gaining of sexual stimulation by exposing the genitalia. Unlike other forms of sexual deviation there is no attempt to establish further contact with the 'victim'. In some instances the exhibitionist may derive satisfaction in a sadomasochistic way by evoking fear in a witness. Some become highly sexually aroused and masturbate during or shortly after the exposure. *Frotteurism* describes the achievement of sexual arousal by rubbing against a stranger, often in crowds.

Paedophilia describes sexual activity with children in preference to adults. Usually a paedophile will be attracted either to boys or to girls but not to both. It is recognized almost exclusively in men.

Factors sometimes associated with sexual deviations include disturbed rearing and parental disharmony leading to difficulties in establishing stable adult relationships and personality disorders particularly in those who are inadequate or psychopathic. The role of low IQ, alcohol abuse and mental illness (manic depressive illness and schizophrenia) should also be considered in the clinical assessment of a case.

Problems with gender identity reflected in cross-dressing behaviour (*transvestism* and *transsexualism*) may reflect a number of quite distinct sexual problems. For some men the wearing of female clothes is sexually arousing and the clothes are objects of fetishism. A homosexual of either sex may cross-dress out of preference but in the absence of any genuine gender confusion or desire to be of the opposite sex. Finally there are genuine transsexuals of either sex who often since early childhood have been aware that their psychological sex is opposite to their anatomical sex. These transsexuals may proceed to successful surgical sexual reassignment.

D. Blackwood

SHOULDER
See JOINTS, AFFECTIONS OF.

Skin hardening

Hardening of the skin is the principal feature of *scleroderma*. This occurs in localized and progressive systemic forms. Localized scleroderma, or *morphoea (Fig.* S.20), usually begins in patients under the age of 30 years of age as asymptomatic, round or oval, firm, smooth, reddish plaques many centimetres in diameter. They are commonest on the trunk and may have a lilac or telangiectatic border. After several years the centre of lesions may become atrophic and hyperpigmented. More rarely morphoea appears in linear form either in paramedian distribution on the scalp (*coup de sabre*) or along the line of a limb. Sclerosis in linear morphoea is very marked, and there can be associated atrophy of underlying bone or muscle. The linear type shows little tendency to spontaneous resolution. At times the whole of a limb or one side of the head may be affected in a child, resulting in a deforming hemi-atrophy. Even more rarely very large areas of skin may be involved in a *generalized morphoea.*

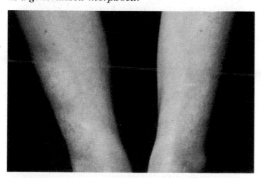

Fig. S.20. Morphoea. (*Westminster Hospital.*)

The progressive type of scleroderma is a systemic disease. It begins with symptoms of Raynaud's phenomenon and gradually the skin of the fingers and hands hardens and loses its mobility (*Fig.* S.21). The feet are similarly affected. The skin of the face may become hard, tight and immobile and on palpation the lower eyelids prove difficult to evert. Systemic manifestations follow in many cases, involving the digestive tract,

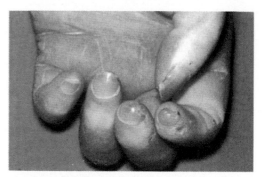

Fig. S.21. Scleroderma. (*Westiminster Hospital.*)

kidneys, lungs and heart. The skin of the extremities often shows areas of pigmentation and subcutaneous calcification may occur.

In addition to scleroderma, hardening of the skin may occur in various other conditions. Hardening of the lower legs is simulated by tense oedema but true sclerotic hardening may follow the recurrent subacute cellulitis associated with *venous stasis*. A similar pseudo-scleroderma can be seen in the lower legs with *vascular insufficiency, lymphoedema* and rarely with the *carcinoid syndrome*.

Hard bead-like infiltration of the skin is seen with *lipoid proteinosis* and this is particularly noticeable around the eyelid margins. Hardening of the skin of the chest can follow secondary infiltration with *scirrhous carcinoma*. A tender, hard plaque appearing on the head and face at the site of inoculation by 'kissing' bugs can occur with *Chagas' disease* in South America. In the West pseudo-scleroderma of facial skin is seen in patients with *porphyria cutanea tarda*.

Localized hardening and hypertrophy of scars is seen with *keloids*. These occur chiefly in young Negroes on the face (*See Fig.* K.1) and upper chest (*See Fig.* K.2), but can also occur 'spontaneously' around an acne folliculitis on the back of the neck—keloid acne (*See Fig.* K.3.)

Richard Staughton

Skin, pigmentation of

Increase in pigmentation of the skin is most commonly due to an increase in melanin deposition, which can be localized, confined to sun-exposed areas, or generalized; deposition of haemosiderin and other chemicals also simulates hyperpigmentation.

1. LOCALIZED HYPERPIGMENTATION

Many skin disorders appear to be able to cause a non-specific post-inflammatory hyperpigmentation. This is particularly seen following *lichen planus* (Fig. P.7) and a *fixed drug eruption* (Fig. S.22), where the condition can be diagnosed retrospectively from the distribution of the pigmentation. In some chronic conditions pigmentation forms part of the spectrum of diagnostic physical signs, for example, *atopic dermatitis*, *morphoea* (Fig. S.20), *urticaria pigmentosa (Fig. W.1)* and *acanthosis nigricans* (Fig. S.23). In a *berloque dermatitis* an acute photo-toxic reaction occurs to perfume or eau de cologne, due to the psoralens they contain. In its most florid form the condition can be dramatic and even bullous but patches of hyperpigmentation on the sides of women's necks are extremely common. A similar hyperpigmentation can follow a photo-toxic reaction to plant chemicals—a *photophytodermatitis*, as seen with primulae. Macular pigmented skin conditions, e.g. freckles and chloasma, are considered on p. 404.

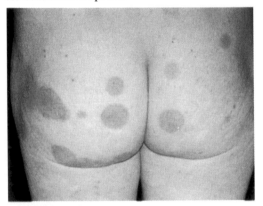

Fig. S.22. Fixed drug eruption.

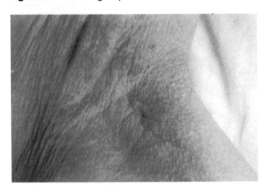

Fig. S.23. Acanthosis nigricans.

2. HYPERPIGMENTATION OF EXPOSED AREA

An annual sun-bathing holiday is becoming routine for more and more individuals, thus a sun-tan is an almost universal finding at certain times of the year. The tendency to such hyperpigmentation is accentuated by certain *drugs*, e.g. thiazides, sulphonamides, amiodarone, nalidixic acid, tetracyclines, chlorpromazine, VP 16; certain deficiencies, e.g. *pellagra*; and certain metabolic disorders such as *porphyria cutanea tarda*.

The sun-tan of a patient with *Addison's* disease is said to last longer than normal and a persistent sun-tan is a feature of *anorexia nervosa*.

3. GENERALIZED HYPERPIGMENTATION

Search should be made in buccal mucosae, gingival margins, in palmar creases, on the nailbeds, and in the bathing costume area to determine if generalized pigmentation is present. Such pigmentation is, of course, physiological in individuals with pigmented *parentage*. It is also extremely common during and after *pregnancy*, and is possibly increased in those taking the contraceptive pill. The traditional medical cause is *Addison's disease*, examples of which are remarkably uncommon in clinical practice. *Ectopic hormone-secreting tumours* are, however, becoming increasingly recognized; for example, various lung carcinomas secrete peptides, some of which have MSH-like (melanocyte-stimulating hormone) properties. Similarly ACTH, for intramuscular injection, is often contaminated with similar peptides and can cause hyperpigmentation (*Fig*. S.24). Diffuse pigmentation can be a feature of *malignant cachexia*, the late wasting phase of HIV disease and can be very marked in those dying with a heavy tumour load of secondary *malignant melanoma*, sometimes accompanied by melanuria (*see* p. 602).

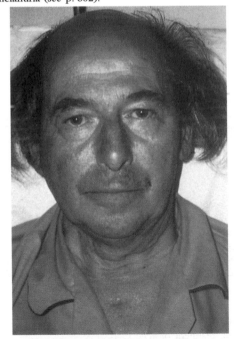

Fig. S.24. Ectopic ACTH-secreting bronchogenic tumour. (*Addenbrooke's Hospital.*)

4. HAEMOSIDERIN

Haemosiderin, which has a greyish-brown appearance in the skin, is often chronically present following local haemorrhage. It is a particular feature of *stasis dermatitis*, and is seen around various purpuric dermatoses such as *Schamberg's disease*. It can also be seen at the site of intramuscular *iron injections*. Generalized deposition of haemosiderin is seen in *haemochromatosis* (bronze diabetes).

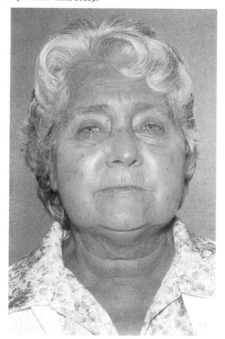

Fig. S.25. Argyria. (*Westminster Hospital.*)

5. OTHER CHEMICALS

Obstructive hepatopathy causes acute or insidious *jaundice* of differing hue, e.g. the greenish colour of primary biliary cirrhosis. *Carotinaemia* results in a yellowish or orange discoloration of the skin, sparing the sclerae, and follows ingestion of large quantities of carrots, oranges and other vegetables. Yellowing of the skin can be caused by drugs, particularly *mepacrine*. In *alcaptonuric ochronosis* the pigment precursor tyrosine cannot be catabolized, and a bluish-black pigment accumulates, particularly in cartilaginous tissues of the ears, sclerae, joints and vertebral column. The urine becomes black on standing for 24 hours. A generalized bluish discoloration is seen with *methaemoglobinaemia* which can be drug-induced, e.g. by dapsone. A deeper colour is induced by deposition of silver in *argyria* (Fig. S.25). High-dose long-term treatment of acne or rosacea with minocycline can result in pigment deposition within acne scars and sometimes more widely. Zidovudine (AZT) can cause linear pigmentation of nails (melanonychia striata) and sometimes diffuse hyperpigmentation.

Richard Staughton

Skin tumours

Cutaneous tumours are growths on the skin larger than nodules (*see* p. 458). They may be firm, fleshy, cystic, multilobulated or ulcerated. The chief causes are neoplasms, both benign and malignant (*see Table* S.7).

Table S.7. Skin tumours

Malignant
a. Secondary deposits
b. Kaposi's sarcoma (Fig. A.19)
c. Primary malignant tumours
   i.   Squamous-cell carcinoma (Fig. S.26)
   ii. Malignant melanoma (Fig. S.27)
   iii. Rodent ulcer (basal-cell carcinoma) (Fig. S.28)
   iv. Mycosis fungoides (cutaneous T-cell lymphoma) (Fig. S.29)
   v. Xeroderma pigmentosum (Fig. S.32)

Benign
Sebaceous cyst
Lipoma
Seborrhoeic keratosis (basal-cell papilloma)
Cutaneous horn (Fig. S.31)
Pyogenic granuloma (Figs. N.43, S.32)
Adnexal tumours

Malignant tumours

a. *Secondary deposits* commonly occur late, as multiple, hard, fleshy nodules of any colour. Subcutaneous secondaries can masquerade as benign lesions and a high level of suspicion should be maintained. Even infectious lesions can be simulated, for example by carcinoma erysipeloides on the chest of a patient with breast cancer. Certain areas are predisposed to metastases, including the scalp (breast, lung and genitourinary tract carcinoma), the chest wall (breast cancer), and the abdominal wall especially around the umbilicus (carcinoma of the stomach and the colon). The skin is sometimes infiltrated by leukaemia or lymphoma.

b. *Kaposi's sarcoma* is a malignant proliferation of vascular endothelial cells giving rise to superficial, subcutaneous or deeper vascular tumours. Tumours do not metastasize but are multi-site in origin. They are probably due to infection with an as yet unidentified viral strain. Tumours flourish when immunity is depressed, e.g. HIV, post-transplant, old age. Classical lesions first described in patients of Jewish or Italian descent living in Vienna in the 1870s are probably acquired on the genome and expressed in old age. Endemic Kaposi's sarcoma was first recognized in the 1950s as a common tumour in sub-Saharan Africa, in younger patients and following a much more aggressive course. The epidemic Kaposi's sarcoma was described in New York in the 1980s. It seemed to spread by sexual intercourse (usually but not exclusively in HIV-positive homosexual men).

Individual lesions begin as pink vascular macules, often in multiple sites, which gradually enlarge and become palpable. They darken with time. Draining oedema is often prominent. The vascular lesions can simulate granulomata, histiocytomata or haemangiomata. Internal lesions can occur chiefly in the gastrointestinal tract and lungs. If immunity improves tumours may shrink.

c. *Primary malignant skin tumours*

i. *Squamous-cell carcinoma (Fig. S.26)* is usually single and as a rule fairly slow growing, extending peripherally and infiltrating deeply while ulcerating at its centre. Sooner or later the lymphatic nodes draining the affected area become involved and enlarged. The usual sites for squamous-cell carcinoma are the lips, especially the lower lip and sun-exposed areas, as well as glans penis and vulva. Solar keratoses, X-ray scars and lupus vulgaris may all undergo malignant squamous change. The main diagnostic features are its origin as a single growth, its craggy hardness, its slow development and the metastases to neighbouring lymph nodes.

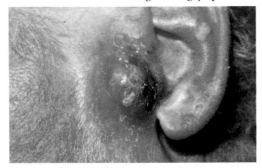

Fig. S.26. Squamous-cell carcinoma. (*Westminster Hospital.*)

ii. *Malignant melanoma (Fig. S.27)* can arise anywhere on the skin surface at any age, often in a simple pigmented or non-pigmented mole. It is rare in blacks and increases in frequency with the fairness of the skin and the amount of previous sun exposure. Patients with a history of severe sunburn in childhood, more than 50 moles on their skin, more than five unusually large moles or a family history of malignant melanoma, are at increased risk.

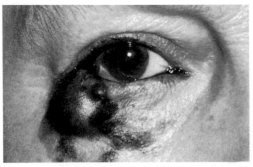

Fig. S.27. Malignant melanoma. (*Addenbrooke's Hospital.*)

It may occur on the scalp, under a nail or on anogenital skin.

Occasionally melanomas lose the capacity to produce pigment—amelanotic melanoma. The characteristics of malignant melanoma are its rapid development and growth, its deepening colour, its ulceration, areas of depigmentation, bleeding and crust formation and its rapid metastases. Sometimes multiple metastases occur in the skin itself. The disease is highly malignant but early diagnosis and excision is curative. Prognosis depends on the thickness of the primary at the time of excision.

iii. *Rodent ulcer (basal-cell carcinoma)* usually affects the face (*Fig.* S.28) and is dealt with on p. 207. These are the commonest primary skin malignancies. They do not metastasize though local invasive destruction can be extensive if lesions are neglected.

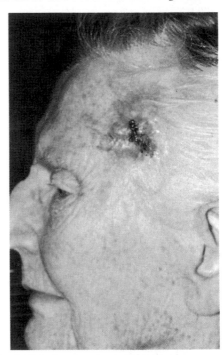

Fig. S.28. Rodent ulcer, basal-cell carcinoma.

iv. *Mycosis fungoides* (cutaneous T-cell lymphoma) is a rare, chronic, slowly fatal disease which is characterized in its final stage by tomato-like neoplasms which may ulcerate. For many years a 'pre-mycotic' non-specific red, scaly rash is present, later (sometimes 30 years plus) forming red plaques of differing hue, and finally neoplasms (*Fig.* S.29).

v. *Xeroderma pigmentosum* is an extremely rare disorder of nuclear protein repair inherited as a recessive trait. It presents in childhood as a proneness to sunburn and early gross sun damage with elastosis, atrophy, telangiectasia and finally multiple skin tumours (squamous-cell carcinoma, rodent ulcer, malignant melanoma, kerato-acanthoma) (*Fig.* S.30).

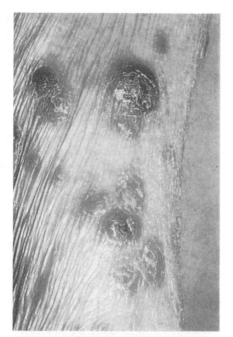

Fig. S.29. Mycosis fungoides. (*Westminster Hospital.*)

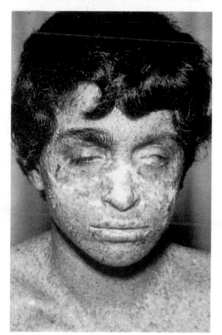

Fig. S.30. Xeroderma pigmentosum. (*Westminster Hospital.*)

Benign cutaneous tumours

Sebaceous cysts, commonest on the back, face, scalp and scrotum, are of variable size, cystic on palpation, and with a minute orifice (punctum) to be found somewhere on their surface. *Lipomas* are usually multiple subcutaneous nodules which may be lobulated, and found on any part of the body. They occur as a

familial trait but can often not be discerned until adulthood. *Seborrhoeic keratosis* (basal-cell papillomas) are extremely common and start as papules in middle age, growing into larger, flat, greasy, warty pigmented neoplasms. They are sometimes unkindly called senile keratoses.

A *cutaneous horn* is a peculiar cutaneous neoplasm surmounted by a spectacular horny overgrowth (*Fig.* S.31). The nature of the underlying neoplasm can only be safely diagnosed by examining the histopathology, e.g. actinic keratosis, squamous-cell carcinoma, viral wart, keratoacanthoma and seborrhoeic wart (basal-cell papilloma).

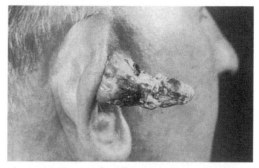

Fig. S.31. Cutaneous horn: keratoacanthoma.

A *pyogenic granuloma* (granuloma telangiectaticum) is a fairly common skin neoplasm (*Fig.* S.32). It often develops at the site of a recent injury and is composed of proliferating capillaries in a loose stroma. This produces a rapidly growing vascular neoplasm which bleeds easily when traumatized. It is distinctive, being bright red, 0·5–1 cm in diameter, often pedunculated and surrounded by a collar of thickened epidermis. The common sites are the fingers, upper chest, lips and toes. It must be differentiated from amelanotic melanoma, and glomus tumour. Kaposi's sarcoma in HIV-infected patients can accurately mimic pyogenic granuloma and for this reason histological analysis after curettage or excision is advisable.

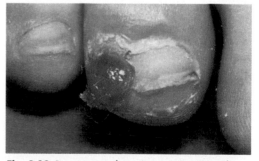

Fig. S.32. Pyogenic granuloma. (*Westminster Hospital.*)

Adnexal tumours. The superficial dermis contains many specialized tissues, some of ectodermal and some of mesodermal origin, forming the various adnexal structures, e.g. hair, sebaceous glands, sweat glands, etc. Benign, or rarely malignant, neoplasms of all these specialized tissues can occur, for example *leiomyoma, hydradenoma, neurofibroma, sebaceous adenoma, tricho-epithelioma* and *glomus neoplasm*. The diagnosis of these rare neoplasms requires many years' experience and is often first made by the pathologist.

Richard Staughton

Sleep, disorders of

The most common complaint is of insomnia although some patients will seek advice on account of too much sleep (hypersomnia) or occasionally for abnormal events which occur during sleep (the parasomnias) (*Table* S.8).

Table S.8. Disorders of sleep

Insomnia

Normal variant
Physical illness (pain, respiratory disease, delirium)
Mood disorder
  Depression
  Anxiety
  Mania
  Post-traumatic stress disorder
Drugs
  Stimulants (including coffee, tea, nicotine,
    amphetamine)
  Alcohol
  Sedative withdrawal

Hypersomnia

Sleep apnoea/hypopnoea syndrome
Intracranial space occupying lesions
Metabolic disorder
  Uraemia
  Hepatic failure
Narcolepsy
Kleine–Levin syndrome
Idiopathic (sleep drunkenness)
Drugs
  Benzodiazepines
  Barbiturates
  Phenothiazines
  Tricyclic antidepressants

Poor sleep is a very common complaint, more so amongst women than men and especially in the elderly. Self-reports from patients are frequently inaccurate because patients typically overestimate the time taken to get to sleep and underestimate the total duration of sleep. Patients generally sleep longer than they think. Complaints of poor sleep come from people who are under stress at home or at work or who have anxious personalities. Such people tend to be highly aroused and stay awake thinking about stressful situations and planning how to cope. In others their reports of poor sleep may be due to stimulants such as coffee, tea or smoking cigarettes and there is a high rate of reported poor sleep in patients with an alcohol pro-

blem. The normal requirement for sleep varies widely and a small number of individuals require only 3–4 hours of sleep each night. During a painful physical illness or in a person with respiratory difficulties the causes of disturbed sleep will be obvious. Poor nutritional status and low weight may also be accompanied by diminished sleep.

Change in sleep pattern is extremely common in all forms of mood disturbance. The manic patient may remain cheerful and active throughout the night showing little sign of fatigue whereas the anxiety prone patient may have difficulty falling to sleep because of worrying thoughts. In depression there may be initial, middle and late insomnia, early morning wakening being one of the features of endogenous or melancholic depression. Such subjects may wake 2 to 3 hours earlier than normal feeling depressed and dreading the coming day.

Hypersomnia may be the complaint of someone who lacks a day time schedule and has no motivation to rise. Poor motivation and the effects of medication can account for the apparently increased sleep of some psychiatric patients especially those with a schizophrenic defect state.

In *narcolepsy* the person experiences bouts of drowsiness leading to short periods of sleep of a few minutes duration recurring two or three times a day. The condition may be associated with cataplexy, a sudden loss of muscle tone lasting for a few seconds, often triggered by strong emotions. Other features of the condition include sleep paralysis, in which the subject is momentarily paralysed and unable to move (as happens sometimes with normal people awaking from a bad dream) and hypnagogic hallucinations which may be auditory, visual or tactile. Usually the diagnosis of narcolepsy is made from the clinical history and EEG findings that on falling asleep the patient goes spontaneously into REM sleep without passing through a non-REM stage.

A rare form of hypersomnia usually in young men is the *Kleine–Levin syndrome*. The patient sleeps excessively by day and night but is rousable. Such patients often eat excessively. *Organic lesions of the mid brain or hypothalamus* may also cause increased hunger, weight gain and drowsiness. The abrupt onset of daytime sleepiness or drowsiness however should immediately alert the clinician to the possibility of an intracranial space occupying lesion.

Parasomnias. When unusual behaviour patterns during sleep develop suddenly in a patient a drug effect should be first excluded. *Nightmares* are a normal phenomenon with no psychiatric significance. Frequent nightmares may occur during anxiety states and depression, post-traumatic stress disorders, with alcohol abuse or following a change of hypnotic. *Sleep walking* and *night terrors* may be familial and can be precipitated by drugs including antidepressants, anticonvulsants, analgesics, lithium and phenothiazines. These sometimes follow a febrile illness. A child experiencing a night terror which usually occurs within the first 2 hours of sleep may sit up with an expression of fear and remain oblivious to the surroundings for a few minutes before dropping soundly to sleep again. The child will have no memory of the event in the morning. Sometimes *sleep walking* occurs during a night terror. Usually patients will sleep walk in a calm, gentle way but sleep walkers are at high risk of injuring themselves by falling downstairs or through windows. The subject is in a state of automatism and may walk some distance and carry out quite complicated series of actions. Both night terrors and sleep walking are more frequent during times of stress and families will require reassurance.

Bruxism, the grinding of teeth during the night causes dental problems and can be provoked by psychotropic medication. *Nocturnal enuresis* is common and multifactorial sources of stress should be sought in a family when this develops in a child after a period of established bladder control.

Sleep apnoea/hypopnoea syndrome

The major complaint of patients with the sleep apnoea/hypopnoea syndrome is usually daytime sleepiness which may vary in severity from trivial to dangerous, many patients falling asleep during driving, working or in mid-conversation (*Fig.* S.33). The patient is usually unaware of the hundreds of brief awakenings per night which result in the daytime sleepiness, although around a third of patients are aware of awaking occasionally at night with choking episodes. The sleep disruption results from total or partial occlusion of the upper airway at the level of the soft palate or tongue each time a patient goes to sleep. This produces apnoeas or severe hypopnoeas which are only terminated when the patient awakens briefly, perhaps, due to the fall in arterial oxygen levels. The awakening is so brief that the patient is not aware of it but is sufficient to increase the tone to the upper airway opening muscles and breathing resumes for a few seconds until the patient goes back to sleep and becomes apnoeic or hypopnoeic again. Patients do not find nocturnal sleep satisfying and sometimes awaken with a headache. Their bed partners report very loud snoring punctuated with breathing pauses and that the patient is a very restless sleeper often thrashing around the bed.

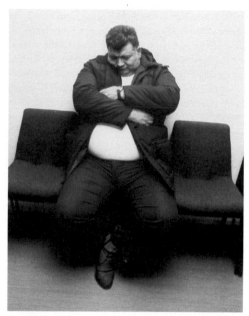

Fig. S.33. A sleepy patient with the sleep apnoea/hypopnoea syndrome.

This condition affects around 1 per cent of adults, 85 per cent of patients are male and half are overweight. Severe long-standing cases, particularly in patients with coexisting lung disease, may be complicated by cyanosis (*see* CYANOSIS) and right heart failure.

Neil J. Douglas

Smell as a physical sign

Of the numerous odours, mostly unpleasant, to which clinicians are exposed, very few are of diagnostic significance. There are better ways of diagnosing *gangrene* in a limb than by the foul smell emitted, the foetid breath of the patient with *acute ulcerative gingivitis* is important only if it makes the clinician recoil from making a proper examination and the offensive sputum produced by some patients with *bronchiectasis* is largely a thing of the past. However, in the latter case, and whenever a purulent exudate has a strong faecal odour, anaerobic infection should be suspected and appropriate microbiological investigations carried out. Uraemia cannot be recognized by smell but the *ammoniacal odour of stale urine* of incontinent patients, who may be in renal failure, has led some to regard this as the smell of uraemia.

Almost the only common condition in which the smell of the patient may be of critical diagnostic importance is *diabetic keto-acidosis*. Unfortunately, the ability to detect the sickly-sweet smell of acetone in the breath is very variable and about 20 per cent of clinicians are quite unable to do so. This is not a serious disability as testing the urine for acetone, and other substances, should be routine in any stuporose or comatose patient. It is sensible for medical students to discover their own ability, or otherwise, to detect the smell of acetone. They need not wait until they see a case of keto-acidosis. In a children's surgical ward on operating day, they will find many children whose breath smells of acetone as a result of pre-operative *starvation*.

Of the other conditions in which a typical smell may be detected, *hepatic failure* is characterized by hepatic foeter—like the smell of a freshly opened corpse; this is said to be due to the presence of mercaptans in the expired air. Very rarely, a diagnosis of *maple-syrup urine disease* will be made in children in the early months of life by the characteristic burnt sugar odour of maple-syrup; this results from the excretion in the urine of branched-chain oxo-acids.

Some substances, ingested by a patient or absorbed in other ways, can cause a typical smell. Of these, by far the most common is *alcohol* although it is unwise to assume that an unconscious patient smelling of alcohol is 'dead drunk'; head injury or hypoglycaemia are much more likely to be responsible for his condition. *Paraldehyde* imparts an easily recognized smell to the patient but is rarely used today. Some industrial chemicals, to which a patient may be exposed, can cause a typical smell. *Selenium*, used in the steel industry, is excreted as a compound which has a garlic-like smell.

A *melaena* stool is, of course, recognized by its appearance but it has a characteristically unpleasant smell different from the usual odour of faeces.

Peter R. Fleming

Smell, abnormalities of

Abnormalities of the sense of smell fall into three main categories, namely: (1) Too great sensitivity to smells which actually exist (hyperosmia); (2) Deficient sensitivity to smells which actually exist (hyposmia); (3) Subjective sensations of smells which do not exist externally (parosmia).

1. *Too great sensitivity to existing smells* is sometimes a nuisance to the individual, but is not a sign of disease. There are great differences in the powers of perception of different sensations in different persons, and just as some can appreciate more than others very slight differences in sounds, so too can some detect smells that are not discernible by others. This is a natural idiosyncrasy, and it is sometimes experienced in pregnancy. In general, sensitivity is reduced in heavy smokers.

2. *Deficient sensitivity to actual smells* is often only the obverse of the above and not a sign of disease.

It may however, be a detriment to the individual, especially in certain commercial activities in which varying qualities of products are judged partly by smell. When the power of smell, having been normal, becomes deficient or totally absent, the change may affect one nostril only, or both. The condition may be transient or persistent. The commonest cause of transient anosmia is acute nasal catarrh, whether the result of an ordinary cold, or of other affections such as hay fever, or oncoming measles. Drugs such as potassium iodide or arsenic can rarely have similar effects. Transient anosmia is occasionally present during an attack of migraine.

Persistent anosmia may be due to:

a PARTIAL OR TOTAL BLOCKAGE OF THE NOSE
   Adenoids
   Polyps
   Hypertrophic rhinitis
   Deviated septum
   Syphilis
   Tumour
b DISEASE OF THE OLFACTORY MUCOUS MEMBRANE WITHOUT BLOCKAGE
   Atrophic rhinitis
   Leprosy
   Paralysis of the 5th nerve, leading to dryness of the mucosa
c ABNORMALITIES OF THE OLFACTORY NERVES AND UNCUS
   Congenital absence
   Rupture of nerve filaments from head injury
   Tabes and general paralysis
   Basal meningitis
   Tumour of the frontal lobe and uncus; meningioma of the olfactory groove
   Raised intracranial pressure with hydrocephalus
d HYSTERIA

Common causes of anosmia include head injury and local nasal infection. When a case is being investigated it is important to examine the nose carefully through a speculum and to test the patency of the airway through each nostril. Hyposmia most commonly results from local nasal disorders.

PERVERSIONS OF SMELL

Parosmia is a perverted sense of smell which is characteristically unpleasant and usually occurs after damage to the olfactory nerves. Common causes include head injury, tumours and nasal infection. Olfactory hallucinations represent a common and striking symptom of partial seizures originating in the medial aspect of the temporal lobe (uncinate seizures). These hallucinations tend to be pungent, sometimes likened to burning rubber, or a smell of gas. Olfactory hallucination is not uncommon in psychosis, when unpleasant smells may be attributed either to the patient himself or to others. A similar subjective sensation of a smell which does not exist externally may be described by patients with offensive or purulent inflammation of the nose or sinuses.

N. E. F. Cartlidge

Sneezing

Sneezing is usually initiated by irritation of the nasal mucosa, especially that of the anterior end of the nasal septum or the middle turbinates. The sneeze reflex is protective in nature and essentially similar to the cough reflex. It is a sudden and involuntary expulsion of air through the nose and mouth and is controlled by a reflex through the 5th and 10th cranial nerves.

At present the record for the longest bout of sneezing is held by Miss Patricia Reay, aged 12 at the time, who sneezed continually from 15 October 1979 until 25th April 1980, a total of 194 days. Sneezing may be caused by:

1 Local irritation
2 Hyperalgesia of the nasal mucosa which may occur—
   a. When the nerve endings are unduly sensitive
   b. Due to susceptibility to particular stimuli
   c. Due to defective control of the nerve centres or to a combination of these factors

The early viral stage of the common cold is, of course, probably the commonest cause of sneezing which subsides once the bacterial secondary infection supervenes with a thicker nasal discharge. Sneezing is common in the prodromal stages of measles and the other infectious fevers but is not common in the more chronic nasal infections.

Fine dusts and powders cause sneezing. Snuff (finely powdered tobacco), sawdust, fine pollens and irritant gases all fall into this group. Riot control gas and war gasses irritate the eyes as well as the nasal mucosa; lacrimation, nasal discharge and sneezing may be incapacitating to those exposed.

Hyperalgesia of the nasal mucosa has the effect of sensitizing individuals to both changes of temperature and to light. Many people sneeze once or twice on their first exposure to bright light. Sneezing on meeting specific pollens is characteristic of seasonal nasal allergy or pollinosis. Prolonged bouts of sneezing occur much more commonly in cases of specific nasal allergy (pollens, house-dust or, commonly, the house-dust mite) than in vasomotor rhinitis.

There are many time-honoured country cures for sneezing, such as rebreathing into a brown paper bag, etc. Certainly modern medical science has little to add to these country cures other than the use of a Beconase nasal spray prior to going into situations where known irritants exist.

A. G. D. Maran

Snoring

(*see also* SLEEP, ABNORMALITIES OF)

Snoring is a disorder of sleep which is especially common in obese people. It is commoner in men than women and in people over the age of 40. It is probably due to air turbulence, secondary to partial airway obstruction during inspiration, causing vibration of the soft tissues in the pharynx.

Habitual snorers have a higher incidence of pulmonary hypertension and apparently simple snorers can develop obstructive sleep apnoea after ingestion of alcohol. It is now considered that a continuous spectrum probably exists between uncomplicated simple snoring and the obstructive sleep apnoea syndrome (*see* SLEEP, DISORDERS OF).

Until recently the only treatment for snoring was to tell the patient to lose weight and to try nasal surgery where it seemed appropriate for a deviated septum or nasal polyps.

In 1981, however, the uvulo-palato-pharyngo-plasty was introduced. This operation abolishes or improves uncomplicated snoring in over 90 per cent of adult patients. Unfortunately it only cures about 20 per cent of patients with sleep apnoea, and it may compromise later CPAP treatment of the sleep apnoea.

It is still difficult to classify snoring and if a snorer is going to have surgery then it is essential for them to be fully investigated with sleep studies to see if there is any co-existing sleep apnoea.

A. G. D. Maran

Speech, abnormalities of

(*see also* DYSPHASIA)

The production of speech depends on three separate components:

1. *The creation of sound (phonation)*. The creation of a sound requires air to be passed over the vocal cords, the control of which is mediated via the recurrent laryngeal branches of the vagus nerve.

2. *The creation of recognizable sounds (articulation)*. The sound created from the vocal cords is manipulated as the air passes over the structures of the upper pharynx and mouth. Structures involved in creating recognizable sounds or phonemes, are the pharynx, palate, tongue and lips. The muscles involved are innervated by the cranial nerves 7, 10 and 12 (the so-called bulbar cranial nerves).

3. *Programming*. The programming of the bulbar cranial nerves and muscles to create language is dependent on the dominant cerebral hemisphere and in particular the speech areas of Broca and Wernicke.

Disorders of speech can occur from abnormality of function of any of the three components listed above. In addition, psychogenic or functional disorders may be associated with abnormalities of speech. Finally, a separate group of speech abnormalities may be seen as the result of developmental disorders.

Dysphonia

Dysphonia occurs when there is an abnormality of function of the vocal cords. This may be neurogenic but can occur as an hysterical manifestation. The latter is readily differentiated from organic disorder by the patient's ability to cough. Structural disorders of the vocal cords themselves may also be associated with dysphonia.

Neurological causes of dysphonia are divided into two separate categories:

SPASTIC DYSPHONIA

Upper motor neurone disorders affecting the vagus, and hence the recurrent laryngeal innervated muscles, may produce a spastic dysphonia, though this is often associated with spastic dysarthria (*see below*). The speech has a strangled quality as occurs in pseudobulbar palsy.

FLACCID DYSPHONIA

Lower motor neurone damage to either the vagus nerve, the recurrent laryngeal nerve or the muscles moving the vocal cords, will be associated with the more common flaccid dysphonia. In this, the patients have not only an abnormality of speech but also the so-called bovine cough. This type of dysphonia most commonly results from isolated damage to one of the recurrent laryngeal nerves. It may also be seen in poliomyelitis, motor neurone disease, cranial polyneuropathies, myasthenia gravis and some rare forms of muscle disease.

Dysarthria

Disorders of articulation are seen when there is impairment of function of the muscles which manipulate those structures which shape the phonemes—the building blocks of speech. They include the pharynx, palate, tongue and lips. These structures are innervated by the facial, vagus and hypoglossal nerves. The controlling area of motor cortex is at the lower end of the precentral gyrus, and neurones here link to the cranial nerve nuclei via the corticobulbar pathway. Four separate types of dysarthria may be recognized.

SPASTIC DYSARTHRIA

Involvement of the upper motor neurone pathway to the bulbar cranial nerves produces spastic dysarthria. Bilateral involvement of either the cortex or descending pathways is necessary to produce such a dysarthria. This is seen in patients who have suffered bilateral strokes, and in motor neurone disease, multiple sclerosis and cerebral palsy. The speech has a strangled quality, often because of associated spastic dysphonia and it is often slow and 'thick'.

FLACCID DYSARTHRIA

Involvement of the lower motor neurone supply to the bulbar muscles produces this type of speech which is often of nasal quality because of air escaping through the nose resulting from palatal weakness. The lesion may be sited in the cranial nerve nuclei, the cranial nerves themselves, the neuromuscular junction or the bulbar muscles. Thus this type of speech disorder may be seen in motor neurone disease, cranial polyneuropathies, myasthenia gravis or those forms of muscle disease which involve the bulbar muscles such as oculopharyngeal muscular dystrophy.

CEREBELLAR DYSARTHRIA

Diffuse cerebellar disorders are associated with imprecise articulation resulting in so-called slurring dysarthria. This may be seen in multiple sclerosis, cerebellar degeneration and vascular disorders of the cerebellum.

EXTRAPYRAMIDAL SPEECH DISORDERS

Two separate types of speech disorder may be seen in extrapyramidal diseases.

In Parkinson's disease, the speech is typically slow and monotonous. In the early stages the only abnormality might be a slight loss of the musical quality of speech whereas in the late stages of Parkinson's disease the speech may be virtually inaudible (so-called hypokinetic dysarthria). Palilalia is occasionally seen. It is characterized by the repetition of a phrase which the patient reiterates with increasing rapidity.

In the dyskinetic types of extrapyramidal disorder, such as chorea, oro-facial dyskinesia and athetosis, the articulation of sound is interrupted by involuntary movements producing jerky and irregular speech.

Disorders of programming—aphasia

The terms aphasia and dysphasia for all practical purposes are interchangeable and indicate a disorder of programming of speech and language such that the speech content in terms of words, syllables and/or sentences does not correspond accurately to the patient's own expected linguistic abilities. The programming of speech is a function of the dominant hemisphere. In 99 per cent of the population who are right handed, the dominant hemisphere is the left, whereas in left-handed individuals there is something like a 50 per cent chance that either the left or the right hemisphere will be dominant.

Table S.9. The differing clinical features of specific forms of aphasia

Aphasia	Spontaneous speech	Fluency	Comprehension	Repetition	Naming
Broca's	Hesitant; agrammatic	Poor	Good	Poor	Poor
Pure motor	Phonetic errors	Impaired	Good	Impaired	Impaired
Global	Sterotypic utterances	Poor	Poor	Poor	Poor
Wernicke's	Paraphasic, jargon	Good	Poor	Poor	Poor
Word deaf	Normal	Good	Poor	Poor	Good
Conduction	Phonemic errors	Good	Good	Poor	Good
Transcortical sensory	Normal to semantic jargon	Good	Poor	Good	Poor
Transcortical motor	Scant, mute	Poor	Good	Good	Impaired
Isolation	Mute	Poor	Poor	Good	Poor
Anomic	Circumlocutory	Good	Good	Good	Impaired

A number of separate speech areas in the cortex have been recognized and it is generally held that a series of separate types of dysphasia may be recognized, based on localized lesions at separate sites within the dominant hemisphere. Some of these are listed in Table S.9.

Two separate speech areas are readily recognized:

BROCA'S AREA

Broca's area is the association area for the lower part of the motor cortex representing the bulbar musculature. In simple terms, Broca's area carries the programme to manipulate the motor cortex and hence the muscles that create recognizable sounds, words and sentences.

A Broca's aphasia is associated with hesitancy of speech and the other features listed in Table S.9.

WERNICKE'S AREA

Wernicke's area is the auditory association cortex of the dominant hemisphere in the superior temporal gyrus. It can be regarded as the memory store for words where words and perhaps sentences or even phrases are understood.

Wernicke's aphasia is associated with a striking loss of comprehension of the spoken word and the other features listed in Table S.9.

An important pathway is the arcuate fasciculus or superior longitudinal fasciculus. Damage to this produces so-called conduction aphasia. Another important area in the control of speech is situated in the parietal lobe, posterior to the lateral fissure and near the supramarginal and angular gyri of the dominant hemisphere—the parietal speech area. Disorders of reading and writing, dyslexia and dysgraphia, may accompany a variety of different forms of dysphasia and may rarely occur in isolation. They are most commonly seen with damage to the parietal speech area.

The musical quality of speech is a function of the non-dominant hemisphere and disorders of this side of the brain may be associated with monotonous speech referred to as dysprosody.

Psychogenic disorders

Stammering or stuttering tends to occur in highly strung individuals although it is not invariably a psychogenic disorder. Psychogenic dysarthria is rare as is hysterical dysphasia. Mutism may occur in psychiatric disorders such as schizophrenia, catatonia or depression and may also be seen in hysteria.

There is some debate as to the cause of lisping and dyslalia as these may be a manifestation of a developmental disorder rather than a psychological disturbance.

Development Disorders of Speech

This term is used to describe those conditions in which the acquisition of speech is retarded, or in some other respect abnormal, as a result of a defect in the nervous system dating from birth. It therefore includes the wide range of abnormalities encountered in the mentally retarded. Before concluding that a child has a developmental disorder of speech, it is important to exclude hearing impairment or emotional blocking as a cause of the defect. A number of very specific developmental syndromes have been described, such as developmental word-deafness (congenital auditory imperception) and developmental word-blindness (developmental alexia). Children who fail to develop normal articulation are often described as dyslalic.

D. A. Shaw

Spine, curvature of

An abnormal curve in *flexion* is called a 'kyphosis' and where this presents as an acute angle the hump of bone is called a 'gibbus'. The extension curve constitutes a 'lordosis'. The lateral spinal curve is called a 'scoliosis' in the thoracic and lumbar regions and in the neck the wry neck is described as a 'torticollis'. The scoliosis is designated 'left' or 'right' according to the direction of the convexity of the curve. There is often a combination of curves and a kyphoscoliosis is frequently seen. A scoliosis or lateral curvature of the spine is always associated with some rotational deformity.

Scoliosis

There are two fundamental types of scoliosis: postural and structural.

POSTURAL SCOLIOSIS

A postural scoliosis disappears when the patient is observed from behind and asked to flex forward to touch his toes. The spine then reverts to its straight position and there is no associated rotation or rib hump. This postural scoliosis is seen in a variety of conditions—the short lower limb will produce a functional compensatory scoliosis convex to the side of the short leg. The poor stance of a child frequently produces this postural scoliosis which is of little importance and can always be corrected by appropriate instruction and discipline.

STRUCTURAL SCOLIOSIS

There are many causes of a structural scoliosis both congenital and acquired. The major classification is divided into (1) osteopathic; (2) neuropathic and (3) myopathic.

With a structural scoliosis there is always rotation of the spine in association and this produces the characteristic rib rotation or hump. The scapula may be elevated on one side and the hip may project on the concave side of the curve (*Fig. S.34*).

Types of structural scoliosis

CONGENITAL

A wedge-shaped hemi-vertebra is present. This produces a kypho-scoliosis which is seen at birth and continues through life. There may be some increase in the curvature around the congenital deformity in the teenage years. Spina bifida will also produce abnormal curves seen at birth and is progressive through the first decade.

INFANTILE SCOLIOSIS

This scoliosis develops before the age of three. It is differentiated from congenital scoliosis by the absence of abnormalities of the vertebral bodies or the ribs at birth. In most cases it resolves spontaneously and only in a few will the curve progress. There is associated plagiocephaly and sometimes a postural adduction contracture of one hip.

IDIOPATHIC ADOLESCENT SCOLIOSIS

This refers to the structural scoliosis whose aetiology is unknown. It constitutes 80 per cent of patients with a structural scoliosis and occurs from the age of 10 years to the end of skeletal growth.

This type of scoliosis is familial. The child usually presents with a high shoulder or prominant hip and it is rare to complain of associated pain or fatigue. Later in life pain may be present from the degenerative changes which occur in the curved segment. In severe scoliotic curves the pressure of the ribs against the iliac crests may produce some discomfort. Respiratory and later cardiac abnormalities may occur in the patient with a severe curve.

The examination of the child with a scoliosis must include the general posture, the alignment of the spinous processes and the level of the shoulders. Rotation producing deformity of the rib cage is best observed in the patient bending forwards and the 'rib hump' then becomes apparent. General and neurological examination of the patient must also be undertaken, for the differential diagnosis between an idiopathic adolescent curve and that present in neurofibromatosis or neurological deficit is important in assessing the prognosis.

Causes of scoliosis

Neuromuscular causes of scoliosis
Neurofibromatosis
Cerebral palsy with spastic paralysis
Poliomyelitis
Syringomyelia
Intraspinal tumour
Friedreich's ataxia
Muscular causes of scoliosis
Muscle dystrophies
Arthrogryphosis multiplex congenita
Other myopathies
Scoliosis due to other abnormalities of the spinal column
Osteochondrodystrophies
Osteogenesis imperfecta
Fracture-disclocations
Tumours such as osteoid osteoma

Kyphosis

This indicates a forward flexion deformity of the spine producing a hump-back or a hunch-back. It may be diffuse over the whole spine or angular in which a gibbus is present. The kyphosis may be congenital or acquired.

CONGENITAL CAUSES (*Fig. S.35*).

There may be a generalized abnormality of the skeleton such as a mucopolysaccharidosis. In Morquio's disease and also Hurler's disease (gargoylism) a kyphosis is present frequently with a gibbus.

ACQUIRED CAUSES

Tuberculosis of spine or Pott's disease
(Fig. S.36).
The child is ill and holds his spine stiffly. The dorsal spine is most commonly affected and an angular prom-

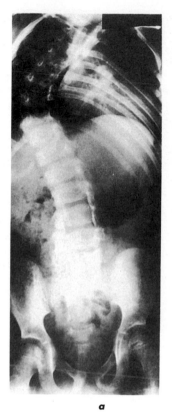
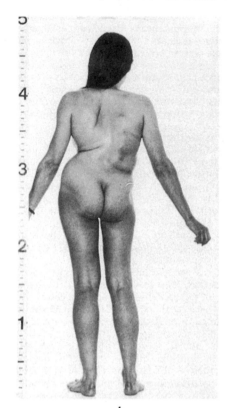

a   b

Fig. S.34. Scoliosis with rib rotation and hump. *a*, X-ray. *b*, Clinical photograph.

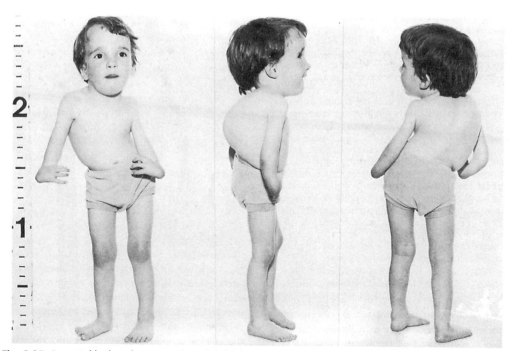

Fig. S.35. Congenital kyphoscoliosis. Note the radial club hands due to absence of the radii.

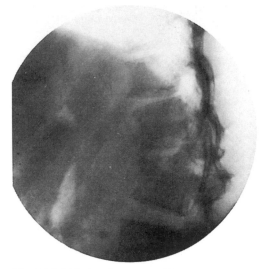

Fig. S.36. Old tuberculous osteomyelitis.

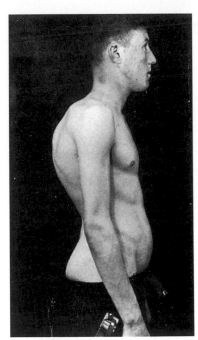

Fig. S.37. Smooth thoracic Kyphosis due to longstanding Scheuermann's disease.

inence is felt when the infection has produced bone destruction and wedging of the vertebral bodies. An abscess frequently occurs around the diseased vertebrae and later may present in the lumbar triangle or in the groin as a cold abscess in the psoas sheath. Spinal cord compression may occur—Pott's paraplegia.

Crush fracture of the vertebral body

An angular kyphosis may be present at the site of a wedge crush fracture. In the osteoporotic, osteomalacic or rachitic patient, multiple wedge-shaped crush fractures may occur producing a smooth kyphosis in the thoracic region.

Scheuerman's disease or adolescent kyphosis

There is a fixed kyphosis developing at about the time of puberty. A wedge-shaped deformity of one or more vertebrae occurs. The cause is not known and the diagnosis is confirmed radiologically where there are multiple wedge-shaped vertebrae and excessive fragmentation of the vertebral end plate epiphyses.

The patient presents with poor posture and there may be aching and pain especially after exercise. The condition is seen in the thoracic spine in 75 per cent (*Fig.* S.37) and the thoracolumbar region in most of the remainder. A purely lumbar Scheuermann's disease is rare.

Paget's disease (osteitis of deformans)

This produces a uniform curve with consequent stooping without a compensatory lordosis (*Fig.* S.38). It is irreducible and the curvature first makes its appearance after middle age. There is usually evidence of the disease in other parts—progressive increase in the size of the head and thickening and bowing of the

tibias and femurs. The disease may be pronounced in long bones long before the spine is affected.

Ankylosing spondylitis

In this condition some patients have a straight, stiff spine, but others are bent forwards with greater or lesser degrees of kyphosis, sometimes associated with scoliosis. The neck is frequently flexed and the hips and shoulders may become involved. It is most common in the younger man and usually starts in the twenties.

Osteoarthritic changes

These occur in the vertebral bodies with advancing age. A fixed stoop occurs and the whole spine including both dorsal and lumbar regions becomes affected.

Porters carrying heavy weights may develop a kyphosis with osteoarthritis in the upper thoracic region. There is frequently a bursa over the 7th cervical spinous process ('Porter's bursa' or 'Porter's hummy').

Lordosis (hollow-back)

A lordosis occurs in the lumbar region and the lower dorsal area. It is an exaggeration of the normal lumbar contour and it usually occurs in compensation for some fixed flexion deformity of the hips. This is frequently seen in untreated bilateral congenital dislocation of the hips.

General muscle weakness as seen in muscle dystrophy frequently produces a lordosis.

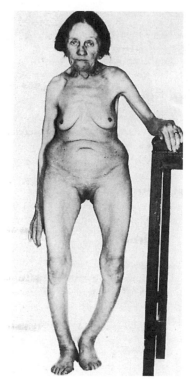

Fig. S.38. Paget's disease showing the kyphosis, bowing of the legs and apparently over-long arms, with increase in the size of the head. (*Dr. C. Baker.*)

SPONDYLOLISTHESIS

The slipping forwards of one vertebral body on the next is seen most commonly at the L5/Sl level. The spondylolisthesis is usually due to trauma and to a fracture through the pars interarticularis. The gradual slip of one vertebral body on the next may produce an increasing hollow of the lumbar region and in severe slips a step may be palpated at the unstable level.

Torticollis (wry neck)

CONGENITAL MUSCULAR TORTICOLLIS

Unilateral contracture of the sternomastoid muscle results in a deformity of the head and neck in which the head is tilted to the side and the chin rotated to the opposite side (*Fig.* S.39). The cause of this deformity is within the sternocleidomastoid muscle in which there is contracture and shortening. It may be due to birth trauma with a bleed into the muscle within its closed compartment and subsequent infarction and then fibrosis of the muscle belly. In the neonate the sterno-mastoid muscle may present a lump in its mid zone (sternomastoid tumour). This is the site of the devel-oping fibrosis and gradually the sternomastoid muscle contracts and as the torticollis continues the face and

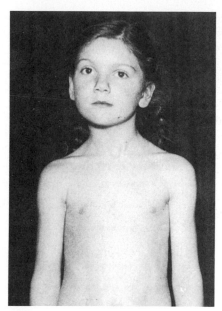

Fig. S.39. Congenital torticollis, with left sternomastoid contracture.

the facial skeleton become flattened on the affected side.

KLIPPEL–FEIL SYNDROME

This is a rare cause of a torticollis in which there is a congenital fusion of two or more vertebrae in the cervical region. There is also hemi-vertebral malforma-tions of the cervical vertebral bodies. The curvature may be severe and fixed and the facial asymmetry is often less than that seen in the congenital muscular type. Klippel-Feil syndrome may be associated with other deformities such as a congenital high scapula (Sprengel's deformity).

Paul Aichroth

SPINE, DEFORMITY OF
See SPINE, CURVATURE OF.

Spine, tenderness of

(*See also* BACK, PAIN IN)

Tenderness of the spine is usually due to local disease of or injury to the tissues at the site of tender-ness. Such tenderness is always deep, but may be associated with cutaneous hyperalgesia as well. In a second and less important group the tenderness is partly or entirely cutaneous, and is a referred pheno-menon found in visceral disease. In testing for spinal tenderness it is therefore desirable to differentiate between cutaneous and deep tenderness and, in the case of the latter, between tenderness elicited by pressing upon the spinous processes and tenderness in the adjacent muscles, since spinal disease is usually accompanied by local muscular spasm and the muscles thus affected become tender although they are not themselves the site of the disease. Failure to allow for this fact is the usual explanation of the mistakes— sometimes serious—which are so often made in attributing muscle tenderness to a strain or to a rheumatic condition when in reality it is due to local spasm in response to disease of the vertebrae, intervertebral discs, or to the spinal cord and its membranes.

The chief conditions in which spinal tenderness occurs are summarized in the following table:

1. **Diseases of the overlying skin and subcutancous tissue**
   These are rare and clinically obvious.

2. **Diseases of the vertebral column.**

   a. INFLAMMATORY
Pott's disease	Ankylosing
Staphylococcal	spondylitis
spondylitis	Actinomycosis
Typhoid spine	Hydarid cyst
	Paget's disease

   b. DEGENERATIVE
Spondylosis	Herniation of
Osteochondritis	nucleus
(rare)	pueposus

   c. NEOPLASTIC
Secondary deposit	Myelomarosis
Sarcoma	Leukaemic deposits

   d. TRAUMATIC
Fracture	Disc herniation
Dislocation	Spondylolisthesis

   e. EROSION BY AORTIC ANEURYSM

3. **Diseases of the spinal cord and meninges**
Metastatic epidural	Meningitis serosa
abscess or tumour	circumscripta
Meningioma	Tumour of the
Neurofibroma	spinal cord
Herpes zoster	Syringomyelia

4. **Hysteria and malingering:**
   Compensation neurosis

5. Metabolic disorders: osteoporosis, osteomalacia, hyperparathyroidism

The investigation of spinal tenderness requires an exhaustive case history, a careful examination and certain special investigations. The history is of particular importance, because not only will it disclose the duration, site and severity of the spinal symptoms, but it will also indicate whether the spinal cord or nerve roots are involved (root pain, girdle sensations, paraesthesiae in the limb, muscular weakness or stiffness, sphincter disturbances). A systematic interrogation as to general health, previous diseases, and symptoms referable to the other systems of the body may bring out facts relevant to the spinal condition. There is no laboratory procedure which can give this information, and a further advantage of the historical approach is that it provides a guide to the patient's mental and emotional conditions which is invaluable in assessing the reality and severity of the spinal symptoms.

The second step, physical examination, must cover the whole body in a search for factors which may throw light on the spinal tenderness. Reference has already been made to the need for care in determining that the tenderness is really in the spine itself, and not in the adjacent muscles or the overlying skin. The extent of the tenderness and the presence or absence of limitation of movement must be established. Acute tenderness of organic origin is always associated with limitation of movement in one or more directions. The examination of sensation, power, and reflexes below the level of tenderness is important, for significant neurological abnormalities may be found in the absence of any subjective symptoms. Attention must be paid to the chest, cardiovascular system, abdomen and prostate. The long bones should receive attention, and the skull must not be forgotten, because in carcinomatosis painless secondary deposits may be found in the latter. Of the special investigations, X-ray examination of the spine takes the first place, but evidence of local disease may be long delayed and it is dangerous to assume that a negative finding is conclusive; further radiographs, taken at a later date, may tell a different tale, CT scanning of the spine gives very accurate delineation of the spinal anatomy. X-ray examination of the chest, aorta, skull and long bones may be necessary. The cerebrospinal fluid should be examined, not only to see whether there is a raised protein and presence of leucocytes such as may be present in disease within the spinal canal, but also to exclude the possibility of a spinal block (Queckenstedt's test). A rise in the acidphosphatase of the serum will suggest the presence of a secondary growth from the prostate, and a high alkaline phosphatase is found in Paget's disease. A raised serum calcium may suggest hyperparathyroidism.

Pain and tenderness in the spine are sometimes functional. There is usually an organic nucleus to this either in the form of a long-past injury to the back or some minor physical abnormality. Marked spinal tenderness, especially in the thoracic spine, is frequently associated with current stress. Patients with spinal osteoarthritis and ankylosing spondylitis, for instance, are seldom tender over the spine unless anxiety or other mental overtones become superimposed.

Tenderness in the spine due to disease in other parts of the body
Superficial tenderness over the spine is a common association of visceral disease, and the tenderness is

situated over the portion of the spine corresponding to the segmental innervation of the affected viscus. The tenderness is not associated with local rigidity, and there is invariably well-marked evidence of the visceral disease, so that such tenderness is unlikely to be taken for a manifestation of spinal disease. On the other hand, spinal disease which gives rise to local tenderness and to a root pain in the chest or abdomen is easily mistaken for visceral disease.

Harold Ellis

Splenomegaly

An enlarged spleen may present because it is causing pressure symptoms or it may be found on examination of a patient who is generally unwell. Occasionally splenomegaly may be found on routine medical examination, in an individual who is asymptomatic, e.g. pre-employment or for insurance purposes. In this instance, particularly in a young person without other abnormal physical signs and a normal blood count, it can sometimes be extremely difficult to reach a diagnosis. A mass in the left hypochondrium, apart from a spleen may be an enlarged kidney, tumour of the splenic flexure of the colon or of the stomach or may arise from a retroperitoneal structure. Good medical practice dictates that an explanation should be found in all individuals for the splenomegaly; on occasions it will be necessary to proceed to laparotomy in an attempt to make a diagnosis.

The causes of splenomegaly are set out in Table S.10. and the most likely diagnosis varies considerably with the age, geographical location and social habits of the patient. Almost all causes of lymphadenopathy may be associated with splenomegaly and failing positive findings in other investigations, biopsy of an enlarged lymph node often renders a diagnosis.

Patients with splenomegaly may present with the symptoms and signs of pancytopenia due to hypersplenism which may occur with only a modest enlargement of the organ. There is usually an approximately parallel reduction in erythrocytes, leucocytes and platelets although on occasions there may be a more marked reduction of only one cell line. In the presence of such haematological abnormalities it is important to demonstrate normal or hyperplastic bone marrow morphology. In addition to the cellular elements being pooled and preferentially destroyed in the spleen the cytopenias are often exacerbated by a consistent increase in plasma volume.

Many diseases may result in enlargement of the spleen by several different mechanisms. For example in schistosomiasis the spleen may be enlarged because of chronic infection as well as portal hypertension secondary to portal fibrosis. A grossly enlarged spleen

Table S.10. Causes of splenomegaly

Acute infections
(*See* LYMPHADENOPATHY, p. 402)

Chronic infections
(*See* LYMPHADENOPATHY, p. 402)
Malaria
Kala-azar
Schistosomiasis

Congestion
Hepatic cirrhosis
Portal vein obstruction
Splenic vein obstruction
Budd–Chiari syndrome
Cardiac failure

Haemolytic anaemias
Haemolytic anaemia
Hereditary spherocytosis
Thalassaemias
Red cell enzyme defects
Immune-mediated haemolysis

Haematological malignancies
Chronic myeloid leukaemia
Acute leukaemias
Chronic lymphatic leukaemia
Macroglobulinaemia
Polycythaemia rubra vera
Myelofibrosis
Essential thrombocythaemia
Lymphomas
  Hodgkin's disease
  Non-Hodgkin's disease
Hairy-cell leukaemia

Connective-tissue disorders
Systemic lupus erythematosus
Felty's syndrome

Storage disorders
Gaucher's disease
Niemann–Pick disease
Histiocytosis X

Space-occupying lesions
Abscess
Metastatic tumour
Cysts
  Hydatid
  Haemangioma
  Dermoid

has a vastly increased blood supply and portal hypertension may result from high blood flow. In myelofibrosis with gross splenomegaly, for example, such a high flow of its own accord may cause portal hypertension such that ascites develops. When this is observed the prognosis is usually poor and splenectomy should be considered.

Investigation

A careful history and examination along with a full blood count and liver function tests will often provide a short differential diagnosis. If an infection is suspected appropriate microbiological tests will need to be carried out. When difficulty is encountered it is usually necessary to undertake fairly wide-ranging investigations. These should start by confirming that the mass palpated is spleen and not another pathology. Although traditionally a plain abdominal X-ray may delineate the splenic outline, other more recently developed techniques are now more informative. An ultrasound examination will confirm the presence of a mass and also provide accurate dimensions; it is usually possible to distinguish between spleen and the other causes of a left hypochondrial mass, e.g. enlarged kidney. Furthermore, it may be valuable for detecting space-occupying lesions, e.g. cysts or abscesses. An isotope liver and spleen scan will confirm splenomegaly and this investigation is particularly useful for detecting diffuse parenchymatous disease in the liver which may be causing portal hypertension, e.g. cirrhosis, or may be due to an infiltrate which could also be affecting the spleen. An abdominal CT scan will delineate the size and consistency of the spleen and is the investigation of choice if a lymphoma is suspected as it is useful for delineating retroperitoneal and mesenteric lymph nodes.

C. A. Ludlam

Sputum

Normally about 100 ml of bronchial secretion is removed daily by ciliary action from the airways of the lung through the larynx and disposed of into the alimentary tract by unconscious acts of swallowing. Sputum consists of bronchial secretions in excess of the amount that can be disposed of in this way; of pathological secretions, exudates and pus from abnormal bronchi, bronchioles and alveoli, or from abscesses, cavities or cysts in the lung; or of material derived from morbid processes in pleura, lymph nodes, mediastinum, oesophagus, subphrenic space and liver which have ulcerated into the lung. It may be mixed with saliva and secretions from the upper respiratory tract, but should be distinguished from these.

The patient's account of its mode of production, quantity and quality of the sputum, and the physician's observations, especially the naked-eye appearances, often give information at least as important as that derived from laboratory procedures.

Although the production of sputum is usually associated with cough, some chronic bronchitic patients deny cough, regarding the expectoration of mucus or even mucopus in the mornings as so 'normal' that they refer to it as 'clearing the throat'. Other patients, who evidently raise excess secretions from their lower respiratory tracts by cough, deny producing sputum because they habitually swallow the material expectorated.

Sputum arising from the bronchi may be mucoid, mucopurulent or frankly purulent. It is important to remember that in asthmatic patients a yellow sputum does not necessarily indicate the presence of pus—i.e. neutrophil polymorphs; it may be due to eosinophil polymorphs, associated with allergic reactions rather than infection.

In acute pulmonary oedema the material expectorated is derived largely from the oedema fluid transuded into the alveoli; it is thin, frothy, and may be pink from uniform bloodstaining.

When sputum is profuse and purulent, it is likely that it arises from a localized abnormality, such as *bronchiectasis, lung abscess* or *empyema with pleuro-bronchial fistula*. Inquiry should be made about the effect of posture upon it; the patient may have noticed that certain postures lead to cough and expectoration; the posture that he adopts for sleeping may be significant since it may have been chosen because it does not lead to cough. The sudden production of a large volume of sputum suggests the evacuation of a localized collection of liquid into a bronchus from a *pleural empyema*, a *cyst* (infected or otherwise), a *lung abscess* or a *mediastinal, subphrenic* or *intrahepatic* abscess. An episode of this sort may be followed by persistent expectoration or may cease temporarily when the bronchial communication becomes occluded, and recur later. Rupture of a *hydatid cyst* in the lung may result in the sudden expectoration of a large amount of thin watery material, which may be accompanied or followed by an anaphylactic reaction.

The uniformly purulent sputum of a patient with a localized source of suppuration in the lungs or pleura is generally distinguishable from that of a patient with a *diffuse mucopurulent bronchitis* with or without *bronchiectasis*; it is often evidently thinner with little or no viscid mucoid secretion mixed with it, and flows easily.

Sputum may be odourless and this gives no indication of the likely pathogens; but if it has a sickeningly offensive smell it is virtually certain that there is an infection with anaerobic organisms as may occur in some types of lung abscess, empyema with pleurobronchial fistula and severely infected bronchiectasis. The pus in acute specific lung abscesses due to *Staphylococcus aureus* or *Klebsiella pneumoniae*, and in empyemas due to these organisms, to pneumococcus or to *Streptococcus pyogenes*, is not malodorous.

In addition to the yellow of pus or eosinophil pseudopus, other colours may be observed in the sputum. A uniformly purulent sputum may be green rather than yellow, either because of degeneration of leucocytes in specimens that have been left standing, or because of infection by *Pseudomonas aeruginosa*. The ulceration of an amoebic liver abscess into the lung gives rise to the expectoration of reddish-brown so-called 'anchovy-sauce' pus. Sputum may be stained with fresh or altered blood, or mixed with larger quantities of blood; this is considered under HAEMO-PTYSIS. The sputum of those exposed to dust will contain the dust that has settled on the bronchi, often aggregated by ciliary streaming to give a mottled appearance. The sputum of coal-miners contains coal-dust. In coal-miners with complicated pneumoconiosis, the confluent collagenous masses incorporating coal-dust that constitute progressive massive fibrosis sometimes liquefy centrally; when this occurs, the liquid black contents are expectorated, resulting in an episode of expectoration of inky black material, or 'melanoptysis'.

Formed elements may be visible in sputum. Although careful search by floating the sputum in water may reveal fragments which are evidently casts of small parts of the peripheral bronchial tree in patients with asthma or with diffuse bronchitis, large casts with multiple branching are rarely seen. They occur in the very rare plastic or fibrinous bronchitis; the patient, often an asthmatic, suffers recurrent febrile illnesses with collapse-consolidation of a lobe or lobes of the lung, re-expanding after expectoration of the cast. Much more frequent is allergic bronchopulmonary aspergillosis, in which the sputum may contain 'plugs', generally about 4–5 mm in diameter and 15–20 mm long. Usually they are roughly spindle-shaped, without the multiple branching of bronchial casts, though occasionally there is a single bifurcation at one end. They consist mainly of tough mucus, containing many eosinophils, and with a little *Aspergillus mycelium* in the centre, usually demonstrable only by special staining. This disease occurs in extrinsic atopic asthmatics, and the sputum may also have the microscopic features seen in asthma (*see below*). Careful search in the sputum of asthmatic patients suspected of allergic aspergillosis may be required to demonstrate the 'plugs', but patients on inquiry will often be found to have noticed the presence from time to time of a tough fragment in the sputum. Very rarely, a patient with a bronchial carcinoma coughs out a gross fragment of the tumour. Another rare event is the expectoration of a fragment of calcified caseous material from an old tuberculous focus, either in lung or in a bronchopulmonary lymph node. If a previous chest radiograph is available, it is sometimes possible to see that one of the calcified foci evident in it has disappeared in a subsequent film.

The principal laboratory examinations to which sputum should be submitted are microscopy and bacteriological culture.

The presence of pus can be microscopically confirmed by the finding of large numbers of neutrophil polymorphs. As already noted, it is important to distinguish the eosinophil pseudopus which appears in the sputum of some asthmatics from true pus. Additionally, in the mucoid sputum of asthmatics, many eosinophils may be present. This finding is of especial importance in the differential diagnosis between late-onset intrinsic asthma and chronic bronchitis. The sputum of asthmatic patients may also contain Curschmann's spirals and Charcot–Leyden crystals. Curschmann's spirals consist of whitish, twisted threads of mucus, often including eosinophils; Charcot–Leyden crystals are colourless, elongated octahedrons which appear to be associated with eosinophils. Occasionally, small clumps of desquamated bronchiolar epithelial cells, the so-called 'Creola bodies', may be seen in the sputum of asthmatic patients, especially after a severe attack or during a prolonged attack.

Examination of the sputum for cancer cells is an important investigation in the diagnosis of bronchial carcinoma. This is a specialized procedure, its reliability depending very much upon the skill and experience of the cytologist. Clinicians should be aware of some possibly confusing factors. In asthmatic patients a report that clumps of adenocarcinoma cells have been seen should be interpreted in the knowledge that the 'Creola bodies', mentioned above, may mimic such cells very closely; and in patients with chronic tuberculous or other cavities in the lung, which may be lined with metaplastic squamous cells, these cells may be desquamated and prove difficult to distinguish with certainty from squamous carcinoma cells.

After haemoptysis from any cause and in the presence of pulmonary congestion associated with heart disease, iron-containing macrophages or siderocytes may be seen in the sputum. They also appear in the sputum in idiopathic pulmonary haemosiderosis, but are not of specific significance in this disease.

Persons who have been exposed to asbestos dust produce 'asbestos bodies' in their sputum. These consist of very thin, needle-like fibres of asbestos surrounded by a clear brownish coating of proteinaceous material containing iron, often arranged in an irregular beaded distribution or with a terminal bead or beads causing the whole to resemble a drumstick or dumb-bell. The presence of these bodies indicates only exposure to asbestos and is not necessarily associated with pulmonary *asbestosis*. Apart from this, microscopy of the sputum gives no specific information in pneumoconioses. Similarly, although oil-containing macrophages may be found in the sputum of patients with *exogenous oil inhalation pneumonia*, they may also be found in users of oily nasal drops—but without pathological consequences in the lungs.

In pulmonary *alveolar proteinosis* microscopy of the sputum shows amorphous eosinophilic PAS-positive material while electron microscopy shows the presence of lamellar bodies, presumably derived from type II pneumocytes, which may be diagnostic.

Microscopy of suitably stained sputum-smears is an essential part of the examination of the sputum for *mycobacteria*. It has been estimated that sputum specimens must contain as many as 100 000 bacilli per ml if acid-fast bacilli can be reliably demonstrated in them by microscopy after Ziehl–Neelsen staining. Examination by fluorescence microscopy after suitable staining has a somewhat higher sensitivity. Appropriate methods of culture demonstrate *mycobacteria* in specimens containing far fewer organisms but there is a delay of several weeks before the result can be available. For this reason, persistent attempts should be made to find acid-fast bacilli by microscopy in any patient who is acutely ill with an inflammatory process in the lung that might be tuberculous. In this interpretation of negative findings it is important to remember that failure to find acid-fast bacilli in a scanty mucoid sputum in a patient with acute pneumonic changes without cavitation militates very little against a diagnosis of tuberculosis: whereas in a patient with a cavitated inflammatory process and frankly purulent sputum, repeated negative findings are much more significant.

Microscopy of Gram-stained smears of sputum is of value in acute pneumonias—e.g. a preponderance of Gram-positive diplococci suggests a *pneumococcal infection*, or of clumps of Gram-positive cocci a *staphylococcal infection*—but in bacterial infections culture is generally required both to identify organisms and to provide information about their sensitivity to antibiotics. Sputum is usually cultured only aerobically. Culture of expectorated sputum anaerobically is useless because the sputum is inevitably contaminated by oropharyngeal organisms which include many anaerobic species. If infection with anaerobic organisms is suspected specimens must be obtained from the lower respiratory tract either by transtracheal aspiration or at fibreoptic bronchoscopy using a sheathed brush to obtain the specimens.

In patients suspected of *pneumocystis pneumonia*, specimens of alveolar secretion may be obtained by alveolar lavage and examined by immunofluorescent staining techniques for *pneumocystis carinii*. It should be remembered that in the sputum of patients receiving broad-spectrum antibiotics, organisms other than the original pathogens often become predominant. These may be organisms that rarely become pathogenic, such as *Proteus* and *coliform* organisms, as well as some that can assume independent pathogenicity, such as *Pseudomonas pyocyanea* and *Candida*. Even with the latter, it is often difficult to be certain whether or not they are truly pathogenic in an individual case of chronic mucopurulent bronchitis.

Sporing organisms, such as *Aspergillus* species, the spores of which are frequently present in the air, appear as contaminants in a proportion of all sputum cultures. For this reason, the finding of an *Aspergillus* species in the sputum is of no significance unless supported by clinical and immunological evidence. When infection with other pathogenic fungi is suspected special culture media are required; such cultures can, if positive, be highly infectious and a laboratory hazard.

Peter Emerson

Squint (Strabismus)

Squints may be classified, according to their *direction,* into convergent, divergent or vertical; and according to their *cause,* into paralytic and non-paralytic (concomitant). The diagnosis between paralytic and non-paralytic squint is, as a rule, easy. In a paralytic squint the degree of deviation of the two eyes varies, as the farther the eyes are moved in the direction of the action of the paralysed muscle, the greater will be the angle of squint. In a concomitant squint the eyes always bear the same relative position to each other in whatever direction they are turned. Concomitant squint is characteristically a disorder of childhood, while paralytic squint more frequently occurs later in life.

The diagnosis of the cause of a paralytic squint is discussed under Diplopia.

Concomitant squints are usually the sequel to disharmony of the accommodation–convergence synkinesis (as with high hypermetropia, poor development in the power of fusion or anatomical fascio-muscular abnormalities) the eyes—all of which may have a congenital basis. They may be aggravated by any sensory or central impediment to the acquisition of the binocular fixation reflex (e.g. poor vision from a congenital cataract, or poor coordination from mental deficiency).

S. T. D. Roxburgh

Stature, short

Patients can be described as suffering from 'short stature' when they are shown to be below the 3rd centile of a normal population of their sex and age. The term 'dwarfism' should not be used as it is insulting. Charts have been devised by Tanner and Whitehouse (*Fig.* S.40) for a normal British population, but these are not necessarily applicable to people of a different ethnic origin. Most short British children are so because they have small parents, are socially deprived or are suffering from delayed puberty, whereas in developing countries of the world common causes of short stature are malnutrition and chronic debilitating disease in childhood. Rarer causes include skeletal deformities and hormonal deficiencies. The causes of short stature are listed in *Table* S.11.

Table S.11.   Causes of short stature

1. **Normal genetic short stature**

2. **Growth delay**

3. **Chromosomal abnormalities**
    (a)   Gonadal dysgenesis
          Turner's syndrome
          Noonan's syndrome
    (b)   Autosomal anomalies
          Trisomy 21 (Down's syndrome, Mongolism)
          Trisomy 18 (Edward's syndrome)
          Trisomy 13 (Patau's syndrome)

4. **Disease in childhood**
    Calorie deficiency (marasmus)
    Protein malnutrition (kwashiorkor)
    Vitamin D deficiency (rickets)
    Tuberculosis
    Bronchiectasis
    Cystic fibrosis
    Chronic asthma (particularly when treated with steroids)
    Gluten enteropathy (coeliac disease)
    Other malabsorption syndromes
    Hookworm infection
    Malaria
    Cyanotic congenital heart disease
    Chronic renal disease
    Congenital syphilis
    Glycogen storage disease
    Thalassaemia major

5. **Psychological causes**

6. **Skeletal abnormalities**
    Congenital
    (a)   Achondroplasia, hypochondroplasia
    (b)   Morquio's disease (chondro-osteodystrophy)
    (c)   Dysostosis multiplex (gargoylism or Hurler's syndrome)
    (d)   Chondrodystrophia calcificans congenita (Conradi's syndrome)
    (e)   Epiphysial dysplasia multiplex
    (f)   Chondro-ectodermal dysplasia (Ellis–van Creveld syndrome)
    (g)   Osteogenesis imperfecta (fragilitas ossium)
    (h)   Approximately 50 others
    Acquired
          Rickets (*see below*)
          Tuberculosis and other infections of the spine
          Deformities secondary to neurological and joint diseases (e.g. poliomyelitis, Still's disease)

7. **Endocrine abnormalities**
    Hypothalamic/pituitary dysfunction
       Destructive lesions
          Craniopharyngioma
          Pituitary tumour
          Tuberculosis
          Meningitis
          Sarcoidosis
          Toxoplasmosis
          Histiocytosis X
          Trauma
          Intracranial irradiation
       Pituitary agenesis
       Isolated growth hormone deficiency
       Idiopathic hypopituitarism
          Fröhlich's syndrome
          Laurence–Moon–Biedl syndrome
          Somatomedin deficiency (Laron type)
          Somatomedin resistance (Pygmies)
    Hypothyroidism
       Thyroid agenesis
       Solitary TSH deficiency
       Dyshormonogenesis
       Auto-immune thyroiditis
       Ectopic thyroid tissue
    Sexual precocity
       True precocity
          Physiological precocious puberty
          Space-occupying lesions of the central nervous system
          Congenital and acquired hypothalamic lesions
       False precocity
          Congenital and adrenal hyperplasia
          Cushing's syndrome
          Adrenocortical tumour
          Interstitial cell tumour of testis
          Granulosa cell tumour of ovary
    Pseudohypoparathyroidism and pseudopseudohypoparathyroidism
    Rickets
       Vitamin D deficiency
       Renal impairment
       Vitamin D resistance

8. **Intra-uterine maldevelopment**
    Small-for-dates babies
    Fetal alcohol syndrome
    Russell–Silver syndrome
    Progeria (Hutchinson–Gilford syndrome)
    Cornelia de Lange syndrome ('Amsterdam dwarfism')
    Cockayne syndrome
    Prader–Willi syndrome

9. **Drugs**
    Glucocorticoids
    Androgens
    Anabolic steroids
    Oestrogens
    Thyroid hormones
    Anti-thyroid drugs
    Vitamin D

1.   Normal genetic short stature

Most children who present with short stature are short because they have small parents. This can be readily ascertained by plotting the child's height on a growth chart (*Fig.* S.40) and comparing the parents' heights with it. The parents' heights are marked on the right-hand side of the chart, 13.0 cm being subtracted from the father's height when plotting on a girl's chart and 13.0 cm being added to the mother's height when plotting on a boy's chart. The mid-point between the parents' centiles is then found and a vertical line is drawn to 8·5 cm above and 8·5 cm below the mid-point. This line will cover two standard deviations above and below the mean and there will be only a 5 per cent chance of a normal child falling outside these centiles.

The short child whose centile falls within his parents' normal range should be seen in 6 months' time, to make sure that the growth velocity is normal.

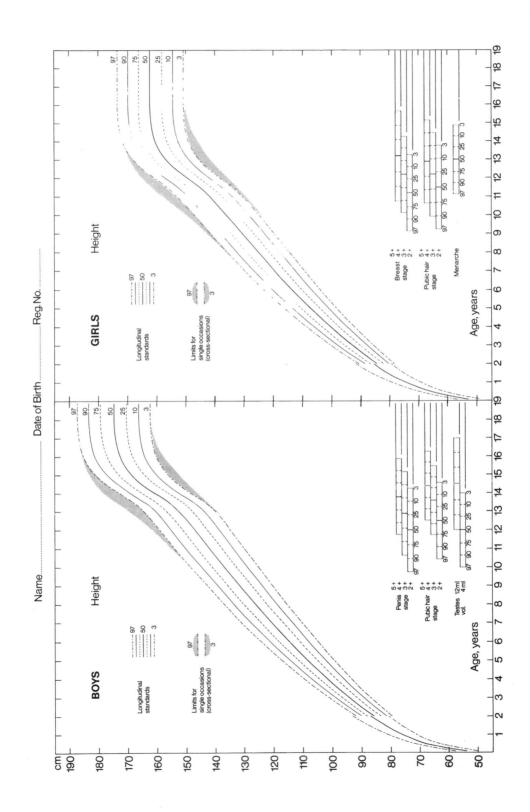

Name.................................... Date of Birth.................... Reg. No....................

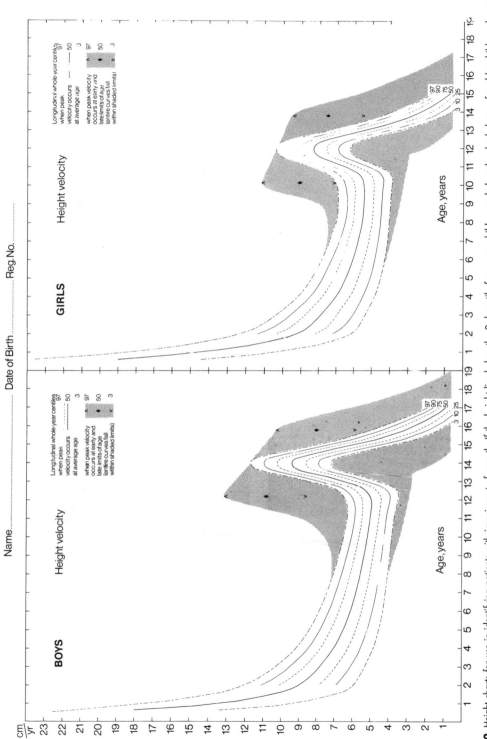

Fig. S.40. Height charts for use in identifying patients with impairment of growth. If the height lies below the 3rd centile for young children or below the shaded area for older children, the patient should be investigated. Velocity charts show the individual growth rate at different ages. (Charts constructed by Professor J. M. Tanner and Mr. R. H. Whitehouse of the Department of Growth and Development, Institute of Child Health, London. Published with copyright permission by Castlemead Publications, Swains Mill, 4a Crane Mead, Ware, Hertfordshire, UK.)

2. Growth delay

Growth delay, often associated with delayed puberty, is a common cause of short stature. There is often a family history of both. The bone age, assessed from a radiograph of the wrist and hand, will usually be delayed by 3 years or more. Ultimately normal growth and sexual development is the rule.

3. Chromosomal abnormalities

The two most common chromosomal abnormalities are Turner's syndrome and Down's syndrome.

TURNER'S SYNDROME. Turner's syndrome occurs in girls and is characterized by gonadal dysgenesis, lack of sexual development and short stature. It occurs with a prevalence of 1 per 3000 female births. The karyotype is 45/XO and the buccal smear will show no Barr bodies. The average height reached is 140 cm and rarely is a height above 152 cm achieved. However, about a quarter of all patients with Turner's syndrome have mosaicism, such as XO/XX or XO/XXX and they may grow to a greater height. These patients may show one or, in the latter case, even two Barr bodies on buccal smear. It is wise in such circumstances to perform a full chromosomal analysis.

Because the ovaries are represented only by a fibrous streak, no oestrogens are secreted and so both internal and external genitalia remain infantile. No breast development occurs and there is primary amenorrhoea. In addition, there are various physical abnormalities that are not hormonally mediated. The short stature is in contrast to most other types of primary hypogonadism, in which tall stature, due to lack of epiphysial fusion, is a feature. There may be webbing of the neck (*Fig*. S.41) and a low hair line at the back of the neck (*Fig*. S.42). There is an increased carrying angle at the elbows (cubitus valgus), shortened 4th and/or 5th metatarsals and metacarpals, Madelung's deformity of the wrist (abnormal carpal angle), a shield-like chest and abnormal fingerprints (dermatoglyphics). Pigmented naevi are often present on the skin and intestinal telangiectasia sometimes occurs. Congenital cardiovascular anomalies exist in about one-fifth of cases and consist of coarctation of the aorta, aortic stenosis and both atrial and ventricular septal defects. Renal abnormalities such as horseshoe kidney or double ureter may occur. Hypertension is not uncommon. Subcutaneous oedema may be present in infancy. Minor abnormalities of the facies frequently draw attention to the diagnosis. The features include a flattened bridge to the nose, wide separation of the eyes (hypertelorism) and epicanthic folds. Osteoporosis may develop late in life due to the lack of oestrogens. Auto-immune thyroid disease is more common

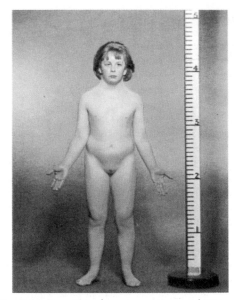

Fig. S.41. Turner's syndrome in a patient aged 23 years. Note the height, which is below 5 feet, webbing of the neck, increased carrying angle at the elbows, failure of breast development and scanty growth of pubic hair. (*Courtesy of the Gordon Photographic Museum. Guy's Hospital.*)

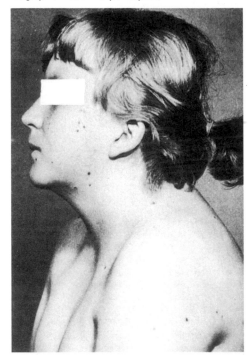

Fig. S.42. Turner's syndrome Showing the low hair line at the back of the neck.

in patients with Turner's syndrome than it is amongst the general female population.

NOONAN'S SYNDROME, which may occur in boys as well as girls, is somewhat like Turner's syndrome. The prevalence is 1 in 8000 births. In both boys and girls the karyotype is normal. Short stature is perhaps not so marked as in Turner's syndrome, but there may be webbing of the neck with a low hair line and a shield-like chest with widely spaced nipples. Pectus excavatum is present in 50 per cent. The face shows some typical features: an antimongoloid slant of the eyes, which are widely spaced, may have epicanthic folds and show ptosis; the face may be triangular in shape, the ears low-set (*Fig.* S.43) and the brow prominent. A high-arched palate is not infrequently present. The cardiovascular abnormalities differ in frequency from those of Turner's syndrome. Although coarctation of the aorta and aortic stenosis have been described, the characteristic cardiac diseases have been pulmonary stenosis in approximately half the cases and atrial septal defect. Sometimes both conditions occur together. Ventricular septal defect and persistent ductus arteriosus have also been associated with Noonan's syndrome. Cubitus valgus is common and mental retardation may be a feature. In males undescended testes are common (*Fig.* S.43) and androgen deficiency may manifest itself at puberty. Girls usually show delayed puberty but eventually normal ovarian function develops.

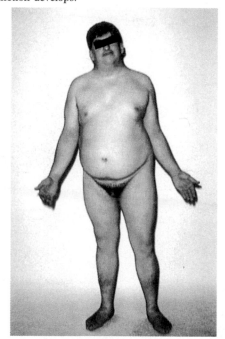

Fig. S.43. Noonan's syndrome. Note the low-set ears and the webbed neck. The testicles are undescended.

DOWN'S SYNDROME (Mongolism, Trisomy 21) is the commonest autosomal abnormality leading to short stature. There is disordered growth of the skull and long bones. The mouth and ears are small, the tongue is large and tends to protrude and there are epicanthic folds on the eyes. There is invariably mental retardation.

Auto-immune thyroiditis is much more common than in the general population.

The second most common autosomal condition is TRISOMY 18 (Edward's syndrome), which is characterized by a small face and cardiac malformations which nearly always lead to an early death. It occurs with a prevalence of 1 per 8000 births.

TRISOMY 13 (Patau's syndrome) is much more rare, occurring only once in 20 000 live births; death tends to occur in the first year of life.

4. Malnutrition and chronic debilitating disease in childhood

General calorie deficiency (marasmus) or protein deficiency (kwashiorkor) are common causes of short stature in underdeveloped parts of the world. *Rickets*, now unusual in the indigenous population of Britain, but relatively frequent among Asian children resident in this country, leads to retarded bone age and short stature.

The existence of *chronic debilitating disease* is readily apparent on taking the history or doing the physical examination. *Tuberculosis* and *bronchiectasis* are not nearly as common as they used to be in the developed countries. *Cystic fibrosis* occurs in approximately 1 in 1700 live births among Caucasians, but is much rarer in other ethnic groups. Recurrent pulmonary infections are usually the predominant feature. *Chronic asthma*, particularly when treated with steroids, leads to stunting, probably because excess glucocorticoids block the action of growth factors at the cellular level.

Malabsorption of food may lead to short stature. *Gluten enteropathy (coeliac disease)* is the commonest, occurring in approximately one in 2000 children. Although characteristic symptoms of chronic diarrhoea, pale bulky stools, anorexia and cramping abdominal pain may be present, they are by no means invariable. Sometimes the only clue in a short child is a rather protuberant abdomen and scanty subcutaneous fat (*Fig.* S.44). If other causes of short stature have been excluded, a small bowel biopsy to show flattened villi is a useful investigation, for once the diagnosis has been confirmed and a gluten-free diet instituted, normal growth should occur. Less common causes of malabsorption include cystic fibrosis (*see above*), lactose intolerance, Crohn's disease and infection with *Giardia lamblia*.

Children who either live in the tropics or have recently returned from there may have *hookworm infestation* or *malaria*. *Thalassaemia major* may be associated with short stature and delayed puberty.

Cyanotic congenital heart disease and *chronic renal failure* are usually obvious clinically as causes

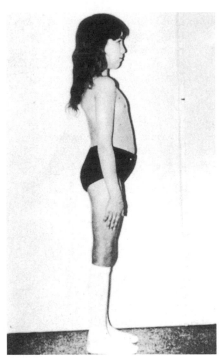

Fig. S.44. Gluten enteropathy. This girl presented with short stature. Note the protuberant abdomen, in contrast with the thin limbs. (*Dr Mary Rossiter.*)

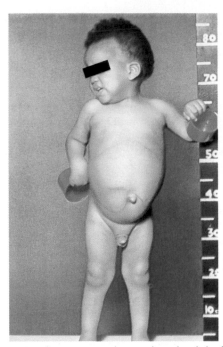

Fig. S.45. Glycogen storage disease. Almost the whole of the abdomen is occupied by the enlarged liver. (*Dr Mary Rossiter.*)

of growth failure. Less commonly seen are *congenital syphilis* and *glycogen storage disease* (Fig. S.45).

5. Psychological causes

An adverse psychological environment, with emotional deprivation and child abuse, is a very important cause of failure of growth. This has been shown to be due to suppression of growth hormone secretion by the pituitary and is reversible when the child is removed to happier and more secure surroundings.

6. Skeletal disorders

CONGENITAL SKELETAL DISORDERS

These are rare and many of them are inherited. The commonest is *achondroplasia* (*chondrodystrophy*) (Fig. S.46). The condition, dominantly inherited, is caused by a disturbance of endochondral ossification in which the growth cartilages are invaded by connective tissue. The trunk is of normal length, but the limbs are shortened. The fingers are short and are of equal length. The head is large, the forehead being particularly prominent, but the nose is small and the bridge is flattened. There is often a marked lumbar lordosis and the buttocks are prominent. Delayed puberty is not a feature.

Hypochondroplasia is similar to achondroplasia,

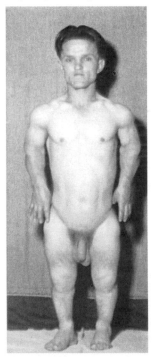

Fig.S.46. Short stature due to achondroplasia. Showing the large head and short extremities. The proximal segments of the limbs are relatively more affected than the distal and there is slight curvature of the tibiae.

but the face is usually normal. Again the inheritance is dominant.

Morquio's disease (chondro-osteo-dystrophy) is

a rare type of skeletal deformity affecting both the limbs and the spine. It is often familial. The epiphyses are deformed or fragmented and a variety of deformities of the long bones have been described. The glenoid fossae and acetabula are poorly formed. The intervertebral spaces are widened and, owing to the irregularity, flattening or wedge-shaped deformity of the vertebral bodies occurs and there is a dorso-lumbar kyphosis and shortening of the neck, the head appearing to be pushed down on the shoulders. Many cases show a gross pigeon-breast deformity and the short stature is further accentuated by limitation of extension of hips and knees. Characteristic changes are seen on X-ray examination (*Fig. S.47*).

Chondrodystrophia calcificans congenita (Conradi's syndrome) is a rare autosomal recessive condition in which the epiphysial centres of the long and small bones ossify and fuse during early childhood.

Epiphysial dysplasia multiplex can be transmitted as an autosomal dominant or as a recessive type of inheritance. It manifests itself in older children (usually under the age of 10) as a disorder of gait and short stature. The pathology lies in the epiphyses, which are fragmented.

Chondro-ectodermal dysplasia (Ellis–van Creveld syndrome) causes short stature because of a reduction in length of the extremities. The fingers are also short and there may be polydactyly. Hypoplasia

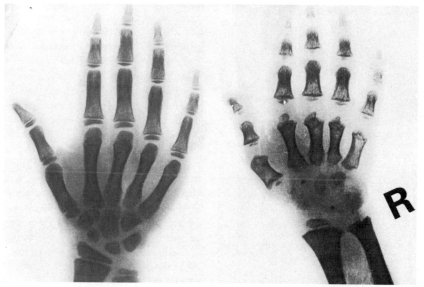

Fig. S.47. Chondro-osteo-dystrophy (Morquio's disease). X-ray of the hand on the right shows wide joint spaces and deformity of the epiphyses. On the left is a normal hand at the same age. (*Professor R. W. B. Ellis.*)

Dysostosis multiplex (gargoylism or Hurler's syndrome) shows similar bony deformities to the above, though a peculiar sabot-shaped deformity of the 2nd and 3rd lumbar vertebral bodies appears more constantly, giving rise to angular kyphosis. The skull commonly is conical (oxycephalic) or hydrocephalic and there may be enlargement of the pituitary fossa. The face shows widely spaced eyes (hypertelorism), a prominent forehead and a large tongue and lips (*Fig. S.48*). The liver and spleen may be enlarged. Mental retardation, corneal opacities and deafness are the rule. Distortion of the heart valves and thickening of coronary arteries are frequent findings. The condition is inherited as an autosomal recessive and is due to the deposition of the mucopolysaccharides heparan sulphate and dermatan sulphate. Infantilism may be associated with the short stature, but this is not always the case. However, most children do not survive longer than about the age of 14.

of the teeth, nails and hair occurs and there may be both cardiac and renal abnormalities.

Osteogenesis imperfecta (fragilitas ossium) is characterized by extreme brittleness of the bones. The multiple fractures which occur during intrauterine life or in childhood, coupled with the fragility of the spine, result in gross deformity and short stature (*Fig. S.49*). The disease is inherited as an autosomal dominant trait and there may be a family history of otosclerosis. The patient may have slaty-blue sclerae. Radiographically the long bones are seen to be both shorter and more slender than normal, poorly calcified, with extreme thinning of the cortex. The appearances are quite distinct from those of rickets.

There are many other rare disorders of growth due to congenital skeletal disorders.

ACQUIRED SKELETAL DISORDERS

Any disorder leading to damage of the long bones or spine will lead to stunted growth. *Rickets (see p. 70)*

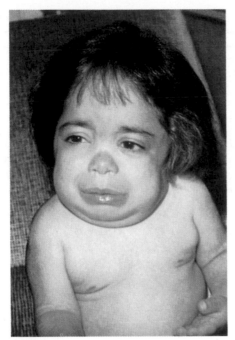

Fig. S.48. Dysostosis multiplex (Gargoylism. Hurler's syndrome). Showing the prominent forehead and lips and the widely spaced eyes. (*Dr Mary Rossiter.*)

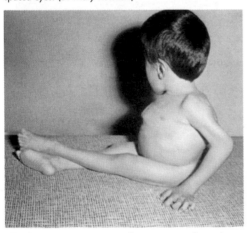

Fig. S.49. Osteogenesis imperfecta. Stunting of growth owing to skeletal deformities. (*Dr Mary Rossiter.*)

is not uncommon amongst Asian immigrant communities in Britain, particularly those who are vegetarians. *Tuberculosis of the spine (Pott's disease, spinal caries)* is much less common than it used to be. It is recognized by pain and tenderness localized to one or more of the vertebrae, associated with angular kyphosis. Radiographs show destruction and collapse of the affected vertebral bodies and there may be evidence of a 'cold abscess'. These features serve to distinguish spinal tuberculosis from congenital abnormality of the vertebrae and kyphosis or scoliosis from other causes, e.g. poliomyelitis, in which weakness of the muscles of

the back, perhaps unrecognized, is liable to result in a severe degree of postural deformity.

Still's disease (chronic juvenile arthritis, see p. 348) may lead to stunting of growth because of premature fusion of epiphyses in affected joints.

7. Endocrine disorders

The commonest endocrine causes of short stature are solitary growth hormone deficiency, which may be partial rather than total, and hypothyroidism. Less common are adrenal disorders and the remaining causes listed on p. 619 are much more rare.

Solitary growth hormone deficiency, secondary to lack of hypothalamic growth hormone releasing hormone, occurs in one per 10 000 live births in Britain and is four times more common in boys than girls. There seems to be a hereditary element, since 3 per cent of those affected have a sibling with growth hormone deficiency. There is also an association with breech delivery, the use of forceps, prematurity and maternal haemorrhage. The cause is probably secondary to anoxic hypothalamic damage. The children tend to be fat and may have small genitalia (*Fig.* S.50). They have delayed bone age and delayed puberty, but enter puberty when their bone age is appropriate. Half the children with growth hormone deficiency may have deficiency of other hormones. Destructive lesions involving the pituitary and hypothalamus may cause pan-hypopituitarism (*Fig.* S.51). They include tumours, of which the commonest in childhood is a craniopharyngioma, but other causes are meningitis (e.g. tuberculous), sarcoidosis, xanthomas (e.g. Hand–Schüller–Christian syndrome, histiocytosis X), trauma (especially basal fractures) and following intracranial irradiation.

Fröhlich's syndrome is mentioned if only to be dismissed. Fröhlich originally described a patient with obesity, somnolence, retarded skeletal and sexual development and optic atrophy. The pathology in this case was a suprasellar tumour pressing on the hypothalamus, and clearly pituitary hormone deficiencies secondary to hypothalamic damage were likely to have been present. Unfortunately the term 'Fröhlich's syndrome' tends to be attached to any short, fat boy with delayed sexual development and small genitalia. It is best forgotten.

Laurence–Moon–Biedl syndrome may sometimes be associated with short stature. The condition is autosomal recessive. Clinical features include obesity, retarded sexual development, mental retardation, retinitis pigmentosa and either polydactylism or syndactylism.

The rare *Laron type* of short stature is due to a deficiency of the growth factor somatomedin. Growth

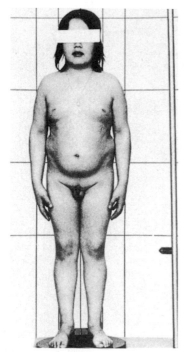

Fig. S.50. Solitary growth hormone deficiency in a boy aged 15. Note the associated obesity and retarded sexual development. (*Dr Charles Brook.*)

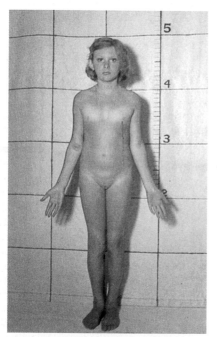

Fig. S.51. Pan-hypopituitarism. This girl aged $16\frac{1}{2}$ shows short stature and complete lack of sexual development.

hormone levels are high and it is presumed that the primary defect is lack of growth hormone receptors. The condition may be autosomal recessive or, in some

instances, sporadic. In some patients a different disorder exists in which growth hormone is biologically ineffective and somatomedin levels are low. They respond to exogenous growth hormone.

The pygmies of Africa have normal growth hormone and somatomedin levels, but abnormally low levels of an insulin-like growth factor. Absence of somatomedin receptors has been postulated.

Hypothyroidism is a common cause of short stature. Somatomedin levels are below normal. One in 3300 babies in Britain is born hypothyroid, usually due to thyroid agenesis. The diagnosis is now made early by neonatal TSH screening. However, it must be noted that neonatal hypothyroidism may be secondary to isolated TSH deficiency. This will be missed on TSH screening, but will be diagnosed if serum thyroxine is measured.

Dyshormonogenesis, which may be due to one of six defects in the synthesis of thyroid hormones, tends to lead to goitre and hypothyroidism in early life, though those with partial defects may present later.

After the age of round about 6 years auto-immune thyroiditis begins to become an increasingly important cause of hypothyroidism (*Fig.* S.52). A goitre is usually palpable and thyroid antibodies are present in blood. Sometimes at the time of puberty an ectopic, often sublingual, thyroid may be the cause of hypothyroidism.

Sexual precocity. When precocious sexual devel-

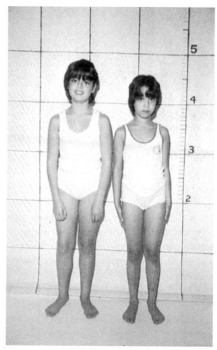

Fig. S.52. Hypothyroidism due to auto-immune thyroiditis has caused the short stature of the girl on the right who can be compared with her euthyroid identical twin sister.

opment occurs the production of sex hormones causes initially an acceleration of growth, but bone maturation is more rapid than normal, fusion of the epiphyses takes place and the final stature is shorter than would be expected from parental height (*Fig.* S.53). Precocious sexual development is five times more common in girls than in boys and in the majority of girls the cause is some unknown triggering mechanism in the hypothalamus which initiates a normal, albeit early, physiological puberty. In boys, on the other hand a pathological cause is found in about half the cases.

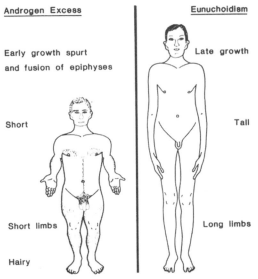

Fig. S.53. Comparison of short stature due to early closure of epiphyses and tall stature due to late closure of epiphyses because of hypogonadism, but with normal growth hormone secretion. (*Courtesy of the Departments of Medical Illustration. Guy's and Westminster Hospitals.*)

It is important to separate true precocity from false precocity. In true precocity puberty is 'physiological' and thus follows the pattern of normal development. While the majority are constitutional, it is important to look for space-occupying lesions of the central nervous system. These include craniopharyngioma, pineal tumour, hamartoma, neurofibroma, astrocytoma and cysts of the third ventricle. Hypothyroidism may cause the premature release of follicle stimulating hormone from the pituitary. Tuberose sclerosis, McCune-Albright syndrome (polyostotic fibrous dysplasia with cutaneous pigmentation), encephalitis and hydrocephalus may all lead to true precocity. On the other hand, 'false' precocity is due to the action of sex hormones produced by the gonad or by the adrenals. The common causes are congenital adrenal hyperplasia due to a 21-hydroxylase defect and Cushing's syndrome (*Fig.* S.54). Testicular and ovarian tumours are very rare. The subject is covered in more detail under PUBERTY, PRECOCIOUS p. 524).

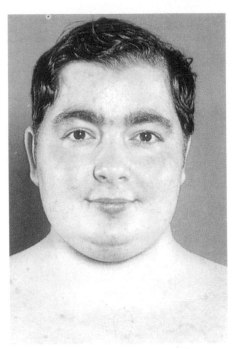

Fig. S.54. Facial appearance of Cushing's syndrome in a 12-year-old boy. (*Dr Charles Brook.*)

Pseudohypoparathyroidism is a disorder in which the renal tubules are resistant to the action of parathyroid hormone. As a result production of 1·25 dihydroxyvitamin D by the kidneys is reduced and as a consequence absorption of calcium from the gut is diminished. The patient is usually short and mentally retarded, has short 4th and 5th metacarpals and may have cataracts and ectopic subcutaneous calcification with ulceration (*Fig.* S.55). Serum calcium levels are low and parathyroid hormone levels are increased. Some patients have the short stature and skeletal abnormalities but with a normal calcium level. This is called 'pseudo-pseudohypoparathyroidism'.

Rickets may lead to stunting of growth and bowing of the legs. The commonest cause is vitamin D deficiency due to lack of ultraviolet light so that the precursor of the vitamin, 7-dehydrocholesterol, is not converted into vitamin D. The normal British diet contains very little vitamin D. Groups particularly at risk are Indian and Pakistani immigrants, especially if they are vegetarian (*Fig.* S.56). Small bowel and biliary diseases also cause malabsorption of vitamin D.

Other rarer causes of rickets are congenital renal tubular defects and 25-hydroxyvitamin D-1-α-hydroxylase deficiency (vitamin-D resistant rickets).

8. Intrauterine maldevelopment

Most small-for-dates babies subsequently grow at a normal rate, though they may not achieve a final stature

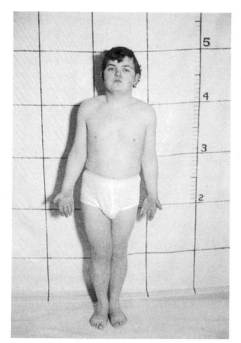

Fig. S.55. Pseudohypoparathyroidism. The patient has short stature and mild mental retardation. His 4th and 5th metacarpals are short.

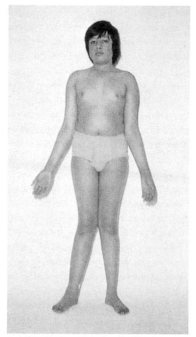

Fig. S.56. Rickets in a vegetarian Indian boy. Note the genu valgum

appropriate for their parents' centiles. Some, however, fail to grow normally and may be examples of specific syndromes, of which the commonest is the Russell–Silver syndrome. This is characterized by lack

of subcutaneous fat, a triangular face with large forehead, small jaw, low-set ears and a turned down mouth. There is incurving and shortening of the 5th fingers.

The fetal alcohol syndrome is being increasingly recognized; this is probably related to the rising consumption of alcohol. In addition to growth retardation there is mental subnormality and a characteristic facial appearance. This consists of a small jaw, short nose, underdeveloped upper lip and a reduction in length of the palpebral fissures. More serious conditions are congenital heart defects and flexion contractures.

Progeria (Hutchinson–Gilford syndrome) is characterized by premature ageing and death usually occurs before the age of 20. Appearances are normal at birth but growth ceases, owing to epiphysial closure, within a period ranging from a few months to 3 years. There is no subcutaneous fat, the nose is beaky and the ears prominent. There may be premature baldness, some mental retardation, periarticular fibrosis and arteriosclerosis.

Cornelia de Lange syndrome (Amsterdam 'dwarfism') is characterized by poor growth, mental deficiency, a small head with a flattened occiput, abnormal lips and mouth, bushy eyebrows that meet in the middle, short nose with anteverted nostrils and abnormalities of the extremities, particularly of the upper limbs. Hirsutism may be a feature (*see Fig.* H.28).

Patients with *Cockayne syndrome* have a somewhat similar appearance to that of progeria, except that mental retardation is more marked, there is retinal degeneration, photosensitive dermatitis, deafness, unsteady gait and tremor.

The Prader–Willi syndrome is characterized by poor growth, obesity, hypogonadism, cryptorchidism, hypotonia and mental retardation. Hands and feet are small compared with the rest of the body.

9. Drugs

The administration of various drugs, particularly in high doses, may lead to stunting of growth in a child. *Glucocorticoids*, used particularly in asthma and Still's disease, may cause short stature due to interference with growth at the cellular level. The dosage should therefore be kept to the minimum possible and should preferably be given on alternate days.

Anabolic steroids have sometimes been used to try to increase the height of a short child. The danger is that they accelerate bone age, cause epiphysial fusion and may thus actually decrease potential height. The same may happen when androgens or oestrogens are used in boys and girls respectively to bring about sexual maturation. Specialist advice should be sought before using any of these drugs in children.

Lack of thyroid hormone (hypothyroidism) causes

delayed bone maturation and short stature, but it must be remembered that the condition may be iatrogenic, when too much anti-thyroid drug is given, and that iodides may lead to goitre formation and hypothyroidism in some individuals who are predisposed to autoimmune thyroid disease. Conversely, overtreatment of hypothyroidism in childhood with thyroxine will lead initially to a growth spurt due to stimulation of somatomedin production by the liver, but, by accelerating bone maturation, may reduce potential stature in the long term.

Vitamin D preparations, given to children for conditions such as hypoparathyroidism, pseudohypoparathyroidism and rickets, may give rise to hypercalcaemia, which, if chronic, will cause renal failure. If the renal failure is severe enough stunting of growth will result. Vitamin D treatment should always be monitored with regular measurement of the serum calcium.

Ian D. Ramsay

Stature, tall

A patient is usually defined as exhibiting tall stature if the height is above the 97th centile for the normal population. The term 'gigantism' should no longer be used. In most cases tallness is inherited from tall parents; pathological causes are much less common. However, a child may be below the 97th centile, but still be inappropriately tall compared with the parents. If a period of observation shows that the growth velocity is greater than normal the appropriate investigations should be carried out. The classification of tall stature is listed in *Table* S.12.

Table S.12. Causes of tall stature

1.	**Constitutional**
2.	**Overnutrition**
3.	**Endocrine abnormalities** Sexual precocity and virilizing syndromes Hypogonadism Thyrotoxicosis Pituitary acidophil over-activity ('gigantism')
4.	**Chromosomal abnormalities** Klinefelter's syndrome (47 XXY) 'Supermale' (47 XYY) 'Superfemale' (47 XXX)
5.	**Miscellaneous** Marfan's syndrome Homocystinuria Cerebral 'gigantism' (Sotos' syndrome) Brain damage Lipodystrophy Beckwith–Wiedemann syndrome

1. Constitutional

Constitutional tall stature can be identified by plotting the patient's height relative to age on a growth-develop-ment chart (*Fig.* S.40.) and comparing it with the heights of the parents in the way described on p. 619.

Some children who enter puberty relatively early may initially become taller than their contemporaries because of an early growth spurt, but their epiphyses will also fuse earlier and so the ultimate adult height attained will be appropriate for their family.

2. Overnutrition

Overnutrition leading to obesity in early childhood may lead to accelerated linear growth but fusion of the epiphyses at an earlier age than usual normalizes the final height.

3. Endocrine abnormalities

The commonest *endocrine* causes of tall stature in childhood are true precocious puberty and false precocious puberty (*see* p. 524). True precocious puberty is either physiological (which is the commonest) or is due to space-occupying or other lesions affecting the hypothalamus. False precocious puberty can be caused by either adrenal disease (congenital adrenal hyperplasia, e.g. 21-hydroxylase defect, and adrenocortical tumour) or by very rare hormone-secreting testicular or ovarian tumours. The increased amounts of sex hormones produced in these various conditions lead to an increased maturation of bone, with an acceleration of growth so that the child is inappropriately tall compared with peers of the same age-group. Unfortunately epiphyses fuse early and a normal adult height is not achieved. A similar growth acceleration is seen in *thyrotoxicosis* (*Fig.* S.57) and in hypothyroid patients who are over-treated with thyroxine. Somatomedin levels are high. Thyrotoxic children are usually round about the 75th centile for height. However, tall stature is rarely a presenting feature in these children and ultimate stature is not usually abnormal because the epiphyses fuse early.

Hypogonadism will cause increased stature with long arms and legs (eunuchoidism), because of delayed fusion of the epiphyses, so long as normal amounts of growth hormone and thyroid hormone are present.

Disease of the hypothalamus, pituitary or gonad may cause hypogonadism leading to tall stature. *Solitary deficiency of the hypothalamic gonadotrophin releasing hormone* is well recognized. When it is associated with anosmia due to agenesis of the olfactory bulbs it is called 'Kallmann's syndrome' (*Fig.* S.58). *Pituitary deficiency of luteinizing hormone* has been described in males. There is little or no testosterone production by the testes and the seminiferous tubules are immature. However, full maturation of both secondary sexual characteristics and of the seminiferous

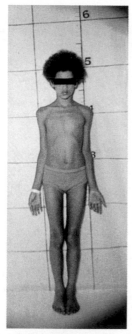

Fig. S.57. Thyrotoxicosis. A boy of 12 years of age with tall stature due to growth acceleration.

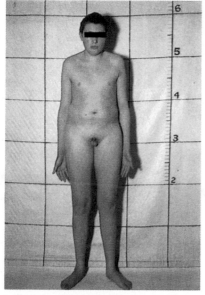

Fig. S.58. Hypogonadotrophic hypogonadism with anosmia (Kallman's syndrome). Note the long arms and legs compared with the trunk. The genitalia are underdeveloped and there is a rather female distribution of body fat.

tubules can be achieved by means of human chorionic gonadotrophin injections, hence accounting for the alternative title of the *'fertile eunuch syndrome'*.

In primary gonadal disorders leading to hypogonadism the characteristic biochemical feature is high serum gonadotrophins. *Anorchia* is a rare congenital

cause in males. More usual causes are *trauma, tuberculous orchitis* or *oophoritis* and *radiation damage to the gonads*. Rarely there may be *auto-immune ovarian failure*; this is usually associated with other auto-immune disease such as Addison's disease. Boys with *Klinefelter's syndrome (XXY)* are usually tall and have abnormally long limbs before puberty, but if testosterone levels are low in the middle to late teens an element of hypogonadism is added (*see below*).

Either *adenoma* or *hyperplasia* of the *pituitary acidophil cells* can lead to the excessive secretion of growth hormone and the rare condition of *'gigantism'*. Sometimes the adenoma may be of chromophobe cells or of mixed cell type. If the condition arises before puberty then the main feature is excessive growth of the long bones, resulting in a wide span and an increased lower segment to upper segment ratio. Heights of over 8 feet have been recorded. If hypogonadism does not supervene then the epiphyses may fuse and acromegalic features may begin to develop. Acromegaly means enlargement of the extremities; the bones of the hands and feet become broadened and the soft tissues become thicker, so that it is difficult for the patient to get shoes and gloves to fit. The facial appearance gradually changes (*Fig.* S.59), the skin and subcutaneous tissues becoming thicker, so that the skin folds are more prominent, the nose enlarged and the general impression is one of coarsened features. The frontal air sinuses enlarge and so the supraorbital ridges are more prominent. The lower jaw elongates and causes prognathism; dental malocclusion may become a problem. Radiographs may show enlargement of the pituitary fossa, but by no means always. Characteristic tufting of the terminal phalanges and widening of the joint spaces may be seen on hand radiographs. Increased heel pad thickness is usually demonstrated on radiographs. If it is above 23 mm acromegaly is possibly present, if above 27 mm acromegaly is certain.

Enlargement of the tongue, lips and ears occurs. Thickening of the vocal cords leads to deepening of the voice. Overgrowth of soft tissues at the wrist causes carpal tunnel syndrome in 35 per cent of cases, Evidence of a proximal myopathy is found in a third of patients. Persistent sweating is a common problem and girls may be troubled by hirsutism. Persistent headaches caused by stretching of the diaphragma sellae by the enlarging adenoma are a feature in a third of the patients. Other local pressure effects include visual field loss due to the tumour encroaching upon the optic chiasm. A very early feature may be loss of central vision for red objects, then the classic bitemporal hemianopia develops and may lead on to optic atrophy and total blindness.

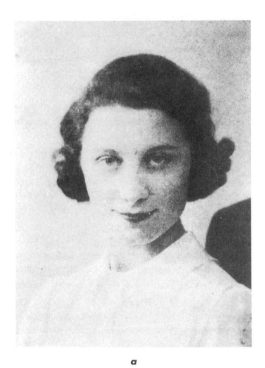
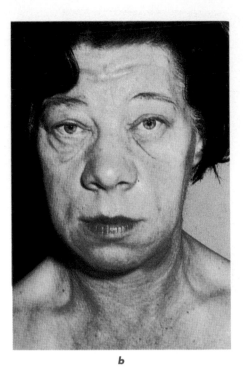

a   *b*

Fig. S.59. Acromegaly. Note the gradual change in appearance over 30 years. In *b* the nose has become broadened and the skin folds coarsened.

All organs enlarge, particularly the heart and liver. A cardiomyopathy may be present and hypertension is a common feature. Frank diabetes mellitus is present in 10 per cent of cases and a further 33 per cent have impaired tolerance to oral glucose. Goitre may be present and thyrotoxicosis occurs in 3 per cent of patients. Galactorrhoea due to excessive prolactin secretion may be a feature. In long-standing cases hypopituitarism develops in about 50 per cent.

A resting growth hormone in the fasting state of more than 10 mU/l (5 ng/ml) which does not suppress to less than 2 mU/l (1 ng/ml) after 75 g of oral glucose is diagnostic of acromegaly or 'gigantism'. Most patients have much higher fasting levels than this and they may even show a rise in growth hormone levels following glucose.

4. Chromosomal abnormalities

The most commonly recognized *chromosomal anomaly* leading to tall stature is *Klinefelter's syndrome*. This syndrome, occurring once in every 500 live male births, is caused by an extra X chromosome giving a karyotype of 47 XXY. The patient is tall and has eunuchoid proportions (*Fig.* S.60). The tallness may not be particularly apparent in childhood but becomes noticeable during the teens because the hypogonadism delays epiphysial fusion. The testes are small and firm and histology shows tubular sclerosis and hyalinization.

Variable numbers of Leydig cells may be present which accounts for the fact that the serum testosterone may be frankly low or be in the low normal range. FSH is elevated and LH usually so, but not if the testosterone is normal. There is a female escutcheon of pubic hair and facial and body hair is usually diminished. Gynaecomastia is a usual finding. Infertility is the rule but occasional exceptions have been described.

Another syndrome, the *supermale* with a karyotype of 47 XYY also occurs, with a frequency of one per thousand live male births. These individuals are usually very tall. The testes may be normal or small; in the latter case the testosterone level is low and FSH and LH are elevated. In some cases mental retardation and a tendency to aggressive behaviour are noted.

The *superfemale* (47 XXX) tends to have long legs and long fingers, but with a relatively normal span. The face is long and narrow, there is sometimes amenorrhoea and the secondary sexual characteristics may be poorly developed. Mild mental subnormality is a feature.

5. Miscellaneous

There is a group of miscellaneous causes of tall stature in children of which *Marfan's syndrome* is the most commonly recognized. The child is usually within the normal height range for his age-group but may be inappropriately tall for his family. The extremities are

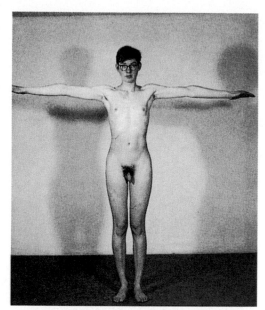

Fig. S.60. Klinefelter's syndrome. The arms and legs are long in proportion to the trunk and there is gynaecomastia.

long and thin and the fingers and toes are spider-like (*arachnodactyly*). The joints are hyperextensible. There may be dilatation of the aorta, aortic regurgitation, dislocation of the lenses of the eye, a high arched palate and long patellar ligaments. Although the skeletal proportions appear 'eunuchoidal', bone maturation, in fact, proceeds at a normal rate. From a radiograph of the hands the metacarpal index can be calculated by dividing the mean of the lengths by the mean of the widths. An index of more than 8·4 indicates arachnodactyly.

Patients with *homocystinuria* are rather similar in appearance to patients with Marfan's syndrome. The condition is an autosomal recessive disease. Additional features are mental retardation, a tendency to spontaneous thromboses in arteries and veins and the presence of homocystine in the urine.

Cerebral 'gigantism' (Sotos' syndrome) is characterized by accelerated growth in the first few years of life, but it then slows down and a normal adult stature is achieved. The hands and feet are large and the appearance is somewhat acromegalic, though growth hormone levels are normal. Mental subnormality is common.

Some children who may have suffered *brain damage* and mental retardation from birth trauma become excessively tall. The cause is unknown.

Lipodystrophy is a rare condition with absent fatty tissue, hyperlipidaemia and diabetes; there may be increased growth hormone levels and tall stature is a feature.

The *Beckwith–Wiedemann syndrome* is rare and

consists of accelerated growth, enlarged tongue, omphalocele and hypoglycaemia secondary to islet cell hyperplasia and raised insulin levels.

Ian D. Ramsay

Stomach, dilatation of

(*See also* ABDOMINAL SWELLINGS).

Dilatation of the stomach presents itself clinically under two totally different aspects: (1) *Acute*; (2) *Chronic*.

1. Acute dilatation of the stomach

This is generally a serious complication or even a fatal catastrophe arising in the course of some other condition, especially after operations (notably laparotomy), or after abdominal injury.

The diagnosis is generally easy. The abdomen is distended and tympanitic; there is constant effort to bring up wind, sometimes in vain, sometimes with copious and recurrent eructations, often with intractable hiccoughs. Sometimes immense quantities of blackish-brown of greenish-brown fluid flow effortlessly from the mouth and nostrils. The dilatation itself is of the nature of an acute paralysis of the stomach. Diagnosis is confirmed, and indeed treatment initiated, by the passage of a stomach tube which deflates the gastric dilatation.

2. Chronic dilatation of the stomach

This is due to conditions which cause stenosis at, or more commonly on either side of, the pylorus.

CAUSES OF STENOSIS

Peptic ulcer, particularly of the duodenum
    although much less commonly a benign gastric
    ulcer at the pylorus or in the antrum may be
    responsible
Carcinoma of the pylorus or antrum
Other tumours in this region; these include
    leiomyoma, leiomyosarcoma, infiltration with
    Hodgkin's disease or lymphosarcoma or invasion
    from an adjacent carcinoma of pancreas or gallbladder
Congenital pyloric septum
Adult hypertrophy of the pylorus
Heterotopic pancreatic tissue
Adhesions of the duodenum to the liver bed
    following cholecystectomy

The history in an established case of pyloric stenosis may be absolutely typical. In the case of a peptic ulcer there may be a long preceding story of ulcer pain. Vomiting is an important symptom and occurs in at least 9 out of every 10 patients. Typically copious amounts of vomitus are produced in a projectile manner and the patient will recall (but often only on direct questioning) that he has noticed fragments of food, particularly vegetable or fruit debris, which had been ingested one day and vomited up the next,

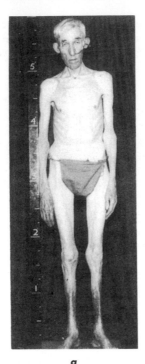
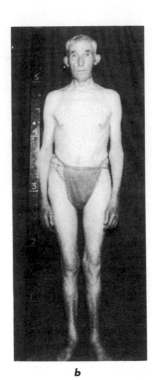

a   *b*

Fig. S.61. *a,* Typical appearance of a patient with longstanding pyloric stenosis due to a duodenal ulcer. The patient demonstrates the drawn, anxious facies, gross dehydration and wasting. *b,* Note the dramatic change following vagotomy and pyloroplasty.

or even two or three days later. There is really no condition other than obstruction to the gastric outlet in which this state of affairs obtains. Obstruction due to carcinoma, in contrast, often has a shorter history, perhaps of only a few months, and pain is completely absent in about one-third of patients. Examination of the patient often reveals features of importance. There may be evidence of dehydration and loss of weight; indeed the classic 'ulcer facies' applies only rarely to uncomplicated examples of peptic ulcer but is perfectly mirrored in the usual appearance of the victim of long-standing stenosis (*Fig.*S.61). A gastric splash which is present 3 or 4 hours after a meal or drink is elicited in two-thirds of patients with benign stenosis. Often the patient when asked directly will agree that he himself has noticed a splashing sound when walking or moving about. Visible gastric peristalsis, passing from left to right, is present much less frequently, and still less often the loaded and hypertrophied stomach may actually be palpable as well as audible and visible (*see* PERISTALSIS, VISIBLE). About half the patients with malignant obstruction will reveal a palpable tumour at the pylorus. Such a mass may, it is true, be felt rarely in the benign case, when a large inflammatory mass is present around the first part of the duodenum. Because of the more rapid progression in the malignant case, gross dilatation of the stomach is much less often

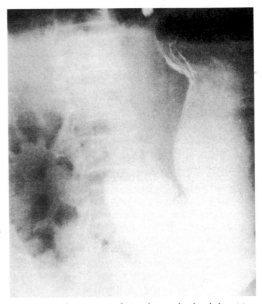

Fig. S.62. Pyloric stenosis due to chronic duodenal ulcer. Note three layers: air, gastric juice and barium.

seen than in benign obstruction, so that a gastric splash and visible peristalsis may not be elicited.

Radiological investigation in these cases is mandatory. The findings can be divided into two groups: the first confirms the presence of an obstruction at the

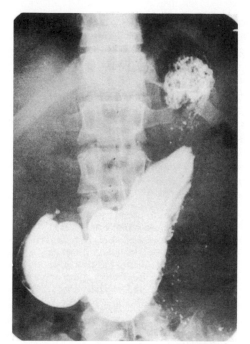

Fig. S.63. Pyloric stenosis due to chronic duodenal ulcer. The picture was taken 3 hours after a barium meal; note the considerable residium of barium. (*Dr Keith Jefferson.*)

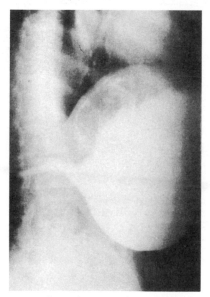

Fig. S.64. Pyloric obstruction due to extensive antral carcinoma.

within the stomach shown after taking a few mouthfuls of barium. Instead of the normal appearance of the barium running down the lesser curvature, the particles of barium can be seen to sink through a layer of fluid and then to rest at the bottom of the greater curve like a saucer. In the erect position three layers can be seen; the air bubble above, then the layer of gastric juice, and finally the lowermost layer of barium (*Fig.* S.62). In the early phase of pyloric stenosis giant peristaltic waves may be seen passing along the gastric wall, but in late decompensated obstruction the stomach is a large atonic bag. Obstruction of the gastric outlet is confirmed by taking further films at 4–6 hours when it will be seen that a large residium of barium remains in the stomach (*Fig.* S.63). Under normal circumstances the stomach is all but empty at the end of 2 hours. It is not always easy to tell the exact cause of the pyloric obstruction. Radiological evidence that a duodenal ulcer is responsible is given by the presence of an active ulcer crater or severe scarring in the duodenal cap. If the obstruction is situated in the antrum of the stomach it is most probable that the diagnosis is cancer (*Fig.* S.64) but occasionally a similar appearance is given by a penetrating benign gastric ulcer. A further sign of duodenal bulb obstruction that we have found to be useful is abnormal dilatability of the pyloric canal which may be seen on screening to dilate up to 2·5 cm or more in width and then contract down again to its usual size proximal to the point of stenosis.

Gastroscopy by means of a fiber-optic endoscope may visualize the obstructing ulcer and allow a biopsy to be performed, but often adherent gastric contents obscure the view.

The less common causes of pyloric obstruction mentioned above which may be associated with chronic dilatation of the stomach are rarely diagnosed before laparotomy. However, since obstruction of the gastric outlet almost invariably requires surgical intervention the elucidation of the exact cause preceding operation is a luxury rather than a necessity for the experienced surgeon.

Harold Ellis

Stools, mucus in

gastric outlet and the second indicates its pathology. A plain radiograph of the abdomen may itself be at least suggestive of pyloric stenosis by demonstrating a large gastric gas bubble with considerable quantities of retained food particles as demonstrated by patchy translucent areas. A sign of obstruction at the gastric outlet on the barium meal is the large residue of food

Mucus in the stools is not pathognomonic. It occurs in *malignant disease of the colon* as a clear glairy substance, often bloodstained, and it has the same character in *intussusception*; the obstruction in both these conditions accounts for the absence of faecal colouring. Large amounts of mucus may be secreted by extensive *benign papillomatous tumours* of the colon and rectum. Since this material is rich in potassium, profound potassium depletion may occur in this condition, leading to weakness, paraesthesiae and even paralysis and vascular collapse. The volume of fluid passed may amount to 2 or 3 litres daily. Mucus is often seen with *constipated motions*, the hard faeces having led to irritation of the large bowel with consequent increased secretion of mucus as a defensive mechanism against misguided therapy, especially intestinal lavage. In severe cases a motion may consist almost entirely of coagulated shreds with little faecal matter. In other cases, complete casts of the bowel formed of coagulated mucus are passed; they may be a foot or more in length. They may have become broken into fragments which the patient describes as skins, looking not unlike segments of tape-worm for which indeed they are on inadequate examination easily mistaken. Patients passing this variety of mucus are said to have *membranous* or *spastic colitis*, an incorrect term, for no inflammatory process occurs. The term 'irritable colon syndrome' is also used for this disorder, which is characterized by colonic abdominal pain, abnormal stools and alteration in bowel habits. It is more common in females aged 15–45 years but may occur in either sex under conditions of emotional tension. The patients on examination often appear anxious and tense and perspire excessively. Curiously enough, this hypersecretion of mucus has almost disappeared during the past 30 years, although the general symptomatology is still recognized. It may be added that the popular treatment of lavage to remove the mucus will be responsible for its continued secretion as a protest against irritation of the mucosa. In the more acute varieties of inflammation of the bowel the mucus passed is jelly-like and semi-liquid, of varying colour according to the amount of faecal staining. In *polyposis coli* and severe cases of *ulcerative colitis, Crohn's colitis, enteritis* and *dysentery* the motions consist of nothing but mucus and blood. One cannot differentiate between the numerous varieties of enteritis and colitis upon the basis of the mucus in the stools alone.

Harold Ellis

Stools, pus in

Pus in the stools in sufficient amount to be recognizable by the naked eye indicates the rupture of an abscess into the intestinal tract. Such recognition is, however, unusual; for even when a large appendicular abscess perforates into the caecum the pus becomes indistinguishable either from admixture with the faeces, the patient believing he simply has diarrhoea, or on account of digestion and decomposition. The less the pus is mixed with other intestinal contents, the nearer to the anus must the site of rupture have been; but the diagnosis of the source of the abscess needs to

be determined upon other grounds, particularly the history and the results of examination, including that of the rectum and vagina. Abscesses most apt to cause a discharge of pus with the stools are of the appendicular, pericolic, pelvic or other local peritoneal types; of prostatic or perirectal origin; or a pyosalpinx.

Microscopical quantities of pus in the stools may be due to any of the causes already mentioned and, in addition, to affections of the mucous membrane itself. These comprise acute or chronic ulcerative colitis, Crohn's colitis; dysentery; cholera; dengue; malignant, tuberculous, typhoidal, carcinomatous or venereal ulceration of the bowel. The pus cells may be recognizable as such under the microscope. Examination with the sigmoidoscope, followed by a barium enema X-ray, is invaluable in deciding the diagnosis.

Harold Ellis

Strangury

Strangury differs somewhat from mere pain on micturition, in that, in addition to severe pain before, during or after the act, the patient is troubled constantly by urgent and repeated necessity to pass his urine, sometimes as often as every few minutes, yet without satisfactory relief to his discomfort. The condition is also spoken of as 'vesical tenesmus'. Very little urine is passed each time; sometimes the desire and the necessity are urgent when there is no urine in the bladder at all. The causes resolve themselves into five groups, as follows:

1. Nervous conditions, especially:

Hysterisa
Anxiety state
Tabes dorsalis (vesical crises)

2. Obstruction to the urine outflow

Urethral stricture
Enlarged prostate
Prostatic calculus
Carcinoma of the prostate
Retroverted gravid urethra
Uterine fibroid
Ovarian cyst   } impacted in the pelvis
Ovarian carcinoma
Extreme prolapse of the uterus and bladder
Calculus impacted in the urethra
Inflamed urethral caruncle
Gonorrhoea
Urethritis other than gonococcal
Periprostatic abscess
Ischiorectal abscess

3. Local affections of the bladder wall

Injury
Acute cystitis
Chronic cystitis
Interstitial cystitis (Hunner's ulcer)
Tuberculous cystitis
Calculus irritating the trigone

Carcinoma
Bilharziasis
Infiltration by—
          Carcinoma of the uterus
          Carcinoma of the rectum
Acute vesiculitis

4. Reflex conditions

Inflamed haemorrhoids
Tuberculous kidney, before the bladder is involved
E. Coli bacilluria   } even before there is infection of
Pyelitis   } the bladder wall

5. The effects of certain drugs, especially:

Cantharides
Oxalic acid
Turpentine
Hexamine and its derivatives

Most of the conditions mentioned above, and the methods of distinguishing between them, are discussed in the article on MICTURITION, FREQUENCY OF

Interstitial cystitis (Hunner's ulcer) is probably not an infectious disease. Histologically there is inflammatory infiltration of the bladder wall, unifocal or multifocal with mucosal ulceration and scarring, leading to contraction of smooth muscle, diminished capacity and frequent painful micturition with haematuria. The patients are usually middle-aged women.

Another point that merits attention is the strangury produced by certain drugs. *Cantharides* is familiar in this respect, but more from its prominence in textbooks upon forensic medicine than from its occurrence in actual practice. The same applies to *oxalic acid* and to *turpentine*. Hexamine and similar drugs derived from it are important. These have been employed in the treatment of pyuria, as well as other conditions, but have now been largely replaced by sulpha drugs and antibiotics. If given for pyuria, when there may have been frequent and painful micturition already, the increased frequency and pain that sometimes ensue when any of the above drugs are administered are apt to be attributed to an increase in the cystitis or other genitourinary lesion, and the dose of the drug may be increased instead of diminished. The important point is that hexamine and other drugs of like nature may be responsible for such strangury as may simulate local disease of the bladder, and unless this is borne in mind an erroneous diagnosis is liable to be made.

Harold Ellis

Striae atrophicae

Striae or 'stretch marks' are unsightly linear marks due to disruption of the dermal support tissue, e.g. collagen

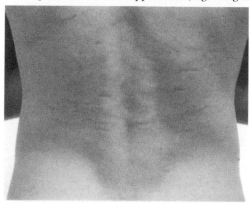

Fig. S.65. Spontaneous striae in the lumbosacral region at puberty. (*St Stephen's Hospital.*)

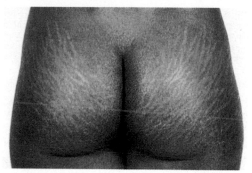

Fig. S.66. Spontaneous striae of the buttocks at puberty. (*St Stephen's Hospital.*)

and elastic fibres. Although initially reddish-purple they later fade to an opalescent whitish colour. They commonly occur following rapid distension, e.g. during the growth phase of adolescence (lumbosacral region in boys (*Fig.* S.65) and thighs, buttocks (*Fig.* S.66) and breasts in girls) and during pregnancy (breasts and abdomen). They are also caused by corticosteroids, which reduce the bulk of dermal support tissue, e.g. Cushing's syndrome (flexures), and after steroid therapy, both systemic and topical. They are usually only a cosmetic problem but can, if extensive, ulcerate, particularly following trauma.

Richard Staughton

Stridor

Stridor is a harsh noise produced during breathing, typically heard as a high-pitched inspiratory wheeze audible at a distance. It is commonly caused by obstruction affecting the larynx or extrathoracic trachea. The intensity of sound is accentuated by inspiratory negative pressure tending to collapse the extrathoracic airways. Stridor may not be evident on quiet breathing,

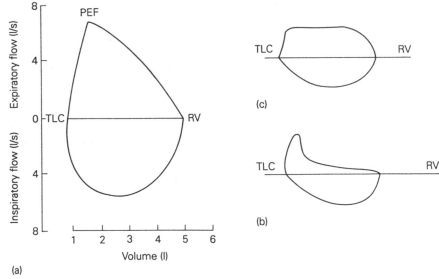

(a)

Fig. S.67. Maximum flow–volume curves represented diagrammatically for a normal subject (a) and for patients with intrapulmonary airflow obstruction (chronic obstructive pulmonary disease) (b) or obstruction of the upper (extrathoracic) trachea (fixed upper airway) (c). In extrathoracic tracheal obstruction the reduction in inspiratory flow is equal to or greater than the reduction in expiratory flow, whereas in intrapulmonary airways obstruction maximum expiratory flow is reduced more than maximum inspiratory flow. TLC, total lung capacity; RV, residual lung volume; PEF, peak expiratory flow.

and is best heard after exercise or during hyperventilation through the open mouth. On auscultation a fixed inspiratory wheeze is heard over the trachea becoming fainter over the lungs. When narrowing affects the portion of the trachea within the thorax, the carina or main bronchi, stridor tends to be louder on expiration because the intrathoracic airways partially collapse due to the expiratory rise in intrathoracic pressure. In this situation it may be difficult to differentiate stridor from abnormal noisy breath sounds commonly present on quiet breathing in widespread airflow obstruction. These differences, and also the distinction between main airway narrowing and diffuse distal airway narrowing, as in asthma or chronic obstructive pulmonary disease, may be demonstrated by flow-volume loops (*Fig.* S.67).

Stridor is generated by vibration of the walls of critically narrowed airways, and the pitch is dependent upon the speed of airflow and the density of the inspired air. Low density gas mixture (helium and oxygen) produces much less turbulence and stridor than conventional nitrogen and oxygen mixtures and therefore may provide useful temporary relief of symptoms in critically breathless patients. With extreme degrees of tracheal narrowing, violent ineffectual respiratory effort, cyanosis and sudden death may result when a relatively minor additional insult, such as a mucous plug, occludes the narrowed trachea.

In children the onset of stridor is usually alarmingly sudden and due to acute infective conditions (*Table* S.13), whereas in adults the onset tends to be insidious and may be confused with late onset bronchial asthma, chronic bronchitis, or other chronic pulmonary disorders. (*Table* S.14).

Table S.13. Causes of acute inspiratory stridor in infants and young children

1. Congenital
Choanal atresia—in newborn
Congenital laryngeal paralysis in newborn

2. Inhaled foreign body
Small plastic toys in crawling children
Peanuts in older children

3. Croup syndrome
Diphtheria—any age
Acute laryngotracheobronchitis—usually in 2 year olds
Acute epiglottitis—usually in 2–7 year olds
Acute pseudo-membranous croup
Upper airway burns
Angioneurotic oedema
Infectious mononucleosis

Table S.14. Causes of stridor in adults

1. *Causes above the larynx*
   Retropharyngeal abscess
   New growths of the pharynx
   Lingual angio-oedema

2. *Causes inside the larynx or trachea*
   Mucus or mucopus in patients enfeebled by illness or in whom a defect of the cough mechanism (laryngeal or respiratory muscle paralysis) leads to inability to expel these secretions

3. *Affections of the wall of the larynx or trachea*
   a. *Inflammatory*

i. Acute diphtheria, acute laryngitis, due to exposure to irritant gases.
ii. Chronic tuberculous or syphilitic laryngitis with stenosis
iii. Wegener's granulomatosis
iv. Sarcoidosis

b. *Traumatic or post-traumatic*
Injuries of larynx or trachea
Post-traumatic stenosis of larynx or trachea, e.g. after tracheostomy, after attempted suicidal 'cut-throat' and after prolonged use of a cuffed endotracheal tube with or without tracheostomy

c. *Neoplastic*
Carcinoma of larynx
Carcinoma of trachea
Benign tumours of larynx or trachea

d. *Oedema of the glottis*
Burn injuries
Angio-oedema
Inhalation of toxic gas

e. *Ankylosis of crico-arytenoid joint in rheumatoid arthritis*

f. *Tracheopathia osteoplastica*

4. **Compression of larynx or trachea from without**
Goitre, especially haemorrhage into an adenomatous goitre. Hashimoto's disease, intrathoracic goitre
Riedel's thyroiditis
Carcinoma of the thyroid
Aneurysm of the arch of the aorta
Malformations of the aorta—double aortic arch
Mediastinal new growths, including metastatic involvement of mediastinal lymph nodes
Mediastinal Hodgkin's disease and other reticuloses
Carcinoma of oesophagus invading the trachea
Malignant disease of lower cervical lymph nodes
Cellulitis of neck
Ludwig's angina
Tuberculous nodes in mediastinum
Fungal infections
   Histoplasmosis
   Coccidioidomycosis
   Blastomycosis

5. **Laryngeal nerve palsies**
Bulbar or pseudobulbar palsy
Bilateral lesions of recurrent laryngeal nerves (post-operative or inflammatory)

6. **Narrowing of both main bronchi**
Bronchial carcinoma arising in main bronchus or metastasizing to subcarinal lymph nodes
Mediastinal tumours
Tuberculous strictures of main bronchi
Strictures of main bronchi in sarcoidosis
Amyloidosis
Bronchopathia osteoplastica
Tracheomalacia

In many patients the cause of stridor is obvious, for instance when it is caused by secretions lodging in the larynx or trachea in seriously ill patients or in patients in coma from any cause. In others, local examination of the upper respiratory tract and larynx will provide the diagnosis without much difficulty.

Fibre-optic laryngoscopy and bronchoscopy will often be diagnostic. The greatest difficulty is likely to be encountered in children in whom the possibility

of stridor of acute onset being due to diphtheria should never be forgotten, and in less acute cases retro-pharyngeal abscess must be borne in mind. Foreign bodies in the larynx or the main air passages are also a possible source of difficulty in children who are often too young to provide a clear history.

Inspiratory stridor is common in early childhood. The most frequent cause is acute viral laryngotracheobronchitis (croup), but it is essential to consider the full differential diagnosis if tragic and preventable death from acute airway obstruction is to be avoided (*Table* S.14).

Acute laryngotracheobronchitis is the common cause of croup in the second year of life. Males are affected most frequently. The main pathogens are para-influenza virus (50 per cent), respiratory syncytial virus, influenza A and B, rhinovirus, adenovirus and measles. It is usually preceded for 1 or 2 days by an upper respiratory tract infection before developing a harsh, barking cough and hoarse voice due to inflammatory swelling of the subglottic region. With more severe airway obstruction chest wall recession occurs and stridor may be inspiratory and expiratory. Fever, restlessness, hypoxia, tachypnoea, tachycardia and eventually cyanosis herald the risk of sudden collapse and death.

Acute epiglottitis is often mistaken for acute laryngotracheobronchitis but its pathology and clinical course are quite different. The onset is usually rapid and the patient pyrexial and lethargic complaining of sore throat. Within a short time upper airway obstruction becomes obvious with a soft inspiratory stridor and expiratory sound resembling a snore. The child prefers to sit upright, mouth breathe and often drools saliva. Acute epiglottitis is an acute life-threatening form of laryngeal obstruction due to oedema and hyperaemia of the epiglottis, aryepiglottic folds and hypopharynx which results in considerable oedema around the laryngeal inlet obstructing respiration and swallowing. The changes do not extend below the vocal cords. Septicaemia is invariably present, the usual organism being *Haemophilus influenza* type B. The clinical features are similar to acute obstructive laryngotracheobronchitis except that there is rapid onset of dysphagia and drooling saliva as well as respiratory distress with stridor and a thick muffled voice.

The child is toxic and complete respiratory obstruction may supervene very quickly. No attempt should be made to examine the pharynx with a tongue depressor as this may precipitate complete obstruction. Because of the risk of laryngeal obstruction, immediate transfer of the child to a hospital with appropriate facilities should be arranged for full assessment with a view to nasal or oral intubation and appropriate antibiotic treatment (*see also* WHEEZE).

P. R. Studdy

STUPOR
See CONSCIOUSNESS, DISORDERS OF.

Succussion sounds

Succussion sounds may be heard when a viscus or cavity that contains both liquid and air or gas is shaken whilst the ear or the stethoscope is applied over it. The sounds may be loud enough to be audible at a distance from the patient. A good example of succession is often afforded by the normal stomach after a quantity of liquid has been swallowed. Gastric succussion sounds are not necessarily evidence of abnormality, they merely indicate that the viscus contains liquid and gas. Succussion sound may be heard in the chest in cases of *hydropneumothorax* when the patient oscillates his trunk to and fro. Less often, succussion sounds may be produced by a pyopneumothorax or a haemopneumothorax, the difference between these being decided by a pleural tap. Other succussion sounds are uncommon.

The following is a list of all possible causes:

1. Causes of succussion sounds in the thorax

Hydropneumothorax
Pyopneumothorax
Haemopneumothorax
Diaphragmatic hernia
Subdiaphragmatic abscess communicating with the stomach or duodenum, or infected with *E. coli*: in either case, gas and pus are present
Hydropheumopericardium
Pyopneumopericardium

2. Causes of succussion sounds in the abdomen

The normal stomach
Dilatation of the stomach
Gross dilatation of the caecum
Gross dilatation of the colon
Pneumoperitoneum due to: (*a* Perforated gastric ulcer; (*b*) Perforated duodenal ulcer; (*c*) Perforated typhoid ulcer of the intestine; (*d*) Perforated carcinoma of the colon; (*e*) Production of gas by *E. coli*, either in a local abscess (e.g. appendicular or subdiaphragmatic) or in the general peritoneum
Subdiaphragmatic abscess communicating with the interior of the stomach
Air and urine in the bladder (*see* PNEUMATURIA)
Gas-production by *E. coli* in a large pyonephrosis
Infection by a gas-producing micro-organism of an ovarian cyst or other collection of fluid.

Succussion sounds in the chest

It is almost unknown for a *tuberculous cavity* to give succussion sounds. Should it do so, the situation would be subapical rather than basal, and thus distinguishable from most cases of hydro-or pyopneumothorax. *Hydro-* and *pyopneumopericardium* are also rare: they are identified by the churning sounds made by the heart beating within the mixture of air and liquid. The cause is generally a tumour of the oesophagus or bronchus opening the pericardium from behind, a foreign body such as dental plate ulcerating through from the oesophagus, the opening of an air-containing subdiaphragmatic abscess through the diaphragm into the pericardium or infection of the pericardial sac by a gas-producing organism.

A *subdiaphragmatic abscess* containing air due to communication with a hole in a gastric or duodenal ulcer may elevate the diaphragm so high that the condition may be mistaken for hydro- or pyopneumothorax. Decision may be impossible until the position of the diaphragm is ascertained by X-rays and ultrasonography. When the pathology is subdiaphragmatic the tendency is to displace the heart upwards rather than towards the opposite side of the chest; the contrary is usual in the case of pneumothorax.

Diaphragmatic hernias, if large and if the stomach is herniated into the thorax, will show the effect of eating and drinking upon the physical signs and may point to the diagnosis. X-rays will demonstrate the condition on barium meal.

Most cases of *hydropneumothorax* present little difficulty in diagnosis although it may not be easy to ascertain its cause. If the onset has been sudden with acute pain in the affected side of the chest, cyanosis and dyspnoea, the most likely cause is *tuberculosis*. In some instances, an injury or a ruptured emphysematous bulla may have been responsible, but injury seldom produces hydropneumothorax unless a tuberculous or other lesion in the lung was present at the time of the accident. Hydropneumothorax may result from *paracentesis thoracis*; if bleeding occurs during the puncture, *haemopneumothorax* will be produced. This too is common after bullet wounds of the chest. Either a hydro- or a haemopneumothorax may become infected with pyogenic organisms and converted into a *pyopneumothorax*. Pyopneumothorax may develop in cases of gangrene of the lung, obstruction of a bronchus by a foreign body or a tumour, the breaking down of an infective bronchopneumonia or pulmonary infarct, or the conversion of a pleural haematoma into a mixture of pus and gas as the result of infection by gas-gangrene organisms after gunshot or other wounds of the chest. Fluid often collects in the pleural cavity when an artificial (therapeutic) pneumothorax has been induced, giving succussion sounds.

Succussion sounds in the abdomen

The first point in the differential diagnosis of succussion sounds in the abdomen is to decide whether the sounds are or are not of gastric origin. This is usually obvious but any doubt can be at once resolved by a barium meal. Dilatation of the stomach has three causes, namely atony, non-malignant pyloric or duodenal obstruction, especially by a healed simple ulcer, and malignant pyloric obstruction by primary gastric carcinoma (*see* PERISTALSIS, VISIBLE). The presence of visible peristaltic waves or the occurrence of vomiting will indicate some degree of pyloric obstruction. Such obstruction will usually result in periodic vomiting, when the particles of food eaten a day or more previously can be recognized. Visible peristaltic waves corresponding to the stomach are another confirmatory feature. The most certain method of detecting gastric outflow obstruction is by means of a barium meal examination.

If there are well-marked abdominal succussion sounds that can be definitely shown to be of non-gastric origin there are generally other signs and symptoms to assist the diagnosis. Succussion sounds in the peritoneal cavity are exceedingly rare, for even though this cavity should contain both gas and liquid—for instance after perforation of a typhoid ulcer—the coils of bowel prevent the sounds from being readily produced. The most common cause is iatrogenic, occurring when air is introduced into the peritoneum, when ascites is tapped or when carbon dioxide is introduced at laparoscopy in the presence of ascites. It would clearly be next to impossible to diagnose most of the conditions listed above unless the previous state of the patient was known or without a laparotomy. *E. coli* produces gas so that intra-abdominal abscesses, appendicular and otherwise, are occasionally resonant; the occurrence, however, of marked non-gastric succussion sounds in the abdomen of a patient who is not acutely ill will support the conclusion that there is distension with gas and liquid of some part of the large bowel, especially the caecum or the sigmoid colon. This distension is generally the result of either chronic constipation or intestinal stenosis. In cases of idiopathic dilatation of the colon, volvulus of the sigmoid colon or Hirschsprung's disease, the sigmoid dilatation may be so extreme that this part of the intestine bulges up as far as the diaphragm.

Ian A. D. Bouchier

Sweating, abnormalities of

Hyperhidrosis, or excess of sweating, may be either generalized or local (*see Table* S.15).

Generalized hyperhidrosis

The sweat glands are controlled via the sympathetic nerves by thermoregulatory centres in the hypothalamus. Sweating is the normal response to exercise or excessive heat, though there is marked physiological variation between individuals. Fever and sweating accompany *infections* and drenching sweats usually occur with fall of temperature. Sweat regulation can be unbalanced by pyrogens and sweating may occur out of phase with the fever, e.g. in some cases of tuberculosis, brucellosis and lymphoma. Generalized hyperhidrosis may also be produced by *drugs*, e.g. alcohol, pilocarpines and tricyclic antidepressants.

Table S.15. Hyperhidrosis

Generalised	Local
Exercise	Organic nerve lesions,
Raised ambient	brain tumours, spinal
temperature	cord injuries
Anxiety	Palms/Soles
Infections/Pyrogens	Pachydermoperiostosis
Drugs	Granulosis rubra nasi
alcohol, pilocarpines,	
tricyclic antidepressants	
Hypoglycaemia	
Dumping syndrome	
Alcohol/Drug withdrawal	
Shock/Syncope	
Intense pain	
Rickets	
Infantile scurvy	
Pink disease	
Hyperthyroidism	
Hyperpituitarism	
Acromegaly	
Phaeochromocytoma	
Carcinoid	
Gout	

A 'cold and clammy skin', where sweating is associated with cutaneous vasoconstriction, occurs in *hypoglycaemia*, the *dumping syndrome*, *alcohol and drug withdrawal*, *shock* and *syncopal states*, and also in *intense pain*. Increased sweating is seen in many endocrinological disturbances—*hyperthyroidism*, *hyperpituitarism* and *acromegaly*. It has also been described with *phaeochromocytoma*, the *carcinoid syndrome* and *gout*. Sweating is a feature of *rickets*, *pink disease* and *infantile scurvy* (*Barlow's disease*).

Local hyperhidrosis

Local increase in sweat production is seen with organic *neurological lesions*, e.g. brain tumours and spinal cord injuries, and can help to localize the neurological defect. Local hyperhidrosis of palms, soles and/or axillae is not uncommon, and occurs in patients who are otherwise perfectly normal; the sweating increases with embarrassment, anxiety and during the summer months. Sweat can literally drip from the hands, making paper-work extremely difficult. The keratin of the soles becomes macerated, and secondary infection causes an offensive odour (osmidrosis). In *pachydermop-*

eriostosis local hyperhidrosis occurs over the skin folds of forehead and extremities.

Granulosis rubra nasi is a rare genetically determined disease where profuse sweating of the tip of the nose is associated with a diffuse erythema and the formation of minute dark red papules. The disorder usually begins in early childhood and subsides at puberty. It must be distinguished from rosacea, lupus erythematosus and lupus vulgaris.

Miliaria

Miliaria are lesions caused by blockage and rupture of sweat ducts; they are most often seen in tropical conditions of heat and high humidity, which are simulated in the UK by polythene occlusion of the skin, or in neonatal nurseries. There are three forms depending on the depth of duct obstruction.

1. *Miliaria crystallina* (sudamina). Superficial blockage causes 'crystal' clear vesicles just below the epidermal surface with little inflammatory reaction and few symptoms. These are often seen on the trunk during febrile illnesses.

2. *Miliaria rubra* (prickly heat). The rupture occurs in mid-epidermis resulting in tiny intensely pricking red papules. These may erupt widely in persons recently arrived in tropical conditions or be confined to friction areas and flexures.

3. *Miliaria profunda* (mamillaria). The blockage occurs within the dermis. Lesions are easily overlooked as they are not red or uncomfortable but appear as firm papules (1-3 mm) on the body or limbs. They may follow repeated attacks of miliaria rubra. The natural history of miliaria depends on environmental factors; if sweating continues lesions continue to erupt, but if sweating is arrested, e.g. by entering an air-conditioned or cool area, healing can commence.

Anhidrosis

Anhidrosis is much less common than hyperhidrosis; sweating may be either diminished or totally suppressed and either the whole skin or only some particular area be affected. Lack of sweat glands may occur with skin dystrophies (e.g. *congenital ectodermal dysplasia*) or atrophy (e.g. *scleroderma*). The sweat gland population may also be diminished in ichthyosis and *Anderson–Fabry's* disease. In these situations heat regulation may be impaired. Suppression of sweating is characteristic of *heat-stroke*, though the mechanism of heat stress and acclimatization is still poorly understood. Organic *brain damage* at any level, especially of the hypothalamus, can result in complete anhidrosis. Localized anhidrosis can follow spinal cord lesions, e.g. syringomyelia or neuropathy of diabetes or leprosy. It can thus help in localizing neurological lesions. Sympathectomy abolishes sweating.

Generalized decreased sweating and dry skin is a well-known sign in myxoedema. Blockage of sweat ducts can occur in *atopic eczema*, *psoriasis* and *lichen planus* and be associated with crises of itching, as in miliaria rubra.

Osmidrosis

Osmidrosis is foul smelling sweat. Eccrine sweat is usually odourless but various substances may be excreted in sweat, e.g. garlic, drugs (e.g. dimethyl sulphoxide) and arsenic. Past physicians remarked on the particular odour of sweat; in diabetes, gout, scurvy, typhoid, uraemia (*see also* SMELL AS A PHYSICAL SIGN). Hyperhidrosis, especially of the soles, is commonly accompanied by foul odour due to bacterial overgrowth. Imaginary osmidrosis is a well-recognized paranoid delusional symptom. Personal body odour is largely determined by apocrine gland secretion.

Chromhidrosis

Chromhidrosis is usually due to coloured apocrine rather than eccrine sweat. Perhaps 10 per cent of normal people have coloured apocrine sweat (blue, yellow or green) and rarely areas of ectopic apocrine glands can give rise to areas of discoloured skin, where it is possible to see tiny beads of coloured sweat. The pigments are lipofuscins. In pseudo-chromhidrosis colourless sweat becomes coloured on the surface of the skin, due usually to chromogenic bacteria. Occasionally workers in the chemical industry can develop coloured eccrine sweat which can be shown to contain dyes. Certain drugs may give rise to coloured sweat, e.g. rifampicin.

Urhidrosis

The urea content of sweat increases with serum urea concentration. Uraemic sweat has a particular odour and after evaporation leaves a visible deposit of urea crystals on the skin—*uraemic frost.*

Richard Staughton

SYNCOPE
See FAINTS.

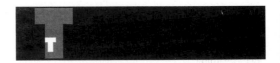

Tachypnoea

Tachypnoea signifies an increase in the rate of breathing, as may occur normally during exercise or abnormally with a number of clinical disturbances, especially those associated with hypoxia. In most clinical situations, tachypnoea is associated with symptoms of breathlessness (*see* DYSPNOEA, p. 163).

In health, both the rate and depth of respiration are controlled by brain stem respiratory centres to maintain a constant arterial blood oxygen level. The relationship between ventilatory rate and depth, demands for oxygen uptake and requirements for CO_2 elimination is controlled by complex interaction between: (1) mechanoreceptors in the airways and lung parenchyma; (2) peripheral chemoreceptors in the carotid and aortic bodies; and (3) central chemoreceptors mostly located on or beneath the ventral surface of the medulla. The automatic control system situated in the brain stem is concerned primarily with oxygen, carbon dioxide and acid-base homeostasis. When metabolic requirements are modest this automatic system can be over-ridden by the voluntary control system which arises in the cerebral cortex to allow other activities such as talking, coughing and singing to occur. A low arterial Po_2, high arterial Pco_2 or acid pH all stimulate ventilation.

There are many causes for tachypnoea. The increased metabolic demands of fever or circulatory shock from myocardial infarction, haemorrhage, trauma or pulmonary embolism, often manifest clinically with rapid breathing. Stimulation of the central chemoreceptors by metabolic acidosis in uncontrolled diabetes mellitus, renal or hepatic failure or acute circulatory collapse as well as salicylate overdose may all cause tachypnoea. Stimulation of lung stretch receptors with reflex increase in ventilatory drive may follow acute pulmonary emboli, acute pneumonias, asthma, aspiration of gastrointestinal contents, pulmonary fibrosis or bullous lung disease and provoke tachypnoea out of proportion to hypoxia so commonly associated with these conditions. Neurological causes of tachypnoea include cerebral haemorrhage, meningitis, encephalitis, head injury or primary abnormalities in the brain stem.

Breathing is under voluntary control and deep inspiration in excess of ventilatory requirements can be taken to anticipate exercise or facilitate talking or singing. Inappropriate hyperventilation is common and may present with complaints of breathlessness, associated with lightheadedness, dizziness, peripheral paraesthesiae, headache or anxiety. Even tetany may occur if a significant respiratory alkalosis results from overbreathing.

Clinical features suggesting the diagnosis of the hyperventilation syndrome (HVS), include complaints of breathlessness at rest for no apparent reason, paradoxical absence of significant breathlessness on exercise, and marked variability of symptoms. Clinical examination with routine respiratory investigations including a chest radiograph may reveal no abnormality, although the occasional patient does exhibit a sighing, irregular pattern of breathing. The most common cause of this condition is anxiety.

P. R. Studdy

Taste, abnormal perception of

The appreciation of taste is a function of the tongue; fibres from the anterior two-thirds pass via the chorda tympani to the geniculate ganglion, passing from there to the pons by the nervus intermedius. Fibres from the posterior third pass ventrally via the glossopharyngeal nerve. In the pons taste fibres pass into the tractus solitarius and from the nucleus of this tract a gustatory lemniscus is formed which, after decussating, passes upwards near the midline to the thalamus and from there to the cortical centre for taste at the foot of the postcentral gyrus. The 'taste' of food is made up of a combination of smell and taste proper; a patient with anosmia will complain that food is 'tasteless' because the normal tongue can only distinguish sweet, salt, sour and bitter. Consequently, both the sense of smell and the sense of taste must be tested in every case. Both may be lost in acute upper respiratory infection with a coated tongue and inflamed nose. Loss of taste proper is found in disease of the tongue itself, of the chorda tympani, of the glossopharyngeal nerve and of the glossopharyngeal nucleus in the medulla. Loss of smell by itself occurs in inflammatory conditions of the nose, in tumours of the anterior fossa which compress the olfactory nerves, and frequently as a result of fractures of the cribriform plate.

Disorders of taste

1. Impairment or loss of taste (ageusia)

A. AFFECTIONS OF THE MOUTH
Coated tongue
Epithelioma
Glossitis
Sjögren's syndrome

B. AFFECTIONS OF THE NERVES
Lesion of lingual nerve
Lesion of glosso-pharyngeal nerve
Lesion of chorda tympani
Bell's palsy

C. DRUGS, e.g. D-penicillamine

2. Perverted taste (parageusia)

Pregnancy
Glossitis
Hysteria

3. Hallucinations of taste

Psychogenic
Lesion of uncus
Uncinate epilepsy

4. Foul taste of mouth (cacogeusia)

A. LOCAL CONDITION OF THE MOUTH
Caries
Stomatitis
Gingivitis
Epithelioma
Glossitis
Gumma

B. GASTROINTESTINAL DISEASE
Gastric carcinoma
Pyloric stenosis
Gastritis

C. SEPTIC LUNG CONDITIONS
Bronchiectasis
Abscess or gangrene
Tuberculous cavitation

From the diagnostic point of view, impairment of taste sensation is important only when it is persistent or recurrent, and even then it is usually a symptom of secondary interest due to a more obvious primary condition of the mouth, nose, lung or gastrointestinal tract. In the absence of some such explanation, diagnosis becomes difficult, and the cause must be looked for in the nervous system.

The most common neurological cause of loss of taste is Bell's palsy, in which it often occurs as an early and transient feature, the loss being confined to the anterior two-thirds of the tongue on the same side as the facial paralysis.

A similar but more permanent combination of facial palsy and loss of taste may result from spread of inflammatory disease from the middle ear to the Fallopian canal. Taste may disappear as a result of bulbar disease, but in some cases it is overshadowed by more important symptoms and signs. Organic lesions of the uncinate gyrus (glioma, pituitary tumour, syphilis, perhaps arterial thrombosis) give rise to *uncinate fits*, characterized by episodic attacks in which the patient experiences a hallucination of smell or taste, usually unpleasant, followed by salivation, champing or sucking movements of the mouth and jaws, and a disturbance of consciousness which usually amounts to little more than a 'faraway' feeling but may go on to unconsciousness, with or without a generalized convulsion. The uncinate hallucination may occur by itself—a brief, discontinuous experience which is repeated from time to time, and in such a case it may be mistaken for the hallucinations of smell which are a significant symptom of delusional insanity. In the latter, however, the hallucination is more persistent and less episodic, the other features of the uncinate fit do not

occur, and there are usually other features of a primary psychological illness. The perversions of taste which occasionally occur during pregnancy are neither delusional nor hallucinatory, but their origin is not understood. The sensation of taste is no exception to the rule that anything can occur in hysteria, but disturbances of smell or taste are uncommon manifestations of hysteria. Complete loss of taste and smell occasionally occurs during an attack of migraine; it is analogous to the hemiplegia and other focal disturbances which sometimes occur in this condition. Patients taking D-penicillamine may lose their sense of taste, which returns some little time after stopping treatment.

Ian Mackenzie

TELANGIECTASIS
See ANGIOMA AND TELANGIECTASIA.

Testicular Atrophy

Apart from the physiological atrophy of the testes which occurs with advancing age and may begin as early as the age of 50, the causes of testicular atrophy can be classified under the headings hypothalamic/pituitary conditions, testicular conditions, adrenal disorders, general disease and drugs.

Hypothalamic/pituitary conditions

The testes contain two main components, the seminiferous tubules, responsible for the production of spermatozoa, and the interstitial tissue containing Leydig cells which secrete testosterone. Spermatogenesis is under the control of one gonadotrophin, follicle stimulating hormone (FSH), and testosterone secretion is stimulated by the other gonadotrophin, luteinizing hormone (LH), both being produced by the pituitary gland in response to the secretion of the hypothalamic hormone gonadotrophin releasing hormone (GnRH). It follows from this therefore that any hypothalamic or pituitary condition (*Table* T.1) which reduces GnRH or gonadotrophin secretion is likely to lead to testicular atrophy. Probably the commonest hypothalamic condition is a congenital lack of GnRH which when associated with anosmia is called *Kallmann's syndrome*. In this condition there is a midline defect with agenesis of the olfactory bulbs and other midline anomalies such as cleft palate and hare lip. The patients are sexually immature and are tall, with eunuchoidal skeletal proportions, having long arms and legs relative to the trunk (*see Fig.* S.58). Kallmann's syndrome is an autosomal dominant condition with variable penetrance and it occurs in 1/10 000 male births and 1/50 000 female births.

Table T.1. Causes of testicular atrophy

Physiological
Old age

Hypothalamic/pituitary conditions
Gonadotrophin releasing hormone deficiency (e.g.
  Kallmann's syndrome)
Hypopituitarism
Isolated LH deficiency
Hyperprolactinaemia
Haemochromatosis
Laurence–Moon–Biedl syndrome

Testicular conditions
Trauma*
Disturbances of blood supply
  Bilateral torsion of testes
  Inguinal hernia
  Ill-fitting truss
  Hydrocele
  Haematocele
  Varicocele
  Postoperative
  Elephantiasis
Destructive lesions
  Orchitis or epididymitis
    Mumps*
    Lymphocytic choriomeningitis virus
    Echovirus
    Arbovirus
    Chickenpox
    Tuberculosis
    Syphilis
    Gonorrhoea
    Typhoid fever
    Brucellosis
    Leptospirosis
    Lepromatosis leprosy
    Autoimmune orchitis
  Congenital lesions
    Cryptorchidism
    Klinefelter's syndrome*
    XX male
    Reifenstein's syndrome
    Noonan's syndrome
    Dystrophia myotonica
    Sertoli-cell only syndrome
    Haemochromatosis
  Tumour
    Feminizing tumour

Adrenal disorders
Cushing's syndrome
Congenital adrenal hyperplasia
Feminizing (oestrogen secreting) tumour

General disease
Alcoholism*
Cirrhosis of liver*
Renal failure
Sickle-cell anaemia

Drugs
Gonadotrophin releasing hormone analogues
Oestrogen therapy
Spironolactone
Marijuana
Cyclophosphamide
Chlorambucil

* The most common causes.

Isolated LH deficiency is a rare condition causing the 'fertile eunuch syndrome'. There is little or no testosterone production by the Leydig cells and the seminiferous tubules are immature because an adequate concentration of intracellular testosterone is necessary for this development and for the production of spermatozoa. The patients are sexually immature and have eunuchoidal skeletal proportions. They can be made sexually mature by treatment with human chorionic gonadotrophin, which has LH-like activity, and this also fully develops the seminiferous tubules.

The Laurence–Moon–Biedl syndrome is an uncommon condition which is an hereditary autosomal recessive disorder with variable penetrance. There are low levels of gonadotrophins with consequent retarded sexual development, obesity, mental retardation, retinitis pigmentosa and either polydactylism or syndactylism.

Raised prolactin levels produced in men by macroprolactinomas of the pituitary or as a consequence of drug therapy (phenothiazines, metoclopramide, haloperidol, pimozide, methyldopa, reserpine, cimetidine) lead to reduced gonadotrophin secretion by the pituitary and consequently to impotence, infertility and testicular atrophy.

Testicular conditions

Conditions affecting the testes directly (*see Table* T.1) are a much commoner cause of atrophy than are those secondarily related to hypothalamic or pituitary disorders. Trauma, such as being struck in the testicles by a cricket ball or falling astride a fence, may lead to an intratesticular haematoma which causes pressure necrosis of the seminiferous tubules and eventual atrophy of the testis. Any disturbance of the blood supply to the testes (*see Table* T.1), particularly torsion, can lead to testicular atrophy.

Mumps occurring in males after the age of 13 is an important cause of testicular atrophy. Permanent atrophy may occur in 36 per cent of cases. A wide range of other infections (*see Table* T.1) may do the same thing.

Testes which have been situated in the inguinal canal (cryptorchidism) or ectopically in the superficial inguinal pouch, perineum or upper thigh may fail to develop properly and remain small. Cryptorchidism which is unilateral in 84 per cent of cases occurs in 3 per 1000 of the adult male population. Cryptorchidism may be associated with Kallmann's syndrome (*see above*), but, more importantly, also with *Klinefelter's syndrome* (*see Fig.* S.60). This condition is relatively common, occurring in 1 per 500 male births. It is due to the presence of an extra X chromosome giving a karyotype of 47XXY, though sometimes mosaicism occurs with a karyotype of 46XY/47XXY. The patients are tall with eunuchoidal proportions and they have small, firm testes, which, if biopsied, show tubular sclerosis and hyalinization. Variable numbers of Leydig cells are present. There is invariably gynaecomastia and there is a tendency to low intelligence. The gonadotrophins LH and FSH are increased.

Patients with partial androgen resistance (*Reifenstein's syndrome*) may present with small testes, though there is usually also hypospadias and a small penis. The condition is an X-linked recessive with a 46XY karyotype.

Noonan's syndrome (*see Fig.* S.43) may present with atrophic testes, though more commonly the testes are undescended. Noonan's syndrome occurs in 1 in 8000 births. The karyotype is normal but the patient has somatic features rather like those of a female with Turner's syndrome. For this reason it is sometimes called 'male Turner's syndrome'. There is short stature, though this is not nearly so marked as in Turner's syndrome, there is webbing of the neck with a low hair line, a shield-shaped chest and cubitus valgus. There is pectus excavatum in 50 per cent of cases. The face has a characteristic appearance. It is triangular with low set ears and widely spaced eyes with an antimongoloid slant. There may be mental retardation. Congenital cardiac abnormalities are common. Pulmonary stenosis and atrial septal defect occur in about 50 per cent of cases, but ventricular septal defect, persistent ductus arteriosus, coarctation of the aorta or aortic stenosis may be present.

Dystrophia myotonica (*Fig.* T.1) is an autosomal dominant condition with a considerable degree of penetrance. Though it commonly appears to present in early middle-age, careful studies have shown that evidence of it is usually present in adolescence. Testicular atrophy, cataract and baldness are usual features accompanying the muscular features which consist of atrophy of the sternomastoids, facial muscles and distal muscles of the limbs and the characteristic delay in the ability to relax the muscles, exemplified in the prolonged handshake. In addition the patient usually displays progressive intellectual and psychological impairment.

Haemochromatosis leads to iron deposition in many tissues, including the pituitary and testes. The patient usually has testicular atrophy secondary to low levels of gonadotrophins. The patient has slate-grey skin and may have an enlarged liver and spleen.

Feminizing tumours of the ovary or adrenal are extremely rare, but may cause atrophy of non-tumourous testicular tissue because of oestrogen secretion. The patient usually also displays gynaecomastia.

Adrenal disorders

Cushing's syndrome may lead to some degree of testicular atrophy because the high levels of plasma cortisol

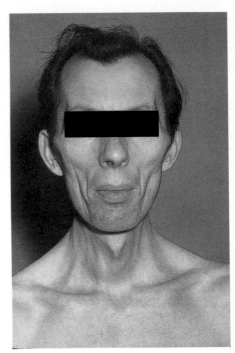

Fig. T.1. Patient with dystrophia myotonica showing wasting of facial muscles and sternomastoids and also frontal balding.

reduce LH secretion. Similarly children with congenital adrenal hyperplasia have small testes, despite development of the penis and secondary sexual hair, because the raised concentrations of androgens suppress the gonadotrophins.

General disease

Alcohol abuse and cirrhosis of the liver are important causes of testicular atrophy. Alcohol impairs gonadotrophin release from the pituitary but also has a direct effect on the testes, lowering testosterone synthesis. Spermatogenesis is also impaired. Testicular atrophy is found in 10–50 per cent of alcoholics without liver disease. Cirrhosis of the liver causes decreased testosterone secretion and an increased conversion of testosterone to oestrogen. This leads to an increase in the carrier protein, sex hormone binding globulin, which binds more avidly what testosterone there is and the level of free testosterone falls even further. Between 30 and 75 per cent of alcoholics with cirrhosis have testicular atrophy.

Approximately a third of males with sickle-cell anaemia have testicular atrophy, presumably secondary to impairment of blood supply or infarction of testicular tissue.

Drugs

Drugs used in the treatment of carcinoma of the prostate lead to testicular atrophy. Oestrogen therapy was commonly used in the past, but recently long-acting analogues of gonadotrophin releasing hormone have been used. They act by exhausting the pituitary gonadotroph cells and lowering the levels of gonadotrophins so that a medical 'orchidectomy' occurs.

Chemotherapy, particularly with cyclophosphamide and chlorambucil, leads to testicular damage. Pubertal, but not prepubertal boys, seem most vulnerable. Marijuana has a direct effect on the hypothalamus, pituitary and testis, and spironolactone not only impairs testosterone synthesis but also antagonizes the action of testosterone.

Ian D. Ramsay

Testicular pain

Pain in the testicle of varying degree may be present in many conditions, which may be discussed under separate headings as follows: (A) *Diseases of the body of the testis or epididymis*; (B) *Affections of the coverings of the testicle*; (C) *Affections of the spermatic cord*; (D) *A retained or misplaced testicle*; (E) *Pain from lesions remote from the testis.*

A. Diseases of the body of the testis or epididymis

Inflammatory lesions

Inflammatory lesions may attack the testis proper, or, as is more common, may begin in the epididymis. The investing tunica vaginalis distends with inflammatory exudate to form a secondary hydrocele. This tender mass may be mistaken for a swelling of the testis proper and the condition is frequently labelled an 'acute epididymo-orchitis'. However, surgical exploration and histological study reveal that the testis proper is rarely implicated and it is accurate, therefore, to speak of 'acute epididymitis'. An inflammatory affection of the testicle may be acute, subacute or chronic, the last often being the terminal result of the others.

An acute epididymitis arises most commonly by spread of infection to the organ from the urethra via the vas deferens or by the lymphatics accompanying the vas. When any inflammation has reached the prostatic portion of the urethra the orifices of the vasa deferentia may become infected, and inflammation spreads along the duct to the epididymis.

CAUSES OF ACUTE EPIDIDYMITIS

Causes of urethral origin
Urethritis due to *N. gonorrhoeae*
Urethritis due to *C. trachomatis*
Septic urethritis
Passage of catheters
Urethral instrumentation
Infection behind a stricture

Ulceration about an impacted calculus
Injections into the posterior urethra
After operations on the prostate
Urinary infections
Non-specific epididymitis

CAUSES OF ACUTE ORCHITIS
Fevers:
  Parotitis (mumps)
  Typhoid
  Lymphocytic choriomeningitis
  Scarlet fever
Injury

CAUSES OF CHRONIC EPIDIDYMITIS
Tuberculosis
Resolving acute epididymitis

SYPHILITIC DISEASE OF THE TESTIS
Diffuse interstitial orchitis
Gummatous orchitis

OTHER DISEASES
Malignant tumours of the testis
Torsion of the testis
Cysts of the epididymis

Acute epididymitis begins as a painful thickening of the epididymis associated with febrile symptoms. Before any actual pain is noticed in the testis there is often a sense of discomfort and weight over the external abdominal ring and inguinal canal due to the inflammatory process extending along the vas deferens. The swelling of the epididymis increases, and with it there is a secondary effusion of exudate into the tunica vaginalis (secondary hydrocele), causing swelling of its body and increase of pain. The whole organ thus becomes enlarged, and it is often exquisitely tender, the touch of the clothes or the most gentle examination causing pain. The swollen gland is often flattened on the outer and posterior aspect from pressure against the adductor muscles of the thigh; the vas deferens and tissues of the spermatic cord are thickened.

By far the most common cause of an acute epididymitis was formerly an *acute gonorrhoeal urethritis*; under the more effective modern antibiotic treatment of gonorrhoea it occurs much less often. During the disease the prostatic portion of the channel frequently becomes infected, when the orifices of the ejaculatory ducts may share in the inflammation, and infection be conveyed by the vas deferens to the testicle. Infection may also arise following an attack of non-specific urethritis, acquired as a result of sexual intercourse with a partner suffering from non-specific genital infection. Non-specific urethritis today is the commonest sexually transmitted disease in the Western world and at least 1 per cent of all male cases develop epididymitis. *C. trachomatis* is commonly found and appears to be the cause in around 50 per cent of cases. The gonorrhoeal form of acute epididymitis usually resolves slowly, and shows little liability to suppurate, whereas the inflammation resulting from a staphylococcal or streptococcal infection may break down into a testicular abscess.

Acute epididymitis may also arise from septic processes in the urethra following the *passage of catheters*, of *instruments* for vesical operations, transurethral prostatic resection or lithotrity for example, from infection behind a *urethral striction* or about a *calculus* in the prostatic urethra, occasionally after the *instillation of strong solutions* into the posterior urethra in the treatment of a chronic urethritis, or after operations on the prostate, especially prostatectomy, or as a complication of a urinary infection by *E. coli* or other organisms. It may follow prostatic massage. In any case the onset of pyrexia with pain and rapid swelling of the testis should lead to suspicion of a urinary tract infection. Bacteriological examination of any urethral discharge and of the urine is essential (*see* URETHRAL DISCHARGE).

In *non-specific epididymitis* there may be no evidence of urethral infection and bacteriological studies are entirely negative; the condition sometimes arises after unaccustomed exercise and has been attributed to a reflux of urine down the vas. The testicle becomes painful, and enlarges rapidly in the same manner as in acute inflammation from urethral infection, and under appropriate conservative treatment by means of a scrotal support gradually resolves. Less frequently testicular inflammation may occur after a direct injury to the organ, such as a *blow* or *squeeze*.

The pain in an acute inflammation is generally of an aching character at first, felt not only in the testis but also at the external abdominal ring, and often as a heavy dragging pain in the inguinal or iliac areas of the affected side. As the testis enlarges the local pain becomes more severe, so that the swollen gland is exquisitely tender to pressure or to the touch. After a few days the pain subsides to a large extent, but remains as a dull ache until the swelling becomes greatly reduced, and it usually does not disappear entirely until the organ returns to the normal size. In a few cases in which a fibrous scar remains in the epididymis pain may remain and cause some difficulty in the diagnosis from an incipient tuberculous lesion, but the earlier history of acute inflammation will help in forming an opinion. In other cases the persistence of the pain and swelling may indicate the formation of an abscess in the testicle, when, after decreasing at first, the swelling increases, the skin covering it becomes reddened and oedematous, and a soft area becomes evident in one aspect of the organ.

Acute orchitis

Acute orchitis may complicate *acute specific parotitis* (mumps), especially when this occurs in adolescents or adults. Both testes may be affected and the result may be testicular atrophy. Much less often the testis may be affected in *typhoid*, *scarlet fever* or *influenza*. Infection with *C. trachomatis* may cause epididymoorchitis.

Tuberculosis of the testicle

Tuberculosis of the testicle is comparatively common today in many parts of the world, including India and the Far East, but is comparatively rare in Great Britain. It arises with extreme rarity as a primary disease but more commonly as secondary to tuberculous disease of the kidney, bladder, prostate or seminal vesicles. It is most frequently seen in young adults. It begins as a localized deposit in almost all cases, causing a rounded, firm nodule in the epididymis, usually in the lower pole. This nodule may remain unaltered for many months, or may enlarge, soften, become adherent to the skin and coverings of the testicle, or actually ulcerate through them to form a discharging sinus in the scrotum. The small nodule in the epididymis is usually painless at first and may be found by accident, but later, as it gradually enlarges, it causes an aching pain in the organ. There may be an associated hydrocele of the tunica vaginalis. Other nodules may be formed in the epididymis, or the body of the testis may become involved, while commonly small shot-like thickenings may be felt in the course of the vas deferens, or a progressively increasing thickening as it is traced down to the epididymis. In the more advanced stages nodules may be felt upon rectal examination in the seminal vesicles or prostate, or there may be some in the epididymis of the other side.

Tuberculous disease of the testicle usually presents some difficulty in its diagnosis from non-specific epididymitis, particularly when it has an acute onset, as sometimes happens. In an early case the occurrence of one or more nodules in the epididymis, which are painful on pressure and which have not resulted from a preceding acute epididymitis, should always suggest a tuberculous focus, and a careful search should be made for other tuberculous lesions in the body. The urine is cultured for *M. tuberculosum* and intravenous pyelography performed. If no evidence of tuberculosis is found the gradual subsidence of the lesion under careful observation will indicate that it was a non-specific epididymitis. In later stages the diagnosis is less difficult; the gradual enlargement of the nodules, their craggy or bossy feel, the infection of the vas or other genito-urinary organs with tuberculosis, and above all the tendency of the focus in the epididymis to soften and to become adherent to the scrotal coverings and to produce an indolent sinus, are points to be looked for.

Syphilitic disease of the testis

Syphilitic disease of the testis, once common, but now a rarity, causes very little pain in the organ, but there is often a sense of dragging or heaviness. Syphilis may attack the testicle in several different ways, producing:

IN ACQUIRED SYPHILIS
Diffuse interstitial orchitis
Localized gummatous orchitis

IN CONGENITAL SYPHILIS
Interstitial orchitis
Localized gummatous orchitis

The outstanding feature of syphilitic disease of the testicle is that it affects the body of the testis rather than the epididymis, thus differing in a marked degree from tuberculous disease. In the interstitial form there is thickening of the intertubular connective tissue, with an infiltration of spindle cells, which, forming young connective tissue, yield fibrous tissue. The subsequent contraction of this fibrous tissue may cause atrophy of the testis. The testis may, on section, show small gummas in addition to the diffuse orchitis, or if the inflammation is more localized, gummas may be the main feature, these varying in size from that of a pea to that of a walnut, or larger. The epididymis is affected but rarely, though cases are on record of a nodular swelling in the epididymis during the secondary stage of syphilis which disappears rapidly under anti-syphilitic treatment.

In congenital syphilis, both the interstitial and gummatous forms exist; they usually occur in childhood or in young adult life, and in many cases the affection is bilateral. Syphilitic inflammation of the testicle may be accompanied in either the acquired or the congenital form by a vaginal hydrocele. A gummatous testis may ulcerate through the scrotum, usually in front, producing a circular 'punched-out' ulcer with a slough in the base.

There is a sense of weight in the scrotum rather than pain, and often an aching or dragging feeling in the inguinal or lumbar region. On palpation, the body of the testis feels enlarged and nodular with the gummatous deposits, but the epididymis can usually be distinguished from the testis and found to be unaffected. Testicular sensation is lost. The tissues of the cord remain unthickened. Tertiary syphilitic lesions of the testicle give rise to very little tenderness on palpation.

The diagnosis of syphilitic disease of the testis is usually simple. There may or may not be a history of syphilis, but other signs of the disease should be looked for—thus, in the acquired form, any scar of previous ulceration or periosteal thickening, or, in the congenital variety, signs in the teeth, eyes or ears. Syphilitic disease is distinguished from *tuberculous disease* of the testis by the fact that the epididymis is usually free; that the cord, prostate and vesicles remain normal; and that pressure applied directly to the testicle gives little or no pain. Tuberculous deposits tend to soften and to involve the scrotal coverings in spite of treatment. From haematocele it is differentiated by the history of injury or by the absence of the history or signs of syphilis. From *malignant tumours of the testis* it is distinguished by the history of syphilis, the tendency of syphilitic disease to be bilateral, the slow enlargement, and positive serological tests. In malignant disease, the increase in the size of the testicle is more rapid, while the tumour often shows areas of varying consistence; the cord is often thickened in malignant or in tuberculous cases, but seldom in syphilitic.

It should be pointed out that gumma of the testis is so rare in Great Britain today, compared with its former frequency, that it is safer to regard any solid swelling in the testicle itself as the much more common and more likely malignant tumour of the testis, and treat it as such by orchidectomy. In the unlikely event that a gumma is thus removed, the surgeon can comfort himself with the fact that a functionally useless organ has been excised.

Malignant tumours of the testis

Malignant tumours of the testis may give rise to pain in the organ, but as a rule pain is experienced only in the later stages of the disease, as testicular sensation is completely lost. Although benign tumours of the epididymis may occur, nearly all tumours of the testis are highly malignant. They fall into two main pathological varieties, *seminoma* and *teratoma*, the latter including the subgroups of *chorionepithelioma*, *dermoid* and *fibrocystic disease*. The *seminoma* (*Fig.* T.2) is a soft vascular solid growth composed of large spheroidal cells derived from the germinal epithelium of the seminiferous tubules. It occurs at about the age of 40 and is less malignant but more radiosensitive than teratoma. It tends to retain the shape of the testis as it enlarges.

The *teratoma* (*Fig.* T.3) or mixed tumour is a solid or multilocular cystic growth in which one or other of the germinal layers may preponderate. Dermoids, containing hair or teeth, are less common than in the ovary but sometimes occur in childhood and are relatively benign.

Fibrocystic disease pursues an even more benign course and may be present for 10 or more years before exhibiting its malignant characteristics by sudden rapid growth and the formation of metastases. Most cases of teratoma occur at the age of 25–30; they give a

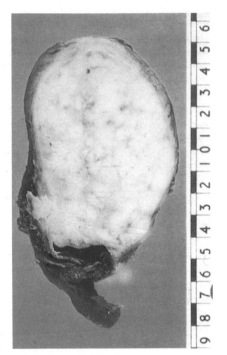

Fig. T.2. Seminoma of the testis.

in the urine; in seminoma the pituitary gonadotrophic hormone is sometimes found in the urine. Either type may follow injury in a significant proportion of cases although it is likely that trauma merely draws attention to the testicular mass. The undescended testis is more prone to develop malignant disease than is the normally placed one. The testis which has been initially undescended and subsequently brought down into the scrotum maintains this higher tendency to malignant change, estimated at about ten times that of the normal organ.

A testicle that is the seat of a malignant growth enlarges slowly or rapidly, but as pain is at first absent there may be nothing to arouse the patient's suspicions. As long as the tunica albuginea remains intact the swelling retains the shape of the testis, but when perforation of the fibrous covering takes place nodular projections appear and render the tumour irregular. These projections are softer than the remainder of the growth, and form a valuable point in the diagnosis. A rapidly growing malignant tumour of the testis may be so soft as to appear to be a fluid collection in the tunica vaginalis. Generally, however, although a growth may be accompanied by a small amount of fluid in the tunica vaginalis, the more solid mass can

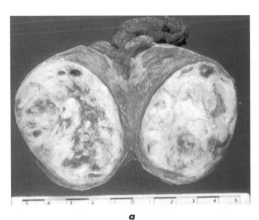

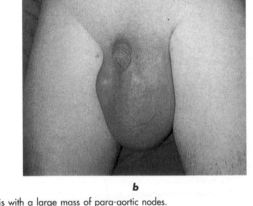

a   b

Fig. T.3. a, Teratoma of the testis. b, Teratoma of the left testis with a large mass of para-aortic nodes.

short history, are more resistant to X-ray treatment, and show early metastases. There may be enlargement of the breasts and chorionic hormone may be present

be felt through the fluid on careful examination; this fluid is often blood-stained. The epididymis may become incorporated in the growth so that it cannot be distinguished, and the tissues of the cord become thickened. The coverings of the testis become stretched over the tumour; the mass does not become adherent to the scrotal skin until late in the disease. Clinically it is impossible to distinguish between a teratoma and a seminoma. In both types the para-aortic lymph nodes become enlarged, and may be felt in a thin subject to one or other side of the epigastric area, and pain due to the pressure of these nodes upon nerve structures may become marked (*Fig.* T.3*b*). The inguinal nodes are usually not enlarged unless the scrotal skin is affected; retrograde spread may then occur to the iliac nodes which may be felt at the brim of the pelvis. In advanced cases, the left supraclavicular lymph nodes are involved and become palpably enlarged. Mediastinal or pulmonary metastases are frequent, the latter giving the characteristic radiological appearance of 'cannon-ball' secondaries. The diagnosis of malignant disease of the testis may be quite easy in the case of rapidly growing tumours, but in others, especially in the early stages, it may present great difficulty. Rarely an *interstitial-cell tumour* occurs in a child and produces sexual precocity. Differential diagnosis must be made between malignant tumours and the following:

Gummatous orchitis may be confused with the more slowly growing forms of tumour. In both the swelling may have followed an injury, and in both there may be a syphilitic history. Gummatous orchitis is, however, either more acute or more chronic; it retains more the oval shape of the testis, and does not present the rounded, slightly raised bosses which are commonly present in a malignant testis. In orchitis the epididymis is usually distinguished more easily, and the cord is not so thickened as with a growth. In any case of doubt it is a wise course to advise exploration. (*See above.*)

Tuberculous disease is usually diagnosed easily from malignant disease by the tendency of tubercle to attack the epididymis, to caseate, suppurate and to become adherent to the scrotal skin comparatively early. Tuberculosis occasionally attacks the body of the testicle first, however, forming an oval, smooth tumour of the organ; the epididymis and vas deferens may be unaffected for a time, and if no deposit is found in the prostate or vesicles the differential diagnosis between tubercle and growth may be far from easy before operation. Tuberculosis most frequently occurs in young adults.

The diagnosis between a *haematocele* and a malignant tumour of the testis may present considerable difficulty. In both, the swelling may date from an injury, while the indistinct fluctuation obtained in the soft areas of a growth, accompanied sometimes by some fluid in the tunica vaginalis, may simulate a haematocele. The latter feels heavy to the hand, but is usually softer in its whole mass and more regular than a growth. Care must be taken not to place too much reliance upon the withdrawal of a few drops of blood from the tumour by means of a trocar and cannula, a result which may happen equally with growth or haematocele. A haematocele may cease to enlarge, or even diminish in size, whereas, in growth, increase in size is progressive. The cord remains unaffected with haematocele, and testicular sensation is more likely to be lost in growth.

Ultrasonography of the testis can be very useful in localizing the exact site of the mass and in differentiating between a solid and a cystic mass. If any doubt exists it is advisable to excise the testis, dividing the cord at the internal ring. Incision into a testis which is the seat of a growth is almost invariably followed by rapid recurrence. If necessary, a radical operation can be done after the histology is known, or radiotherapy can be given. (*See also below.*)

A *hydrocele* of very long standing with an irregular, nodular surface, and absence of translucency due to the thickened tunica vaginalis and the thick contents of the sac, may simulate a new growth, but the long history of the case, and the absence of progressive increase in size of the swelling, will prevent a mistake of this kind. (*See also below.*)

Torsion of the testis

Torsion of the testis on its vascular pedicle may occur in a testis which has a mesorchium or in one which is ectopic. It occurs most commonly in youths soon after puberty, or in infants; the exciting cause may be some mild exertion or movement such as crossing the legs or turning over in bed. There may be a history of repeated minor attacks before complete torsion takes place, and the other testis may have suffered similar incomplete attacks or be found to be unduly mobile or horizontally placed. At the moment of torsion there is severe sickening pain which may be felt at first in the abdomen but is quickly localized to the testis; the boy may even say that his testicle has twisted. There is usually nausea and sometimes vomiting. The testis forms a tense tender swelling in the upper part of the scrotum or at the external abdominal ring, and the scrotum below is empty. This sign serves to distinguish the condition from a strangulated hernia or an inflamed lymph node. In acute epididymitis the testis is in its normal position and there may be evidence of urethral discharge or of a urinary tract infection. Because of the initial abdominal pain and vomiting the condition has been mistaken for acute appendicitis, but adherence to the rule of examining the scrotal contents in all abdominal cases should prevent this error.

Cysts of the testis

Cysts of the testis occur most frequently in connection with the epididymis, very rarely with the body of the testis. These cysts are quite different from hydrocele of the tunica vaginalis, and are often spoken of as a spermatocele, although all do not contain spermatozoa and the term is thus better avoided. They cause a swelling of varying degree in the scrotum, and usually an aching in the testicle, groin or lumbar region. They may arise as retention cysts of the tubules of the epididymis or from one of the fetal remains which occur about the globus major of the epididymis. These cysts are usually placed above and to the outer side of the testis, occasionally behind it. They move with the organ, and can usually be distinguished from the latter by the test of translucency. They may be multiple and are frequently bilateral. Their increase in size is very slow, but they may cause aching pain in the testicle by pressure upon, or stretching of, the tissues of the epididymis. They can be distinguished from hydrocele of the tunica vaginalis by the position of the swelling relative to the testicle, and by the fact that the fluid contained in them is colourless or slightly opalescent from the contained spermatozoa, in distinction from the straw-coloured clear fluid of a vaginal hydrocele.

B. Affections of the coverings of the testis causing pain in the organ

The only common lesions of the coverings of the testis are *hydrocele* and *haematocele*: new growths of the testicular tunics are so rare as to render them surgical curiosities and they rarely cause pain.

Hydrocele

Hydrocele may occur occasionally as an acute affection accompanying an acute epididymitis, injury to the scrotum or in the course of acute specific fevers such as mumps. Acute hydrocele has been described in conjunction with acute lesions of other serous membranes, e.g. polyserositis. The more usual form of hydrocele is the chronic variety, which may be due to some disease of the testicle, but for which, in the majority of cases, no ascertainable cause can be found (primary or idiopathic hydrocele).

A hydrocele may cause some aching in the testicle, but more frequently it causes a dragging sensation in the inguinal or iliac areas from the mechanical effect of its weight. It forms a swelling on one side of the scrotum, oval with smooth uniform surface; it gives a distinct sense of fluctuation. The swelling is limited

above from the cord or external abdominal ring, and gives no sense of impulse on coughing; with a good light it can be found in most cases to be translucent, the testicle occupying a posterior and low position in the swelling. The diagnosis of hydrocele is usually easy, but difficulty may be experienced in old-standing cases in which the walls are much thickened. A hydrocele must be diagnosed from: (1) A scrotal hernia; (2) Haematocele; (3) New growth and; (4) A cyst of the epididymis.

Scrotal hernia. Usually a hernia gives an impulse on coughing, can be reduced into the abdomen with a sudden slip or gurgle, and varies in size with the position of the patient. A hernia comes from above and descends into the scrotum. In a large irreducible hernia, some part of it is usually resonant from the contained intestine, the swelling is not limited above, and the testis can be distinguished at the bottom of the scrotum. A hydrocele is distinctly limited above so that the examining fingers can meet above it, gives no impulse on coughing, is translucent, and the spermatic cord can be distinguished easily. The testis in a hydrocele cannot usually be distinguished in the scrotum as in a hernia. Difficulty may arise between the two conditions when the hydrocele extends along the funicular process in the inguinal canal and thus gives an impulse on coughing, or if the translucency is lost owing to the thickness of the walls of the sac. A scrotal hernia in an infant may be translucent.

Haematocele is distinguished from hydrocele by the absence of translucency and the rapidity of the onset, usually after an injury or puncture (*see also below*).

New growths of the testis. A hydrocele is of much slower rate of increase in size, of smooth surface and uniform consistence, and is translucent.

Cyst of the epididymis. (*See above*.)

In cases of doubt, **ultrasonography** of the swelling usually enables accurate anatomical delineation of the mass to be made and distinguishes between a cystic and a solid swelling.

Haematocele

Haematocele may occur from puncture of a vein in the sac or of the testicle as the result of tapping a hydrocele, or by the occurrence of bleeding into a hydrocele. It may occur quite independently of a hydrocele, usually after direct injury. As a rule there is a rapid onset of swelling in the scrotum following the injury, with ecchymosis of the scrotal skin; the resulting tumour resembles a hydrocele in its clinical symptoms, save that it is not translucent. In other cases the swelling arises more slowly, when a pyriform or oval swelling is present in one side of the scrotum covered by normal skin; the surface of the swelling is smooth, and gives a sense of fluctuation and elasticity. There is no translucency, and on tapping, dark blood-stained fluid is withdrawn.

The diagnosis in the less acute cases often presents a difficulty, especially with regard to *malignant disease of the testicle* (*see above*); this is particularly so when the haematoma is organized. From *hydrocele* it is distinguished by the absence of translucency; from *hernia* by the same points, except translucency, mentioned above in the diagnosis between hydrocele and hernia.

C. Affections of the spermatic cord causing testicular pain

An inflammatory affection of the cord secondary to urethral infection is not uncommon. Tuberculous infection of the cord is practically never present without corresponding infection of the epididymis. New growths of the cord, lipomas, sarcomas (extremely rare) and hydroceles of the cord cause no pain in the testis. A *varicocele*, especially if large, in a pendulous scrotum, is a frequent cause of a dull, aching pain in the testicle; it is nearly always left-sided, although the reason for this is obscure. The characteristic feel of the enlarged veins in the erect position, and the slight impulse and thrill on coughing, will readily point to the correct diagnosis.

D. Retained or misplaced testis

This, in its various situations, may give rise to pain. A testis may be arrested in its descent at the external abdominal ring, in the inguinal canal, may remain inside the abdomen, or may pass upwards and outwards from the external abdominal ring into the superficial inguinal pouch where it can be felt readily. It is doubtful if a testis retained within the inguinal canal is ever palpable. Occasionally it passes into the perineum after traversing the inguinal canal, to the upper part of the thigh via the crural ring, or to the root of the penis in front of the pubis. In one fifth of all cases, the undescended testes are bilateral.

In the various situations in which an undescended or ectopic testicle is placed it may be attacked by the several diseases which affect the normally placed organ, and thus give rise to pain; but in addition, owing to the effect of recurrent muscular strains and the comparative immobility of the organ, it is particularly liable to attacks of inflammation, especially when the testis is retained in the inguinal canal; in the intra-abdominal position it remains protected from muscular injury, while ectopic testicles have a greater range of mobility than has one that is retained in the inguinal canal and are thus especially prone to torsion. The

inflammation of an undescended testicle may be so acute as to lead to gangrene of the organ, with or without torsion of the cord. The pain may be complained of first when the testes begin to enlarge at puberty, at which time an undescended right testicle may produce symptoms which can be easily mistaken for appendicitis.

The diagnosis of undescended testicle rests upon the following points: the fact that one side of the scrotum is empty; the outline and situation of the swelling in the superficial inguinal region or elsewhere; the testicular sensation upon pressure; and the recurrent attacks of pain. An undescended testicle may give rise to acute pain from inflammatory lesions or from acute torsion of the organ, and may if it is in the inguinal canal give rise to symptoms suggesting a strangulated hernia. A partially descended testicle is often accompanied by an inguinal hernia. The misplaced testis is especially liable to become the seat of malignant disease.

It should be remembered that an imperfectly descended testis is a small and poorly developed organ and the spermatogenesis from the gland may be absent or only last for a short time after puberty.

E. Testicular pain from lesions other than in the testicle

Complaint may be made of testicular pain when on clinical examination the testis is found to be normal. After an acute inflammation of the organ, even when no palpable nodule remains, the resulting cicatrization may cause aching in the organ, especially after *sexual excitement* or prolonged desire. Apart from former testicular disease pain may be felt in the organ if a *calculus* is present *in the pelvis of the kidney* or *upper ureter*, or from stimulation of the peripheral nerves by *secondary deposits in the bodies of the lumbar vertebrae*, pressure from an *extramedullary intraspinal tumour* such as a neurofibroma, meningioma or ependymoma, or the pressure of an *aneurysm* in this situation. Pain in the testicle is occasionally present in *appendiceal inflammation* when the appendix turns down into the pelvis. Finally when no organic cause of any sort is present the condition is usually called *neuralgia testis*; this is pain of an aching character which may occur in patients of a neurotic tendency.

Harold Ellis

Testicular swelling

(*See also* TESTICULAR PAIN.)

It is first essential to prove that the swelling is really testicular. This is done by grasping the root of the scrotum between the thumb and index fingers to determine whether any of the swelling extends along the cord into the inguinal region. True scrotal swellings may arise in: (1) skin; (2) the various connective-tissue coverings of the testicle; (3) tunica vaginalis; (4) testicle; (5) epididymis; (6) the lower end of the spermatic cord; (7) the urethra; (8) the bones of the pubic arch. Of these the swellings in the cord, testicle, epididymis and tunica vaginalis are the commonest and most important.

1. Swellings affecting the skin

The nature of these is usually obvious. The only common ones are sebaceous cysts. Much less common are soft sores, chancre, warts and epithelioma. The last-named soon ulcerates and was once commonly seen in sweeps or in those who work in tar, tar products or petroleum. It is now relatively rare.

2. Swellings of the various connective-tissue coverings

These are rare, but occasionally a fibrosarcoma may occur. These swellings are movable upon the testicle. The symmetrical enlargement called *elephantiasis scroti* (*Fig.* T.4), due to *Wuchereria bancrofti*, is limited to the tropics, though sometimes a similar state of scrotal distension and overgrowth results in Great Britain from lymphatic obstruction due to pelvic cellulitis or to congenital abnormality. The enlarged scrotum resulting from acute generalized oedema in acute or chronic renal disease is seldom difficult to recognize; the penis and prepuce are generally distended by oedema at the same time as are the legs, loins, eyelids and other parts, and the diagnosis is confirmed by the albumin and tube-casts in the urine.

Gross oedematous scrotal swelling also occurs with ascites or inferior vena caval thrombosis, and may accompany the abdominal swelling of pellagra and infantile kwashiorkor.

Neurodermatitis affecting the scrotum may produce a considerable amount of scrotal oedema, as does moniliasis (candidiasis).

3. The tunica vaginalis

The tunica vaginalis may become distended with serous fluid, blood or pus: distension with fluid may be primary, the ordinary vaginal hydrocele, or secondary to disease of the testis or epididymis. *Vaginal hydrocele* usually arises slowly, though some follow injury and give a short history. The patient is well, with no pain or urinary complaint, and merely complains of the lump or of the drag it causes. The swelling is large, heavy, ovoid, tense and elastic rather than fluctuating, though fluctuation can be proved if the swelling is fixed by an assistant or the patient; neither testis nor

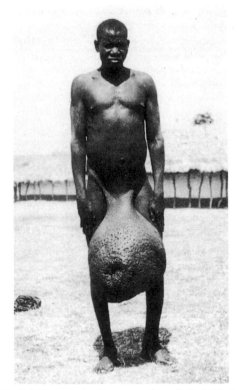

Fig. T.4. Elephantiasis of the scrotum due to filariasis. (*Dr C. J. Hackett, Wellcome Museum of Medical Science.*)

epididymis can be felt apart from the swelling. A hydrocele can be transilluminated, but it needs a dark room and a strong light (*Fig.* T.5): when transilluminated the testicular shadow will be noticed at one edge of the swelling, usually behind. Tapping withdraws a golden fluid of soapy feel, with a specific gravity of about 1030, that coagulates solid on boiling. *Secondary hydrocele* follows disease of the testis or epididymis: the amount of fluid is usually small, and the swelling lax, so that the finger can be passed through it to touch the testis. The complaint is of the causative disease rather than of the hydrocele, which is usually discovered on examination. Transillumination will confirm the presence of fluid. A *haematocele* has the physical characters of a hydrocele except that it is not translucent. Vaginal hydroceles vary very much in this respect, for their wall becomes thicker from fibrosis or deposition of fibrin, particularly after repeated tapping, and the fluid becomes stained with blood-pigment and hazy with cholesterol crystals, so that the strongest light may only just be perceptible across them. Tapping may be required to establish the presence of blood. Haematocele is due to injury, torsion or growth of the testis, and its discovery is therefore the indication for exploration, unless the history of trauma is recent and definite, for example, as the result of tapping a hydrocele. A *pyocele* is merely part of a suppurative process arising in the testis or the epididymis. The differential diagnosis of hydrocele is from translucent swellings in the epididymis and cord—cyst of the epididymis and encysted hydrocele.

vomiting, are moderate enlargement of the testicle, tenderness, the presence of a small haematocele and the appearance after a few hours of oedema of the scrotal wall on the affected side. Recurring subacute torsion of the testicle is not uncommon, and in these

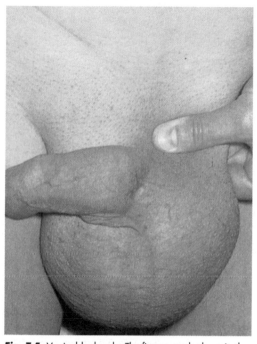 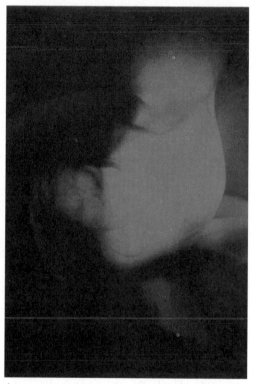

Fig. T.5. Vaginal hydrocele. The fingers reach above it, thus excluding inguinoscrotal hernia. It transilluminates brilliantly.

Ultrasonography has proved to be invaluable in the investigation of at testicular mass, in particular in determining whether or not there is underlying testicular disease in a patient with hydrocele.

4.   Swellings of the testicle

These usually affect either the body or the epididymis, rarely the two together. The first group includes torsion, mumps, gumma and new growth; the second tuberculosis, gonorrhoea, *Esch. coli* infection and cysts. Determination of the anatomical site of the swelling will therefore go some way towards settling its pathological nature.

SWELLING OF THE BODY OF THE TESTICLE

Torsion is met with as an acute condition accompanied by abdominal pain and vomiting, and it often occurs in the undescended testis (*see* INGUINAL SWELLING). Torsion of a fully descended testis, giving rise to a scrotal swelling, is seldom seen except in small boys; the local signs, in addition to the abdominal pain and

cases the signs and symptoms are less pronounced than in the acute variety into which they eventually pass.

The main points of distinction between the less acute enlargements of the corpus testis may be tabulated as in *Table* T.2.

It is often difficult to distinguish syphilitic enlargement of the testicles from that due to growth; but a course of anti-syphilitic therapy and the serological reactions may settle the matter. Gumma of the testis, once common, is now a clinical rarity in Western communities, so that today a solid mass in the testis is highly suspicious of a neoplasm. Malignant new growth nearly always grows steadily, and being entirely within the tunica albuginea it maintains the shape and smooth surface of the testicle until it reaches a size much larger than that of a syphilitic testicle.

The pathology of malignant tumours of the testicle has proved a fertile ground for debate, but nothing can be gained by discussing their classification since the differentiation depends upon examination of sections from the removed specimen and is impossible on clinical grounds. Both the teratomas, which may con-

Table T.2. Swellings of the body of the testicle

	Mumps	Syphilis	Tumour
Age	Puberty or adolescence	Any age, but usually 18 to 30	Any age, commoner after 20
History and other symptoms	Short history with pyrexia. Previous contact with mumps. Parotids enlarged	Previous history of exposure to venereal disease; usually has had chancre and rash. Gumma or tertiary rashes may be found elsewhere	Onset insidious. History of months
Scrotum	Normal or red and hot	Normal or adherent in front. Later, ulcer with sharp edges and slough at base, or hernia testis	Normal or merely stretched till growth is size of tennis ball, when it may be invaded
Testis Size and shape	Moderately enlarged, shape normal	Enlarged up to two or three times normal. May be nodular	Increases steadily and may reach diameter of 10–13 cm. First smooth, later nodular
Sensation	Tender and painful. Testicular sensation present	Not tender or painful. Testicular sensation lost	Painful, but not tender. Testicular sensation lost late in disease
'Weight'	This test is hoary with tradition, but it is quite valueless. It will be found that the specific gravity of a cubic centimetre of each of the pathological tissues is identical		
Tunica vaginalis	Slight hydrocele in most	Hydrocele in 60 per cent	Hydrocele in early stages: later haematocele
Epididymis	Unaltered	Usually unaltered	Flattened
Cord	May be tender	Normal	Usually normal, but may have nodules of growth in lymphatics
Nodes	Not characteristically enlarged	Not characteristically enlarged	Drainage to para-aortic nodes at kidney level. These may form very large mass. Eventually left supraclavicular nodes involved. Inguinal nodes not enlarged unless scrotal skin is invaded

tain structures representing the three layers of the embryo, and the seminomas, supposedly derived from the germinal elements, may give rise to metastases in the lymphatics to the para-aortic nodes and the bloodstream. (See *Figs*. T2 and T3.)

5. The epididymis

The epididymis may become enlarged as the result of inflammation, new growth or cystic degeneration. Primary new growth of the epididymis is excessively rare and need not give rise to much concern in differential diagnosis; it will generally be regarded as tubercle until after operation and microscopical examination of the tissue excised.

Inflammatory swellings are characterized by being elongated in a vertical direction; by their relation to the testicle, which they overlap at its posterior border and its upper and lower poles; and by being flattened from side to side. Inflammatory swellings may be: (*a*) tuberculous; (*b*) due to *Escherichia coli* (certain cases of epididymitis, indistinguishable clinically from *E. coli* infection, are of very obscure aetiology: some say that

they are due to irritation by urine passing by reflux up the vas, others that a virus is responsible; they are grouped as 'non-specific' epididymitis, and they tend to settle spontaneously in about three to four weeks); (*c*) *C. trachomatis*; (*d*) gonorrhoeal; (*e*) septic, secondary to some infection of the urethra. The main points of the distinction are shown in *Table* T.3.

It will be seen that *E. coli* epididymitis may bear a close resemblance to a tuberculous lesion, particularly when the acute infection has been partially aborted by antibiotic therapy, but lacks any distant or constitutional evidence of the disease. Support of the testicle in a suspensory bandage and the administration of suitable antibiotic therapy will cause marked improvement in a few days and thus settle the diagnosis. Apart from the history and an increased liability to suppuration in septic epididymitis, there is little to distinguish the latter from the gonococcal variety.

Cysts of the epididymis may be solitary or multiple, and may be bilateral. A cyst of the epididymis is placed above and behind the testicle, from which it is distinct; though attached to the epididymis, it is

Table T.3. Inflammatory swellings of the epididymis

	Tuberculosis	Esch. coli and 'non-specific'	Gonorrhoeal	Septic
History	Previous tuberculous infection, especially urinary	Usually none	Recent infection, with gleet, and pain on micturition	Recent catheterization or operation on bladder or prostate
Other signs and symptoms	? Cough, wasting. ? Evidence of phthisis in lungs. ? Tubercle bacilli in urine	Usually none. Urine may smell fishy and contain *Esch. coli*	Urethral discharge. Gram-negative diplococci: other manifestations such as joints	Pus in alkaline urine
Scrotum	May be adherent behind. May have sinus discharging thin pus	Normal	Red, hot, swollen and tender	Red, hot, swollen and tender. May suppurate
Testes	Usually normal	Normal	Normal, but outline obscured by surroundings	Normal, but outline obscured by surroudings
Tunica vaginalis	Hydrocele in 30 per cent	Normal	Small hydrocele usually present	Hydrocele or pyocele
Epididymis	Nodular enlargement of globus minor, less commonly globus major or whole epididymis. Nodules, hard and very tender. Later break down to abscess, with sinus	No local nodules or much enlargement, but affected part hard and tender. Changes usually involve globus minor or whole epididymis. Does not break down	Whole epididymis large, hard and broad; hot and tender	Globus minor or whole epididymis enlarged and broad; hot and tender
Cord	Oedema of cord. Vas may be thickened. Beading of vas excessively rare	Normal	Whole cord tender and swollen	Whole cord tender and swollen
Prostate and seminal vesicles	Vesicle on affected side may be hard and tender	Normal	Prostate may be hot and tender. Tenderness along vesicles	Swollen and tender. Vesicles may be felt

rounded, but being thin-walled it does not feel as tense as a hydrocele; it tends to have several rounded projections rather than a simple surface; and the fluid withdrawn by tapping is milky or opalescent, of low specific gravity, containing little albumin but showing numerous cells under the microscope, some of which may be spermatozoa. *Multiple cysts* occur in men past middle age, and are probably analogous to cystic degeneration of the breast. They are painless and increase in size very slowly. These swellings are usually strikingly translucent.

6. Swellings of the lower end of the cord

The most important swelling of the lower part of the spermatic cord is *varicocele*. It is apt to be mistaken for an inguinal hernia, but this mistake should never be made because of the characteristic feel of the varicocele (like a bag of worms), and the reappearance of the swelling after it has been completely reduced by elevation of the scrotum and the finger is firmly pressed on the external abdominal ring. Varicocele is far commoner on the left than the right.

7. Urethral conditions

Occasionally a *peri-urethral abscess* may form a swelling in the scrotum. Tenderness, oedema and fluctuation, together with the history and evidence of urethral disease, serve to make the diagnosis clear. *Primary epithelioma of the urethra*, which is rare, is distinguished by the great pain and urethral obstruction that it engenders.

8. Diseases of the pubic bones

Inflammatory products may travel into the scrotum from diseases of the bones of the pubic arch, especially from the neighbourhood of the symphysis pubis. *Acute necrosis* of these bones is sufficiently indicated by the grave constitutional symptoms which always accompany it. *Caries* gives rise to more difficulty.

Harold Ellis

Tetany

(See also CRAMPS, TIC, VERTIGO.)

Tetany is a condition where abnormal muscle cramps are caused by increased neuromuscular excitability induced by a fall in the concentration of ionized calcium; important precipitating factors include a low calcium diet, pregnancy and lactation. Early symptoms of acute tetany include paraesthesiae and numbness of the extremities and around the mouth. Then muscle cramps may occur, particularly in the extremities. The wrist and elbow may become flexed, the fingers flexed at the metacarpophalangeal joint, but extended at the terminal interphalangeal joint and the fingers all pressed together, with the thumb adducted into the palm of the hand so that the whole hand forms the 'main d'accoucheur' (obstetrician's hand). When the legs are affected the knees and ankles are extended, the foot is arched and inverted and the toes flexed and pressed together. The cramps may be painful and last from several minutes to a couple of hours. In severe cases face and neck muscles may be involved and laryngospasm may cause respiratory obstruction and lead to loss of consciousness and death. Generalized epileptic convulsions may occur, especially in children.

Latent tetany may be revealed by special signs:

1. CHVOSTEK'S SIGN. Twitching of the muscles of the upper lip may be elicited by tapping on the facial nerve in front of the ear. However, note that this sign can be present in some people with normal calcium levels.

2. TROUSSEAU'S SIGN. Spasm of the fingers and hand to form the 'main d'accoucheur' is induced by obstruction of the brachial artery for up to 3 minutes by a sphygmomanometer cuff.

Additional features which may be present in patients with chronic tetany include:

1. ECTODERMAL CHANGES (particularly in idiopathic hypoparathyroidism). The skin is dry and scaly, the tongue atrophic, the hair sparse and brittle and the nails ridged; cataracts may be present.

2. CENTRAL NERVOUS SYSTEM CHANGES. General fatigue, irritability, anxiety, depression, paranoia and epilepsy. Papilloedema is sometimes found.

Causes of tetany

The causes of a reduced serum calcium are:

1. *Hypoparathyroidism*: (*a*) Following thyroid or parathyroid surgery; (*b*) idiopathic, either sex-linked recessive or auto-immune.

2. *Pseudohypoparathyroidism*. This is a rare disorder in which the hypocalcaemia is due to end organ resistance to the actions of parathyroid hormone

(PTH), the concentration of which is raised. The patients have certain phenotypic characteristics (*See Fig. S.55*). They are short, have a round face and short metacarpals and metatarsals. They are usually obese, mildly mentally retarded, may have subcutaneous bone formation, cataracts and basal ganglia calcification.

3. *Vitamin D deficiency*. Skin irradiation is the most important source of vitamin D, blood levels of which rise in the summer and fall in the winter. Elderly people and certain ethnic groups who do not venture outside very much are most at risk for vitamin D deficiency. It is difficult to provide enough vitamin D from even a normal diet. Vitamin D is found in wheatgerm, eggs and fish. Margarine and milk is fortified with vitamin D in some countries. Malabsorption syndrome of all types may cause vitamin D deficiency. Since vitamin D has to be hydroxylated in the liver and kidney in order to create its most potent form, diseases of these organs may lead to hypocalcaemia. The problem of vitamin D deficiency is always exacerbated by prolonged lactation.

4. *Magnesium deficiency*. This leads to reduced secretion of PTH and to peripheral resistance to the actions of PTH. It occurs in: (*a*) Patients on prolonged intravenous therapy who are not receiving magnesium supplements; (*b*) Severe diarrhoea; (*c*) Malabsorption syndrome; (*d*) Small bowel resection or bypass; (*e*) Chronic alcoholism; (*f*) Diuretic phase after recovery from renal tubular necrosis; (*g*) Hyperaldosteronism.

5. *Acute pancreatitis*. Hypocalcaemia may occur early on in acute pancreatitis. The mechanism is not clearly understood, but part of it may be due to the formation of calcium soaps.

6. *Renal failure*. In acute renal failure hypocalcaemia may occur secondary to phosphate retention and the formation of insoluble calcium compounds. In chronic renal failure calcium levels may fall due to a fall in the renal hydroxylation of vitamin D.

7. *Alkalosis*. Alkalosis from any cause, which may be associated with hypokalaemia, can lead to a decrease in the ionized fraction of calcium and cause tetany. The causes of alkalosis are: (*a*) the excessive ingestion of alkali; (*b*) frequent vomiting; (*c*) hyperventilation, especially hysterical; (*d*) hyperaldosteronism, where magnesium deficiency also plays an accessory role.

Ian D. Ramsay

Thinking, disorders of

Disorders of thinking are commonly considered under two separate headings: (1) *Disorders of the content of thinking*—these include adherence to delusional beliefs as found in psychotic individuals and the presence of unwelcome, intrusive obsessional thoughts found in patients with obsessional neurosis. These are discussed in other sections (DELUSIONS, OBSESSIONS). (2) A second category are disorder of the thinking process including abnormalities of the *flow* and the *form* of thoughts. A person's thought processes can only be inferred from their words and actions. We may consider that a person's thoughts are racing when they have pressure of speech or flight of ideas as in *mania*. Here there are logical connections between the ideas expressed but the subject's thinking is so speeded up that it tends to jump from topic to topic often in response to environmental distractions. The speaker is difficult to interrupt, loud, emphatic and may use clang associations when the choice of words is governed by their sound rather than by a logical relationship. Sentences may be linked by rhyming and punning often with amusing consequences. The above description is typical of mania but lesser degrees of increased flow of thinking may be found in acute reactions to stress, major depressive illness with marked features of anxiety, and occasionally in schizophrenia and organic mental disorders. A reduced flow of speech may reflect *poverty of thought* when the subject makes no spontaneous conversation and responds to questions with only brief unelaborated replies in a flat monotonous tone. In its most severe form it may lead to muteness and this occurs frequently in major depressive episodes, schizophrenia and the dementias. However, when assessing a mute patient *hysteria* should always be considered as a possible cause.

Disorders in the *form* of thinking (formal thought disorder) are of enormous importance in the diagnosis of schizophrenia but similar features may also occur in normal subjects who are tense or fatigued and in patients with organic brain diseases. An important symptom in schizophrenia and one which can often be observed in patients with long-standing chronic disability is *loosening* of association of thoughts leading to *incoherence* of speech. These characteristic changes may be accompanied by other so-called *negative symptoms* of schizophrenia including a degree of apathy with diminished drive and volition which may be the principal feature of the disease after the more florid symptoms of delusions and hallucinations have resolved in response to antipsychotic medication. *Loosening* of association describes a thought disorder characterized by speech in which ideas shift from one subject to another completely unrelated topic without the speaker being aware that the topics are disconnected. Unlike flight of ideas the flow of talk may be normal or even reduced. *Derailment* is a description sometimes used for such idiosyncratic moves from one frame of reference to another and if severe, speech becomes *word salad* and totally incoherent. In very

severe schizophrenia thought disorder the speech has some of the characteristics of a fluent aphasia (schizophasia) becoming a series of totally incomprehensible sentences often admixed with *neologisms*. *Thought blocking* is expressed as an interruption in the normal flow of speech, usually in a patient with schizophrenia. The subject, moreover, is aware and will spontaneously describe how their train of thought was suddenly stopped and they had no control over it. The symptom is quite different from mere absentmindedness and sometimes the patient may elaborate the paranoid delusion that an external force is responsible for taking their thoughts away. *Concrete thinking* again is a term frequently applied to schizophrenic patients but is also observed in patients with low IQ, who are brain damaged and in autistic individuals. It describes a difficulty in handling abstract and symbolic language leading, for example, to very literal interpretations of proverbs. When mild this feature has no diagnostic value as it reflects cultural, educational and personality factors. In *perseveration*, found in organic brain disorders and in schizophrenia, the patient continues to hold ideas long after they have ceased to be appropriate so that the same word or idea will crop up in the patient's speech many times in a few sentences. It may be quite marked, for example, 'I think I'll put on my hat, hat, hat, hat', when the term logoclonus or syllable repetition would apply.

Obsessional and anxious people may betray aspects of their thinking by *circumstantiality*. Here speech may be produced in a slow stream but with a great excess of unnecessary detail which can entirely obscure the main answer to the question. Circumstantiality, however, is commonly found in those with no mental illness.

D. Blackwood

Thoracic wall veins

Venous blood from the posterior chest wall muscles, skin and vertebral venous plexuses drains into eleven posterior intercostal veins. On the right side the second, third and often fourth posterior intercostal veins unite to form the right superior intercostal vein which then drains directly into the azygos vein. The lower posterior intercostal veins individually drain into the azygos vein. On the left side the second, third and sometimes fourth posterior intercostal veins unite to form the left superior intercostal vein to open directly into the left innominate vein. The lower left posterior intercostal veins drain individually into the hemiazygos vein to then cross the midline behind the mediastinal structures to the azygos vein and on to the superior vena cava just above the pericardium. The superior vena cava arises from the innominate, jugular and azygos veins.

The thoracic wall veins may become distended in a number of conditions, usually associated with partial or complete obstruction of blood flow in the innominate or vena cava to cause a rise in pressure in the azygos, hemiazygos or jugular venous systems.

Superior vena caval (SVC) syndrome

This may be caused by either partial or complete obstruction of the superior vena cava. The condition was first described by William Hunter in 1757 in a patient whose SVC was obstructed by a syphilitic aortic aneurysm. The signs and symptoms can be subtle and may evolve slowly over a few weeks. Characteristic signs include cyanosis, oedema, venous engorgement of the head, neck and arms, chest and upper abdomen, brawny non-pitting oedema of the neck and dysphonia due to laryngeal oedema. Symptoms, which frequently worsen when the patient lies down or leans forward, include facial congestion and swelling, breathlessness, cough, dysphagia, headache, stupor, seizures and syncope. Malignant disease accounts for most cases, especially from small cell carcinoma involving the right upper lobe and causing paratracheal gland enlargement and mediastinal infiltration. Lymphomas, malignant thymomas, germ cell tumours, and to a lesser extent, metastatic carcinomas may also give rise to SVC obstruction. Benign lesions account for about 5 per cent of cases. Aneurysms of the ascending aorta and innominate artery are now rare.

Large retrosternal goitres or chronic fibrous mediastinitis account for some cases, the latter being secondary to tuberculosis, histoplasmosis, coccidioidomycosis, blastomycosis or filarial mediastinal lymphadenitis.

In a proportion of patients the cause of mediastinal fibrosis remains obscure. Iatrogenic causes of SVC obstruction include thrombosis following the introduction of subclavian lines for venous access or the insertion of temporary pacemaking wires. Superior venal caval obstruction is seldom a medical emergency, but does warrant prompt investigation and treatment. Whenever possible a histological diagnosis should be obtained, either by bronchoscopy, mediastinoscopy or thoracotomy, to facilitate effective treatment for lymphoma, small cell carcinoma, other tumours or non-malignant conditions.

Lesser degrees of localized chest wall venous distention may occur secondary to axillary vein thrombosis. This is not an uncommon condition and may occur after vigorous use of the arm, allowing the vein to be compressed and damaged between the clavicle and first rib. Painful congestion and oedema of the affected arm follow with collateral vein distension on the upper chest. The condition usually settles over 3 months.

Thrombophlebitis of the superficial veins of the breast and anterior chest wall (Mondor's disease) are also encountered. This condition may also affect the arm. The essential characteristic physical sign is an indurated subcutaneous thrombophlebitic cord about 3 mm in diameter. The cause is uncertain and the condition gradually subsides over a few months.

P. R. Studdy

Thrills

(*See also* HEART, MURMURS IN.)

A thrill is a palpable vibration of vascular origin. It indicates vascular turbulence close to the site where it is felt. Thrills can be divided into those of cardiac origin, which can be regarded virtually as palpable heart murmurs, and those which arise in the extracardiac vessels. Cardiac thrills are discussed along with heart murmurs on page 284. Extracardiac thrills are usually accompanied by an audible component, termed a bruit.

Carotid thrills usually arise from turbulence generated at the aortic valve rather than from a local carotid stenosis. This is perhaps because turbulence in the relatively small carotid vessel generates a high frequency sound which is more easily heard than felt. A slow-rising carotid pulse with a thrill is virtually pathognomonic of aortic stenosis, and this is confirmed by hearing an aortic ejection systolic murmur and demonstrating aortic valve disease by ultrasound. It must be remembered that intracardiac and carotid lesions may coexist.

Subclavian thrills may be generated locally or arise from the aortic valve. A difference in timing of the pulse at the two wrists, and unequal blood pressures in the arms should be sought. A subclavian aneurysm may cause a thrill, but these are rare.

Periscapular thrills are a feature of aortic coarctation, and are due to dilatation and increased flow in the periscapular vessels as these form part of an anastomotic circulation round the aortic obstruction. There is often an associated bruit, together with upper segment hypertension and delayed or absent femoral pulses.

Cimino-Brescia arteriovenous fistulae created surgically in the vessels of the forearm (less commonly the leg), to allow easy venous access for haemodialysis in patients with renal failure, are probably the commonest cause of peripheral vascular thrills in modern practice. The presence of a thrill indicates that the anastomosis remains functional. Sometimes these fistulae enlarge excessively, and have adverse haemodynamic effects.

Congenital arteriovenous fistulae are much less common. In children they may cause excessive lengthening of a limb. There is usually conspicuous dilatation of superficial vessels.

Abdominal thrills are uncommon. An arteriovenous malformation in the liver, or a very vascular tumour such as an angiosarcoma, may cause a palpable thrill usually accompanied by a bruit.

Femoral artery thrills are usually the result of iliac atheroma, and are accompanied by a bruit and evidence of peripheral vascular disease elsewhere. Very occasionally they may be due to a femoral arteriovenous fistula, which is a rare complication of cardiac catheterization by the femoral route.

D. De Bono

Throat, sore

Sore throats are common and affect all age groups but are most common in children and young adults. Most sore throats are part of the spectrum of viral upper respiratory infections but they may be caused by bacterial infections in younger patients. Prolonged pain in the throat in middle-aged or elderly adults is cause for concern, especially if they are heavy smokers or drinkers. In this situation one must consider the presence of a neoplasm. The complaint of a sore throat demands a thorough physical examination of the oral cavity, oropharynx, hypopharynx, larynx, thyroid gland and neck. Pain is sometimes referred to the throat from the oesophagus, stomach or heart.

When the diagnosis is not immediately obvious on physical examination, routine cultures for bacteria and viruses, routine haematological studies, lateral X-rays of the neck, barium studies of the pharynx, oesophagus and stomach and CT scanning of the neck may be required. If pain in the throat is initiated or accentuated by exertion, then cardiac assessment is needed. Frequent recurrent infections of the pharynx may be an expression of immunodeficiency as seen in the diGeorge syndrome or AIDS. It is also seen in subclass deficiencies of immunoglobulins.

The causes of sore throats are shown in *Table* T.4.

The present thinking about tonsillitis is that there is a resident Epstein–Barr virus in the tonsil which is activated by physical factors. There then occurs a viral tonsillitis which causes a mild malaise and mild sore throat but its importance lies in the fact that the tonsil no longer secretes immunoglobin A and is, thus, prone to secondary opportunistic bacterial infections. This may cause a bacterial tonsillitis, which presents with an elevation of temperature, pain in the throat, trismus, difficulty in eating and speaking, and is often accom-

Table T.4. Causes of sore throats

Tonsillitis
  Bacterial—streptococcal
  Viral—mononucleosis
Viral Pharyngitis
  Rhinovirus
  Coxsackie
  Epstein–Barr
  Adenovirus
  Herpes, Type I and II
Vincent's angina
Fungal pharyngitis
  Candida
  Phycomycetes
  Blastomyces
Syphilis
AIDS
Aphthous ulcers
Pemphigus
Erythema multiforme
Eagles's syndrome
Glossopharyngeal neuralgia
Carotidynia
Cervical spine pain
Blood dyscrasias
Thyroiditis
Reflux oesophagitis
Lymphoma
Carcinoma
  Tonsil
  Tongue base
  Soft palate
  Supraglottic larynx
Minor salivary gland tumours

panied by cervical lymphadenopathy (*Fig.* T.6). There is usually a good response to antibiotics. Tonsillitis may go on to spread outside the capsule of the tonsil, resulting in a peritonsillar abscess or even into the parapharyngeal space in the neck causing a parapharyngeal abscess.

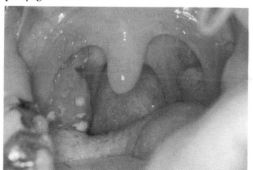

Fig. T.6. Acute tonsillitis on the right side showing the tonsillar crypts filled with pus.

Viral pharyngitis can be caused by the influenza virus, herpes simplex virus, adenovirus, rhinovirus, Coxsackie virus and the Epstein–Barr virus. The patient usually complains of severe pain with comparatively mild clinical findings. There will probably be redness and oedema of the pharynx, especially along the pillars of the tonsil and the posterior pharyngeal wall. Lymphoid aggregates in the pharyngeal mucosa swell, causing a nodular appearance on the posterior pharyngeal wall.

Vincent's angina, or trench mouth, is a contagious disease of the oral cavity and pharynx which is more frequent in young adults and is caused by *Treponema microdentium* and a fusiform bacterium. There is extensive smelly, painful bleeding ulceration covered in grey, nectrotic membrane along the margins of the gum.

Fungal pharyngitis due to candida infection is not uncommon in debilitated adults or in diabetic or immunosuppressed patients. Less common is infection with the phycomycetes and blastomyces fungi and it is usually confined to selected geographic areas.

Aphthous lesions are painful superficial ulcers occurring on the mucosa of the oral cavity. They occur episodically and may be recurrent. They are often associated with regional ileitis and the patient must be investigated for this coexisting condition.

Eagle's syndrome, or stylalgia, is a controversial symptom. It consists of pain in the tonsil or fossa which is usually unilateral and is presumed due to an elongated styloid process. It is difficult to distinguish between this and glossopharyngeal neuralgia.

Acute or subacute thyroiditis can cause pain in the neck or throat. In the acute phase of the disorder, the patient has no difficulty in localizing the problem to the neck. Patients with subacute thyroiditis, however, frequently complain of a persistent soreness in the throat. Discomfort is constant and is aggravated by swallowing and is associated with the sensation of a lump in the throat. Patients are intolerant of constriction of the neck by shirt collars, etc.

Reflux oesophagitis usually causes vague symptoms of soreness in the throat or a sensation of a lump in the throat. The patient may have chronic hoarseness or a constant feeling of wanting to clear his throat. The pain may be aggravated after meals or at night-time when the patient is recumbent.

Lymphoma rarely causes pain in the throat and usually presents as enlargement of one tonsil. Carci-

noma in the area of the base of tongue, tonsil, soft palate, or upper part of the larynx produces a deep pain in the throat which is quite often difficult to diagnose because it remains hidden and is usually of an ulceral infiltrative variety. Most minor salivary gland tumours in this area are malignant, the adenoid cystic variety being the commonest (*Fig.* T.7).

A. G. D. Maran

Thyroid enlargement

(*See also* NECK, SWELLING OF THYROID, PAIN IN.)

An enlarged thyroid gland gives rise to a swelling in the front of the neck, medial and deep to the sternomastoid muscles and medial to the carotid vessels, which, if the swelling is large enough, are displaced laterally and backwards. The gland is connected intimately with the larynx so that it rises and falls with the larynx and trachea during deglutition. This sign alone is generally sufficient to establish the diagnosis of enlarged thyroid gland. The only other lump in the neck which moves on swallowing is a thyroglossal cyst, which characteristically, and in addition, moves upwards when the patient protrudes the tongue. This is because of the attachment of the cyst by a fibrous strand extending to the foramen caecum of the tongue. (*See Fig.* N.31.)

Inspection with the patient at rest and on swallowing may alone be enough to render a diagnosis of thyroid swelling extremely likely. Palpation will confirm this, and is usually best performed while standing behind the patient. The lateral lobes are palpated with the appropriate sternomastoid muscle relaxed, and, if the enlargement is only slight, help may be obtained by displacing the trachea towards the side being examined, when it is possible to introduce the fingers under the relaxed sternomastoid to feel the posterior border of the lobe. The trachea and larynx may of course already be the subject of pathological displacement by pressure of the enlarged gland and this should be determined at the time of palpation. The larynx should also be examined with a mirror for paralysis or asymmetry of the vocal cords. Vocal cord paresis will usually be accompanied by alteration in the voice and, if both cords are affected, possibly with dyspnoea and stridor as well.

The possibility of pressure effects always requires investigating, and these may be enumerated as follows:

(i) Pressure on the trachea causing deviation or compression or both, with varying degrees of dyspnoea and stridor.

(ii) Pressure on the oesophagus causing dysphagia.

(iii) Pressure on nerves, usually the recurrent laryngeal nerves, producing various forms of vocal

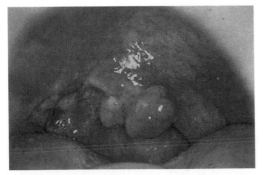

Fig. T.7. Carcinoma of the tongue.

cord palsy with or without alteration in the voice, dyspnoea, stridor and 'brassy' cough. The cervical sympathetic is occasionally involved, as shown by contracted pupil and ptosis (Horner's syndrome). Such nerve palsies are almost invariably associated with invasive tumours of the thyroid gland.

(iv) Pressure on veins giving rise to engorgement and setting up of anastomotic channels, as a result of superior mediastinal obstruction from a large retrosternal extension of the gland.

Acute pressure symptoms may arise, or those already present may become acutely aggravated, by haemorrhage into a cystic space in a goitre.

Retrosternal prolongation of the thyroid should not be forgotten, and may be recognized by dullness on percussion over the manubrium, but this sign is unreliable. When the patient is asked to swallow or cough it is sometimes possible to feel the lower limit of the gland as it rises; at the end of deglutition it slips back behind the sternum ('plunging goitre'). The thyroid in the neck may occasionally appear of normal size in the presence of a retrosternal enlargement, and in a few rare cases the whole gland lies behind the sternum. Pressure symptoms are liable to be great when part or the whole of the gland is in this position, and sometimes the result of pressure on the great veins is seen in the presence of dilated anastomotic skin veins over the upper anterior part of the thorax.

Radiographic examination is a most useful adjunct in the diagnosis of thyroid enlargement, showing both the presence of retrosternal prolongation and tracheal displacement and compression. Other aids may be apparent with individual cases.

Varieties of enlargement and their differential diagnosis

PHYSIOLOGICAL ENLARGEMENT

Occurs at puberty and during menstruation and pregnancy, usually symptomless

INFLAMMATORY ENLARGEMENT

1. Acute

Acute thyroiditis, symptoms include the usual signs of acute inflammation; condition is rare

2. Chronic

Tuberculosis, syphilis, Riedel's disease; all rare; lymphadenoid goitre (Hashimoto's disease)

SIMPLE GOITRE

(Endemic and sporadic.) Parenchymatous goitre, colloid goitre, nodular goitre, solitary (fetal) adenoma

HYPERTHYROID (THYROTOXIC) GOITRE

Primary hyperthyroidism (*Fig.* T.8).
Secondary hyperthyroidism

GOITRE OF THYROID DEFICIENCY

Cretinism
Myxoedema
Drugs, e.g. resorcinol, phenylbutazone

MALIGNANT GOITRE

Carcinoma
Sarcoma (rare)

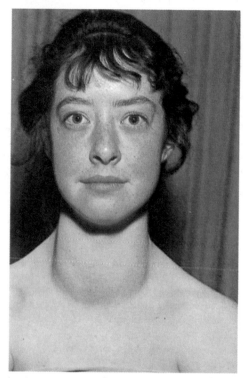

Fig. T.8. Primary hyperthyroidism. Note the even thyroid swelling and exophthalmos. (*Courtesy of the Gordon Museum, Guy's Hospital.*)

These conditions can be regrouped for diagnostic purposes as follows:

THYROID ENLARGEMENT WITH HYPERTHYROIDISM

Primary hyperthyroidism (enlargement general)
Secondary hyperthyroidism
   Localized enlargement—Toxic adenoma (rare)
   Generalized enlargement—Nodular goitre in which one nodule may be so large as to suggest a solitary adenoma, occasionally parenchymatous or even malignant goitre.

THYROID ENLARGEMENT WITH SIGNS OF DEFICIENT SECRETION

Congenital
Cretinism

Acquired

Myxoedema (mild deficiency may be exhibited by colloid or malignant goitre), Hashimoto's disease

THYROID ENLARGEMENT UNCOMPLICATED

Localized enlargement

One large nodule in a small nodular goitre, cyst, adenoma, Riedel's disease (early stages), malignant disease (early stages)

Generalized enlargement

Parenchymatous goitre, colloid goitre, nodular goitre, lymphadenoid goitre, Riedel's disease (late stages), malignant goitre (late stages)

The thyroid gland is in a continual state of fluctuating activity and the structure varies not only at different times but in different parts of the same gland. When enlarged, even more diversity of structure may be present. This may render clinical distinction of the various pathological types of simple goitre impossible. Parenchymatous, colloid and diffuse nodular goitre will therefore be grouped together.

Thyroid enlargement with hyperthyroidism

Primary thyrotoxicosis or hyperthyroidism is characterized by the presence of symptoms of hyperthyroidism from the onset of the disease; in secondary thyrotoxicosis these symptoms develop after a simple goitre has been present for a variable period, often many years. The diagnostic points of each condition are tabulated below (and see Table T.5).

Various eye signs are described in connection with exophthalmos, of which the following are the best known:

von Graefe's sign—Lagging behind of the upper lid as the patient looks downward

Dalrymple's sign—Retracted lids causing a wide palpebral opening

Stellwag's sign—Diminished frequency of blinking

Moebius' sign—Inability to maintain convergence for close vision

Dalrymple's sign is fairly constantly present, but may be found in other conditions, while the other signs are neither constantly present nor confined to exophthalmic goitre. Indeed, lid retraction alone may be found without true exophthalmos.

Cretinism

Usually the thyroid is atrophic in this condition, but a goitre is occasionally present, especially in a long-standing case. An untreated patient is easily recognizable, but one seldom seen nowadays. Slow development, either physical or mental, should rouse a suspicion of thyroid deficiency, remembering other possible causes of backward development such as rickets, renal rickets, achondroplasia, etc. The diagnosis of cretinism will not be detailed more as it is barely relevant.

Myxoedema

As in cretinsm, the thyroid is only occasionally enlarged, and here again a detailed account will not be given. The characteristic symptoms of hypothyroidism include slowed mentality, coarse features, dry skin, brittle nails and sparse coarse hair, and a gain in weight, often gross. (See THYROID, FUNCTION TESTS.)

Certain drugs, e.g. resorcinol as an external application and phenylbutazone by mouth, may occasionally be associated with thyroid enlargement with signs of hypothyroidism reversible on stopping drug administration. Occasionally a moderately enlarged gland may increase in size during treatment with an antithyroid agent, e.g. neomercazole.

Table T.5. Diagnostic points of hyperthyroidism

	Primary hyperthyroidism	Secondary hyperthyroidism
Age of onset	Young	Middle aged
Onset	Acute	Insidious
Thyroid swelling	Not present before onset. Generalized soft elastic and vascular swelling, enlargement not gross. May harden if iodine has been given	Present before onset. Enlargement may be considerable; frequently nodular
Exophthalmos	Generally present, often gross	Rare, and if present slight
Heart	Tachycardia, but fibrillation and heart failure not common except in late or severe cases	Tachycardia. Cardiovascular failure most prominent symptom. Atrial fibrillation fairly common
Tremor and general excitability	Marked	Slight
Loss of weight	Marked	Present, not so marked
Increased perspiration	Marked	Present, not so marked
Results of iodine medication	Often striking improvement	Improvement, but of a lesser degree
Thyroid function tests	Raised	Raised
Radio-iodine uptake	Raised	Raised

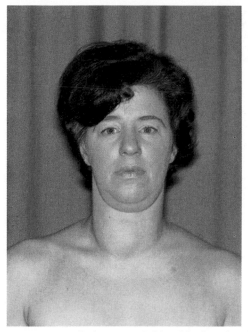
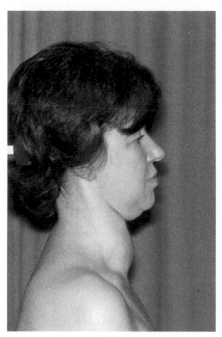

Fig. T.9. Large colloid mass in right lobe of the thyroid producing an asymmetrical enlargement of the gland.

Lymphadenoid goitre (Hashimoto's disease)

In this disorder the thyroid gland becomes infiltrated with lymphoid tissue as a result of an auto-immune reaction. It is a disease occurring in women in middle life and usually produces a uniform, firm enlargement of the thyroid with evidence of hypothyroidism. The gland is often H-shaped. Laboratory tests for thyroid function show low levels. There is an increased serum cholesterol, a raised erythrocyte sedimentation rate, and auto-immune antibodies are present in the blood. Occasionally, lymphadenomatous goitre will occur with normal thyroid function and, very exceptionally, with hyperthyroidism. In the past, diagnosis has often been made after operation as a result of histological section of the tissue removed, but with careful investigation this should not be necessary in a typical case.

Carcinoma of the thyroid may cause confusion, but this condition is practically never associated with hypothyroidism in an untreated case.

Riedel's disease

This is an interesting and rare condition where an intense sclerosing fibrosis starts in one area of the gland and spreads first to the whole gland and then to surrounding structures. The progress is slow as a rule, but gradually the trachea, the oesophagus, and the great vessels all suffer from constriction while the recurrent laryngeal nerves are affected early. The diagnosis from malignant disease is very difficult, but the condition should be suspected when an intensively hard goitre with pressure symptoms out of all proportion to its size is found in a young adult. Diagnosis is confirmed by histological examination of biopsy material.

Uncomplicated thyroid enlargement

A true *adenoma* is an uncommon condition, but a particularly large nodule in an otherwise small nodular goitre forming an asymmetrical swelling in the thyroid tissue is common (*Fig.* T.9). It may be cystic or solid but palpation is not always reliable in determining this. *Nodular goitre* may give rise to a uniform enlargement, as also may *colloid goitre*. This last condition may present a smooth surface, as it is usually the case in *parenchymatous* enlargement. A *simple cyst* is quite common and may suddenly enlarge from haemorrhage into it.

Malignant disease starts in one area and spreads to involve the whole gland, finally breaking through the capsule to invade surrounding structures. Movement on deglutition may be lost, the recurrent laryngeal nerve is involved early, and the growth tends to surround the carotid bundle rather than push it back, as is the case with large simple goitres, so that pulsation of these vessels may be impalpable in the middle of the neck. The sympathetic chain is often involved late in the disease, with a resultant Horner's syndrome. The swelling is usually hard, as in Riedel's disease, but tends to be much greater in size and more rapid in growth. Pressure symptoms are early and pain is often a marked feature, particularly on swallowing. Bone and lung metastases are not uncommon. One type of thyroid carcinoma, namely the papillary carcinoma, deserves special mention. This typically occurs in the 4th and 5th decades and metastasizes to the lymph nodes. The secondary deposits may be much larger than the primary which cannot be detected, so that these cases often present with soft lumps in the side of the neck which used to be called, erroneously, 'lateral aberrant thyroids'. Thyroid tissue so situated is always a secondary deposit from a small primary in the thyroid which has completely replaced the lymphoid tissue in which it germinated.

Harold Ellis

Thyroid, pain in

A painful thyroid swelling is not a common clinical situation. The following conditions may give rise to this symptom:

1   Inflammatory:
     Acute (suppurative) thyroiditis
     Subacute thyroiditis (De Quervain's disease)
     Inflammation of a thyroglossal cyst or fistula
2   Haemorrhage into a cyst of the thyroid
3   Hashimoto's disease (rarely)
4   Carcinoma of the thyroid in its late stages

Acute (suppurative) thyroiditis

This is a rare condition which is nearly always bacterial in origin. Fungal and parasitic causes can be regarded as medical oddities. The usual organisms producing this condition are *Staphylococcus aureus, haemolytic Streptococcus, Pneumococcus*, and occasionally *Salmonella* and *E. coli*. In two-thirds of cases, there is pre-existing thyroid disease. The sexes are equally affected.

The source of the bacterial invasion is either extension from an adjacent infection or bacteraemia secondary to a distant focus. Commencing as an acute inflammation, the condition usually progresses to suppuration.

The clinical features are a sudden onset with severe pain in the neck which may be referred to the ear, the lower jaw or the occiput and which is aggravated by swallowing and movement of the neck. There is associated malaise and fever.

Examination reveals a febrile patient (the temperature in the range 38–40°C), and tachycardia. Swelling, tenderness and redness in the region of the thyroid generally appears later; more characteristically, only one lobe of the thyroid is involved. Regional lymphadenopathy is variable. The neck is held flexed and neck movement is painful. Fluctuation is not usually elicited because of induration of the surrounding tissues. There

is leucocytosis and, untreated, the mass progresses to the formation of an obvious abscess.

Subacute (non-suppurative) thyroiditis (De Quervain's thyroiditis)

This is probably viral in origin. Any age may be affected, ranging from 3–76 years, although the fifth decade is commonest. Females are far more often affected than males. Usually the condition involves a previously normal gland.

The illness is preceded frequently by an upper respiratory infection and the thyroid symptoms are often anteceded by muscular aches and malaise with fever (in the region of 39°C) and weight loss. Pain then develops in the thyroid gland and the pain may radiate to the ears. It is aggravated by movement of the neck and by swallowing. Usually both lobes are enlarged, although in one-third of cases one lobe is involved first and the inflammation then spreads to the opposite side. Examination of the neck reveals a tender, firm or hard enlargement of the thyroid gland.

Quite often there are accompanying symptoms and signs of hyperthyroidism.

Laboratory tests reveal a raised white count and ESR. Usually the T_4 is raised and this elevation lasts for 1 to 3 months.

The condition runs a variable course of weeks or months and even if untreated usually subsides without sequelae. Rarely it is followed by clinical hypothyroidism. As its name implies, it does not proceed to frank suppuration.

Inflammation of a thyroglossal cyst or fistula

The typical thyroglossal cyst lies in the midline of the neck, usually at the cricothyroid space, less commonly at a higher or lower level, although it may deviate somewhat to one or other side of the midline. It usually presents in children or young adults and characteristically moves upwards on protrusion of the tongue as well as on swallowing (*see* NECK, SWELLING OF). Infection of the cyst is not uncommon and then presents as an obvious inflammatory mass above the anatomical region of the thyroid gland. A thyroglossal fistula is occasionally congenital but may follow infection or inadequate removal of a thyroglossal cyst. The fistula discharges mucus and is frequently the site of recurrent attacks of inflammation.

Thyroid cyst

Haemorrhage into a pre-existing thyroid cyst produces a sudden, painful enlargement of a lump in the thyroid gland which may or may not have already been noted by the patient. Its danger is that it may also produce

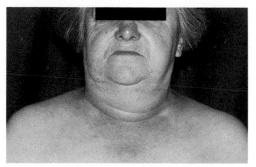

Fig. T.10. An advanced carcinoma of the thyroid in an elderly lady. The sternomastoid muscle and regional nodes are involved. The gland is painful and tender.

sudden and dangerous compression of the trachea with respiratory obstruction. The symptoms may require urgent surgical treatment but, if less severe than this, the swelling gradually subsides over the succeeding few days.

The cystic nature of the swelling can be confirmed by ultrasound examination of the mass.

Hashimoto's disease

This condition (*see* p. 665) is usually painless, but from time to time the thyroid enlargement may be painful and tender.

Carcinoma of the thyroid

Poorly differentiated (anaplastic) carcinomas of the thyroid usually occur in elderly patients. In their advanced stages, they produce a tender and painful infiltrating mass in the neck, usually with local lymphadenopathy (*Fig.* T.10). Clinical diagnosis is not usually in doubt but can be confirmed by needle biopsy.

Harold Ellis

Tic

(*See also* TETANY; VERTIGO)

Tics or habit spasms are the terms which cover a variety of twitching or jerking movements which occur irregularly and which tend particularly to involve the muscles around the eyes, the face and the shoulders. These are voluntary movements and usually patients obtain relief from tension by the repetitive performance of these movements. In many instances, the affliction is clearly related to anxiety. Often with the passage of time the movements become so habitual as to be almost involuntary.

In most instances the movement is the same and repeated in an identical fashion. Multiple tics may occur in the syndrome of Gilles de la Tourette. In this syndrome the multiple tics may be accompanied by involuntary utterances and grunts. Although tics in isolation are thought to be functional in nature, there

is some evidence to suggest that this particular syndrome has an organic neural basis. Multiple tics need to be differentiated from involuntary movement disorders such as chorea.

D. A. Shaw

Tinnitus

Tinnitus is a term which denotes a ringing or whistling sound in the ears but is customarily applied to other sounds described by patients such as hissing, throbbing, buzzing or roaring. It has been known since the time of Hippocrates and is one of the most irritating auditory sensations. Some patients can cope with it but, in many others, it represents a severe strain and in some may even cause severe psychological disorders and suicide. It seems to be a symptom that is on the increase and, in the 1980s and 1990s, tinnitus has been in the position of fever a century ago. It is something which can now be reasonably quantified and there are a plethora of treatments advocated. As with fever, however, it is essential not to consider the entity in itself but rather the underlying cause. Most subjective tinnitus is considered to arise in the cochlea—one of the most inaccessible parts of the human body. Determination of the underlying cause, therefore, is inevitably by indirect methods and by extrapolation. It has been shown that the sensitive hair cells, which change sound waves into electrical impulses in the cochlea, are in constant mechanical vibration. The reason for this is probably because a completely passive system would not be sensitive enough to pick up the very quietest sound the normal ear can hear. Experiments with normal hearing adults show that everyone can hear this background hair cell vibration if they are in quiet enough surroundings (e.g. an anechoic chamber). One might refer to this as the 'sound of silence' or 'physiological tinnitus'. The normal vibration of hairs on these hair cells in the inner ear can be measured using a sensitive microphone placed in the outer ear canal. In some cases of low-frequency tinnitus, extra loud hair cell vibrations, or cochlear emissions as they are called, can be detected by this method. On many occasions, however, the tinnitus experienced by the patient is quite different to the cochlear emissions which can be recorded so this is not the whole answer. In addition, these cochlear emissions cannot at present be recorded from those with a hearing loss greater than 40 dB, so a different explanation has to be found for those with deafness and tinnitus.

One explanation could be that the hearing centres in the brain control, to some extent, the function of the internal ear. Cochlear efferents act as a gain control, constantly adjusting the function of the inner ear. In a noisy environment the gain control would be turned down, resulting in less spontaneous vibration, and this might explain why tinnitus is often less noticeable in the presence of environmental noise.

Another theory is that certain forms of tinnitus are related to abnormal phase locking of discharges in groups of auditory nerve fibres. The normal nerve, in situations of total quietness, transmits random messages which are interrupted as the absence of external noise. The ear responds to sound by synchronizing with firing of adjacent fibres in the auditory nerve and this, together with the change of pattern of firing, is interpreted by the brain as a sound from the outside.

The character of the sound may give some clue to the cause. Thus a pulsatile or rhythmical sound may be produced by the flow of blood through an atheromatous internal carotid artery, which in its course through the carotid canal is separated from the tympanum only by a thin plate of bone. Internal carotid thrombosis should be suspected if the pulse in one carotid artery is absent or greatly diminished. The noise in the ear may be heard on the opposite side on account of compensatory dilatation. Other symptoms of this condition may be intermittent headache, often over one eye, transitory hemiparesis, transitory loss of vision in one eye, temporary aphasia and fits. Digital compression of the carotid on the sound side may precipitate such phenomena, which also include hemiparaesthesia. A carotid arteriogram (*Figs T.11, T.12*) is diagnostic. Tinnitus is common in cases of arteriosclerosis, and conditions associated with high blood pressure: it may also occur when there is severe anaemia; the noises heard may be variously described by patients as humming, hissing, rhythmic thumping, roaring, whistling or musical. A crackling noise may be produced by cerumen, or a foreign body, in the external auditory canal. A bubbling noise may be due to catarrhal exudation in the middle ear. A crackling or clicking sound may be caused by spasmodic contraction of the dilator tubae and salpingopharyngeus muscles which are attached to the Eustachian tube. A clicking sound may be caused by intermittent contraction of the tensor tympani. In rare cases the tinnitus may be associated with a carotid artery murmur, which is detected on examination of the neck with the stethoscope.

Though tinnitus is very common in diseases of the ear, yet serious lesions of the middle ear, internal ear or auditory nerve may be present without this symptom. There is no constant relation between tinnitus and deafness. The former may be present with good hearing, but when long continued the hearing tends to become impaired. The sounds may persist when a patient has become totally deaf.

Tinnitus may occur from the following diseases of the ear:

1. The presence of *cerumen, aural polyps* or *a foreign body* in the external auditory meatus coming in contact with the drum. Removal of the offending body leads to the cessation of the tinnitus.

2. In any *inflammatory disease, acute or chronic, suppurative or non-suppurative, of the middle ear*. In catarrhal inflammation of the middle ear, the noise frequently has the character of bursting bubbles, and is due to movements of the viscid exudation in the ear itself. Low-frequency vibratory clicks, pops and roaring noises arise almost always from the middle ear and Eustachian tube. Chronic sinusitis may be the underlying cause. In *otosclerosis*, tinnitus is a very prominent and usually early symptom. It may occur before any alteration in hearing is present.

3. In diseases of the *internal ear* tinnitus may be severe and intractable; especially in *Ménière's disease, syphilitic disease* of the internal ear, and in those lesions of the internal ear which may arise in the course of *typhoid* and other *specific fevers. Extension of suppuration to the labyrinth* from the middle ear is also an important cause; and tinnitus, usually associated with deafness, may persist after *fracture of the base of the skull*.

Perhaps the commonest cause of an inner ear tinnitus is from the cochlear damage caused by exposure to excessive noise.

Paget's disease of the skull may be associated with tinnitus, often intermittent, and sound may be conducted to the ear from a congenital intracranial aneurysm, an arterial angioma or a carotico-cavernous fistula.

Persistent unilateral tinnitus with progressive internal-ear deafness and vertigo raises suspicion of *acoustic nerve tumour*. Unilateral tinnitus with a ringing or bell-like quality and reduced hearing suggests cochlear involvement. High-pitched tonal non-vibratory tinnitus strongly suggests disease of the cochlea and 8th nerve.

'Noises in the ears' are complained of in many general diseases with or without a lesion of the ear; thus, they are frequent in *anaemia, leukaemia*; some *cardiac lesions*, especially aortic regurgitation, may be found in the pulsatile variety of tinnitus. *Chronic nephritis, uraemia* and *arteriosclerosis* with high blood pressure may also be responsible for tinnitus, and it may occur during attacks of *neuralgia* or of *migraine*. Quinine, salicylates and streptomycin may cause tinnitus.

Tinnitus masking remains by far the best treatment for those patients who have any useful hearing. The masking noise is usually quite different to the

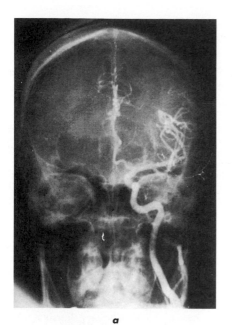

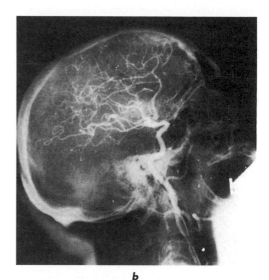

Fig. T.11. Normal left-sided cerebral arteriogram. a, Anterior view. b, Lateral view. (Dr R. D. Hoare.)

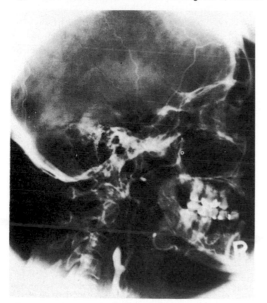

Fig. T.12. Arteriogram showing occlusion of internal carotid artery. (Dr R. D. Hoare.)

tinnitus and may well be at a much lower intensity. Since it is an external noise it is often easy to adapt to, rather like the noise of passing traffic in the street. The sort of noise used in maskers has also been used for producing sleep, relaxation and even anaesthesia under different circumstances. So, far from being irritating, many tinnitus sufferers find this noise soothing as well as effective in masking their tinnitus. In about half of those who are effectively masked, there will be the phenomenon of residual inhibition. This means

that the tinnitus is turned 'off' or turned 'down' for a period of time after the masker is removed.

There are no medical drugs that will make tinnitus disappear. Those who are getting psychological problems from their tinnitus are best treated with antidepressants.

A. G. D. Maran

Tongue, discoloration of

The mucous membrane of the tongue is covered mainly by filiform papillae which cover the major portion of the tongue and vary in length from 1–3 mm. Fungiform papillae are found at the apex and along the lateral aspect of the tongue. They are barely visible but on occasions even in the normal patient may be red, large, smooth and round.

Discoloration of the tongue has much less of a diagnostic role in gastrointestinal disease than in the past. Changes that are thought to take place with constipation, appendicitis and other gastrointestinal diseases are insignificant and unreliable. On the other hand, there are more important changes which are associated with infectious diseases, deficiency states and metabolic disorders.

The tongue surface may be dry, brown and slightly furred in patients who are *mouth breathers* or who are *dehydrated*. A brown, dry tongue is common in *tobacco smokers*. Furring of the tongue is due to heaping up of the squamous epithelium on the filiform papillae probably from inadequate cleansing of the tongue which ordinarily occurs during chewing. The term 'geographic tongue' is used when an area of filiform papillae is lost from the dorsum of the tongue. Smooth, pink mucosa is seen which contrasts sharply against that mucosa which is covered with normal papillae. A feature of the condition is that the appearance of the tongue will change from day to day, creating a 'wandering rash' across the surface of the tongue. This condition can be regarded as a variant of normal.

Very marked overgrowth of the filiform papillae produces a black, hairy tongue. This rare condition is encountered in patients on antibiotic therapy and some smokers. Hypertrophy of the fungiform papillae in *scarlet fever* produces the classic 'strawberry' or 'raspberry' tongue.

Leucoplakia describes white patches on the surface or lateral aspect of the tongue. These, on histology, show hyperkeratosis, acanthosis and dyskeratosis. The white areas may be seen as a patch or a raised plaque and are usually painless. Leucoplakia is regarded as a precancerous lesion as is the asymptomatic red, velvety lesion which may sometimes be seen on the ventrolateral aspect of the tongue. 'Hairy' leucoplakia is unique to *HIV infection* and is found particularly along the side of the tongue although it may occur anywhere in the mouth. The lesions are slightly raised, poorly demarcated, and show a corrigated white 'hairy' surface which does not rub off and which are asymptomatic. Histology is distinctive showing keratin projections, parakeratosis, acanthosis, and a characteristic ballooning change in the pickle-cell layer. The significance of this lesion is that it is a strong predictor of AIDS for 80 per cent of patients will develop the full syndrome within 1 year.

Mucosal infection with the yeast *Candida albicans* produces the clinical picture of *moniliasis*, or candidosis or thrush. Creamy white curd-like patches occur on the tongue and other areas of the buccal mucosa. When scraped they reveal a raw bleeding area. The lesion can be quite painful and is found particularly in sick infants, debilitated patients, or those receiving broad spectrum antibiotics or high doses of corticosteroids. Candidiasis is a common manifestation of *immunodeficiency* and over 50 per cent of HIV antibody positive patients with this infection will develop the AIDS syndrome within 2 years. In infants thrush is distinguished from milk curds by the difficulty with which the former are removed leaving an underlying patch of inflamed mucosa.

The tongue will appear blue in patients who are centrally *cyanosed* and pale in *anaemic* patients. Many anaemic patients however have a red, painful, bald tongue. This is the consequence of complete atrophy of the papillae which may occur in *pernicious anaemia*, severe *iron-deficiency anaemia*, and/or *deficiency states involving other B vitamins*. The red, painful tongue may be associated with other evidence of mucosal atrophy in the mouth and fissuring at the corner of the lips known as angular stomatitis. The mucosal lesions of folic acid deficiency are often more marked than those encountered in vitamin B_{12} deficiencies. Other terms which have been used to describe the colour changes taking place in vitamin B deficiencies are the 'beefy red' tongue of *pellagra* and the 'magenta' tongue of *riboflavin deficiency*. The *Plummer-Vinson* (or *Patterson-Kelly*) syndrome describes the iron-deficiency state in which the tongue is painful, reddened and smooth. There is cheilitis, postcricoid webs and koilonychia.

Pigmentation of the tongue may be found in *Addison's disease* and *acanthosis nigricans* in which the tongue undergoes hypertrophy of the filiform papillae to produce a shaggy, papillomatous dorsum. *Acrodermatitis enteropathica* is a rare autosomal recessive disorder related to zinc deficiency. Intraoral features include a white coating to the tongue and buccal mucosa with marked halitosis. There is chronic diarrhoea, hair loss, severe dermatitis and failure to thrive. The condition may also occur in patients on maintained hyperalimentation who become deficient in zinc.

In *hereditary haemorrhagic telangiectasia* (Osler–Weber–Rendu syndrome) telangiectasia occur throughout the gastrointestinal tract. The most commonly occur in areas of the oral cavity including lips, gingiva, buccal mucosa and tongue. The lesions are dilated capillary vessels and small arterioles. The pigmentary changes involving *Peutz-Jeghers syndrome* and *pseudoxanthoma elasticum* do not normally involve the tongue. Granulomatous involvement of the tongue and buccal mucosa in *Crohn's disease* produces raised, smooth, red nodules and hyperplastic ridges on the tongue. These may appear erythematous. A number of dermatological diseases may affect the mouth including *erythema multiforme, lichen planus, pemphigus* and *pemphigoid*, but involvement of the tongue in these conditions is rare.

Ian A. D. Bouchier

Tongue, pain in

Pain in the tongue may be attributable to some obvious lesion, usually with breach of surface such as an epithelioma. Such conditions are discussed under the heading of TONGUE, ULCERATION OF. On the other hand, pain in the tongue or soreness of the tongue may be an insistent complaint when there is no superficial evidence of abnormality. The conditions that have to be considered include the following:

1   *When the pain complained of is not on the dorsum,
    tip or sides of the tongue but underneath or deeper:*
    Injury to the frenulum linguae
    Ranula
    Calculus in the duct of a submandibular salivary
      gland
    Foreign body in the tongue
    Myositis
    Trichinosis
2   *When the pain complained of appears to be upon the
    surface of the tongue, even if it also affects the tongue
    as a whole:*
    Bitten tongue
    After an anaesthetic (mouth-gag)
    Injury by tooth or dental plate
    Antibiotic glossitis, associated with lichen planus,
      Behçet's disease or pemphigus vulgaris
    Congenital fissured tongue
    Geographical tongue
    Median rhomboid glossitis
    Moeller's glossitis
    Glossitis of deficiency disease
    Smoking
    The effects of over-hot beverages or foodstuffs
    The effects of pungent condiments such as
      cayenne pepper
    Minor viral diseases
    Carcinoma

The differential diagnosis depends upon the following considerations:

1. Pain underneath the tongue or deeper

Injury to the frenulum linguae may cause visible abrasion or a definite ulcer. The most injured spot is tender as well as painful, the diagnosis depending on careful attention to the appearance and to the site of greatest tenderness. The cause may be injury by a fish-bone or other sharp or puncturing object. In violent coughing bouts as in whooping cough the protruded tongue may be forced against the lower incisor teeth with such violence that the frenulum becomes abraded, inflamed or ulcerated.

Ranula is not painful unless it becomes inflamed. It is an asymmetrical red smooth cystic swelling in the floor of the mouth under the tongue on one or other side of the fraenum. It may result from obstruction of the duct of one of the sublingual salivary glands but more often it is a retention cyst arising in one of the many mucous glands in the floor of the mouth.

Calculus in the duct of a submandibular salivary gland is not necessarily painful. It may produce discomfort or more or less severe pain recurrent or constant according to the degree of inflammation. The stone may be very small and difficult to detect either with a probe or by X-rays, but its existence may be suspected by the situation of the discomfort, or by the corresponding salivary gland swelling when the patient begins to eat, the stone interfering with the free passage of the increased flow of saliva. The calculus can frequently be palpated bimanually in the floor of the mouth and is occasionally seen to protrude through the duct orifice. An X-ray will confirm the diagnosis.

Foreign body in the tongue is uncommon, though a fish-bone may become impacted in it. More often the foreign body injures the tongue, itself escaping but leaving pain behind. The diagnosis depends on the accuracy of the story obtained or the discovery of the foreign body by palpation or by radiography.

Myositis of the tongue is seldom if ever a localized condition; it may, however, be a prominent feature in *polymyositis* or in *trichinosis*, in which the embryo trichinellae have a special predilection for the muscles at the base of the tongue which become stiff, painful and tender. The diagnosis of trichinosis is difficult especially as it will hardly be thought of unless there is an epidemic at the time. The blood exhibits eosinophilia, but the only way of clinching the diagnosis is by demonstrating the trichinellae embryos microscopically in portions of the muscles excised.

2. Pain upon the surface of the tongue

Bitten tongue will usually present an obvious lesion but pain may persist after a tongue-bite even when no obvious bruising or breach of surface can be detected. The patient may be unaware of having accidentally inflicted the bite, if the accident occurred during sleep or during an epileptic seizure. Indeed, the occurrence of a local painful area in the tongue suggesting the effect of tongue-bite may be the first indication that the patient is an epileptic. In tetanus, traumatic glossitis is common and may cause airways obstruction.

After general anaesthetics, patients often complain of soreness of the tongue resulting from the use of tongue forceps or of a mouth-gag.

Injury by a tooth or *dental plate* may cause a local painful place upon one side of the tongue, often fairly far back, the pain being increased by movements of the tongue in speaking, eating or swallowing. Fear of cancer is usual until the cause is found in the jagged edge of the adjacent tooth, or of the dental plate at the corresponding site. The condition needs to be watched carefully to be certain that the lesion disappears after the offending irritant is smoothed down or removed, and to allay any anxiety that the jagged tooth or plate may have initiated an epithelioma. Tuberculosis of the tongue, presenting as a painful deep persistent ulcer, is now rarely seen.

Antibiotic glossitis. A common cause of diffuse soreness of the tongue is the taking of antibiotics by mouth. The pain is sometimes due to infection with *Monilia albicans* which can be grown from the surface. Its preponderance is favoured by the wide-spectrum antibiotics. In other cases of antibiotic glossitis no such cause can be found and the change is attributed to vitamin deficiencies arising from suppression of normal gut flora. The tongue is clean, red and very sensitive to heat (*Fig.* T.13). Glossitis occurs in deficiency of vitamin B$_{12}$, and folic acid, in pellagra, malabsorption syndrome and the Plummer–Vinson syndrome but seldom causes acute pain in these conditions.

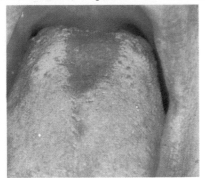

Fig. T.13. Glossitis due to oral antibiotic. (*Professor Martin Rushton.*)

Lichen planus affecting the tongue may be confused with monilia glossitis because both produce small whitish patches on the surface. The lichen tends to produce lines or a mesh of pearly dots and to favour the cheeks near the occlusal line of the molars.

The tongue may also become inflamed and painful in Behçet's disease, erythema multiforme or pemphigus vulgaris.

Congenital fissured tongue (*Fig.* T.14) or 'scrotal tongue' is thick, deeply fissured and usually symptomless. If food particles lodge in the fissures infection may arise and thus cause pain.

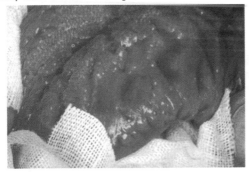

Fig. T.14. Congenital fissuring of the tongue. (*Professor Martin Rushton.*)

Geographical tongue (*Fig.* T.15) shows red denuded patches of irregular outline which often change their position. It causes anxiety rather than pain.

Median rhomboid glossitis (*Fig.* T.16) is a rare congenital abnormality due to persistence of the tuberculum impar between the two halves of the tongue.

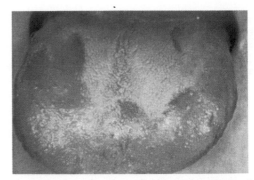

Fig. T.15. Geographical tongue. (*Professor Martin Rushton.*)

It occupies the middle third of the dorsum and is smooth, shiny and red. It carries no filiform papillae. Opalescent nodules may be scattered over the surface. The area may become inflamed and thus cause soreness and often unfounded fear of cancer.

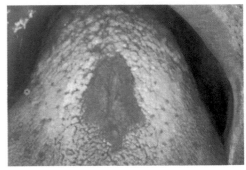

Fig. T.16. Median rhomboid glossitis. (*Professor Martin Rushton.*)

Moeller's glossitis (*Fig.* T.17), often confused with Hunter's glossitis of pernicious anaemia (q.v.), presents atrophic sharply defined red patches on the dorsum and sides: the atrophy in pernicious anaemia is evenly spread and the mucosa pale and dry. Spiced food causes pain. The condition may be met in allergic states, nutritional deficiencies and with certain drug eruptions (e.g. reserpine).

Glossitis of deficiency disease occurs with avitam-

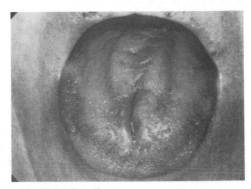

Fig. T.17. Moeller's glossitis.

inosis, particularly of the B group, as in pellagra, but also with iron deficiency and pernicious anaemia.

Smoking and the effects of tea or other *hot liquid* or *food* may cause acute pain in the tongue lasting for days after the cause has ceased to act. *Pungent condiments* such as capsicum, cayenne pepper, ginger and the like may similarly be responsible.

Minor viral diseases. Foot-and-mouth disease may rarely be contracted by humans from infected farm animals or consumed milk or milk products from infected herds, vesicles appearing in the mouth and on the tongue. In the so-called 'hand-foot-and-mouth disease', probably due to Coxsackie A viruses, children are affected. Vesicular stomatitis contracted from horses, cattle and pigs occurs in North and South America.

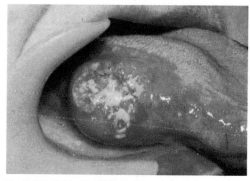

Fig. T.18. Carcinoma of the tongue.

Carcinoma of the tongue (*Fig.* T.18) starts as a nodule, fissure, or ulcer, usually on the lateral border of the organ. At first painless, it becomes painful as it invades and becomes grossly septic. The pain often radiates to the ear, being referred from the lingual branch of the trigeminal nerve supplying the tongue along its auriculotemporal branch. Ulceration is accompanied by bleeding; hence the typical picture of late disease is an old man spitting blood into his handkerchief with a plug of cotton-wool in his ear.

Harold Ellis

Tongue, swelling of

Swelling of the tongue is a condition the nature of which is generally obvious on inspection and palpation, if the history is taken into account at the same time. Many causes given in the following list need little detailed discussion:

1. Causes of acute swelling of the tongue

A bite or sting

Injury, for instance by a fish-bone, or by biting during an epileptic fit

Corrosives or acute irritant applications

Acute oedema, secondary to:

a. Inflammatory conditions within the mouth–stomatitis (p. 677)
b. The effects of certain drugs, e.g. mercury, rarely aspirin
c. Erythema bullosum or pemphigus (p. 425)
d. Variola
e. Serum injections and other conditions liable to cause giant urticaria
f. Angioneurotic oedema (angio-oedema)

Haemorrhage into the substance of the tongue, as in scurvy, leukaemia and other haemorrhagic states.

2. Causes of chronic or persistent swelling of the tongue

Where the swelling is general

Macroglossia
Cretinism
Myxoedema
Mongolism
Acromegaly
Primary amyloidosis

Where the swelling is local or asymmetrical

Irritation of a dental plate or decayed tooth
Epithelioma
Gumma
Leucoplakia (chronic superficial glossitis)
Tuberculous infiltration
Actinomycosis
Ranula
Calculus in a sublingual salivary gland
Suprahyoid cyst
Haemangioma or lymphangioma
Sarcoma
Lipoma

If the nature of the tongue enlargement is not obvious from the history and simple inspection and palpation—as will probably be the case when it is due to a *bite, sting, injury, corrosive* or *irritant* application, after the use of *serum, mercury, aspirin* or other drugs, *variola, pemphigus* or *erythema multiforme*—it may be so from the concomitant symptoms, as in the case of *cretinism, acromegaly, mongolism* or *myxoedema*.

Simple *macroglossia* is rare; when it does occur the history is that it dates from youth or childhood and the patient may otherwise be perfectly normal, unless he also has some other congenital peculiarity, such as macrocheilia (blubber-lips).

The chronic local lesions associated with swelling are in many cases accompanied by superficial ulceration, and the difficulties, that may arise in distinguishing *simple, syphilitic* and *epitheliomatous* ulcers are discussed under TONGUE, ULCERATION OF. *Tuberculous* and *actinomycotic glossitis* are both rare, and may be mistaken for malignant or syphilitic disease. Tuberculous lesions are usually painful and this cause should always be thought of when considering the possible causes of a painful swollen tongue, particularly as the manifestations of tuberculosis of the tongue may assume unusual and bizarre forms. *Ranula* and *sublingual salivary gland calculus* or *cyst* both cause swellings that are beneath the front part of the tongue rather than in its substance, generally bulging up one side of the floor of the mouth near the frenulum linguae. A ranula is a distended mucous gland, and after enlarging slowing to perhaps the size of a chestnut, it often ceases to grow further; it does not fluctuate in its dimensions in relationship to meals as a salivary gland swelling often does.

A *suprahyoid cyst* is situated in the root of the tongue posteriorly, where it arises from remains of the embryological thyroglossal duct. It is seldom large; its nature is suggested by its situation.

An *angioma* of the tongue is rare (*Fig.* T.19): sometimes, however, after remaining latent for years, it grows with rapidity and necessitates an operation. The diagnosis may be suggested by the colour of the tumour, but histological examination subsequent to removal may be required before one can be sure whether the tumour is a simple angioma, an angiosarcoma or a *sarcoma*.

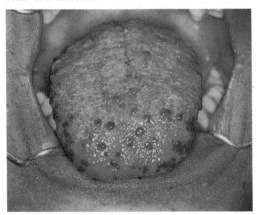

Fig. T.19. Angioma of the tongue.

A *lipoma* occurs not infrequently in the tongue and its lobulated form generally breaks surface and presents like a cluster of soft white cherries.

Haemorrhage into the substance of the tongue, with swelling and inability to speak or eat, may result from certain blood disorders, such as acute leukaemia or primary or secondary thrombocytopenic purpura (*see* PURPURA).

Acute oedema of the tongue may be due to *severe stomatitis, angioneurotic oedema of the tongue* and *Ludwig's angina.* This is an acute inflammatory condition, often streptococcal in origin, affecting the floor of the mouth and tongue, and spreading rapidly through the deeper structures of the mouth, throat and neck, causing extreme swelling of the adjacent tissues.

Angioneurotic oedema of the tongue is rare, but it is important because it may, rarely, prove fatal. As a rule there is a history of previous similar attacks in other parts of the body and other members of the family may have had similar episodes. Tracheostomy may, though very rarely, be necessary as a life-saving measure, the diagnosis becoming clear only when the oedema of the tongue and adjacent parts subsides almost as rapidly as it came on, and the patient develops similar (angio-oedema), probably in other parts, on subsequent occasions.

Harold Ellis

Tongue, ulceration of

To enable a good view to be obtained of the affected part the patient should be seated in a good light and the protruded tongue gently dried with a piece of gauze. The presence of an ulcer being ascertained, its nature may be considered under the following heads: (1) *Carcinomatous*; (2) *Syphilitic*; (3) *Dental*; (4) *Tuberculous*; (5) *Ulcer in connection with stomatitis.*

1. Carcinomatous ulcer

Carcinomatous ulcer is much more common in men than in women. It is very unusual before the age of 30, and rarely starts before 45. The foul smell of the breath and the ill and wearied expression of the patient may awaken suspicion before the tongue is seen, for the sloughing ulcer is usually heavily infected, and the toxic absorption combined with pain and loss of sleep have a rapid and marked effect upon health. The tongue in a normal individual can be protruded from three to four centimetres beyond the teeth; if the protrusion is limited, or if the tongue is not protruded straight, it can generally be inferred, except in cases of paralysis, that there is some tumour binding it down (ankyloglossia). The position of the ulcer is to be studied and its relation to any sharp and carious tooth. An epithelioma is usually on the side of the tongue, but it may be anywhere on the upper, lateral or undersurface or on the floor of the mouth, but is hardly ever exactly in the midline.

As regards the ulcer itself, the typical appearance when fairly developed may be described as irregular, deep, foul, sloughy, with raised nodular everted edges and a surrounding area of induration. Other types associated with minimal ulceration of the mucous membrane are the scirrhous, where there is an excessive fibroblastic reaction, and the affected part of the tongue is shrivelled up as in the similar atrophic scirrhous cancer of the breast; and the nodular, where the lesion is mostly buried within the substance of the tongue and, like an iceberg, broaches the surface over a deceptively small area. In addition, the papilliferous type and multiple ulceration are not uncommon. Lastly there is the fissure carcinoma associated with leucoplakia (*Fig*. T.20). Except in early cases some of the lymphatic nodes are enlarged and hard, and they may be fixed. The submandibular group is generally the first affected, but the disease sometimes misses these and invades the jugular and even the supraclavicular nodes. Examination, therefore, should not be concluded before the whole of the neck has been palpated. The diagnosis should have been made, however, before the disease has developed thus far; in its earliest stages an epithelioma may be represented by a superficial ulcer no more than a sixteenth of an inch in diameter, by a crack or a small lump, without any enlargement of the nodes. In all these conditions, however, the ulcer is already hard and very resistant to any form of simple topical treatment. Any ulcer of the tongue occurring in a middle-aged man, and lasting for more than 2 or 3 weeks, should always awaken suspicion. (*Figs*. T.21, T.22).

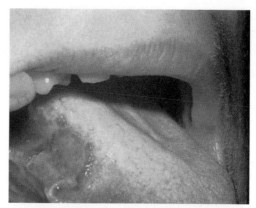

Fig. T.21. Carcinomatous ulcer of the tongue. Surprisingly, the patient was a girl of 17, with no demonstrable aetiology.

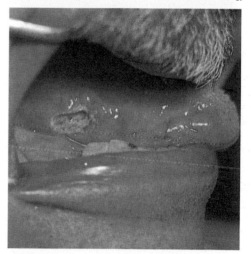

Fig. T.22. Ulceration from epithelioma of the tongue. (*Courtesy of the Gordon Museum, Guy's Hospital*)

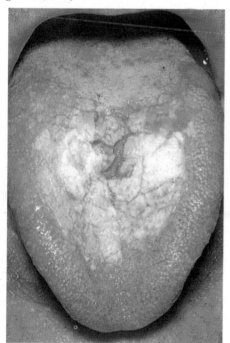

Fig. T.20. Non-syphilitic leucoplakia of the tongue.

DIAGNOSIS FROM SYPHILITIC ULCER. This may be a very real difficulty, owing to the fact that the two conditions may exist side by side (*Fig*. T.23), and that the syphilitic leucoplakia may be the actual precursor of a cancer. Positive serological reactions, therefore, are not proof that an epithelioma is not present. If a well-formed gumma is present, antisyphilitic remedies soon make a great change in its appearance. Although a biopsy is necessary for a definite diagnosis, certain clinical criteria are characteristic and a putative diagnosis of gumma may be made when the ulcer is centrally situated, painless, serpiginous in outline, and has the steep-cut edges and wash-leather slough base typical of syphilitic ulcers elsewhere.

DIAGNOSIS FROM DENTAL ULCER. The ulcer in this case is caused by a carious or otherwise jagged tooth, and therefore is in a corresponding position on the tongue. Further, the ulcer is soft to the touch and heals rapidly when the offending tooth is stopped or extracted. There is seldom difficulty in differentiation except when the ulcer is of very long standing.

2. Syphilitic ulcer

This may be primary, secondary or tertiary.

PRIMARY SYPHILIS or CHANCRE is certainly rare on the tongue and, owing partly to its rarity and partly to the fact that it is unexpected, it is frequently missed.

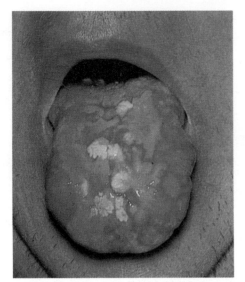

Fig. T.23. Leucoplakia of the tongue (syphilitic) with extensive carcinomatous charge.

It is more common in men than in women, but it may occur even in children. It starts as a small pimple which ulcerates and becomes indurated, though the induration is not so marked as when it is situated on the glans penis. The appearance of a secondary rash with general enlargement of the lymphatic nodes would indicate the true diagnosis. Further proof is supplied by positive serological tests, and the detection of spirochaetes in serum from the sore. Furthermore, the sore heals rapidly under the influence of treatment.

SECONDARY SYPHILIS manifests itself by the formation of mucous patches and superficial ulcers. The latter are almost always multiple, and situated along the edges and tip of the tongue, and with them are also found similar sores on the mucous membrane of the cheek, lips, palate and tonsil, and at the edges of the mouth. The ulcers are small, round, painful, with sharply cut edges and a greyish floor. Other secondary symptoms will be present to make the diagnosis clear.

TERTIARY SYPHILIS or GUMMATOUS ULCERATIONS. These lesions, now extremely rare, are divided into superficial and deep. *Superficial* gummas begin as small round-celled infiltrations in the mucous and submucous tissue. The ulcers are usually shallow, often irregular and associated with chronic glossitis, fissures and leucoplakia. Though rare today they are extremely important, for they may be followed by epithelioma. The ulcers themselves are not at first indurated, but if surrounded by interstitial fibrosis may appear hard; a histological examination is essential if there is the least doubt. A *deep* gumma starts as a hard swelling in the substance of the tongue. It is usually situated in the midline, and in the posterior half. Later it softens, breaks down and shows itself as a deep cavity with

irregular soft steep-cut walls, and a wash-leather-like slough at its base. It is not painful, and does not increase progressively in size. The important thing is to distinguish it from epithelioma and tuberculous disease. Unlike epithelioma it does not infiltrate widely or fix the tongue, its history is short and it causes no pain. Furthermore, it yields rapidly to anti-syphilitic treatment.

3. Dental ulcer

Dental ulcer is due to repeated small injuries from the sharp edge of a decayed tooth or damaged denture and is situated opposite the tooth, generally on the side of the tongue. The ulcer is small, superficial and not indurated unless it is of long standing. It is therefore not easily mistaken for any other kind of ulcer, or if doubt arises it is allayed by the healing of the ulcer on appropriate dental treatment: failure to heal within a fortnight suggests that it is an epithelioma.

There is a form of dental ulcer which is found on the fraenum of the tongue in children suffering from whooping cough; during the violent expiratory spasms peculiar to the illness, the undersurface of the tongue may suffer from rubbing over the lower incisor teeth.

4. Tuberculous ulcer

This is rare in the Western world, but it occurs at that period of life during which tuberculous disease of the lung is common, between the ages of 15 and 35. It is due to infection with tubercle bacilli brought up into the mouth. The ulcer itself is usually on the tip of the tongue or the side in its anterior half and is generally painful, although sometimes entirely painless. The outline is irregular. The edges are usually thin and undermined, and the base is covered by pale granulations, or excavated clearly down to the underlying muscle-fibres; less commonly the edges are raised, though never everted or hard, and the base is nodular, sloughy or caseous. It has often been mistaken for epithelioma or gumma. The fact that it is not hard, that is usually painful, and that pulmonary tuberculosis is present should point to the true diagnosis. Negative serological tests exclude a syphylitic gumma, though histological proof may be necessary by biopsy, and cultures carried out for bacteriological confirmation. A further example of tuberculous ulceration is the so-called 'truncated tongue'. In this type there is an oedematous infiltration of the parenchyma of the tongue, causing it to become swollen and almost 'woody', and there is a shallow ulceration of the tip, giving an appearance as if part of the tongue had been amputated. In fact the clinical manifestations of tuberculosis of the tongue are so protean that this disease should always be suspected in unusual lesions, especially if associated with pain.

5. Ulcers in connection with stomatitis (ulcerative stomatitis)

Septic infection of the mouth due to a variety of causes, such as irritation from decayed teeth, alkalis, acids or mercury, may be accompanied by the formation of small vesicles which, on bursting, give rise to superficial ulcers (*Fig.* T.24). They are not limited to the tongue, but appear as well on the mucous membrane of the cheeks and gums. Aphthous stomatitis commonly occurs in conjunction with the febrile diseases of childhood. It is characterized by the formation of whitish spots on the buccal mucous membrane; and by the shedding of epithelium small superficial ulcers may be formed. The ulcers of the tongue here occur in the course of a general inflammation of the mouth. One type that may be resistant to treatment is produced by Vincent's angina organisms; bacteriological tests give the diagnosis, but it may be suggested by the extreme foetor of the breath.

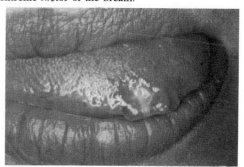

Fig. T.24. Aphthous ulcer. (*Professor Martin Rushton.*)

When ulceration of the tongue, and at the same time, very probably of the inside of the mouth generally, occurs in such conditions as *chickenpox, pemphigus* and other conditions that may affect the buccal mucosa as well as the skin, the diagnosis depends, not upon the appearances of the ulcers or the tongue, but upon the concomitant skin eruption.

Harold Ellis

Tonsils, enlargement of

The tonsils consist of lymphoid tissue with minor salivary glands and a covering of squamous epithelium. They lie encapsulated between the anterior and posterior pillars of the pharynx and intermingle with the lymphoid tissue at the base of the tongue. There is a physiological increase in size between the ages of 4 and 6 and subsequently the tonsils shrink. At this age, the tonsil enlargement is usually accompanied by enlargement of the adenoids. This can lead to the sleep apnoea syndrome which can vary from snoring to respiratory obstruction. It is not thought to occur early enough to be accountable as a cause of cot death. These patients improve dramatically with removal of tonsils and adenoids.

Large tonsils in young adults, especially if accompanied by malaise, are due to a glandular fever. The types of fever that cause the most marked tonsillar swelling are mononucleosis and especially toxoplasmosis.

Bacterial tonsillitis make the tonsils enlarge. A peritonsillar abscess means the infection has passed through the capsule of the tonsil so that there is oedema between the superior constrictor muscle and the capsule of the tonsil. This pushes the tonsil medially on one side and causes trismus, difficulty in speaking and marked elevation in temperature and malaise. There is dramatic relief when the pus is evacuated.

Lymphoma also occurs in young adults and presents with unilateral enlargement of the tonsil. This may, or may not be, accompanied by enlargement of the cervical lymph nodes.

In adults, salivary gland tumours can cause tonsillar enlargement in two ways. Firstly, an ectopic pleomorphic adenoma can occur in a tonsil, causing unilateral tonsillar enlargement, as can a malignant minor salivary gland tumour such as an adenoid cystic carcinoma or a mucoepidermoid carcinoma. Secondly, a tumour arising in the deep lobe of the parotid lies in the parapharyngeal space and can push the tonsil medially. Other lesions in the parapharyngeal space, such as chemodectoma, glomus vagale, schwannoma or a parapharyngeal space abscess, can cause the same tonsillar displacement and apparent enlargement of the tonsil.

A. G. D. Maran

Tracheal deviation

The trachea extends downwards from the lower border of the cricoid cartilage to the bifurcation into the two main bronchi at the level of the fifth thoracic vertebra. In normal individuals the upper half of the trachea lies in the midline of the neck, while the lower intrathoracic portion inclines slightly to the right of the midline. Palpation of the trachea in the neck may provide information about the position of the mediastinum provided the thoracic spine is straight and the thyroid gland not enlarged.

Displacement of the trachea from the mid-sternal line will usually signify disease of the pleura, lung or occasionally the mediastinum. In conjunction with conventional physical examination of the chest to assess chest wall movement, air entry, percussion note, vocal fremitus and breath sounds, the position of the trachea should be carefully palpated. Deviation of the trachea away from the abnormal side will suggest volume displacement, perhaps due to a large pleural effusion, pneumothorax under tension, bullous emphysema, or rarely, a massive lung or mediastinal tumour. Deviation towards the abnormal side will suggest collapse of the underlying upper lobe or lung. In adults, deviation of the trachea towards the affected side in conjunction with flattening of the upper anterior chest raises the possibility of long-standing fibrotic contracture of the lobe or lung, possibly with associated pleural thickening, secondary to healed pulmonary tuberculosis.

The trachea is not displaced by consolidation without collapse of the underlying lung. It may remain centrally positioned when carcinoma has caused a combination of lung collapse with pleural effusion.

A confirmatory chest radiograph should be taken if the physical signs suggest underlying lung or pleural disease.

P. R. Studdy

Tremor

Tremor may be defined as a more or less regular, rhythmical oscillation of one part of the body from a fixed point usually in one plane. Two separate categories may be recognized: normal or physiological tremor and abnormal or pathological tremor. The former is present in all muscle groups and throughout the waking state. The movement is so fine that it can barely be seen by the naked eye and then only if the fingers are held outstretched. Certain abnormal tremors, namely the metabolic varieties of postural or action tremor and at least one type of familial tremor, are believed by some to be variants or exaggerations of physiological tremor.

Abnormal or pathological tremor preferentially affects certain muscle groups and is present only in the waking state. The following are the common types of tremor:

PARKINSONIAN (REST) TREMOR

This is a coarse rhythmical tremor which is most often localized in one or both hands and less frequently in the feet, jaw, lips or tongue. It occurs when the limb is at rest and is usually suppressed or diminished during willed movement.

The tremor takes the form of flexion/extension or abduction/adduction movements of the fingers or hand and there may be superadded pronation/supination, giving the appearance of a so-called compound tremor. Flexion/extension of the fingers in combination with abduction/adduction of the thumb leads to the classically described pill-rolling tremor. The parkinsonian tremor usually continues whilst the patient walks and may be exaggerated by movement of the contralateral limb. Emotional stress may increase the tremor. Although embarrasing, the tremor interferes surprisingly little with voluntary activity largely because it is suppressed during movement. Within the various parkinsonian syndromes, tremor is most often a manifestation of true Parkinson's disease and it is less common in postencephalitic, drug-induced or other forms of parkinsonism.

INTENTION (ATAXIC) TREMOR

This tremor occurs during the most demanding phases of active movement and as such usually at the extremes of movement. The tremor is absent when the limbs are inactive and during the first part of voluntary movement, but as the action continues and fine adjustments of the movement are required (for example in touching the tip of the nose or the examiner's finger) a rhythmical side-to-side oscillation appears, interfering with the final stage of the intended movement. This type of tremor may seriously interfere with the patient's performance of any skilled movement. Tremors of this type invariably indicate disease of the cerebellum or its connections. Severe tremors of this type usually indicate disease of the brain stem and particularly the dentato-rubral thalamic tract. Most commonly this is seen in multiple sclerosis and it may also occur in Wilson's disease.

POSTURAL OR ACTION TREMOR

This type of tremor is present when the limbs and trunk are actively maintained in certain positions, such as holding the arms outstretched, and it persists throughout the active movement. The tremor is absent when the limbs are relaxed. It is accentuated as greater precision of movement is demanded but never approaches the degree of accentuation seen in intention tremor. There are many different types of action tremor. One type seems to be a mere exaggeration of normal or physiological tremor and is a characteristic of anxiety, hyperthyroidism, toxic states of withdrawal from alcohol and sedative/hypnotic drugs. A tremor of this type is also observed in certain families constituting one form of familial tremor. A second variety of familial action tremor is of lower frequency. It is often inherited as an autosomal dominant trait and is referred to as benign essential tremor, essential tremor or, if it becomes evident in later years, senile tremor. Such tremors always spare the lower limbs.

A curious factor about essential or familial tremor is that it may be suppressed by alcohol and it often responds also to the beta-adrenergic antagonist propranolol or to barbiturates.

Other action tremors may be seen in disorders such as meningoencephalitis and in certain intoxications.

HYSTERICAL TREMOR

Tremor is a rare manifestation of hysteria but it may simulate a variety of organic tremors. It is usually restricted to a single limb and is often exceedingly gross.

TREMORS OF MIXED TYPE

Not all tremors correspond exactly to the types described above; for example, in some parkinsonian patients the tremor is exaggerated rather than diminished by active movement and in others the tremor may be absent at rest and only become obvious with movement.

A rest component to the tremor may be seen in certain families with so-called 'familial tremor'.

Tremors need to be differentiated from asterixis, myoclonus, polymyoclonus and clonus.

D. A. Shaw

Trismus (lockjaw)

(*See also* FACE, ABNORMALITIES OF APPEARANCE AND MOVEMENT). Trismus, or lockjaw, signifies a maintained muscular spasm tending to closure of the jaws so that the mouth cannot be opened. The term does not include mechanical inability to open the jaws owing to such affections as mumps, alveolar abscess with surrounding inflammatory oedema, injury, Ludwig's angina, quinsy or severe tonsillitis, an odontoma, epithelioma of the mouth, myositis ossificans or cervicofacial actinomycosis. There are two conditions which may not at first sight be obvious, but may lock the jaws together and simulate true trismus—*impaction of a wisdom tooth* and *arthritic changes in the temporomandibular joint*. These are diagnosed by careful local examination of the teeth and of the joint respectively; in the latter case there may be arthritic changes in other joints also. X-ray examination may be required to detect the joint changes or the impacted wisdom teeth (*Fig.* T.25).

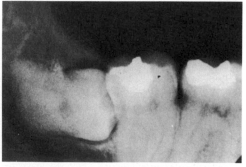

Fig. T.25. Radiograph showing impacted third molar.

Circumstantial evidence will generally serve to distinguish trismus due to *hysteria* or to *facial neur-algia*; any doubt at first experienced is dispelled if the patient is watched for a while. Convulsive seizures in a hysterical patient with trismus can generally be distinguished from those due to tetanus or to strychnine poisoning by their polymorphous character, and by the fact that touching the patient, and other similar stimulation, does not bring them on so certainly as would be the case with strychnine or tetanus.

In fits, for example epilepsy, the trismus is of short duration and offers no difficulty in diagnosis.

MALINGERING may sometimes take the form of lockjaw, and it may be a little while before the fraud can be detected. In sleep the malingerer's muscles relax completely.

TRICHINIASIS is rare, but if infected pork is eaten raw, or insufficiently cooked, the larvae of the parasites find their way to many different muscles, and they show predilection for those of the tongue, mouth and jaws. The resultant irritation, pain and stiffness can cause trismus, the origin of which may be difficult to determine unless the history points to pork. The patient is very ill in the earlier stages, with high fever, and the condition may be fatal. The malady may be epidemic. The blood exhibits eosinophilia. The final criterion of the diagnosis is the discovery of the typical parasites coiled up in their little oval cysts among the affected muscle fibres.

HYDROPHOBIA (RABIES) and TETANY seldom exhibit trismus as a prominent symptom. The former, though now almost unknown in Great Britain, would suggest itself if a convulsive illness developed after a bite by a dog, fox or other similar animal, particularly if the spasmodic muscular difficulty is markedly increased by efforts at swallowing. The symptoms may not develop for weeks or months after the bite, so that the patient may fall ill when he has come from a country overseas where rabies is endemic. *Tetany*, also rare, is at once distinguished by its typical carpopedal contractions; trismus, almost constant in tetanus, is nearly always absent in tetany.

STRYCHNINE POISONING gives rise to generalized twitchings and convulsions long before trismus, the lateness of the development of the latter serving to distinguish it from tetanus. Furthermore there is complete muscular relaxation between spasms. There may be evidence of strychnine having been taken or administered, either by the mouth or hypodermically; the symptoms develop very acutely, and are often rapidly fatal.

TETANUS is the cause *par excellence* of trismus. The diagnosis is often obvious if the illness develops in an otherwise healthy person, with stiffness starting usually in the neck muscles, spreading to those of the face and jaw, and thence to the rest of the trunk and limbs, with extremely painful exacerbations on the slightest stimulation even by a stroke with a feather or the banging of a door; dysphagia; risus sardonicus; opisthotonos; no complete relaxation of the stiff muscles unless an anaesthetic be given; a duration of days rather than hours; especially if all these things follow a few days, or a week or more, after a small penetrating wound which becomes septic. It may be possible to demonstrate the presence of the drum-stick bacilli in films prepared from the deeper parts of the wound. The chief difficulty arises when there is no clear history, or when the wound has been so small that it has healed or cannot be found; even then, most cases are so typical that they can be diagnosed as tetanus without difficulty. Unnecessary anxiety arises chiefly in cases of an impacted wisdom tooth, or of hysteria, where tetanus may be suspected at first; the subsequent course of the malady soon serves to exclude this. Involvement of the temporomandibular joint in a *serum reaction*, especially if prophylactic tetanus antitoxin has been given, may lead to the belief that tetanus has in fact set in.

Trismus may be simulated by *scleroderma* of the face. But here the condition is rather one of fixation of the skin than of the muscles; the skin becomes like parchment so that one cannot pick it up between the fingers, it feels firm or almost hard, and the patient becomes unable to open the mouth properly. The disease is of slow onset and gradual progress, so that there is seldom difficulty in diagnosis.

Ian Mackenzie

Underactivity

The causes of underactivity are listed in *Table* U.1.

Underactivity will most commonly be a normal response to *fatigue* and *insomnia*. The complaint of underactivity may also come from someone suffering an *adjustment reaction* from recent severe stress such as marital or business problems or chronic illness. The response to stress may include anxious and depressed mood, physical complaints, disturbance of conduct including antisocial behaviour or it may take the form of withdrawal from normal activities without any clear evidence of mood change. Timely intervention with counselling may help the situation to resolve.

Feelings of tiredness, fatigue and lack of drive accompany almost every form of debilitating illness and a complaint of underactivity may be due, for example, to anaemia, endocrine disorders such as

Table U.1. Causes of underactivity

Common causes
Insomnia and physical fatigue
Physical illness
   Hypothyroidism
   Addison's disease
   Chronic infections
   Cardiac, renal, hepatic failure
   Anaemias
   Undernourishment
Adjustment reaction
Uncomplicated bereavement
Depressive illness
Organic brain disease
Frontal lobe syndrome
Causes of confusion (*see* pp. 114, 115)
Schizophrenia
Drug abuse
   Opioid
   Barbiturate
   Cannabis
   Inhalent intoxication
Post head injury

Less common causes
Obsessive compulsive disorder
Psychogenic stupor

hypothyroidism or Addison's disease; cardiac, renal or hepatic impairment; chronic infections; postviral states. Malnutrition caused by malabsorption will similarly cause symptoms related to debility. However, in people who are malnourished and also living in conditions of poverty and extreme deprivation, there can develop a profound state of apathy and underactivity as a result of a combination of adverse physical and social factors.

Many drugs of abuse are taken because they generate euphoria and underactivity. These include opioids, cannabis, hallucinogens (LSD, mescaline, magic mushrooms), barbiturates, benzodiazepines and other hypnotics and sedatives.

In *depression* patients may show a slowing of all motor activity including speech, gestures and facial movements. There is usually retardation of thinking and complaint of difficulty in initiating and executing all voluntary acts. Severe *depression* with retardation may pose diagnostic problems in an elderly person when a gradual onset may lead the clinician to erroneously diagnose dementia in a patient whose apparent memory loss and cognitive impairment is due to their slowness in performing the tasks rather than to real cognitive change. *Depressive pseuodementia* often responds well to antidepressant treatments and it is important to bear in mind that during the early stages of treatment retardation may improve more quickly than the mood state and there is a high risk of a patient making a suicide attempt. Depression is undoubtedly the commonest cause of retardation and even when retardation develops in a patient with another condition such as schizophrenia or obsessional illness, depression may be an important contributing factor. In *obsessive compulsive disorder* (*see* OBSESSIONS, p. 463) some patients are so preoccupied by obsessional thoughts and inner rituals that they appear uncommunicative and slow in all their activities. In *schizophrenia* underactivity may be the result of several different processes. *Catatonic schizophrenia* describes a relatively uncommon presentation of the psychosis, in which motor disorders dominate the picture. Patients may become mute or stuperose and in rare cases adopt strange postures, exhibiting a disturbance of muscle tone by which their limbs will remain in any new position, however uncomfortable for minutes at a time (waxy flexibility). They may show automatic obedience, responding to all requests without question; negativism, responding in exactly the opposite way to that requested; or sometimes they will remain mute and unresponsive, unwilling to engage at all with the interviewer. A detailed history and follow-up assessment is the only way that the diagnosis can be confirmed.

A rather more common type of underactivity affecting many patients with schizophrenia occurs with so-called 'negative' symptoms. These patients lose their sense of drive and volition become apathetic and careless about their appearance. They have paucity of speech and emotional blunting which limits the full enjoyment of anything. They are poor time-keepers at work and will be described as lazy, egotistical and inconsiderate by family and friends who are not made aware of the true nature of the condition. Depressive symptoms are common in chronic schizophrenia and may exacerbate the underlying slowness and apathy. The side-effects of anti-psychotic medication is a further cause of slowness in these patients since higher doses of most anti-psychotic drugs cause a combination of motor and psychological slowing which adds to the negative symptoms.

Stupor describes a state in which a subject is fully conscious but makes no spontaneous movements and does not respond to stimuli. Occasionally this may be *psychogenic* in origin in which case the onset is sudden and stress-related and the patient may sit motionless for long periods without moving or talking although their muscle tone, posture and eye movements indicate that they are not asleep or unconscious.

Patients with damage to their *frontal lobes* show changes in behaviour, mood and volition, typically with loss of initiative and spontaneity and a marked reduction in motor behavior. Such people have particular difficulties in starting any new initiatives. Despite their mood which can be euphoric, they perform tasks slowly and incompetently. A frontal lobe syndrome may follow *head injury*, be due to vascular or space-occupying lesions, or other pathologies such as demyelination involving the frontal lobes.

D. Blackwood

Urethral discharge

The causes are as follows:

1. Gonorrhoea
2. Non-specific urethritis
3. Trichomoniasis
4. Bacterial:
   E. coli
   Ducrey's bacillus (Haemophilus ducreyi)
   Tuberculosis
5. Chemical
6. Traumatic:
   Instrumental
   Accidental
7. New growth
8. Foreign bodies

Any inflammatory process in the urethra causes a discharge. Although often the result of infection by the *gonococcus*, by no means every urethritis is of this nature, and bacteriological examinations show that other organisms besides the gonococcus may produce a urethral discharge and the same symptoms as gonorrhoea. Further than this, a purulent discharge may occur in which no micro-organisms can be found; for instance, when the urethra has been injured or subjected to irritation by the injection of strong solutions, or when it contains a foreign body, such as a calculus or a retained catheter.

There is no doubt that an acute *non-specific* urethritis may be caused by other organisms than the gonococcus, and is today more common than gonococcal urethritis. These cases may cause complications in the genito-urinary organs similar to those due to the gonococcus, such as prostatitis, epididymitis or cystitis. They may arise by the infection of the urethra by septic instrumentation, or after connection with a woman with trichomoniasis. A careful bacteriological examination should always be made in order to determine the causative organism. An acute urethritis may accompany a haematogenous urinary infection; for instance, an acute infection of the upper urinary tract due to *E. coli* may be followed by acute cystitis, prostatitis and urethritis, in which no other organism but *E. coli* can be found. *Non-specific (non-gonococcal) urethritis* is due probably to several infective agents, such as *Chlamydia trachomatis* and *Trichomonas vaginalis*. It is usually a venereal disease contracted in coitus. A watery, whitish penile discharge in males may be associated with mild dysuria and lower abdominal discomfort. The discharge may be so slight as to be overlooked, but there is a tendency for exacerbations and remissions to occur, and the urethral discharge is sometimes purulent, serous or mucopurulent. In Reiter's disease there is arthritis and sometimes conjunctivitis and uveitis in addition (see p. 351). In such cases although the urethritis may respond to tetracycline therapy, the arthritis does not. Reiter's disease, although commonly venereal in origin in Great Britain, may follow bacillary dysentery.

GONORRHOEAL URETHRITIS

This is due to the infection of the urethra by the gonococcus (*Neisseria gonorrhoeae*). The gonococcus is seen in a stained specimen to be *intracellular*, penetrating not only the leucocytes but also the epithelial cells found in a smear preparation, and, although the cocci may be found also between the cells, their appearance in the cells is strong evidence of their specific nature.

In any case presenting a purulent discharge from the urethra it is necessary, in order that appropriate treatment may be carried out, first to make a smear of the discharge for bacteriological examination, and secondly to make a culture of the discharge in order to determine drug sensitivity of the organisms, and also to confirm the smear test.

A gonococcal complement fixation test (GCFT) is not useful in diagnosis of early cases as it is associated with many false-negative results. It must be established that the pus comes from the urethra and not from beneath the prepuce. For the purposes of clinical investigation the urethra is divided into anterior and posterior portions, separated by the membranous urethra, the anterior comprising the bulbous and penile urethra, and the posterior the prostatic portion. A urethritis is also, according to its clinical aspect, acute or chronic, the acute form being characterized by a thick, creamy, purulent discharge, with pain, and the chronic by a thin, greyish, muco-purulent discharge. Acute gonorrhoea affects not only the superficial layers of the urethral mucous membrane, but also the subepithelial tissues and the glandular elements, causing a leucocytic infiltration. The tendency of the inflammation is to spread backwards along the canal so that the prostatic urethra may become infected even in the acute stage, though most frequently this occurs at a later period; the prostatic and the ejaculatory ducts may become infected, and the inflammation may spread to the seminal vesicles and epididymes. In the acute stages of the disease the infection of the anterior urethra is accompanied, as a rule, by redness of the external meatus, scalding pain during micturition, and painful emissions. These patients have described the pain on micturition as like passing red-hot fish-hooks through

the urethra. Occasionally all pain is absent, especially in patients previously infected with gonorrhoea. If the anterior urethra alone is infected and the urine is passed into two glasses, the first portion will be turbid from admixture with the urethral discharge, whilst the second portion may remain clear.

When the posterior urethra becomes infected in the acute stages the symptoms are much more severe. Micturition is more painful and greatly increased in frequency, both by day and by night, the patient often being obliged to pass urine every half-hour. It may follow that a prostatic abscess develops to complicate posterior urethritis, in which case micturition becomes very painful, or a painful retention of urine may occur. There is usually an associated high fever and rigors. On rectal examination the prostate is found much swollen, hot to the touch, and extremely tender, while with an abscess a soft fluctuating area may be felt. An acute posterior gonorrhoea is only rarely accompanied by infection of the bladder, cystitis supervening on the urethritis.

With successful antibiotic treatment the purulent urethral discharge will disappear within 24 hours and the patient will be symptom-free in 2–3 days.

NON-SPECIFIC URETHRITIS

Non-specific urethritis (NSU) is now the commonest sexually-transmitted disease in the UK. The urethral discharge tends to be thinner and more mucopurulent than the thick creamy pus of the typical gonococcal urethritis. However, it may be clinically impossible to distinguish between gonorrhoea and NSU and, indeed, some patients may have a mixed infection with the gonococcus and one of the other organisms which may have caused NSU.

Among the causative organisms of NSU are:

1 *Chlamydia trachomatis*
2 *Ureaplasma urealyticum*
3 *Trichomonas vaginalis*
4 *Secondary bacterial infections* from coliforms, anaerobes, yeasts, etc.

Chlamydia trachomatis is the predominant cause of NSU infections and the organism can be seen on microscopy or isolated from something like half the patients with NSU. The organism proliferates within epithelial cells and this produces characteristic large intracytoplasmic inclusion bodies which stain with specific fluorescent antibody techniques.

Ureaplasma urealyticum (T strains of mycoplasma) are found in the genital tract of many sexually active individuals without clinical evidence of infection but occasionally clinical urethritis is probably caused by these organisms.

Trichomonas vaginalis may colonize the male urethra and may in some cases produce urethritis.

Reiter's syndrome may complicate NSU in a small proportion of patients. Symptoms include conjunctivitis, uveitis, arthritis and pustular hyperkeratosis on the soles of the feet.

A urethral discharge may in rare cases be gonorrhoea or non-specific urethritis, and as difficulty may arise if one of these cases is met with it is necessary to mention them.

Herpetic Urethritis. The mucous lining of the urethra may be affected by herpes in the same manner as other mucous membranes. There is irritation of the urethra during micturition, and a slight mucopurulent discharge from the meatus. The small vesicles may be seen by the endoscope, and may be associated with herpes of the prepuce or glans penis.

Soft sores in the urethra (**Chancroid**) are distinctly uncommon. They occur in the terminal portion of the urethra, and cause painful micturition and a profuse, thin, purulent discharge, which contains no gonococci; Ducrey's bacillus (Haemophilus ducreyi) may be found. There may be other sores on the glans penis, and an ulcerated surface will be seen on endoscopic examination. They occur within a few days of infection, and, if extensive, may produce narrowing of the urethra on healing. Lymph nodes in the groins may be enlarged and tender.

Syphillis may affect the urethra either as a hard chancre or as a gumma.

The *chancre* occurs in the terminal inch of the urethra, forming a firm indurated mass which can be felt readily on external palpation. The meatus is oedematous and swollen, so that the introduction of an endoscopic tube is impossible; there is a thin, purulent, and often blood-stained discharge from the meatus. A urethral chancre must be diagnosed carefully from peri-urethral infiltration due to urethritis; the period of incubation from time of infection, the presence of small, hard inguinal nodes, the occurrence of secondary lesions of syphilis, and positive serological tests will point to the diagnosis. The *Treponema pallidum (Spirochaeta pallida)* may be found in the fluid expressed from the surface of the sore

Gumma of the urethra is now extremely rare; it gives rise to a watery urethral discharge when it ulcerates. It may ulcerate through the canal and form fistulas, but may usually be recognized on careful examination.

PAPILLOMAS OF THE URETHRA

These may occur either in the anterior or posterior portion, as small, pedunculated tumours in the canal, and frequently as a sequel to a chronic gonorrhoea.

They may arise, however, in the urethra of a patient who has never had urethritis. They cause a thin, scanty discharge together with spontaneous urethral bleeding; they are seen readily through the endoscope and some are often visible when the lips of the meatus are retracted (*see Fig.* H.8).

CARCINOMA

Carcinoma of the urethra is very rare as a primary disease, and many of the cases recorded have been in association with stricture. It forms a tumour in the urethra palpable from the exterior, and causes painful micturition with a blood-stained discharge, and enlargement of the inguinal nodes. Suspicion of carcinoma should arise if a hard, irregular tumour is felt in the course of the urethra, without gonorrhoeal infection, in an elderly patient. Carcinoma of the urethra may also occur as an extension from carcinoma of the bladder or prostate or as a malignant change in urethral papilloma; the papillary type will not be palpable from the exterior. The final diagnosis depends on histological examination of a portion of the growth, removed for biopsy through an endoscope. An irrigating posterior urethroscope or panendoscope is the best instrument for this purpose.

TUBERCULOSIS OF THE URETHRA

This is always secondary to disease elsewhere in the genito-urinary tract, usually of the prostate or seminal vesicles; it is very rare. Tubercle bacilli may be found in the urethral smear.

FOREIGN BODIES IN THE URETHRA

These may cause a purulent urethral discharge if they remain for any length of time. They may be introduced through the meatus by intent—matches, pins, etc.; or a piece may be detached from a damaged catheter; or a small calculus may come down from the bladder and be arrested; in the latter case the history is usually clear—sudden stoppage of the stream of urine during micturition, with penile pain; a calculus may be felt from the exterior or seen through the endoscope.

Harold Ellis

URETHRA, PAIN IN
See PENIS, PAIN IN.

Urethra, faeces passed through

Faeces or faecal fluid are passed per urethram only when the bladder is in fistulous communication with some part of the bowel, or with an abscess infected with *Escherichia coli*, PNEUMATURIA (q.v.) may occur at same time. The chief causes are as follows:

> Diverticular disease of the sigmoid colon with a fistula into the bladder (the commonest cause).

Carcinoma of the bladder opening into the rectum or into some loop of bowel which has become adherent to the bladder.

Carcinoma of
the rectum
the sigmoid
colon
the caecum } opening into the bladder either directly or through the medium of an intervening abscess.

Carcinoma of the uterus opening both into the bladder and into the rectum.

Crohn's disease of large or small bowel with vesical fistula.

Prostatitis or prostatic abscess opening into the rectum.

Rectovesical fistula from injury and sloughing, particularly after childbirth.

Appendicular abscess opening into the bladder

Pelvic actinomycosis.

The passage of faeces into the urine may be simulated by some cases of very foetid cystitis due to infection by *E. coli*, especially in diabetic subjects.

If the symptom is due to carcinoma it matters little which viscus is the primary site by the time the growth has involved both bladder and bowel. The differentiation resolves itself, therefore, between malignant and non-malignant conditions. If malignant disease is not obvious it will nearly always be advisable to resort to surgical measures in the hope of discovering some curable primary condition—rectal, appendicular, prostatic or otherwise. The diagnosis will be suggested by the history and confirmed by local examination or exploration.

Harold Ellis

Urine, abnormal colour of

The normal amber colour of urine is due mainly to urochrome; the depth of colour naturally varies with the concentration and very dilute urine is nearly colourless. In very concentrated urine the depth of colour may raise suspicions of biliuria. Several substances can alter the colour of the urine. This is usually of no pathological significance although a patient may seek an explanation; in a few conditions the colour is characteristic and of diagnostic significance.

Bile pigment imparts a deep *orange* colour to the urine; in high concentration the appearance resembles beer. Senna and rhubarb ingestion can produce a similar colour.

A *red* colour in the urine can be due to a number of substances. Haemoglobin is the most important, either in intact red cells when the urine has a turbid or 'smoky' appearance or as free pigment when the urine is clear. If large amounts are present and, particularly, if some of the haemoglobin has been oxidized to methaemoglobin, the colour may be brownish-black. In porphyrinuria the colour is typically that of 'port wine' but it may be pink or red. Myoglobinuria may give

a red or brown colour in the urine. Other substances causing red urine include beetroot, blackberries, phenolphthalein in purgatives (if the urine is alkaline) and certain aniline dyes in sweets. Eosin produces a pink colour with a green fluorescence and uro-erythrin often contributes to the red colour of abnormal urine; it is of no pathological significance and is mainly seen adsorbed on deposits of urate ('brick-dust' deposit).

Apart from methaemoglobin, a *dark brown* or *black* urine may be due to phenol (carboluria), melanin, homogentisic acid or p-hydroxy-phenyl pyruvic acid. In carboluria, due to phenol poisoning, the urine may be greenish-brown. Melanin or melanogen is found in the urine in some cases of disseminated malignant melanoma; the urine may be of normal colour when passed but turns black on standing, from above downwards. A similar colour change on standing occurs in the urine in alkaptonuria in which homogentisic acid is excreted. This substance also accumulates in the cartilage of the ear and in the sclera, which may become black, and in joint cartilage causing severe arthritis; this syndrome is known as ochronosis. The urine may also darken in air in the very rare tyrosinosis in which *p*-hydroxyphenyl pyruvic acid is excreted. The antimicrobial drug metronidazole also causes the urine to become dark brown.

Due to the presence in normal urine of urochrome, any blue compound in low concentration may produce a green colour. *Green* and *blue* urines are most commonly due to biliverdin in long-standing obstructive jaundice or to methylene blue in pills or sweets. Indigo-carmine and indigo-blue can also colour the urine. The former may rarely be present after exposure to industrial dyes and the latter is the consequence of oxidation of indican. Indicanuria is due to intestinal malabsorption of tryptophan which is metabolized to indole by intestinal bacteria in such conditions as coeliac disease and Hartnup disease.

Peter R. Fleming

Urine, incontinence of

Incontinence is the involuntary loss of urine from the bladder at times and in places which are inappropriate and inconvenient. Preservation of continence depends on the integrity of the lower urinary tract, both anatomically and physiologically. Incontinence secondary to an anatomical abnormality occurs congenitally, as in ectopic ureter, or is acquired, as in vesico-vaginal fistula; physiological disturbance occurs because of imbalance between the tone of the detrusor muscle and that of the external urethral sphincter.

Sphincter weakness results in genuine stress incontinence, sometimes called simply stress incontinence; detrusor incontinence occurs when detrusor activity is sufficiently enhanced to overcome the resistance offered by a normal sphincter mechanism. Overflow incontinence occurs when the detrusor is flaccid so that urine trickles out when the fully distended bladder can hold no more, in much the same way that water trickles over the lip of a dam.

The common causes of incontinence of urine can be divided into: (1) Sphincter damage; (2) Neurological lesions.

1. Sphincter damage

Mechanical damage to the sphincter is the commonest cause of genuine stress incontinence. Broadly speaking, the sphincter apparatus in both sexes consists of three components: the bladder neck, which is a muscle group derived from the detrusor muscle of the bladder wall; the intrinsic urethral apparatus, which consists of muscle components from both bladder neck and external sphincter together with fibrous and vascular components; and the external sphincters, which consist of the striated muscle of the pelvic floor.

In women, all three components can be affected by stretch or direct damage during the passage of the fetal head during labour, giving rise to stress incontinence.

In men, prostatectomy is a common cause of stress incontinence; the bladder neck has been ablated inevitably during prostatectomy itself, but there is additional damage to the intrinsic apparatus and even occasionally to the external sphincter. Prostatectomy inevitably implies internal sphincter ablation and considerable resection of the intrinsic apparatus but provided this procedure is limited to the zone proximal to the verumontanum the remaining intrinsic urethral mechanism and the external sphincter together will allow preservation of continence. Incontinence is almost inevitable following total prostatectomy carried out for carcinoma of the prostate. Sphincter involvement by malignant extension from prostatic carcinoma is rarely enough in itself to give rise to stress incontinence as the simultaneous obstruction produced by the enlarged malignant gland will compensate for loss of sphincter tone.

The pelvic floor can be injured by trauma, such as gunshot wounds, and is particularly vulnerable to injury when the pelvis is fractured. A dual mechanism is often responsible for incontinence in the latter as direct damage to the pelvic floor is compounded by damage to its nerve supply, particularly the pudendal nerves.

STRESS INCONTINENCE

Genuine *stress incontinence in women* is related to sphincter damage during childbirth and to the weakening of the supporting pelvic floor muscles. The sphincter apparatus falls below the level at which it can be protected by transmitted pressure during coughing and other activity so that the intra-abdominal pressure acts in an unopposed manner on the bladder dome. Increases in abdominal pressure produce a simultaneous leak of urine. The condition is usually associated with anterior and posterior vaginal wall prolapses, manifested as cystocele or rectocele respectively, but this is by no means invariable. Supporting the bladder neck by inserting the index and middle finger against the anterior vaginal wall and pushing upwards will control the leaking. This test mimics the effect of a successful surgical procedure. Genuine stress incontinence also occurs in some congenital abnormalities, such as the short urethra, the wide urethra and epispadias.

Some degree of *stress incontinence in men* is usual after prostatectomy but clears up as the prostatic cavity heals and infection is eradicated. If there has been sphincter damage as a result of the procedure, the resulting incontinence improves slowly with time. A period of some 12 months must elapse before the degree of remaining incontinence can be judged permanent.

URGE INCONTINENCE

Incontinence after prostatectomy also usually relates to the irritability of the bladder base related to the oedema of the healing zone. This incontinence is called urge incontinence, where the desire to micturate is so strong that it overrides all attempts of the sphincters to retain urine. Urge incontinence is frequent in both sexes and is the major differential diagnosis from genuine stress incontinence. The detrusor contracts in an abnormal manner and, as it does so, it opens the bladder neck and thus decreases the outflow resistance. This kind of incontinence is sometimes called 'unstable bladder' incontinence. It is not related to any neurological factor but is seen in association with acute cystitis, chronic cystitis, post-radiotherapy, in tuberculous cystitis, interstitial cystitis, in the presence of a foreign body in the bladder, when a stone is impacted at the uretero-vesical junction, in outflow tract obstruction secondary to posterior hypertrophy and bladder neck stenosis. In most cases, no specific aetiological feature can be discovered. It is difficult to distinguish from genuine stress incontinence on clinical grounds as, during the circumstances of examination, the first cough may not precipitate incontinence but subsequent coughing on request may initiate a detrusor contraction which is strong enough to open the sphincter.

2. Neurological lesions

Incontinence related to neurological causes may be due to upper or lower motor neurone lesions. In upper motor neurone lesions the central inhibitory impulses to the micturition centre in the sacral segments are lost. Sudden contractions of the detrusor muscle occur, resulting in unheralded precipitate micturition. The volume of urine lost in upper motor neurone lesions is almost always greater than that lost in simple detrusor instability. The condition is associated with disseminated sclerosis, follows cerebrovascular accidents, is seen in some cases of Parkinson's disease, syringomyelia, and in fact any condition which affects the conducting pathways in the upper part of the spinal cord. The reflex centre in the cord is intact so that the stretching of the bladder wall causes reflex detrusor spasm and micturition. The difficulty arises because the sphincter mechanism is also subject to a similar degree of spasm. The result is bladder wall hypertrophy with trabeculation, formation of saccules and diverticula and the presence of a urine residue. If the patient is paraplegic, management becomes extremely difficult as sepsis, excoriation of the genitalia and perineum, and areas of pressure necrosis occur.

In lower motor neurone lesions which affect the afferent and efferent portions of the sacral reflex arc as well as the reflex centre itself, the bladder is cut off from this spinal regulatory centre. As the pathognomonic feature of an upper motor neurone lesion is spasticity, so is flaccidity the feature of a lower motor neurone lesion. The detrusor muscle becomes flaccid, often insensitive to stretch, and the bladder distends enormously. The concomitant weakness of the sphincter mechanism eventually leads to overflow incontinence where urine trickles through the urethra. The bladder is readily palpable, is asymetrical, often enormous, not tender and relatively soft; from the side,

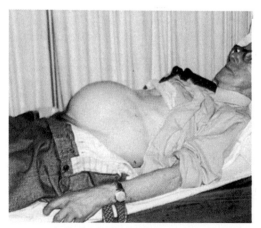

Fig. U.1. Swelling in the lower abdomen caused by chronic retention of urine due to enlarged prostate.

the huge bulge above the symphysis pubic is readily apparent and unchanging, during respiration while the upper abdomen adopts a scaphoid shape (*Fig.* U.1). Pressure on the bladder dome often results in the expression of urine, a diagnostic test which, in itself, can sometimes be adapted as a therapeutic technique to promote bladder emptying.

Lower motor neurone lesions are also associated with peripheral neuritis, as in diabetes or tabes. In diabetes, a selective peripheral neuropathy can affect bladder behaviour, and the mechanism of erection in the male, without any peripheral signs of such a neuropathy. Damage to the autonomic supply to the bladder also follows pelvic surgery, especially abdomino-perineal excision of the rectum, Wertheim hysterectomy and radical cystectomy. Operations which spare the autonomic supply to the pelvis and genitalia have been developed.

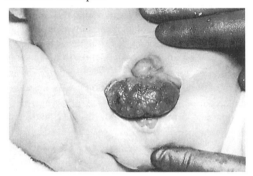

Fig. U.2. Ectopia vesicae in a boy of 6 months. The bladder mucosa protrudes and urine drips constantly from the ureters.

A similar picture of incontinence with overflow is also seen in chronic outflow obstruction, almost always secondary to prostatic enlargement or bladder neck stenosis. Enuresis is a pathognomonic clinical feature of this condition.

All the conditions described so far present as incontinence of an intermittent variety. Continuous incontinence, day and night, is found in some congenital abnormalities. The most severe of these is *ectopia vesicae* (bladder extrophy) where there is failure of development of the abdominal wall and anterior wall of the bladder so that the mucosa of the bladder is exposed and the two ureteric orifices can be seen with urine dripping from them (*Fig.* U.2). There is wide separation of the two pubic rami (pubic diastasis).

An *ectopic ureter* occasionally opens into the vagina in the female or into the urethra beyond the sphincter apparatus in either sex. Urine leaks continually. The ectopic ureter usually drains a duplex kidney and when a pyelogram shows a duplex system in a case of incontinence an ectopic ureter should be sought. The opening is often extremely difficult to find, but the intravenous injection of indigo-carmine

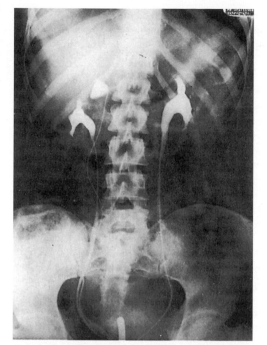

Fig. U.3. Pyelogram in a case of incontinence of urine in a woman. There is a duplex kidney on the right; the ureter from its upper segment drained into the vestibule.

or methylene blue will facilitate its location. The rule in duplex kidneys is that the ureter of the lower moiety is orthotopic, the ureter of the upper moiety always heterotopic and opening inferior to the orthotopic ureter. The upper moiety ureter will always be the ectopic ureter and the affected moiety is usually hydronephrotic; it may drain only one calicine system (*Fig.* U.3).

Incontinence from a *fistula* is usually continuous, but if the abnormal opening is between the ureter and vagina leakage may appear to be intermittent. Fistulae from the urinary tract may communicate with the uterus (in which case urine can be seen escaping from the cervical os), or with the vagina (when the fistulae can usually be seen on speculum examination of the anterior vaginal wall). Uretero-vaginal fistula may arise in the female from erosion of a calculus into one of the vaginal fornices, and also after gynaecological surgery. Vesico-vaginal fistulae are secondary to malignant processes within the upper vagina or in the posterior bladder wall, invading anteriorly or posteriorly respectively. They may follow surgery.

The investigation and diagnosis of incontinence when there is no overt cause such as fistula or congenital abnormality depends on urodynamic assessment of the patient. The study consists of three phases:

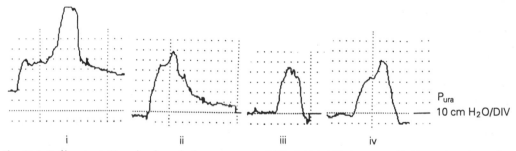

Fig. U.4. Profilometry. i, Normal male urethral pressure profile (UPP). ii, Male UPP showing no bladder neck peak, as after prostatectomy or α-blockage. iii, Female UPP showing sphincter incompetence (predicted normal pressure = 100 – patient's age). iv, Female UPP showing distal urethral stenosis. P_{ura} = urethral pressure.

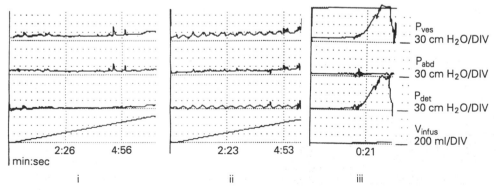

Fig. U.5. Cystometry. i, Normal cystometrogram (CMG). ii, CMG showing detrusor instability. iii, CMG showing a voiding contraction. P_{ves} = intravesical pressure; P_{abd} = abdominal pressure; P_{det} = detrusor pressure; V_{infus} = volume of infusion.

1. *Sphincterometry*, where the pressure exerted by the sphincter apparatus is measured and the configuration of the sphincter complex observed. When there is sphincter incompetence the pressure is low, and when the sphincter is in spasm, as in an upper motor neurone lesion, the pressure is high (*Fig*. U.4).

2. *Cystometry*, where bladder pressure is monitored during filling. Two parameters are measured, the intra-abdominal pressure through a vaginal or rectal transducer and the total bladder pressure through a bladder transducer. Electronic subtraction of the former from the later gives a reading of true or intrinsic bladder pressure.

The bladder is a perfectly compliant organ in that intrinsic bladder pressure does not rise as the bladder fills. The normal curve is observed in genuine stress incontinence. In enuresis and in minor degrees of bladder disturbance secondary to upper motor neurone lesions, a 'delayed voiding contraction' is seen, the bladder contracting vigorously near capacity. When the bladder is extremely irritable, as in acute cystitis, or when there is an upper motor neurone lesion affecting the bladder to a considerable degree, an uninhibited pattern of behaviour is seen. The 'unstable detrusor' is manifest as waves of contraction of a pressure which exceeds 10 cmH$_2$O. In lower motor neurone lesions, or in bladders affected by chronic retention, filling goes on and on with little alteration in intrinsic bladder pressure. (*Fig*. U.5).

3. *Voiding pressure and flow rate*. During the void phase, the bladder voiding pressure and the flow rate are measured. When there is sphincter incompetence voided pressure is low while flow rate is often abnormally high; in obstruction the voiding pressure will be high and the flow rate low.

Lynn Edwards

Urine, retention of

Retention of urine is the inability to empty the bladder completely; the end result is the acute or gradual accumulation of urine within the bladder. In *acute retention* there is a sudden inability to pass urine. The condition is painful and presents as a surgical emergency. In **chronic retention** there is a gradual increase in bladder size; it can often reach enormous proportions, occasionally reaching as high as the xiphisternum (see *Fig*. U.1). Pressure effects on the upper tract are not uncommon and an elevation of the blood urea, in association with bilateral hydronephrosis and hydroureters, is observed; the condition is a medical emergency in that stabilization of the biochemical changes is a pre-requisite precursor to surgical correction of the cause. Retention of the urine must be distinguished from anuria, when the kidneys fail to

secrete urine. In retention, whether acute or chronic, the kidneys still function and urine continues to collect in the distended bladder.

Acute retention

Acute retention produces severe pain. The bladder is palpable some two fingers' breadths above the symphysis pubis. It is central, tense and tender. The commonest cause is outflow tract obstruction in the male, secondary to *prostatic enlargement* or *bladder neck stenosis*. It should be noted that the severity of outflow tract obstruction bears no relation to the size of the prostate, a tiny prostate often being responsible for an acute retentive episode, the largest prostate often remaining asymptomatic.

Acute retention from **urethral stricture** alone is uncommon but secondary spasm and congestion proximal to the stricture, especially involving the sphincter apparatus, may result in retention.

Acute retention may be precipitated by exposure to *cold*, overindulgence in *alcohol*, the administration of *anticholinergic agents* in order to relieve the urinary frequency which the patient almost invariably has, and *bronchodilating agents*, thus explaining the increased frequency of acute retention in elderly men with chronic bronchitis in winter when their chests need treatment. Under some circumstances, particularly delay in the act of micturition beyond reasonable limits, a feat often accomplished while the patient is 'anesthetized' with alcohol, the prostate becomes acutely congested and retention follows. The retention is relieved by catheterization, the congestion subsides and normal micturition can be re-established, to recur with the next bout of excess.

Acute retention in women is sometimes associated with *pregnancy*, especially when the *gravid uterus is retroverted*, while large uterine *fibroids* may produce the same effect. In young women, *herpes genitalis*, acquired as a sexually transmitted disease, may also precipitate acute retention, not only because of the urethral oedema associated with the herpetic lesions, but also by neurological involvement of the sacral reflex arc in such a way that detrusor activity is lost. *Herpes zoster* may give rise to acute retention in both sexes; in this case the pathognomonic herpetic eruptions will be seen over the buttock area or the sacrum.

Chronic retention

Chronic retention is insidious in its onset and symptoms develop so slowly that the patient may deny urinary difficulty. It is only in retrospect and after surgical correction that the patient admits that there were significantly lower urinary track symptoms preoperatively. Enuresis (bed-wetting) is a frequent presenting feature.

Retention secondary to *urethral stricture* can be related to previous episodes of sexually transmitted diseases, chlamydia trachomatis being a potent cause of extensive stricture formation. Primary infection with gonorrhoea is now almost exclusive to the male homosexual population in the UK, but the heterosexual male may acquire gonorrhoea as a result of sexual contact overseas.

The history in stricture is of a gradual increasing difficulty with micturition, slowing of the stream, and dribbling after micturition; this last symptom occurs because of the column of urine which is trapped between the sphincter apparatus and the stricture. An important distinction between stricture and prostatic obstruction is that straining assists urine flow in the former and reduces flow in the latter. The investigation of choice is urethrography (*Fig* U.6). but if instrumentation is undertaken as a primary investigation direct vision urethroscopy is obligatory; the stricture may then be visualized before it has been traumatized and divided appropriately by direct vision urethrotomy.

Prostatic enlargement is unusual below the age of 50 but **bladder neck stenosis** can occur much earlier. The condition which has been recently recognized is that of *detrusor-sphincter dyssynergia*, where contraction of the detrusor is not accompanied by reflex relaxation of the bladder neck. The presenting features of both conditions are similar, the patient having increased frequency of micturition, especially at night, hesitancy, reduction in flow, dribbling postmicturition and sometimes urgency.

On rectal examination, prostatic enlargement may be found. The gland may be smooth, uniform in consistency, elastic and movable within the pelvis when the enlargement is benign. A nodular, hard, irregular prostate may indicate *carcinoma*, while fixation to either side of the pelvic walls implies malignant extension well beyond the confines of the capsule. With bladder neck stenosis and detrusor-sphincter dyssynergia, the prostate is of normal size.

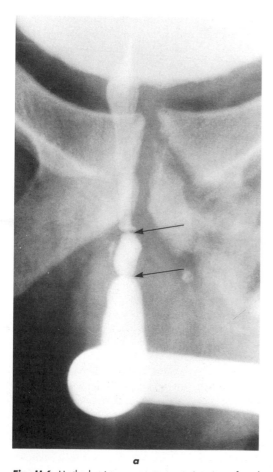
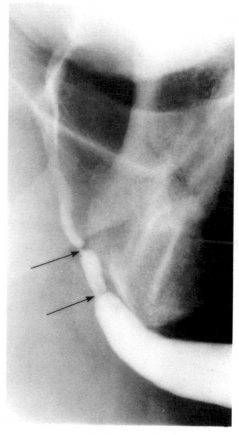

a   *b*

Fig. U.6. Urethral stricture. *a*, anteroposterior view of urethrogram showing two strictures (arrows) of a male urethra, one submembranous, one bulbar. *b*, Same strictures (arrows); lateral view.

When retention of urine follows *acute prostatitis* or a prostatic abscess, a history of recent urethral discharge will be obtained. The patient will be obviously ill, with a fever, rigors, frequency of micturition, pain on micturition, and perineal and pelvic discomfort.

Acute retention of urine secondary to urethral intra-luminal causes is most commonly caused by the *impaction of a calculus* in the urethra. A calculus may impact at the site of a stricture, when it can often be felt on examination of the penis, or at the external urethral meatus, in which case it can usually be seen. The history in such a case is dramatic in that a normal flow of micturition is quite suddenly interrupted, causing a sudden pain along the urethra, a feeling similar to receiving a blow in the bladder area and the dribbling of a few drops of blood.

As transurethral resection is now the favoured procedure for correction of prostatic enlargement, and the removal of all the resulting chips often difficult, especially if there are bladder diverticula, 'chip retention' is a relatively new but not uncommon phenomenon, having the same symptoms as retention secondary to impaction of a stone.

Blockage of the bladder neck by the free-floating area of a *pedunculated bladder tumour* is rare; the growth is forced into the orifice during micturition, causing obstruction.

Complete *traumatic rupture of the urethra* leads to acute retention of urine. It almost always follows rupture of the pelvis but may follow a blow to the perineum, for example from a boot or from falling astride a bar. There will be history of injury and blood will appear at the external urethral meatus; perineal haematoma may not be too evident in pelvic fracture but will certainly indicate local urethral trauma. If urethral rupture is incomplete, the patient should be encouraged not to pass urine as extravasation may occur and cause a haemato-urinoma in the perineum. (*Fig.* U.7).

Prolapse of an intervertebral disc will occasionally cause acute neurological urinary retention from direct pressure on the nerve roots. Retention may occasionally be the presenting feature of the condition which, from the spinal point of view, remains asymptomatic.

Acute retention is a fairly common complication of *operations on the rectum* and neighbouring organs. It also seems to follow operations on the hip (in both sexes) and hernia repairs. The mechanism in these cases must be reflex spasm of the sphincter apparatus. When there is dual pathology, for example, hernia or haemorrhoids in the presence of benign prostatic enlargement, it may be as well to combine the two

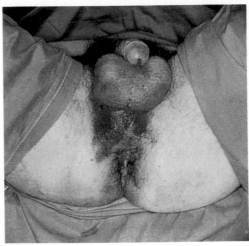

Fig. U.7. Traumatic rupture of the urethra showing blood from meatus and perineal haematoma limited by attachment of Colles' fascia.

surgical procedures to avoid the acute retention that the hernia or haemorrhoid operation may cause. It is particularly important to record prostatic size in all male patients with rectal carcinoma requiring abdomino-perineal excision of the rectum. If acute retention follows such a procedure it is no longer possible to assess prostatic size accurately and inform the patient regarding the prostatectomy technique that will be employed, in that a large gland will be beyond the reasonable range of resection (limit of some 80 gm). This failure to give the patient full information may, of course, change as abdominal ultrasound assessment of prostatic size becomes more accurate. (Transrectal ultrasound assessment is impossible, of course, after excision of the rectum.)

Acute retention of urine may be a manifestation of *hysteria*, but in common with all other diagnoses, medical and surgical, an organic cause should be sought and excluded before any psychogenic element is ascribed to the diagnosis. Hysterical retention usually occurs in children and in young women. Retention due to psychiatric illness is more usually a complication of therapy as tricyclic antidepressants are powerful anticholinergic agents which suppress detrusor activity to the extent that retention, either acute or chronic, may occur.

Acute retention in female children is unusual but it not infrequently occurs in males. While the male infant is still wearing nappies, *ammoniacal ulceration of the foreskin*, or of the meatus if circumcised, can give rise to acute retention because micturition is so painful that the child refuses to allow the act to continue. Retention in the presence of a tight *phimosis* is unusual but the pathognomonic feature will be ballooning of the foreskin during micturition. *Meatal stenosis* following ulceration secondary to circumcision can occasionally lead to acute retention in young males; when micturition is attempted, the urethra can be often felt as a distended and rigid band on the ventrum of the penis. Retention may also follow the inadvertent insertion of a *foreign body*, such as a beam or screw, into the anterior urethra.

Lynn Edwards

Vagina and uterus, prolapse of

Prolapse is essentially a condition in which the supports of the vagina fail to hold it in place, with the result that it tends to turn inside out and to bulge externally at the vulva. Because the uterus is inserted into the vagina vault, if the upper part of the vagina descends the uterus comes down with it as a uterine prolapse or vaginal vault prolapse. The vagina is normally held in place by the transverse cervical ligaments (of Mackenrodt), the pubo-cervical and the utero-sacral ligaments. At a lower level the vagina is supported by the pelvic floor or levatores ani muscles. During pregnancy the supporting ligaments are softened and stretched and during childbirth the opening in the pelvic floor is enlarged. Prolapse therefore occurs mainly in women who have had children, but the vaginal vault may prolapse with projection of the cervix through the vulva in nulliparous women. Prolapse does not usually occur until the menopause and the patient complains of a swelling at the vulva giving rise to a feeling of bearing down and discomfort on walking or straining. The swelling and the symptoms disappear when the patient lies down. If the patient is examined in the left lateral or Sims' position, with a Sims' speculum holding back first the posterior and then the anterior vaginal wall, it is possible to determine which part of the vagina is prolapsing. Low down anteriorly is a *urethrocele*, which is associated with stress incontinence of urine. At a higher level prolapse of the anterior vaginal wall contains the bladder to give rise to a *cystocele*. Straining may cause kinking of the urethra with inability to micturate. The bladder does not empty completely and basal cystitis with urinary frequency is common. *Uterine (or vaginal vault) prolapse* occurs in three degrees. In the first degree the cervix descends to the vulva; in the second it protrudes through the vulva; and in the third, which is a *procidentia*, the whole of the uterus is outside the vulva. Sometimes there is much elongation of the supravaginal portion of the cervix, the vagina is turned completely inside out, but the body of the uterus remains within the pelvis. If the vagina in relation to the posterior fornix prolapses it is related to the pouch of Douglas to give rise to an *enterocele* containing loops of small gut or a *pouch of Douglas hernia*. Lower down the vagina posteriorly is the rectum and prolapse of this part gives rise to a *rectocele*. It is possible to hook the finger into the rectocele through the anus. Patients often find difficulty in emptying the rectum because the faeces tend to go forward into the pouch of the rectocele. Prolapse of the vaginal wall has to be differentiated from other swellings which protrude at the vulva. These include: a *fibroid polyp* which has a pedicle passing through the hard rim of the cervix into the uterine cavity where it is attached; *chronic inversion of the uterus*, a rare condition in which the uterus turns inside out, the fundus passing through the cervical rim leaving a cup-shaped depression where the uterine body should be; a long tongue-shaped *endometrial polyp*; a large *mucous polyp of the cervix*; a *vaginal cyst*; and a *malignant growth* of cervix of vagina.

N. Patel

Vagina, discharge from

The normal discharge from the vagina is a mixture of those from the uterine body, cervix, and vaginal wall; that from the uterine body is watery and small in amount; that from the cervix is thick and mucoid, but clear and transparent, like unboiled white of egg; that from the vagina is merely a transudation of plasma from the vessels, mixed with desquamated vaginal epithelium, and in virgins looks like unboiled starch mixed with water; it is small in amount. The bulk of the discharge found in the vagina comes from the cervix; there are more glands there than in any other part of the genital tract; there are no glands in the vagina. The cervical secretion is alkaline, consisting of mucus with a pH of 6·5. The secretion varies during the menstrual cycle, being abundant, clear, and almost free from leucocytes at the time of ovulation. At this time its elasticity is greater than one inch (*Spinnbarkeit*) and it is more easily penetrated by the spermatozoa. At other times of the month the cervical mucus is scanty, opaque, and tenacious. The secretion from

Bartholin's gland, thin and mucoid, may be copious under sexual excitement, but under normal conditions it is scanty, and so does not contribute to a vaginal discharge. The vaginal mixed secretion is acid in reaction, owing to the presence of lactic acid produced by Doderlein's bacillus from the glycogen in the basal cells of the vaginal epithelium. This bacillus is normally found in the vagina from puberty to the menopause. The pH of the vagina is 4·5, the vaginal acidity being a bar to vaginal infection; unmixed uterine secretion is alkaline.

Normally, the amount of mixed vaginal discharge should do no more than just moisten the vaginal orifice; when the amount is so great as to moisten the vulva and consequently stain garments, the discharge is pathological. *Excess of the normal discharge (leucorrhoea)* may be due to (1) such conditions as anaemia, tuberculosis, chronic nephritis, indeed any debilitating state; (2) any condition causing increased pelvic congestion such as constipation, provoked but unsatisfied sexual desire, masturbation; (3) chronic passive congestion of heart disease or cirrhosis of the liver; (4) endocrine disorders resulting in hypersecretion of the cervical glands, the result of excessive oestrogen stimulation. This is not uncommonly found in those suffering from functional uterine bleeding; (5) no abnormality may be found. In many normal women a premenstrual mucoid discharge is seen, and in pregnant women leucorrhoea, the result of passive congestion or endocrine factors, is commonly encountered. Occasionally a congenital erosion may be responsible.

Girls before puberty and women after the menopause do not have the protection of an acid secretion in the vagina. Non-specific infection is liable to occur and discharge is complained of. A foreign body may be the precipitating factor in young girls. Oestrogen withdrawal is the cause in post-menopausal women, when the condition is referred to as *atrophic (or senile) vaginitis.*

The composition of an abnormal discharge varies according to the source from which it comes and the acuteness of the inflammation; a frankly purulent discharge indicates acute inflammation, whereas a mucopurulent discharge indicates chronic inflammation involving the cervix.

1. The mucopurulent discharge

This, the commonest type, is a thick, white or yellow discharge. It contains must mucus, many leucocytes, masses of epithelium from the vagina (squames) and various bacteria: diphtheroids, streptococci, staphylococci, *Streptococcus faecalis, E. coli.* Doderlein's bacillus will not be found. This discharge is typically produced by endocervicitis and cervical erosions. When endometritis is present as well, which is uncommon, the discharge becomes thinner and white, yellow, brown or even bloodstained. Microscopically, the films made from the mixed cases show proportionally less mucus, but otherwise the constituents are the same.

2. The frankly purulent discharge

This discharge occurs in:

A.   ACUTE CERVICITIS

Due to gonorrhoea or sometimes following puerperal or post-abortal infections; the cervix is red, swollen and oedematous, being bathed in pus. There is nothing characteristic of gonorrhoeal discharges visible to the naked eye. The detection of the gonococcus can alone decide the question. This is often a matter of difficulty, because it is only in the few days immediately after infection that the organism can be found in the discharge. In chronic cases the gonococcus must be looked for in one of three places—in the interior of the cervical canal, in the urethra and Skene's tubules which open posterolaterally at the entrance to the urethra, or in discharge squeezed from the orifices of Bartholin's glands. Discharge from the cervical canal should be taken on a platinum loop after carefully wiping away discharge from the os uteri with sterile wool, using a vaginal speculum. This discharge should be spread on to two glass slides and put by to dry. Two other films should then be made by massaging the urethra from above downwards and collecting any discharge thus made to appear at the urinary meatus. It is important that micturition should not have taken place for several hours beforehand. Finally two films should be taken from the orifices at Bartholin's glands after squeezing the glands between the finger and thumb. After drying in the air the films should be fixed by passing through a flame and then stained by Gram's method, followed by neutral red as a counter stain. In films thus prepared gonococci are strained red (Gram-negative) while organisms which retain Gram's stain appear deep violet or black (Gram-positive). The gonococci are found as diplococci in the cytoplasm of the polymorphonuclear leucocytes and epithelial cells. Cultures of the discharge should also be taken and grown on a suitable medium such as chocolate agar.

B.   GRANULAR VAGINITIS

The discharge is copious and purulent. It is associated with trauma of the vagina from the irritation of rubber, or poorly fitting ring pessaries, or actual ulceration as in decubitus ulcers on prolapsed portions. Practically no mucus is found in such discharge unless the cervix shares in the inflammatory process.

C. TRICHOMONAS VAGINITIS

Due to a flagellate parasite, this produces a frothy purulent discharge causing local pain and soreness and being extremely irritating to the external genitalia. The discharge is green or greenish-yellow with small bubbles of gas in it and has a characteristic odour. The protozoon is to be found by diluting some of the vaginal discharge with normal warm saline and examining with a high-power lens, when the parasite, which is about the size of a leucocyte, will be found actively mobile, being propelled by its flagellae. The trichomonas live in the vagina in symbiosis with the micrococcus *Aerogenes alcaligenes*, which organism forms the froth or bubbles so characteristic of the discharge, It is a Gram-negative micrococcus, smaller than the gonococcus. The vaginal walls have a typical red stippled appearance.

D. MONILIA VAGINITIS

Common during pregnancy, giving rise to white patches of thrush on the vagina walls. It is a common cause of pruritis vulvae. It may complicate diabetes and the urine should always therefore be tested for sugar. If the white patches are scraped off the vaginal walls they leave raw bleeding areas. Vaginitis rarely exists alone, but when it does occur the discharge is thick and pasty if it is a simple catarrhal condition— pasty on account of the large admixture of vaginal squamous epithelium. Specimens of the discharge should be taken for recognition of the mycelium and spores of *Candida albicans* in stained smears and for culture.

E. NON-SPECIFIC VAGINITIS

Some patients with a purulent and offensive discharge who do not have trichomoniasis have large numbers of *Gardnerella vaginalis* (*haemophilus*) and anaerobic bacteria in the vagina. The pH is 5·0 or more and the treatment similar to that of a trichomonas infection.

3. Offensive-smelling vaginal discharge

This discharge is associated with decomposition; the discharge itself may decompose because it cannot escape fast enough from the passage, or the source of the discharge may be a decomposing substance like a *sloughing fibroid* or necrotic *carcinoma of the cervix*; in the two latter cases the discharge is copious, watery, and bloodstained, with a horribly fetid smell. When the discharge itself is decomposing it is usually thick and purulent as when a retained foreign body

such as a ring pessary, an internal tampon or contraceptive cap is the cause. Infected retained gestation products, a faecal fistula or a pelvic abscess rupturing into the vagina (*E. coli*) may occasionally be responsible. In elderly women a foul discharge may come from the interior of the uterus, a *pyometra*; in which case pus can be made to flow from the os uteri by squeezing the uterus or passing a sound; it is due to *senile endometritis*, or it may be associated with carcinoma of the uterine body or cervix.

4. Watery blood-stained discharge

Watery blood-stained discharge, not offensive occurs with *carcinoma of the body of the uterus* in early *carcinoma of the cervix*, with *mucous polyps, placental polyps, hydatidiform mole* and *new growths of the Fallopian tubes*. Other causes such as endometrial hyperplasia, rupture of the membranes in early pregnancy, or an intermittent hydrosalpinx may be responsible. The differential diagnosis of these conditions cannot be made from the discharge alone, but must rest upon physical examination combined with the use of the microscope upon materials removed from the uterus. The use of vaginal smear tests (Papanicolaou) may help in the diagnosis, as in some cases cancer cells may be found in the discharge, but if malignancy is suspected reliance should not be placed on this test alone. Whenever there is any blood in the discharge the patient should be examined under anaesthesia and biopsies taken of the endometrium and cervix in case of malignancy.

Smears of the cervix and vagina may be taken with a wooden spatula (Ayre) for cytology. Malignant cells may be found in symptomless women with apparently normal cervices. Colposcopy and cervical biopsy is used to make the decision of cervical intra-epithelial disease. This condition is found in about 5 in every 1000 women examined over the age of 30 years. Its discovery and removal from the population may lead to the reduction in incidence of invasive carcinoma of the cervix but the hoped-for abolition has not been realized due to failure of screening programmes and the fact that a small proportion of invasive growth seems to pass through a carcinoma-in-situ phase.

Vaginal casts may be composed of coagulated surface epithelium, the result of astringent injections or applications, and are recognized easily with the microscope. Membranous flakes may be passed with discharge in cases of *membranous vaginitis*; they consist of vaginal epithelium entangled in coagulated blood plasma, and present quite a different appearance from casts of coagulated epithelia layers. These membranous masses may be seen lining the whole vagina, and are generally due to special organisms. The *diph-*

theria bacillus has been found to be the causal agent in some; in others the *Escherichia coli*.

N. Patel

Vagina, swelling in

Inflammatory

Gonorrhoeal
Non-specific; (*a*) streptococcus; (*b*) staphylococcus;
  (*c*) E. coli
Trichomonas
Monilia
Senile
Chemical

New growth

1   Innocent:
    a. Cystic: (i) cysts of Gartne's duct; (ii) implantation cysts; (iii) endometriomas
    b. Solid: (i) fibroma; (ii) adenomyoma
2   Malignant. Primary carcinoma, primary sarcoma, secondary carcinoma

The vagina is resistant to infection because of its lining of stratified epithelium and the absence of glands; further protection is brought about by the action of Doderlein's bacillus on the glycogen in the vaginal cells, producing lactic acid where keeps the pH of the vagina at about 4·5. This acidity inhibits the growth of most organisms during the menstrual life of a woman; before puberty and after the menopause this protection is non-existent.

Trichomonas vaginitis is very common and gives rise to a typical red stippling of the vaginal walls, particularly in the fornices. The discharge is frothy, greenish-yellow in colour, and has a rather characteristic unpleasant smell. A discharge of sudden onset with soreness of the vulva is often due to trichomonas vaginitis. Sometimes *Gardnerella vaginalis (haemophilus)* and anaerobic bacteria are found.

Monilial infection may occur in the debilitated subject, but is most typically seen in diabetes. The discharge is thick, white, curdy and adherent to the vaginal walls. An accompanying vulvitis that has the appearance of raw beef steak with a rather abrupt edge is characteristic; pruritus is the leading symptom.

Gonorrhoeal vaginitis is most frequently seen in the young child. It is not common in the adult because of the vaginal resistance to infection.

The non-specific forms of vaginitis, due to *E. coli, Staph, aureus* and streptococci, are usually associated with the retention of some foreign body, such as tampons, or a ring pessary. It may also occur before puberty or following childbirth or abortion.

Chemical. Occasionally a too-hot vaginal douche or the use of strong chemicals, such as potassium permanganate, may be responsible. The characteristic signs of inflammation, with vaginal discharge, are present.

Senile vaginitis. This is a common condition occurring after the menopause when the protective mechanism of the vagina is lost. The vaginal epithelium is thinned, and, in places, minute areas become completely denuded of epithelium, and appear as red points, giving a somewhat spotted appearance to the vagina. These areas may adhere and cause vaginal adhesions; they also cause a thin blood-stained watery discharge. On breaking down the adhesions with the finger, frank bleeding may take place. Senile vaginitis is most marked in the upper part of the vagina.

Cysts of Gartner's duct are cystic growths of the remains of the Wolffian duct, which has failed to be obliterated. They are always found in the anterolateral wall of the vagina. They may be small but sometimes grow to a large size, protruding outside the vaginal orifice and occluding the vaginal cavity. The characteristic position and cystic feel serve to differentiate them from the various types of vaginal prolapse. *Small implantation cysts* may be seen at the vaginal orifice posteriorly; they are small, and may follow operations on the perineum, or lacerations at childbirth. Occasionally an *endometrioma* may burrow through into the posterior vaginal fornix from the floor of the pouch of Douglas, forming nodular growths which tend to bleed at the time of menstruation. This condition may be confused with a primary carcinoma of the vagina, but it is not friable. Microscopic section will settle its nature.

Benign tumours. Sessile and pedunculated swellings arise in the vaginal wall which on histology are found to be papilloma, fibroma or lipoma. They are uncommon.

Primary carcinoma of the vagina is rare. It occurs in the posterior fornix, often following the retention of a pessary which has been forgotten for a number of years. It usually takes the form of a typical epitheliomatous ulcer eventually producing a rectovaginal fistula. Its friability and vascularity make the diagnosis clear, which should be confirmed by biopsy. A rare form of adenocarcinoma occurs in the vagina of teenage girls whose mothers took large doses of stilboestrol during their pregnancies. It has to be differentiated from benign adenosis vaginae in which there are numerous small swellings in the mucosa with a profuse discharge of mucus.

Secondary carcinoma usually spreads to the upper part of the vagina from the cervix. Occasionally metastases spread from carcinoma of the body of the uterus; they occur constantly at the lower end of the vagina in the midline anteriorly about half an inch behind the urethral meatus. Curettage reveals the uterine growth and biopsy the nature of the metastasis. Secondary growths have been described as occurring at the same site from primary carcinomas in the ovary and colon and also from hypernephroma of the kidney. They may ulcerate, causing bleeding. Microscopical examination will reveal their true nature.

Sarcoma of the vagina is rare, but occasionally the grape-like tumour sarcoma botryoides (or embryonal rhabdomyosarcoma) may appear to originate in the vagina rather than in the cervix. It occurs in infants and young children and is one of the causes of vaginal bleeding before puberty. It has a characteristic appearance, like a bunch of grapes, and microscopic section proves its nature.

In the normal adult the healthy vaginal transudation will be found to contain many cornified cells and few, if any, leucocytes. This is due to the normal circulation of oestrogen. Excessive oestrogen stimulation leads to a multiplication of the layers of the vaginal epithelial cells with an increase in their glycogen content. At the menopause, due to lack of oestrogen stimulation, the transudation contains few cornified cells but many nucleated cells and leucocytes. It is thus possible, by examining a smear of vaginal cells obtained from the pool of discharge in the posterior vaginal fornix and rolled on to a slide with a swab-stick, to obtain some idea of the excess or deficiency of oestrogen. The healthy vaginal walls take on a deep brown colour if painted with Lugol's iodine solution, due to the abundance of glycogen in the vaginal cells. This is also an indication of oestrogen sufficiency.

As carcinoma is an exfoliative disease cancer cells can be found in preparations of vaginal and cervical smears in some cases of carcinoma of the cervix or corpus uteri. The taking of smears is simple but the correct interpretation of the findings requires experience. It can be of the greatest use, however, as a positive smear test for cancer cells, the absence of any symptoms or obvious signs of carcinoma of the uterus, calls for a thorough examination of the cervix with a colposcope and the uterine cavity by curettage. In about 5 cases per 1000 of women examined the biopsy shows disease of the cervix. Invasive cancer can be prevented in these cases by cauterization, laser treatment or cone biopsy. If the disease persists after treatment and positive smears are obtained, a cone biopsy or hysterectomy is indicated.

N. Patel

Veins, varicose abdominal

The point at which distension of veins becomes varicosity is arbitrary; most conditions that produce undoubted varicosity of the veins of the abdominal wall in some cases merely dilate them in others. When this dilatation is considerable (*Fig.* V.1) it nearly always has much diagnostic significance, particularly if the direction of blood flow is reversed.

Veins, however, may seem to be dilated when they are but unduly visible owing to wasting of the subcutaneous fat; or they may, in rare cases, be simply varicose, like veins in the leg, owing to idiosyncrasy or hereditary predisposition. In neither of these cases however, is the blood current in them reversed. To test the direction of blood flow, part of a vein should be chosen where there are no side branches, and the blood should be expressed from it by means of two fingers pressed gently down on the vein close together and then drawn apart whilst pressure over the vein is maintained by each; when a length of the distended vein has been emptied in this way, one of the two fingers is taken off, and the time taken by the vein in refilling is noted. The procedure is repeated, the other finger being taken off this time; it is then generally easy to decide whether the vein fills from below upwards or from above downwards. Normally, the blood flows from above downwards in the veins of the lower two-thirds of the abdominal wall; when the blood flow is from below upwards there is almost certainly obstruction to the inferior vena cava, the blood which is unable to return by it finding a collateral circulation via the abdominal parietes to the superior vena cava.

Obstruction to the inferior vena cava is due to one or other of three main groups of conditions, namely:

1 *Great general increase in the intra-abdominal tension*, owing to such conditions as: ascites, ovarian cyst, great splenic or hepatic enlargement.
2 *Thrombosis* without external obstruction.
3 *Obstruction by local compression*, especially by secondary deposits in the retroperitoneal lymph nodes.

When the obstruction of the inferior vena cava is due not to the vein itself being thrombosed or invaded by new growth but to the *general intra-abdominal pressure* becoming so great that the vein is, so to speak, flattened out, the varicosity of the veins upon the abdominal wall is but a late symptom, and the diagnosis of the cause of the great abdominal distension, generally ascites or a large tumour, will already have been made. If there is marked varicosity of the superficial veins early in a case of ascites the probability is that both are due to malignant disease.

When the inferior vena cava is obstructed by 'simple' thrombosis, the clotting will probably have started, not in the inferior vena cava itself, but below it, either in the legs or in the pelvis; oedema of the legs will be pronounced, and it may be ascertained that one leg became oedematous and painful before the other; when this is so it suggests thrombosis starting

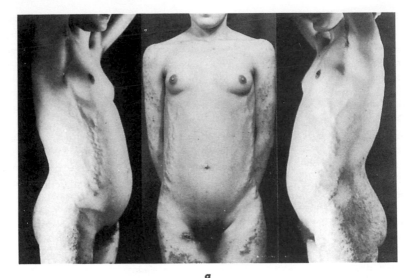

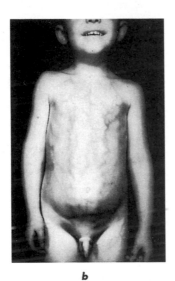

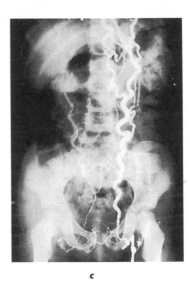

Fig. V.1. Inferior vena caval obstruction showing greatly dilated collaterals by means of surface and infra-red photography and by venography. (*Dr R. G. Ollerenshaw, Manchester Royal Infirmary.*)

in the calf or femoral vein of one side, the other leg becoming affected later when the clot has spread up through the iliac veins of the one side to the inferior vena, and thence down the iliac veins of the other side. The higher the thrombosis extends the higher up the back will the oedema spread; and when the renal veins have been reached, albuminuria, with tube casts, haematuria and ascites, may ensue, and acute nephritis may be simulated. Distension or varicosity of the veins of the abdominal wall assists in distinguishing such a case from one of acute or sub-acute nephritis; besides which there will be no oedema of the eyelids or face.

If there is no very tense distension of the abdomen; if the way the case began does not suggest

thrombosis in one leg, or in the pelvis, extending upwards; and if, nevertheless, there is marked varicosity of the veins of the lower part of the abdominal wall, with the blood flow in them reversed, so as to be from below upwards, the history being a relatively short one—the probability is that the inferior vena cava is being obstructed by something that is in immediate contact with it. There will very likely be symmetrical oedema of the legs, and possibly albuminuria and haematuria. It is remarkable how seldom an aortic aneurysm or other non-malignant mass obstructs a large vein sufficiently to produce this collateral varicosity; hence, the presumption is that such varicosity indicates *malignant disease*. It is worthy of note that carcinoma of the kidney is prone to extend into the renal veins and thus into the inferior vena cava by direct extension—sometimes the malignant clot reaches as far as the right atrium, and may produce therein a pedunculated polyp. In such cases there has generally been haematuria or other renal symptoms before evidence of inferior vena caval obstruction arises, whereby cases of growth in the kidney invading the inferior vena cava may be distinguished from cases of secondary growth in the retroperitoneal nodes, which if they produced haematuria at all, would do so by first obstructing the inferior vena cava, and thence involving the renal veins. In such cases there are often other symptoms pointing to primary growth in some organ from which lymphatics drain into the retroperitoneal nodes; the testes and ovaries should not be overlooked in this respect.

It is said that *cirrhosis of the liver* leads to varicosity of the veins around the umbilicus—the *caput medusae*; most cases of cirrhosis of the liver cause no distension of the superficial abdominal veins until the general intra-abdominal tension has been greatly increased by the tenseness of the ascites which occurs late. Not even the telangiectases that occur so commonly in men past middle age around the lower part of the chest, in a line with the attachment of the diaphragm, indicate cirrhosis; they are quite as common in cases of emphysema without cirrhosis.

Varicosity of the superficial abdominal veins generally indicates either thrombosis of the inferior vena cava, secondary to direct spread of thrombosis up to it from veins in the pelvis or in the leg, or else stenosis of the vena cava by secondary malignant disease.

Harold Ellis

Vertigo

(*See also* FAINTS)

The term 'vertigo' implies by derivation a subjective sense of rotation, either of one's self or of the surroundings, but it is helpful to include within the term simply a feeling of being off-balance, without any sense of rotation, which some patients with Menière's disease experience between the more usual spinning attacks. Likewise the sensation which some people experience when looking down from a height or in the presence of diplopia might also be described as vertigo. It can then be concluded that vertigo, as more broadly defined, must always mean some involvement of the vestibular apparatus, either in its peripheral pathways or central connections.

Vertigo due to affections of the *external auditory meatus* must be very rare, if indeed it occurs at all, but removal of wax is said to have cured vertigo on occasion. *Disease of the middle ear and blockage of*

the Eustachian tubes by catarrh or new growth may be accompanied by vertigo but probably the labyrinth is affected too in all such cases. Thus otitis media can cause either a serous or a purulent labyrinthitis, and otosclerosis may spread to involve the inner ear. If infection has caused a fistula into the internal ear, vertigo can occur either spontaneously or by increasing the pressure in the external meatus (the fistula sign), or even by the pressure changes within the Eustachian tubes during swallowing. These conditions of the middle ear are usually accompanied by deafness and tinnitus, and by auroscopic evidence of disease.

Disease of the internal ear is the most common source of paroxysmal vertigo. Labyrinthine causes may be listed under six subheadings:

1 *Spread of disease* from the middle ear as described above.
2 *Ototoxicity* with salicylates, quinine, streptomycin and acute alcoholism.
3 *Allergy* to foods, a very rare cause.
4 *Haemorrhage* into the semicircular canals, as in any disease accompanied by purpura or by a bleeding diathesis.
5 *Menière's disease*: a common affection due to degenerative changes in the membranous labyrinth with hydrops of the endolymph and characterized by paroxysms of vertigo which last minutes or hours and are often accompanied by pallor, prostration, vomiting, slight mental confusion and pain behind the ear or a more generalized headache. Vestibular nystagmus occurs during the vertigo but is not present between attacks. Tinnitus and nerve deafness ultimately supervene but are often slight or absent in the early stages of the disease.
6 *Positional* vertigo, which may arise when the head is placed in a particular position, can result either from a peripheral or from a central lesion.

If peripheral, the condition is commonly attributed to disease of the otolith organ and severe vertigo is experienced when the head is lowered so that the affected otolith organ is undermost. The vertigo will eventually pass off if the head is maintained in this position and there will be increasingly less vertigo as the manoeuvre of lowering the head with the affected otolith organ undermost is repeated. The vertigo may or may not be accompanied by nystagmus. This condition may develop after head injury, possibly as a result of nearby infection or for no apparent reason.

Positional vertigo may also arise, however, from central lesions such as multiple sclerosis or cerebellar neoplasm, often metastatic, and in such cases there is no adaptation but the vertigo is present and persists for as long as the head is held in the critical position.

Affections of the vestibular component of the 8th nerve are an infrequent source of vertigo so far as is known at present. In vestibular neuronitis there is intense vertigo with which a patient may waken and which may be accompanied by vomiting unless he lies absolutely still. There is no associated deafness or tinnitus but the caloric responses are abnormal in one or both ears. The intense vertigo usually passes off within a few days but there remains a liability to brief vertigo on head movement which may persist for weeks or even months. In many cases there is evidence of infection in the nose, sinuses; or tonsils. There is no pathological evidence as to its nature, but the term 'vestibular neuronitis' serves as a convenient label pending further clarification of the subject. In some cases the discomfort falls short of obvious vertigo, amounting to no more than an intermittent sense of inequilibrium which is aggravated by moving the head or by walking.

Less common than the above are *gross lesions of the 8th nerve*, notably *acoustic tumours, syphilitic and other inflammatory affections of the cerebello-pontine recess, tumour of the petrous temporal bone, and gliomas and haemangioblastomas at the point where the nerve enters the pons*. The most important of these is the *neuroma*, a benign tumour which is easy to remove when small but which constitutes a formidable surgical hazard once it has grown large enough to produce the 'classic' signs—deafness, loss of the corneal reflex, facial weakness, homolateral cerebellar signs, and raised intracranial pressure with papilloedema. Fortunately, early diagnosis is now practicable in many cases at the stage of moderate deafness, with or without vertigo, and long before the facial or trigeminal nerves are affected, intracranial pressure is raised or the internal auditory meatus is expanded by the growth. In cochlear lesions the deafness is characterized by the fact that once the threshold of hearing is reached, sounds are heard as well as in the normal ear—and may even appear louder. This phenomenon is called *recruitment* and it is absent in deafness due to affections of the nerve itself. That is to say, in an 8th nerve tumour the affected ear will hear less than the normal side at all ranges of sound intensity. The best test, however, is the MRI scan with gadolineum enhancement. It is essential, therefore, to have tests carried out in all cases of vertigo and deafness for which no satisfactory explanation can be found.

Affections of the *medulla and lower pons* can cause vertigo. It may be paroxysmal or continuous, but generally speaking the diagnosis depends less upon the quality of the giddiness than on satellite symptoms and signs arising from simultaneous involvement of structures adjacent to the vestibular fibres and Deiter's vestibular nucleus. There is seldom tinnitus or deafness, because the auditory and vestibular pathways diverge after the 8th nerve enters the pons, but long tracts may be involved and nystagmus is present even when the patient is not actually feeling vertiginous; in labyrin-

thine and vestibular nerve lesions it usually ceases between attacks. Moreover, the nystagmus changes character: in labyrinthine and nerve lesions the quick component is always towards the affected side, whereas in central affections it is towards the left when the patient looks to the left and to the right when he looks to the right. (This is an oversimplification of a complicated subject, but it is a useful working rule, valid for most cases.) The diseases which produce vertigo in this situation include *multiple sclerosis*, thrombosis of the *posterior inferior cerebellar artery*, atheromatous *stenosis* of the basilar artery, *tumours* and *syringobulbia*. A condition notable for its extreme rarity and for its popularity amongst collectors of the recondite is *cysticercosis of the 4th ventricle*, which has been known to cause vertigo when the head is moved.

Cerebellar disease and injury can give rise to vertigo, more especially if the lesion is acute, as in penetrating injuries and infarction, but generally speaking chronic lesions cause a sense of disequilibrium rather than a sense of movement. In the case of tumours, however, a true vertigo may occur either through direct pressure on the vestibular centre in the brainstem, or from *a rise of intracranial pressure* (which is communicated to the labyrinth through the ductus endolymphaticus), or perhaps from traction on the 8th nerve. It is apposite to remark that *transient vertigo can be caused by any rise of intracranial pressure*, irrespective of the nature or position of the lesion.

Disease of the cerebral hemispheres seldom causes vertigo. It can occur as the aura of an *epileptic fit*, and is occasionally seen in *migraine*, but it is uncommon in supratentorial tumours unless the intracranial pressure is high.

The relationship between 'giddiness' and *head injuries* requires separate treatment, because it is seldom possible to ascertain the anatomical seat of the trouble. Following either minor or major cerebral contusion, the patient is apt to complain of dizziness on quick movements of the head or movements of the head in space. Occasionally it amounts to a true vertigo, but more often it falls short of this and is described as dizziness or giddiness. In a minority of cases there is evidence of damage to the labyrinth, or to the 8th nerve, but usually there is no such evidence and the patient comes to the doctor with complaints not only of dizzy spells but of nervousness, irritability, incapacity for mental and physical effort, and dislike of loud noises—a story liable to be mistaken for neurosis by the uninformed. There is evidence that such cases react abnormally to labyrinthine tests, but it is not clear whether the site of the damage is in the

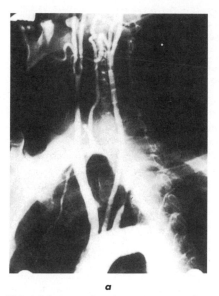 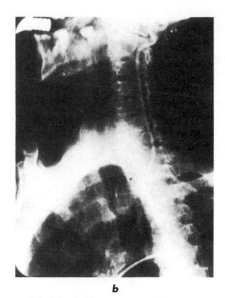

a   b

Fig. V.2. Subclavian steal syndrome. Aortogram showing (*a*) occlusion of the left subclavian artery and (*b*) some 6 seconds later showing filling of the distal portion of the subclavian artery by means of retrograde flow in the left vertebral artery.

semicircular canals or in the afferent conducting system. The main interest of this work is to confirm what neurologists have believed for many years, viz. that there is an organic basis for 'dizziness' and vertigo after head injury. The fact that patients are sometimes encouraged by circumstances to prolong these symptoms for gain does not invalidate this view.

Vertigo also occurs in *anaemias*, in *hypertension* and in *hypotensive states*. Anaemia, whether acute or chronic, can not only aggravate vertigo due to other processes but can also cause either lightheadedness or transient mild attacks of vertigo. With regard to hypertension, the position is confused by the circumstance that hypertension, atheroma and labyrinthine disease are all found in the same age-group. While it is true that hypertensives sometimes complain of vertigo, there is no evidence that the raised blood pressure is directly to blame and it is wiser to avoid this facile diagnostic alibi. The 'giddiness' of which so many hypertensives complain often resolves itself, on cross-examination, into a sense of confusion or faintness or lightheadedness rather than a true vertigo, and of those whose testimony survives interrogation some turn out to have labyrinthine disease and other are clearly suffering from focal or diffuse vascular lesions of the brain. Atheromatous stenosis of the basilar artery is frequently accompanied by vertigo presumably from reduction of blood supply to the brainstem.

A further interesting cause of vertigo is the 'subclavian steal syndrome' (*Fig.* V.2). In this there is severe stenosis or occlusion of the subclavian artery before the origin of the vertebral artery and the blood pressure

in that arm is considerably reduced. Characteristically, when the arm is used the distal part of the subclavian artery is supplied by reverse flow by the vertebral artery, thus rendering the hindbrain ischaemic and causing vertigo.

Vertigo induced by turning the head in a particular way, sometimes known as 'cervical vertigo', can occur in subjects suffering from atheromatous stenosis of the carotid artery, or a similar narrowing of the vertebral arteries. It is thought that the flow of blood to the brain is obstructed by the movement of the head, and there is some evidence that the vetebral artery may also be compressed within its bony canal by the bulging intervertebral discs of spondylosis. Unlike positional vertigo, it is a movement of the neck, and not the position of the head, which determines the symptoms. In place of vertigo there may be syncope or merely a feeling of lightheadedness.

Hypertensive encephalopathy, i.e. cerebral symptoms of brief duration accompanying an exacerbation of an already high blood pressure, is said to include vertigo amongst its protean manifestations; this may be so, but it is always difficult to be sure of this diagnosis. Any sudden fall or cardiac output, whether from a haemorrhage, cardiac infarction, cardiac arrhythmia, or a prolonged fit of coughing (laryngeal vertigo), can cause vertigo, either by itself or as a prelude to complete syncope. The common faint is often preceded by vertigo, but it is usually coupled with sensations of lightheadedness, nausea, and tinnitus.

Hypotensive drugs used in the treatment of hypertension may produce faintness and occasional vertigo, particularly after sudden changes of posture from recumbency to the erect position.

Finally, there is no evidence whatsoever that true vertigo, as defined here, can be 'psychogenic'. On the other hand, vertigo is a frightening and unsettling experience which, when persistent or recurrent, can cause anxiety and loss of morale even in the most stable of persons, and its effect on neurotic subjects can be cataclysmic. Indeed, the emotional and visceral disturbances may come in time to overshadow the organic nucleus of the illness.

A. G. D. Maran

Vesicles

A vesicle is a circumscribed elevation of the skin varying in size from that of a pin's head to that of a small pea, containing free fluid. Vesicles larger than 5 mm in diameter are usually called 'bullae' (blisters). The fluid in vesicles or bullae may be lymph, serum, extracellular fluid or blood. If vesicles become purulent they are termed *pustules* (*see* p. 540). They may be of any shape, but are usually round. While some dermatoses produce both vesicles and bullae, others show predominantly one or other type of lesion. The dermatoses discussed in this section are chiefly vesicular.

Vesicles may be *grouped* together e.g. herpes, or be scattered more widely apart. The *scattered* lesions may be *generalized* e.g. chickenpox, or occur in particular areas, e.g. hands in cheiropompholyx (*see Table* V.1).

Grouped vesicles

Herpes simplex may occur anywhere on the body—the face (*Fig.* V.3) and genitalia being the most common sites. *Primary* attacks are more severe than the more familiar recurrent *secondary* attacks which appear at the original site or close to it. Type II herpes simplex virus usually causes more severe lesions, with increased toxicity and more likelihood of recurrent disease. Recurrent herpes lesions can be precipitated by fever (cold sores), sunburn, friction and by gastrointestinal or emotional upset. Lesions begin with a patch of burning itchy erythema; on this a group of clear tiny vesicles soon forms. These dry up and form yellowish crusts, which after a few days detach sometimes leaving tiny grouped scars. On the mucous membranes the course of the disease is slightly different; vesicles become macerated and the roofs rub off, leaving painful round erosions or shallow ulcers.

In the crusted stage facial herpes may resemble *impetigo*, but the rapid course herpes runs, its limited distribution and failure to spread elsewhere on the face or body, and the fact that in impetigo the lips

Table V.1. Vesicles

Grouped vesicles
 Herpes simplex (*Fig.* V.3)
 Eczema herpeticum (*Fig.* C.50)
 Herpes zoster (*Fig.* V.4)
 Acute dermatitis
 Lymphangioma circumscriptum
 Dermatitis herpetiformis
 Familial benign chronic pemphigus

Scattered discrete vesicles

Generalized
 Varicella
 (Smallpox)
 Scabies (*Fig.* V.5)
 Allergic vasculitis

Hands, feet and mouth
 Hand, foot and mouth disease

Hands and feet
 Pompholyx (*Figs* B.44, V.6)
 Vesicular id

On exposed skin
 Porphyria cutanea tarda
 Hydroa aestivale
 Plant dermatitis
 Insect bites (*Fig.* B.42)
 Photodermatitis

are seldom affected, should suffice to differentiate them. It must be remembered that a healing herpetic lesion can become secondarily impetiginized.

The commonest sites for *herpes genitalis* are the glans penis, the inner side of the prepuce, the labia or the cervix uteri. Genital herpes cannot be mistaken if it is seen before rupture of the vesicles occurs. In some cases there may be doubt as between herpes genitalis and syphilitic chancre. The points for differentiation are in herpes the absence of induration, the less considerable and more transitory lymph node enlargement, the group of small vesicles leading to ulcers and particularly the intense burning and itching, a chancre being absolutely painless. Occasionally herpes can be responsible for a 'whitlow' (*see* Fig. F.39). This usually occurs as a primary attack after inoculation of the virus into the finger, e.g. a nurse carrying out oral toilet on a patient with a cold sore.

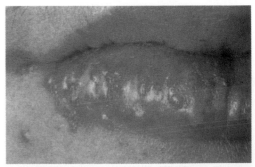

Fig. V.3. Herpes labialis. (Westminster Hospital.)

There is intense pain and a multilocular vesicle will be associated with draining lymphadenopathy.

Eczema herpeticum occurs in children or adolescents with atopic dermatitis. A primary or secondary attack of herpes simplex can spread from a confined area, e.g. near the mouth, to form large sheets of innumerable uniform-sized umbilicated vesicles superimposed on patches of dermatitis. There is usually associated toxicity and prostration and in the very young the condition can be fatal.

Herpes zoster causes a band of vesicles along a dermatome (*Fig.* V.4). It is caused by a secondary activation of *varicella* virus lying dormant in nervous tissue following primary (chickenpox) infection, sometimes as long as 60 years previously. The condition is rare in childhood and more common with increasing age. It also occurs in those immunosuppressed by drugs or HIV disease, systemic illness or malignancy, where it may be accompanied by toxicity and disseminated chickenpox lesions.

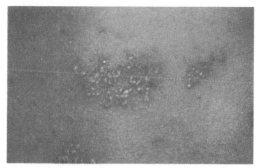

Fig. V.4. Close up of vesicles of herpes zoster. (*St Stephen's Hospital.*)

Pain usually precedes obvious skin changes by up to 48 hours. The first sign in the skin is erythema on which grouped clear vesicles appear, which later become umbilicated and haemorrhagic (*Fig.* V.4). Smears from the base of vesicles show multinucleated giant cells. The limitation to one side of the body, the distribution in one or more dermatomes and the pain usually suffice to distinguish zoster from erythema multiforme and dermatitis herpetiformis. When the trunk is affected the preceding pain may be mistaken for pleurisy or some intra-abdominal condition. The pain may also simulate myocardial infarction, slipped disc, orchitis or venous thrombosis depending on the site affected. When the second division of the trigeminal nerve is affected involvement of the tip of the nose with vesicles indicates infection of the nasociliary branch of the ophthalmic nerve and hence is a sign that keratitis may occur.

Vesicles are the hallmark of *acute dermatitis*. Dermatitis is an inflammatory response of the skin to a variety of irritants, allergens or other stimuli. It is characterized in its *acute* stage by irregular, poorly outlined patches of erythema and oedema on which are superimposed closely spaced, non-umbilicated vesicles. These readily rupture, exuding serum and forming crusts. In some instances the vesicle is so minute as not to be obvious, and only tiny red weeping papules can be seen; in others, e.g. plant dermatitis, large vesicles or bullae occur. The more acute the dermatitis the greater the degree of erythema, swelling and vesiculation. When the disease becomes chronic vesicles subside and papules become scaly, but biopsies of such lesions reveal continuing microscopical vesiculation (spongiosis).

Dermatitis can be due to externally applied irritants or to allergy to substances applied externally or acting internally. *Primary irritants* include acids, alkalis, solvents, tars and abrasive dusts. Site and configuration give clues to the contact agent. *Contact allergens* include plants, drugs, cosmetics, metals, plastics, fabrics, dyes and handled foods.

A careful history of the daily routine often gives valuable clues to the diagnosis, which can be confirmed by patch tests. If the responsible allergen can be avoided a cure can be achieved. A vesicular eruption can occur around a patch of infected skin due to an allergic reaction to a component of the infectious agent, e.g. superficial fungus infection, molluscum contagiosum, secondarily infected leg ulcer, etc. Widespread vesicular dermatitis can occur due to allergy from absorbed and circulating substances: e.g. drugs; inhalants—pollens, chemicals; bacterial and fungus products—id reaction.

Groups of vesicles are seen in *lymphangioma circumscriptum*. These congenital abnormalities of lymphatics are not visible at birth but appear in early childhood on the proximal portion of the extremities, axillae, scapular region, mouth, pharynx. They are more common on the left than the right hand side of the body. Small glaring vesicles, which may become haemorrhagic, appear recurrently at the same site.

Dermatitis herpetiformis is more common in males and is characterized by intense itching groups of vesicles on the scalp, elbows, knees, shoulders, buttocks and natal cleft which can erupt over many years until the diagnosis is made. Postinflammatory hyperpigmentation is marked and weals are occasionally seen. Itching is so intense that vesicles are quickly excoriated. The itching dramatically ceases following treatment with dapsone. Histologically the vesicle is subepidermal and direct immunofluorescence shows diagnostic deposits of IgA in the dermis. There is usually associated gastrointestinal gluten hypersensitivity but clinical signs of malabsorption are not pronounced.

Familial benign chronic pemphigus (Hailey-

Hailey disease) (Fig B.47) is a familial tendency for persistent recurrent vesicular dermatitis on the sides of the neck, axillae, groins and sometimes lips. The vesicles soon rupture leaving crusted erosions resembling impetigo—the histology is diagnostic.

Scattered vesicles

GENERALIZED

In *varicella* (chickenpox) the main feature is the eruption of vesicles; these only rarely become pustules. They are usually preceded by a faint macular erythema and, while they may arise anywhere on the body and mucosae, the commonest sites are the face, chest, back and scalp and the mucous membranes of the palate. After an incubation period of 2–3 weeks the rash develops within the first 24 hours and is accompanied by only the mildest constitutional disturbance. The vesicles appear in crops during the first 3 days and when some have dried up to form crusts fresh ones will continue appearing, so that there are lesions of all ages present at the same time.

In *variola* (smallpox), cases of which are no longer seen, the pustules were usually multilocular and most importantly occurred in one crop. Thus lesions were all at approximately the same stage of development at any one time. A generalised vesicular or pustular eruption was a very rare sequel to vaccination and usually appeared on about the eighth day and continued for several weeks.

The lesion of *primary vaccination* begins as a papule on an erythematous base which quickly becomes a vesicle and then a pustule. Later a crust forms which falls off to leave a small scar. Occasionally primary vaccination is an accidental occurrence from contact with a recently vaccinated person.

In *scabies* a minute discrete vesicle is often present at one end of the burrow (*Fig.* V.5) that is the characteristic of the disease. All other lesions are the result of scratching and may consist of papules, pustules and crusts. Pustules are common on the hands especially in the finger webs, but only occur on the palms in infants. In men a solitary papule can usually be observed on the glans or shaft of the penis and this is almost diagnostic in itself. Similar papules may be found on the breasts and areolae of women. The face is never affected except in early infancy. Itching is more pronounced at night and a history of contact with a known case is usually obtained.

Allergic vasculitis usually causes purpuric papules but the lesions may become vesicular and occasionally differentiation from chickenpox is difficult. The condition is more common in boys and affects ankles, lower legs and buttocks, rather than the chest

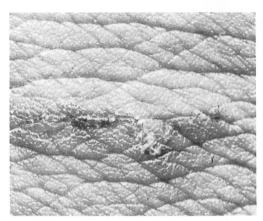

Fig. V.5. Scabies burrow.

and back as in chickenpox. There is usually accompanying arthralgia and there may be abdominal pain and rarely nephritis. Biopsy reveals diagnostic leucocytoclastic vasculitis.

VESICLES ON HANDS AND FEET

Discrete oval grey vesicles with an erythematous halo are scattered sparsely along the sides of fingers, on the ankles and over the tongue in *hand, foot and mouth* disease—a Coxsackie virus infection, commonest in children and young adults. Vesicles scattered on hands and feet are seen in *pompholyx* (dysidrosis) (*Fig.* V.6). The vesicles are deeply embedded in the skin and show through the epidermis like boiled sago grains. The palms and sides of fingers are symmetrically affected and there may be lesions on the soles and toes. The vesicles often later unite to form bullae. The condition may cause great irritation and be recurrent, e.g. each spring. Similar lesions can follow allergy to localized dermatophyte infection—a vesicular id—and this should always be carefully excluded.

VESICLES ON EXPOSED SKIN

In *porphyria cutanea tarda* vesicles and bullae occur on exposed skin in response to trauma and sun exposure. There is usually associated underlying liver disease, e.g. alcoholic cirrhosis, but identical lesions appear in familial *porphyria variegata*. In *hydroa aestivale* deep-seated umbilicated vesicles develop on exposed skin of face, dorsa of hands and lower limbs. Healing occurs to leave large varioliform scars. It is the rarest of the photodermatoses and begins in early childhood, persisting to early adult life. *Plant dermatitis* causes streaks of vesicles and bullae on areas of exposed skin brushed by leaves, e.g. those of primulas (*see* p. 89). Vesicles are sometimes caused by the *bites* and *stings* of gnats, mosquitoes, pets' fleas and other insects.

A *photosensitive* dermatitis can occur spontaneo-

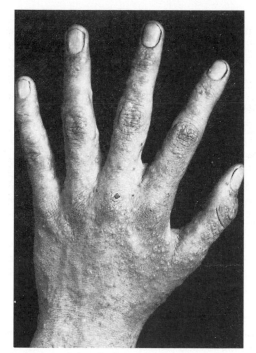

Fig.V.6. Pompholyx (dysidrosis).

usly (e.g. polymorphic light eruption), following external sensitizers (e.g. cologne, citrus fruits, tars) or due to absorbed circulating photosensitizers (psoralens, nalidixic acid, thiazides, sulphonamides).

Richard Staughton

Vision, defects of

(*see also* EYE, BLINDNESS OF.)

The subject may be considered under the following headings: (A) *Normal vision*; (B) *Amblyopia*; (C) *Impairment of the visual field*; (D) *Complete blindness*; (E) *Defects in colour vision*; (F) *Abnormal sensations of size*; (G) *Night-blindness*.

A. Normal Vision

1. VISUAL ACUITY

Vision comprises the perception of form, colour and brightness; and the perception of space and distance. It is necessary to distinguish between peripheral and central vision; between merely seeing a thing and looking at it. An object is seen by any portion of the retina that has visual perception, but an object is only looked at when its image falls upon a particular portion of the retina, the macula, at the posterior pole of the globe top to the temporal side of the optic disc. The act of so directing the eye that the image of a given object falls upon its macula is termed 'fixation', vision obtained by the fixation of the eye is termed 'central

vision', and owing to the anatomical structure of the retina at the macula, the vision here is the most acute of which the eye is capable. In the normal eye, central vision is capable of distinguishing two points or parallel lines which are separated by a space subtending an angle of about 1 minute of a degree, or the diameter of a small coin at 200 feet—and it is on this basis that ordinary test-types are constructed. Central vision, however, though acute, is very limited in extent; the field of acute vision is only about the size of the thumbnail held at arm's length, all vision outside this area being comparatively indistinct. This limitation of the field of acute central vision is barely appreciated in ordinary circumstances, owing to the speed with which the retina receives consecutive visual impressions, and the constant movements of the eyes. In comparison, peripheral vision is relatively poor, though it is of extreme value, since without it locomotion is almost impossible, since one cannot see one's position in relation to surrounding objects, the peripheral portion of the field of vision being responsible for the automatic appreciation of these. On the other hand, a person deprived of central vision can see to get about quite well, though unable to read, recognize people when looking at them, or do any work in which fine vision is required.

2. COLOUR VISION

A person with normal colour vision can recognize the colours of the solar spectrum, and is able to appreciate many hundreds of varieties of colour caused by mixtures of them, and the colour perception of the normal person is most acute in the central portion of the field.

3. BRIGHTNESS PERCEPTION

In ordinary illumination the central portion of the field is the most efficient, but not in a weak illumination; in other words, there is in dim light a relative central scotoma or loss of vision. Thus, in viewing stars of low magnitudes, vision is much better if they are not looked at directly, the Pleiades being a well-known example; more of these stars can be counted when the vision is directed to a point to one side, and the same holds good of vision for any object in a dim light. These facts are correlated with the anatomical structure of the retina; in the region of the macula— the area of the retina endowed with acute vision— the cones are numerous, with few rods; towards the periphery of the retina the cones become fewer and the rods more numerous. The cones function in light of considerable brilliance, are capable of extremely acute vision for small objects, and are also concerned with the perception of colour. The rods, on the other hand, have no perception of colour; their perception of form is poor compared with that of the cones; but in very weak lights their visual acuity is greater than that of the cones, and the retinas of owls and nocturnal animals are more fully provided with rods than cones.

B. Amblyopia

Amblyopia is the term applied to defective vision, in cases where there is no evidence of any organic defect. The commoner forms of amblyopia are:

1. AMBLYOPIA EX ANOPSIA

This arises when an impediment to a clear retinal image prevents the development of full acuity. Thus in high refractive errors, especially high astigmatism or hypermetropia which have not been corrected in early life, it may be found that visual acuity is below normal even after correction of the refractive error, or that its return to normal is delayed. This is especially marked in the defective eye when one eye differs markedly from the other in refraction (anisometropic amblyopia). In childhood squints there is some suppression of one retinal image in order to avoid diplopia; if uncorrected this suppression becomes permanent ('strabismic amblyopia'). Severe ambylopia may result from obstruction of the light pathway to the retina from birth e.g. congenital cataract, ptosis (stimulus deprivation ambylopia).

2. TOXIC AMBLYOPIA

Due to tobacco, alcohol, ethambutol, isoniazid, streptomycin, chloramphenicol, quinine, etc.

In tobacco amblyopia there is a central loss of vision for colours, green only in the earlier stages, subsequently green and red, and in extreme cases even a central scotoma for white. The patient may state that he sees better in a dull than in a bright light, and that he is incapable of reading or writing. In mild cases of toxic amblyopia the fundus appears normal; optic atrophy is evident if gross. In quinine amblyopia the retinal vessels also become constricted and the field of vision is progressively diminished peripherally, though the blindness often precedes any ophthalmoscopic signs.

3. HYSTERICAL AMBLYOPIA

Hysterical amblyopia may, like other hysterical affections, take various forms such as loss of visual acuity, a loss of colour vision, or diminution in the visual field. The characteristic form of the visual field in hysteria is either a spiral contraction or an extreme concentric limitation. The symptoms, however, vary much at different examinations, a point of importance in diagnosis.

C. Impairment of the visual field

This may be: (1) *hemianopia*; (2) *central scotoma*; (3) *peripheral constriction*; (4) *quadrantic and asymmetrical defects*.

1. HEMIANOPIA

See p. 292.

2. CENTRAL SCOTOMA

A scotoma is a localize defect in the visual field, and may be either central or peripheral. It may also be a *negative* scotoma where the defect of vision exists, but where the patient is unaware of it; sight is merely absent over that area, e.g. the blind spot in the field of vision caused by the exit of the optic nerve, or the sequel to damage to parts of the retina or optic nerve.

A *positive* scotoma is one in which the patient is aware of a dark spot or cloud which obscures the vision in some part of the visual field. Such positive scotomas are usually due to opacities in front of the retina.

Scotomas frequently exist in the peripheral portion of the field of vision without being noticed, and not discovered unless looked for carefully. A central scotoma, on the other hand, is noticed at once, however minute, because it affects direct vision and lowers the visual acuity. A central scotoma may be either relative or absolute, and may exist for colour only or for form. Central loss of vision for colour, more particularly red and green, is associated with *tobacco poisoning*, and vision in such cases is generally better in a dull than in a bright light. The scotoma is not always truly central, but may be paracentral or centrocaecal, i.e. between the fixation point and the physiological blind spot.

' Central scotomas are common in optic nerve disease, e.g. optic neuritis and certain forms of hereditary optic atrophy such as Leber's Optic Atrophy and macular disease. The diagnosis of hereditary optic atrophy depends on the history of a similar affection among a family of relations and its usual incidence in early adult life. *Optic neuritis* usually occurs in young adults and attacks only one eye. Its onset is gradual, vision failing within a few days; in most cases vision commences to return after a week or two and is ultimately restored in 3–4 weeks. Most cases of optic neuritis are due to multiple sclerosis. The diagnosis of a *hereditary optic atrophy* (Leber's atrophy) depends upon the history of a similar affection among family relations and its usual incidence in early adult life. *Retrobulbar neuritis* usually occurs in young adults, commonly attacks one eye only, and is gradual in its onset, the vision failing within a few days; in most cases vision commences to return after a week or two, and is ultimately restored in 3–4 weeks. Most cases of retrobulbar neuritis without apparent cause are due to multiple sclerosis. The most common cause of central scotoma due to macular disease are aged related macular degeneration and diabetic maculopathy. The central visual loss known as eclipse blindness arises from a thermal burn of the macula resulting from gazing at the sun without protection. The effect is permanent and the lesion is visible ophthalmoscopically.

3.   PERIPHERAL CONSTRICTION

Peripheral constriction of the visual field occurs commonly in affections such as primary open angle of glaucoma, *optic atrophy, chorioretinitis, retinitis pigmentosa* and various *functional conditions*. The constriction of the visual field in *glaucoma* is usually most marked on the nasal side, and it is associated with atrophy and cupping of the optic disc (*See Fig. O.5*). Central vision may remain good, even though the field of vision is extremely limited. The peripheral vision is progressively limited in *retinitis pigmentosa*, where the failure of sight is associated with night-blindness and characteristic ophthalmoscopic appearances comprise a small, ill-defined, pale waxy-looking disc, slender retinal vessels, and diffuse superficial pigmentation of the equatorial zone of the retina in patches resembling Haversian bone corpuscles (*See Fig. O.25*). The condition is hereditary and transmission can be autosomal recessive, autosomal dominant, or X-linked recessive. A limitation of the field and fundus changes similar to that of retinitis pigmentosa is often met with in cases of *chorioretinitis* with consequent optic atrophy; but may be distinguished from it by evidence of deeper changes in the retina and choroid. Constriction of the field of vision may also occur in certain *functional states*, recognized by its variable character and the absence of all evidence of organic, ocular or general nervous disease.

4.   QUADRANTIC AND ASYMMETRICAL DEFECTS

A homonymous quadrantic defect is normally cortical in origin; unilateral and asymmetrical defects must be due to a cause situated in front of the chiasma.

D.   Complete blindness

Total loss of vision, blindness, or amaurosis, may be: (1) *Bilateral*; (2) *Unilateral*.

1.   BILATERAL BLINDNESS

Total blindness in both eyes may be congenital or acquired. Congenital blindness may be due either to absence of the eyes themselves, *congenital anoph-*

thalmos or to *congenital defects* in the development of the eyes.

Retrolental fibroplasia (the end result of severe retinopathy of prematurity), in which a mass of whitish tissue is seen occupying the vitreous of an infant, was an increasingly common cause of blindness (usually bilateral) in infants, until it was shown to be the sequel to administration of oxygen (over 40 per cent) to premature babies. Since the cause was demonstrated (by Ashton in 1953) and the administration of oxygen to premature babies has been rigidly controlled the condition virtually ceased to arise. However as smaller birth weight premature infants are now surviving, the incidence of retinopathy of prematurity and blindness secondary to it is increasing.

Adult blindness may be caused by bilateral primary glaucoma, optic atrophy or lesions of the optic chiasma. It is seldom due to lesions of the optic tracts, as this would only be caused by a bilateral lesion totally destroying the optic tract on both sides.

Transient blindness may be due to microemboli from an artheromatous plaque on the carotid artery ('amaurosis fugax'). This may occur in cases of quinine or lead poisoning, in epilepsy, migraine or eclampsia. The loss of sight in a patient suffering from 'giant-cell arteritis' may be complete and permanent. It is to be noted that no cataract ever causes total blindness; provided that the rest of the eye is normal, a patient with the densest cataract can always perceive light, and also has the power of projection (the recognition of the direction from which the ray of light is coming).

2.   UNILATERAL BLINDNESS

Unilateral blindness is always due to some lesion in the eye itself, or to one between the eye and the optic chiasma. Lesions of the optic tract above the chiasma do not cause monocular blindness, but bilateral defects. Monocular blindness may be either sudden or gradual.

Gradual blindness may be due to such progressive diseases as optic atrophy or glaucoma, and in the elderly to cataract and macular degeneration (these are often restricted to one eye for many years, and constitute overall the two commonest causes of certifiable blindness).

Sudden blindness in one eye may be due to one of the following causes:

Detachment of the retina (*See Fig. O.23*)
Occlusion of the central retinal artery
Occlusion of the central retinal vein (*See Fig. O.14*)
Vitreous haemorrhage
Acute glaucoma (*See Fig. O.5*)
Injury to the optic nerve
Ischaemic optic neuritis
Optic neuritis
Migraine
Hysteria

The diagnosis of most of these causes is simple, owing to the characteristic appearances. The only cases which present problems are those in which there is sudden loss of vision without visible ocular changes. These are usually due to retrobulbar neuritis, an acute demyelination of the optic nerve, characterized by rapid loss of sight, with some pain on movement of the eye. In most patients vision returns entirely; if there is permanent defect it takes the form of a paracentral scotoma.

Monocular blindness may also occur in *migraine*, but it seldom lasts more than 10 minutes and is usually followed by the characteristic headache, sickness and fortification figures.

E. Defects in colour vision

Defects in colour vision may be either congenital or acquired; in congenital colour blindness there is inability to recognize in the spectrum one or more of the six or seven distinct colours which may be apparent to a normal eye. The common causes of colour blindness are those who have a selective dulling of red and green (about 1 in 12 of our male population, and 1 in 200 of the females).

Cases of congenital colour blindness can be recognized by examination with testing charts of 'pseudoisochromatic' dots, or with more precision and certainty by the 100 hue test.

Acquired disturbances of colour vision are generally the sequel to damage to the retina and optic pathways by a wide variety of poisons. The rainbow-coloured haloes around lights are the classic feature of acute glaucoma, associated with corneal oedema, a shallow anterior chamber, mid-dilatated pupil, and increased tension in the eyeball. Indefinite haloes may be produced by a film of mucus, from a conjunctivitis; but these disappear on blinking. Haloes may also be due to lens opacities but these are less bright and generally colourless.

F. Abnormal sensations of size

Objects may appear to increase or diminish rapidly in size in the preliminary stages of an attack of epilepsy; and this variation in size of objects is occasionally noted by normal children, adult neurotics, and in the slight delirium of infantile febrile disorders. An elevation of wrinkling of the retina by haemorrhage or tumour of the choroid which causes mechanical crowding or separation of the retinal elements may give rise to a corresponding abnormal sensation size.

G. Night blindness

Night blindness, or *nactalopsia*, is commonly a congenital defect, having no organic ocular changes; it may also be associated with lack of vitamin A. It occurs most frequently in retinitis pigmentosa, diagnosable at once on ophthalmoscopic examination by reason of the pale optic disc, thin arteries and veins, and the characteristic spider-like pigment patches seen in the fundus.

S. T. D. Roxburgh

Vision, subjective disturbances of

There are a few common subjective disturbances of vision which have not been mentioned elsewhere.

The most dramatic are the flashes, sparks, colours, scotomas and fortification spectra which are a frequent accompaniment of an attack of *migraine*. Occasionally (as 'phosphenes') they occur in healthy eyes after sudden movements, or as evidence of retinal traction (which may anticipate retinal detachment).

Spots Before the Eyes

These may be considered under the headings of: (1) floating and (2) fixed.

Floaters (MUSCAE VOLITANTES) are an almost universal complaint, although manifest only against a bright background; they often appear quite suddenly, and then very gradually fade away. They are probably due to condensations in the vitreous gel, in which even minor 'degenerative' changes may cause such symptoms. The usual outcome is for them to break up and disappear, or alternatively to sink and thus pass out of recognition. A far more serious cause of vitreous floaters is uveitis, when the particles represent an inflammatory exudate, possibly with a cellular element. They are also very common in the degenerative changes of high myopia. A rare cause of complaint of floating spots is the presence of small aggregations of mucus on the cornea, maybe in conjunctivitis but sometimes without apparent cause. Their movement or actual removal by the act of blinking reveals their origin. In all cases where floaters are complained of, careful examination is indicated in order to discover whether there is any underlying pathology.

FIXED SPOTS may be due to one of a variety of causes. The limited central loss of vision caused by a macular lesion, especially the senile type, may be called a 'spot' by the patient. A fixed opacity in the vitreous may cast a shadow on the retina as may also, rarely, one in the lens or cornea. The paracentral scotoma of early chronic simple glaucoma must not be forgotten on account of its extreme importance. The larger scotomatous areas in the visual field caused by such conditions as detachment of the retina and neoplasm of the choroid are not properly described as spots except perhaps rarely in the very early stages.

Partial loss of field due to a central lesion, though

hardly to be described as a 'spot', may also be so regarded and described by the patient. Sometimes a patient may become aware of the normal 'blind-spot' which is due to the presence of the non-sensitive area where the optic nerve leaves the eye, especially if he is one-eyed, when the area is not covered in the binocular field by the corresponding sensitive area of the fellow eye. A reassurance that this is a normal phenomenon should put the complainant's mind at rest.

S. T. D. Roxburgh

Voice, disorders of

The larynx consists of an outer skeleton and an inner mucosal framework. The skeleton consists of the hyoid bone, the thyroid cartilage and the cricoid cartilage. The arytenoid cartilages sit on top of the lamina of the cricoid cartilage and the vocal cords are attached to both the arytenoid cartilage and the prominence of the thyroid cartilage. Males have a longer vocal cord than females and the extra length is made up by the development of the thyroid prominence or Adam's apple. The vocal cords are supplied by the recurrent laryngeal nerves. On the left, the nerve is long and has an intrathoracic component, while on the right it is short.

To understand how sound is produced, it is necessary to understand the Bernoulli effect. This principle states that during the steady flow of a fluid or a gas, the pressure is less when the velocity is greater. In other words, when air passes from one large space to another (i.e. from lung to pharynx) through a constriction (the glottis), the velocity will be greatest and the pressure least at the site of the constriction.

When we wish to phonate, the recurrent laryngeal nerves set the vocal cords into the adducted position but, because the vocal processes are slightly bulkier than the membranous cord, a slight gap exists between the membranous cords. The lungs then expel air and the airstream passes through this chink between the vocal cords. According to the Bernoulli principle, therefore, there is a drop of pressure at this site and this causes the mucosa of the vocal cords to be drawn into the gap, thus blocking it. At this time the subglottic pressure rises, causing another stream of air to flow through the cords with another resultant pressure drop and closure of the gap. As this process is repeated, a vibratory pattern develops at the vocal cords and the resulting sound is what we appreciate as voice. The change of this sound into speech is accomplished by the tongue, teeth, lips and palate.

There are, thus, only two vocal symptoms, namely dysphonia or hoarseness and aphonia or loss of voice. Dysphonia is caused when the cords meet with an abnormality of the mucosa which causes a roughness in the voice and aphonia occurs when the cords do not meet and air flows between the edges of the vocal cords without voice being produced. In some circumstances when there is a large lesion on the vocal cord, there can be a mixture of dysphonia and air wastage.

The conditions causing abnormalities of the voice are shown in *Table* V.2.

Because of the relative simplicity of the two symptoms, some idea of the cause of the voice disorder can be gained while taking the history from the patient. The next stage is to carry out laryngoscopy. This can be done with a mirror and a headlamp or with rigid Hopkin's rod attached to a fibreoptic light source. It can also be performed with a flexible laryngoscope although this is very uncomfortable for the patient since it needs to be passed through the nasal cavity. Since carcinoma of the larynx is relatively common and since the results of treatment are so good, it is essential that any patient who is hoarse has the larynx visualized so that carcinoma can be diagnosed early if it is, indeed, present.

Carcinoma of the larynx is a disease of smokers. It is not as common as carcinoma of the lung in Northern Europe but in Southern Europe it is commoner than carcinoma of the lung in smokers. The presenting symptom is hoarseness and this will occur when the tumour is only a few millimetres in size. This is why it is very important to examine the larynx and visualize the vocal cords in anyone who is hoarse. The tumour will gradually expand along the length of the cord but even when it occupies the whole length of one vocal cord, it will only be 2 cm long. Once it spreads into the tissues of the vocal cords then the prognosis is not nearly so good. Most early carcinomas can be cured with radiotherapy but when they are larger, the patient will need either a partial or a total laryngectomy (*Figs.* V.8, V.9).

Vocal cord nodules occur in people who abuse their voice. These are virtually 'corns' on the vocal cords and are caused by abnormal vibratory patterns. The patient who gives a loud shout or who has the vocal cords traumatized by intubation, can develop a vocal cord polyp on the edge of the cord. Polyps can also be the way that benign tumours such as neurilemomas, myoblastomas, etc. can present. TB and sarcoid look like carcinoma in presentation. Myxoedema looks like gross oedema of the vocal cords and can look like a large polyp. A similar condition known as Reinke's oedema can occur sometimes related to myxoedema but often times not.

Depending on the cause, vocal cord paralysis may be unilateral or bilateral, complete or incomplete,

Table V.2. Causes of voice disorders in adults

Inflammatory

Acute
  Acute laryngitis following an upper respiratory

  Herpetic laryngitis
  Acute epiglottitis

Chronic
NON-SPECIFIC
  Vocal abuse
  Tobacco and alcohol
  Pachydermia (*Fig.* V.7)
  Polypoid degeneration (Reinke's oedema)
  Vocal nodules (Singer's nodes) (*Fig.* V.7)
SPECIFIC
  Tuberculous
  Lupus vulgaris
  Syphilis
  Leprosy
  Scleroma
  Mycoses
    Actinomycosis
    Candidiasis
    Coccidioidomycosis
    Rhinosporidiosis
  Sarcoid
  Wegener's granuloma

Tumours

Benign
  Vocal polyps
  Retention cysts
  Single papilloma
  Fibroma, haemangioma and neurofibroma

Neoplastic
  Leucoplakia (*Fig.* V.7)
  Carcinoma of the larynx (*Fig.* V.9)—growth on
    the cord
  Growths of the laryngo-pharynx

Traumatic
  Foreign bodies
  Intubation damage
  Burns
  Chemical, from inhalation
  External injury with oedema and haematoma

Neurological
  Recurrent laryngeal nerve (especially the left side as
    this nerve has the longest course through neck
    and chest)

Palsy due to
  Surgical injury
  Peripheral neuritis
    Diphtheria
    Viral
    Chemical. Lead
    Vitamin B deficiency (beriberi)
  'Idiopathic'
  Carcinoma of thyroid or upper oesophagus
  Carcinoma of lung—primary or lymph nodes (left)
  Aneurysm of subclavian or aorta
  Cardiac enlargement

Vagus nerve
  Poliomyelitis
  Ascending polyneuritis
  Vascular accidents in brain-stem
  Aneurysm of cartoid artery
  Malignant disease of nasopharynx
  Syphilis

Various
  Allergic oedema (Quinke's oedema or 'angio-
    neurotic oedema')
  Rheumatoid arthritis of crico-arytenoid joints
  Myxoedema
  Myasthenia gravis
  Functional aphonia

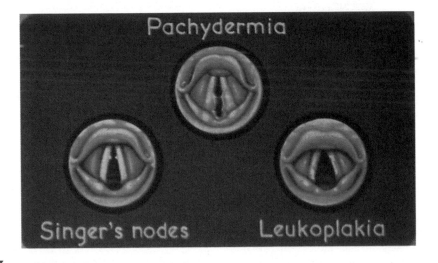

Fig. V.7.

giving four possible combinations, namely: (*a*) unilateral abductor; (*b*) unilateral adductor; (*c*) bilateral abductor; (*d*) bilateral adductor. Each of these presents a different clinical picture and each requires different management (*Fig.* V.10).

The conditions that affect either vagus nerve are: (*a*) tumours of the base of the skull, e.g. glomus jugulare tumours and nasopharyngeal carcinoma; (*b*) bulbar paralysis; (*c*) peripheral neuritis due to influenza, herpes or Epstein–Barr virus; (*d*) high neck injuries;

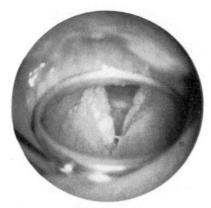

Fig. V.8. Carcinoma of the vocal cord.

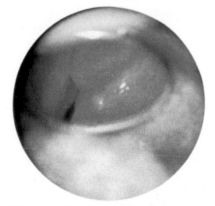

Fig. V.9. Advanced carcinoma of the larynx.

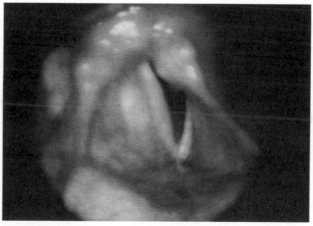

Fig. V.10.

gland; (*d*) operative trauma from thyroidectomy, radical neck dissection, pharyngeal pouch removal, cricopharyngeal myotomy, ligation of a patent ductus, and other cardiac and pulmonary surgery; (*e*) mediastinal nodes or tumour, e.g. Hodgkin's disease; (*f*) any enlargement of the left side of the heart; (*g*) peripheral neuritis; (*h*) aortic aneurysm.

The lesions affecting the right recurrent laryngeal nerve are: (*a*) carcinoma of the thyroid gland; (*b*) operative trauma from thyroidectomy, pharyngeal pouch removal or myotomy procedures; (*c*) carcinoma of the oesophagus; (*d*) carcinoma of the apex of the right lung; (*e*) peripheral neuritis; (*f*) subclavian aneurysm.

In unilateral adductor paralysis, the cord lies in the cadaveric position and cannot reach the midline. Normal voice cannot be produced unless the vocal cord is brought towards the midline, either by surgery to medialize the cord or by a Teflon injection. Unilateral abductor paralysis means that the cord is in the midline and the good cord comes across to meet it and so the patient has a voice and no treatment is usually required. In bilateral adductor paralysis, the cause is usually a fatal neurological condition and the patient often dies from aspiration.

Bilateral abductor paralysis is when both vocal cords lie in the mid-position. This is sometimes seen after nerve injury, subsequent to thyroid gland surgery. The patient will have a normal voice but will have stridor. The treatment of this condition is either a

e.g. trauma or surgical complication of radical neck dissection; (*e*) metastatic node involvement; (*f*) basal meningitis; (*g*) vagal tumours, e.g. glomus vagale or neurilemoma.

Lesions affecting the left recurrent laryngeal nerve (which has an intrathoracic course) include: (*a*) carcinoma of the bronchus; (*b*) carcinoma of the cervical or thoracic oesophagus; (*c*) carcinoma of the thyroid

permanent tracheostomy or an arytenoidectomy which allows one cord to be pulled laterally. The patient then has a breathy voice but does not have the inconvenience of a tracheostomy.

A. G. D. Maran

Vomiting

Vomiting is the forceful ejection of gastric contents through the mouth. It results from a forceful, sustained contraction of the abdominal muscles and pelvic floor against a closed glottis. The pylorus is contracted and the open cardiac is herniated through a contracted diaphragm.

A vomiting centre is present in the medulla oblongata and is stimulated by raised intracranial pressure, brain lesions, hydrocephalus, posterior fossa lesions and vestibular disorders. The vomiting centre is also stimulated via a chemoreceptor trigger zone in the floor of the fourth ventricle which is responsive to drugs and metabolic abnormalities including electrolyte disorders, ketoacidosis or high fever. It is possible that other centres in the brain may be sensitive to emetic drugs or metabolic disturbances. While vomiting of a non-psychogenic mechanism is usually reflex, pathological vomiting of a voluntary nature can take place. Dopamine and opiate neurotransmitters may influence from both a central effect and also a peripheral effect. Thus brain gut peptides which influence gastric motility and emptying include motilin, cholecystokinin and neurotensin (increased motility) and secretin (decreased motility). Gut motility is also influenced by disorders of the autonomic nervous system at either peripheral or central levels. Stimuli carried to the brain by the somatic nerves can also elicit vomiting, for example, if there is severe pain such as in myocardial infarction or colic of one kind or another or pancreatitis.

Vomiting must be distinguished from *regurgitation* which is the effortless expulsion of food from, or the return of food to the mouth. In a restricted sense it describes the expulsion of contents from the oesophagus only; but patients are often unable to distinguish between regurgitation, gross oesophageal reflux and vomiting. The absence of a bitter or acid taste helps to distinguish regurgitation from vomiting. *Rumination* is the repeated return of small quantities of food to the mouth where it is chewed and swallowed again. It is uncommon and usually occurs in patients who are psychiatrically disturbed. In order to ruminate the patient increases intra-abdominal pressure thereby regurgitating food into the mouth. In *retching* there is forceful contraction of the stomach wall muscle, of the diaphragm, and the abdominal muscles similar to that which takes place in vomiting. There is, however, no relaxation of the cardiac sphincter and no food returns to the mouth. Retching is also known as 'dry heaves' and is seen most characteristically in the gastritis associated with alcohol abuse when the patient complains of early morning nausea and dry heaves. The causes of vomiting are listed in *Table V.3.* below.

Investigation of vomiting may include some or all of the procedures in *Table* V.4.

Vomiting is one of the commonest symptoms in clinical medicine. It may represent the beginning of a minor illness or herald a severe disease process. It may be associated with significant complications. The cause of the vomiting is helped if a number of associated features are questioned and elucidated.

1. THE NATURE OF THE VOMITUS: Bright red or altered blood suggests bleeding anywhere from the mouth to the duodenum. The quantity varies according to the speed of bleeding but it must be remembered that the volume of blood is often overestimated by the patient for the red blood is diluted with the volume of gastric contents. 'Coffee-ground' is usually taken to indicate blood altered by gastric juice. A coffee-ground appearance to the vomit is therefore taken to indicate that there is blood in the material but sometimes this is not so and a coffee-ground appearance can be given by altered food mixed with bile. Vomiting of bile occurs after *gastric surgery* and in *high small bowel obstruction*. Repeated vomiting in the absence of bile, particularly in children, suggests that the obstruction is proximal to the second part of the duodenum. The presence of food taken hours or days previously suggests that *gastric statis* is present. This may be due to reflect atony or may reflect long-standing gastric outflow obstruction such as in *pyloric stenosis*. Vomit which has a faecal smell suggests that there is *small bowel obstruction* or an *ileus*, or the presence of a *gastro-colic fistula*. Occasionally faecal-smelling vomit is seen in patients with *bacterial overgrowth* in the proximal small bowel.

2. TIMING OF THE VOMIT: Vomiting occurring during or soon after a meal can occur in patients with a *peptic ulcer* in the pyloric channel but it is also a feature of *psychoneurotic vomiting*. Early morning vomiting before breakfast occurs characteristically in *pregnancy, alcoholic gastritis* and *uraemia*. Patients who have *postnasal drip* or who have *chronic bronchitis* and who swallow their sputum may also vomit at this time. Patients with chronic bronchitis who cough a great deal in the early morning may follow a bout of coughing with vomiting.

3. RELIEF OF PAIN BY VOMITING: This is a feature of *peptic ulcer* disease particularly.

4. PROJECTILE VOMITING: This term is used to describe vomit which is ejected forcefully from the mouth. It is said to occur in *raised intracranial pressure* and also in patients who have *gastric outflow obstruction*. The description is however a poor one as many other causes of vomiting may be of a projectile nature while not every patient with raised intracranial pressure or gastric outflow obstruction will have vom-

Table V.3. Causes of vomiting

Gastrointestinal diseases
Gastritis, alcoholic, campylobacter and other causes
Peptic ulceration
Colic, biliary and renal
Cholecystitis
Appendicitis
Pancreatitis, acute and relapsing
Gastric outflow obstruction
Intestinal obstruction, small and large
Gastric cancer
Postgastrectomy syndrome
Acute liver failure
Amyloidosis
Hollow visceral myopathy
Chronic intestinal pseudo-obstruction

Acute infections
Urinary tract infections
Viral gastroenteritis
Viral hepatitis
Measles
Whooping cough
Pneumonia

Drugs
Aminophylline
Aspirin
Cytotoxic agents
Digoxin general anaesthetic agents
Iron preparations
Metronidazole
Narcotic analgesics
Oestrogens
Sulphasalzine
Sulphonamides

Metabolic/endocrine
Pregnancy
High fevers
Diabetic ketoacidosis
Uraemia
Hyperparathyroidism and other causes of
   hypercalcaemia
Addison's disease
Acute intermittent porphyria

Neurological
Meningitis
Raised intracranial pressure
Migraine
Menière's disease
Labyrinthine disorders
Autonomic neuropathy or diabetic
Gullaine–Barre syndrome
Chaga's disease
Tabetic crisis
Autonomic epilepsy
Paraneoplastic neuropathy

Psychogenic
Bulimia
Functional
Anorexia nervosa

Other
Cardiac failure
Myocardial infarction
Hypertensive encephalopathy
Irradiation
Food intolerance
Diffuse malignant disease
Acute glaucoma

Table V.4. Tests that may be necessary in unexplained vomiting

Full history and physical examination
Haematological and biochemical screen
Drug screen
Hormone tests
Protein electrophoresis
Plain X-ray abdomen
Gastric intubation
Endoscopy
Upper and lower GI tract barium examination
Intravenous urography
Computed tomography
Gastric emptying tests
Oesophageal manometry
Psychiatric assessment
Laparotomy with full thickness muscle biopsy

iting. Most patients who vomit will have preceding nausea but in the case of projectile vomiting this is often absent.

MEDICAL HISTORY

It is very important to take a complete history in attempting to elucidate the cause of vomiting. Details of previous surgery are important as is information relating to childhood health and any psychiatric disease. A social history is also of significance. Information is required about the patient's marriage, occupation, work satisfaction, and other issues relating to his personal life. This is the opportunity to explore phobias and fears and inappropriate anxiety situations.

PHYSICAL EXAMINATION

This is of importance not only to attempt to identify the underlying cause but also to elucidate whether or not complications of the vomiting have developed. A succussion splash and visible peristalsis, particularly when it passes from left to right in the anterior abdomen, is of value. Increased bowel sounds will be observed if there is small or large bowel obstruction. The features to observe are abdominal distension, an abdominal mass, the presence of weight loss and evidence for disease in other body systems.

COMPLICATIONS OF VOMITING

These can be considered under two headings, those related to damage to the gastrointestinal tract and those associated with metabolic disorder. Movement of the stomach through the oesophageal hiatus can cause damage to the mucosa resulting in severe haemorrhage. These tears at the gastro-oesophageal junction are known as the *Mallory-Weiss syndrome*. Rupture of the oesophagus can take place, the *Boerhaave's syndrome*. Aspiration of the vomitus can cause a *chemical pneumonitis*. This topic has received prominence as a complication of women who vomit as they go into labour with consequent severe pulmonary oedema due to the chemical pneumonitis. Prolonged vomiting may be associated with the following electrolyte changes, potassium deficiency, alkalosis, hypernatraemia, hypotension, decreased blood volume and haemo concentration. Subsequently renal failure may develop, paralysis due to potassium depletion may occur and malnutrition may become severe.

1. Gastric causes

Most *corrosive* and *irritant poisons* cause vomiting immediately after swallowing, accompanied by intense burning pain in the epigastrium. The vomit contains food, blood, mucus and may have the characteristic odour of the poison. With some irritant poisons, e.g. arsenic or phosphorus, the vomiting may be delayed and resemble that of an acute gastritis. The diagnosis depends on chemical analysis of the vomit, as well as the associated signs and symptoms. Shreds of gastric mucosa may be seen or even a large portion of the mucosa forming a partial or complete cast of the interior of the stomach (*gastritis membranacea*). Many drugs medicinally employed may cause vomiting if administered in excess, and, in the case of susceptible persons, even in ordinary pharmacopoeial doses, iron preparations being a good example.

In *acute viral gastroenteritis* repeated vomiting is usually very severe and attended by abdominal pain. It occurs shortly after taking food and leads to some relief of pain. The vomited matter consists at first of food ingested, later of mucus and bile. There are often accompanying diarrhoea and febrile disturbances, especially in children.

In *chronic gastritis* pain is of variable degree. The vomited matter consists of partially digested food, mucus, and a considerable quantity of sour-smelling liquid. Hydrochloric acid is usually reduced, or entirely absent. When *dilatation* of the stomach is present, the quantity of liquid ejected is often very large; portions of food taken many hours previously may be recognized.

'*Hour-glass*' *contraction* is a rare condition and is due to transverse constriction of the stomach by fibrous tissue, may be a cause of vomiting which resembles in most respects that associated with dilatation. Examination with a barium meal will generally establish the diagnosis.

In adults, the vomiting due to *gastric outflow obstruction* presents no characteristics other than those associated with the dilatation of the stomach which it usually produces. The cause of the obstruction may be either irreversible fibrosis and stenosis (*pyloric stenosis*) or remedial oedema of the pyloric canal. Radiographic evidence that there is a large residuum in the stomach 8 hours after the intake of the barium is the most direct method of demonstrating pyloric stenosis. The absence of free hydrochloric acid and the presence of blood in the vomit would favour the diagnosis of carcinoma. Persistent vomiting in young male infants, especially if breastfed, attended by wasting and constipation, arouses suspicion of *hypertrophic stenosis of the pylorus*. The vomiting in these cases is very forcible, usually shortly after a feed. Visible gastric peristalsis and the presence of a small tumour in the epigastrium would complete the diagnosis.

Vomiting is by no means universal in cases of non-malignant *gastric ulcer*. Pain as a rule occurs within an hour of taking food and is relieved by vomiting. The vomit consists of food more or less digested, a variable but generally at least normal quantity of free hydrochloric acid, and sometimes blood.

2. Intestinal, peritoneal and general visceral causes

In *intestinal obstruction* vomiting sets in after an interval the length of which may depend on the situation of the obstruction. The higher this is situated in the intestinal canal the earlier and more severe the vomiting. The contents of the stomach are returned first, and later mucus, bile and intestinal contents, often of a dull brown colour and thin fluid consistence; obvious pieces of faecal matter are rarely distinguishable. Faecal vomiting should be recognizable by its odour.

Vomiting is an early symptom in *appendicitis* and may persist to resemble that met with in intestinal obstruction.

Intestinal worms may cause vomiting in children, probably owing to reflex irritation. A round-worm is sometimes found in the vomit.

Enemas induce vomiting in certain individuals and rare cases have been described where liquid injected per rectum has been returned by the mouth.

Vomiting is a common symptom in the condition known as *Henoch–Schönlein purpura*. The vomit may contain blood from the mucous membrane of the stomach. It is usually accompanied by abdominal pain, sometimes of an acute and agonizing character closely simulating that occurring with intestinal obstruction, in consequence of haemorrhage into the intestinal wall or the mesentery, occasionally simulating or even giving rise to intussusception. Recurrent attacks of vomiting and abdominal pain associated with arthropathies affecting one or more joints for a few days at a time, haematuria and a purpuric eruption particularly on the buttocks in a child would point to this not uncommon disease.

In *acute peritonitis*, vomiting is an early symptom; rarely the vomit may have a faecal odour. The history, together with the rigidity and immobility of the abdominal wall, generally indicates the need for early laparotomy.

Epidemic vomiting is caused by a number of viruses including the Norwalk virus. Characteristically there is sudden onset of severe vomiting, headache, dizziness, aches and pains, sweating and fever. In *biliary* and *renal colic* the vomiting accompanying the attacks of agonizing pain presents no special features. The pain in the upper right part of the abdomen distinguishes biliary colic from that due to renal calculus in which the pain is in the loin or the lower abdomen shooting down towards the groin and testicle and often followed by haematuria. True biliary colic results from a stone obstructing the cystic duct. Jaundice is absent if the gallstone is in the cystic duct. A gallstone in the common bile duct causes more prolonged pain rather than the waves of colic which accompany cystic duct obstruction.

Acute pancreatitis may closely simulate intestinal obstruction in that it is attended by nausea and vomiting, constipation and severe abdominal pain. The vomit is, however, not faecal in character; there is usually localized tenderness over the pancreas. There may be discoloration of the skin of the abdominal wall as described by Grey Turner. If laparotomy is performed (on account of the urgency of the symptoms), fat necrosis is usually found in the omentum and mesentery.

Severe nausea and vomiting may occur with acute myocardial infarction. It may be caused by the drugs administered for pain.

3. Affections of the central nervous system

In all cases of vomiting with the least suspicion of an intracranial lesion a full examination of the central nervous system with X-ray of the skull, ophthalmoscopy for papilloedema or optic atrophy, and computed tomography are necessary. Instances occur when attacks of vomiting may be the only symptom of an intracranial tumour long in advance of any other symptom or sign of increased intracranial pressure.

Cerebral haemorrhage may be attended by vomiting especially when the cerebellum is the part affected or when the haemorrhage is subarachnoid.

Menière's syndrome is characterized by recurrent paroxysms of vertigo, vomiting, tinnitus and progressive nerve deafness. Vomiting tends to follow the attack of vertigo. Characteristically there is rotatory nystagmus and unsteadiness of stance and gait during an attack. *Vestibular neuronitis* and *benign recurrent*

vertigo describe a clinical syndrome commonly occurring in the middle-aged associated with abrupt onset of vertigo, nausea and vomiting without any impairment of hearing. The attack lasts only for a few days and is followed by a brief period of mild positional vertigo.

Functional or *hysterical vomiting* may not be attended by nausea or pain, and although the vomiting may be a frequent occurrence the general state of nutrition often remains good. It is by no means unusual for a subject to vomit, and return to complete a meal. Other hysterical manifestations are generally present in these patients and detailed interrogation may elicit a psychological cause to encourage the conclusion that the act symbolizes a (possibly subconscious) feeling of disgust. Some people are prone to vomit on the slightest psychological disturbance as a means of expressing their emotions. In *bulimia* there is gorging followed by self-induced vomiting. Vomiting can also occur in *anorexia nervosa* but failure to eat is the prominent feature of the disease.

The *gastric crises* in tabes dorsalis are attacks of vomiting usually accompanied by severe epigastric pain. Occasionally, vomiting may be an isolated symptom. The attacks usually last for several days, and tend to recur at irregular intervals. During the intervals alimentary functions may be completely normal. The diagnosis would be supported by the characteristic Argyll Robertson pupil and the loss of the knee-jerks, but, in some cases, visceral crises are the only manifestation of tabes and a mistaken diagnosis of an abdominal catastrophe is by no means easily avoided. The absence of abdominal rigidity is an important feature.

Blood and CSF tests are necessary for *Treponema pallidum* haemagglutination (TPHA) and a fluorescent test of treponemal antibody (FTA-ABS).

Disease of the labyrinth such as may be associated with drugs or viral infection is associated with nausea, vomiting and vertigo of the peripheral type. Hearing is almost invariably affected.

Disorder of the autonomic nervous system may alter gut motility and cause vomiting. Autonomic system degenerations occur in primary idiopathic hypotension and the Shy–Drager syndrome as well as diabetes mellitus. In the Shy–Drager syndrome, the basic lesion lies in the basal ganglia as well as degeneration of the autonomic nervous system. Neuromuscular disorders that cause vomiting require careful investigation of the central nervous system, the autonomic nervous system and an evaluation of gut smooth muscle. The latter may be achieved by manometry but frequently a full thickness biopsy is required.

Ian A. D. Bouchier

Vulva, swelling of

The differential diagnosis of vulval swellings includes not only tumours of the vulva itself, but also swellings which appear at the vulva as a result of the displacement of other structures as in cases of uterine prolapse and cystocele. Inflammatory lesions and ulceration of the vulva may be accompanied by swelling of the vulva due to oedema. These conditions are considered under VULVAL ULCERATION. Conditions presenting with itching of the vulva as the main complaint are described under PRURITUS VULVAE.

Vulval swellings may be tabulated as follows:

Inflammatory swellings

Warts
Condyloma acuminatum
Bartholin's abscess

Cystic swellings

Bartholin's cyst
Sebaceous cyst
Mucous cyst
Implantation cyst
Dermoid cyst
Hydrocele of the canal of Nuck
Vestigial (mesonephric) cyst

Blood cysts

Varicocele
Traumatic haematoma
Endometrioma

Benign new growths

Caruncle
Fibroma
Fibromyoma
Lipoma
Hidradenoma
Papilloma
Lymphangioma
Myxoma
Angioma
Melanoma
Neuroma

Malignant new growths

Squamous-cell carcinoma
Rodent ulcer
Adenocarcinoma
Sarcoma
Melanoma
Chorioncarcinoma

Hernia

Inguinal
Hernia of the pouch of Douglas (enterocele)

Displacement

Prolapse of the urethral mucosa
Prolapse of the vaginal vault and uterus
Cystocele
Rectocele
Chronic inversion of the uterus

INFLAMMATORY SWELLINGS. Warts on the vulva are usually multiple. They are caused by a virus of the papovirus group and may be transmitted sexually (*venereal warts*). They may spread up into the vagina and a careful inspection of the vaginal walls with the aid of a speculum should always be made in the presence of vulval warts. In pregnancy, or in the presence of much sweating, vulval warts proliferate and may become macerated. They are then referred to as *condyloma acuminata*.

BARTHOLIN'S ABSCESS presents as an extremely painful swelling in the region of the Bartholin (greater vestibular) gland. Pressure on the gland causes much pain, but a bead of pus can be seen escaping from the mouth of the Bartholin duct just below the lateral attachment of the hymen. If not incised, the abscess usually bursts through the skin of the posterior aspect of the labium majus with consequent relief of pain. Recurrence is common until the gland is removed surgically.

CYSTIC SWELLING. The commonest one is a Bartholin's cyst. This is usually a swelling in the duct of the Bartholin's gland producing a swelling in the posterior third of the labium majus which projects medially so as to encroach on the vaginal entrance causing dyspareunia. It is not particularly tender unless it becomes infected forming an abscess. The cyst tends gradually to increase in size, causing local discomfort until marsupialization is performed.

Sebaceous cysts are fairly common affecting the labia majora as a rule. They may occur in groups. Mucous, inclusion and implantation cysts also occur, as do vestigial cysts of mesonephric origin (Gartner's duct cysts). The true nature of these cysts is not usually known without histological examination.

VARICOCELE of the vulva occurs mainly in pregnancy giving rise to the characteristic 'bag of worms' feel to palpation. Since the veins are close to the skin, there is a bluish discoloration. The patient is conscious of an uncomfortable swelling on standing. The veins seldom rupture during delivery. Varicocele must be differentiated from an *inguinal hernia* extending into the labium majus and from a *cyst of the canal of Nuck* (the processus vaginalis which has failed to become completely obliterated). Both the latter tend to involve only the anterior parts of the labium majus, but all these conditions extend to the groin. Whereas a hernia is reducible as a rule, a cyst of the canal of Nuck is not. Inguinal hernias usually disappear as pregnancy progresses, but varicoceles become worse. If a hernia contains bowel, it is resonant to percussion. A strangulated hernia will not be reducible, but the accompanying acute symptoms and the history should make the diagnosis clear.

A *haematoma* of the vulva may follow delivery or occur as the result of direct trauma. It is recognized as a bluish swelling which is painful and tender and spreads up into the pelvis by the side of the vagina. The appearance is characteristic and the diagnosis is made on the history. An endometrioma is a rare cause of a blood-containing cyst on the vulva.

BENIGN NEW GROWTHS. Both *fibroma* and *lipoma* are seen in the vulva and may become pedunculated. They may occur at any age, are soft, oval or rounded and covered by vulval skin. They may grow slowly to reach the size of a fist. A lipoma is usually broader based than a fibroma. Several other benign swellings are found on the vulva. They are usually solitary and small (about 1 cm or so in diameter) and their nature is arrived at on histology. A *papilloma* is a sessile benign tumour of the skin of the labia in women of middle or old age. A *hidradenoma* is a tumour of sweat gland origin which may be solid or cystic and which may ulcerate to allow a red papillomatous growth to be extruded. When ulcerated it may suggest the diagnosis of carcinoma clinically. Biopsy solves the problem. Less commonly there are found fibromyoma, myxoma, angioma, lymphangioma, benign melanoma and neuroma, each distinguished by microscopic examination.

TUMOURS AT THE URETHRAL MEATUS. *Urethral caruncles* are frequent, especially in older women. A caruncle appears as a small reddish sessile growth arising from the posterior wall of the urethral meatus causing bleeding and painful micturition. It is often very tender but may be symptomless. It is usually granulomatous, but may be polypoidal and papillomatous. It has to be distinguished from *prolapse of the urethral mucosa* in which there is a ring of protruding red tissue all round the urethral opening.

MALIGNANT NEW GROWTH. *Squamous-cell carcinoma* (epithelioma) is the most important of these. It occurs mainly in elderly women over 60 or 70 years of age. In about half the cases, it is preceded by pruritus vulvae for several years due to hyperplastic vulval dystrophy (*see under* PRURITUS VULVAE). It commonly arises in the anterior part of the vulva in the skin of the labia majora, or is in the region of the clitoris. Usually there is a single lesion, but there may be two opposite each other, so-called 'kissing cancers'. It begins as a raised intracutaneous nodule which ulcerates to give rise to a hard-based ulcer with raised everted edges. The proliferative type presents with an irregular friable mass of growth. A biopsy and histology establish the true nature of the lesion. Spread occurs to the inguinal nodes which should always be felt for

enlargement and hardness. In advanced cases the nodes ulcerate through the skin of the groin and become fixed to the deeper tissues. *Other malignant tumours* found in the vulva include rodent ulcer (basal-cell carcinoma) forming a flat plaque with its characteristic rolled edge, malignant melanoma (pigmented and non-pigmented), adenocarcinoma arising in Bartholin's gland or in the urethra, and sarcoma. Metastatic tumours from primaries in the cervix, uterine body and ovary rarely occur. Chorioncarcinoma has also been described. The *displacements* given in the list above are dealt with under the heading VAGINA AND UTERUS, PROLAPSE OF.

N. Patel

Vulva, ulceration of

Ulceration of the vulva may be due to:

Squamous-cell carcinoma (epithelioma)
Rodent ulcer
Other malignant tumours (melanoma, sarcoma, adenocarcinoma, etc.)
Vulval dystrophy (hypoplastic and hyperplastic)
Carcinoma-in-situ (intra-epithelial carcinoma)
Bowen's disease
Paget's disease
Herpes genitalis
Behçet's syndrome
Soft sore (chancroid)
Granuloma inguinale
Lymphopathia (lymphogranuloma) venereum
Syphilis
Yaws
Tuberculosis
Furunculosis
Diptheria
Vincent's infection
Diabetic vulvitis
Mycotic vulvitis

MALIGNANT AND PREMALIGNANT ULCERATION

Malignancy of the vulva produces a localized swelling which becomes ulcerated. The various lesions are dealt with under VULVAL SWELLINGS, *above*. Vulval dystrophies are chronic conditions which cause intense itching of the vulva. They are dealt with under PRURITUS VULVAE. Hyperplastic dystrophy with atypia seen under the microscope should be regarded as premalignant and excised. Intra-epithelial carcinoma (Bowen's disease) and Paget's disease also cause chronic pruritus. They give rise to thickening of the vulval skin which is dusky red in colour with patches of white due to hyperkeratosis and superficial ulceration from rubbing and scratching. Biopsies are needed for diagnosis, as they are both premalignant.

ACUTE MULTIPLE ULCERS

These may occur as the result of *herpes genitalis infection* transmitted sexually. Primary infection occurs 2–7 days after inoculation. Prodromal symptoms of tingling or itching are followed by vesicular eruptions which rapidly erode resulting in painful, shallow ulcers all over the vulva. They give rise to dysuria, bilateral inguinal lymphadenopathy, fever and malaise. Herpes virus can be obtained from the vesicular fluid in the early stages, 85 per cent being due to the herpes virus, type 2. The lesions, which are very painful, persist for 2–6 weeks before healing occurs and antibody appears in the blood. The ulcers tend to recur at intervals of weeks or months and the virus may be recovered from them. Coitus with a non-immune partner will pass on the infection. The disease is self-limiting in time and the lesions eventually heal spontaneously.

Behçet's syndrome is a rare disorder of unknown cause characterized by oral and vulval ulceration. Iridocyclitis, arthritis and nervous system involvement are complications of severe cases.

SEXUALLY TRANSMITTED INFECTIONS

Syphilis is the most important of these. Between 10 and 90 days after contact with an infectious lesion, the Hunterian chancre develops at the portal of entry. It is an indurated firm painless papule or ulcer with raised edges. In the case of a vulval lesion, the inguinal nodes are enlarged and firm and painless. Genital lesions in women often escape notice because they are hidden inside the vagina or on the cervix. The lesion has to be differentiated from an epithelioma. The serum from a chancre contains the spirochaete *Treponema pallidum* which can be seen under a microscope with the aid of dark ground illumination. If an epithelioma is suspected the ulcer and swelling should be excised and examined microscopically. The chancre persists for 1–5 weeks, but serological tests for syphilis do not become positive for about 4–6 weeks after the appearance of the chancre. The serological tests most commonly performed are the VDRL slide test and the FTA-ABS (fluorescent treponemal antibody absorption) test which have replaced the Wassermann, Kahn and TPI (treponemal immobilization test). To exclude primary syphilis, serological tests have to be done every week for 6 weeks after the appearance of the chancre. Two weeks to 6 months after the chancre has healed, the generalized cutaneous eruption of secondary syphilis appears. Numerous moist flat-topped papules occur on the vulva and round the anus. They are known as 'condyloma latum'. In only one-third of untreated cases does tertiary syphilis occur, but not until some years after the primary lesion.

Spreading ulceration on the vulva is a rare manifestation which has to be differentiated from an epithelioma on histology.

Granuloma inguinale is a chronic venereal infection with a tendency to ulceration and massive granulation tissue affecting the vulva and groins. It is almost non-existent in Great Britain, but is seen in India, Brazil and the West Indies, islands of the South Pacific, Australia, China and Africa. It starts as a raised papilloma which soon ulcerates, the ulcer having a typical serpiginous outline. The granuloma in the groin rarely suppurates but much scarring develops. Scrapings from the ulcers reveal the causative organism, the Donovan body, a small bacterium encapsulated in mononuclear leucocytes with a curved rod-like nucleus.

Lymphogranuloma venereum is another sexually transmitted disease found in the tropical and subtropical regions of Africa, Asia and south-eastern USA. It is due to *Chlamydia trachomatis*. It begins with a vesicopustular eruption on the vulva which soon disappears but there follows painful suppuration in the inguinal glands with hypertrophy and ulceration of the groins, vulva and perineum. Later scarring may cause anal stricture or severe dyspareunia. The diagnosis may be made by isolating the organism, by the intradermal injection of virus antigen when a cutaneous reaction develops (Frei test) or by a complement fixation test.

Chancroid (soft sore) occurs 3–5 days after coitus. It begins as a vesicopustule which becomes a punched-out ulcer with a red base or as a saucer-shaped, ragged ulcer. The lesion is extremely tender and produces a heavy foul discharge which is contagious. It contains the causative organism, Ducrey's bacillus (*Haemophilus ducreyi*) a Gram-negative rod. The lesion may be solitary or there may be several ulcers. Usually there is a painful inguinal adenitis which may break down and discharge. Syphilis, herpes, granuloma inguinale and lymphogranuloma venereum must be ruled out and attempts made to isolate the organism from the ulcers or from the buboes in the groin.

OTHER CONDITIONS

Yaws occurs in tropical countries and produces a lesion similar in appearance to the condyloma latum of secondary syphilis. *Tuberculous ulcers* are very uncommon on the vulva. They are very indolent and can only be diagnosed with certainty on microscopical section. *Furunculosis* (boils) due to staphylococcal infection of the hair follicles are common, affecting the labia majora in particular. *Diphtheria* produces ulceration with a characteristic membranous exudate. *Vincent's infection* of the vulva is the cause of indurated ulceration with an exudate containing fusiform bacilli and spirochaetes. *Mycotic and diabetic vulvitis* (thrush) cause soreness and pruritus of the vulva with redness, excoriation and oedema of the skin and a characteristic white curd-like discharge containing the mycelium of *Candida albicans*.

N. Patel

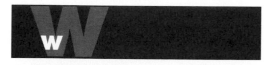

Weals

Weals are the characteristic lesion of *urticaria*. They are flat-topped evanescent elevations of the skin, the result of local oedema in the skin. They may occur as a physiological response to trauma, e.g. caning or whipping.

Urticaria is a common condition where weals arise in the skin spontaneously—it varies in severity from minor itchy blemishes to a severe, even life-threatening angio-oedema of the laryngeal tissues. Lesions begin as red intensely itchy areas, which become raised and show central pallor over a few minutes. Characteristically they vanish without trace within 6 to 12 hours, though new neighbouring weals may continue cropping. The weals are due to focal oedema following dilatation and increased permeability of cutaneous capillaries. Sometimes deeper vessels are involved resulting in more massive subcutaneous *angio-oedema*. Rarely weals arise so violently that the overlying epidermis blisters (bullous urticaria). Weals can be produced experimentally by intradermal injection of histamine and are largely blocked by antihistamines; the release of histamine from dermal mast cells is the suggested mechanism in most cases, though other inflammatory mediators may be involved, e.g. acetylcholine, kinins, prostaglandins and platelet activating factor.

Urticara is very common (probably 10 per cent of the population will experience an attack at some stage) but the majority of cases are of unknown cause—*idiopathic urticaria*.

We will consider first those varieties when an underlying cause can be found:

1 *Physical urticaria*. Weals occur in response to various physical stimuli, the commonest of which is *dermographism*, where firm stroking of the skin results in wealing. This is seen in 3-5 per cent of the population, yet only a proportion of such individuals complain of itching. In *pressure urticaria* deep painful swelling occurs after sustained pressure, e.g. on buttocks or soles. Swelling may be delayed several hours after pressure, and lasts 24–48 hours. Temperature change may provoke wealing in some individuals, e.g. *cold urticaria*, which may be reproduced by application of ice cubes to the skin. Such wealing can occur in the presence of cryoglobulins in patients with *lupus erythematosus, syphilis* or *paraproteinaemia*. Occasionally collapse due to massive histamine release follows immersion in cold water, e.g. swimming. Tolerance can be induced by regular cold showers, but is seldom pursued. Exposure to local heat, e.g. hot water bottle and ultraviolet radiation (*solar urticaria*), can produce wealing in susceptible individuals, and it has recently been established that contact with water, irrespective of temperature, results in urticaria in a surprising number of people (*aquagenic urticaria*).

2 *Cholinergic urticaria* is a distinctive condition where numerous intensely itchy pin-head papules develop some 10 minutes after sweating. Susceptible individuals show an exaggerated reaction to the introduction of acetylcholine derivatives into the skin. Severe attacks are followed by a refractory period of 24–48 hours (*Fig. W.1*).

3 *Drugs*. Some chemicals cause release of histamine from mast cells, and all varieties of urticaria may be improved by avoiding them. Salicylates, and opiates such as codeine and morphine, are common examples, but food preservatives, e.g. benzoates and dyes, such as tartrazine and azodyes, can cause similar reactions. Careful history taking may identify such patients, but a proportion of those with *idiopathic* urticaria can be improved by the adoption of a diet free of preservatives and food dyes.

4 *Allergy* Some acute urticarias can be truly allergic in origin, e.g.
   —food urticarias: shellfish, strawberries, nuts, etc. (*Fig. W.2*).
   —drug urticarias: penicillin, sulphonamides
   —infestations: parasitic worms, trichinosis, loiasis and scabies
   —infections: candidiasis

5 *Serum sickness*. Type III hypersensitivity causes weals of longer duration. Wealing is a rare feature of several general medical conditions and infections. In *thyrotoxicosis* and *lymphoma* other signs and symptoms can be found, but in early stages of *systemic lupus erythematosus* urticaria may be the only clinical abnormality, the weals often persist for an unusually long time, e.g. 2–4 days, and may cause bruising. *Viral hepatitis* can begin with urticaria, the fever and icterus following 2–3 days later. A particular urticarial eruption appearing dramatically each evening often accompanies adult *Still's disease*.

Weals can be the presenting feature of other dermatoses, e.g. *pemphigoid, dermatitis herpetiformis* or *vasculitis*. In a few *atopic* individuals a *contact urticaria* occurs soon after the skin is touched by, for example, certain grasses, animal hair or saliva, or foods such as fish or fruits. Contact allergic urticaria is also seen, especially to rubber gloves in health care personnel.

Hereditary angio-oedema is a dominantly inherited lack of the enzyme C_1 esterase inhibitor. Affected family members suffer severe attacks of weals accompanied by abdominal colic and glottic oedema. Treatment is now available.

In the great majority of patients, however, none of these associated conditions can be found, and by

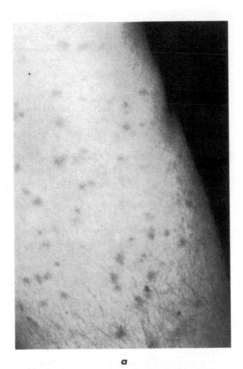 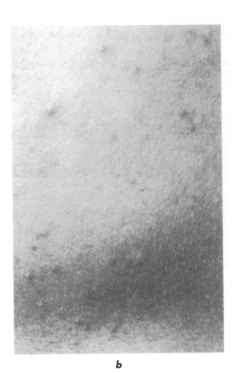

a   *b*

Fig. W.1. *a*, Urticaria pigmentosa. *b*, Cholinergic urticaria.

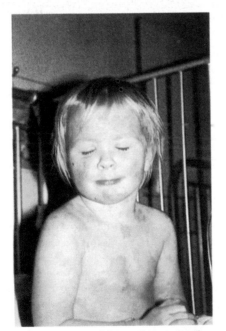

Fig. W.2. Acute urticaria following the ingestion of peanuts.

exclusion are at present classified as *idiopathic urticaria*. More common in women, with a peak incidence in 20–40 year-olds, the condition is slow in onset. Eventually crops of weals may appear daily. Weals recur over periods of weeks, sometimes months, but spontaneous remission occurs within 6–8 months in the vast majority. Recurrences do occur and some unfortunate individuals are prone to indefinite urticaria. In a third of patients episodes of angio-oedema occur, with asymmetrical swelling of cheeks, lips, eyelids and floor of mouth. If the larynx or pharynx is involved the airway can be prejudiced. Angio-oedema sometimes occurs as the only manifestation of urticaria.

Richard Staughton

Weight gain

Table W.1 highlights the major causes of weight gain. Although it is usually simple to differentiate the major causes, especially where pregnancy or oedema are apparent, a scientific assessment of fat and muscle mass can be made by using skinfold-thickness measurements or by electrical impedance method. Overweight and obesity refer to conditions where body fat is in excess. The term 'overweight' is used when weight is 110–119 per cent above the upper limit of an acceptable range (which is itself defined as 100 per cent), the term 'obesity' referring to a weight 120 per cent or above. The acceptable range is based on life assurance figures of mortality, drawn up for height and weight. Originally this included frame size, but because this is so awkward to quantify it has now been discarded. Often in the literature the degree of obesity is expressed as the body mass index (BMI)

Table W.1. Causes of weight gain

Pregnancy

Excess fluid retention
Cardiac failure
Liver failure
Renal failure
Nephrotic syndrome
Periodic oedema
Hypoproteinaemic states

Lymphatic obstruction
Milroy's syndrome
Elephantiasis
Metastatic carcinoma

Excess muscle
Precocious puberty
Androgenic steroids
Growth hormone
Athletes, especially weightlifters

Fat excess—obesity

Organ enlargement
Ovarian cyst

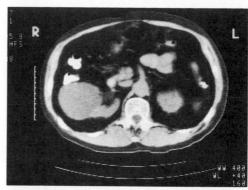

Fig. W.3. CT scan showing predominantly intra-abdominal fat in an obese male patient.

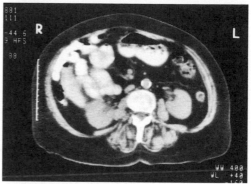

Fig. W.4. CT scan showing that in females with 'apple' or central obesity, the excess fat is mainly deposited subcutaneously.

which is calculated from the equation weight (in kilograms) divided by height^2 (in metres). A BMI of 25–29·9 is graded as overweight (Garrow Obesity Scale I), 30–40 as Grade II obesity and greater than 40 as morbidly obese (Grade III).

Recent surveys have indicated the enormity of the problem in Western society. Both sexes show a rapid increase in weight in their mid-20s. Males tend to become progressively heavier until they reach their 50s, whereas in women, weight remains fairly static until the menopause when there is a substantial weight gain. By the age of 25 years about 30 per cent of males and females are overweight, whereas at 60 years of age about half have a weight problem considered a risk to health. In the 1990 census in the UK, 8 per cent of males and 12 per cent of females had a BMI of 30 or above. Although the risk to health increases with the degree of obesity, the configuration of adipose tissue may be an independent risk factor associated with an increased risk of hyperinsulinaemia, hyperlipidaemia, hypertension, ischaemic heart disease, cardiovascular events and death (*Figs.* W.3, W.4). Comparison of the circumference of waist and hip indicates that a ratio of over 0·8 in females and 0·95 in males is hazardous to health.

The cause of obesity in everyone is an energy intake in excess of energy expenditure. The scientific arguments arise over whether some individuals with a predisposition for obesity have a lower energy expenditure at the outset. Recent reports suggest a degree of variability in energy expenditure in any obese population and if this is matched by a similar variability in appetite, then possibly this explains in a simple manner the aetiology of obesity. Studies of twins indicate a degree of genetic involvement in the development of obesity but there is no doubt that the cause is multifactorial with environmental influences playing a major role. Much emphasis has been made for an aetiological role for brown fat, which is a potent thermogenic tissue in rodents. Certainly in adults brown fat is present, but is thought to contribute little to daily energy expenditure and could not by itself account for the variations in energy expenditure reported.

Although the vast majority of obese individuals could be said to have 'idiopathic' or 'simple' obesity, it is always worth while considering the other rare causes of obesity (*Table* W.2).

Table W.2. Causes of obesity

Idiopathic or simple
Energy intake in excess of energy expenditure; multifactorial causes

Genetic
Prader–Willi syndrome
Laurence–Moon–Biedl syndrome
Alstrom
Morel syndrome
Morgagni syndrome
Morgagni–Stewart–Morel syndrome
Carpenter's syndrome

Cohen's syndrome
DIDMOAD

Hypothalamic
Trauma
Tumours
   Craniopharygioma
   Astrocytoma
Inflammation
   Meningitis
   Encephalitis
   Tuberculosis
   Syphilis
Infiltration
   Sarcoidosis
   Histiocytosis X

Endocrine
Hypothalamus
   Hypogonadotrophic hypogonadism
   Growth hormone failure
Pituitary
   Laron dwarf
   Hyperprolactinaemia
   Cushing's disease
   Nelson's syndrome
   Hypopituitarism (Fröhlich)

Thyroid
Cretin
Primary and secondary hypothyroidism
Rare cases of thyrotoxicosis

Parathyroid
Pseudohypoparathyroidism
Pseudo-pseudohypoparathyroidism

Adrenal
Cushing's syndrome (ectopic source, adenoma,
   carcinoma)

Pancreas
Nesidioblastoma
Insulinoma
Beckwith–Wiedemann syndrome

Ovaries
Polycystic ovarian syndrome
Postmenopausal

Testes
Primary hypogonadism

Inactivity
Mental retardation, e.g. Down's
Physical disability, e.g. spina bifida

Drugs
Insulin
Cessation of smoking
Sulphonylurea agents
Corticosteroids
Oestrogen
Alcohol excess (pseudo Cushing's)
Cyproheptadine

Abnormal fat distribution
Multiple lipomatosis
Partial lipodystrophy

Painful fat
Dercum's disease

Hypothalamic lesion. Any hypothalamic lesion which destroys the ventromedial nucleus (classical 'satiety' area) may result in obesity. Some have suggested that the mechanism is by a stimulation of excess insulin secretion by the pancreas causing hyperphagia as has been shown with similar lesions in rodents, nevertheless, truncal vagotomy in man does not appear successful on a long-term basis. Others have shown a reduction in sympathetic outflow in similarly damaged rodents reducing brown fat and other thermogenic influences but whether this plays a part in the development of obesity in the hypothalamic-damaged person has not as yet been shown. Often other hypothalamic manifestations may be present in such patients. They include panhypopituitarism, diabetes insipidus, also lethargy and somnolence. If the condition arises in childhood, then the genitalia are usually poorly developed. In Fröhlich's original case, a craniopharyngioma was pressing upon the hypothalamus and hence such obesity associated with a hypogonadal state and poor growth are often referred to as Fröhlich's syndrome. Most boys in whom the diagnosis of Fröhlich's syndrome is entertained are in fact suffering from 'simple' obesity in whom prepubertal genitalia are buried in a pubic pad of fat (*Fig.* W.5).

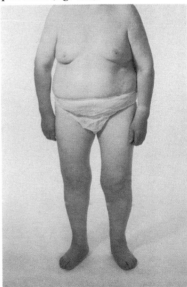

Fig. W.5. Fröhlich's syndrome—showing short stature, marked abdominal obesity and panhypopituitarism.

Hypothyroidism leads to weight gain due to both a reduction in the metabolic rate and to the deposition of hydrophilic mucopolysaccharides all over the body. Most cases are due to thyroid gland dysfunction and in such serum TSH is elevated. Hypothalamic pituitary lesions can result in a similar dysfunction (known as *secondary hypothyroidism*) with a low serum TSH and an absent or delayed TSH response to TRH. Weight loss can be rapid following the introduction of replacement thyroxine therapy in severely hypothyroid patients. Nevertheless, in those whose obesity precedes the development of mild hypothyroidism weight loss can be slight with thyroid replacement, a source of disappointment to many, but indicative of an underlying 'simple' obese problem. In most cases of thyrotoxicosis, weight decreases due to an increase in energy expenditure. In some rare cases of thyrotoxicosis the increase in appetite produces an energy intake in excess of the rise in energy expenditure, hence resulting in an increase in weight.

Pseudohypoparathyroidism is associated with some degree of obesity. These patients are short with stubby hands and feet due to the shortening of one or more (which can include all five) metacarpals and metatarsals. Ectopic calcification, including basal ganglia calcification, and cataracts have been reported. The cause appears to be due to a peripheral resistance to the metabolic effects of parathyroid hormone producing serum hypocalcaemia. This is most likely as a consequence of a deficiency in the membrane regulatory or coupling proteins (known as N or G). This membrane protein dysfunction can extend to other hormone receptors, hence explaining the abnormalities in secretion and in the effects of thyrotrophin, prolactin, gonadotrophin, vasopressin, glucagon and insulin sometimes encountered in this syndrome. There is also a variant disorder of similar phenotype but normal biochemistry called *pseudo-pseudohypoparathyroidism* which can occur independently or in relatives of patients with pseudohypoparathyroidism.

Cushing's syndrome is rare, but can be differentiated from 'simple' obesity by its four cardinal signs, namely, thin skin, conjunctival oedema (chemosis), frontal balding, most notably in women, and proximal myopathy. In a florid case obesity is central with thin arms and legs due to muscle wasting and a moon plethoric face; aptly but ingraciously termed 'a lemon on matchsticks with a cherry head' (*Fig.* W.6). Oedema, hypertension, diabetes mellitus, and severe osteoporosis are usually present. The latter often results in spontaneous rib and spine fractures resulting in loss of height and kyphosis. The latter must also be distinguished from the buffalo hump associated with fat over the upper thoracic spine. Acne, virilism, hirsutism and spontaneous bruising are often present. In children this disease slows growth unlike simple obesity where growth is accelerated in the early years. Striae can be found in Cushing's syndrome (*Fig.* W.7), but the absence does not exclude the condition. Striae is not pathognomic of Cushing's syndrome, for it is often found in healthy individuals who have had a rapid weight change.

In mild cases of Cushing's syndrome, the diagnosis from simple obesity is not easy. If suspected then 24-hour urine samples should be measured for free cortisol as this is elevated in Cushing's syndrome. Some

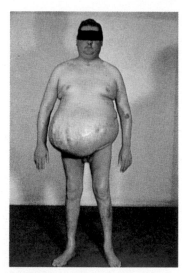

Fig. W.6. Cushing's syndrome showing moon face, central obesity, wasted arms and legs, abdominal striae and bruising.

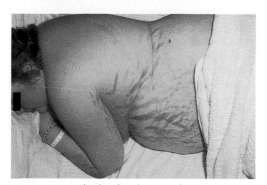

Fig. W.7. Steroid-induced Cushing's syndrome.

use an overnight 1 mg dexamethasone test, the drug being taken at midnight and a blood cortisol value measured at 9 a.m. the next morning; a value of less than 100 nmol/1 being considered normal. Although the simple overnight dexamethasone test is helpful, no test is ever totally reliable and if still clinically suspicious more investigations should be carried out on an inpatient basis. Alcohol can mimic Cushing's both in clinical features and by increasing urine free cortisol output and this situation is termed *pseudo Cushing's*. Admission to hospital with a total ban on alcohol will eventually result in normal cortisol values.

Patients with *insulinoma* are said to be mildly obese as insulin stimulates appetite. Hyperinsulinaemia due to islet cell hyperplasia can occur in the rare abnormality of *Weidmann–Beckman syndrome*. These children grow more rapidly, have an enlarged tongue, omphalocele and tend to be mildly obese.

In the *polycystic ovarian syndrome* over half the patients are obese. The reason for this is not known, but obesity tends to perpetuate the syndrome because

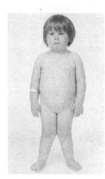
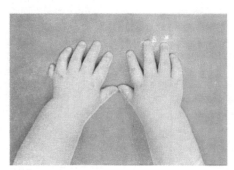
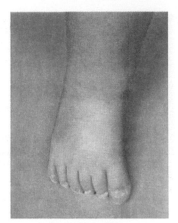

Fig. W.8. Laurence–Moon–Biedl syndrome. Showing obesity, genu valgum and polydactylism (supplementary little finger on the left hand and six toes on the foot). (*Courtesy of Professor C. Chantler, Guy's Hospital, London.*)

of the conversion in adipose tissue of ovarian androstenedione to oestrone. The other features of the syndrome are oligomenorrhoea or menorrhoea, infertility, hirsutism and enlarged polycystic ovaries. Biochemically, serum LH is elevated in comparison to FSH, associated with a raised serum testosterone and androstenedione. Many have wondered whether *hyperprolactinaemia* induces weight gain, for the clinical impression is that many such woman are obese. One survey disputed whether obesity was more prevalent in hyperprolactinaemia, but the impression still remains.

Males with *hypogonadism* of whatever cause tend to be slightly obese. The distribution of fat is of a female distribution over the lower abdomen, hips and thighs. *Growth hormone failure* in children is associated with mild obesity, as is the rare *Laron dwarf* who has a deficiency of the growth factor somatomedin. There are various other congenital syndromes associated with obesity. The *Prader–Willi* syndrome is characterized by muscular hypotonia, short stature, small body and feet, mental retardation, hypogonadism and gross obesity. Hyperappetite appears to be the principal cause of their obesity although a hypothalamic thermic abnormality has been reported. Recently deletions of chromosome 15 have been implicated as the cause of this condition. In *Laurence-Moon-Biedl* syndrome obesity is associated with short stature (in some), retarded sexual development, mental retardation, retinitis pigmentosa, and either polydactylism or syndactylism (*Fig.* W.8).

In *Alström's* syndrome there is obesity, diabetes mellitus, nerve deafness, retinal degeneration and cataracts producing childhood blindness and late onset nephropathy. Many patients with *Down's syndrome* are obese as are many children with mental or physical retardation, possibly due to inactivity associated with too high an energy intake.

Morgagni-Stewart-Morel is a combination of the

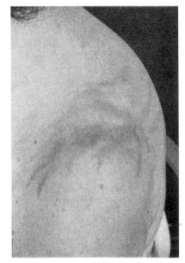

Fig. W.9. Livid striae in the left shoulder produced by glucocorticoid excess.

syndromes described by Morel and Morgagni. In *Morel's syndrome* there is obesity, hyperostosis of the frontal bone, headache, nervous disturbance and a tendency to mental disorder. In *Morgagni syndrome*, the obesity is associated with internal frontal hyperostosis and virilism.

Carpenter's syndrome is associated with acrocephaly, polydactyly and syndactyly, mental retardation, male hypogonadism and mild obesity. In *Cohen's syndrome* obesity is associated with severe mental retardation, microcephaly and short stature and facial abnormalities.

DIDMOAD is an acronym for the major features of the syndrome namely diabetes insipidus, diabetes mellitus, optic atrophy and deafness. Most are associated with mild obesity as well as bladder and ureter atonia.

Some *drugs* may cause obesity or a worsening

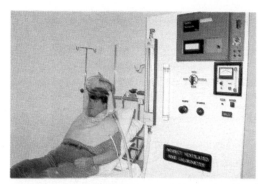

Fig. W.10. Energy expenditure measured by ventilated hood calorimetry. In this machine housed at Ninewells Hospital, Dundee, air is pumped from inside the hood and analysed for oxygen consumed by paramagnetic analysis and carbon dioxide exhaled by infrared analysis. A computer attached analyses the output, takes into account temperature and saturated vapour pressure, producing minute-by-minute readout of energy expended.

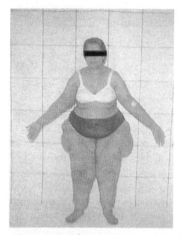

Fig. W.11. Lipomatosis. Showing symmetrical distribution of fat deposits over the lower half of the body.

of a pre-existing weight problem. Insulin given to diabetics tends to lead to weight gain, as do the sulphonylurea drugs, but usually this is not seen with the biguanide metformin. Weight gain noted when glycaemic control is improved with insulin is partly due to a reduction in both energy expenditure and urine glucose losses. Glucocorticoids in excess rapidly cause weight gain and produce iatrogenic Cushing's syndrome (*Fig.* W.9). Oestrogen can also induce weight gain. Although water retention has been implicated, a reduction in energy expenditure in the second half of the menstrual cycle due to a lack of ovulation also plays a role. A frequent finding is of weight gain on cessation of smoking. Recent work has shown that a smoked cigarette increases sympathetic drive and on average one cigarette increases energy expenditure by about 9 kcal. Hence, if smoking is ceased then energy intake must be appropriately reduced to prevent weight gain. Nevertheless, many tend to overeat on cessation of smoking which exacerbates the problem (*Fig.* W.10).

An abnormal distribution of fat occurs in *lipodystrophies* which comprise a group of disorders ranging from generalized lipo-atrophy to partial forms. *Partial lipo-atrophy* (lipodystrophia progressiva) is characterized by a symmetrical loss of subcutaneous fat over dermatone areas of the face and upper body, with a normal or even excessive amount of adipose tissue below the waist. Occasionally the atrophy is confined below the waist without upper body involvement (*Fig.* W.11). This condition, which mainly affects females, is associated with hyperglycaemia, hyperinsulinaemia, marked insulin resistance, hyperlipaemia and hepatosplenomegaly. In *Dercum's* disease obesity is generalized but there is pain and tenderness in the more prominent fatty deposits for reasons as yet unknown.

Roland T. Jung

Weight loss

Loss of weight may be the result of inadequate food intake, absorption or retention. It may also be due to increased utilization. It is important to distinguish between those patients who lose weight in spite of normal food intake and those whose calorie intake is diminished. In children, the commonest causes are malnutrition from injudicious feeding and gastrointestinal disease (*see* MARASMUS, p. 406); in adults, when loss of weight is considerable, with no definite physical signs and little relevant history, one thinks first of *malignant disease*, a chronic infection such as *tuberculosis*, or *hyperthyroidism, diabetes mellitus, anorexia nervosa* or some other *psychiatric disturbance*.

Research indicates that in 35 per cent of patients losing weight no specific cause is usually found. In the others a serious underlying cause is discovered, 10 per cent having a psychiatric aetiology, the others having a physical disorder, the commonest being cancer, gastrointestinal disease, heart failure, alcohol abuse, obstructive airways disease, poorly controlled diabetes mellitus and thyrotoxicosis. Patients who have nausea, vomiting, alterations in appetite or cough are likely to have a physical cause whereas those who maintain the same level of physical activity during loss of weight and are non-smokers are not. The single most helpful investigation is a chest radiograph which often reveals masses, infiltrates, heart failure or lymph node enlargement.

Weight loss with adequate food intake

1. Increased utilization

Hyperthyroidism
Chronic infections (e.g. pulmonary tuberculosis)

Anxiety states, food phobias
Drugs: thyroid, amphetamine

2. Diminished absorption

Intestinal insufficiency states
Intestinal hypermotility states
Chronic pancreatitis
Carcinoid
Short-circuit operations
Post-colectomy and post-gastrectomy states
Chronic hepatic disease
Dysphagia, e.g. scleroderma
Whipple's disease
Lymphatic obstruction
Drugs, purges

3. Abnormal calorie loss

Diabetes mellitus
Fistulas
Intestinal parasites

Weight loss with diminished food intake

1. Psychogenic

Depression
Anorexia nervosa
Psychoses

2. Gastrointestinal

Peptic ulcer
Malignancy
Chronic colitis
Hepato-biliary disease

3. Malignant conditions

Lymphoma
Leukaemia
Carcinoma
Sarcoma

4. Uraemia

5. Chronic infections

6. Chronic non-infective inflammatory conditions

Rheumatoid arthritis
Systemic lupus erythematosus
Dermatomyositis
Polyarteritis nodosa
Giant-cell arteritis
Systemic sclerosis

7. Chronic intoxications

Alcohol
Additive drugs
Heavy smoking
Lead

8. Advanced crippling from any cause

9. Endocrine disease

Addison's disease and some cases of hypopituitarism (Simmond's disease)
Phaeochromocytoma
Gut hormone tumours (e.g. vipoma)

10. Faulty diet

Food faddism
Food intolerance

11. Chronic cardiac conditions

12. Chronic lung conditions

(e.g. obstructive airways disease)

13. AIDS (acquired immune deficiency syndrome)

Young persons may lose weight as the result of change of surroundings, for instance from school life to work in a city office; depression, anxiety, sorrow, disappointment in love, too strenuous a life of pleasure, irregularity of meals, overlong hours of work are familiar causes of what at the time may appear to be ominous loss of weight. In some patients an accompanying loss of appetite and inadequate food intake supply a plausible explanation. In other cases it appears that the nervous disturbance is in itself responsible. Many young girls taking up a new occupation such as nursing lose weight initially, and regain it as they adapt to their new life.

Any affection of the alimentary tract interfering with intake, digestion and absorption of food may produce a loss of weight—gastric or duodenal ulcer, inflammatory bowel disease in its many forms, excessive smoking, or drinking, monotony of food or of circumstances, carious teeth, ill-fitting dental plates, pyorrhoea alveolaris, and the abuse of purgatives may contribute to the wasting. When gastric symptoms are prominent it may be difficult initially to tell whether the condition is nervous in origin or due to organic disease. Weight loss also may occur after partial or total gastrectomy or colectomy, when a new 'normal' is created for the patient.

Any malady which produces *sleeplessness* or *persistent pain* may lead to serious loss of weight.

Chronic infections may not be obvious in themselves, and yet may produce loss of weight by interfering with general nutrition. This is seen in many who have returned from the tropics after infection by dysentery, yellow fever, malaria, dengue, hepatitis; chronic affections of the joints, the skin or the alimentary tract may produce loss of weight in a similar way.

Chronic pyelonephritis is often missed through neglect of bacteriological examination of the urine.

Liver disorders may affect general nutrition, and loss of weight may occur in some sufferers from cirrhosis, though in the early stages the patient may be fat and towards the end, loss of weight may be masked by deceptive increase due to ascites. Malignant change in cirrhotic livers is not uncommon, carcinoma (hepatocellular) being seen most often in haemochromatosis and hepatitis B virus infections. In drug addiction and AIDS weight loss is often considerable.

The effect of *alcohol* upon bodyweight is variable, some persons becoming stout, others thin, and others changing little. This depends greatly on food (calorie) intake, beer-drinkers tending to become obese and pot-bellied. Broadly speaking it is heavy spirit drinkers who lose weight, and in some cases serious doubts may arise whether the loss in such a patient is due to alcoholic habits alone or whether there is not in addition some cancer or tuberculous infection. When alcoholism leads to peripheral neuropathy there is often rapid and extreme loss of weight. In chronic crippling disorders such as rheumatoid arthritis, multiple sclerosis or hemiplegia marked loss of weight may occur, as it may in chronic congestive heart failure, where oedema may mask the wasting.

The loss of weight in *old age*, due to diminished intake of and lessened interest in food, is usually gradual and slow: if otherwise, neoplasia or chronic infection, such as tuberculosis, depression, giant-cell arteritis or some other cause should be suspected.

Diabetes mellitus, especially in the young, may have loss of weight as its earliest symptom.

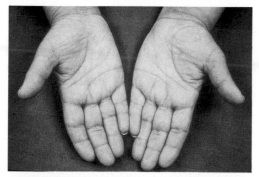

Fig. W.12. Crease pigmentation indicated Addison's disease in this patient who had noted progressive and rapid weight loss associated with diarrhoea and lassitude.

Addison's disease is another affection in which, besides the progressive asthenia, loss of weight may be marked. There may or may not have been attacks of syncope or of diarrhoea; the diagnosis is suggested by brown pigmentation of the skin, particularly in the flexures and groins (*Fig.* W.12), but also beneath the mucous membranes, particularly of the mouth, inside

the lips, or within the cheeks where it is a grey colour. The blood pressure is usually low with a marked postural fall.

Loss of weight is a prominent feature in cases of *hyperthyroidism*; it may be the first symptom to attract attention preceding tachycardia, nervousness, excessive perspiration, fine tremor of the outstretched fingers, exophthalmos, and symmetrical enlargement of the thyroid gland.

Anorexia nervosa is a condition in which wasting is the prominent symptom (*see* p. 32), but amenorrhoea often occurs very early in the disease.

Roland T. Jung

Wheeze

Wheezes are continuous, musical sounds with a definite pitch, typically loudest during expiration, which may be heard at the mouth or with the aid of a stethoscope. These sounds are generated by vibration of an airway, not only narrowed, but almost closed to allow the walls to touch lightly. Air accelerating through the narrowed airway generates pressure fluctuations causing the airway walls to oscillate rapidly producing a musical wheeze. The pitch of the wheeze depends upon the speed of vibration rather than the length or calibre of the airway. Four clinical types of wheeze may be identified:

1. Expiratory polyphonic wheeze

This is a complex musical sound commonly associated with widespread airflow obstruction due to chronic obstructive pulmonary disease or bronchial asthma. The wheeze, together with a background of loud noisy breathing, is audible at the mouth. When listened to on the chest wall the higher frequencies of the breath sounds are filtered out and the wheezes dominate. Polyphonic wheeze present during tidal breathing is a reliable sign of severe airways obstruction. Normal subjects can generate polyphonic wheezes but only on forced expiratory effort.

2. Fixed monophonic wheeze

When a bronchus is narrowed by stenosis of an intrabronchial tumour, a low-pitched monophonic wheeze may be heard, often on inspiration in association with noisy breathing. The low note of the wheeze is related to the tumour mass, which is set in slow oscillation by high velocity gas flow. The pitch can be varied within a narrow range by altering the velocity of gas flow. Stridor is a special example of this sound.

3. Random monophonic wheeze

A particular variety of wheeze distinct from the polyphonic expiratory sounds may be heard in widespread airflow obstruction, overlapping throughout inspiration and expiration with varying duration, timing and pitch.

4. Sequential inspiratory wheeze

In patients with lung restriction due to pulmonary fibrosis, oedema or infiltration a brief high-pitched wheeze can frequently be heard late in inspiration in association with inspiratory crackles. The musical note may repeat from breath to breath, or disappear and reappear at different times. These sounds occur in deflated areas of lung, and are therefore heard in various forms of pulmonary fibrosis, especially extrinsic allergic alveolitis.

The paradoxical absence of wheezing may be of great clinical importance, indicating severe and widespread airflow obstruction. The production of a wheeze requires an airway on the point of closure and an optimum velocity of gas flow at the site of stenosis to set the bronchial walls in oscillation. In patients with severe ventilatory failure, wheezing may be absent because the velocity of flow is too slow to oscillate the airways on the point of closure. For the same reasons, deteriorating asthmatic patients may become less wheezy and eventually develop a silent chest indicating ominous airways obstruction.

(*See also* STRIDOR, p. 637.)

P. R. Studdy

WRIST
See JOINTS, AFFECTIONS OF
XANTHOMA
See NODULES; PAPULES

Yawning

Yawning is such a commonplace physiological occurrence that very little is known about its aetiology. It is a reflex action whose pathways reach no higher in the central nervous system than the basal ganglia. The act itself consists of a tonic contraction of several muscle groups resulting in a deep inspiration, dilatation of the pharynx, and depression of tongue and lower jaw. The physiological effects of the deep inspiration include an increase in venous return to the heart and, probably more significant, the opening of pulmonary alveoli which may have closed during a prolonged period of quiet breathing. If yawning is impossible, as in a patient on a ventilator, disseminated alveolar collapse may occur; this is the cause of the veno-arterial shunting and arterial hypoxaemia seen in this

situation. The 'purpose' of the associated facial contortions is less easy to determine. It has also been noticed that the sense of smell is more acute during a yawn; this is probably as a result of a large bolus of air being brought into contact with an unusually exposed nasopharynx. The importance of an acute sense of smell for wild animals is clear and it has been postulated that this reflex may have had a survival value for primitive man.

The stretching of arms, commonly associated with yawning, is known as 'pandiculation' and is also a reflex act. This information comes as a surprise to some but is conclusively proved by the fact that the paralysed arm in hemiparesis may demonstrate pandiculation even when no voluntary movement is possible.

It remains to give an account of the afferent side of this reflex arc. This can be based only on personal experience and everyday observations. Boredom and drowsiness certainly provoke yawning as does the sight or sound of someone else's yawn. This remarkable contagiousness of yawning is well known but no satisfactory explanation for it appears ever to have been offered.

Very occasionally yawning, especially when occurring very frequently, may be evidence of organic disease. It may be an epileptic phenomenon or occur following attacks of encephalitis along with other disturbances of respiration such as hyperventilation and Cheyne–Stokes breathing. Paroxysms of yawning may also be caused by cerebral tumours, especially those situated in the posterior fossa, and yawning can be regularly produced in an opiate addict by the injection of a narcotic antagonist.

Peter R. Fleming

APPENDIX

ACID–BASE HOMEOSTASIS

The maintenance of extracellular hydrogen ion (H^+) concentration within narrow limits is essential for normal cell function. Around 20,000 mmol of CO_2 are produced during metabolism over a 24 h period. This CO_2, through its ability to combine with H_2O and form carbonic acid (a weak acid), is the major source of H^+ from metabolism. The ability to excrete CO_2 normally through the lungs is necessary to avoid build-up of H^+ and the possibility of acidosis of respiratory origin. In addition, a much smaller amount of non-volatile acid (normally less than 100 m. equivalents per 24 h) is produced from the incomplete oxidation of fat and carbohydrate (producing ketone bodies and lactate, respectively), from acid in foodstuff and from metabolism of S-containing amino acids. Excretion of this acid requires normal renal function.

Thus, retention of CO_2 in acute respiratory acidosis will, by the law of mass action, lead to a movement of the equation to the right and the generation of H^+ (i.e. an acidosis). Renal compensation depends on the secretion of H^+ in the distal nephron. For each H^+ secreted a HCO_3^- anion is generated which is added to the ECF compartment. Hence, the plasma $[HCO_3^-]$ will rise in a chronic respiratory acidosis. In a respiratory alkalosis, the fall in PCO_2 will lead to a movement of the equation to the left, with a decrease in $[H^+]$ (i.e. an alkalosis). In chronic respiratory alkalosis, where compensation has occurred, the $[HCO_3^-]$ will fall.

In a metabolic acidosis, the accumulation of H^+ (or loss of HCO_3^-) will lead to a fall in plasma $[HCO_3^-]$. Any potential increase in pCO_2 accompanying H^+ retention is more than compensated by the stimulation of the respiratory centre by H^+, so that pCO_2 is typically decreased. Conversely, in a metabolic alkalosis the loss of H^+ (or gain in HCO_3^-) will lead to an increase in plasma $[HCO_3^-]$. There is a tendency for pCO_2 to

Table APP.1 Arterial blood analysis

Analysis	Reference range	Units
Bicarbonate	21–27.5	mmol/l
Hydrogen ion	36–44	nmol/l
Pa_{CO_2}	4.4–6.1	kPa
Pa_{O_2}	12–15	kPa
Oxygen saturation	Normally >97	%

Most disorders of H^+ homeostasis lead to acidosis, either through failure to excrete CO_2 (respiratory acidosis) or the accumulation of non-volatile acid as a result of renal disease, overproduction of non-volatile acid or loss of buffer (metabolic acidosis). Metabolic acidosis sometimes results from the ingestion of acids or substances metabolized to acid. Respiratory and metabolic alkaloses are less common.

The assessment of acid–base status is critically dependent on correct blood sampling. Clearly, the acid–base composition of venous blood is variable, reflecting the metabolic activity of the organ through which the blood has passed. For this reason, it is essential to obtain a sample of arterial blood. Furthermore, analysis must be carried out promptly, preferably on a cooled arterial sample, to avoid spurious results due to the metabolic activity of the cellular elements of blood. A further requirement is to collect the sample anaerobically.

In the interpretation of disorders of H^+ homeostasis, the following equation is helpful in explaining the changes of $[H^+]$, $[HCO_3^-]$ and pCO_2 which can be measured in the different types of disorder:

$$CO_2 + H_2O \rightleftharpoons H_2CO_3 \rightleftharpoons H^+ + HCO_3^-$$

increase to compensate for the alkalosis, though this is strictly limited by the reduction in alveolar ventilation and fall in pO_2 which is a necessary consequence of CO_2 retention.

BLOOD GASES

In this section a brief summary of one approach to the interpretation of arterial blood acid–base status will be explained. Such an approach should allow the general category of disorder (if present) to be understood. Having established this, the appropriate section or sections should be consulted for possible specific differential diagnoses. The interpretation of the pO_2 status is considered separately, for simplicity, but should clearly be a part of any assessment of any possible acid–base pathology. An alternative method of determining the general category of disorder is to use an acid–base diagram.

Arterial [H+] normal

1. *pCO_2 normal.* If both $[H^+]$ and pCO_2 are normal, then $[HCO_3^-]$ must be within normal limits from the

relationship which exists between them according to the Henderson equation:

$$[H^+] = \frac{K^1.pCO_2}{[HCO_3^-]}$$

Hence, *there is no acid–base problem*.

2. *pCO_2 increased*. The possibilities are a *fully compensated respiratory acidosis* or *a mixed respiratory acidosis/metabolic alkalosis*. In both conditions, unlike above, the arterial blood [HCO_3^-] will be elevated. Additional clinical information is necessary to distinguish between these two possibilities.

3. *pCO_2 decreased*. This is the converse of above and may result from *a fully compensated respiratory alkalosis* or *a mixed respiratory alkalosis/metabolic acidosis*. The arterial blood [HCO_3^-] will be decreased in both states and cannot be used to distinguish between them.

Arterial [H+] increased

1. *pCO_2 normal*. The situation is one of a *simple metabolic acidosis*, confirmed by the decreased arterial blood [HCO_3^-].

2. *pCO_2 increased*. The patient must have a *respiratory acidosis* confirmed by the high normal or elevated [HCO_3^-]. If the [HCO_3^-] is low, then the picture is consistent with *a mixed respiratory acidosis/metabolic acidosis*.

3. *pCO_2 decreased*. The patient has a *metabolic acidosis/respiratory alkalosis*. The metabolic acidosis is clearly dominating the picture (since [H+] is increased), and the respiratory alkalosis is likely to be *compensatory in origin*. The [HCO_3^-] will be low.

Arterial [H+] decreased

1. *pCO_2 normal*. The patient has a *metabolic alkalosis*. The [HCO_3^-] will be increased.

2. *pCO_2 increased*. A small increase in pCO_2 is most likely to be *a compensatory response to a metabolic alkalosis*. Clearly, CO_2 retention is limited by the associated hypoventilation and reduced pO_2, so that pCO_2 barely rises above the upper limit of the reference range if the response is compensatory. Higher increases in pCO_2 would be consistent with *a mixed metabolic alkalosis/respiratory acidosis*, with the metabolic alkalosis component dominating. The [HCO_3^-] will be increased in both situations.

3. *pCO_2 decreased*. The patient has a respiratory alkalosis. The [HCO_3^-] will be low. If the [HCO_3^-] is high then a *mixed respiratory alkalosis/metabolic alkalosis* is likely to be present.

Specific types of acid–base disorder

a. Respiratory acidosis

The CO_2 retention which is a feature of respiratory acidosis can be subdivided into three categories. It may arise from a failure of the respiratory centre to drive respiration, from pathology in the mechanics of chest movement (neuromuscular lesions or gross structural problems) or from intrinsic lung disease.

1. Respiratory centre disturbances

Especially important in this regard are drugs which depress the respiratory centre, including *opiates, barbiturates, anaesthetic drugs* and *benzodiazepines*. The respiratory centre may be involved in *cerebral trauma* or *tumour*. *Respiratory arrest* may be present.

2. Neuromuscular or gross structural lesions affecting respiration

A variety of neurological conditions or toxins can interfere with respiration. Central or cord lesions resulting from *cervical* or *head injury* or conditions such as *motor neurone disease, poliomyelitis, acute ascending polyneuritis* or *acute porphyria* may lead to CO_2 retention. Interference with neuromuscular transmission in *myasthenia gravis*, or with *tetanus* or *botulinum toxins*, or *muscle relaxant drugs* (e.g. in *suxamethonium sensitivity*) can produce the same effect. Muscle disease in the *muscular dystrophies* or gross structural deformities, as in *traumatic 'flail' chest injury, ankylosing spondylitis* or *severe kyphoscoliosis* may also lead to CO_2 retention and respiratory acidosisis. In the *hypoventilation-obesity syndrome* (*'Pickwickian syndrome'*) extreme obesity can lead to mechanical impairement of ventilation.

3. Intrinsic lung disease

The most common intrinsic lung disease associated with CO_2 retention is *chronic bronchitis and emphysema*. A feature of these conditions, in part related to a raised CSF bicarbonate buffering the CSF against increased acidity, is the depressed respiratory response to CO_2. Retention of CO_2 may also be a feature of *severe asthma*. It may also be found in more extreme states of ventilation/perfusion imbalance (see section on O_2 transport), including *bronchopneumonia, severe pulmonary fibrosis or infiltration* or *pulmonary collapse*. *Obstruction of the large airways* should also be remembered.

b. Respiratory alkalosis

The following should be considered if the picture is one of respiratory alkalosis:

1. Mechanical overventilation

in patients on respirators.

2. Psychogenic hyperventilation

in response to pain, anxiety or voluntarily.

3. Stimulation of the respiratory centre

This may result from:

i. Hypoxia. Low arterial pO_2 is a potent stimulus to the respiratory centre below a certain level. Hence, *hypoxia of high altitude, right-to-left shunts, CO poisoning* and certain types of pulmonary disease *(e.g. alveolar capillary block)* will stimulate respiration and perhaps lead to lowered pCO_2.

ii. Reflex hyperventilation in response to conditions such as *pulmonary embolism* or *pulmonary oedema*.

iii. Miscellaneous conditions which include respiratory stimulants such as *salicylates*, in *acute liver failure* and with *local cerebral lesions* involving the respiratory centre.

c. Metabolic acidosis

The metabolic acidoses are sometimes divided into *increased anion gap* and *normal anion gap* acidoses. The anion gap is defined as the difference between the sum of the principal cations and the sum of the principal anions in plasma, viz.,

$$([Na^+] + [K^+]) - ([Cl^-] + [HCO_3^-])$$

In many types of acidosis H^+ is produced along with an unmeasured anion (e.g. H^+ and lactate in a lactate acidosis). Under these circumstances the normal anion gap of 10–20 mmol/l is increased as HCO_3^- is used up in buffering, with the unmeasured anion maintaining charge balance. In contrast, when the metabolic acidosis results from loss of HCO_3^-, electroneutrality is maintained by a rise in plasma $[Cl^-]$ and the anion gap is unaffected.

It is important to note that Cl^- is not measured routinely in some laboratories, limiting the value of this approach.

The many different reasons for the occurrence of metabolic acidosis can be considered under the following headings:

1. Ingestion of acidic or acid-producing substances

Included under this heading are the poisons *methanol* and *ethylene glycol*, which are metabolized to formic and oxalic acids, respectively. *Salicylate* itself is acidic, but may also increase endogenous production of acid (lactate and keto-acids). Salicylate also stimulates the respiratory centre, so the picture is often a mixed one of respiratory alkalosis and metabolic acidosis. *Paraldehyde* poisoning can also produce a metabolic acidosis. NH_4Cl, used by mouth in tests of urinary acidification, produces a normal anion gap acidosis (all the other examples in this section produce an increased anion gap acidosis).

2. Endogenous excessive acid production

i. Lactate acidosis. Lactate is produced during anaerobic glucose metabolism and is removed from the circulation, especially by the liver. *Severe exercise* may produce a transient physiological lactate acidosis, returning rapidly to normal levels at the end of the period of exercise.

Pathological lactate acidosis is usually divided into types A and B. In type A, the appearance of lactate is generally associated with poor tissue perfusion, with or without hypoxia. This is not the case in type B, where impaired lactate utilization may be more important.

Type A lactate acidosis includes *all states of shock* (haemorrhagic, traumatic, septicaemic or cardiogenic) and hypoxia associated with *severe anaemia* or *CO poisoning*, for example.

Type B lactate acidosis is exemplified by *biguanide-induced* lactate acidosis (e.g. with *metformin therapy*, where impaired utilization and increased production of lactate may contribute). The condition is also seen in *severe liver disease* and *ethanol ingestion*, after *paracetamol poisoning, infusion of sorbitol, fructose* or *xylitol* and in a number of *inherited metabolic defects*.

ii. Keto-acidosis. This occurs as a component of the normal physiological response to *starvation* and pathologically in *diabetic ketoacidosis*. The condition may also be found following *ethanol intoxication* or as a component of the acidosis produced by *biguanides and salicylate* (also see *i* above).

iii. Other endogenous acids. A variety of inborn errors of metabolism can lead to overproduction of organic acids (usually higher keto-acids). Although generally rare, such conditions should always be considered in any unexplained paediatric metabolic acidosis.

3. Failure of normal excretion of H+

This is most commonly a feature of the impaired acid excretion of *chronic* and *acute renal failure*, whatever the aetiology. Acidosis may be specifically of tubular origin in, for example, the *Fanconi syndrome*. Alternatively, it may be largely glomerular in origin. Thus, the glomerular filtration rate is reduced in *renal circulatory insufficiency, hypotensive states* or *true glomerular disease (e.g. acute glomerulonephritis)* leading to the potential for acid retention.

A specific renal lesion in acid excretion exists in *distal renal tubular acidosis*, where there is an inability to achieve the lower limit of urinary pH of approximately 4·6, thereby restricting H+ excretion. This condition may be primary or secondary to conditions such as vitamin D intoxication, amphotericin B therapy and some hypergammaglobulinaemic states.

4. Excessive loss of HCO₃ from the body

Metabolic acidosis will result from excessive loss of extracellular HCO₃ buffer. Since intestinal, pancreatic and biliary secretions contain appreciable quantities of HCO₃, this situation can arise in *severe diarrhoea* and *fistulous drainage of intestinal, pancreatic* and *biliary secretions*. Reclamation of HCO₃ from the glomerular filtrate is impaired in patients treated with *carbonic anhydrase inhibitors* and in *proximal renal tubular acidosis*. Again, proximal renal tubular acidosis may be primary or secondary to one of the causes of the *Fanconi syndrome (see above)*.

d. Metabolic alkalosis

The occurrence of metabolic alkalosis can be linked to either excessive loss of H+ or to the addition of alkali, typically NaHCO₃ by infusion or ingestion.

1. Loss of H+

This ion can be lost from the GI tract (gastric juice) or in the urine.

An important cause of loss of gastric contents is *pyloric stenosis* (whether congenital, or resulting from outlet obstruction from gastric carcinoma or the scarring associated with peptic ulceration) or in *excessive gastric aspiration*. The loss of Cl⁻ in *congenital chloride diarrhoea* may occasionally be a cause.

Excessive losses of H+ in urine can occur for a variety of reasons. Any state of increased mineralocorticoid activity will lead to H+ loss (in exchange for Na+). This may be *iatrogenic* in *steroid therapy* or may be observed in *primary or secondary hyperaldosteronism, hyperreninaemia* or *adrenocortical defici-*

ency of 11- or 17-hydroxylase enzymes (with overproduction of deoxycorticosterone with mineralocorticoid activity). External agents or drugs with mineralocorticoid-like activity, such as *liquorice* or *carbenoxolone*, should also be considered.

An important reason for extracellular alkalosis is K+ *deficiency* (see section on K+). Loss of K+, with intracellular K+ deficiency, leads to movement of H+ into cells to maintain charge balance in the cell. Furthermore, K+ deficiency means that more H+ is lost in exchange for Na+ reabsorption in the distral tubule, also contributing to the alkalosis. *Thiazide and 'loop' diuretics* by increasing Na+ delivery to the distal tubule, promoting K+ loss and possibly contracting the intravascular volume (with secondary aldosteronism) are especially likely to produce a metabolic alkalosis.

2. Addition of alkali to body fluid

This may occur as *NaHCO₃*, either orally (as an antacid) or when used intravenously. Fluids containing *Na lactate, Na citrate* or *Na acetate* are alkaline (salts of weak acids and a strong base) and may produce a metabolic alkalosis.

Disorders of oxygen transport

Routine assessment of acid base status on an arterial blood sample also includes measurement of pO₂. An abnormally low pO₂ value may be clinically of greater significance than an abnormal arterial blood [H+] or pCO₂.

Increased arterial blood pO₂

Such a situation may be found in patients on O₂ therapy. If the pO₂ value achieved is abnormally low in relation to the percentage O₂ in the inspired gas, it is likely that the arterial blood pO₂ will be abnormally low if the patient is breathing air.

Decreased arterial blood pO₂

Oxygen saturation of haemoglobin remains high until the pO₂ falls below 8·0 kPa, when the curve relating pO₂ to haemoglobin saturation falls quite steeply. Hence, arterial pO₂ values below 8·0 kPa will be of marked clinical significance and patients, by definition, have respiratory failure.

In general terms, low arterial pO₂ may result from alveolar hypoventilation, right-to-left shunting of blood, impaired diffusion or ventilation/perfusion mismatch. Alveolar hypoventilation will clearly be associated with retention of CO₂ (i.e. raised pCO₂) in addition to low pO₂. However, for the other causes of low pO₂, theroretical considerations allow for pCO₂ values to be normal or even lower than normal. Thus in conditions such as pulmonary oedema, O_2 exchange is more readily hindered than CO_2 exchange (since CO_2 is more water soluble and diffuses much more readily than O_2). Moreover, haemoglobin is typically 95 per cent saturated with O_2 and blood can carry very little extra O_2 if respiration increases.

These different possibilites for the pCO_2 value have led to the classification of respiratory failure into types I and II. In type I, the low pO_2 is accompanied by a normal or even low pCO_2 whereas the low pO_2 in type II failure is accompanied by CO_2 retention with an elevated pCO_2.

Type I respiratory failure

In this category are included conditions associated with diffusional defects in gas exchange, such as *pulmonary oedema, fibrosis* and *infiltration*. This picture may also be found in association with localised ventilation/perfusion defects, as in *lobar pneumonia* or localised *pulmonary collapse*. Severe collapse, fibrosis or infiltration may be associated with a type II picture.

Type II respiratory failure

The problem here is either *generalized alveolar hypoventilation, extensive airways obstruction (e.g. chronic obstructive airways disease, severe asthma), bronchopneumonia* or *more severe pulmonary fibrosis or collapse*. Retention of CO_2, unless compensation is complete, will be accompanied by acidaemia.

ADRENAL STEROIDS AND RELATED ANALYTES

a. Basic biochemistry

The adrenal cortex secretes three classes of steroid hormone: glucocorticoids; mineralocorticoids and sex steroids.

Cortisol is the principal glucocorticoid in man. Ninety-five per cent of circulating cortisol is *bound to plasma proteins*, the most important of which is transcortin. Because of this high level of protein binding excessive venous stasis during sampling should be avoided and total serum (or plasma) concentrations of cortisol must be interpreted with caution. In particular, high oestrogen states (including pregnancy) are associated with high levels of transcortin (and therefore high total cortisol concentrations), whereas in low protein states (e.g. nephrotic syndrome) the converse is true. The small proportion of total cortisol that is unbound by protein can be filtered by the glomerulus and is assayable as urinary free cortisol. It is also possible to measure salivary cortisol as an index of circulating free hormone levels.

The secretion of cortisol by the adrenals follows a *nychthemeral rhythm*, peak levels occurring at about 8 a.m. and troughs around midnight. Cortisol levels rise in response to *stress*. The production of cortisol by the adrenal cortex is stimulated by *adrenocorticotrophic hormone (ACTH)* which arises from the anterior pituitary, the secretion of ACTH itself being induced by the hypothalamic factor, *corticotrophin-releasing hormone (CRH)*. Both the nychthemeral rhythm of glucocorticoid release and the stress response are mediated through these hypothalamo-pituitary mechanisms. Glucocorticoids (including synthetic substances) exert a *negative feedback* action at the level of the hypothalamus. The activity of the entire hypothalamo-pituitary-adrenal axis is *pulsatile*. Because of these factors *random serum cortisol estimations are rarely of any diagnostic value*.

Cortisol is metabolized in the liver to a variety of derivatives, many of which are excreted as conjugates in the urine. Assays of groups of these metabolites (e.g. 17-oxogenic steroids and 17-hydroxycorticoids) in urine are rarely performed nowadays, having been superseded by measurements of individual steroids (including cortisol) in serum and urine. However, chromatographic profiles of steroid precursors and metabolites are important in the study of inborn errors of steroid biosynthesis.

Fluorometric methods for cortisol assay are notoriously non-specific and subject to interference by many metabolites and drugs (especially spironolactone). Assay by competitive protein binding using transcortin as the binding agent is more specific but cross-reactions with 11-deoxycorticosteroids, 17α-hydroxyprogesterone and some synthetic steroids do occur. *However, most laboratories now employ radio-immunoassay or non-isotopic immunoassay for the determination of serum and urine cortisol. These methods are of high specificity, although prednisolone and prednisone (but not dexamethasone) cross-react with most cortisol antibodies in current use.* In most circumstances so-called 'direct' (i.e. without solvent extraction) assays of serum are satisfactory but in renal failure anomalous results may be obtained due to the accumulation of steroid metabolites unless an extraction procedure is used. Similarly, in urine (even in the absence of renal failure) steroid metabolites and conjugates can lead to the overestimation of urinary free cortisol by direct radio-immunoassay and many authorities recommend extraction for this purpose.

Aldosterone is the principal mineralocorticoid in man. Secretion is stimulated by sodium deprivation and depletion of the extracellular fluid compartment, these effects being mediated in part through the renin-angiotensin system. Potassium loading (another stimulus to aldosterone release) probably affects the adrenal directly. Aldosterone is largely metabolized in the liver to various compounds which are excreted in the urine. One such metabolite, aldosterone 18-glucuronide, can be assayed as so-called 'urinary aldosterone'.

Adrenal androgens (including *androstenedione* and *dehyroepiandrosterone sulphate*) are important in the development of certain secondary sexual characteristics in the female. Assays of these substances, which are generally only available in specialist centres, may be of value in certain conditions presenting with abnormal virilization or precocious puberty.

b. Adrenocortical hypofunction

Failure of the adrenal cortex may be either *primary* (e.g. Addison's disease) or *secondary* to pituitary or hypothalamic dysfunction. Random serum cortisols are of virtually no diagnostic value in this context, with the possible exception of a suspected Addisonian crisis (in a shocked patient with intact adrenal glands the serum cortisol concentration should be either high normal or frankly elevated). The resuscitation of a patient with a possible Addisonian crisis should not await the results of steroid assays. Steroid cover in this situation may be given in the form of dexamethasone since this does not interfere with radio-immunoassays for cortisol. It may be useful to store a sample for possible ACTH assay (with due attention to sample handling requirements) before steroids are administered since this may be of value in differentiating between primary and secondary adrenal failure, should adrenocortical hypofunction be confirmed by other procedures. *The most useful screen for potential adrenocortical failure is the short tetracosactrin (synacthen) test*. In this procedure a dose of soluble tetracosactrin (usually 250 micrograms Synacthen) is given intramuscularly after taking a baseline sample for serum cortisol estimation at 9 a.m. Further samples are taken at 30 and 45 minutes after the injection. Because cortisol assays are somewhat method-dependent, ideally this test should be interpreted with local reference data. In general, however, in patients with hypoadrenalism a low basal level of serum cortisol is obtained, together with a poor or absent response to tetracosactrin. A normal result excludes adrenal failure but abnormal outcomes should be followed up by more extended testing with a depot preparation of tetracosactrin. Such *'long' Synacthen tests are useful in confirming abnormalities found in the short screen and may help discriminate between primary adrenocortical hypofunction (in which the response remains flat) and adrenal failure secondary to hypothalamo-pituitary disease (in which the adrenal response to repeated stimulation with tetracosactrin may increase over a few days)*. It may be appropriate to investigate pituitary function more fully in the latter situation. Characteristically, in Addison's disease ACTH levels are high, whereas in secondary adrenal failure levels are low.

Although in hypoadrenalism an early feature is loss of the nychthemeral rhythm (the morning cortisol being inappropriately low) the finding of an apparently intact rhythm should not be taken to exclude adrenal insufficiency and a tetracosactrin test should be performed in all suspected cases.

In the West tuberculosis has given way to auto-immune disease as the commonest cause of Addison's disease, assays of anti-adrenal auto-antibodies being available in specialist centres.

Adrenal function may also be inadequate as a result of inborn effors of steroid biosynthesis, such as 21-hydroxylase deficiency, which is the commonest cause of *congenital adrenal hyperplasia (CAH)*. The adrenal hyperplasia is induced by high levels of ACTH. This condition may present in the neonatal period as a salt-losing crisis, or with ambiguous genitalia in females (due to high concentrations of adrenal androgens). Assay of serum *17α-hydroxyprogesterone* has largely superseded the measurement of urinary pregnanetriol in the investigation of CAH. However, it should be noted that *increased levels of 17α-hydroxyprogesterone occur in disorders other than CAH and caution is particularly necessary in sick preterm infants. 17α-hydroxyprogesterone should not be assayed in samples taken within the first 48 h of life* because placental transfer renders the results uninterpretable. The site of the enzyme block can be confirmed by studying the urine steroid profile by gas-chromatography/mass spectroscopy. Antenatal diagnosis in families containing an index case is possible by analysis of the steroid patterns in amniotic fluid. Late onset forms of CAH may present as pseudoprecocious puberty in males, or hirsutism and/or infertility in females. It may be useful to measure serum 17α-hydroxyprogesterone concentrations in response to tetracosactrin in these late presentations. In monitoring replacement therapy, assays of 17α-hydroxyprogesterone (taking into account the ACTH-dependent nychthemeral rhythm), androstenedione and renin may all be helpful.

c. Cushing's syndrome

Obesity, hypertension and impaired glucose tolerance are all common, whereas non-iatrogenic Cushing's syndrome is rare. The approach for investigation therefore employs simple screening tests to identify potential cases worthy of more detailed assessment. Where appropriate, these preliminary procedures are followed by tests designed first to confirm the presence of Cushing's syndrome and second to establish its cause. The term *Cushing's disease* refers specifically to those cases of *Cushing's syndrome* due to an ACTH-secreting pituitary tumour.

Two tests which have proved of value as screens are the *overnight dexamethasone suppression test* and the measurement of *urinary free cortisol* excretion, both of which can be performed on an outpatient basis.

In the overnight dexamethasone test the patient takes either 1 or 2 mg of dexamethasone at 10 p.m. on the evening before the clinic attendance, at which a blood sample is taken for cortisol estimation at 9 a.m. Because the degree of suppression accepted as normal depends on a variety of factors, local reference data should be used. Although normal suppression in this test makes Cushing's syndrome unlikely (but not impossible), *failure to suppress can occur in a number of conditions other than genuine Cushing's syndrome including alcohol abuse, endogenous depression, simple obesity, severe illness and other stress, and consumption of drugs leading to the rapid metabolism of dexamethasone (e.g. phenytoin, phenobarbitone and rifampicin).*

Urinary free cortisol can be assayed in timed urine collections (usually 24 h) or is early morning samples, the results then being expressed as a cortisol:creatinine ratio. As with the overnight dexamethasone suppression test, there are several causes of increased urinary free cortisol other than true Cushing's syndrome so that abnormal results should lead to further investigation. *Urinary cortisol excretion is unreliable as an indicator of adrenocortical hyperfunction in renal failure and in the presence of significant proteinuria.*

Confirmatory tests for the presence of Cushing's syndrome include the low-dose dexamethasone suppression test and insulin hypoglycaemia. In the low dose dexamethasone test the patient is given 0·5 mg dexamethasone 6-hourly for 2 days. In most patients with Cushing's syndrome endogenous cortisol production (usually assessed by sequential 9 a.m. serum cortisol levels) is not suppressed. Causes of false-positive results are similar to those described for the overnight dexamethasone suppression test. The normal response to insulin-induced hypoglycaemia is an increase in serum cortisol (and ACTH) levels but in Cushing's syndrome no such rise occurs. *Patients with endogenous depression who fail to respond to dexamethasone may give a normal result with insulin hypoglycaemia.* In true Cushing's syndrome midnight cortisol levels are typically elevated but this is not a specific finding.

The differential diagnosis regarding the cause of Cushing's syndrome usually lies between pituitary-dependent disease, the ectopic ACTH syndrome and a primary adrenal tumour (either an adenoma or a carcinoma). *Several biochemical tests may be valuable in establishing the aetiology of Cushing's syndrome (Table APP.2).*

In the *high dose dexamethasone suppression test* the patient is given 2 mg of dexamethasone four times daily for 2 days. In pituitary-dependent disease, typically endogenous cortisol production (usually monitored by sequential 9 a.m. serum cortisol levels) is suppressed, whereas in the ectopic ACTH syndrome and in primary adrenal tumours such suppression does not generally occur.

In both pituitary disease and the ectopic ACTH syndrome, *ACTH concentrations* tend to be elevated, by contrast with the low levels characteristically found in adrenal tumours.

Metyrapone is a drug capable of inhibiting cortisol biosynthesis at several steps, the predominant effect being on 11B-hydroxylase. The normal response to metyrapone comprises elevated levels of ACTH (due to reduced negative feedback by cortisol), increased serum concentrations of cortisol precursors (including 11-deoxycortisol) and increased urinary excretion of their metabolites (including 17-oxogenic steroids). In pituitary-dependent disease the normal response to metyrapone is exaggerated, whereas in the ectopic ACTH syndrome and primary adrenal disease the response is diminished or absent. The metyrapone test has been used less frequently in recent years, partly because assays of the appropriate biochemical endpoints (ACTH, 11-deoxycortisol and 17-oxogenic steroids) are not readily available. It should be noted that the measurement of serum cortisol is not a satisfactory method for assessing the effect of metyrapone.

A recent addition to the range of tests used in establishing the cause of Cushing's syndrome is the *CRH stimulation test.* In this procedure the pituitary response to exogenous CRH is assessed either directly (in terms of ACTH release) or indirectly (in terms of serum cortisol). Patients with pituitary disease tend to give an exaggerated response in contrast with the reduced or absent effect obtained in cases of the ectopic ACTH syndrome and primary adrenal disease.

It is important to appreciate that false positives and negatives occur with all these investigations so that the diagnosis should be made on the basis of a combination of several biochemical tests, together with imaging techniques. In practice, the discrimination between the ectopic ACTH syndrome and pituitary-dependent Cushing's disease is often especially difficult to make. Although patients with the former

Table APP.2 Tests of value in establishing the cause of Cushing's syndrome

	Pituitary dependent disease	Ectopic ACTH syndrome	Primary adrenal tumour
High-dose dexamethasone	Suppression	No suppression	No suppression
Plasma ACTH	High	High	Low
Metyrapone test	Exaggerated response	Absent response	Absent response
CRH test	Exaggerated response	Absent response	Absent response

Note: Atypical responses in these tests are not unusual.

condition may present with the weight loss of malignancy (rather than the obesity of Cushing's syndrome) and weakness associated with a hypokalaemic alkalosis, it has been increasingly recognized in recent years that ectopic ACTH-producing tumours (including carcinoids) may present insidiously with a clinical picture indistinguishable from classical Cushing's disease. A variety of specialized techniques, including selective venous catheterization for ACTH and the assay of tumour markers other than ACTH may be helpful in these difficult cases. A further complication is that Cushing's syndrome may be cyclical (i.e. producing intermittent abnormality).

Although Cushing's syndrome is rare in childhood, in young children primary adrenal tumours are relatively common as compared with pituitary-dependent disease. Adrenal tumours (especially malignant cases) may produce features attributable to excessive sex steroid activity (e.g. pseudoprecocious puberty and hirsutism).

d. Conn's syndrome

Conn's syndrome (primary hyperaldosteronism) presents with *hypertension* and *hypokalaemic alkalosis*. There may be associated muscle weakness, paraesthesiae, polyuria and polydipsia. Renal potassium wasting occurs despite the hypokalaemia, this process being unaffected by sodium loading. Conn's syndrome is usually due to an adrenal adenoma, although bilateral adrenal hyperplasia sometimes occurs. Adrenal carcinoma is a very rare cause. Treatment of hypertension with diuretics should be remembered as a cause of hypokalaemia in this context. Liquorice derivatives (e.g. carbenoxolone) can induce a picture similar to Conn's syndrome. Hypermineralocorticoidism can also arise as a consequence of certain defects in steroid biosynthesis, including deficiencies of 17α-hydroxylase and 11B-hydroxylase. *The diagnosis of Conn's syndrome depends on the finding of an inappropriately elevated plasma or urinary aldosterone associated with a low renin level.* This is in contrast with the hyperreninaemia characteristic of secondary hyperaldosteronism (e.g. in cardiac failure, nephrotic syndrome, cirrhosis, Bartter's syndrome, renal artery stenosis and renin-secreting tumours). To yield clinically useful information, samples must be collected with rigorous attention to details of posture and electrolyte intake. *Certain drugs (including diuretics) render these measurements useless* and such agents must be withheld for an appropriate period of time (up to 4 weeks) before measurements are undertaken. Claims have been made that assays of aldosterone precursors, including 18B-hydroxycorticosterone, may also be helpful but these tests are not widely available. Imaging techniques and selective venous catheterization are of value in establishing the cause of Conn's syndrome.

ALBUMIN

Albumin is the most abundant plasma protein from about 20 weeks' gestation onwards. In the adult around 55–65 per cent of total plasma protein is made up of albumin. Synthesis occurs in the liver, is dependent upon an adequate supply of amino acids and is probably also subject to feedback regulation by the absolute level of plasma albumin. At neutral pH the albumin molecule is negatively charged and binds almost 50 per cent of the plasma calcium and a significant proportion of plasma magnesium. In addition, it binds unconjugated plasma bilirubin, free fatty acids, urate and certain hormones, which include thyroid hormones, cortisol and aldosterone, and a variety of drugs.

Abnormalities in plasma [albumin] are common; a raised plasma [albumin] level is of little significance in itself, except that it may draw attention to a clinically significant problem, such as dehydration. On the other hand, a low plasma [albumin] can lead to clinically detectable oedema which may be extreme in severe hypoalbuminaemia.

Around 20 genetic variants of albumin are described with no associated disease states. The most striking of these, on serum electrophoresis, is the condition of *bisalbuminaemia*, in which two distinct bands of albumin are observed; it is entirely benign.

The effects of posture on plasma [total protein] equally apply to plasma [albumin] — *see* Plasma Total Protein.

Raised plasma [albumin]

There are no known pathological causes for a raised plasma [albumin]. If an increase is measured, then one of the following is likely:

1. DEHYDRATION. This is also reflected in an increase in plasma [total protein], a raised haematocrit and appropriate clinical features.
2. VENOUS STASIS.
3. ALBUMIN INFUSION.

Decreased plasma [albumin]

1. INCREASE IN PLASMA H₂O. This occurs as a part of the physiological response in *pregnancy*. It may also arise from *the excessive infusion of intravenous fluids* or with H₂O *retention* which is a feature of the *syndrome of inappropriate ADH secretion*. In *glucocorticoid deficiency* there is impaired ability to excrete an H₂O load.
2. DIMINISHED SYNTHESIS. Any cause of *generalized protein malnutrition* will ultimately be reflected in a low plasma [albumin]. Worldwide, a diet which is *deficient in protein nitrogen* is the commonest cause, but the problem may also arise through *protein malabsorption*, as in *coeliac disease, tropical spruce, Crohn's disease* or *cystic fibrosis*, for example. A specific inability to synthesize albumin (and some other plasma proteins) is found in *chronic liver disease*. In *hereditary analbuminaemia*, there is a marked impairment of albumin biosynthesis with plasma [albumin] levels which are typically very low. Rather surprisingly, this condition is without symptoms, apart from intermittent, mild oedema.
3. INCREASED CATABOLISM. This is a feature of the *hypercatabolic state*. An important feature of the hypercatabolic state is the stress-related stimulation of glucocorticoid production; these hormones are known to stimulate protein catabolism. Conditions such as *fever, trauma, major surgery, severe sepsis* and *malignant disease* may all be associated with varying degrees of hypoalbuminaemia.
4. LOSSES OF ALBUMIN FROM THE BODY. Sites of excessive albumin loss are the *GI tract, kidneys* and *skin*.

BILIRUBIN

Bilirubin (strictly, bilirubin IXα) is derived from protoporphyrin IX; the tetrapyrrole ring remaining after removal of iron from haem. The major haem-containing protein is haemoglobin and about 85 per cent of the daily bilirubin production is from haemoglobin released from senescent erythrocytes and taken up by the reticulo-endothelial cell system (chiefly, the spleen). The remaining bilirubin is derived from the destruction of red cell precursors in the bone marrow (ineffective erythropoiesis) and from the catabolism of other haem-containing proteins such as myoblobin, cytochromes and peroxidases.

Unconjugated bilirubin is lipophilic and poorly water-soluble. It is carried in plasma bound to albumin. In its unconjugated form and associated with albumin, bilirubin is not significantly filtered at the glomerulus and does not readily enter most tissues. However, the liver possesses a carrier-mediated, active transport mechanism. Within the hepatocyte, the unconjugated bilirubin is bound to a number of non-specific, anion-binding proteins, including a basic glutathione S-transferase enzyme (ligandin), possibly also involved in the active transport mechanism. After conjugation, chiefly to glucuronic acid, the water-soluble bilirubin conjugates are excreted in the bile.

These conjugates are not significantly absorbed after entry into the intestinal lumen. Deconjugation and eventual reduction, principally in the colon, leads to the formation of a group of colourless tetrapyrroles, collectively termed urobilinogen. Spontaneous oxidation of urobilinogen to urobilin is responsible for the brown coloration of the stool. Around 20 per cent of the urobilinogen is reabsorbed; this is mostly taken up and re-excreted in the bile by the liver (enterohepatic circulation). A small quantity of the reabsorbed urobilinogen appears in the urine. It is self-evident that complete biliary obstruction will lead to the disappearance of urinary urobilinogen, whilst urinary excretion of urobilinogen will be greater with increased production of bilirubin (e.g. in haemolytic anaemia).

Bilirubin is most often measured as the total bilirubin (i.e. unconjugated plus conjugated). On occasion it may be helpful to quantitate these separately. The water-soluble, conjugated bilirubin reacts *directly* with the colour reagent used for its assay, whereas the unconjugated fraction only reacts after further chemical treatment. Hence, the unconjugated fraction is determined *indirectly* as the difference between the total [bilirubin] and the direct reacting [bilirubin]. The terms direct and indirect bilirubin are often used to refer to the conjugated and unconjugated fractions, respectively. It should be noted that a small amount of unconjugated bilirubin (σ-bilirubin) is covalently bonded to albumin and reacts directly with the colour reagent. The upper limit for direct bilirubin is less than 15 per cent.

Low plasma [bilirubin]

Low plasma [bilirubin] is generally of no significance. It may be observed in patients treated with *phenobarbitone*. It will not be discussed further here.

High plasma [bilirubin]

Increases of plasma [bilirubin] beyond 17 µmol/l (the upper limit of the *adult* reference range) will be discussed under this heading. An abnormal increase in plasma [bilirubin] may be present without clinical jaundice, which only becomes apparent at levels exceeding about 50 µmol/l. It should also be remembered that the reference ranges at birth and in the first few days of life are different, with the upper limit of the reference range well into the range where clinical jaundice is evident. Pathological jaundice in the neonatal period and in childhood will be summarized after this first section on high plasma [bilirubin].

Physiological increase

1. In the newborn

mild jaundice most often reflects a combination of normal postnatal haemolysis and immaturity of the hepatic conjugation system. Unusually early, or severe or prolonged jaundice clearly demands further investigation (see 'Neonatal jaundice' below). This is also the case if the conjugated bilirubin fraction is increased, since unconjugated bilirubin is largely responsible for this form of physiological jaundice.

2. Other reasons

for small increases in plasma [bilirubin] include *pregnancy*, *severe exercise* and *adaptation at high altitude*.

Pathological increase

It is convenient to subdivide the pathological increases in plasma [bilirubin] into prehepatic, hepatic and posthepatic causes. Even so, considerable overlap is possible, as illustrated by the hepatic parenchymal cell damage resulting from prolonged cholestasis due to extrahepatic obstruction.

a. Prehepatic hyperbilirubinaemia

Any cause of *increased bilirubin production* will produce the picture of prehepatic hyperbilirubinaemia. Levels of plasma [bilirubin], especially the unconjugated form, are increased. Urinary urobilinogen loss increases as biliary excretion of bilirubin is greater than normal. The possibility of pigment stone formation in the biliary tract increases for the same reason. Since the conjugated bilirubin levels are relatively unaffected, urine coloration does not markedly increase, in contrast to obstructive jaundice.

Prehepatic hyperbilirubinaemia may result from *ineffective erythropoiesis (e.g. pernicious anaemia)* and is sometimes observed in patients after the *transfusion of stored blood*. An important cause is *excessive haemolysis* which is best considered under two headings, namely *intrinsic red cell defects* and *factors extrinsic to the red cell*. The following is a summary of the more important causes of haemolysis and, therefore, hyperbilirubinaemia under these headings. The list is not intended to be comprehensive:

1. Intrinsic red cell defects

Under this heading are included the *haemoglobinopathies*, whether resulting from qualitative haemoglobin defects (e.g. *sickle cell anaemia*) or defective haemoglobin production (e.g. *β-thalassaemia major*). In the case of *β-thalassaemia major*, ineffective erythropoiesis also contributes. Other conditions include *hereditary spherocytosis*, *hereditary elliptocytosis* and *red cell enzyme defects*, such as *glucose-6-phosphate dehydrogenase deficiency* (see (2) below) or *pyruvate kinase deficiency*. Under this heading should also be included *paroxysmal nocturnal haemoglobinuria* in which the red cells show increased osmotic resistance to hypotonic saline.

2. Extrinsic factors

Extrinsic factors leading to intravascular haemolysis with increased unconjugated [bilirubin] may be conveniently divided into immune and non-immune causes.

Immune causes

Autoimmune haemolytic anaemia may be of the *warm-antibody* or *cold-antibody type*. The warm-antibody type is either idiopathic or associated with some underlying disorder, most commonly systemic lupus erythematosus, chronic lymphocytic leukaemia or Hodgkin's disease. Similarly, the cold-antibody type can be idiopathic or in association with an underlying illness such as a histiocytic lymphoma. A variety of drugs can give rise to a *drug-induced autoimmune haemolysis* (e.g. *methyldopa*).

Non-immune causes

Extrinsic factors under this heading include the many causes of *microangiopathy* associated with fibrin deposition and mechanical damage to the red blood cells. Also included are a number of *infective causes* such as the haemolysis sometimes observed in *malaria* (especially due to *Plasmodium falciparum*) or in *Clostridium welchii septicaemia*. In *septicaemia due to gram negative organisms* intravascular haemolysis may result from disseminated intravascular coagulation (i.e. a microangiopathic cause). Mechanical red cell damage is also possible from *valve prostheses*.

Drugs, in conjunction with the intrinsic red cell

deficiency of *glucose-6-phosphate dehydrogenase*, specifically lead to haemolysis in susceptible individuals (e.g. *quinidine, nitrofurantoin* and *antimalarials*). Dose-dependent haemolysis is found in *arsenic poisoning*.

Where significant intravascular haemolysis occurs in the conditions described under (1) and (2), in addition to unconjugated hyperbilirubinaemia, there will be haemoglobinaemia, haemoglobinuria and reduced levels of haptoglobins. Typically, a reticulocytosis will be present with evidence of marrow hyperplasia and reduced lifespan of radiolabelled red blood cells.

b. Hepatic hyperbilirubinaemia

This results from a defect in the hepatic handling of bilirubin. Specific failure to take-up unconjugated bilirubin, conjugate it to glucuronic acid or excrete the conjugate into the bile are considered under (1), (2) and (3) below. A more generalized derangement of hepatocyte function may interfere with one or more of these basic processes; this is considered under the hepatic causes from (4) onwards.

Specific defects

1. Decreased uptake
of bilirubin is found in *Gilbert's disease*. This is an inherited, benign, unconjugated hyperbilirubinaemia which affects around 2–3 per cent of the population. Levels of bilirubin are generally <50 μmol/l. Although the exact cause is unknown, the primary defect may actually be in bilirubin conjugation, with the decreased uptake a secondary defect. Impaired bilirubin uptake may also occur in *severe cardiac failure, portacaval shunt* and is also described with the antituberculous drug, *rifampicin*.

2. Impaired hepatic conjugation
occurs in the *Crigler–Najjar syndrome*, a familial condition in which there is complete (type I) or partial (type II) deficiency of the conjugating enzyme, bilirubin-UDP-glucuronyltransferase (UDPGT). The condition is a cause of neonatal jaundice (q.v.), which is lethal in type I. *High levels of 3-α-20-B-pregnanediol in breast milk*, with inhibition of UDPGT activity, is an uncommon cause of neonatal, unconjugated hyperbilirubinaemia.

3. Defective transfer of conjugated bilirubin
to the biliary canaliculus is a feature of the two familial conditions known as *Dubin–Johnson syndrome* and *Rotor syndrome*. The Rotor syndrome is characterized also by increased urinary coproporphyrin excretion, whilst a dark pigment is demonstrable in the liver in Dubin–Johnson syndrome.

17-Substituted 19-norsteroids (*synthetic androgens*

and *oestrogens*) can specifically interfere with canalicular excretion of bilirubin.

Generalized hepatic dysfunction
In those conditions associated with generalized hepatic dysfunction there is often impairment of secretion of bilirubin conjugates into the canaliculus leading to conjugated hyperbilirubinaemia. However, defective uptake and/or conjugation may also be a feature, leading to an increase in the unconjugated fraction.

The liver damage associated with hyperbilirubinaemia may be acute (4, 5 and 6) or chronic (7).

4. Acute liver damage of infective origin
Predominant liver damage is a feature of infection with *type A, type B, type C* and *delta viruses*. Jaundice is also a feature of *yellow fever*. Mild hepatitis, with modest increases in plasma [bilirubin] is sometimes found in *infectious mononucleosis* and occasionally in other viral infections. Systemic infection with *rickettsial, fungal* and *mycoplasma organisms* may involve the liver, with consequent hyperbilirubinaemia. The same is true of *septicaemia* with *liver abscess formation*.

5. Acute liver damage from drugs, chemicals and toxins
There are many *drugs* which can lead to liver damage with hyperbilirubinaemia. Most bring about this problem in an unpredictable way, not necessarily dose related. This is not true of *paracetamol* and some other drugs, where liver damage (in the case of paracetamol overdose) is predictable. Although it is not possible to be comprehensive in this section, a few examples will be chosen from the unpredictable group. *Monoamine oxidase inhibitors* and *para-aminosalicylic acid* can produce a hepatic necrosis which resembles viral hepatitis. This is also true of *halothane* and other anaesthetic agents, though severe hepatic necrosis has an incidence less than 1 : 20 000, in the case of halothane. Other drugs, including *tricyclic antidepressants, phenothiazines, benzodiazepines* and *oral hypoglycaemic agents*, may lead to a situation resembling cholestatic hepatitis. Prolonged treatment with *methyldopa* and *isoniazid* can produce a picture which resembles chronic active hepatitis. *Methotrexate* can lead to hepatic fibrosis, sometimes progressing to cirrhosis (i.e. chronic liver damage; see (7)).

A number of *chemicals* and *toxins* can lead to liver damage and hyperbilirubinaemia. Examples of hepatotoxic chemicals include *chlorinated hydrocarbons* such as *trichloroethylene, carbon tetrachloride* and *dicophane (DDT)*. *Phosphorus* and *iron* are also hepatotoxic. Although *ethanol* may lead to jaundice as a result of chronic alcoholic liver disease, *acute alcoholic hepatitis* from a bout of heavy drinking is also possible. Some naturally occurring hepatotoxins are also described, such as the *mycotoxin* from *Amanita phalloides* and *aflatoxin* present in food contaminated by *aspergillus species*.

6. Other causes of acute liver damage

with hyperbilirubinaemia include the hepatocellular necrosis sometimes observed in *acute left ventricular failure*. Jaundice may also occur in *acute fatty liver of pregnancy*. Abnormal liver function tests, sometimes with raised plasma [bilirubin] and usually temporary, are not uncommon during *total parenteral nutrition*.

7. Chronic liver damage

Jaundice may, of course, be a feature of *cirrhosis*, though cirrhosis (which is a histopathological definition) may be present without jaundice. Amongst the many causes of cirrhosis, the *infective (especially resulting from hepatitis B virus infection), autoimmune (primary biliary cirrhosis* and *chronic active hepatitis)* and *toxic* causes (especially alcohol) are important. *Biliary obstruction* and a number of metabolic, inherited disorders (e.g. *Wilsons' diseases, haemochromatosis* and α₁*antitrypsin deficiency*) can also produce cirrhosis with jaundice. Cirrhosis may also be *cryptogenic*.

Primary and secondary liver tumours may lead to raised plasma [bilirubin], as may *granulomatous diseases* or infiltrative disorders (e.g. *amyloidosis*).

c. Post-hepatic hyperbilirubinaemia

Cholestasis leading to hyperbilirubinaemia may occur within the liver ('medical jaundice') or be due to extrahepatic obstruction to the outflow of bile ('surgical jaundice').

1. Intrahepatic cholestasis

Since this phenomenon is frequently associated with hepatocellular damage, it is impossible to completely separate it from hepatocellular jaundice discussed in (B) above. Biochemically, it is suggested by relatively large increases in plasma alkaline phosphatase (liver isoenzyme), with more moderate increases in the transaminases (of hepatocellular origin), as compared to acute hepatitis where cholestasis is minimal. Lipoprotein abnormalities may be present, often with the appearance of lipoprotein X and an increase in the conjugated bilirubin fraction. Intrahepatic cholestasis leading to hyperbilirubinaemia is often present in *primary biliary cirrhosis* and may be the predominant picture in other cases of cirrhosis. Likewise, some cases of viral hepatitis may present with a predominantly cholestatic picture. It sometimes occurs following treatment with certain *drugs*, especially the *phenothiazines*. It may be due to *intrahepatic space-occupying*

lesions, most commonly *primary* or *secondary tumours*.

2. Extrahepatic cholestatis

Although chemical tests do *not* allow accurate diagnosis of extrahepatic cholestasis ('surgical jaundice'), complete obstruction to the outflow of bile will lead to the absence of urobilinogen from a dark urine containing bilirubin, with the passage of a pale stool.

Obstruction may arise *within the bile duct lumen*, most commonly from *gallstone(s)*, though a number of *parasites*, including *Opisthorus tennicollis, Clonorchis sinensis* and *Ascaris lumbricoides* may also obstruct.

The bile duct lumen may be partially or totally obstructed from *pathology of the duct wall itself*. Included under this heading are *biliary atresia* in the newborn, *bile duct carcinoma* and cicatricial contraction of the bile duct system in *chronic pancreatitis*. Alternatively, the bile duct system may be compressed from without in *carcinoma of the head of the pancreas* or *carcinoma of the ampulla of Vater*. Rarer causes under this heading would include *peritoneal adhesions, enlarged portal lymph nodes* and *hepatic artery aneurysm*.

Jaundice in the neonatal period and childhood

Although several of the causes of jaundice in early life have been considered above, it is helpful to summarize the conditions which can give rise to this problem in the neonatal and childhood periods. What follows is, of necessity, a summary.

As explained previously, mild jaundice is common in the newborn and in the great majority of cases is self-limiting and requires no further investigation. *Early (at birth or during the first 24 hours), severe (>250 µmol/l) or prolongd (>14 days) jaundice* all require further investigation. This is also the case if the *conjugated bilirubin* is increased.

1. Prehepatic jaundice

Immunological damage to red blood cells is an important cause of haemolysis in the neonatal period. *Rhesus disease* or *ABO* or other blod group incompatibility is the usual cause. *Drugs* may increase susceptibility to haemolysis. Thus, *vitamin K3* will deplete cells of NADPH and glutathione, leading to Heinz body formation and haemolysis. *Oxytocin* is reported to increase osmotic fragility.

Also included in this category are the *haemoglobinopathies* and *thalassaemia*, hereditary red cell defects such as *spherocytosis* or *elliptocytosis* and *enzyme defects*, such as *glucose-6-phosphate dehydrogenase* or *pyruvate kinase deficiency*.

Bilirubin production may be increased after *haematoma formation* or after *swallowing blood* during birth.

Bacterial sepsis may be the cause (also see (3) below).

2. Specific defects of bilirubin metabolism

Most specific defects of bilirubin metabolism result from *inherited disorders*; these have been considered above. It is also important to remember that *hypothyroidism* is associated with defective synthesis of the enzymes involved in bilirubin conjugation and excretion. This is an important condition in the differential diagnosis of early jaundice.

3. Hepatic damage (early)

The term *'neonatal hepatitis' syndrome* is used to describe liver damage, usually with hyperbilirubinaemia, in the first few weeks of life. Although infective causes are important in the causation of this syndrome, a number of metabolic conditions are also important.

Antenatal infections include viral infections due to *rubella, cytomegalovirus, herpes simplex*, in addition to *hepatitis B*. Infection with *Toxoplasma gondii* and *syphilis* are also possiblities. The syndrome is also described with peri- and postnatal infections, notably in the presence of *bacteraemia*.

Inherited metabolic causes include α_1-*antitrypsin deficiency* and *galactosaemia*. Other conditions to be excluded are *hereditary tyrosinaemia* and *lipid storage diseases* (e.g. *Gaucher's disease*). *Hereditary fructose intolerance* is also a cause but typically presents at weaning when fructose is introduced into the diet.

Biliary atresia is also conveniently included in this section.

4. Hepatic damage (late)

Chronic liver disease in childhood includes *chronic active hepatitis*. Chronic liver damage may result from neonatal hepatitis or be associated with *cystic fibrosis* or *chronic inflammatory bowel disease*. A number of the metabolic causes of neonatal hepatitis may also lead to chronic liver disease, including *galactosaemia*. *Wilson's disease* typically presents in later childhood or early adult life, since time is required for copper to accumulate and cause liver damage. *Indian childhood cirrhosis* also comes under this heading.

CALCIUM

Plasma calcium measurements are usually *total* measurements, made up of both diffusible calcium (just over 50 per cent of total) and a non-diffusible component (just under 50 per cent) which consists of calcium bound to protein (largely albumin). Of the diffusible calcium, a small fraction (less than 10% of *total*) is complexed with anions such as phosphate and citrate, leaving just under 50% of *total* calcium as the physiologically active, 'free' fraction. Some laboratories report a 'free' calcium (Ca^{2+}) by undertaking measurements with a Ca^{2+}-specific electrode but problems with this method limit its use. Because of its binding to albumin, total calcium measurements can be greatly affected by changes in albumin concentration. It is important to realize that significant hypoalbuminaemia may be accompanied by hypocalcaemia without there necessarily being any abnormality in calcium homeostasis (i.e. free Ca^{2+} concentration is within normal limits). A similar argument applies in hyperalbuminaemia, where the finding of hypercalcaemia need not necessarily reflect any increase in the free Ca^{2+} concentration.

Maintenance of the free Ca^{2+} concentration within normal limits is essential for normal neuromuscular activity. A fall in free Ca^{2+} concentration can lead to tetany and convulsions whilst an increase can delay neuromuscular conduction and impair muscle activity; effects on cardiac muscle function are also important. It is important to recognize clinically and biochemically if the free Ca^{2+} concentration is abnormal and to know the differential diagnosis if appropriate treatment is to be instituted.

In the following section, [calcium] will refer to the total calcium concentration, whilst [Ca^{2+}] will refer to the physiologically active, 'free' concentration of calcium.

Raised plasma [calcium]

a. Spurious hypercalcaemia

Any condition in which plasma [albumin] is increased can potentially lead to a measured increase in plasma [calcium] but where the underlying [Ca^{2+}] is typically normal.

The commoner reasons include:

1. Blood sample taken with *undue venous stasis*.
2. *Dehydration*.
3. *Albumin infusion*.
4. Occasionally, levels may be high in *multiple myeloma*, where a high concentration of the abnormal immunoglobulin binds Ca^{2+}. More usually a raised [calcium] in this condition reflects an increase in [Ca^{2+}] and is pathological.

b. True hypercalcaemia – commoner causes

There are many causes of true hypercalcaemia in which the increased [calcium] reflects a pathological increase in [Ca^{2+}]; some are relatively common and will be discussed here, whilst many are rare.

1. Neoplastic disease

Included under this heading are malignant tumours with metastatic deposits in bone (e.g. Carcinomas of breast and bronchus). The tumour deposits produce locally active factors which stimulate osteoclast activity, leading to erosion of bone matrix and movement of Ca^{2+} into the extracellular fluid.

Carcinoma without metastatic deposits in bone (humoural hypercalcaemia of malignancy) is also described. This is a feature of some *bronchial carcinomas* and *solid tumours of the head and neck*. A number of humoural factors have been identified which stimulate osteoclast activity, including epidermal growth factors and transforming cell growth factors. PTH-related peptide has also been identified as an important cause of humoural hypercalcaemia. True ectopic PTH productin is rare.

Some *haematological tumours*, notably *multiple myelomas* and also *HTLV-associated lymphoma*, may also elevate [Ca^{2+}]. Hypercalcaemia is rare in other haematological tumours.

2. Primary hyperparathyroidism

Hyperparathyroidism is the term applied to any condition in which circulating parathyroid hormone (PTH) level is raised. In primary hyperparathyroidism, autonomous overproduction of PTH occurs (c.f. secondary hyperparathyroidism, when the increased plasma PTH is secondary to a hypocalcaemic stimulus). Primary hyperparathyroidism is the commonest cause of hypercalcaemia in *fit-patient screening*. In contrast, malignant disease is the commonest cause for hypercalcaemia if a hospital population is screened. A high plasma [calcium] (and [Ca^{2+}]) is accompanied by an inappropriately high [PTH].

c. True hypercalcaemia – other causes

As compared to malignant disease and primary hyperparathyroidism, these are uncommon or rare causes of hypercalcaemia.

1. Vitamin D related

Excess intake of vitamin D can produce hypercalcemia (usually iatrogenic). In *sarcoidosis*, levels of calcitriol are sometimes increased, leading to enhanced Ca^{2+} absorption from the intestine, hypercalciuria and sometimes hypercalcaemia. There may be excessive conversion of calcifidiol to calcitriol, possibly by the granulomatous tissue.

2. Excessive calcium intake

(in milk), accompanied by excessive base intake, is a feature of the hypercalcaemia of the milk-alkali syndrome. The alkali component is believed to reduce calcium excretion and to contribute to in the pathogenesis of the condition.

3. Tertiary hyperparathyroidism

This refers to the situation in which a chronic hypocalcaemia stimulus to PTH secretion (i.e. secondary hyperparathyroidism) leads to an eventual state of autonomous PTH hypersecretion and hypercalcaemia. It is observed in cases of *longstanding chronic renal disease* or *malabsorption* and also after correction of the hypocalcaemia (which usually accompanies chronic renal disease — see below) following *renal transplantation*.

4. Bone derived (other than malignancy)

In *Paget's disease* there is a characteristic increase in bone turnover, occasionally, but not normally, accompanied by hypercalcaemia. Similarly *prolonged immobilization* can sometimes lead to hypercalcaemia (bone resorption exceeds formation), especially during adolescence when increased bone mass and raised bone turnover is present.

5. Endocrine disorders

Raised plasma [calcium] has been reported in association with both *hypoadrenalism* and *Cushing's syndrome*, in *phaeochromocytoma, acromegaly* and in *thyrotoxicosis*. All are rare causes.

6. Drugs

A mild degree of hypercalcaemia can develop with *thiazide diuretics* which interfere with renal calcium excretion. *Chronic lithium therapy* may be a cause, possibly as result of stimulation of PTH secretion.

7. Hypercalcaemia in childhood

Hyperparathyroidism is rare in childhood. In the neonatal period *phosphate depletion* may lead to hypercalcaemia in premature neonates. In the *infantile hypercalcaemia (Williams') syndrome* children usually present within the first 3 years with hypercalcaemia, characteristic facies and aortic stenosis.

8. Familial hypocalciuric hypercalcaemia

is an uncommon disorder transmitted by an autosound dominant gene. Patients have hypercalcaemia, unaccompanied by hypercalciuria and do not benefit from parathyroid surgery. The parathyroid glands are believed to have an altered set-point at which they respond to extracellular calcium.

Low plasma [calcium]

The differential diagnosis of hypocalcaemia can be considered in a similar way to hypercalcaemia.

a. Spurious hypocalcaemia

Again this term is applied to measured hypocalcaemia in which there is no pathology in the physiologically active 'free fraction'. The low plasma [calcium] simply reflects a reduced plasma albumin, for whatever reason. It is very important to remember this fact since hypoalbuminaemia is a relatively common finding. The differential diagnosis of hypoalbuminaemia is considered under albumin.

b. True hypocalcaemia – commoner causes

Having excluded a spurious cause, it is necessary to determine the cause of the reduced [Ca²⁺]. In developed countries *chronic renal disease* is an important reason but worldwide *dietary deficiency of calcium and vitamin D* is important.

1. Chronic renal disease

This is frequently accompanied by hypocalcaemia. The kidney is the site of conversion of 25-hydroxycholecalciferol (calcifidiol) to 1,25-dihydroxycholecalciferol (calcitriol); parenchymal destruction leads to a reduced activity of the 1-hydroxylase enzyme with reduced calcitriol levels and calcium malabsorption. High phosphate levels may also interfere with the 1-hydroxylation step.

2. Deficiency of vitamin D (and calcium)

Vitamin D availability depends upon both dietary sources and adequate exposure to sunlight. Inadequate sunlight exposure and poor diet (e.g. *the elderly confined indoors in temperate climate*), or a diet deficient in both calcium and vitamin D (*malnutrition*) can lead to hypocalcaemia. The importance of cultural and geographical factors is illustrated by the susceptibility of the immigrant Asian population in Northern Europe to osteomalacia and rickets.

Malabsorption of vitamin D with hypocalcaemia may be due to *gastrointestinal, pancreatic* or *hepatobilary disease*.

c. True hypocalcaemia — other causes

1. Iatrogenic

Removal or serious damage to the parathyroid glands (e.g. interference with vascular supply during neck surgery) can produce hypoparathyroidism and hypocalcaemia. *Anticonvulsant drugs* (e.g. phenytoin) appear to antagonize the peripheral actions of calcitriol. *Diphosphonate drugs*, used in the treatment of metabolic bone disease (e.g. Paget's disease) can also have this effect. *Massive transfusion with citrated blood* can lead to complexing of citrate anion with calcium and development of hypocalcaemia. *Treatment with corticosteroids* may occasionally be a cause.

2. Hypoparathyroidism

Unlike primary hyperparathyroidism, primary hypoparathyroidism is relatively rare. Failure to secrete PTH may result from surgery (iatrogenic — see (1) above) or may be *familial* or *sporadic* in origin. *Defective end-organ responsiveness* is the cause in *pseudohypoparathyroidism* (types I and II) where PTH levels are, if anything, elevated.

Occasionally the parathyroid glands are suppressed as a result of *magnesium deficiency* (normal magnesium levels are necessary for PTH release) or in neonates as a consequence of *maternal hypercalcaemia*.

3. Neonatal and childhood hypocalcaemia

In addition to neonatal PTH suppression (see (2)) early hypocalcaemia (24–48 hours) is much more commonly a result of *prematurity* or found in the *offspring of diabetic mothers*. The mechanism is complex but may relate to impaired Ca²⁺ mobilization in the face of high neonatal levels of calcitonin and cortisol, withdrawl of maternal Ca²⁺ supplies and the time required for PTH secretion to respond. The *late hypocalcaemia* observed at 5–10 days in full-term as well as premature infants is usually associated with *hyperphosphataemia* from the high phosphate content of cows' milk feeds or *neonatal renal disease*.

The most important cause of childhood hypocalcaemia is vitamin D deficiency (see (B)), typically of nutritional origin. Rickets may also rarely arise from defective vitamin D metabolism (see (4) below) or as a result of *phosphate wasting* in *familial hypophosphataemic rickets* or in the *Fanconi syndrome*.

4. Rarer causes of vitamin D-related hypocalcaemia

Reduced availability of calcifidiol may sometimes be a feature of *liver disease* or the *nephrotic syndrome*. In *vitamin D-resistant rickets* (type I) deficiency of the renal 1-hydrosylase may be responsible for the reduced plasma calcitriol levels and hypocalcaemia. In contrast in vitamin D-resistant rickets (type II) there is probably end-organ resistance to calcitriol, whose levels are elevated in conjunction with hypocalcaemia.

CREATININE

Creatine is synthesized in the liver, kidneys and pancreas and transported to its sites of usage, especially muscle and brain. In muscle, the enzyme creatine kinase converts creatine to its high energy phosphate form, creatine phosphate. About 1–2 per cent of the total muscle creatine pool is converted daily to *creatinine* through the spontaneous, non-enzymatic loss of H_2O.

Creatinine appears in the plasma and is excreted in the urine. Although largely filtered unchanged by the kidney, a small amount undergoes tubular reabsorption, whilst a larger amount (approx. 7–10 per cent of total urine creatinine) appears as a result of tubular secretion.

If creatinine production remains constant, then plasma [creatinine] is inversely related to creatinine clearance. In turn, creatinine clearance approximates to GFR, so that a rising plasma [creatinine] indicates a falling GFR. Hence, the value of plasma [creatinine] as a test of renal function.

Decreased plasma [creatinine]

1. Reduced muscle bulk

Since creatinine production is determined by the size of the creatine pool, it is evident that the smaller the muscle mass, the lower the daily creatinine production. Hence, a low plasma [creatinine] may be found in children and values are, on average, lower in women than men (in the absence of renal disease). Abnormally low values may be found in starvation and wasting diseases and also in patients treated with corticosteroids, where muscle mass may be reduced.

2. Pregnancy

Although creatinine synthesis is increased in pregnancy, this is more than offset by the physiological rise in GFR. Thus, creatinine levels may be low.

Increased plasma [creatinine]

a. Non-renal causes

As explained above, levels will be higher, on average, in individuals with increased muscle mass. This fact should always be borne in mind in interpreting a raised plasma [creatinine].

1. High meat intake

A diet rich in meat, which itself contains creatinine, can elevate plasma [creatinine] by 25 per cent or more.

2. Exercise

A transient, usually small, increase may be observed in more severe exercise.

3. Drugs

By competing with creatinine for the tubular transport mechanism, certain drugs will reduce the tubular secretion of creatinine and elevate plasma levels (e.g. salicylate).

4. Analytical overestimation

Certain widely used analytical methods are not entirely specific for creatinine, but also measure endogenous and exogenous interfering substances. Thus, *increases in plasma [acetoacetate] and [pyruvate]* can lead to artefactual increases, as can certain *cephalosporin antibiotics*.

b. Renal causes

In most patients, excluding the reasons listed in (A) above, an increase in plasma [creatinine] reflects impaired renal function. Renal causes would include any disease where there is impaired renal perfusion (e.g. fluid depletion, reduced BP, renal artery stenosis), loss of functioning nephrons (e.g. chronic renal failure, from whatever cause), or acute renal shutdown, or where pressure is increased on the tubular side of the nephron (e.g. urinary tract obstruction due to prostatic enlargement). The following points should be remembered:

1. Absolute plasma levels may show considerable individual-to-individual variation for reasons discussed above.
2. With this proviso, serial measurements of plasma [creatinine] within an individual should reflect time-dependent changes in renal function.
3. At very low levels of GFR, non-renal excretion routes (e.g. the gut) make an increasingly important contribution to total excretion.

ENZYMES

Amylase

Amylase is responsible for splitting α-D-glucose units linked through carbon atoms 1 and 4 on adjacent residues in polymers such as starch. Although found in quite a wide range of organs, the highest activities occur in the pancreas and salivary glands.

It is possible to distinguish between the salivary and pancreatic forms using immunological or electrophoretic methods, although this is rarely carried out in practice.

Increases in plasma amylase occur in the following conditions:

1. Acute pancreatitis

Activity rises in 2-12 hours, reaching a peak after about 24 hours, thereafter declining to normal over the next few days. Peak values tend to be higher in this condition than the other causes of a raised amylase, but this need not always be the case. Also, the height of the amylase activity does not necessarily reflect the severity of the attack.

2. Other acute abdominal conditions

A variety of other acute intra-abdominal conditions may be associated with a raised amylase activity. As a general rule, the elevation is usually less than five times the upper limit of the reference range (cf. acute pancreatitis, where it may be more than 10 times the upper limit). These conditions include *biliary tract disease, acute appendicitis, aortic aneurysm (with dissection) and ruptured ectopic pregnancey*.

3. Disease of the salivary glands

Significant increases may be observed in *mumps, maxillofacial surgery* and following *irradiation of the salivary glands*.

4. Other conditions

A number of other conditions are associated with a raised plasma amylase and may cause diagnostic confusion. In *macroamylassaemia*, an increase in the molecular mass of amylase, probably through complex formation with immunoglobulins, leads to reduced renal excretion and an elevated plasma amylase activity. Similarly, levels may be increased in any *renal disease* in which clearance may be reduced. *Opiate drugs*, by causing spasm of the sphincter of Oddi, can elevate plasma amylase activity and increased activity may also occur in *diabetic ketoacidosis, acute alcohol intoxication, burns* and *traumatic shock*.

Alkaline phosphatase

Alkaline phosphatase activity, typically measured as the ability to split off phosphate from a synthetic substrate at alkaline pH, is shown by a number of tissue-specific enzymes. These isoenzymes can be separated in plasma using methods such as activity staining after electrophoresis. Although alkaline phosphatase activity is widespread, the clinically important sources of plasma activity are liver, bone, placenta and intestine.

Alkaline phosphatase is found in many tissues attached to cell membranes. A good example is the liver, where the enzyme is located predominantly on the parenchymal cell membrane which forms the biliary canaliculus and on the sinusoidal aspect of the cell. Despite considerable study of this enzyme its precise function is unclear in liver, bone and other tissues.

Increases in plasma activity occur under the following circumstances:

1. Physiological

In *infancy and childhood*, especially during the adolescent growth spurt, levels may be as much as four times the adult value. The source of activity is bone, where alkaline phosphatase is released from osteoblasts during bone growth.

In *pregnancy*, levels may reach two times the normal adult value in the 2nd and 3rd trimesters; the placenta is the source of activity.

Small increases in the intestinal form may occur after eating, especially after a *fatty meal*. This problem can be avoided by collecting the blood sample from a fasted subject.

2. Liver disease

Plasma activity is increased in association with *cholestasis*, where both enzyme induction and solubilization (with release into the plasma) contribute to the elevated levels. Levels are especially likely to be high in extrahepatic obstruction (e.g. from a stone in the common bile duct or carcinoma of the head of the pancreas), often greater than three-fold the upper limit of the reference range. Intrahepatic cholestasis (e.g. malignant infiltration or drug-induced) will also lead to elevation in plasma alkaline phosphatase, but generally of lesser degree than is the case for extrahepatic obstruction. Similarly, increases are normally less in disorders which principally affect the parenchymal cells. It must be remembered that these are only generalizations subject to individual exceptions.

3. Bone disease

Any situation in which osteoblast activity is increased can be associated with a raised plasma alkaline phosphatase. In *Paget's disease* there occurs a marked increase in bone turnover (formation and resorption both increased) leading to plasma alkaline phosphatase activities which are often very high. *Primary or secondary hyperparathyroidism* increases osteoblast activity and may lead to raised plasma alkaline phosphatase activity. In *osteomalacia and rickets* where both secondary hyperparathyroidism and vitamin D deficiency occur, the increased osteoblast activity leads to raised plasma alkaline phosphatase activity.

Osteoblast activity is also increased during *repair of fractures* and as a reparative response to the osteolytic activity associated with *malignancy* (either local, bony deposits or humoral hypercalcaemia of malignancy).

4. Miscellaneous

In addition to the increased bone alkaline phosphatase activity described in malignant disease, some *malignant tumours* independently produce tumour-specific activity, although increases in plasma activity are often slight. For example, *bronchial carcinomas* sometimes produce a heat-stable alkaline phosphatase, closely resembling the placental enzyme.

It is sometimes helpful to determine the particular origin of a raised alkaline phosphatase activity. This is possible through the use of isoenzyme separation techniques such as electrophoresis. Alternatively, other organ-specific enzymes may assist the diagnosis. For example, a concomitant increase in γ-glutamyl transferase would suggest a hepatic origin for the increased activity.

γ-Glutamyl transferase

This enzyme is involved in the transfer of the terminal glutamate residue, joined through the γ-carboxyl group in a peptide such as glutathione, to a receptor (e.g. an amino acid or another peptide). The enzyme has a predominantly membrane location and is found in high activity in kidney, pancreas, biliary tract and liver. Since the renal enzyme is not released into the plasma, increased activity generally reflects disease of the liver, biliary tract or pancreas.

Increases in this enzyme are observed in the following circumstances:

1. Liver disease

γ-Glutamyl transferase is a sensitive indicator of hepatic disease. Increases are observed in a wide range of hepatic disorders, with the highest increases (5–30 times normal) being observed in cases of *intra- and extrahepatic cholestasis*. γ-Glutamyl transferase is a more sensitive indicator of cholestasis than alkaline phosphatase; activity increases earlier and lasts longer. High levels are often observed in *primary or secondary malignant disease*. The increases observed in infectious hepatitis are generally considerably smaller. It is inferior to alkaline phosphatase in separating hepatocellular from cholestatic disease.

Induction of liver γ-glutamyl transferase by a variety of drugs is a well-recognized phenomenon. This occurs especially with the anticonvulsant drugs, *phenytoin and phenobarbitone*, and also with the antituberculous drug, *rifampicin*. Increases occur in the majority of *chronic alcoholics*.

Since the activity is not increased in bone disease, measurement of γ-glutamyl transferase often assists the interpretation of a raised alkaline phosphatase.

2. Pancreatic disease

Levels may be increased in both *acute and chronic pancreatitis* and sometimes in *pancreatic malignancies*, although associated hepatobiliary obstruction may be more important in the latter.

3. Other diseases

Increases are sometimes seen following myocardial infarction and in other illnesses. It is probable that secondary hepatic involvement (e.g. venous congestion) may be the underlying reason for the increase observed in these circumstances.

Creatine kinase

This enzyme catalyses the reversible phosphorylation of creatine by ATP. Highest activity is found in striated muscle, cardiac muscle and brain. The enzyme is dimeric, made up of two distinct subunits, the products of two distinct structural genes, termed M and B. This situation leads to the occurrence of the three major isoenzymes, CK-MM, CK-MB and CK-BB. A fourth and immunologically distinct form is found in a mitochondrial location. In addition, high molecular mass forms are sometimes encountered in plasma.

An important feature of creatine kinase, for diagnostic purposes, is that the distribution of the major isoenzyme forms is variable. Thus, CM-MM makes up the majority of activity in skeletal and cardiac muscle, but cardiac muscle contains 20–30 per cent CK-MB, as opposed to the <2 per cent generally found in skeletal muscle. It should be noted that the proportion of CK-MB in skeletal muscle sometimes exceeds this level. This may be the case, for example, in muscle disease and in athletes undergoing training. Other tissues which contain significant amounts of CK activity (e.g. brain) contain predominantly CK-BB.

Plasma values of CK-BB are typically low, even with brain disease, so that increases in total CK activity are generally of cardiac or skeletal muscle origin. Exceptions to this rule sometimes occur (see (3) below).

An *increased* total CK value is found under the following circumstances:

1. Skeletal muscle origin

The largest increases in plasma total CK are observed in patients with *muscular dystrophy*, particularly the *Duchenne sex-linked form*. Levels may actually fall as the patient becomes older and the functional mass of muscle tissue reduces. Increases may also be observed in a variety of conditions where *ischaemic, inflammatory or metabolic damage* occurs. Levels are often high in *malignant hyperpyrexia* and *rhabdomyolysis*. Variable increases are observed *after surgery* or *intramuscular injections*.

2. Myocardial infarction

Several types of heart disease, including angina pectoris and congestive cardiac failure typically have normal plasma total CK values. A notable exception is *myocardial infarction*, where elevated total CK is an important diagnostic indicator. Levels may also be raised after *cardiac trauma*, including the trauma associated with heart surgery and in *myocarditis*.

In the absence of skeletal muscle disease, there is no specific requirement to measure the CK-MB activity. However, under some circumstances (e.g. after major surgery) measurement of CK-MB may be helpful. If the CK-MB isoenzyme contributes 6 per cent or more to the total value, this is consistent with myocardial infarction.

There has also been recent interest in isoforms of CK in the diagnosis of myocardial infarction. CK-MM is released into plasma as CK-MM3. A carboxypeptiolase, present in plasma, splits a terminal lysine from one of the two polypeptide chain of CK-MM3 to produce the CK-MM2 isoform. The CK-MM1 isoform results when the terminal lysine has been split from both chains. It has been suggested that the CKMM3/CKMM1 ratio, which increases after myocardial infarction, may have diagnostic value.

3. Other conditions

Increases may be seen in *hypothyroidism* (the thyroid contains mostly CK-BB), though *not* typically in hyperthyroidism. Increases are sometimes observed after *head injury* or *actue cerebrovascular disease*. Increases are also occasionally found in the CK-BB isoenzyme

during normal childbirth and in tumours of the GI tract, prostate, bladder, breast, ovary and kidney.

Aspartate aminotransferase

The aminotransferases are enzymes which catalyse the transfer of amino groups between amino acids and keto acids. One amino group donor/recipient pair is invariably glutamate/α-ketoglutarate, respectively. In the case of *aspartate aminotransferase (AST)*, the other pair is aspartate/oxaloacetate. In contrast, in the case of *alanine aminotransferase (ALT)*, the corresponding donor–recipient pair is alanine/pyruvate.

AST shows a wide tissue distribution with highest activity present in heart, skeletal muscle, liver, kidney and red blood cells. Two major isoenzymes exist, cytoplasmic and mitochondrial, but the distinction between these forms has not proven useful clinically.

1. Myocardial damage

Increased levels are found in *myocardial infarction*. The widespread distribution of the enzyme means that this is clearly not a particularly specific diagnostic test for this condition. Nevertheless, in conjunction with the clinical and ECG evidence, its measurement may be valuable. The concentration of ALT in cardiac muscle is considerably less than AST, so that ALT levels may be normal, despite the AST increase (cf. liver disease).

2. Liver disease

Both AST and ALT are increased in a variety of liver diseases. The largest increases, 20–100 times normal, are observed in acute hepatocellular damage due to *viral hepatitis* or *toxic* liver damage (e.g. *paracetamol overdose*). In contrast to aminotransferase release after myocardial infarction, levels of ALT are generally higher than AST with acute hepatocellular damage or necrosis. Other types of liver disease may be associated with elevated AST levels, although levels are generally lower than is the case for hepatitis/toxic damage. Moderate increases can be observed in *cholestatic jaundice*, *cirrhosis* (often modest, upto twice normal) and in *primary* and *secondary malignant disease*.

3. Other conditions

A variety of other conditions may be associated with raised AST levels. Increases are seen in *muscular dystrophy* (relatively much smaller than creatine kinase), in *acute pancreatitis, acute renal disease* and *pulmonary infarction*. Because of its location in the red blood cell, levels can rise in *haemolytic states* and may be *artefactually increased* for the same reason in *haemolysed samples*. The increases observed in these conditions are usually much less than is the case for acute hepatocellular damage/necrosis and less than for myocardial infarction.

Alanine aminotransferase

Increases in ALT activity often follow those of AST. As explained above, levels tend to be lower than AST in myocardial infarction but higher in acute hepatocellular disease of viral or toxic aetiology. With these provisos, the statements listed under (1) and (2) above (AST) cover the important reasons for elevated ALT levels.

As is also the case for AST, the wide tissue distribution means that a variety of other diseases can be associated with increases in plasma ALT, including muscle disease, acute renal disease and acute pancreatitis.

Lactate dehydrogenase

This enzyme catalyses the reversible oxidation of lactate to pyruvate, using NAD as hydrogen acceptor. The enzyme is present in a cytoplasmic location in all body cells. Hence, the measurement of total lactate dehydrogenase (LD) activity lacks specificity and increases may be observed in a wide variety of conditions.

One method to improve diagnostic specificity is to take account of the different tissue distribution of the major isoenzymes of LD. The enzyme is a tetramer made up of all possible combinations of the two subunits known as H and M. Thus, there exist H_4, H_3M, H_2M_2, HM_3 and M_4 isoenzymes, also referred to as LD_1, LD_2 ... LD_5, respectively. The LD_1 and LD_2 forms predominate in heart and red blood cells, whilst LD_4 and LD_5 isoenzymes are particularly found in liver and skeletal muscle. Other tissues show no particular predominance of one or more forms.

It is possible to measure the activity of the LD_1 and LD_2 isoenzymes by making use of the fact that, as compared to the other isoenzymes, activity is present using 2-oxobutyrate as substrate ('hydroxybutyrate dehydrogenase'). Alternatively, the fact that LD_1 and LD_2 are relatively unaffected by the presence of urea, which inhibits the other isoenzymes, allows measurement of LD_1 and LD_2 as 'urea-stable LD'. LD isoenzymes may also be separated by electrophoresis and the different isoenzymes quantified by densitometric scanning after activity staining.

Increases in the 'hear-specific' (so-called) LD_1/LD_2 activity are found under the following conditions:

1. Myocardial infarction

The 'heart-specific' isoenzyme is often used as a diagnostic test of myocardial infarction. Levels rise more slowly than creatine kinase or AST, with peak values at 48 hours, thereafter declining over several days. This fact makes it quite valuable in the late presentation of suspected myocardial infarction.

2. Haematological disease

As stressed above, LD has a very wide distribution, with LD_1/LD_2 present in many tissues other than heart; the term 'heart-specific' is clearly misleading. In particular, levels of these isoenzymes are high in red blood cells. Consequently, increased activity of the 'heart-specific' LD activity is found in haematological conditions such as *haemolytic states, megaloblastic anaemias* and *leukaemias*. Also, *artefactual increases* may be observed in *haemolysed blood samples*.

3. Other conditions

Levels may be increased in *acute renal damage*, sometimes in *liver disease*. As a rule, activity rises higher in (1) and (2) above.

Acid phosphatase

Acid phosphatase activity is shown by a number of isoenzymes present both in lysosomes and in an extralysosomal location. Greatest activity is shown by the prostate gland, but significant activity is found in liver, spleen, bone, platelets and red blood cells. The main clinical value of the measurement is in the detection and follow-up of patients with prostatic carcinoma. The method can be made to be more specific by measuring the prostatic form. A method which is still in use is based on the fact that the prostatic acid phosphatase is selectively inhibited by *l*-tartrate and to report the 'tartrate labile' activity. Immunoassay methods for measuring the mass of the prostatic form are also in use.

Increases in acid phosphatase activity are observed as follows:

1. Prostatic origin

Increased plasma activity is observed in only a minority of patients with *carcinoma* confined to the prostate. Spread beyond the gland or more distant spread leads to an elevated level in up to 80 per cent of patients. The activity is also increased under a number of other circumstances. *Rectal examination* can achieve this; blood for acid phosphatase measurement should ideally be taken *before* rectal examination. Likewise, increases can be observed with *acute retention of urine* or *after passage of a urethral catheter. Prostatic inflammation* or *necrosis* may also increase acid phosphatase in plasma.

2. Other conditions

By measuring the prostatic activity (as the 'tartrate labile' form or by immunoassay or other methods) increases in activity can mostly be accounted for by the list in (1) above. Where the total activity is determined levels may be increased in a number of other conditions which include: *bone disease* (especially *Paget's disease, hyperparathyroidism* and *metastatic malignant bone disease*). The same is also true in *liver disease, Gaucher's disease* (probably derived from the Gaucher cells) and in the platelet lysis found in some types of *thrombocytopenia. Artefactually increased* levels may be observed in *haemolysed specimens.*

Prostate-specific antigen is an anzyme (a serine protease) which is located in the prostatic epithelial tissue. It is a particularly sensitive marker of prostatic cancer and its measurement is likely to supersede that of acid phosphatase. Nevertheless the test lacks specificity for prostatic carcinoma, since it is often elevated in benign prostatic hypertrophy.

GLUCOSE

Glucose is the main energy source for man and, as such, its plasma concentration is closcly regulated, despite wide fluctuations in glucose intake and utilization. Glucose homeostasis is a complex phenomenon involving the interplay of many factors, but central to its regulation is the hormone insulin. Insulin secretion from the pancreatic beta-cells is stimulated by an increase in plasma [glucose] and, in turn, enhances glucose uptake and utilization by tissues such as muscle, liver and adiposc tissue.

In considering *hyperglycaemia* the following classification depends upon the extreme clinical importance of idiopathic diabetes mellitus, and follows the accepted nomenclature for this condition, viz; types I, II and III. Consideration of the secondary causes of diabetes mellitus then follows.

Hyperglycaemia

Criteria for hyperglycaemia and the diagnosis of diabetes mellitus have been laid down by the WHO Study Group on diabetes mellitus (1985) and the criteria for venous plasma are:

	Fasting	2 hours after oral glucose (75 g)
1. Diabetes mellitus	$\geq$ 7·8 and/or	$\geq$ 11·1 μnol/l
2. Impaired glucose tolerance	< 7·8 and	$\geq$ 7·8–<11·1 μnol/l
3. Normal	< 7·8 and	< 7·8 μnol/l

Diabetes mellitus

This condition results from the complex metabolic and other consequences following defective insulin secretion or action and is characterized by fasting hyperglycaemia (see list above). Traditionally it is divided into types I and II, with a type III category recently added.

1. Type I

This is the so-called juvenile-onset or insulin-dependent diabetes mellitus, in which insulin secretion is severly defective, with a proneness to develop ketosis.

Type Ia shows a HLA association, often with transient islet cell antibodies present at an early stage which later disappear. In contrast, type Ib is associated with persistent islet-cell antibodies and is probably autoimmune in origin.

2. Type II

This group is typically characterized by onset in middle or later life (hence maturity onset) and is generally non-insulin dependent. One form is associated with obesity, in contrast to non-obese type II illness which probably has a different aetiology.

3. Type III

The association here is with malnutrition. This may take the form of childhood malnutrition (J-type) or relate to Cassava consumption, together with malnutrition (Z-type). Some endogenous insulin secretion is probably maintained.

Other causes of diabetes mellitus

4. Pancreatic diseases

These include *chronic pancreatitis, pancreatectomy* and *haemochromatosis.*

5. Hormonal

A variety of endocrine disorders are associated with impaired glucose tolerance or diabetes mellitus. In general, an excess of one or more hormones which have an anti-insulin action is (are) present. This is the situation in *glucocorticoid excess, thyrotoxicosis* (occasionally), *growth hormone excess, phaeochromocytoma* or with a *glucagon-secreting tumour.*

6. Drugs

A number of drugs produce impaired glucose tolerance, sometimes frank diabetes mellitus. These include *thiazide diuretics, oestrogen-containing oral contraceptives, β-blockers* and *catecholaminergic drugs* (such as salbutamol).

7. Miscellaneous

Included in this category are *insulin-receptor abnormalities*, together with a variety of genetic disorders which include *type I glycogen storage disease, Down's syndrome, Turner's syndrome, Huntington's chorea* and the syndrome of diabetes insipidus, diabetes mellitus, optic atrophy and deafness (DIDMAOD syndrome).

Hypoglycaemia

The definition of hypoglycaemia is usually taken as a venous plasma glucose concentration of less than 2·2 mmol/l, measuring the [glucose] by a specific, enzymatic method. Despite this, symptoms may often relate more to the rate of fall in [glucose] than the absolute value. There are many causes of hypoglycaemia, most of which are rare or relatively rare. The commonest causes are those of *insulin excess in the treatment of diabetes mellitus, sulphonylurea therapy* and *insulin-secreting tumours*.

It is useful to subdivide causes of hypoglycaemia into reactive and fasting. In reactive hypoglycaemia an identifiable external agent (e.g. drug or poison) can be found to be responsible, whereas some endogenous factor is responsible for fasting hypoglycaemia.

a. Reactive hypoglycaemia

1. Drug or poison-induced

The important causes in this group are *insulin, sulphonylurea drugs* and *alcohol*. Insulin excess may be due to its therapeutic use in diabetes mellitus or it may be self-administered to induce illness. *Salicylates* can produce hypoglycaemia (factitious hypoglycaemia) in children and *quinine* (in treatment of malaria) has also been implicated.

A number of poisons are known to produce hypoglycaemia, including liver poisons such as *phosphorus, chloroform* and *paracetamol overdose*, and the toadstool, *Amanita phalloides*.

2. Post-prandial

Although this may be *idiopathic*, it is also established that *alcohol* and *gastric surgery* may lead to this problem. In the case of alcohol ingestion, there occurs an enhancement of the insulin response to a carbohydrate load. Rapid gastric emptying or the release of insulinotropic hormones from the gut may contribute to the hypoglycaemia following gastric surgery.

3. Inherited metabolic disorders

See section on hypoglycaemia in childhood for consideration of *galactosaemia* and *fructose intolreance*, where hypoglycaemia is provoked by lactose or fructose ingestion, respectively.

b. Fasting hypoglycaemia

This may arise either because of impairment of glucose mobilization from glycogen by the liver or because of enhanced glucose utilization by the tissues during starvation.

1. Defective glucose production

Severe *starvation and malnutrition* may be accompanied by failure to maintain blood glucose levels. This is also a feature of some *inborn errors of metabolism* (see section on 'Hypoglycaemia in Childhood' below).

The ability of the *liver* to maintain blood glucose levels, despite extensive disease, is moderately good (at least in the adult). As discussed above, acute liver necrosis (incduced by poisons such as choloroform) may produce hypoglycaemia ('reactive hypoglycaemia'). Low blood glucose has been reported in *hepatic carcinoma*; also in *portal cirrhosis* and *congestive cardiac failure*, where passive venous congestion may be the mechanism.

Occasional fasting hypoglycaemia is a feature of terminal *renal disease*, but the mechanism is not fully understood. One possible factor may be the contribution of the renal cortex to maintenance of blood glucose levels through the occurrence of gluconeogenesis in this tissue.

A number of *endocrine disorders* may be associated with hypoglycaemia. Cortisol promotes hepatic gluconeogenesis and deficiency of the hormone in *adrenocortical insufficiency* may lead to hypoglycaemia. Similarly, deficiency of growth hormone and ACTH in *pituitary insufficiency* may be a cause. Hypoglycaemia is also described in *hypothyroidism*.

2. Enhanced glucose utilization

Endogenous overproduction of insulin (as opposed to exogenous use — see 'Reactive hypoglycaemia') is a feature of *pancreatic insulinoma*, whether benign or malignant. The tumour may be a part of the *MEN I* syndrome.

A number of non-pancreatic tumours are known to be associated with hypoglycaemia, typically in patients with advanced malignant disease. *Large sarcomas*, especially in a retroperitoneal or pleural location may do this, as may *primary hepatomas, adrenal carcinomas* and *carcinoid tumours*. Some of the larger tumours may consume excessive amounts of glucose, but there is also evidence for the production of hormonal insulin-like substances (NSILA — non-suppressible insulin-like activity).

Hypoglycaemia in childhood

Although all of the causes of hypoglycaemia discussed above may be relevant to the child, there are a number of causes specific to this age-group which require mention.

Neonatal hypoglycaemia

The criteria for hypoglycaemia are different in the newborn compared to adult. A value of less than 1·6 mmol/l would be regarded as abnormal in a term newborn, though a more realistic figure for a premature or small-for-dates neonate would be less than 1·1 mmol/l.

Neonatal hypoglycaemia (as defined above) has been divided by Cornblath *et al.* into the following categories:

1. Early, transitional hypoglycaemia refers to an exaggerated physiological fall in the blood glucose after birth, readily responding to feeding. The problem is more likely in babies of *diabetic mothers* or in association with *erythroblastosis fetalis*, in both of which islet cell mass may be increased.
2. Secondary to *asphyxia, respiratory distress syndrome, severe infection* or *brain damage*.
3. In *small-for-dates babies* and *prematurity*.
4. Recurrent, postnatal hypoglycaemia (see next section) may also present in the neonatal period, particularly if due to an inborn error of carbohydrate or amino acid metabolism.

Postneonatal hypoglycaemia

Ketotic hypoglycaemia may occur in the postneonatal period. Disorders can be divided into a group with raised fasting plasma [lactate] and a group with normal fasting [lactate].

The first group is made up of a number of inborn errors of metabolism including *glycogen storage disease type I* (deficiency of glucose-6-phosphatase), *fructose-1-6-diphosphatase deficiency* and occassionally in *organic acidaemis*.

The second group also includes a number of inborn errors of metabolism, notably *glycogen storage diseases types III* and *VI*. Also in this group are included a variety of endocrine disorders such as *hypopituitarism, isolated deficiency of growth hormone* or *ACTH, glucagon deficiency* and *adrenal insuffiency*. Ketotic hypoglycaemia with normal plasma [lactate] may also occur with *emotional deprivation* or be *idiopathic*.

Non-ketotic hypoglycaemia is also described in this period. It may result from *elevated plasma insulin levels* from an *islet cell tumour*, as in the adult. In the condition known as *nesidioblastosis* the increased insulin levels are associated with a developmental abnormality of the endocrine pancreas, with islet cell hyperplasia and duct overgrowth. Where insulin levels are normal, the absence of ketosis may result from a *disorder of fatty acid oxidation*.

Hypoglycaemia in childhood may also result from *liver disease. Acute liver failure* in childhood is often associated with hypoglycaemia. A number of inborn errors of metabolism lead to liver disease with accompanying hypoglycaemia. These include *galactosaemia* (resulting from deficiency of galactose-1-phosphate uridyl transferase), *hereditary fructose intolerance* (deficiency of aldolase) and *hepatorenal tyrosinaemia* (tyrosinosis type 1).

Finally, malnutrition (e.g. due to *starvation, kwashiarkor, malabsorption, chronic diarrhoea*) may lead to hypoglycaemia, as may toxic conditions (e.g. *insulin overdose, Reye's syndrome*).

IMMUNOGLOBULINS

Immunoglobulins are produced by plasma cells and function as antibodies. Plasma cells are formed through the differentiation of B lymphocytes. Each immunoglobulin molecule has a basic structure, comprising two identical light chains (kappa or lambda) and two identical heavy chains (gamma, alpha, mu, delta or epsilon), cross-linked by disulphide bridges. Immunoglobulins are divided into five classes (IgG, IgA, IgM, IgD and IgE) on the basis of the identity of the heavy chain. In addition, IgG and IgA molecules fall into four and two subclasses respectively, which have differing structural and functional properties. IgM usually exists in the form of a pentamer of the basic immunoglobulin structure, whereas IgA is either dimeric (in secretions) or monomeric (in serum). IgG, IgE and IgD are monomeric.

Table APP.3 summarizes some of the characteristics of the immunoglobulin classes.

There are important changes in immunoglobulin concentrations with age in normal individuals. During the final stages of pregnancy maternal IgG is actively transported across the placenta into the fetal circulation, resulting in high serum IgG levels in normal, full-term neonates. As maternal IgG is lost after birth, total

Table APP.3 Properties of immunoglobulin classes

Class	Heavy chain	Molecular weight (Da)	Approximate mean adult serum concentration	Placental transfer
IgG	Gamma	150 000	10 g/l	+
IgA	Alpha	160 000	2 g/l	−
IgM	Mu	950 000	1 g/l	−
IgD	Delta	175 000	30 mg/l	−
IgE	Epsilon	190 000	Trace	−

serum IgG levels fall until about 6 months, by which stage the infant's own IgG synthesis is appreciable, resulting in increasing serum levels. Normal serum concentrations of IgM and IgA at birth are low, and adult levels are not reached until about 12 months and 12 years respectively. However, salivary IgA approaches normal adult concentrations by about 6 weeks of age.

There are significant differences in normal serum immunoglobulin levels between different racial groups so that care must be taken in the use of reference data.

1. Low immunoglobulin levels

Immunoglobulin deficiencies can be described as primary (i.e. an abnormality in the development of the immune system) or secondary (i.e. the consequence of the effect of another disease on a normally developed immune system). Serum immunoglobulin levels should be determined if either a primary or a secondary immunodeficiency is suspected, and in difficult cases it may be appropriate to assay serum IgG and IgA subclasses and to measure IgA levels in saliva.

a. Selective immunoglobulin deficiencies

Selective IgA deficiency, which is relatively common in the West but virtually unknown in the Third World, may lead to repeated infections of the respiratory tract and other mucosal surfaces. Many people with IgA deficiency, however, remain entirely well. In most cases of IgA deficiency both subclasses, IgA1 and IgA2, are affected in parallel. However, because IgA1 is the dominant subclass in serum, whereas IgA2 predominates in external secretions, a deficiency in secretory IgA may coexist with a normal total serum level, and assay of the IgA subclasses may be justified in cases of recurrent respiratory tract infections where no other cause has been found. Because of the length of time taken to attain normal adult levels in serum, some authorities recommend salivary measurements for the investigation of suspected IgA deficiency in children.

Selective deficiencies in IgG (and its subclasses) and IgM do occur but are rare. Because IgG1 is the dominant subclass in serum, selective deficiencies in the other IgG subclasses may exist despite a normal total IgG concentration.

b. Non-selective immunoglobulin deficiences

Primary generalized immunoglobulin deficiency is rare. In *Bruton's disease*, which is inherited as an X-linked recessive, there is a total absence of immunoglobulins and affected children suffer from recurrent bacterial infections. Primary immunoglobulin deficiency may be part of a wider inherited or developmental problem. Infants with severe combined immunodeficiency have both inadequate antibody production and poor cell-mediated immunity. In *DiGeorge's syndrome*, which is an embryopathy affecting the third and fourth pharyngeal pouches, hypogammaglobulinaemia is associated with thymic and parathyroid hypoplasia. Severe neonatal hypogammaglobulinaemia, which is commoner in premature babies, may be transient.

Secondary deficiencies in immunoglobulin production are relatively common, especially in *malignant disease*, including *myeloma*, *lymphoma* and *leukaemia*. *Cytotoxic drugs* may also contribute to low immunoglobulin levels found in cancer. Other causes of secondary immunoglobulin deficiency include *nephrotic syndrome*, *malabsorption* and *protein-losing enteropathy*, *marrow hypoplasia* and *myelosclerosis*, and severe *renal failure*.

Normal concentrations of serum immunoglobulins do not exclude all abnormalities of humoral immunity. The possibility of IgA and IgG sub class deficiencies has already been mentioned. Failure to respond to specific antigenic stimulation is sometimes seen in patients with normal levels of IgG, IgM and IgA in serum. Investigation of non-specific immunity (including complement) and cell-mediated immunity should also be considered in patients with multiple infections.

2. High immunoglobulin levels

a. Polyclonal and oligoclonal hyperimmunoglobulinaemia

Stimulation of the immune system by antigen results in immunoglobulin production by plasma cells. Initially IgM is produced but subsequently synthesis is usually switched to either IgG or IgA, according to circumstances. Generally antibodies are produced by many different clones of plasma cells and on serum electrophoresis a diffuse increase in the gamma region is seen. Occasionally multiple discrete bands are found, indicating a response by a restricted number of clones. The same phenomenon occasionally occurs in other body fluids and so-called oligoclonal bands are found in the cerebrospinal fluid of most patients with multiple sclerosis.

Many different *infections* result in polyclonal antibody production but quantitation of the total IgG, IgM and IgA concentrations is rarely of value in this context. Tests for specific antibodies, however, are often extremely valuable in identifying particular infective agents. Paradoxically, high serum levels of immunoglobulin may be found in some immunodeficient states, such as HIV infection.

Polyclonal increases in serum immunoglobulins also occur in a variety of non-infective conditions, including *sarcoidosis, chronic liver diseases, rheumatoid arthritis* and *systemic lupus erythematosus.*

Measurement of total IgM may be useful in certain special circumstances. First a high level of IgM in umbilical cord blood or in blood taken during the first week of life suggests the possibility of antenatal infection, although a similar intrauterine immunological response can be induced by maternal antigens. Second, high IgM levels occur in a variety of tropical diseases including *malaria* and *trypanosomiasis.* Third, serum IgM levels are raised in most cases of *primary biliary cirrhosis.* Antimitochondrial antibody should be assayed if this condition is suspected.

The indications for determining IgE levels deserve special consideration. In the West measurement of IgE is usually performed in suspected *atopic allergy.* Although most atopic persons have elevated total IgE levels and although the finding of a high IgE concentration in an infant increases the likelihood of an atopic disorder developing, the clinical value of these measurements is debatable. There are several complicating factors. The distribution of IgE concentration in the non-atopic population is markedly skew and overlaps the range of values found in atopy, although the discrimination between atopic and non-atopic individuals on the basis of total IgE concentration is clearer in children than in adults. IgE is not a specific test for atopy and, indeed, in the Third World high levels are usually due to parasitic disease, such as hookworm (*Table* APP.4). Many allergic phenomena are not mediated via IgE and in some IgE-dependent allergies total IgE levels may be normal. None the less, knowledge of the total serum IgE level may be of value in selecting candidates for allergen-specific IgE measurements.

The assay of allergen-specific IgE by radioallergosorbent tests (RAST) or similar techniques is a controver-

Table APP.4   Disorders associated with high serum IgE levels

Atopy (asthma, eczema, rhinitis, food allergy)
Parasites (including hookworm and schistosomiasis)
Pulmonary allergic aspergillosis
Churg–Strauss syndrome
Wiskott–Aldrich syndrome
Hyperimmunoglobulin E syndrome
Pemphigoid
Systemic sclerosis
Lymphoma (including Hodgkin's disease)

sial matter and a WHO report has suggested that such measurements are not essential in any clinical situation. These tests are extremely expensive and may yield irrelevant or misleading information unless used in a discriminatory manner, taking into account the clinical history. In most situations specific IgE measurements offer no advantage over skin-prick tests and should probably be reserved for special circumstances such as skin disease, risk of anaphylaxis on antigen exposure (including suspected bee and wasp venom sensitivity, and penicillin allergy), very young children or when skin tests have produced ambiguous results. IgE-mediated allergies with very localized effects, such as allergic rhinitis, commonly produce no detectable specific IgE in serum, whereas some individuals with high levels of allergen-specific IgE in serum have no associated clinical features.

b. Monoclonal hyperimmunoglobulinaemia (paraproteinaemia)

Paraproteins are immunoglobulins produced by monoclonal lines of B-cell origin. They are particularly associated with *multiple myeloma* but sometimes occur in other B-cell malignancies, such as *chronic lymphocytic leukaemia, B-cell lymphoma* and *Waldenström's macroglobulinaemia.* In addition, paraproteins can arise in the absence of evidence of malignant disease, especially in the elderly. *Table* APP.5 lists some points of value in discriminating between malignant and benign paraproteinaemias.

Table APP.5   Typical features of benign paraproteinaemias

Absence of lytic lesions in bone
Paraprotein concentration less than 10 g/l
No increase in paraprotein level on serial measurement
No Bence Jones proteinuria or evidence of
  immunoglobulin fragments
No suppression of other immunoglobulin classes

Most myelomas produce an IgG paraprotein, IgA being the next commonest class. In about 20 per cent of myelomas Bence Jones protein (free light chain) can be demonstrated in the urine in the absence of a serum band. Examination of the urine is mandatory if the diagnosis is being seriously considered. Occasionally paraproteins behave as cryoglobulins and will not be detected unless special procedures are adopted. Paraproteins may also be missed if they co-migrate with a normal serum band on electrophoresis, unless immunochemical detection is used. A variety of other proteins, including fibrinogen (a normal component of plasma but not serum) can give rise to discrete bands on electrophoresis and any unusual bands must be fully characterized, preferably by immunofixation. Measurement of plasma β-2-microglobulin which reflects both tumour mass and renal impairment, has prognostic value in myeloma.

IRON STATUS

No single biochemical test of iron status is satisfactory under all circumstances and haematological data are required for satisfactory interpretation.

Serum ferritin

Serrum ferritin determination is the most satisfactory test of *irton deficiency*, this condition being the only cause of a low ferritin level. However, a ferritin concentration in the lower part of the reference range does not exclude iron deficiency because various factors unrelated to iron status, including acute phase responses and liver injury, tend to increase serum ferritin, and may thereby mask iron deficiency. It is important to appreciate that normal ranges for ferritin are based on individuals who are not anaemic, so that if a patient with an anaemia due to factors other than iron deficiency is to replenish his red cell mass he will need greater reserves of iron than a normal subject. For this reason even in non-iron-deficiency anaemias, ferritin levels in the lower part of the reference range may indicate inadequate iron stores. However, in many types of anaemia (e.g. aplastic, sideroblastic, dyserythropoietic and chronic haemolytic) iron stores are often high.

Increases in serum ferritin concentration occur in *iron overload* of any cause (including haemochromatosis) but elevated levels are found in a variety of other situations including *malignancy*, *thyrotoxicosis*, *inflammatory conditions* and *liver diseases* other than haemochromatosis. In the early stages of haemochromatosis ferritin levels may be within the reference range, even when transferrin saturation is elevated.

Serum iron and transferrin

Serum iron concentrations fall in *iron deficiency*, while transferrin levels (often measured as iron binding capacity) rise. However, serum iron levels and transferrin saturation are unsatisfactory as indicators of iron deficiency for a variety of reasons. Serum iron represents only about 0·1 per cent of the body pool and undergoes rapid turnover. Because of this, serum iron levels may be unrepresentative of body reserves and exhibit marked intraindividual fluctuations unrelated to changes in body iron status. Reductions in serum iron also occur as part of the metabolic response to *acute injury* and in *chronic disease*. The specificity of serum iron concentration for iron deficiency can be improved by relating it to transferrin (or iron binding capacity), which tends to fall in those conditions other than iron deficiency causing reductions in serum iron levels. However, even when expressed in terms of transferrin saturation, serum iron determinations are inferior to ferritin measurements as a test of iron deficiency, partly because transferrin has a relatively long half-life so that acute variations in serum iron levels are directly reflected by similar fluctuations in saturation.

In suspected iron overload, however, the assay of serum iron remains useful in three ways. First, serum iron measurements are essential in the management of *acute iron poisoning*. Secondly in some patients with *early haemochromatosis* the serum iron rises and the transferrin falls (producing an increased saturation) before the serum ferritin becomes elevated. Thirdly, in a proportion of patients with increases in serum ferritin due to causes other than iron overload (e.g. malignancy) the serum iron and transferrin saturation may be normal or reduced, although this is not an invariable finding. In a patient with abnormal liver function tests associated with an increased serum ferritin, therefore, the finding of a low serum iron saturation would make haemochromatosis extremely unlikely.

Transferrin levels are increased in *high oestrogen states* (oral contraceptives, pregnancy) and this must be taken into account in interpreting serum iron levels in these conditions.

LIPID MEASUREMENTS

Apart from non-esterified fatty acids, lipids are transported as lipoproteins, which comprise complexes of triglyceride, cholesterol (free and esterfied), phospholipid and apoproteins. Lipoproteins can be divided into the following classes: chylomicrons (CMs); very low density lipoprotein (VLDL); intermediate density lipoprotein (IDL); low density lipoprotein (LDL) and high density lipoprotein (HDL).

CMs and VLDL are both triglyceride-rich and contain a relatively low proportion of cholesterol. CMs are the form in which triglyceride derived from the diet is transported, while VLDL transports triglyceride synthesized endogenously in the liver. Triglyceride from these particles is taken up by adipose tissue, muscle and the liver. In addition, some triglyceride is transferred to HDL in exchange for esterified cholesterol, by a process involving cholesterol ester exchange protein. As a result of their catabolism, VLDL particles are converted via IDL to LDL, which is secreted by the liver. LDL is cholesterol-rich and accounts for about 80 per cent of the plasma cholesterol concentration. LDL particles are cleared from the plasma by the liver and peripheral tissues through a receptor-mediated process. LDL is important both in centrifugal cholesterol transport (away from the liver to peripheral tissues) and in the centripetal return of cholesterol to the liver. HDL contains about 15 per cent of circulating cholesterol and is synthesized in the liver and, to a lesser extent, in the small intestine. HDL is important in the centripetal transport of cholesterol to the liver but it has become apparent in recent years that the mechanisms by which HDL influences this process are largely indirect, involving the esterification of free cholesterol taken up by HDL, and subsequent transfer to other types of lipoprotein particle.

In clinical terms the importance of lipoprotein metabolism is related to the risk of atheroma in general, and ischaemic heart disease in particular, high levels of total cholesterol (more specifically, LDL cholesterol) being a strong risk factor in this context. Most authorities consider that HDL levels have an independent, inverse relationship to the risk of coronary artery disease. It is uncertain as to whether triglyceride levels have independent significance in atherogenesis, although some hypertriglyceridaemic states (e.g. familial combined hyperlipidaemia) are associated with an increased risk. High levels of triglyceride, however, predispose to lipaemia retinalis and acute pancreatitis.

A number of factors related to life-style influence plasma lipid concentrations. VLDL and LDL tend to be increased in the *obese*, in whom HDL levels are commonly reduced. These abnormalities are reversible by weight reduction. *Physical activity* increases HDL levels and reduces VLDL and LDL. *Diets* rich in saturated fatty acids and cholesterol (to a variable degree) tend to increase LDL concentrations, polyunsaturated fatty acids and soluble dietary fibre having the opposite effect.

Dyslipoproteinaemias can be classified in several ways. In the Fredrickson/WHO system the disorders are described in terms of their biochemical phenotypes (*Table* APP.6), i.e. according to the pattern of abnormality in the various lipoprotein types. It should be noted, however, that the Fredrickson classes do not correspond to disease entities as such, in the sense that various members of families affected by the same

inherited disorder may exhibit different Fredrickson phenotypes, while the same individual may fall into different Fredrickson classes at different times. In the classification introduced by Goldstein *et al* dyslipoproteinaemias are described on a genetic basis which separates metabolically distinct disorders (*Table* APP.7). However, it should be appreciated that most hyperlipidaemia is polygenic and, with certain exceptions (e.g. hyperchylomicronaemia and remnant hyperlipidaemia), a detailed biochemical diagnosis is not required for treatment. In addition, hyperlipidaemia may be secondary to another condition or drug ingestion (*Table* APP.8) and this possibility should always be considered before a primary lipid disorder is diagnosed.

Random (non-fasted) samples generally give a reasonable indication of total cholesterol levels but fasted samples should be obtained if more detailed information is required. The patient should be fasted overnight for 14 hours, triglyceride levels being markedly affected by recent ingestion of fat. There should have been no alteration in the patient's diet or pattern of alcohol consumption for at least a fortnight before venesection and lipo-active drugs should have been avoided for 3 weeks. Excessive venous stasis causes artefactual elevation of blood lipid levels and to avoid orthostatic effects the patient should be seated or recumbent during venepuncture. EDTA is often recommended as anticoagulant, although many laboratories find heparin acceptable. Any abnormal result should be confirmed by at least one further sample before treatment is instituted. Samples taken within 24 hours of a myocardial infarction can be interpreted in the normal way but after this interval LDL and total cholesterol levels fall as part of the metabolic response to injury, lipoprotein metabolism remaining deranged for a variable period up to 3 months.

Plasma lipids should be measured in patients with *premature ischaemic heart disease*, in those with a strong *family history of ischaemic heart disease* or *hyperlipidaemia*, in patients with *xanthomata* or premature arcus, and in those noted to have lipaemic fasting plasma. The case for population screening is unproved and a matter of debate.

Baseline investigation of plasma lipoprotein abnormalities should include the measurement of fasted cholesterol and triglyceride concentrations. If the cholesterol level is high but the triglyceride level is normal, an HDL assay should be performed to identify the occasional patient with mild hypercholesterolaemia due to an increase in HDL. More often, however, isolated hypercholesterolaemia is due to an elevated level of LDL. Combined hyperlipidaemia, in which cholesterol and triglyceride levels are increased to a comparable degree, may be due to elevations in VLDL and LDL

Table APP.6 Fredrickson/WHO classification of hyperlipoproteinaemias

	I	IIa	IIb	III	IV	V
CMs	+	−	−	−	−	+
VLDL	N	N	↑	*	↑	↑
LDL	N	↑↑	↑	↓	N	N
Cholesterol	N	↑↑	↑	↑	N(↑)	N(↑)
Triglyceride	↑↑	N	↑	↑	↑↑	↑↑

N = normal;   = ↑ increased;   = ↓ decreased.

* In type III IDL accumulates, giving rise to a broad beta band on lipoprotein electrophoresis.

Table APP.7 Genetic classification of hyperlipoproteinaemias

Disease	Main lipoprotein abnormalities	Cholesterol	Triglyceride	Fredrickson type
Familial hypercholesterolaemia	LDL	↑↑	N(↑)	IIa (IIb)
Familial hypertriglyceridaemia	VLDL (± CMs)	N(↑)	↑↑	IV, V
Familial combined hyperlidaemia	LDL and/or VLDL	↑	↑	IIb (IIa, IV)
Remnant hyperlipoproteinaemia	IDL	↑	↑	III
Lipoprotein lipase deficiency	CMs	N(↑)	↑↑	I (V)
ApoC II deficiency	CMs	N(↑)	↑↑	I (V)

N = normal;   ↑ = increased

Table APP.8 Secondary causes of hyperlipidaemia

	Hypertriglyceridaemia	Hypercholesterolaemia
Primary hypothyroidism		+
Cholestasis		+
Nephrotic syndrome	+	+
Chronic renal failure	+	+
Corticosteroids	+	+
Oral contraceptives	+	+
Diabetes mellitus	+	+
Alcohol abuse	+	
Thiazide diuretics	+	
Gout	+	
Glycogen storage disease	+	

together, or to an accumulation of IDL (remnant hyperlipoproteinaemia). These two possibilites may be distinguished by lipoprotein electrophoresis. In hyperlipidaemias in which hypertriglyceridaemia is the predominant element it is useful to inspect the plasma after an overnight stand at 4°C, VLDL giving a diffuse opalescence, while CMs float as a creamy layer on the plasma surface. In most hypertriglyceridaemic states the HDL level is reduced but in hypertriglyceridaemia due to alcohol or oestrogen the concentration of this lipoprotein is often increased.

LDL cholesterol concentration may be calculated from the total cholesterol, triglyceride and HDL cholesterol concentrations, assuming that there are no CMs, that the triglyceride concentration does not exceed 4·5 mmol/l and that the patient does not have remnant hyperlipidaemia:

$$\text{LDL cholesterol} = \text{total cholesterol} - \text{HDL cholesterol} - \frac{\text{triglyceride}}{2 \cdot 2}$$

(All quantities in mmol/l)

More specialized investigations include the typing of ApoE variants in remnant hyperlipidaemia, and assays of ApoC II and lipoprotein lipase in fasted chylomicronaemia. The value of $ApoA_1$ and B measurements in routine clinical work has yet to be clearly defined.

MAGNESIUM

Magnesium concentration in serum or plasma is easily determined. If plasma is used, care should be taken to ensure that the anticoagulant is not contaminated with magnesium. In normal plasma, about one-third of the total magnesium content is protein bound, the remainder being either complexed or existing as free ions.

Intracellular concentrations of magnesium, however, are much higher than those found in normal plasma. Magnesium is the second most abundant cation found within cells and is essential for the normal activity of many enzymes including phosphotransferases. Unfortunately there is no simple means to determine intracellular magnesium levels, which vary between different tissue types.

Because of this and because over half the body's magnesium content is located in the skeleton, plasma measurements may not be representative of body reserves, particularly in chronic disorders. There is no consensus on the best test of magnesium status in this situation, although various methods, including formal magnesium balance studies, retention of magnesium after oral or parenteral administration and isotopic techniques have been described.

Measurement of the renal excretion of magnesium is easy to perform and may be of value in distinguishing between renal magnesium wasting and hypomagnesaemia due to other causes. Non-protein-bound magnesium is filterable by the glomeruli, the most important site for magnesium reabsorption being the thick ascending limb of the loop of Henle. In the absence of renal disease, urinary magnesium excretion varies according to the plasma level and when plasma magnesium is reduced, urinary excretion may fall below 0·5 mmol/day. Urinary magnesium excretion shows a circadian rhythm so that renal losses must be determined on 24 hour collections, which should be taken into acid to prevent precipitation of magnesium compounds.

On an average dietary intake of about 10 mmol/day, about 40 per cent is absorbed in the small intestine, although fractional absorption varies inversely with intake. Gastrointestinal secretions are rich in magnesium. The difference between gastrointestinal absorption and secretion is similar to the quantity excreted by the kidneys in a normal individual in magnesium balance. Assay of faecal magnesium may be of value in patients suspected of laxative abuse.

Hypermagnesaemia

This condition, which is rare and often iatrogenic, may cause cardiac and central nervous system depression. Hypermagnesaemia is most likely to occur in patients with *acute or chronic renal failure*, especially after the administration of *magnesium-containing preparations*. Hypermagnesaemia may also occur in *liver failure*.

Hypomagnesaemia

Hypomagnesaemia may produce neuromuscular excitability, tetany and convulsions. There is controversy concerning the role of hypomagnesaemia in the induction of arrhythmias and hypertension. There is evidence that hypomagnesaemia suppresses parathormone secretion and impairs its peripheral action. These factors may explain why hypocalcaemia often coexists with hypomagnesaemia and may contribute to the clinical presentation. Hypomagnesaemia can also cause a hypokalaemia that is relatively refractory to potassium supplementation.

Causes of hypomagnesaemia may be classified as follows:

1. Dietary deficiency (including alcoholoics).
2. Gastrointestinal pathology:
   a. diarrhoea (including steatorrhoea and laxative abuse)
   b. gastrointestinal fistulae
   c. nasogastric aspiration and vomiting
   d. familial hypomagnesaemia (inherited disorder of intestinal magnesium transport).
3. Urinary losses:
   a. drugs (including diuretics and aminoglycosides)
   b. Barrter's syndrome
   c. alcohol abuse
   d. diuretic phase of acute renal failure
   e. diabetes mellitus (including ketoacidosis)
   f. hypercalcaemia
   g. Conn's syndrome
   h. hyperthyroidism.
4. Lactation.

PHOSPHATE

Phosphate, either inorganic or organic, is approximately equally distributed between the extra- and intracellular compartments. Within the cell, most phosphate is organic, existing as a component of phospholipids, phosphoproteins, nucleic acid and energy-rich phosphate compounds such as ATP. Outside the cell, the majority of phosphate is inorganic, existing as a mixture of HPO_4^{2-} and $H_2PO_4^-$ at physiological pH.

Plasma [phosphate] is subject to considerable variation during the day, often related to eating. Reference intervals also change with age. Plasma levels are further influenced by a number of hormones. Thus, parathyroid hormone (PTH) decreases proximal tubular reabsorption of phosphate, decreasing plasma [phosphate], whilst calcitriol promotes the intestinal absorption of *both* Ca^{2+} and phosphate, thereby elevating plasma [phosphate]. Insulin increases the uptake of phosphate into liver and muscle and can contribute to hypophosphataemia.

Consistently low or high plasma [phosphate] should be recognized with a view to treatment, usually of the underlying cause.

Increased plasma [phosphate]

a. Decreased renal excretion

An inportant cause of a consistently elevated plasma [phosphate] is the falling GFR which is a feature of *chronic renal failure. Hyperphosphataemia is also found in acute renal failure.* In the earlier states of chronic renal failure, the phosphate retention may be partially offset by secondary hyperparathyroidism which stimulates urinary phosphate loss, but compensation is later lost with progressive increase in plasma [phosphate].

In *hypoparathyroidism* (and *pseudohypoparathyroidism*) there is reduced renal excretion accompanying the depressed (or, in the case of pseudohypoparathyroidism, ineffective) PTH. Similarly in cases of *hypercalcaemia* (other than PTH excess), plasma [phosphate] tends to be high as PTH secretion is supressed by the hypercalcaemic stimulus.

b. Increased intake

This is a feature of *excessive vitamin D intake* (along with hypercalcaemia), since calcitriol stimulates intestinal absorption of both Ca^{2+} and phosphate. *High phosphate content in the diet* can lead to hyperphosphataemia in young infants fed phosphate-rich cows' milk.

Parenteral administration of phosphate (e.g. during total parenteral nutrition) may sometimes lead to increased plasma [phosphate].

c. Re-distribution

Cellular breakdown may also release inorganic phosphate, as in the hyperphosphataemia which sometimes occurs during the *treatment of malignant disease.*

In *diabetic ketoacidosis* there is tissue catabolism and impaired phosphate uptake (insulin deficiency). Conversely, plasma [phosphate] levels may actually fall during treatment as it is taken up into the depleted cells (see 'Low plasma [phosphate]' below).

d. Miscellaneous

Acromegaly and *lactate acidosis*

Low plasma [phosphate]

Severe degrees of hypophosphataemia may impair cellular energy metabolism and be accompanied by myoglobinuria and renal impairment. As with hyperphosphataemia, causes can best be considered under related headings.

a. Increased phosphate loss in urine

This accompanies the high PTH levels of *primary hyperparathyroidism*. In any situation where there is true *hypocalcaemia* (other than hypoparathyroidism), there will be secondary *hyperparathyroidism* and a tendency for plasma [phosphate] to be low. Excessive urinary phosphate loss may also be a feature of the *Fanconi syndrome* where a generalized proximal tubular defect of multifactorial origin is present and in *familial hypophosphataemic rickets* where a specific defect in phosphate reabsorption is present. Increased excretion may also occur in *hypomagnesaemia* and with *diuretic therapy*.

b. Decreased phosphate intake

This is a feature of *vitamin D deficiency* and may also accompany excessive use of *phosphate binding agents* such as *aluminium hydroxide*. On a worldwide basis *malnutrition* is an important cause. Deficient dietary intake may also contribute to the low plasma [phosphate] often observed in *chronic alcoholism*. Hypophosphataemia may also be observed in generalized *malabsorption*.

c. Redistribution

Hypophosphataemia may appear during *enteral and parenteral feeding* with inadequate phosphate replenishment. Phosphate is taken up and incorporated into the cells during re-feeding and requirements are increased. Movement into the cells also occurs during *glucose infusion* (as would be used in parenteral nutrition) and in the treatment of *diabetic ketoacidosis*. Cellular uptake is also encouraged by β-*adrenergic agents*.

d. Others

A low plasma [phosphate] is also observed in *severe injury and burns*. The cause is probably multifactorial, with redistribution and increased losses contributing.

PORPHYRIAS

The porphyrias are a group of disorders due to abnormal haem biosynthesis. Most of these diseases are hereditary although cutaneous hepatic porphyria (CHP) often occurs as an acquired disorder. *Fig.* APP.1 shows the relevant metabolic pathways. In health, aminolaevulinic acid (ALA) synthase, which catalyses the first step in the sequence, is rate-limiting and in the liver this enzyme is regulated via feedback inhibition by haem. In the porphyrias, enzyme deficiencies in the pathway cause a breakdown in the normal control mechanisms, with the production of abnormal patterns of metabolites and, in some cases, clinical conse- quences. Accurate diagnosis requires a close liaison between the physician and the laboratory since it is essential to interpret the biochemistry in relation to the clinical situation. Because porphyrins and porphob- ilinogen (PBG) are labile it is important that details concerning specimen collection and transport should be discussed with the laboratory. According to the clinical presentation, specimens of urine, blood and faeces may be required for analysis of porphyrins and their precursors and, in certain circumstances, the direct assay of enzymes involved in haem biosynthesis may be helpful (*Fig.* APP.2).

Classification of porphyrias (*Table* APP.9)

The tissues most active in the synthesis of haem are the liver and the marrow, and porphyrias can be described as hepatic or erythropoietic according to the major site of the biochemical abnormality. From a clinical point of view, however, it is more useful to divide porphyrias into the acute and non-acute forms.

Acute porphyrias

The neurovisceral attacks characteristic of these disor- ders are thought to be due to the accumulation of porphyrin precursors. Gastrointestinal symptoms, including acute abdominal pain, vomiting and constipa- tion, are common and are frequently accompanied by elevations in blood pressure and heart rate. Neurolog- ical problems include confusion, psychosis, fitting, autonomic neuropathy and peripheral neuropathy (which may affect ventilation and lead to respiratory failure). A fever often develops and a dilutional hypona- traemia may occur. Red or brown urine may be noted.

Attacks may be precipitated by a wide range of drugs and toxins including barbiturates, oral contraceptives, sulphonamides, anticonvulsants and ethanol.

In the United Kingdom acute intermittent porphyria (AIP) is the commonest acute form. This disorder has no dermatological manifestations. In South Africa there is a high incidence of variegate porphyria (VP), which, in common with the acute porphyria, hereditary copro- porphyria (HC), produces photosensitive skin lesions.

If an acute porphyric episode is suspected fresh

Fig. APP.1. Haem biosynthesis

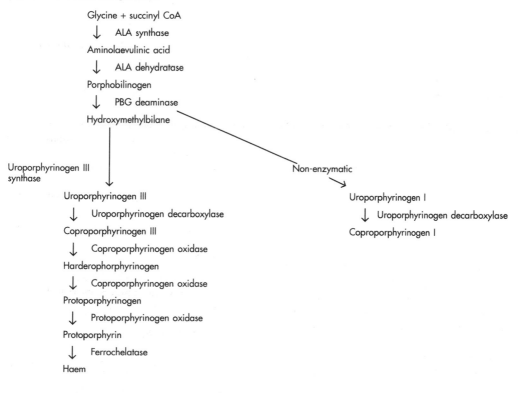

Fig. APP.2. Laboratory strategy for the investigation of suspected porphyria

(a) *Suspected acute attack*

Screen for urinary PBG

Negative	Positive
Excludes acute porphyria (rare exceptions)	1. Quantitation of urinary ALA and PBG by specific method
	2. Faecal porphyrins
	AIP—often normal (sometimes increased proto- and coproporphyrin)
	VP—proto- (and sometimese coproporhyrin) raised
	HC—coproporphyrin raised, protoporphyrin usually normal
	3. Consider requirement for enzyme assays in doubtful cases
	4. Initiate family studies

(b) *Suspected latent acute porphyria*

1. Faecal porphyrins for VP and HC as above
2. Quantitate urinary ALA and PBG by specific method:
   AIP—usually raised
   VP
   HC } usually normal
3. PBG deaminase for suspected AIP

(c) *Patient with skin lesions*

Non-bullous urticaria/erythema	Bullae ± erosions
Consider EP	Test faeces, urine and erythrocytes for excess porphyrins
Measure erythrocyte porphyrin:	If all normal, porphyria unlikely
Normal—excludes EP	If any abnormal, characterize porphyrins fully
Raised—further tests to confirm EP and	In CHP urinary uroporphyrin raised and greater than coproporphyrin
differentiate from lead poisoning, etc.	Isocoproporphyrin present in faeces
	In VP, faecal protoporphyrin (and often coproporphyrin) raised
	Urinary uro- and coproporphyrin sometimes raised
	In HC, faecal coproporphyrin raised (protoporphyrin usually normal)
	and urinary uro- and coproporphyrin often raised
	In CP, erythrocyte porphyrins raised and urine contains excess
	uro- and coproporphyrin

Table APP.9   Classification of porphyrias

Disease	Site of Expression	Enzyme defect	Inheritance	Acute attacks	Skin Lesions
Acute intermittent porphyria	Liver	PBG deaminase	Autosomal dominant	+	−
Variegate porphyria	Liver	Protoporphyrinogen oxidase	Autosomal dominant	+	+
Hereditary coproporphyria	Liver	Coproporphyrinogen oxidase	Autosomal dominant	+	+
Cutaneous hepatic porphyria	Liver	Uroporphyrinogen decarboxylase	Autosomal dominant or acquired	−	+
Erythropoietic protoporphyria	Marrow	Ferrochelatase	Autosomal dominant	−	+
Congenital porphyria	Marrow	Uroporphyrinogen-III-synthase	Autosomal recessive	−	+

urine collected during the attack should be tested for PBG with Ehrlich's aldehyde reagent (paradimethylami-nobenzaldehyde). Repeated extraction with organic solvents after the addition of saturated sodium acetate permits a discrimination between PBG and urobilinogen (*see* p. 774) to be made. An amyl/benzyl alcohol mixture is preferable to chloroform for this purpose, the latter producing more false positive and negative reactions. Irrespective of the solvent used, false positive results are occasionally produced by drugs and their metabolites, and positive screens should be fol-

lowed up by quantitation of PBG and ALA using a specific method. Analysis of faecal porphyrins (by thin-layer or high performance liquid chromatography) is helpful in distinguishing between the various forms of acute porphyria. A negative screen for PBG on a urine sample taken during a suspected attack makes the diagnosis of acute porphyria extremely unlikely, although if there is a strong clinical suspicion quantitative assay of PBG and ALA may be justified.

Occasionally total urinary porphyrins may be increased despite a negative screen for PBG. In these circumstances the urinary porphyrins concerned should be identified, the PBG assayed quantitatively and the faecal porphyrins characterized. HC often underlies this situation.

It is important to appreciate that a negative screen for urinary PBG performed between suspected attacks does not exclude porphyria. In AIP in remission, quantitative determinations of ALA and PBG are often raised even when simple qualitative tests for PBG are negative, although in some cases the urinary excretion of these haem precursors is entirely normal. Assay of red cell PBG deaminase may help here. In quiescent VP and HC quantitative determinations of urinary ALA and PBG excretion are generally normal and analysis of faecal porphyrins should be performed if latent cases of these conditions are suspected.

The first degree relatives of known cases of acute porphyria should be investigated in a similar manner to suspect latent cases.

Non-acute porphyrias

Skin lesions are the most striking characteristic of the non-acute porphyrias (although two of the acute porphyrias, HC and VP, can affect the skin). The laboratory investigation of these patients is complex and may require a combination of measurements on blood, urine and faeces.

In Western Europe and the USA the commonest non-acute porphyria is cutaneous hepatic porphyria (CHP), also known as porphyria cutanea tarda. This disorder is characterized by a bullous dermatosis with hirsutism. There is often evidence of hepatic dysfunction and liver iron stores are increased. Impaired glucose tolerance occurs in about 25 per cent of patients. CHP is often an acquired, rather than an inherited condition. Alcohol abuse is the most important precipitating agent, although other toxins, such as hexachlorobenzene, have caused outbreaks. In untreated cases the urinary uroporphyrin level is increased (and greater than the urinary coproporphyrin concentration, by contrast with what occurs in VP) and the faeces contain isocoproporphyrin. The two erythropoietic porphyrias, erythropoietic protoporphyria (EP) and congenital porphyria (CP) also involve the skin. In addition to its dermatological manifestation EP affects the liver and patients may develop gallstones. A normal erythrocyte porphyrin content excludes this condition but raised levels also occur in lead poisoning and iron-deficiency anaemia, more sophisticated tests being required to make a definitive diagnosis. There is usually an increase in faecal protoporphyrin in EP, although urinary porphyrins are normal. CP (Gunther's disease) is extremely rare and usually presents in childhood. The photosensitivity can be devastating and usually produces severe

scarring. There may be a haemolytic anaemia and splenomegaly. In this disease red cell, urinary and faecal porphyrins are all abnormal.

Other conditions associated with abnormal porphyrin excretion

Secondary abnormalities in haem biosynthesis occur in a wide variety of other disorders, including chronic renal failure, lead poisoning, several types of anaemia, liver disease and alcohol abuse.

POTASSIUM

In contrast to sodium, potassium is the major intracellular cation where it is present at a concentration of around 150 mmol/l. Maintenance of the distribution of Na^+ and K^+ between intra- and extracellular compartments depends upon the energy-dependent Na^+-K^+ ATPase situated in the plasma membrane.

In considering disorders of plasma K^+, the distinction between internal and external K^+ balance is important. External balance refers to the relationship between intake and loss whilst internal balance relates to the distribution of K^+ between intra- and extracellular compartments.

Low plasma [potassium]

a. Altered internal balance: shift of potassium to the intracellular compartment

1. Alkalosis

Movement of K^+ into cells may partly account for the low plasma levels encountered in alkalosis, especially in metabolic alkalosis. However, metabolic alkalosis may also be associated with absolute losses of K^+ in urine, especially in the presence of volume depletion (e.g. pyloric stenosis). This negative external balance is usually more important.

2. High-dose insulin therapy

High doses of insulin will promote the uptake of K^+ by liver and muscle.

3. Beta-adrenergic agonists

These also stimulate the uptake of K^+ into cells. This phenomenon may contribute to the hypokalaemia appearing *before* diuretic therapy in patients after myocardial infarction with raised catecholamine levels. The effect is also observed with catecholaminergic drugs such as salbutamol. *Theophylline* levels may also stimulate K+ uptake by cells.

4. Cellular incorporation

This may be very rapid in states where cell mass rapidly increases. Examples include the *treatment of severe megaloblastic anaemia* with vitamin B_{12} or folate; the *parenteral re-feeding of wasted patients* (especially if insulin is also administered); in *rapidly proliferating leukaemic cells*.

5. Hypokalaemic periodic paralysis

is a relatively rare familial disorder in which a transient re-distribution of K+ from an extra- to an intracellular location occurs, accompanied by characteristic symptoms of muscle weakness.

b. Altered external balance: deficient intake

Prolonged K+ deficiency can lead to a decrease in total body K+, eventually manifesting as hypokalaemia. Situations in which this phenomenon may arise include: *third world poverty; the elderly on deficient diets; anorexia nervosa; prolonged postoperative intravenous nutrition with inadequate K+ replacement*.

c. Altered external balance: excessive losses

Excessive loss of K+ from the body can occur either in the urine or through abnormal GI losses.

1. Renal losses

An important reason for the excessive loss of K+ in urine is in response to the presence of certain diuretics. *Osmotic diuretics*, including *glucose* (in *diabetes mellitus*), *mannitol* and large amounts of *hypertonic solutions* used intravenously can have this effect. In the recovery phase of *acute tubular necrosis*, or *following relief of urinary obstruction*, excessive loss of urea and Na+ can lead to polyuria and K+ depletion. Similarly, many *diuretic drugs* may lead to K+ loss, the exception being certain K+-retaining diuretics acting on the distal tubule (e.g. amiloride). *Thiazide diuretics* and *'loop' diuretics* (e.g. frusemide) lead to increased delivery of Na+ to the distal tubule, promoting K+ loss in exchange for Na+ reabsorption.

K+ loss is stimulated by *metabolic alkalosis*. The loss of *gastric contents* in conditions such as *pyloric stenosis* and *prolonged nasogastric suction* can lead to severe metabolic alkalosis and hypokalaemia (see

also (2) below). An important factor in the urinary K+ losses is the volume depletion and secondary hyperaldosteronism (also see the section on internal balance).

Hyperaldosteronism, whether *primary (Conn's syndrome)* or *secondary*, will lead to Na+ reabsorption at the expense of K+ loss and the possible occurrence of hypokalaemia. *Carbenoxolone* therapy or excessive intake of *liquorice*, through their aldosterone-like action, can achieve the same effect. The use of potent *thiazide* and *'loop' diuretics* may also lead to intravascular volume contraction and secondary hyperaldosteronism, thereby increasing further the potential for K+ loss in the urine.

A number of rarer conditions are also associated with renal K+ wasting. These include *Mg^{2+} deficiency, Bartter's syndrome, Liddle's syndrome, renal tubular acidosis (types I and II)* and *tubular damage* from antimicrobials such as *gentamicin* and *amphotericin B*. The excretion of *urinary lysozyme* in *acute myeloid, monocytic* and *myelomonocytic leukaemias* may also be associated with K+ loss.

2. Gastrointestinal losses

K+ losses may occur in *gastric juice*, with fluid loss in *enterocutaneous fistulae (e.g. postoperatively)* or as a result of *diarrhoea*.

Gastric fluid contains around 5–10 mmol/l K+. However, the urinary loss of K+ (see 1. above) is generally more important in the development of hypokalaemia after gastric fluid loss. The K+ wasting in *diarrhoea* is an important cause of hypokalaemia. On a global scale, the high stool volumes which accompany *cholera* or *enteritis caused by Escherichia coli* are especially important. Nevertheless, any cause of significant diarrhoea may be to blame. In developed countries, more especially in the elderly, *laxative abuse* can produce hypokalaemia. Rarer causes include, *non-insulin secreting islet cell tumours, villous adenoma of the rectum* and *urinary stagnation in ureterosigmoidostomy*.

d. Other causes

1. Artefactual

Collection of a blood sample near to a site of infusion (where the fluid has a low K+ content).

2. Excessive sweating

High plasma [potassium]

High plasma [K+] can also be considered as arising from altered internal balance (movement from intact cells, leakage from damaged cells, restricted entry into cells) or from abnormal external balance (increased intake or decreased excretion).

a. Altered internal balance

1. Acidosis

The effects of acidosis on internal (and external) K+ balance are complicated. As a general rule, *acidotic states* are often accompanied by *hyperkalaemia*, as K+ moves from the cell into the extracellular compartment. Although this is the case for acute respiratory acidosis and both acute and chronic metabolic acidosis, it is more unusual to find hyperkalaemia in chronic respiratory acidosis. It is also important to remember that a *high plasma [K+]* may be accompanied by a *reduced* total body K+. Thus, urinary K+ losses are increased in both chronic respiratory and metabolic acidosis, as illustrated by the excessive K+ losses which accompany diabetic ketoacidosis.

2. Hypertonicity

can contribute to a raised plasma [K+]. The mechanism may be through cellular dehydration with an increase in intracellular K+ concentration promoting K+ efflux. *Infusion of glucose into insulin-requiring diabetics* can lead to hyperkalaemia, especially in the presence of the selective hypoaldosteronism which may be found in diabetics.

3. Insulin deficiency

may restrict cellular K+ uptake and contribute to the hyperkalaemia of *diabetic keoacidosis*.

4. Cellular necrosis

inevitably leads to the release of K+ and the possibility of hyperkalaemia. Extensive cell damage may be a feature of *rhabdomyolysis* (e.g. crush injury), *haemolysis, burns* or in *tumour necrosis* (e.g. in the treatment of leukaemias).

5. Drugs

such as *digoxin* inhibit the Na+-K+-ATPase, leading to increased cellular efflux of K+. Hyperkalaemia is an established feature of poisoning with cardiac glycosides, although therapeutic concentrations have little effect on plasma [K+].

6. Hyperkalaemic periodic paralysis

is a rare familial disorder in which K+ spontaneously moves from an intra- to extracellular location.

b. Altered external balance: increased intake

Increased intake may be enteral or parenteral. The possibility of hyperkalaemia is more likely following injudicious parenteral K+ administration, but either route is more likely to lead to significant hyperkalaemia in the presence of impaired excretion (renal disease). *Excessive oral K+ supplementation*, especially inappropriate administration with a K+-retaining diuretic, *high K+ diet* (notably, in the presence of impaired renal function), *intravenous K+ replacement therapy, infusion of K+- salts of antibiotics* and use of *stored blood* may all lead to hyperkalaemia.

c. Altered external balance: decreased excretion

Decreased K+ excretion arises from *intrinsic renal disease* or as a result of a *defect in the endocrine (aldosterone) mechanism* responsible for K+ secretion by the distal nephron.

1. Intrinsic renal disease

is an important cause of impaired K+ excretion and possible hyperkalaemia. Impaired K+ excretion occurs in *acute renal failure* and the later stages of *chronic renal failure*. In patients with disease which largely affects the renal medulla, hyperkalaemia may occur earlier. This may be because increased K+ secretion from the collecting duct is an important adaptive response in the damaged kidney which is lost earlier in patients with medullary disease.

2. Low aldosterone levels

Together with deficiency of other steroid hormones, this is a feature of *Addison's disease*. In contrast, *selective hypoaldosteronism* is accompanied by normal glucocorticoid production; in this condition, the hypoaldosteronism appears to be the consequence of low renin levels. This condition is recognised in patients with *diabetes mellitus*, where juxtaglomerular sclerosis probably interferes with renin production. The use of *ACE inhibitors*, by reducing AII levels, may lead to an elevation in plasma [K+], but severe problems are only likely at creatinine clearance values of less than 20 ml/min.

3. Failure to respond to aldosterone

This is the case in patients treated with *K+-sparing diuretics* such as *spironolactone* or *amiloride*. A simultaneous high K+ intake, renal insufficiency or selective hypoaldosteronism can all lead to dangerous hyperkalaemia.

Unresponsiveness to aldosterone has also been described in a variety of conditions which include *amyloidosis, renal autografts, sickle cell disease* and *systemic lupus erythematosus.*

d. Miscellaneous causes

1. Delay in blood separation

K+ leaks from the cells on storage of whole (i.e. unseparated) blood. This is a common reason for artefactual hyperkalaemia.

2. Use of K+ EDTA collection tube

K+ EDTA is often used as a preservative for haematological analysis. If a blood sample is collected into this anticoagulant and subsequently decanted into the appropriate collection tube for biochemical analysis, K+ levels will be artefactually high. The low plasma Ca^{2+} (due to its chelation by EDTA) is a useful clue in detecting this error.

3. Collection

of a blood sample near the *site of an intravenous infusion* where K+ is present in the infused solution.

4. Pseudohyperkalaemia

is a spuriously elevated plasma [K+] resulting from its release by lysis from platelets or leucocytes during venepuncture. It has been described in *acute and chronic myeloproliferative disorders, chronic lymphocytic leukaemia* and *severe thrombocytosis.* A *familial form,* in which the red blood cells 'leak' K+ also exists, but there is no underlying proliferative abnormality.

SODIUM

An adult male possesses about 3000 mmol of Na+, with approximately 30 per cent present in bone and the remainder distributed throughout the rest of the body. Most Na+ is extracellular in location where the ECF concentration is around 140 mmol/l. In contrast, the intracellular Na+ concentration is less than 10 mmol/l (cf. K+).

Obligatory Na+ losses are small, and the daily Na+ requirement is less than 5 mmol/day under normal circumstances. The Na+ content in the diet is very variable worldwide, but a typical Western diet provides 100–200 mmol Na+/day. In order to remain in external balance, the excess Na+ (i.e. beyond the obligatory daily requirement) must be lost from the body. The

healthy kidney is able to adjust Na+ excretion over a wide range to achieve this.

In considering disorders of plasma [Na+], potential disturbances in the very large internal turnover of Na+ must be borne in mind. Thus, around 25,000 mmol of Na+ are filtered at the glomerulus over 24 hours, whilst only 100–200 mmol (i.e. less 1 per cent of the filtered load) would appear in the urine, even on the higher Na+ diet of 100–200 mmol Na+/day found western society. Similarly, about 1000 mmol of Na+ per day enters the lumen of the GI tract in the various secretions; the vast majority of this Na+ is subsequently reabsorbed under normal circumstances.

In interpreting disorders of plasma [Na$_2$] it is essential to remember two points:

1. Na+ concentration measures the *ratio* of Na+ to plasma H_2O in that particular sample, so that loss or gain of H_2O can affect the value of [Na+] without there necessarily being net loss or gain of Na+ from the body. Conversely, the plasma [Na+] may be normal, with a total body Na+ content which is abnormal (e.g. haemorrhage in the earlier stages).

2. The interstitial compartment is three- to four-fold larger than the intravascular compartment. Hence the evaluation of *total body* Na+ excess or deficiency cannot be inferred from the amount of Na+ in the intravascular compartment alone. Conversely, knowledge of the total body Na+ (whether excessive or deficient) can greatly assist the interpretation of an abnormal plasma [Na+].

A number of factors which regulate Na+ and H_2O homeostasis have been identified. Two major regulatory hormones which regulate Na+ and H_2O homeostasis are aldosterone and arginine-vasopressin (AVP), also known as antidiuretic hormone:

1. AVP secretion is stimulated by a rise in extracellular osmolality, and the actions of AVP are to promote passive renal reabsorption of H_2O from the distal nephron, thereby returning the extracellular osmolaritry to normal levels (and vice versa). Although H_2O retention is *relatively* ineffective in expanding the intravascular volume (since H_2O distributes freely throughout all body compartments), H_2O retention becomes relatively more important if the circulation starts to fail. The left atrium and large arteries in the chest and neck possess stretch receptors which normally exert a tonic inhibitory effect on AVP secretion. A reduction in intravascular volume will release this tonic inhibitory action, resulting in the stimulation of AVP secretion. Volume deficits approaching 10 per cent are equipotent with osmolality in stimulating the AVP response. Thus, maintenance of osmolality is

temporarily sacrificed to the greater need to restore the circulation. Such H_2O retention would be reflected in a lowering of plasma [Na^+] and this is one of the reasons why hyponatraemia may occur in states of volume depletion.

2. Aldosterone secretion occurs indirectly in response to a reduction in renal blood flow, for whatever cause. A decline in renal blood flow activates the renin–angiotensin II–aldosterone axis. Since aldosterone promotes Na^+ reabsorption in the distal tubule, it is ideally suited to expanding the ECF volume, since Na^+ and its accompanying isosmotic H_2O are confined largely to this compartment.

Low plasma [sodium]

In interpreting a low plasma sodium, it is most convenient to first assess the *total body* sodium status, since this will direct attention to the likely cause(s) and the correct therapy. Careful attention to the clinical history and examination is of great value in assessing whether total body sodium is increased or decreased.

a. Decreased total body sodium

The patient has lost sodium and water in one or more body fluids (e.g. GI tract secretion, urine, inflammatory exudate), leading to characteristic and predictable clinical manifestations, viz. tachycardia, orthostatic hypotension, reduced skin turgor, oliguria, etc. The hypovolaemia will lead to secondary aldosteronism (low sodium content in urine) and a 'volume stimulus' to AVP secretion (oliguria, with a concentrated urine). The water retention contributes to the measured hyponatraemia.

1. Loss of GI secretions

This would include vomiting; diarrhoea; postoperative fistulae.

2. Loss from skin

This would include burns; severe dermatitis. Excessive sweating does deplete total body sodium but relatively much more water is lost leading to hypernatraemia.

3. Renal losses

Diuretic drug therapy or *endogenous osmotic diuretics* (e.g. glucose); *sodium-losing chronic renal disease* ('salt-losing nephropathy'); *mineralocorticoid deficiency* (Addison's disease); *renal tubular acidosis*.

4. Internal or 'third space' losses

There is no overt sodium loss from the body but an excessive accumulation of sodium-containing fluid in an internal location. Examples include *ileus; pancreatitis* or *peritonitis* (with inflammatory exudates into the peritoneal cavity); *muscle trauma*.

b. Normal or near-normal total body sodium

The hyponatraemia results from excessive water retention, itself due to an inability to excrete a water load. Failure to normally excrete water is found under conditions where AVP levels are high. Although this may be contributory in the examples discussed in A (where total body sodium is decreased), this would be inappropriate in the absence of a hypovolaemic stimulus and without evidence of a failing circulation. This is an important point of clinical distinction.

In addition to those conditions associated with inappropriately high AVP, water excreton is impaired in glucocorticoid deficiency and chronic renal disease. Occasionally the osmostat appears to be 'reset' at a lower level of plasma osmolality.

1. High AVP levels

Acute situation
AVP levels are increased after *trauma, major surgery, during delivery* and *post-partum*. This increase is part of the metabolic response to trauma. From the point of view that these situations are associated with real or potential ECF volume depletion, this response appears appropriate. Under circumstances where serious volume depletion *does* occur, patients fall into the category of decreased total body Na^+ (see (**A**) above). The AVP secretion which occurs in response to trauma means that hyponatraemia *after surgery* is a relatively common finding and need not *necessarily* reflect hypovolaemia or Na^+ depletion. A danger under circumstances where AVP levels are acutely increased is that administration of water (e.g. as 5 per cent dextrose intravenously) will lead to acute water retention, cellular swelling and potentially serious clinical consequences.

Acute secretion of ADH with hyponatraemia and a normal body Na^+ is also described in *acute schizophrenia*.

Chronic situation
Plasma sodium can fall to low levels with surprisingly few clinical symptoms if the excess H_2O retention occurs over a prolonged period. In the chronic situation the AVP excess is said to be 'inappropriate' from both the osmotic standpoint and because there is no

significant volume depletion. The causes of 'inappropriate' AVP secretion are varied and include:

a. *Ectopic AVP production* — from *malignant tumours of bronchus, pancreas, prostate* and *thymus*.

b. *CNS disorders* — *intracranial tumours* and *trauma.*

c. *Chest disease* — *pneumonias, tuberculosis, positive pressure mechanical ventilation.*

d. *Drugs* — *Opiates, barbiturates, chlorpropamide, clofibrate, carbamazepine, tolbutamide* and *nicotine.*

e. *Miscellaneous* — *Acute porphyria, Guillain–Barré syndrome; hypothyroidism.*

Before a diagnosis of inappropriate AVP secretion is made, it is important to establish that renal and pituitary causes of H_2O retention have been excluded (see below).

2. Chronic renal disease

The damaged kidneys are unable to achieve normal levels of urine concentration or dilution. Whereas the normal kidney can produce a urine as dilute as 60 mosm/kg (normal plasma 280–300 mosm/kg), in chronic renal disease the lowest osmolality achieved may be as high as 250 mosm/kg. Consequently the ability to excrete a water load is severely impaired and excess water intake (oral or intravenous) readily produces a dilutional hyponatraemia. Note that these patients may be Na^+ overloaded, falling into category (C) below.

3. Glucocorticoid deficiency

Abrupt *withdrawal of chronic glucocorticoid therapy* or *anterior pituitary disease* can lead to selective glucocorticoid deficiency (cf. Addison's disease, where there also occurs mineralocorticoid deficiency). Under these circumstances there may occur an inability to excrete a water load leading to hyponatraemia.

4. Resetting of osmostat

These patients have a plasma sodium chronically in the low range, generally 125–130 mmol/l, and respond normally to a water load. The inference is that the osmostat is 'reset' at a lower level. It has been described in association with *malnutrition, carcinomatosis* and *tuberculosis. Deficiency of intracellular potassium* with reduced intracellular solute has also been cited as responsible for the resetting.

c. Increased total body sodium

The consequence of a significant increase in total body sodium is clinically manifest oedema. This should be

sought for in any patient with hyponatraemia. Patients fall into a number of categories:

1. Renal failure

Excess water intake in a poorly controlled patient with *chronic renal disease*, with pre-existing sodium retention can lead to hyponatraemia. The patient with *acute renal failure* can become sodium and water overloaded. These patients do not normally pose a diagnostic problem.

2. Congestive cardiac failure

The failing heart leads to reduced renal perfusion and an 'apparent' volume deficit, registered by receptors in the left atrium and the great arteries of the chest and neck. The consequent secondary hyperaldosteronism and AVP secretion produce sodium overload, H_2O retention and hyponatraemia.

3. Hypoproteinaemic states

Low plasma protein leads to increased movement of water and low molecular weight solutes from the intravascular to the interstitial compartments. Hence interstitial oedema is accompanied by a reduced intravascular volume, with secondary aldosteronism and stimulation of AVP. Thus hyponatraemia may be found in any of the following hypoproteinaemic conditions: *cirrhosis, nephrotic syndrome* and *severe hypoproteinaemia of nutritional or GI origin.*

d. Other causes

1. Sick cell syndrome

This is a term applied to the circumstance in which cell membrane permeability to intracellular solutes increases, leading to a movement of solute and water from the intra- to the extracellular compartments, with resultant hyponatraemia. It has been described in patients with a *variety of generalized illnesses.*

2. Addition of solute to the extracellular compartment

Where a low molecular weight solute is present to excess in the extracellular compartment, and is largely confined to that compartment, a shift of water from the intra- to the extracellular compartments will occur. Examples occur in patients with *diabetes mellitus* (raised ECF glucose), or following *infusion of mannitol* for the treatment of cerebral oedema.

3. Pseudohyponatraemia

The presence of *increased amounts of protein or lipid,* encroaching on the water space in plasma, can lead to pseudohyponatraemia when plasma [Na⁺] is measured by certain techniques. In this condition the true sodium/water ratio is within normal limits, as reflected in a normal osmolality.

4. Artefactual

Collection of a venous blood sample proximal to the site of administration of intravenous fluid of low or absent sodium content (e.g. 5 per cent dextrose).

High plasma [sodium]

This is generally less common than hyponatraemia. Diagnosis can again be considered in terms of the accompanying change in total body sodium.

a. Decreased total body sodium

In this situation both sodium and water are lost from the body but water loss predominates, i.e. the overall composition of the fluid lost is hypotonic with respect to plasma.

1. Gastroenteritis

Especially in *infants* but also sometimes in adults.

2. Renal losses

in association with *osmotic diuretics.* These would include high osmotic loads of *urea* (e.g. high protein infant food formula or high protein enteral feeds in adults), *glucose* (e.g. in diabetes mellitus) or osmotic agents, such as *mannitol,* used therapeutically. *Note* that mannitol infusion or hyperglycaemia may be associated with hyponatraemia (see section (**d**) 'Other Causes', above).

3. Extreme sweating

4. Peritoneal dialysis

A hypertonic dialysate can lead to significant hypotonic fluid losses via the peritoneal surface.

b. Normal total body sodium

In effect the hypernatraemia in this condition is accounted for by pure water loss.

1. Excessive insensible water losses

This can occur in *hot dry climates* or with *high fever,* sometimes with *thyrotoxicosis,* especially when excessive water losses are not replaced. It is also recognized as a complication of *mechanical ventilation with poor humidification* leading to excessive insensible losses from the lungs.

2. Unconsciousness

Since the patient is unable to respond to the thirst sensation insensible losses are not replaced. The same situation can arise in *very young children* or the *elderly, confused patient.*

3. Diabetes insipidus

Hypothalamic deficiency of AVP or ineffective renal action of AVP leads to excessive urinary water losses, with the potential for developing hypernatraemia if these excessive losses are not replaced.

c. Increased total body sodium

This is relatively uncommon. It is accompanied by expansion of the ECF volume and cellular dehydration. Acutely, pulmonary oedema may develop.

1. Iatrogenic

This refers to excessive intravenous administration of hypertonic sodium-containing solutes, including *sodium bicarbonate solution during resuscitation, 3 per cent and 5 per cent sodium chloride.* It should be remembered that the Na⁺ concentration in *N saline* is higher than plasma.

2. Mineralocorticoid excess

This may be due to endogenous overproduction of aldosterone *(Conn's syndrome)* or in *Cushing's syndrome,* including that resulting from the *therapeutic administration of steroids.*

THYROID FUNCTION TESTS

In recent years there have been major changes in the biochemical tests used to investigate suspected thyroid dysfunction. Although in many respects these developments have facilitated diagnosis, in certain circumstances, particularly in the presence of non-thyroidal illness and in patients with abnormalities of protein binding, potentially misleading results may be obtained. Careful clinical assessment and a sound understanding of thyroid physiology remain essential in the evaluation of these patients.

Physiology

The predominant hormone secreted by the thyroid gland is thyroxine (T_4), which is thought to behave as a pro-hormone for the biologically more active molecule, tri-iodothyronine (T_3). The majority of circulating T_3 is formed from T_4 by de-iodination in peripheral organs such as liver, kidney and muscle. In addition, in some tissues (including brain and pituitary) an important component of nuclear T_3 is derived through local de-iodination of T_4, rather than by extraction of T_3 circulating in the plasma. An alternative fate for T_4 is conversion to the metabolically inert species reverse T_3 (rT_3), levels of which increase in some forms of non-thyroidal illness.

Circulating thyroid hormones are transported bound to plasma proteins. In quantitative terms thyroxine-binding globulin (TBG) is the most important, approximately three-quarters of T_4 and T_3 being bound to TBG. Smaller quantities of thyroid hormones are bound to thyroxine-binding prealbumin (TBPA) and albumin. Less than 1 per cent of total plasma T_3 and T_4 is unbound by protein and it is commonly assumed that only this minute free fraction is metabolically active (although this may be an oversimplification).

Synthesis and secretion of thyroid hormones are stimulated by thyroid-stimulating hormone (TSH) released from the anterior pituitary, which in turn is stimulated by a hypothalamic agent, TSH releasing hormone (TRH). Circulating thyroid hormones exert negative feedback actions on the hypothalamus and pituitary.

In the assessment of suspected thyroid dysfunction the analytes most frequently measured are TSH, total T_3 and T_4, and free T_3 and T_4.

TSH

Radioimmunoassays (RIA) for TSH have to a large extent been replaced by two-site immunometric assays (IMA), which are both more specific and more sensitive than the older techniques. In particular, IMA measurements permit a reliable discrimination to be made between normal and low levels of TSH, this distinction being impossible by routine RIA. IMA methods may employ radiolabels and are then termed immunoradiometric assays, IRMA, although there is increasing interest in the use of non-isotopic labels.

The increase in analytical sensitivity achieved with IMA measurements has been of greatest value in the investigation of *thyrotoxicosis*, in which TSH levels are suppressed, often to undetectable levels. It is important to appreciate, however, that low TSH concentrations occur in a variety of circumstances other than primary hyperthyroidism, including *old age, severe*

intercurrent illness and during treatment with certain drugs (e.g. glucocorticoids and dopamine). It follows that while an undetectable TSH level is consistent with thyrotoxicosis it is not pathognomonic of that diagnosis. Occasionally patients with primary hyperthyroidism are found to have apparently unsuppressed IMA TSH measurements. This situation can arise if the patient's plasma contains interfering anti-mouse antibodies, the monoclonal antisera used in most assays being murine. Methodological modifications have made this problem far less common than it used to be. However, if an unsuppressed IMA TSH result is obtained where there is a strong suspicion of primary hyperthyroidism, a TRH test should be considered. In this procedure TSH is measured before and 20 minutes after an intravenous injection of 200 µg TRH. An increase in TSH concentration in excess of 2 mU/l excludes the diagnosis. The TRH test is also useful in the investigation of thyrotoxicosis if TSH can only be measured by RIA, rather than by IMA, a subnormal response having the same significance as a suppressed IMA TSH result.

In *primary hypothyroidism* TSH levels are characteristically increased, both IMA and RIA measurements being capable of detecting this. However, increases in TSH can occur in a variety of other conditions, including *recovery from severe illness* and *adrenocortical insufficiency*. Occasionally, elevated TSH levels are found in clinically euthyroid individuals with normal T_4 concentrations. Many of these patients have incipient thyroid failure and on follow-up are found to develop frank hypothyroidism.

Although measurement of basal TSH by IMA is probably the most effective single first-line test in the investigation of suspected hyper- and hypothyroidism, it is clear that in neither context is the test infallible. In addition to the problems already discussed, secondary thyroid dysfunction requires special care. In thyroid failure due to *pituitary disease* TSH levels are not raised while in rare cases of hyperthyroidism due to excessive TSH secretion, TSH levels are usually elevated (but occasionally normal).

Total T₄ and Total T₃

Total plasma concentrations of these hormones are commonly determined by RIA, although non-isotopic methods are gaining in popularity.

Elevations in total thyroid hormone levels are found in *hyperthyroidism*. In most cases of thyrotoxicosis total T_3 levels are more obviously raised than those of total T_4 and occasionally total T_3 levels are elevated despite a normal total T_4 concentration ('T_3-toxicosis'). However, levels of total T_3 and/or T_4 may be elevated in several conditions other than thyrotoxicosis. Measurement of TSH by IMA may help in these cases. Increased concentrations of TBG arising either as a result of inheritance or as an acquired trait (e.g. through oestrogen administration or pregnancy) are associated with raised total T_4 and T_3 levels in the *euthyroid state*. Variants of albumin and TBPA with abnormally high affinity for T_4 have been described. Euthyroid patients with these proteins have raised total T_4 levels, although the concentration of total T_3 is usually (but not invariably) normal. Similarly in patients with *autoantibodies to T_4* (which may develop in Hashimoto's disease) a combination of elevated total T_4 and normal total T_3 levels may occur. Hyperthyroxinaemia in the absence of an elevated total T_3 can also arise as a result of impaired deiodination of T_4 to T_3. This is occasionally encountered as a *familial condition* but is more often due to certain forms of non-thyroidal illness or *drug administration* (e.g. amiodarone, propranolol). Resistance to thyroid hormones at the receptor level is an exceptionally rare cause of elevations in both total T_3 and total T_4.

Decreased total T_4 level are characteristic of *hypothyroidism*. In general measurement of total T_4 in this situation is unhelpful, the results often being normal. However, there are several causes of euthyroid hypothyroxinaemia including *congenital TBG* deficiency, *non-thyroidal illness* (both with and without general hypoproteinaemia) and *drug administration* (e.g. phenytoin, salicylate).

Free T_4 and free T_3 levels

The gold-standard technique for the assay of free thyroid hormones is equilibrium dialysis but this is unsuitable for routine use.

An early approach to the question of free hormone levels which is still favoured by some is the calculation of a so-called free T_4 (or T_3) index. This method involves measuring both the the total T_4 (or T_3) level and estimating the plasma protein binding capacity for thyroid hormones by means of an *in vitro* uptake test. Free T_4 indices have proved useful in patients with relatively small abnormalities in TBG (e.g. in pregnancy) but are less reliable in patients with other types of atypical protein binding and in the presence of non-thyroidal illness. A variation on the free T_4 index is to measure TBG directly by RIA and then to determine a total T_4:TBG ratio. Results calculated in this way may be more effective than a free T_4 index in allowing for marked variations in TBG level but in other circumstances offer no advantage.

In recent years analogue radio-immunoassays have been widely employed for the estimation of free T_4 (FT_4) and free T_3 (FT_3) levels. These assays use analogues of T_4 and T_3 which are in principle not bound by plasma proteins but are recognized by antithyroid hormone antisera. In reality, however, some binding by plasma proteins does occur, especially to thyroid hormone binding proteins other than TBG. Because of this there has been a controversy in the literature on the value of these tests, one school of thought suggesting that they have no validity at all. Other authors consider that analogue methods are useful in investigating patients with anomalous total T_4 and /or T_3 levels thought to be due to either high or low levels of TBG. However, potentially misleading results can be obtained in various situations. In general, analogue FT_4 and FT_3 measurements correlate (artefactually) with the plasma albumin concentration. In cases of albumin and TBPA variants with an abnormal affinity for T_4, analogue FT_4 levels are falsely raised, although analogue FT_3 concentrations are often normal or only slightly raised. Likewise, in patients with anti-T_4 autoantibodies analogue FT_4 measurements are commonly spuriously elevated. Drugs affecting the protein binding of thyroid hormones (e.g. salicylates and phenytoin) interfere with analogue methods and are often associated with false depressions in apparent FT_3 and FT_4 concentrations. Perhaps the commonest problem with analogue techniques occurs in non-thyroidal illness when, for diverse reasons (including alterations in plasma proteins and the presence of metabolites affecting protein binding) analogue FT_4 and FT_3 levels often appear abnormal (usually low but sometimes high) under conditions when assays performed by equilibrium dialysis are normal.

It is apparent, therefore, that while analogue assays may be superior to total thyroid hormone measurements in patients with simple TBG abnormalities, in many other situations, including other protein binding abnormalities and non-thyroidal illness, the results must be interpreted with extreme caution. IMA measurement of TSH is often helpful in these difficult cases, although a powerful case can be made for completely avoiding thyroid function tests in patients with any severe intercurrent illness unless there is a very strong clinical suspicion of thyroid disease.

Recently several non-analogue immunoassays have been developed for the assay of free thyroid hormone concentrations. Because they show better agreement with equilibrium dialysis, these methods may become more widely available in the future.

Thyroid function tests in pregnancy

During the first trimester in a minority of euthyroid women IMA TSH levels are undetectable, this phenomenon being thought to be related to the high concentrations of human chorionic gonadotrophin found at this time. Total T_3 and T_4 levels increase during pregnancy because of increased concentrations of TBG. However, although analogue methods compensate for this effect, FT_4 and FT_3 assayed by this technique fall during pregnancy in association with declining plasma albumin levels. For this reason trimester related reference ranges should be employed when analogue results are interpreted.

Thyroid function at the extremes of life

Abnormalities in total and analogue free thyroid hormone assays are common in the elderly in the absence of thyroid disease. This is due, at least in part, to the high incidence of non-thyroidal illness and use of medication in these patients. In addition, IMA TSH levels are commonly reduced in euthyroid geriatric individuals.

In the neonatal period complex and marked changes in the hypothalamopituitary-thyroid axis occur. These variations will not be discussed in detail but they must be taken into account in assessing the results of thyroid screens performed on babies.

Biochemical tests in monitoring the treatment of thyroid disease

This is a controversial area. Some authorities (albeit a minority) consider all chemical tests redundant in this context, while others, who feel that laboratory monitoring does have a role to play, disagree about the choice of analyte.

In monitoring the control of thyrotoxicosis (and overtreated hypothyroidism) it is important to appreciate that the pituitary may remain suppressed for many months after adequate treatment has been instituted. TSH levels are therefore an unreliable index of thyroid status in this situation and an assay of circulating thyroid hormone concentration should be used.

In controlling replacement therapy in hypothyroidism it is probably appropriate to give sufficient thyroxine to restore TSH levels to normal, at which dose FT_4 concentrations are typically high–normal or slightly raised. A complicating factor here is the fact that TSH secretion is determined by both T_3 and T_4 as a result of intrapituitary conversion of T_4 to T_3, whereas many other tissues, being unable to deiodinate T_4, are solely dependent on the uptake of circulating T_3. Because of this it is sometimes argued that the dose of thyroxine should be adjusted to maintain a normal FT_3 level. However, in practice FT_3 concentrations may be normal even when FT_4 is markedly raised, TSH secretion is suppressed and there is evidence of end-organ toxicity as assessed by heart rate, myocardial contractility and urinary sodium excretion. On average it takes about 6 weeks for the thyrotroph response to the

introduction of thyroxine replacement or an increase in dose to stabilize and this should govern the frequency of testing.

Tests related to the aetiology of thyroid disease

Serial measurements of thyroglobulin are useful in the follow-up of known cases of thyroid carcinoma (other than medullarly cell carcinoma). It should be noted, however, that many benign thyroid disorders are associated with raised thyroglobulin levels so that this investigation should not be regarded as a diagnostic test. Neonates with thyroid hypoplasia have low levels of thyroglobulin.

Antithyroid antibodies occur in patients with Hashimoto's thyroiditis. However, similar autoantibodies are found in other auto-immune disorders and in a small proportion of apparently normal people.

TSH-receptor antibodies may be assayed in patients with suspected Graves' disease.

TOTAL PROTEIN

Total plasma protein estimation measures a complex mixture of proteins (more than 300 are known to be present in plasma), of which albumin contributes the greatest amount (in mass terms) to the measured value. Hence, changes in albumin (discussed below) will often produce concomitant changes in the total protein measurement. However, this need not always be the case. For example, a decrease in albumin and an increase in immunoglobulin concentration may lead to hypoalbuminaemia but with a normal total protein value; such may be the situation in chronic liver disease.

In interpreting plasma [total protein], it is important to remember the effects of posture. Thus, redistribution of H_2O within the ECF compartment means that the [total protein] value may be 10 per cent or more higher in the standing as opposed to the recumbent posture. These differences are exaggerated in oedematous patients.

Raised plasma [total protein]

a. Decreased plasma H²O

Loss of plasma H_2O affects the concentration of individual plasma protein species to the same extent, leading to an increase in the measured [total protein] value.

1. Dehydration

2. Prolonged venous stasis

during *blood sampling*. The increase in plasma [total protein] will be accompanied by an increase in albumin and a raised haematocrit.

b. Increases in immunoglobulins

1. Acute and chronic infections

2. Autoimmune diseases

e.g. *rheumatoid arthritis* and *systemic lupus erythematosus*.

3. Chronic liver disease

which may include some diseases with an autoimmune basis (e.g. *primary biliary cirrhosis*).

4. Paraproteinaemia

whether malignant (e.g. *in multiple myeloma, Waldenström's macroglobulinaemia, heavy chain disease*) or *benign*.

c. Increases in other plasma proteins

Since proteins, other than albumin, and to a lesser extent the immunoglobulins, are present at relatively low concentrations, alterations in absolute concentration usually have little effect on the total protein measurement. Increases in the *acute phase proteins* may contribute in a small way to the increase [total protein] observed in infections or malignancy, but the immunoglobulin increase makes a greater contribution (see also (**b**) above).

Decreased plasma [total protein]

a. Increased plasma H²O

1. Overhydration

during *intravenous therapy*.

2. Pregnancy

where plasma volume shows a physiological increase.

b. Any cause of hypoalbuminaemia

The many reasons for a low plasma [albumin] are discussed under this heading.

c. Low immunoglobulin levels

UREA

Urea is synthesized from ammonia which, in turn, is derived from deamination of amino acids. Its formation requires enzymes of the urea cycle which are restricted to the liver. More than 75 per cent of non-protein nitrogen is excreted as urea, largely by the kidneys, but with small losses through the skin or the GI tract.

Laboratory measurement of urea is widespread, reflecting the speed, accuracy and precision of the assay. As a test of renal function, it is inferior to creatinine in a number of ways. Thus 50 per cent or more of filtered urea is passively reabsorbed, and this fraction increases if urine flow rate decreases (e.g. following shock due to blood loss or other causes.). This so-called prerenal uraemia may not be necessarily associated with intrinsic renal disease. Also, urea production will increase on high protein diets or increased protein catabolism (e.g. after major surgery). These factors must always be considered when interpreting plasma [urea].

Reduced plasma [urea]

1. Low protein diet

Less urea is synthesized in the liver following reduced availability of amino acids for deamination. In extreme starvation, urea may rise as a result of increased muscle protein breakdown providing the major source of fuel.

2. Dilution of urea in plasma

Water retention in the presence of *inappropriate AVP secretion* or *dilution with intravenous fluids,* for example, can lower plasma [urea]. An *artefactual* decrease in plasma [urea] may be observed if blood sampling takes place near the infusion site.

3. Liver disease

In more advanced, usually chronic, liver disease, the ability to synthesize urea is impaired and plasma levels will fall.

Increased plasma [urea]

a. Prerenal uraemia

1. Increased production (in the liver)

This occurs on *high protein diets,* or following *increased protein catabolism (e.g. trauma, major surgery,*

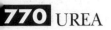

extreme starvation). Levels may rise after upper GI haemorrhage following the 'protein meal' of blood.

2. Impaired renal perfusion

Any situation where renal blood flow falls, leads to reduced urine flow and increased passive tubular reabsorption of urea. Thus, any state of *shock* due to *burns, blood loss or loss of water/electrolytes (e.g. severe diarrhoea),* for example, may be accompanied by an increased plasma [urea]. This is also true in *congestive heart failure* or states of reduced *intravascular* volume (with interstitial oedema) accompanying *hypoproteinaemia* (see below), especially if treated with potent diuretics.

3. Urea infusion

Urea can be used, like mannitol, as a diuretic in the treatment of cerebral oedema.

Since creatinine, unlike urea, is largely excreted without significant tubular reabsorption, it is relatively less affected in (2) above. Hence, plasma [urea] increases relatively more than plasma [creatinine] in prerenal uraemia due to (2), than in renal uraemia (see below), where the two estimations tend to parallel one another.

b. Renal uraemia

Clearly, in *acute or chronic renal failure,* where a reduction in glomerular filtration rate (GFR) occurs, plasma [urea] increases either until a new steady state is reached (at which urea production equals loss in the urine) or continues to rise in the face of near total renal shutdown or end-stage disease. Urea is traditionally measured as a test of renal function. Whilst it may be increased because of renal disease, this need not be the case, for reasons discussed in (a) and (c).

A better test of renal function is plasma [creatinine].

c. Postrenal uraemia

Urine outflow obstruction may occur at different levels (e.g. ureter, bladder, urethra) due for example, to *renal stones, prostatism, schistosomiasis* or *genitourinary cancer.* The obstruction to urine flow leads to a rise in urea (and creatinine). Back pressure on the tubular system enhances back diffusion of urea so that urea rises disproportionately more than creatinine, as with prerenal uraemia.

Of course, both postrenal uraemia and prerenal uraemia due to impaired renal perfusion may themselves lead to intrinsic renal disease (i.e. renal uraemia) and distinction may only be possible by measurement of other parameters such as plasma [creatinine], urine volume and composition, etc.

URIC ACID

The purine bases adenine and guanine are major constituents of the nucleic acids (both DNA and RNA) and contribute to the nucleoside and nucleotide pools of the cell. Uric acid is a major end-product of the breakdown of these compounds, whilst a smaller daily production derives from the breakdown of dietary nucleic acid. The enzymes xanthine oxidase and guanase act on the free bases hypoxanthine (ultimately derived from deamination of the adenine ring in AMP) and guanine, respectively, to produce uric acid. This production of uric acid is moderated by the ability of the cell to reutilize the free bases using a 'purine salvage pathway'.

About 75 per cent of uric acid is excreted in the urine, the remainder being lost chiefly via the GI tract; non-renal routes of excretion may increase if renal excretion is impaired for any reason. Renal handling is complex but the proximal tubule reabsorbs most of the filtered uric acid. Secretion then takes place in the distal tubule with a further postsecretory reabsorption.

Plasma [urate], even in the absence of disease, varies according to a number of social and demographic factors. Thus levels tend to be higher in men than women (though the difference is less after the menopause), higher in obese individuals, those on high protein diets and with high alcohol intake.

Raised plasma [urate]

A large number of conditions can lead to a raised plasma [urate]. In the simplest sense a high value occurs because of increased production or diminished excretion. Clinically, however, a raised [urate] per se becomes important if it is associated with the development of gout. Gout is more likely in primary hyperuricaemia, as opposed to secondary hyperuricaemia where it is relatively rare.

a. Primary hyperuricaemia

This is characterized by a primary defect in the urate biochemistry, either overproduction, underexcretion or a combination of both.

1. Idiopathic

The tendency to raised plasma [urate] and the occurrence of gouty symptoms is characterized by a number of findings:

a. As a population patients with idiopathic gout show

a decreased fractional excretion of urate. Renal function is otherwise apparently normal (c.f. secondary hyperuricaemia due to renal disease), unless impaired by urate deposition in the kidney. About 75 per cent of patients with idiopatric hyperuricaemia show decreased fractional excretion of urate.

b. In up to 25 per cent of patients urate overproduction is believed to occur.

c. Partial deficiency of 'purine salvage' enzymes may be important in a minority of patients.

2. Overproduction due to inherited enzyme defects

The *Lesch–Nyhan syndrome* is a rare X-linked disorder characterized biochemically by elevated plasma [urate] and clinical gout. It is due to deficiency of the purine salvage enzyme hypoxanthine guanine phosphoribosyl transferase with consequent overproduction of uric acid.

Overproduction is also described where purine biosynthesis is increased as a result of *overproduction of the precursor ribose-5-phosphate or overactivity of 5-phosphoribosyl-1-pyrophosphate synthetase.*

b. Secondary hyperuricaemia

In this group of conditions, urate biochemistry is assumed to be normal in the absence of the particular drug or disease causing the derangement in urate production or excretion (cf. (a)). It is convenient to divide the secondary causes into those due to increased urate formation and those resulting from impaired renal excretion. Overproduction is the consequence of increased nucleic acid breakdown due to cell destruction alone or increased cell turnover. Impaired renal excretion arises either because of specific renal disease or the presence of drugs or endogenous metabolites which impair urate excretion.

Increased formation

1. Myeloproliferative syndromes
with increased cell turnover.

2. Chemotherapy
of *malignant tumours*, especially *leukaemias* and *lymphomas*.

3. Psoriasis
with increased turnover of skin epidermal cells.

4. Starvation
and hypercatabolic states with increased cell destruction; production of lactate may also be a factor (next section).

5. Carcinomatosis.

6. Chronic haemolytic anaemias.

7. Ethanol ingestion.
(also see next section).

Decreased renal excretion

1. Renal failure (acute and chronic)
will lead to retention of urate. In the case of chronic renal failure plasma [urate] rises relatively late and is not generally associated with symptoms of clinical gout.

2. Drugs.
A variety of drugs compete with and interfere with distal tubular secretion of urate, including *diuretics* (especially *thiazide diuretics*), *ethambutol, pyrazinamide, ethanol and salicylates (low dosage)*. Salicylates at a high dosage are uricosuric since a competitive interference with proximal reabsorption predominates leading to net increased urate excretion.

3. Organic acids.
Endogenously produced acids such as *lactate, acetoacetate and B-hydroxybutyrate* also compete with urate for the distal tubular secretory mechanism and can lead to increased plasma urate.

4. Tubular poisons
including *lead* and possibly ethanol.

5. Hypothyroidism and hyperparathyroidism.

Decreased plasma [urate]

This is much less common than increased plasma [urate] and though not in itself serious may be a concomitant of serious illness. It may arise from impaired urate production or as a result of increased renal excretion.

Decreased production

1. Severe hepatocellular disease

The size and metabolic activity of the normal liver makes a significant contribution to the daily urate production; this is reflected in the low plasma urate which may be a feature of advanced liver disease.

2. Xanthine oxidase deficiency

This enzyme converts xanthine (on the purine degradative pathway) to uric acid. Hence deficiency leads to increased xanthine excretion, with the possibility of xanthine stone formation, and decreased urate production. In the absence of stone formation the condition may be asymptomatic.

Increased renal losses

1. Acquired or congenital defects in urate reabsorption

Impaired urate reabsorption may be a feature of the generalized proximal tubular defect in *Fanconi's syndrome,* from whatever cause.

2. Drugs

including *high-dose aspirin* and the uricosuric drug, *probenicid.*

TESTS ON URINE

Proteinuria

'Test-tube' tests for proteinuria (e.g. salicylsulphonic acid) and urinary globulins (e.g. Bradshaw's test) are now rarely used, and side-room or outpatients screening for proteinuria is generally performed with indicator strips (e.g. Boehringer BM strips or Ames Albustix). These dipstick tests are based on the 'protein-error-of indicators'. The strips are impregnated with a buffered indicator dye, such as tetrabromophenol blue. Protein present in the sample binds to the dye, inducing a change in its pK_a. In consequence, the protonation of the dye molecules alters, producing a change in colour. These reagents are best regarded as tests for albumin. Sensitivity for some other types of protein, including Bence Jones protein, is lower and can lead to false negative results. False-negative tests can also arise if the sample pH is too low, as may be the case if the urine is (incorrectly) collected into acid. Alkaline urines and samples contaminated with certain disinfectants (e.g. chlorhexidine) may give false positive results. Correct storage of reagent strips, with protection against ambient moisture, light and heat, is essential if reliable results are to be obtained. Fresh urine is preferred, early morning specimens being especially useful since they are more concentrated and free from orthostatic (postural) influences.

There are four mechanisms by which proteinuria can occur: (1) increased glomerular permeability (glomerular proteinuria); (2) defective tubular reabsorption (tubular proteinuria); (3) overflow proteinuria resulting from the presence in the plasma of abnormal quantities of low molecular weight proteins; (4) abnormal protein arising from the post-renal urinary tract.

1. Glomerular proteinuria

In all forms of glomerular proteinuria albumin accounts for a high proportion of the increase in urinary protein. Glomerular proteinuria can be classified both in terms of quantity and selectivity.

In microalbuminuria the urinary albumin excretion is increased but remains below the detection limit of dipstick tests (i.e. about 250 mg/l). The gold standard in this context is the determination of urinary albumin excretion in serial overnight collections, a rate in excess of 20 μg per minute being abnormal. Simpler screening tests include the measurement of urinary albumin concentration (abnormal greater than 25 mg/l) and the urinary albumin/creatinine concentration ratio (abnormal greater than 3·5 mg/mmol). (*See* Table APP.10.) Microalbuminuria occurs in several glomerular pathologies but is of particular interest in *diabetes mellitus*, in which it has prognostic significance for the development of long-term complications (renal and non-renal).

Gross glomerular proteinuria (i.e. several grams per day), associated with oedema and hypoalbuminaemia, constitutes the *nephrotic syndrome*. Many nephrotic patients are hyperlipidaemic and there is often a relative increase in the α_2-globulin peak on serum electrophoresis.

A selective glomerular proteinuria is one in which the protein loss predominantly consists of low molecular weight proteins (e.g. albumin and transferin), while in *non-selective proteinuria* the urine contains, in addition, higher molecular weight proteins (e.g. immunoglobulins and α-$_2$-macroglobulin). Estimation of the differential urinary clearance rate (selectivity index) between high and low molecular weight proteins may be of value in children presenting with the nephrotic syndrome: minimal change glomerulonephritis, which often responds to steroids, tends to produce a selective proteinuria.

Causes of glomerular proteinuria include:

> Glomerulonephritis (most forms)
> Diabetes mellitus
> Systemic lupus erythematosis
> Amyloidosis
> Renal vein thrombosis
> Drugs (e.g. penicillamine and gold)
> Malaria
> Malignancy (including lymphoma)
> Pre-eclampsia
> Subacute bacterial endocarditis

Table APP.10 Reference values for the more common analytes in urine

Analysis	Reference range	Units
Albumin	†	
Calcium	1.2–3.7 (low calcium diet)	mmol/24 h
	Up to 12 (normal diet)	
Copper	Up to 0.6	μmol/24 h
Cortisol	9–50	μmol/mol creatinine
Creatinine	10–20	mmol/24 h
5-Hydroxyindole-3-acetic acid (5-HIAA)	10–45	μmol/24 h
Metanephrines (conjugated)	Up to 3	μmol/24 h
Oxalate		
Male	80–490	μmol/24 h
Female	40–320	μmol/24 h
Phosphate	15–50	mmol/24 h
Porphyrins (total)	90–370	nmol/24 h
Coproporphyrins	150–230	
Uroporphyrins	Up to 40	
*Potassium	25–100	mmol/24 h
Protein	Up to 0.3	g/l
*Sodium	100–200	mmol/24 h
Urate	1.2–3.0	mmol/24 h
Urea	170–600	mmol/24 h

† Albumin : creatinine ratio (ACR) and urinary albumin excretion rate (AER) are used to detect microalbuminuria, ie. excessive albumin excretion in patients with diabetes mellitus (type I) which is of predictive value in identifying patients at risk of progression to diabetic nephropathy. The test should only be carried out in the absence of overt proteinuria (dipstix negative).

ACR
Reference range:	<3.5 mg albumin/mmol creatinine
'Borderline':	3.5–10 mg albumin/mmol creatinine
Positive test:	>10 mg albumin/mmol creatinine

AER
Reference range:	<20 μg albumin/min
Microalbuminuria:	20–200 μg albumin/min

* The urinary output of electrolytes such as sodium and potassium is normally a reflection of intake. This can vary widely, especially on a cultural, worldwide basis. The values quoted are more appropriate to a western diet.

Mild, transient glomerular proteinuria may also occur as a result of many severe illnesses, including *congestive cardiac failure* and *pyrexial conditions*. *Orthostatic proteinuria* (i.e. proteinuria occurring only in the upright position) and exercise-induced proteinuria are often benign.

2. Tubular proteinuria

The proteinuria arising from tubular damage is usually mild and involves low molecular weight proteins which, in health, are reabsorbed and degraded in the proximal convoluted tubule. These substances include β_1-microglobulin. On electrophoresis the urine may show prominent α and β bands. Measurement of urinary β_1-microglobulin may be unreliable as a marker of tubular damage because this protein is unstable in acid media. Tubular proteinuria is often associated with the presence of urinary casts and evidence of other types of tubular malfunction (e.g. renal glycosuria and tubular acidosis). Acute tubular proteinuria is some-

times reversible. Causes of tubular proteinuria include:

Circulatory failure (shock)

Drugs (lithium, phenacetin, non-steroidal anti-inflammatory agents, some antibiotics)

Diabetes mellitus

Chronic pyelonephritis

Heavy metal poisoning (lead, cadmium)

Balkan nephropathy

Sickle cell disease

Sarcoidosis

Irradiation

Hyperuricaemia

Hyperoxaluria

Myeloma (also causes overflow proteinuria)

Various inborn errors of metabolism (cystinosis, Wilson's disease, hepatorenal tyrosinaemia, classical galactosaemia, hereditary fructose intolerance, glycogen storage disease type I).

3. Overflow proteinuria

Bence Jones proteinuria is due to the overflow of monoclonal immunoglobulin light chains into the urine. If this condition is suspected it should be investigated by laboratory analysis (including urinary electrophoresis). Twenty per cent of patients with *myeloma* produce Bence-Jones protein without showing a serum paraprotein band.

Haemoglobinuria (caused by intravascular haemolysis) and Myoglobinuria (due to rhabdomyolysis) both produce positive responses in dipstick tests for blood (e.g. Ames Hemastix or Multistix, or Boehringer BM strips), which are based on the peroxidase-like activity of these haemoproteins. Laboratory methods should be used for further identification. False positive reactions may occur in urine infected with peroxidase producing organisms and in the presence of certain disinfectants. False negatives may occur in urines containing reducing substances, such as ascorbic acid.

4. Postrenal proteinuria

This may be associated with haematuria and/or pyuria. Causes include *calculus, urinary tract infection and malignancy.* The urine does not contain casts.

Bile pigments

Bilirubin

Dipstick tests for bilirubin (e.g. Ames Multistix and Bili-Labstix, or Boehringer BM strips) are based on a coupling reaction with a diazo reagent. They are very sensitive, being capable of detecting about 5–10 μmol/l bilirubin, and are adequate for most clinical purposes. Normal urine contains no bilirubin detectable by such methods and positive results should be investigated further. In the absence of renal damage, free (unconjugated) bilirubin is not excreted by the kidney but the renal threshold for conjugated bilirubin is low. Urinary bilirubin is increased in *obstructive* and *hepatocellular jaundice,* and in the *Dubin-Johnson* and *Rotor syndromes.* Haemolytic jaundice and the jaundice of Gilbert's and Crigler-Najjar syndromes are acholuric.

Occasionally dipstick tests for bilirubin may yield atypical colours due to the presence of bile pigments other than bilirubin. False positive results may be produced by drugs and their metabolities (e.g. chlorpromazine). In these circumstances a further test with ictotest (Ames), which is more specific, may be helpful.

Bilirubin is labile and urine samples should be tested when fresh.

Urobilinogen

Urobilinogen arises as a result of the action of enteric bacteria on bilirubin so that the presence of bilirubin in the intestine can be inferred from the detection of urobilinogen in the urine. Urobilinogen itself is colourless but may undergo conversion to urobilin (which is brown) both *in vivo* and after the collection of urine, which is best examined fresh.

Most screening tests of urobilinogen (e.g. Ames multistix and urobilistix, and Boehringer BM strips) are based on the Ehrlich reaction with *p*-dimethylaminobenzaldehyde in acid. In normal urine, urobilinogen may be present in trace amounts or be undetectable by dipstick tests, which cannot discriminate between low, normal levels and pathological absence of urobilinogen. Various drugs and their metabilites can produce false positives or mask colours. Porphobilinogen may give a positive reaction but urobilinogen strip tests are not a reliable means for the detection of this substance.

Tests for urinary urobilinogen are negative in biliary obstruction, and similar results are commonly obtained in the congenital hyperbilirubinaemias, such as *Gilbert's syndrome.* In *haemolytic disease* urinary urobilinogen is increased. The pattern seen in *hepatitis* is variable: urinary urobilinogen may be increased in the early stages, subsequently becoming undetectable for a period before reappearing during the recovery phase.

Concentration

Measurement

Methods used to assess urinary concentration include: (1) Urinary osmolality; (2) Urinary specific gravity; (3) The urine : plasma urea concentration ratio.

The most satisfactory technique is measurement of urinary osmolality. In normal urines osmolality is linearly related to specific gravity, which can be measured as a side-room test with a urinometer. However, a variety of abnormal urinary components increase specific gravity out of proportion to the effect they exert on osmolality. These substances include glucose, radiological contrast media, artificial colloids and protein. In addition, urinometer measurements are temperature dependent and subject to parallax errors.

Some reagent strips (dipsticks) contain test pads said to measure specific gravity. In fact, these strips respond to ionic strength rather than specific gravity. They depend on the induction of a pK_a change in polyelectrolytes within the strip by the urinary ionic composition, producing a colour change in the indicator.

The urine : plasma urea concentration ratio is discussed under urinary urea.

Interpretation

Urinary osmolality varies between 50 and 1400 mosmol/kg according to the pathophysiological circumstances. It is important to interpret urinary osmolality measurements in conjunction with information concerning the patient's clinical state, urinary flow rate and plasma composition. In some cases it may be helpful to measure plasma osmolality directly but in many situations a satisfactory interpretation can be made from a knowledge of the plasma concentrations of sodium, urea and glucose.

Measurements of urine concentration are of value in the following circumstances: (1) in the differential diagnosis of polyuria; (2) in oliguric patients with suspected acute renal failure; (3) in the investigation of patients thought to have the syndrome of inappropriate antidiuretic hormone secretion (SIADH).

1. In a polyuric patient the finding of a relatively concentrated urine suggests an osmotic diuresis (e.g. due to glucose). In polyuric patients with *chronic renal failure* there is often an inability either to concentrate or to dilute the urine appropriately and in this situation the urinary osmolality is within about 50 mosmol/kg of the plasma value. In *primary polydipsia* and *diabetes insipidus* (both cranial and nephrogenic) the patient produces a high volume urine of low osmolality (often less than 100 mosmol/kg). A water deprivation test may be required to distinguish between these two possibilities. Classically, patients with primary polydipsia have a plasma osmolality that is initially low but rises in response to fluid deprivation, while their urinary osmolality rises to over 800 mosmol/kg. However, in chronic primary polydipsia, dissipation of renal medullary hyperosmolality may necessitate a period of fluid restriction in excess of 24 hours before urinary concentrating capacity is recovered. In diabetes insipidus the urine fails to concentrate despite dehydration (as indicated by weight loss and changes in plasma composition). The administration of desmopression induces urinary concentration in cranial diabetes insipidus. Direct assay of plasma antidiuretic hormone levels is rarely required but may be helpful when osmometry is ambiguous (e.g. in partial forms of diabetes insipidus).

2. In an *oliguric, uraemic patient* the finding of a urine approximately isosmotic with plasma (usually accompanied by a urinary sodium concentration in excess of 20 mmol/l) is indicative of renal tubular damage, whereas the production of a relatively concentrated urine (usually over 600 mosmol/kg and often in excess of 800 mosmol/kg) suggests a prerenal problem likely to resopond to intravenous fluid replacement. Urine from such patients typically contains very little sodium (10 mmol/l or less). An antidiuresis, comprising a low volume urine of high osmolality, is a normal response in the immediate aftermath of trauma and surgery.

3. In the syndrome of inappropriate antidiuretic hormone secretion (SIADH) the urine is not maximally diluted despite a dilutional (hypo-osmolar) hyponatraemia. It is not an absolute requirement that the urine osmolality should exceed that of the plasma for this diagnosis to be made; in many patients with SIADH the urine osmolality is less than that of plasma but nonetheless inappropriately high. However, it is important to exclude renal, adrenal and pituitary pathology before SIADH is diagnosed.

pH

In healthy subjects on a meat-containing diet the urine has an acidic reaction as a result of the excretion of acidic metabolites derived from dietary protein. An alkaline urine may be found in *vegans*, in patients with *urinary tract infections* and in patients *ingesting alkali*. Failure to reduce urinary pH to an appropriate degree (less than about 5·3) in the presence of a metabolic acidosis occurs in *renal tubular acidosis*. An ammonium chloride loading test may be helpful if this condition is suspected. In the treatment of salicylate poisoning by forced *alkaline diuresis,* alkalinization of the urine is more important than the urine flow rate in promoting the elimination of the drug. Paradoxical urinary acidity may occur in the metabolic alkalosis due to *gastric outlet obstruction*. This is due, at least in part, to the increased reabsorption of bicarbonate as a counter-ion to sodium by the kidney, in the face of a relative deficit of chloride.

Urinary pH can be determined approximately by means of reagent test strips (Ames and Boehringer). These double indicator methods permit the determination of pH within 1 unit in the range 5–9. However, laboratory methods are more reliable. Urinary pH may change rapidly after collection and measurements are best made on fresh specimens.

Sodium

In a healthy individual with normal body reserves of sodium, the daily output of sodium is equal to the intake, urinary excretion varying between 5 and over 200 mmol/24 h according to diet. Because of this enormous variability sodium determinations on random samples of urine are rarely of value but may be interpretable in certain special circumstances. Sodium excretion determined on a 24-hour urine collection may be easier to interpret but in evaluating the data it is essential to take into account the plasma sodium concentration and the patient's extracellular fluid volume status assessed by independent means. This is true both when the urinary sodium is being used to help diagnose the cause of a disturbance in body salt and water handling, and when it is being used in planning replacement therapy.

In the hyponatraemic patient with evidence of extracellular fluid volume depletion, continuing natriuresis (urinary sodium greater than 20 mmol/l) suggests one of the following: (1) A defect in the hypothalamopituitary-adrenal axis (including Addison's disease); (2) A salt-losing nephritis; (3) Diuretics.

Natriuresis also occurs in the hyponatraemic states resulting from *acute water intoxication* and the *syndrome of inappropriate antidiuretic hormone secretion (SIADH)*. In these conditions both the extracellular and intracellular fluid compartments are expanded but generally there is no interstitial oedema. In a patient with an uncertain extracellular fluid volume status with a natriuresis it is important to exclude *renal* and *adrenal disease* before instituting treatment for water overload.

A low urinary sodium concentration (less than 10 mmol/l) may occur as an appropriate response in patients with normally functioning kidneys and adrenal glands who are *extracellular fluid volume* depleted as a result of losses via other routes (e.g. skin or gastroinstestinal tract). Such individuals are usually oliguric. A similar pattern is seen immediately after *surgery* or *trauma*. Inappropriate retention of sodium by the kidney occurs in *Cushing's* and *Conn's syndromes*, and in *secondary hyperaldosteronism* (in the absence of diuretics) associated with congestive cardiac failure, liver disease, nephrotic syndrome, etc.

Urea

In health, most urinary nitrogen is excreted in the form of urea and quantitation of urinary urea excretion is helpful in the evaluation of nitrogen balance. Urea excretion in the urine is related both to the protein content of the diet and to the rate of endogenous protein catabolism. Renal clearance of urea is positively correlated with urinary flow rate. The normal 24-hour excretion of urea varies between about 150 and 600 mmol/day. One mmol of urea contains 0·028 g of nitrogen. Urinary nitrogen excretion can then be estimated as follows, assuming that urea accounts for about $\frac{5}{6}$ths of the total:

ammonium ions account for a relatively higher proportion of urinary nitrogen.

Urinary urea excretion is increased in:

> Protein rich diets
> Catabolic states following trauma or surgery
> Hyperthyroidism
> Glucocorticoid excess
> Severe sepsis
> The recovery phase of acute renal failure (under conditions when the plasma urea is falling)

Decreased urinary urea excretion occurs in:

> Normal childhood growth
> Pregnancy
> Severe liver disease (failure of urea synthesis)
> Convalescence from trauma, surgery or other severe illness
> Renal failure (under conditions when the plasma urea is rising)
> Dietary protein restriction
> Contamination of urine with urea-splitting organisms
> Use of anabolic steroids

The urine : plasma urea concentration ratio is related to urinary concentration and flow rate. In oliguric uraemia due to prerenal factors the ratio usually exceeds 10 : 1, whereas in acute tubular necrosis ratios of less than 3 : 1 are common.

Tests for glucose and reducing substances in urine

Tests intended to detect glucose in urine can be classified as specific or non-specific. Non-specific methods (e.g. those using Fehling's and Benedict's reagents) are based on the detection of reducing substances in urine, commonly used procedures depending on the reduction of cupric compounds to cuprous oxide. Fehling's test is rarely employed nowadays but a convenient form of Benedict's reagent is marketed by Ames (Clinitest). In this version of the test urine and water are added to a tablet in a test-tube, the heat

$$\text{Urinary nitrogen loss} = \text{urine [urea]} \times \text{urine volume} \times 0\cdot028 \times \frac{6}{5}$$

$$\qquad\qquad (\text{g}/24\ \text{h}) \qquad (\text{mmol/l}) \qquad (\text{l}/24\ \text{h}) \qquad (\text{g/mmol})$$

$$= \frac{\text{urine [urea]} \times \text{urine volume}}{30}$$

In assessing nutritional requirements, account should also be taken of additional losses through other routes (skin, faeces, fistulae, etc.), which may amount to 2 g of nitrogen per day, or more. In some conditions, particularly those associated with metabolic acidosis,

needed for the copper reduction being generated by the exothermic reaction between water and sodium hydroxide (in the tablet). The manufacturer's instructions should be followed exactly if reliable results are to be obtained.

More specific tests for urinary glucose employ glucose oxidase. The enzyme catalyses the oxidation of glucose to gluconic acid and hydrogen peroxide. Peroxidase is used to accelerate the decomposition of the peroxide to water and oxygen, the latter being detected by one of a variety of indicator reactions involving oxygen acceptors. The specificity of these enzymatic methods is not absolute, false-positive results being obtained if the urine container is contaminated with oxidizing agents such as hydrogen peroxide, hypochlorite or certain detergents. Ascorbate diminishes the sensitivity of these tests.

Any urine giving a positive result with a non-specific method, such as Benedict's reagent, should be further tested by a more specific enzymatic test. If the presence of urinary glucose is confirmed then it is essential to establish whether or not the patient has *diabetes mellitus*. This requires plasma glucose measurements and, should the result of a fasting blood glucose estimation be indecisive, a glucose tolerance test. Non-diabetic causes of genuine glycosuria include a *lowered renal threshold for glucose* (which may be *inherited*, associated with *pregnancy* or due to *renal tubular disease*, such as a *Fanconi syndrome*) and conditions causing so-called '*lag-storage curves*' on glucose tolerance testing (e.g. *severe liver disease, thyrotoxicosis, upper gastrointestinal surgery*).

In adults urinary constituents other than glucose producing a positive reaction for reducing substances are rarely of importance. However, in babies and young children such results should be investigated thoroughly as they may signify an inborn error of metabolism. Thin layer chromatography is a useful first step in this context. Non-glucose reducing substances include *galactose, fructose, lactose*, various *pentoses, homogentisic acid* (in alkaptonuria) and metabolites of *salicylate* (and some other drugs). Very occasionally *uric acid* or *creatinine* may give a positive reaction in concentrated urines, although this is less common with Benedict's reagent than with some other methods for reducing substances.

Inborn errors of galactose and fructose metabolism will be described in more detail because they are of some importance in paediatric chemical pathology.

Galactosaemia

Classical galactosaemia, which is due to galactose-1-phosphate uridyl transferase deficiency, is a serious condition which often presents in the first week of life with vomiting, hypoglycaemia, hepatocellular dysfunction and renal tubular damage. Cataracts may be present. Although in this disease urine may produce a positive Benedict's reaction with a negative glucose oxidase test, it is not unknown for the glycosuria to

occur in the absence of galactosuria in very sick patients. Galactosuria will not occur unless milk is being ingested, while tubular damage may lead to renal glycosuria. A negative test for urinary reducing substances does not reliably exclude this condition and if the diagnosis is being considered the enzyme should be assayed directly in blood. Blood transfusions, however, can cause misleading results. Galactokinase deficiency, by contrast, is a relatively benign cause of galactosuria, the only serious complication being cataract formation. Uridyl diphosphate galactose-4-epimerase deficiency is a rare and benign disorder associated with increased red cell galactose-1-phosphate but normal galactose tolerance.

Fructose intolerance

Hereditary fructose intolerance (fructose-1-phosphate aldolase deficiency) resembles classical galactosaemia but presents later (often in weaning, when sucrose is introduced into the diet). As with galactosaemia, a negative screen for urinary reducing substances does not exclude the diagnosis with certainty. Fruktokinase deficiency is a benign cause of fructosuria. Fructose-1,6-diphosphate deficiency, a disorder of gluconeogenesis, does not generally produce fructosuria but instead presents with attacks of ketotic hypoglycaemia and lactic acidosis.

Tests for ketone bodies in urine

Ketone bodies (3-hydroxybutyrate, aceto-acetate and acetone) accumulate under conditions in which the rate of formation of acetyl-CoA by the oxidation of fatty acids exceeds the supply of oxalo-acetate, which is required if further catabolism through the tricarboxylic acid cycle is to occur. The control of ketogenesis involves several steps. The liberation of non-esterified fatty acids (and glycerol) from triglyceride stored in adipose tissue is regulated by hormone-sensitive lipase, itself under the control of insulin. Circulating non-esterified fatty acids are transported to the liver where they may be either re-esterified or oxidized. Oxidation (leading in part to ketone body formation) is the preferred route of metabolism when the glucagon : insulin ratio is high, as is the case when hepatic glycogen stores are depleted. It is now thought that malonyl-CoA, an intermediate in hepatic lipogenesis, plays a key role in maintaining the reciprocal relationship between ketogenesis and lipogenesis. Malonyl-CoA, the formation of which is increased when liver glycogen stores are replete, appears to control the activity of carnitine acyl transferase I, a crucial enzyme in the transport of fatty acyl moieties, into the mitochondria for β-oxidation.

Aceto-acetate and 3-hydroxybutyrate (which is not

a true ketone) are generated as a physiological adaptation in some circumstances and act as an important energy source in certain tissues (e.g. heart and brain) under conditions of restricted carbohydrate availability. Excessive levels of these metabolites, however, are pathological, leading to metabolic acidosis and the generation of acetone through the non-enzymatic decarboxylation of aceto-acetate.

Physiological increases in ketone body formation occur in fasting, in subjects consuming a diet which is rich in fat and poor in carbohydrates and in parturition. Untrained individuals may develop ketone bodies during prolonged exercise.

In adults, pathological ketosis is most commonly associated with uncontrolled diabetes mellitus. Other causes of ketoacidosis include starvation, severe illness (especially when associated with pyrexia) and alcohol abuse.

In the investigation of hypoglycaemia in children and babies it is often useful to know whether the patient is ketotic or not. In most conditions causing significant hypoglycaemia insulin levels are depressed and ketosis occurs. Absence of ketosis during hypoglycaemia suggests either that hyperinsulinism is the cause of the hypoglycaemia, or that there is a defect in fatty acid oxidation or ketone body formation (including disorders of carnitine metabolism). Hypoglycaemia associated with inherited organic acidaemias and with severe hepatocellular dysfunction may be ketotic or non-ketotic.

Methods for the detection of ketone bodies in urine include Gerhardt's and Rothera's tests.

In Gerhardt's test a couple of drops of 10 per cent ferric chloride solution are mixed with 1 ml of urine. In the presence of aceto-acetate the mixture turns red. However, this test is very non-specific, many different endogenous and drug metabolites giving rise to various colours, some of which (e.g. that obtained with salicylate) may be mistaken for the reaction given by aceto-acetate. For this reason Gerhardt's test is seldom used in adults, although in paediatric chemical pathology the non-specificity of this reaction is sometimes exploited in screening for inherited metabolic disease. However, it must be recognized that a normal result does not exclude an inborn error, while abnormal findings must be followed up by more rigorous analyses, including chromatography for organic acids, amino acids, etc.

In Rothera's test aceto-acetate and acetone react with nitroprusside in alkali to give a purple colour. Convenient forms of this technique include Acetest (Ames), in which the reagents are in tablet form, and stick tests such as Ketostix (Ames) and BM-Test Keton (Boehringer). Although a variety of substances other than ketone bodies (e.g. L-Dopa metabolites) give a similar reaction, in practice false positives are rarely a problem. Certain indicators (e.g. bromsulphthalein (BSP), phenol red and phenolphthalein (PSP)) give a reddish-purple colour in the test, but these colour changes depend solely on the alkaline conditions used and still occur when the nitroprusside is omitted.

TESTS ON CEREBROSPINAL FLUID

CSF protein

The protein content of the cerebrospinal fluid (CSF) depends on the site of sampling, lumbar fluid having a higher concentration (up to 500 mg/l) than ventricular fluid (up to 150 mg/l). In health the most abundant protein is albumin, with beta trace protein (a brain-derived substance) coming second. Normal CSF contains smaller quantities of other proteins including IgG, pre-albumin and transferrin. Tau protein, which is normally present only in the CSF, and not in serum, is thought to be a desialated derivative of transferrin. The normal range for CSF protein concentration is higher during the first year of life (up to 1000 mg/l in lumbar fluid).

In clinical practice two types of protein measurement are of value:

(1) total protein; (2) specific proteins (IgG and albumin).

1. Total protein

The examination of CSF total protein is used mainly to detect increased permeability of the blood–CSF barrier, although total protein concentrations may also be increased in some disorders associated with intrathecal immunoglobulin synthesis. Striking elevations occur in various infective conditions including *bacterial meningitis* (acute pyogenic, tuberculous and syphilitic), and *meningitis due to fungi and parasites*. In general, viral meningitis and encephalitis produce little or no increase in CSF total protein, although in severe cases marked elevations may be seen. These atypical cases tend to be associated with a more pronounced pleocytosis than is usually seen in viral infection, and may produce a fall in CSF glucose (a finding more characteristic of bacterial meningitis). A normal CSF total protein does not exclude bacterial meningitis, particularly in the early stages. An elevation in CSF total protein may also be due to *malignant infiltration* of the meninges, *Froin's syndrome* (mechanical obstruction to the flow of CSF), *Guillain–Barré syndrome, neurosarcoid, brain abscess, brain tumour* or *haemorrhage* into the subarachnoid space. Blood-stained CSF should be collected ino three successive tubes: in a subarachnoid haemorrhage the tubes are

Table APP.11   Cerebrospinal fluid

Analysis	Reference range	Units
Cells	5 (all mononuclear)	cells/mm^2
Chloride	120–170	mmol/l
Glucose	2.5–4.0	mmol/l
IgG index*	<0.65	
Total protein	100–400	mg/l

* A crude index of increase in IgG attributable to intrathecal synthesis.

uniformly red, whereas in blood-staining due to a traumatic puncture successive collections are less contaminated. Blood-stained fluid should be centrifuged to look for xanthochromia in the supernatant. Spectophotometric techniques may detect subtle Xantrochromia invisible to the naked eye.

2. Specific proteins

The blood–CSF barrier

The permeability of the blood–CSF barrier can be quantified by immunochemical measurements of albumin in CSF and serum (samples being collected at the same time). The albumin concentration ratio, CSF : serum, is normally less than 9×10^{-3}, values above this indicating abnormal leakage of albumin into the CSF.

Intrathecal immunoglobulin production

The ancestral test in this field was Lange's colloidal gold curve (now obsolete), which was a crude measure of the ratio of globulin to albumin in the CSF.

Modern tests of intrathecal immunoglobulin are either quantitative or qualitative.

The simplest quantitative test is the assay of CSF IgG concentration (usually performed by an immunochemical technique). However, more useful information is obtained if the CSF IgG level is related to other protein concentrations in CSF and serum, the most commonly used formula being the IgG index:

$$IgG\ index = \frac{[IgG]\ CSF}{[IgG]\ serum} \times \frac{[Albumin]\ serum}{[Albumin]\ CSF}$$

This approach enables some distinction to be made between a high CSF IgG level due to, on the one hand, to leakage across the blood–CSF barrier, and on the other, to local, intrathecal immunoglobulin synthesis.

Electrophoresis or isoelectric focusing of paired CSF and serum samples for so-called oligoclonal bands is a qualitative test of intrathecal immunoglobulin production. This is a more sensitive technique than the IgG index but false positives may occur unless a specific immunochemical method is used to detect the bands.

Evidence of intrathecal immunoglobulin synthesis is usually found in *multiple sclerosis (MS), subacute sclerosing parencephalitis* and *neurosyphilis*. In addition, elevations of the IgG index and/or oligoclonal bands are found in some cases of *systemic lupus erythematosus, neurosarcoidosis, Guillain-Barré syndrome, Behçet's disease, tuberculosis and viral encephalitis.*

The sensitivity of these tests for MS may depend on geographical location: in Europe and North America oligoclonal band analysis is positive in 95 per cent of clinically definite cases of MS whereas in the Far East the incidence of oligoclonal bands in MS may be only about 50 per cent.

CSF glucose

The concentration of glucose in the CSF is highly correlated with the plasma level, which should be determined at the same time. In health the concentration ratio, CSF:plasma, averages about 65 per cent but there is considerable variation about this mean. However, in suspected meningitis a concentration ratio below 40 per cent usually indicates a bacterial (acute pyogenic or tuberculous) or fungal cause. In most *viral infections* of the CNS the CSF glucose is normal but in atypical cases a relatively low glucose concentration may occur in association with a pleocytosis and raised protein. A normal CSF glucose does not exclude *acute pyogenic meningitis* (especially in the early stages) and normal concentrations also occur in some cases of chronic bacterial and fungal infection. *Malignant infiltration* of the meninges may produce a relative reduction in the CSF glucose.

TESTS ON FAECES

Occasional chemical tests on faeces may be of diagnostic value. They include the following:

Faecal occult blood

For this purpose it is useful to employ a test which is relatively insensitive, to avoid the excessive numbers of false-positive tests which would otherwise result. On the debit side, false negatives may occur unless the blood loss is greater than 10 ml/24 h. Oral iron

Table APP.12 Haematological Values

	SI units	Other units
Bleeding time (Ivy)	2–8 min	
Body fluid (total)		50% (obese)–70% (lean) of body weight
Intracellular		30–40% of body weight
Extracellular		20–30% of body weight
Blood volume		
Red cell mass,		
Men	0.027–0.035 l/kg	
Women	0.023–0.029 l/kg	
Plasma volume (both sexes)	0.04–0.05 l/kg	
Total blood volume,		
Men	75 ± 10 ml/kg	
Women	70 ± 10 ml/kg	
Erythrocyte sedimentation rate (Westergren)*		
Adult male	1–10 mm/h	
Adult female	3–15 mm/h	
Fibrinogen	1.5–4.0 g/l	
Folate		
Serum	2.2–18 μg/l	
Red cell	>160 μg/l	
Haemoglobin		
Men	130–180 g/l	
Women	115–165 g/l	
Haptoglobin	0.3–2.0 g/l	
Leucocytes – adults	4.0–11.0 × 10^9/l	
Differential white cell count		
Neutrophil granulocytes	2.0–7.9 × 10^9/l	40–75%
Lymphocytes	1.5–4.0 × 10^9/l	20–45%
Monocytes	0.2–0.8 × 10^9/l	2–10%
Eosinophil granulocytes	0.04–0.4 × 10^9/l	1–6%
Basophil granulocytes	0.01–0.1 × 10^9/l	0–1%
Mean corpuscular haemoglobin (MCH)	27–32 pg	
Mean corpuscular haemoglobin concentration (MCHC)	30–35 g/dl	30–35%
Mean corpuscular volume (MCV)	76–100 fl	
Packed cell volume (PCV) or haematocrit		
Men	0.40–0.54	
Women	0.35–0.47	
Platelets	150–350 × 10^9/l	
Prothrombin time	10.5–14.5 s	
Prothrombin ratio	2.0–4.5	
APTT (heparin control)	1.5–2.5	
Red cell count		
Men	4.5–6.5 × 10^{12}/l	
Women	3.8–5.8 × 10^{12}/l	
Red cell life span (mean)	120 days	
Red cell life span T$_{1/2}$(^{51}Cr)	25–35 days	
Reticulocytes (adults)	25–85 × 10^9/l	0.2–2%
Vitamin B$_{12}$	170–1600 ng/l	

* Higher values in older patients not necessarily abnormal

may produce false positives, as may foods rich in haemoglobin (e.g. liver or foods made from blood).

errors, a 5-day collection is recommended, and the average daily fat loss determined.

Faecal fat

Measurement of faecal fat is the definitive test for demonstrating the presence of steatorrhoea which results from intestinal or pancreatic disease. To reduce

Faecal trypsin and chymotrypsin

These enzymes are present in pancreatic exocrine secretions and, apart from the fraction subject to proteolytic breakdown in the GI tract, appear in the faeces.

Measurement in faeces has been used as a test of pancreatic exocrine function. False negative results (normal values) in mild pancreatic disease appear to be common, whilst false positive results (low values) may occur if stool volume is high.

Faecal electrolytes

Measurements of Na^+ and K^+ may be helpful in deciding on electrolyte replacement therapy, but are probably best restricted to liquid specimens only, where losses are potentially significant.

Faecal porphyrins

Porphyrin measurement may assist in the diagnosis of the porphyrias (see PORPHYRIAS).

NOTES ON INTERNATIONAL SYSTEM OF UNITS (SI UNITS)

(Reproduced with permission from Bouchier, I. A. D. and Edwards, C. R. W. (1995) *Davidson's Principles and Practices of Medicine*, 17th edn. Churchill Livingstone, Edinburgh.)

Examples of basic SI units:

Length	metre (m)
Mass	kilogram (kg)
Amount of substance	mole (mol)
Energy	joule (J)
Pressure	pascal (pa)

Examples of decimal multiples and submultiples of SI units:

Factor	Name	Symbol
10^6	mega-	M
10^3	kilo-	k
10^{-1}	deci-	d
10^{-2}	centi-	c
10^{-3}	milli-	m
10^{-6}	micro-	μ
10^{-9}	nano-	n
10^{-12}	pico-	p
10^{-15}	femto-	f

Volume. The basic SI unit of volume is the cubic metre (1000 litre). Because of its convenience the litre is used as the unit of volume in laboratory work.

Amount of substance ('molar') concentration (e.g. mol/l, μmol/l) is used for substances of defined chemical composition. It replaces equivalent concentrations (mEq/l), which is not part of the SI system. For univalent ions such as sodium, potassium, chloride and bicarbonate the numerical value is unchanged. For divalent ions such as calcium and magnesium the numerical value is halved.

Mass concentration (e.g. g/l, μg/l) is used for all protein measurements, for substances which do not have a sufficiently well defined composition and for serum vitamin B_{12} and folate measurements. The numerical value in SI units will change by a factor of 10 in those instances previously expressed in terms of 100 ml.

Haemoglobin is an exception. It is generally expressed in terms of g/dl.

SI units are not employed for enzymes nor usually for immunoglobulins.

Table APP.13 Reference values in venous plasma for the more common analytes in adults

Analysis	Reference range	Units
α_1-Antitrypsin	1.7–3.2	g/l
Alanine aminotransferase (ALT)	10–40	U/l
Albumin	36–47	g/l
Alkaline phosphatase	40–125	U/l
Amylase	50–300	U/l
Aspartate aminotransferase (AST)	10–35	U/l
Bilrubin (total)	2–17	µmol/l
Calcium	2.12–2.62	mmol/l
Carboxyhaemoglobin	Not normally detectable	%
	Up to 1.5% in non-smokers	
Ceruloplasmin	150–600	mg/l
Chloride	95–107	mmol/l
Cholesterol (total)*		
HDL-cholesterol	0.5–1.6 (M)	mmol/l
	0.6–1.9 (F)	
Copper	13–24	µmol/l
Creatine kinase	Normally <5% of total CK	
(MB isoenzyme)		
Creatine kinase (total)	30–200 (M)	U/l
	30–150 (F)	
Ethanol	Not normally detectable	mmol/l
	65–87 (marked intoxication)	
	87–109 (stupor)	
	>109 (coma)	
Creatinine	55–150	µmol/l
Ferritin	15–350 (M)	µg/l
	8–300 (F)	
Gamma-glutamyl transferase (GGT)	10–55 (M)	U/l
	5–35 (F)	
Glucose (fasting)†	3.6–5.8	mmol/l
Glycated haemoglobin (HbA₁)	4.5–8	%
Immunoglobulin A	0.5–4.0	g/l
Immunoglobulin G	5.0–13.0	g/l
Immunoglobulin M	0.3–2.2 (M)	g/l
	0.4–2.5 (F)	
Iron	14–32 (M)	µmol/l
	10–28 (F)	
Iron binding capacity	45–72	µmol/l
Lactate	0.4–1.4	mmol/l
Lactate dehydrogenase (urea-stable)	100–300	U/l
Lactate dehydrogenase (total)	230–460	U/l
Lead‡	<1.7	µmol/l
Magnesium	0.75–1.0	mmol/l
Osmolality	280–290	mmol/kg
Phosphate (fasting)	0.8–1.4	mmol/l
Potassium (plasma)	3.3–4.7	mmol/l
Potassium (serum)	3.7–5.1	mmol/l
Protein (total)	60–80	g/l
Sodium	132–144	mmol/l
Total CO_2	24–30	mmol/l
Transferrin	2.0–4.0	g/l
Triglycerides (fasting)	0.6–1.7	mmol/l
Urate	0.12–0.42 (M)	mmol/l
	0.12–0.36 (F)	
Urea	2.5–6.6	mmol/l
Zinc	11–22	µmol/l

* Cholesterol (total) ideally	<5.2 mmol/l
mild increase	5.2–6.5 mmol/l
moderate increase	6.5–7.8 mmol/l
severe increase	>7.8 mmol/l

(As defined by the European Atherosclerosis Society.)

† Values quoted for venous plasma or serum

Diagnostic criteria for 75 g oral glucose tolerance test (venous plasma) are as follows:

	Glucose (mmol/l) (fasting)		Glucose (mmol/l) (2 h post 75g glucose)
Normal	<7.8	and	<7.8
Impaired glucose tolerance	<7.8	and	≤7.8–<11.1
Diabetes mellitus	≥7.8	and/or	≥11.1

‡ Up to 1.2 μmol/l in children.

Table APP.14 Concentrations of therapeutic drugs in blood

Drug	Sample time	Therapeutic range	Units
Anticonvulsant drugs:			
Carbamazepine	Just before next dose	17–51	μmol/l
Phenobarbitone	Not critical	65–170	μmol/l
Phenytoin	Not critical	40–80	μmol/l
Valproate	Just before next dose	300–600	μmol/l
Atibiotics:			
Amikacin	Peak: 1 h after i.v. dose	15–30	mg/l
	Trough: pre-dose	5–10	
Gentamycin	Peak: 1 h after i.v. dose	8–12	mg/l
Tobramycin	Trough: pre-dose	<2	
Netilmycin			
Streptomycin	Peak: 1 h after i.v. dose	15–40	mg/l
	Trough: pre-dose	<5	
Vancomycin	Peak: 1 h after i.v. dose	30–40	mg/l
	Trough: pre-dose	5–10	
Others:			
Cyclosporin	Just before next dose	70–300	nmol/!
Digoxin	6–18 h after last dose	1.0–2.6	nmol/l
Lithium	12–18 h after last dose	0.6–1.0	mmol/l
Quinidine	Just before next dose	2–5	mg/l
Salicylate	Just before next dose	Up to 250	mg/l
Theophylline	Just before next dose	55–110	μmol/l

1. Care should be taken in comparing values between different laboratories. This is especially important since drug measurement units can be different. In the above table, both SI *and* non-SI units feature.
2. Drug pharmacokinetics are dependent on the *individual*. For within individual comparison, it is advisable to sample at the same relative time(s) in relation to drug administration.

Table APP.15   Tumour markers

Tumour marker	Application
α_1-Fetoprotein	Hepatoma, teratoma
Acid phosphatase (prostatic isoenzyme)	Prostate
Bence Jones protein	Multiple myeloma
CA 15.3	Breast
CA 125	Ovary
Calcitonin	Medullary carcinoma of thyroid
Carcinoembryonic antigen (CEA)	Colon, GI
Human chlorionic gonadotrophin	Choriocarcinoma, testicular tumours, hepatoma
Prostate-specific antigen	Prostate

Notes:
1. Tumour markers have little place in diagnosis, the exception being HCG in the detection of choriocarcinoma and Bence Jones protein in the detection of multiple myeloma. For this reason, reference ranges have not been given.
2. Measurements are useful in monitoring disease progress and in the diagnosis of recurrence.

Table APP.16   Gastrointestinal, pancreatic and liver data

Test	Reference range	Units	Comments
Faecal fat	<18	mmol/24 h	Average over 5 day collection
Stool weight (wet)	<200	g/24 h	
Xylose excretion	>15% excreted at 2 h (urine) or	%	Use blood xylose test if plasma urea >8.3 mmol/l
(5 g test)	>35% excreted at 5 h (urine)		
	>0.3 (blood concentration at 2h)	mmol/l	
Secretin stimulation	>2 (juice volume)	ml/kg/h	
(pancreatic exocrine	>10 (HCO_3 output)	mmol/h	
function)	>80 (HCO_3 concentration)	mmol/l	
Liver copper	<50	μg/g dry weight	
	>250 (Wilson's disease)		
Liver iron	40–60	μg/100 mg dry weight	
	>1000 (haemochromatosis)		

Miscellaneous:
1. Sweat
   Sweat [Cl]⁻ is *normally* <50 mmol/l (equivocal range 50–70 mmol/l).
   In cystic fibrosis (CF) high values are obtained.
2. Ascites and pleural effusions
   Transudates: total protein <30 g/l
   Exudates: total protein >30 g/l.

Table APP.17   Hormones

Hormone	Reference range	Units	Comments
Adrenocorticotrophic hormone (ACTH)	Up to 20 (07 : 00h–09 : 00h)	mU/L	Nycthemeral rhythm, so sampling time is critical. Avoid stress. Unstable
Cortisol	160–565 (at 08 : 00h) <205 (at 22 : 00h)	nmol/l	Nycthemeral rhythm, so sampling time is critical. Avoid stress
Follicle-stimulating hormone (FSH) (male)	1.5–9.0	U/l	
Follicle-stimulating hormone (FSH) (female)*	3.0–15 (early follicular) Up to 20 (mid-cycle) >30 (post-menopausal)	U/l	
Gastrin	Up to 120	ng/L	Collect after overnight fasting. Unstable
Growth hormone (GH)	Very variable, usually less than 2, but may be up to 50 with stress	mU/l	Avoid stress. Stimulation and suppression tests required
Insulin	Highly variable	mU/l	Levels can only be interpreted in relation to plasma glucose and body habitus
Luteinizing hormone (LH) (female)*	2.5–9.0 (early follicular) Up to 90 (mid-cycle) >30 (post-menopausal)	U/l	
Luteinizing hormone (LH) (male)	1.5–9.0	U/l	
Oestradiol-17β (female)	110–180 (early follicular) 550–1650 (mid-cycle) 370–770 (luteal) <150 (post-menopausal)	pmol/l	
Oestradiol-17β (male)	<200	pmol/l	
Parathyroid hormone (PTH)	10–55	ng/l	
Progesterone (male)	<2.0	nmol/l	
Progesterone (female)	<2.0 (follicular) >15 (Mid luteal) <2.0 (post-menopausal)	nmol/l	
Prolactin (PRL)	60–390	mU/l	Avoid stress
Testosterone (male)	10–30	nmol/l	
Testosterone (female)	0.8–2.8	nmol/l	
Thyroid stimulating hormone (TSH)	0.15–3.15	mU/l	
Thyroxine (free T_4)	10–27	pmol/l	Reference range may change in pregnancy
Tri-iodothyronine (T_3)	1.0–2.6	nmol/l	
TSH receptor antibodies (TRAb)	<7	U/l	

* Luteal phase values similar to follicular phase.

Notes:
1. A number of hormones are unstable and collection details are critical to obtaining a meaningful result. Refer to the local handbook.
2. Values in the table are only a guideline; hormone levels can often only be meaningfully understood in relation to factors such as sex (e.g. testosterone), age (e.g. FSH in women), time of day (e.g. cortisol) or regulatory factors (e.g. insulin and glucose, PTH and [Ca^{2+}]). Also, reference ranges may be critically method dependent.

INDEX

Index